TECHNIQUES IN CLINICAL NURSING

TECHNIQUES IN

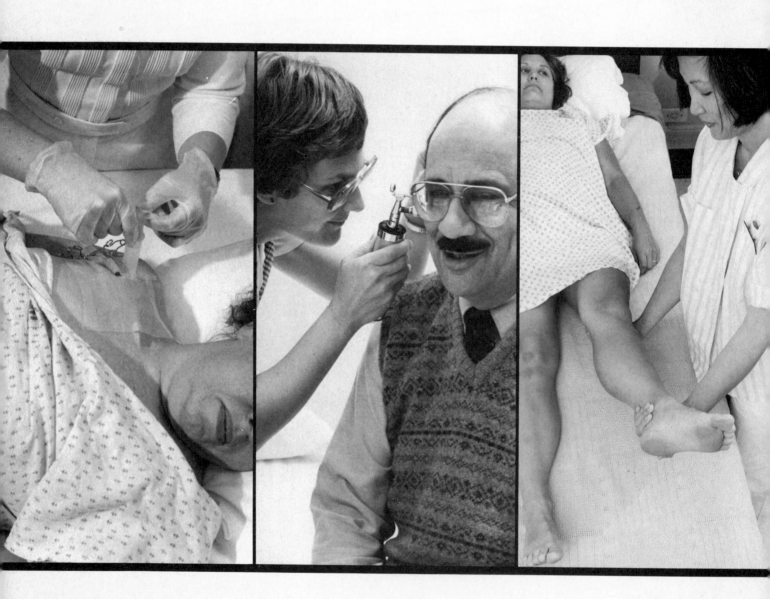

Addison-Wesley Publishing Company
Health Sciences Division, Menlo Park, California

Reading, Massachusetts ▪ Don Mills, Ontario ▪
Wokingham, UK ▪ Amsterdam ▪ Sydney ▪ Singapore ▪
Tokyo ▪ Madrid ▪ Bogota ▪ Santiago ▪ San Juan

CLINICAL NURSING

A Nursing Process Approach

Second Edition

With Appendix of Home Care Variations

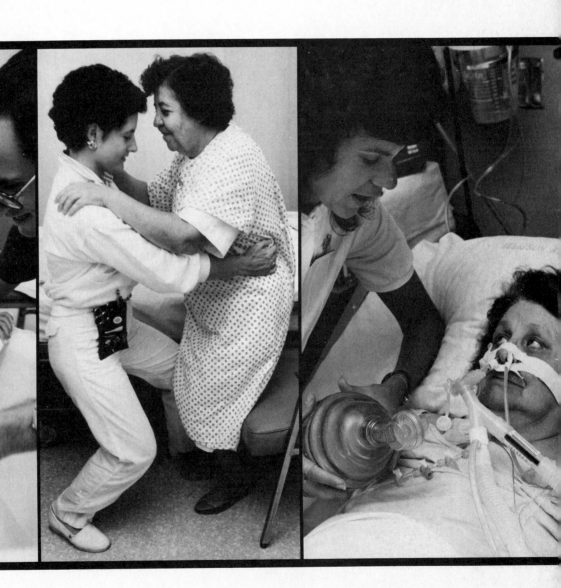

BARBARA KOZIER ▪ GLENORA ERB

BA, BSN, RN, MN   BSN, RN

Illustrations by Jack P. Tandy

Photographs by William Thompson, RN, Limited Horizons ▪
Jeffry Collins ▪ George B. Fry III

Sponsoring editor: Nancy Evans
Production editor: Zipporah W. Collins, assisted by Loralee Windsor
Production supervisor (in house): Judith Johnstone
Book designer: Alice Klein
Cover designer: Michael A. Rogondino
Copyeditors: Zipporah W. Collins and Alice Klein
Proofreader: Katherine L. Kaiser
Page layout: Alice Klein and Nancy Warner
Indexer: Elinor Lindheimer

Photographic credits are given on page 1002.

 Addison-Wesley Publishing Company
Health Sciences Division
2725 Sand Hill Road
Menlo Park, California 94025

Library of Congress Cataloging-in-Publication Data

Kozier, Barbara.
  Techniques in clinical nursing.

  Includes bibliographies and index.
  1. Nursing.   I. Erb, Glenora Lea, 1937–
II. Title.   [DNLM: 1. Nursing process.   WY 100 K88t]
RT41.K723   1986   610.73   86–1084

ISBN 0-201-11755-X

ABCDEFGHIJ–MU–89876

The authors and publishers have exerted every effort to ensure that drug selections and dosages set forth in this text are in accord with current recommendations and practice at the time of publication. However, in view of ongoing research, changes in government regulations, and the constant flow of information relating to drug therapy and drug reactions, the reader is urged to check the package insert for each drug for any change in indications of dosage and for added warnings and precautions. This is particularly important where the recommended agent is a new and/or infrequently employed drug.

CONTENTS

LIST OF TECHNIQUES

■ following a technique title indicates a new technique in this edition.

⌂ following a technique title indicates home care variations are given in the appendix.

Chapter 10 Health Assessment of the Adult

Chapter 11 Special Procedures

Chapter 12 The Hair, Nails, and Feet

Chapter 13 The Mouth, Eyes, and Ears

Chapter 14 The Skin

■ following a technique title indicates a new technique in this edition.

🏠 following a technique title indicates home care variations are given in the appendix.

■ following a technique title indicates a new technique in this edition.

🏠 following a technique title indicates home care variations are given in the appendix.

■ following a technique title indicates a new technique in this edition.
🏠 following a technique title indicates home care variations are given in the appendix.

■ following a technique title indicates a new technique in this edition.

🏠 following a technique title indicates home care variations are given in the appendix.

■ following a technique title indicates a new technique in this edition.
🏠 following a technique title indicates home care variations are given in the appendix.

PREFACE

Clinical nursing skills and techniques underlie the entire scope of day-to-day care of patients. The teaching and learning of these skills can present a major challenge to faculty and students. The first edition of *Techniques in Clinical Nursing* demonstrated that it can help faculty and students successfully meet this challenge. Response to the first edition has been gratifying; educators and students have offered praise and constructive criticism, inspiring us to offer a second edition that is even more current and comprehensive. The new subtitle, *A Nursing Process Approach,* reflects a major revision in the framework of the text: Each technique is described in a nursing process format.

Although updated and revised throughout, the second edition retains the same purposes as the first edition:

■ To help students learn the skills most commonly required in patient care
■ To present these techniques in a format compatible with any nursing curriculum

The text can be used effectively in independent learning situations as well as situations where the instructor actively participates. It can be used as a primary or supplemental text in a skills course and by learners reorienting themselves to clinical nursing.

A complete learning system

In response to comments from instructors, this new edition has been repackaged not as a single text but rather as a complete learning system. In addition to the text itself, the system now includes:

1. A Student Workbook containing performance checklists for each technique and a post-test for each chapter.
2. An Instructor's Manual offering learning activities, answers to the post-tests, and suggested readings.

This method of packaging the components increases the convenience for both student and instructor by reducing the size of the text itself. Thus the student need only carry the checklist/post-test workbook to the clinical setting. Including the post-test answers in the Instructor's Manual allows the instructor greater flexibility in the use of these tests.

New features

1. A total of 237 techniques, 77 of which are new to this edition.
2. New chapters on Health Assessment of the Adult, Tracheostomy Care, and Chest Drainage.
3. A nursing process format for each technique, to help the student individualize care for each patient.
4. A total of 1,028 illustrations—410 photographs and 618 drawings—increase the text's appeal to students and their understanding.
5. A special appendix outlining home care variations for 72 selected techniques. Despite the growing need for home care, students' initial clinical experience is most commonly in a health care setting outside the home. The home care variations are consolidated in an appendix to make them available without complicating the basic technique or confusing the new student. Each technique for which there is an appendix variation is marked with an icon (this symbol of a house 🏠) after the technique title.

Organization

The first four chapters of the text provide the learner with information essential to the techniques described in chapters 5 through 42. Chapters are grouped in units according to categories of techniques, such as asepsis, assessment, and personal hygiene. Within each chapter, techniques are arranged generally from simple to complex. Chapters are designed so that they may be used independently and thus in any order. The inclusive glossary at the end of the text also facilitates flexibility in course organization.

Chapter format

Each chapter has behavioral objectives that are reflected in the technique performance checklists and in the chapter post-test. Selected terms and their definitions, and a relevant theory base are supplied for the techniques. Included in the theory of some chapters are developmental variables, where appropriate, and common health problems.

Each technique applies the five-step nursing process, except where a patient is not involved:

1. *Assessment* data required.

2. Examples of *nursing diagnoses* for which the technique may be implemented if the technique can be an independent nursing function.

3. *Planning,* which includes nursing goals and equipment.

4. *Intervention,* the steps required to implement the technique. *Rationales* are included for selected nursing interventions to help students understand why a certain action is performed. Each technique also includes *examples of specific data to be recorded.*

5. *Evaluation,* which includes examples of expected and unexpected outcomes, recognizing that in practice these outcomes are specific for each patient. An expected outcome may or may not be a "normal" outcome. If, for example, a patient has had copious drainage from a wound for five days, the nurse can expect drainage when the dressing is changed. This would be an expected outcome at this stage. As the drainage decreases in amount, however, an expected outcome would be less drainage and eventually no drainage.

Evaluation tools

A performance checklist for each technique is provided in the workbook. The checklists now follow the nursing process format and are written in a step-by-step format that *coincides* with the sequence in each technique.

A post-test for each chapter is also provided in the workbook. The post-tests now include a patient/clinical study that applies the knowledge of the chapter. Answers to the post-test questions are provided in the Instructor's Guide.

This book is designed to encourage independent learning and self-evaluation, thus enhancing the instructor's role as a resource person.

Barbara Kozier
Glenora Erb

HOW TO USE THIS BOOK

We have tried to make each technique as complete as possible to guide you in clinical settings. Certain nursing actions, however, have been omitted from each technique to avoid repetition. These actions, which are considered basic to safe, competent nursing intervention, are:

1. Carrying out a medical aseptic hand wash before gathering any clean supplies or before implementing a procedure and after contact with a patient, so as not to transmit microorganisms to patients or to others.

2. Carrying out a surgical hand wash before opening any sterile supplies, so that microorganisms are not transmitted to the supplies or to the patient.

3. Identifying the patient appropriately, for example, by reading the patient's Identaband.

4. Explaining the technique to the patient and, in some instances, to support persons, adjusting the explanation to their needs. Explaining what you plan to do reassures people by letting them know what to expect. Explanations are provided in some techniques, where special information needs to be included.

5. Providing privacy for the patient, when any aspect of the procedure could be embarrassing to the patient or to other people, and as an indication of respect for the patient even when he or she is not conscious.

6. Elevating the patient's bed to a working level and lowering the near side rail before starting a procedure. These actions help the nurse maintain good body mechanics.

7. Lowering the bed and raising the near side rail for patients requiring these precautions, following a procedure. These actions are taken for the patient's safety.

8. Ensuring that the patient is comfortable following the technique.

9. Disposing of used and unused supplies according to agency practice. This includes cleaning and/or disinfecting equipment as necessary.

Chapters 1 through 4 provide a brief orientation to some areas of nursing, and it is suggested that these chapters be learned first, so that they can be applied to the remaining chapters. The following guidelines are suggested for each chapter:

1. Read the introductory section, including the chapter outline, to obtain an awareness of the content of the chapter.

2. Review the chapter objectives.

3. Learn the terms and their definitions. A glossary is also provided at the end of the book for your use.

4. Study the theory provided in the chapter.

5. Turn to the technique you need to learn, or to the first technique, and study it.

6. Consult your instructor or an appropriate person to learn about any adjustments for the technique as practiced in a specific health agency.

7. Practice the technique in a nursing laboratory or learning resource area. Audiovisual aids may be available to help you learn the technique. Consult with your instructor about any difficulties you encounter.

8. Using the performance checklist provided in the workbook, evaluate your own practice of the technique, preferably with the assistance of another person.

9. Adjust your performance according to the checklist.

10. After learning all the techniques in the chapter, complete the post-test provided in the workbook.

11. Mark the test using the answers provided in the Instructor's Guide. Review the material you did not know.

12. If you require assistance, discuss your difficulties with your instructor or a reference person.

13. In a clinical area, perform the techniques you have learned, with appropriate assistance. Evaluate your performance.

We hope you find this book helpful in learning techniques.

Barbara Kozier
Glenora Erb

ACKNOWLEDGMENTS

We would like to express our warmest appreciation and thanks to:

- The many nurses—students and teachers—who used the first edition of *Techniques* and who sent suggestions for revisions or additions. These comments have been informative and helpful.
- The nursing educators and practicing clinicians who kept a user's "diary" or who reviewed content for this edition: Erma Bahrenberg, Joy Boarini, Patricia Brown, Barbara Butera, Gail Button, Charles Christoph, Deanna Cross, Elizabeth Cutezo, William Donovan, Diane Ebken, Barbara Gruendemann, Harriet Hecker, Nancy Hilt, Daisy Hines, Jean Hutten, Marguerite Jackson, June Johnson, Lynette Karls, Patricia Lynch, Erroll McCrae, Jacqueline Octavio, Teresa Smith, Nancy Stotts, Betsy Todd, Mary Vandeberg, and Joanne Walker. Their thoughtful and objective critiques were very useful.
- Kris Ziegler, Visiting Nurses' Association, Buffalo, New York, for her assistance in the development of the home care variations for selected techniques.
- Ilka Abbott, librarian at the Registered Nurses' Association of British Columbia, Vancouver, for her invaluable help in obtaining and providing references for this book.
- The talented illustrator Jack Tandy, St. Louis, Missouri, whose superb line drawings make explicit what words alone cannot.
- The creative photographers William Thompson, Palo Alto, California, George B. Fry III, Atherton, California, and Jeffry Collins, Indianapolis, Indiana, whose talents are obvious in the clarity, sensitivity, and realism of the photographs. Special thanks are also due to Pamela Swearingen, author of *The Addison-Wesley Photo-Atlas of Nursing Procedures,* for allowing us to use photographs from that book; and to Kaye Dunbar, RN, and the staff at El Camino Hospital, Mountain View, California, and the staff of Stanford University Hospital, Stanford, California, where many of the photographs for this edition were taken.
- Our typist A. Goldie, Vancouver, British Columbia, who spent many long hours preparing the manuscript and whose patience, expertise, accuracy, and speed helped us meet many deadlines.
- Our indispensable copy and production editor Zipporah Collins, Berkeley, California, who performed the monumental task of coordinating the production of this book. We are grateful for her special qualities of sensitivity, support, flexibility in manipulating schedules, optimism, humor, and high standards. To her associates Alice Klein, Loralee Windsor, and Katherine L. Kaiser, we also wish to say thank you.
- Alice Klein, Berkeley, California, who created the aesthetic page designs and successfully coordinated the illustrations with the text in an inviting way. Thanks also to Nancy Warner, San Francisco, California, who planned the layout of many of the pages.
- Elinor Lindheimer, Ukiah, California, who prepared the index with skill, speed, and judgment.
- Lynn Meredith, Vancouver, British Columbia, who graciously assisted in the compilation of the glossary.
- The staff at Addison-Wesley whose behind-the-scene work was of inestimable value: Nick Keefe, Vice-President and General Manager of the Health Sciences Division, who conveyed interest and instilled confidence and support when it was most needed; Nancy Evans, our sponsoring editor, who solicited so many credible and valuable reviewers; Judith Johnstone and Glenda Epting, who provided production liaison services that helped move the book to completion.
- The staff of Skillful Means Press, who did a fine job of typesetting and paging the book, meeting deadlines even when others were late.
- Our families and friends who have provided much support and encouragement during a demanding and busy time preparing this book.

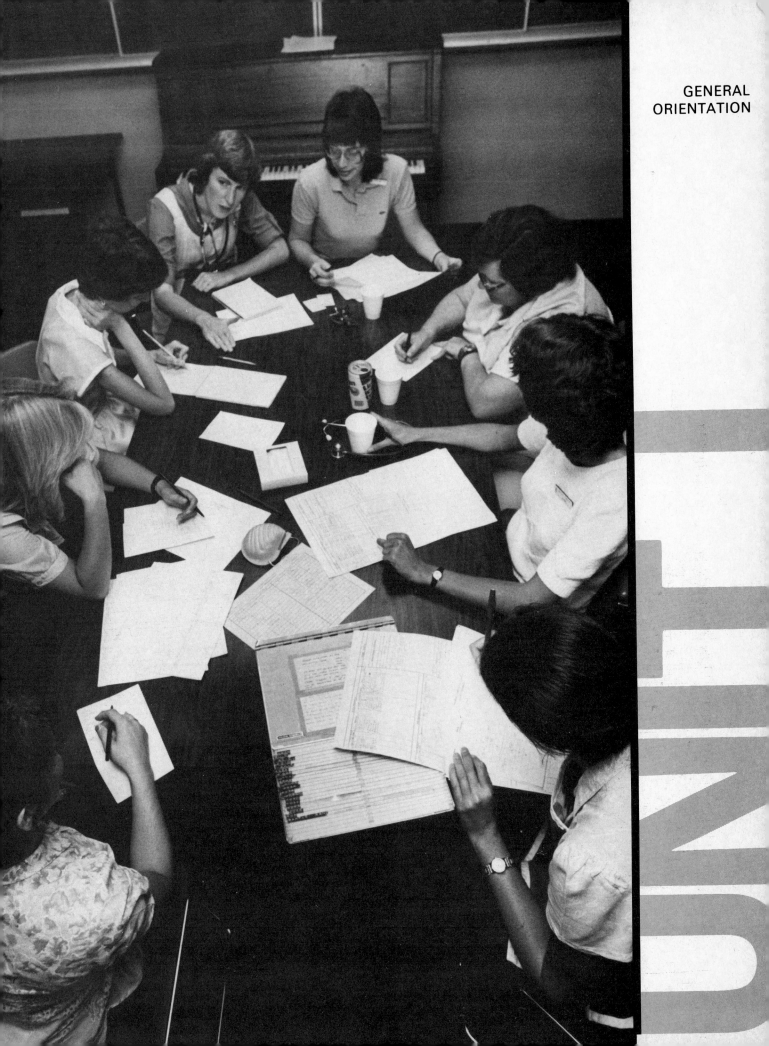

UNIT

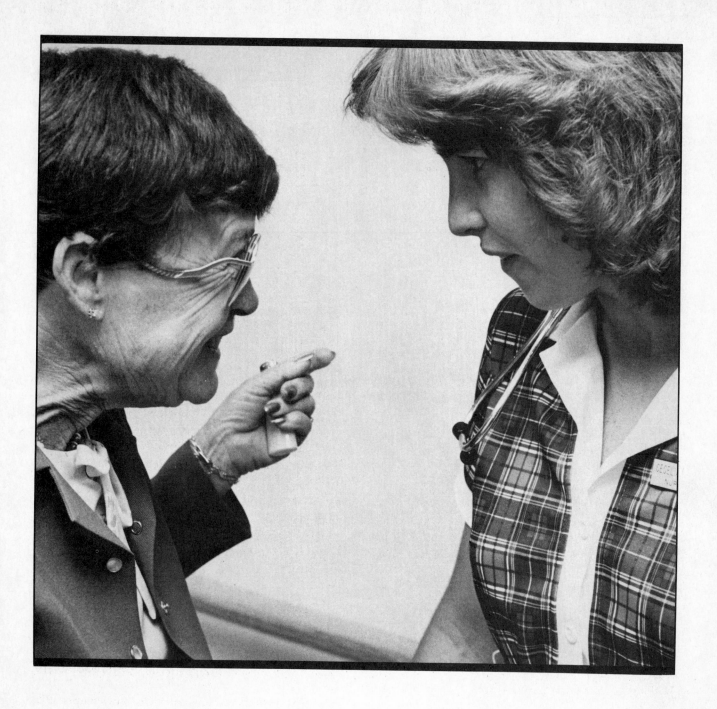

NURSING TECHNIQUES IN CLINICAL PRACTICE

1

The concept of basic needs provides nurses with an approach to understanding people's behavior. Although each individual is unique, certain needs are common to all people.

At a time of illness, patients may require assistance to meet needs that they meet independently when healthy. During an illness, most patients and their support persons experience stresses and behavior changes. Therefore, an important nursing function is to support and comfort individuals throughout the stressful period.

Chapter Outline

Changing Nursing Techniques
    Technologic Development
    Increased Knowledge from the Biologic and
       Social Sciences
    Recognition of Basic Needs

Patients and Illness

Supportive Nursing Interventions

Conveying Nursing Competence

Objectives

Upon completion of this chapter, the student will:

1. Know the essential facts about basic human needs
   1.1 Define selected terms
   1.2 Explain three influences of nursing techniques
   1.3 Outline Maslow's hierarchy of needs
   1.4 Describe Kalish's hierarchy of needs

   1.5 Explain common behaviors of the patient that
       require support
2. Understand ways of assisting people to meet their basic needs
   2.1 Identify nursing interventions that support patients
   2.2 Identify ways in which nurses convey competence

Terms

- anxiety   mental uneasiness
- basic human need   something required by human beings in order to maintain physiologic and psychologic homeostasis
- client   a person who seeks help but is neither ill nor injured
- dependent nursing action   action carried out by a nurse as a result of a physician's order
- egocentricity   concern about oneself
- homeostasis   the tendency of the body to maintain a state of balance while continually changing

- independent nursing action   action carried out by a nurse as a result of the nurse's judgment
- interdependent nursing action   action carried out by a nurse in association with other health professionals
- patient   a person who seeks help because of illness or injury
- regression   reversion to a behavior or state that was acceptable at an earlier age
- stress   a physical or psychologic condition or situation that causes tension in the body
- therapeutic   healing; supportive of health

CHANGING NURSING TECHNIQUES

Nursing techniques are the "hands-on" aspect of nursing practice. A *technique,* also referred to as a *procedure,* is a particular way of doing a task or a series of steps followed in a regular order using special knowledge. Techniques may be implemented as independent, interdependent, or dependent nursing actions. An *independent* nursing action is taken as a result of the nurse's own judgment, eg, turning a patient to a lateral position. An *interdependent* action is carried out in association with other health professionals, eg, holding a patient in the correct position for a lumbar puncture. A *dependent* action is carried out as a result of a physician's order, eg, cleaning a surgical wound.

Nursing techniques are employed in three phases of the nursing process: assessment, intervention, and evaluation. For example, assessing a patient's pulse can be part of assessment and evaluation. Giving an enema or inserting a urinary catheter can be an aspect of intervention. For further information about the nursing process, see chapter 3.

Nursing techniques must be carried out competently and applied to the individual patient's needs. In the past, nursing techniques were often applied in a rote fashion; that is, the technique was memorized by the nurse and then carried out in the same manner for every patient. Some hospitals established routines, such as a bath routine in which specific patients received baths at a specific time whether or not the bath was wanted or needed.

Three major factors influence changes in nursing techniques:

1. Technologic development
2. Increased knowledge from the biologic and social sciences

3. Recognition of the basic needs of patients and their support persons

Technologic Development

Technology is affecting all areas of the health field. New equipment, medical techniques, and drugs have a vast impact on nursing practice. Equipment has become more complex, as well as more efficient. For example, blood pressures that were immeasurable in the past can now be assessed using ultrasound equipment. Patients who years ago would have died because they could not breathe can be kept breathing for days, even years, by respirators. The development of computer technology has made immense changes in the way information about patients is obtained and stored.

As nurses use this complex equipment, they may become preoccupied with the technology itself and "forget" about the patient and support persons. The many nursing techniques that employ new technology require knowledge not only about how the equipment works but also about how it affects the patient's physiologic and psychologic processes.

Increased Knowledge from the Biologic and Social Sciences

At one time nursing actions were taken because they were *thought* to help the patient, but nursing actions today have a sound biologic or social science basis. There is a scientific reason, or rationale, for each significant step in a nursing technique, whether it is the placement of a stethoscope to assess the apical heartbeat or the position of a patient for an enema. As the bodies of knowledge in the biologic and social sciences increase, nursing actions must change to reflect this knowledge.

Nursing techniques usually have a direct relation to body anatomy and/or physiology. For example, to give an intramuscular injection safely, a nurse must know the location of both the specific target muscle and the adjacent structures, such as bones, major blood vessels, and nerves. Furthermore, once the drug has been injected, nurses need to understand the effect it will have on the patient, including the clinical signs of both anticipated and adverse effects.

While the relationship of the biologic sciences to nursing techniques is well understood and accepted, application of the social sciences to nursing techniques does not always receive the same emphasis. The social sciences involve the caring and compassionate aspects of nursing, as well as consideration of the patient as a unique individual. Nursing techniques should always be viewed within the context of a patient's psychosocial needs. Often a technique is frightening to the patient and support persons. Explanations by nurses and communication of

support, warmth, and caring help patients to deal with their fears and enhance their feelings of self-worth.

Recognition of Basic Needs

A *basic human need* is something required by human beings to maintain their physiologic and psychologic homeostasis. *Homeostasis* is the tendency of the body to maintain a state of balance while continually changing. There are a number of lists of basic human needs that are considered common to all people. Maslow's five categories of needs are (1970, p 37):

1. Physiologic
2. Safety and security
3. Love and belonging
4. Self-esteem
5. Self-actualization

Maslow's highest level, self-actualization, is the apex of the fully developed personality; few people are completely self actualized (1968, p 204).

Richard Kalish (1977, p 32) has adapted Maslow's hierarchy and suggests an additional category between physiologic needs and the safety and security needs. This category, stimulation needs, includes sex, activity, exploration, manipulation, and novelty. Kalish emphasizes that children need to explore and manipulate their environments in order to achieve optimal growth and development. He notes that adults, too, often seek novel adventures or stimulating experiences before considering their safety or security needs. Maslow, on the other hand, includes many of the stimulation needs, such as the pursuit of knowledge and aesthetic needs, in the category of self-actualization. See Figure 1–1.

Physiologic needs

The physiologic needs encompass the basic survival requirements of humans. The needs included in this category are for oxygen, water, food, elimination, rest and sleep, pain relief, exercise, and temperature regulation. Generally, when these needs are not met, other needs, such as stimulation and love and belonging, are not aroused.

Nurses frequently help patients of all ages to meet their physiologic needs. In terms of nursing priorities, the physiologic or survival needs of patients generally take precedence over other needs. Nurses should be sensitive to patients' feelings, however, when assisting them with physiologic needs. Adult patients in particular perceive inability to meet their own needs in this area as a disturbing and sometimes embarrassing dependence on others. Deprivation of other physiologic needs is more than embarrassing; for example, the inability to acquire

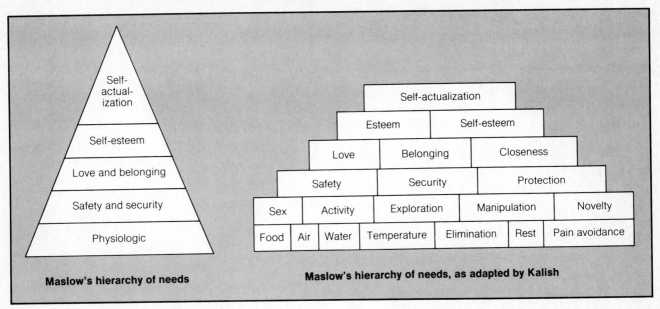

FIGURE 1-1 ■ Maslow's hierarchy of needs and Maslow's needs as adapted by Kalish. (Adapted from Abraham H. Maslow, A theory of human motivation, *Psychological Review*, 1943, 50:370–96. Copyright © 1943 by the American Psychological Association, Inc. Reprinted by permission. From *The Psychology of Human Behavior*, 3rd Ed. by Richard A. Kalish. Copyright © 1973 by Wadsworth Publishing Company, Inc. Reprinted by permission of Brooks/Cole Publishing, Monterey, California.)

sufficient oxygen, feeling suffocated, can be a terrifying experience for any patient.

Stimulation needs

Various stimuli rouse people's minds or spirits, spur them to activity, or prompt them to pursue a goal. As a category of basic needs, stimulation is used in a broad sense, referring to stimulation of the emotions, the cognitive processes, and the senses. A number of things can provide stimulation.

Any change can be stimulating to a person provided the degree of change is appropriate for that person. One person may find moving to another city a stimulating experience that affords opportunities for new activities and growth; another person making the same move may be overwhelmed and feel acutely insecure rather than stimulated. Changes of a lesser degree, such as a new book, new clothes, or a different restaurant, can also be stimulating.

Stimulation can come from a hobby or an activity in which a person is interested. This type of stimulation can balance the routine and problems of daily life. Sensory stimulants, such as a movie, the smell of newly baked bread, a beautiful sunset, or the sound of certain music, can also add interest to life.

Not all stimulation is pleasant. Adults, for example, may feel bombarded by unpleasant acoustic stimuli when a teenager turns music to a high volume. Unpleasant sensory stimuli are familiar to all people. However, even unpleasant stimulation can provoke interest and thus help to meet some people's basic needs.

Nurses should consider a patient's stimulation needs when carrying out nursing techniques. Some of these needs may be met by fostering the patient's active participation in the planning and activity of a technique and by providing explanations that meet the patient's particular need to understand the technique. However, while stimulation is important, it is also important to avoid overstimulating the patient. This should be considered in the timing of techniques.

Safety and security needs

Safety needs are needs to protect oneself from physical harm. The threats to a person's safety can be categorized as mechanical, chemical, thermal, and bacteriologic. Generally, adults meet their own safety needs in daily life, and seldom consider them survival needs, except under unusual circumstances such as war. During an illness, however, patients are frequently less able to protect themselves; their resistance to infection may be lowered, for example, or they may be immobilized.

Patients are not always aware of the threats to their safety in a hospital or health agency. Nurses therefore need to be aware of threatening situations. Explanations to patients and appropriate precautionary measures generally will protect a person adequately. These measures include not only those that prevent accidents but also those that maintain integrity of the skin and mucous membranes.

Precautionary measures integrated into many of the techniques include:

1. Identifying the patient before initiating any technique
2. Performing a medical aseptic hand wash before gathering clean supplies and after completing techniques
3. Lowering the side rail of a bed only when the nurse is present at that side of the bed
4. Leaving a bed in a low position so that the patient can get out of bed more safely
5. Leaving a call signal within easy reach

A feeling of security is a psychologic need and depends on many factors, such as consistency in the behavior of others, awareness of the expectations or limitations of others, familiarity with people and the environment, ability to control matters concerning oneself, ability to communicate, and desire or ability to know or understand what is going on around one.

When caregivers act consistently, patients know to some degree what to expect. When nurses make their expectations and limitations clear, patients know what

FIGURE 1–2 ■ The nurse's facial expression conveys warmth and caring.

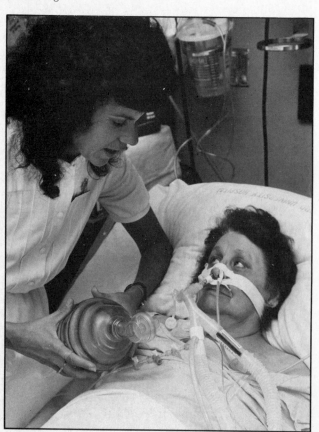

behavior patterns are acceptable in the relationship, and the resulting structure of rules offers security.

It becomes obvious that familiarity with people or places facilitates security when one experiences the opposite feelings upon meeting new people or living in strange places. The ability to communicate in the same language is an important part of this kind of familiarity.

The unknown often produces feelings of anxiety and insecurity. For example, if a patient is having surgery for a tumor that could be cancerous, the person's security is threatened until the diagnosis is known.

In institutional health care settings, people temporarily lose their rights to control personal matters. For example, the time and type of bath that a patient has are often prescribed by hospital policy instead of the person's preference. This lack of control may produce feelings of insecurity.

Nursing actions that help meet a patient's need for security include:

1. Providing adequate explanations about techniques in a language understood by the patient. An interpreter may be necessary.
2. Having consistency of care and, if possible, the same nurse for a period of time.
3. Helping patients to maintain control over what happens to them by encouraging their participation in the planning and performance of techniques.

Love and belonging needs

Nurses can help patients meet their needs for love and belonging by:

1. Conveying through nursing actions that they are profoundly interested in that patient and his or her welfare. See Figure 1–2.
2. Accepting the patient regardless of his or her behavior.
3. Conveying the desire to be present when needed. Although nurses cannot be present all the time, it is important to tell the patient when the nurses are leaving the unit and when they will return. If nurses say they will do something, it is very important for them to follow through or explain why there is a delay.
4. Encouraging the patient to participate in the planning of his or her care.

Self-esteem needs

Self-esteem is often referred to as self-respect, self-approval, or self-worth. Whatever label is used, all people need to think well of themselves. Some psychologists believe that people need to respect themselves before they can respect others. To possess self-esteem, people must respect what they have done and what they can do—that is, they need to think they are worthwhile, needed, and useful.

A person's self-esteem depends on other basic needs being met. If needs such as love or security are not met satisfactorily, the basic need of self-esteem is also threatened.

People's self-esteem is often considerably influenced by their feelings of dependence or independence. Few human beings are entirely independent or self-sufficient, but some have stronger needs for independence than others.

Illness almost always alters the balance of dependence and independence. Even temporary limitations on normal activities can decrease a person's self-respect. It often becomes the nurse's responsibility to make decisions with the patient about balancing needs for dependence and independence in order to hasten recovery. To enhance the patient's self-esteem, nurses can:

1. Permit patients as much control of themselves and their environment as possible.

2. Convey an accepting but nonreactive attitude. An individual's behavior can be accepted without necessarily being approved.

The need for esteem from others is associated with social approval and recognition for achievements. Nurses can help fulfill this need by:

1. Providing recognition of patients' achievements

2. Indicating that patients or support persons are worthwhile people by saying, "It's good to see you again," for example, or by enquiring about family members or activities of interest to the family

Self-actualization needs

According to Maslow (1968) and Kalish (1977), self-actualization is the final level of need (see Figure 1–1). The fully self-actualized person has realized his or her full potential. Such a person has the ability to connect the past and the future to the present while living fully in the present. The self-actualized person is also inner directed and autonomous rather than other-directed and dependent. An inner-directed individual has a few basic values and principles that guide him or her whatever the situation. The autonomous individual is free from parental and social pressures and applies his or her values or principles to behavior in a manner that appears appropriate to the individual. The other-directed, dependent individual is influenced by outside pressures, accepts guidance and direction from others, and adheres to this guidance to gain approval.

Not all people become fully self-actualized. According to Maslow, intelligence is neither required nor sufficient for self-actualization. However, if all the "lower" needs have been met, an individual may aspire to self-fulfillment or self-actualization. The fully self-actualized person may not always be happy, successful, or well adjusted. Maslow viewed many of the subjects he believed to be self-actualized as prideful, vain, and possessing doubts and fears. However, they were able to deal positively with their fears, doubts, and failures.

Nurses can help people become self-actualized by:

1. Providing patients and support persons with the information they require to make decisions

2. Supporting patients when they make decisions regarding health and activities

PATIENTS AND ILLNESS

The *patient* is a person who seeks help, usually because of illness or injury. In some situations, patients are called *clients.* In contrast to patients, clients may not be injured or ill. They are consumers of health care and as such may be seeking preventive care, eg, immunizations, or the promotion of health, eg, weight loss. In many settings *client* and *patient* are used interchangeably. The behavior of patients when they are ill or injured is highly individual and is usually learned from the cultures in which they live, their families, and their social environments. A person from an Italian or Greek background, for example, may express emotions openly, while one from an Oriental, eg, Japanese, culture may be much less expressive and more stoic. There are, however, five common responses to illness:

1. Fear and worry are very common, because patients anticipate an inability to function normally following illness. The fear may focus on the ability to return to work and thus meet financial obligations or the ability to function socially and thus meet obligations to a spouse, children, or friends. Patients are often fearful about their ability to withstand pain, their diagnosis, and how they present themselves. Fear of the unknown is also common when patients find themselves in unfamiliar settings with unknown people and practices.

2. Acute anxiety may cause patients to regress to behavior more appropriate for a younger person. For example, a 10-year-old boy may begin to suck his thumb.

3. Egocentricity is another common behavior. Patients are preoccupied with their own illness and uninterested in other people's concerns or activities. Many patients' interests become narrowed, particularly when they are in the hospital. Two factors that contribute to this are lack of energy and separation from normal interests and responsibilities.

4. Emotional overreactions are also common. Patients cry or get angry more easily than they would normally. They have a greater need for affection and understanding. Patients may show exaggerated concern about small matters, such as how the corner of the bed is made, the type of food served, or a slight delay in an x-ray film appointment.

5. Patients' perceptions of others may change unrealistically. Patients may perceive the nurse as nonsupportive or uncaring; they often see the physician as very powerful.

SUPPORTIVE NURSING INTERVENTIONS

Nurses spend a good deal of time performing techniques that assist patients. These skills are described in detail in chapters 5–42. Before, during, and after performing these techniques, it is important that nurses support patients who are anxious and who show any of the behavior changes described above. The following measures can reduce stress for some individuals. Not all methods are effective for all patients; nurses must be sensitive to a patient's needs and reactions and choose the methods that are most effective for that person.

1. Orient patients and support persons to the agency. People are assisted in their adjustment to change when they become familiar with such matters as visiting hours and mealtimes.

2. By listening attentively, convey caring and understanding to patients and support persons about their situations. This will help them to talk about their worries and needs.

3. Maintain patients' identities by calling them by name and encouraging them to wear their own clothes if agency policy permits this.

4. Provide information when patients and/or support persons have insufficient information.

5. Repeat information you have already given, when it is requested, realizing that anxious people often find it difficult to remember.

6. Encourage patients to participate in some physical activity if it is permitted. Activity often helps to reduce stress.

7. Assist patients to make correct appraisals of events or situations. If, for example, a patient is worried because a urine specimen has been requested, it may reassure him or her to know that specimens are requested of all patients newly admitted to the hospital.

8. Encourage patients to do independently the functions they can handle safely and effectively, such as shaving or bathing.

9. Arrange for patients to meet other compatible patients. When rooms are occupied by several patients, make arrangements for compatible people to share rooms, if possible.

10. Convey nursing competence to patients as much as possible.

CONVEYING NURSING COMPETENCE

The following measures help to convey competence when nurses perform techniques and give a sense of security to patients and their support persons.

1. Follow through with activities. If you will be delayed, explain this to the patient.

2. Review a technique before you start, so that you can carry it out without the guidance of reference material.

3. Gather the required equipment and supplies before starting your nursing techniques.

4. Make your movements firm, smooth, and gentle.

5. Explain beforehand if you will be supervised by someone while carrying out care.

6. If a patient or support person asks you a question that you cannot answer, acknowledge that you do not know the answer, tell the person that you will find out, and follow through.

7. Maintain your composure. Do not exclaim or appear shocked at anything you hear or see, such as a traumatic wound. Do not convey disgust or anger. Be aware that the patient is reading your facial expressions. Purposefully control your verbal and nonverbal responses.

8. Accept criticism or anger from patients objectively. Try to understand the situation from their point of view, and realize that the source of their anger is the illness and what is happening to them, not their feelings toward you personally.

9. If you require assistance during a procedure, tell the patient and explain why assistance is necessary before seeking the assistance.

10. Appear neatly dressed, clean, and well groomed. Dress according to agency policy.

11. Talk with the patient as you carry out care.

12. Handle equipment skillfully. This may necessitate practicing in the laboratory before using the equipment with a patient, eg, opening and closing artery forceps with each hand.

References

Chaska NL (editor): *The Nursing Profession: A Time to Speak.* McGraw-Hill, 1983.

Cowles K: Life, death, and personhood. *Nurs Outlook* (May/June) 1984; 32:168–172.

Kalish RA: *The Psychology of Human Behavior,* 4th ed. Wadsworth, 1977.

Maslow AH: *Motivation and Personality,* 2nd ed. Harper & Row, 1970.

Maslow AH: *Toward a Psychology of Being,* 2nd ed. Van Nostrand Reinhold, 1968.

McCann/Flynn JB, Heffron PB: *Nursing from Concept to Practice.* Brady, 1984.

Schoenhofer SO: Support as legitimate nursing action. *Nurs Outlook* (July/August) 1984; 32:218–219.

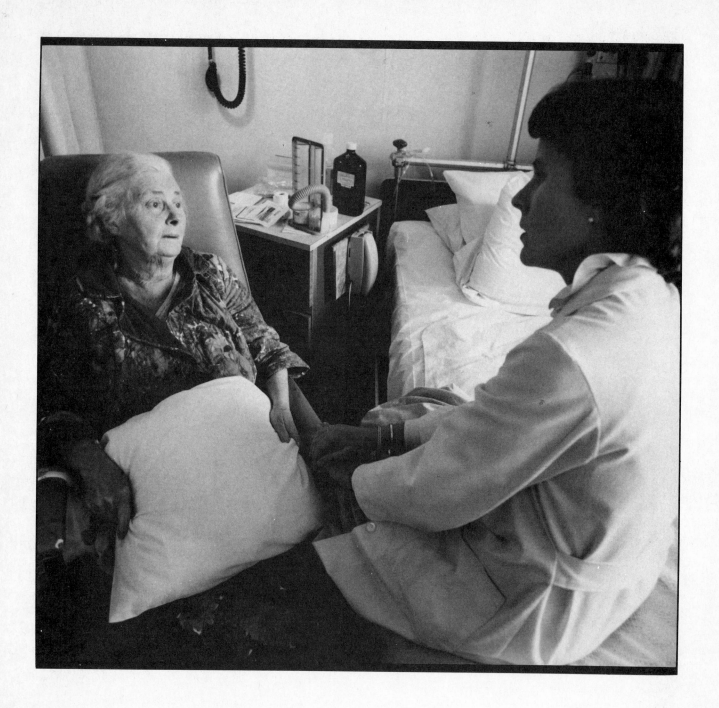

THE HEALTH CARE ENVIRONMENT

2

Nurses care for patients and their support persons in many environments. One of the important functions of a nurse is to provide a therapeutic environment. A helpful or healing environment is also a safe environment.

This chapter includes two aspects of the environment: physical and professional. A physically safe environment protects patients from bodily harm or injury. It also offers physical comfort, security, and when possible a few pleasures. A professionally safe environment is one in which nurses observe ethical standards, uphold the values of the nursing profession, and preserve the personal and legal rights of patients and their support persons.

Chapter Outline

The Physical Environment
    Temperature, Humidity, and Ventilation
    Lighting
    Decor and Design
    Noise
    Odors
    Cleanliness and Neatness
    Common Injuries and Hazards

The Professional Environment
    Values
    Rights
    Law
    Ethics

Objectives

Upon completion of this chapter, the student will:

1. Know the essentials of a physical and professional environment for patients
   1.1 Define selected terms
   1.2 Identify aspects of a physically safe environment
   1.3 Identify four aspects of the professional environment
   1.4 List specific rights of patients as outlined by the American Hospital Association and the National League for Nursing
2. Understand measures that nurses employ to ensure a safe and comfortable environment for patients
   2.1 Explain how various aspects of the physical environment are controlled
   2.2 Identify patients who are at risk for injury
   2.3 Explain ways in which falls and burns are prevented
   2.4 Discuss ways in which electric shock and radiation hazards are minimized
   2.5 Give examples of ways in which nurses convey human values to patients
   2.6 Give examples of nursing actions related to specific health care rights of patients
   2.7 Discuss nursing responsibilities related to specific areas of the law
   2.8 Give examples of ways in which ethics govern nursing action
   2.9 Explain the purposes of nursing licensure
   2.10 Explain informed consent

Terms

■ **accountable** answerable

■ **assault** an attempt or threat to touch another person unjustifiably

■ **battery** the willful or negligent touching of a person (or the person's clothing or even something the person is carrying), without consent, which may or may not cause harm

■ **bill of rights** a summary of fundamental rights and privileges guaranteed to people

■ **consent** permission given voluntarily by a person in his or her right mind; informed consent implies that the individual is knowledgeable about the consent and understands it

■ **contract** a written or verbal agreement between two or more people to do or not do some lawful act

■ **crime** an act committed in violation of societal law

■ **defamation** a communication that is false, or made with careless disregard for the truth, and results in injury to the reputation of a person

■ **ethics** the rules or principles that govern right conduct

■ **humidity** the amount of moisture in the air

■ **libel** defamation by means of print, writing, or pictures

■ **license** a legal document authorizing an individual to offer knowledge and skills to the public

■ **malpractice** professional misconduct or unreasonable lack of professional skill

■ **negligence** the omission of something a reasonable person would do or the doing of something a reasonable person would not do

■ **pathogen** a microorganism capable of producing disease

■ privileged communication   information given to a professional person such as a physician

■ radiation   electromagnetic waves used in diagnostic tests and some kinds of therapy

■ right   a matter to which a person has a just claim

■ slander   unprivileged or false words by which a person's reputation is damaged

■ tort   a wrong committed by a person against another person or the other person's property

■ value   something of worth; a belief held dearly by a person

■ ventilation   the movement of air

■ will   a person's declaration about how his or her property is to be disposed of after his or her death

THE PHYSICAL ENVIRONMENT

A safe physical environment is one in which people can function without injury and feel a sense of security. A comfortable environment is one that is free from unpleasant stimuli to the senses of sight, smell, hearing, touch, and temperature. Although many individuals work in a health care setting, nurses have traditionally assumed and continue to assume considerable responsibility for the safety and comfort of the patient's immediate environment. It is often the nurse who is first aware of a patient's discomfort or possible hazards in the surroundings, such as a slippery floor, a cold room, or electric or fire dangers. Aspects of a safe and comfortable physical environment include:

1. Adequate temperature, humidity, and ventilation
2. Adequate lighting
3. Pleasant decor and safe design
4. Minimal noise
5. Freedom from odors
6. Cleanliness and neatness
7. Freedom from hazards

Temperature, Humidity, and Ventilation

The *temperature* of the environment primarily affects comfort; only in situations of prolonged exposure to extreme heat or cold is safety affected. Because a "comfortable" temperature varies for individuals, it is often a challenge for the nurse to provide the most comfortable temperature for each in a health care setting, especially when several patients are in the same room. Generally, a room temperature between 20 and 25 °C (68 and 77 °F) is considered comfortable by most. The warmer temperature is often needed and preferred by babies, the elderly, and the inactive ill person. Most hospitals are equipped with thermostat controls and air conditioners that allow different temperatures in patient rooms and nurseries. Nurses may also need to use additional means to help patients deal with uncomfortable temperatures. Warm socks, additional bedding, and shawls can provide added warmth, while a sponge bath may refresh and cool a patient who is perspiring excessively on a hot day. When the temperature is controlled satisfactorily or means are provided to deal with it effectively, patients feel more comfortable both physically and mentally. People are often impatient and irritable if the temperature is unsatisfactory; they then have less capacity to deal with the activities of daily living and recovery from illness.

Humidity is the amount of moisture in the air. Generally a range of 30% to 60% is comfortable to most people. A very low humidity, such as 10%, is drying to the skin and mucous membranes of the air passages, and it accelerates the evaporation of perspiration. A high humidity, such as 90%, impedes the evaporation of perspiration and thus interferes with one of the body's major cooling mechanisms. Fortunately, as the temperature increases, the air can hold more moisture. However, when the temperature is high and the air is saturated with moisture, people experience considerable discomfort.

A highly humid environment is sometimes provided as a therapeutic measure. For example, cool air vaporizers or humidifiers may be used for patients with respiratory infections, since increasing the humidity of the inhaled air facilitates breathing. In other situations dehumidifiers are necessary, especially if the individual has an allergy to mold or mildew, since these frequently grow in high-humidity environments. Many air conditioners regulate both temperature and humidity.

Ventilation refers to the movement of air. Air that is still becomes stale and oppressive. Circulating air is refreshing and cooling. Open windows, when weather permits, or air conditioners can provide cooling and comforting ventilation even when high temperatures and humidity cannot be changed substantially. However, nurses need to beware of creating excessive drafts and chilling patients.

Lighting

Most health care facilities are designed to provide adequate natural and artificial light. A bright, sunny room often lifts a person's spirits, but curtains may need to be adjusted or other measures taken to shield patients from direct sunlight. Nurses need to learn patients' preferences regarding lighting. Rooms are generally equipped with overhead fluorescent lights that provide soft and diffused lighting. Lights that are too dim or that glare create mental discomfort and produce sharp, confusing shadows, which cause accidents.

Reading lamps are usually provided for each bed unit so that eyestrain is avoided. In addition, night lights are situated near the floor and, in most instances, beside the head of each hospital bed to illuminate the walking areas without shining in patients' eyes. Although many patients do not require or use night lights, children and the elderly often find them helpful for orienting themselves to strange surroundings at night and for getting to a bathroom. Nurses also use night lights for observing critically ill patients throughout the night. If patients have eye problems or have had eye surgery, nurses may need to dim overhead lights and natural light from the windows in the daytime, since the eyes may be photosensitive. This is also an important consideration for certain patients who are subject to convulsive seizures.

Decor and Design

The traditional all-white, "sterile" decor of hospitals and physicians' offices is being replaced by color combinations that provide a more cheerful environment for patients. Because bright colors stimulate, and many persons have distinct aversions to or preferences for certain colors, subdued pastel colors are most frequently used in examination and patient rooms. However, bright colors are increasingly being used in areas such as cafeterias, children's playrooms, and solariums. In many convalescent hospitals, colorful draperies, carpets, and wallpapers create a more homelike environment. The decor needs to be modest and selected carefully, however. Certain designs in flooring, wall coverings, or fabrics can cause discomfort. For example, tiny squares or parallel lines on the floor may make some people feel dizzy; bold, distinct designs may be associated with unpleasant shapes and objects by others.

Greater attention to the design of a hospital unit is focusing not only on pleasant and functional decor but also on greater safety for patients. Critical care units, for example, are sometimes designed in a circle around the nurses' station, facilitating quick access to all patients. The wall of the room facing the nurses' station often consists of glass or observation windows, so that critically ill patients can be observed constantly. Curtains are usually placed over these windows so that when the patient requires less observation, privacy can be provided. Single rooms for patients requiring protective asepsis (isolation) are sometimes designed with a service area containing needed special equipment.

Noise

People who are ill are frequently sensitive to noises that normally would not disturb them. Health care facilities are generally designed with acoustic tile on the ceilings and resilient floor materials to reduce noise. Drapes and wall-to-wall carpets further absorb sound. However, considerable noise often occurs despite these design efforts. It can be largely attributed to the presence of large numbers of agency personnel, visitors, and other patients. Nurses need to make a concerted effort to maintain a quiet, restful environment for all patients. Some points to consider in noise control are:

1. Reduce talking and laughing to a minimum, especially in long corridors, which tend to conduct sound.

2. Wear shoes with rubber or soundless soles.

3. Handle equipment and trays of dishes carefully to avoid dropping or clattering. Many agencies now use plastic equipment and carts to further reduce noise.

4. Help patients to keep television and radio volumes low. Most agencies supply earphones to prevent disturbance to adjacent patients.

5. Monitor visiting hours and, when necessary, tactfully remind visitors of the need for quiet.

6. Keep all conversations with patients and staff at low volumes.

Odors

Mild odors that normally are innocuous or even pleasant can be unpleasant to the ill person. Many people find that the smell of food cooking produces a feeling of nausea when they have the flu. Common scents that can be unpleasant to patients may arise from refuse, such as dressings, body discharges from patients, the nurse's perspiration or breath, and decayed flowers. Ways to reduce odors include the following:

1. Discard waste and refuse promptly in a utility area away from the patient's bedside.

2. Empty bedpans, urinals, and emesis basins immediately after use, and clean them effectively.

3. Change soiled linen promptly.

4. Remove food trays as soon as possible after meal hours.

5. Remove old flowers, and change stagnant water.

6. Provide adequate ventilation.

7. Make sure your breath is free from cigarette smoke or the odor of strong foods.

8. Keep yourself and your uniform clean.

9. Avoid the use of strong perfumes.

Cleanliness and Neatness

Microorganisms ever present in the environment include pathogens that are a potential source of injury to patients.

A normal person's body defenses generally protect against disease; however, an ill person's defenses are often already weakened by disease and leave the person vulnerable to surrounding pathogens. Cleanliness, which minimizes the number of microorganisms, is therefore an essential component of a safe environment for patients. Although the housekeeping staff is largely responsible for cleaning floors and furniture, the nurse plays a key role in keeping the patient's environment clean and as free from pathogens as possible. Limitation of the spread of microorganisms is referred to as *medical asepsis.* Chapters 6 and 7 discuss specific ways for the nurse to prevent the spread of microorganisms to patients. Throughout this book, however, in all techniques, medical aseptic practices are emphasized.

A neat environment helps to prevent accidents, eg, tripping over a misplaced stool. It also communicates to patients and the support persons that care is being given competently.

Common Injuries and Hazards

The most common injuries to patients in a health care facility result from falls, burns, electric shocks, and radiation.

Falls

Falls occur most commonly among the very young and the very old; they also happen frequently to patients sedated with drugs or anesthetics and to confused patients (who may be elderly or may be emotionally disturbed). Illness itself often weakens a patient; with this unaccustomed lack of strength, an individual can readily lose his or her balance.

Safeguards generally employed to prevent falls include the following:

1. Call signals are placed on patients' beds within easy reach to call for assistance. Calls are answered promptly by the nurse.

2. Articles required by patients are placed nearby so that patients do not need to reach far for them and risk losing their balance.

3. Patients who have had surgery or have been in bed for some time are advised to have assistance when first getting out of bed.

4. Footstools are supplied with rubber feet that do not slip.

5. Wheelchairs and stretchers are stabilized by locking the wheels, and crutches are equipped with rubber tips that do not slip.

6. Adjustable beds are put in the low position when patients are getting in and out of bed and for any patient who is likely to get out of bed.

7. Floors have nonslip surfaces; rugs and carpeting are fixed securely in place so that they will not slip. In some agencies, special nonskid flooring is used in halls and on stairs, and nonskid mats are placed in bathtubs.

8. The environment is kept tidy so that people do not trip over light cords, toys, or misplaced furniture.

9. Most agencies have railings along corridors and in bathrooms to assist ambulating patients.

10. Side rails are attached to the sides of the bed for all patients who are unconscious, confused, or sedated. Some agencies require that side rails be raised on the beds of all patients over 70 years of age, especially at night. Patients who object to the use of side rails may need to sign a written statement releasing the agency from any responsibility if an accident occurs.

11. Restraints are frequently ordered for restless, unconscious, confused, or sedated patients. Crib nets are used for children. See chapter 18. If there is no order, nursing staff members are often required to stay with the patient.

12. Spilled liquids are mopped up quickly, and signs are posted to warn patients and visitors when washed floors are wet.

13. Patients are encouraged to wear shoes with low heels for walking.

Burns

Burns are generally caused by hot water bottles, heating pads, hot water in a tub or shower, spills of hot liquids, and fire.

The risk of patients incurring burns is a continual problem, since patients' ability to protect themselves may be impaired with illness. Body senses, mental orientation, and consciousness levels are frequently altered by illness. Patients particularly at risk are those who:

1. Have neurologic impairments such as paralysis and lack the ability to perceive stimuli such as heat or pain

2. Are unconscious or semiconscious and lack the ability to communicate their perceptions of heat to the nurse

3. Have circulatory problems in their extremities and thus limited sensations of heat

4. Smoke cigarettes when they are confused or sedated and do not extinguish their cigarettes safely

5. Are receiving oxygen and are unaware of the safety precautions necessary to prevent combustion

Safeguards to prevent burns include the following:

1. The temperature of the water used for bathing patients and used by patients in tubs and showers is measured. See chapter 14.

2. Hot water bottles and heating pads are used with discretion and care. See chapter 34. Some agencies do not allow their use.

3. Recommended temperatures are used for hot applications such as sitz baths, soaks, moist packs, and compresses. See chapter 34.

4. Patients who are unable to handle hot liquids such as coffee or tea safely are assisted by the nurse.

5. Regular fire drills, education about the use of fire extinguishers, etc, are conducted so that all health practitioners know what to do in case of fire.

6. Emergency exits are posted, and fire extinguishers are placed in all corridors.

7. Smoking regulations are enforced. Ashtrays from which a burning cigarette cannot fall are provided in areas where smoking is allowed for visitors and patients. Patients who are confused or sedated are supervised when smoking and often have their cigarettes and matches stored away from the bedside, especially at night.

8. The safety precautions required for oxygen therapy, such as "No Smoking" signs, are explained to the patient and support persons and are posted to inform patients and visitors of the potential fire hazards. See chapter 38.

9. Materials that are saturated with combustible solutions, such as cleaning fluids, are stored in a safe place in airtight metal containers. These are a particular hazard to young children and confused patients.

Electric shocks

Electric shock is a potential hazard to patients, but the incidence of actual injury to patients from it is less than from falls or burns. Like homes, health agencies contain much electric equipment, and the best way to prevent accidents is to keep all electric equipment in good repair and working order. Specific precautions to safeguard electric equipment and prevent electric shocks include:

1. Using three-pronged plugs, which have a ground prong, and three-prong receiver outlets.

2. Checking electric equipment before use; avoiding the use of equipment with frayed or broken cords and equipment that overheats or gives off an odor.

3. Removing plugs from wall sockets by grasping the plug rather than the cord.

4. Remembering that water conducts electricity well. Electric equipment should be kept away from water sources such as sinks and bathtubs. For example, radios should not be used in the bathroom. Nurses also should ensure that their hands and feet are dry when they handle electric equipment.

5. Coiling electric cords loosely when storing electric equipment. Severe kinks in a cord can cause broken wires inside the cord.

6. Adhering to specific safety precautions when oxygen therapy is used. For example, materials (such as wool blankets) that generate static electricity are not used around oxygen. See chapter 38.

Radiation

Radiation has recently become more recognized as a cause of injury to patients. Injury can occur from overexposure to radioactive materials used in diagnostic procedures such as roentgenography, fluoroscopy, and nuclear medicine. In fluoroscopy, radioactive materials that have an affinity for specific tissues are taken into the body, usually by ingestion or intravenous routes. Among these elements are calcium, which has an affinity for bones; iodine, which is attracted to the thyroid gland; and phosphorus, which is attracted to blood. Injury can also occur when exposure to radiation to treat specific tissues damages other tissues. Radiation therapy is a common treatment for some forms of cancer.

The following precautions are taken to minimize radiation hazards for patients and nurses:

1. The patient's exposure time to roentgenography and fluoroscopy is kept to a minimum.

2. Health personnel wear lead aprons or shield themselves behind lead partitions when assisting or near patients receiving roentgenography.

3. Policies and procedures are established to guide all individuals in the care of patients who are receiving radioactive materials.

4. Radioactive body discharges are handled with care. Nurses wear rubber gloves and in some instances may place excretions in special containers for disposal.

5. Special rooms are provided for radiation therapies such as cobalt therapy.

6. Special sealed lead storage containers are provided for some radioactive materials. Special instruments are provided for handling them.

7. Nurses are required to wear special badges that record exposure time.

THE PROFESSIONAL ENVIRONMENT

A professional environment is one in which clients expect to feel safe and to some degree comfortable. When patients enter a health care agency such as a hospital, they usually believe they are entering a professional environment. Such an environment has four primary bases: values, rights, law, and ethics.

Values

A *value* is something of worth, a belief held dear by a person. Values are personal and often evolve from personal experience. An individual's real values are shown by consistent patterns of behavior. Values influence everything people do.

Because values can be held both consciously and unconsciously, and because people are frequently not clear about their own values, health education programs are increasingly placing more emphasis on the examination of personal value systems. Nurses need to understand their own values before they can assist patients and their support persons, who may confirm or reject the nurse's values.

Some values, such as compassion and respect for life, are universal—common to all cultures. However, many vary from one culture to another and even from one subgroup to another within the same broad culture. Great differences can be seen, for example, in values about aging, death, rules, authority, family, clothing, material possessions, leisure time, schooling, work, politics, friends, religion, love, sex, and health.

When providing care to patients, nurses reveal their value systems largely through their actions. Some of the ways in which nurses convey values specifically during nursing techniques are:

1. By respecting the patient as a unique individual and conveying interest in him or her as a person.

2. By listening attentively to patients' concerns and giving these priority for attention.

3. By providing privacy for patients.

4. By ensuring minimal exposure of the patient's body.

5. By providing information and explanations about what the nurse plans to do.

6. By allowing patients to participate in their care as much as possible.

7. By handling patients and their property gently and caringly.

8. By answering a patient's questions about a technique truthfully (for example, telling whether a procedure will be painful).

9. By respecting and supporting patients' own values. For example, some cultures dictate that girls and women cannot have their bodies inspected or touched by any strange man, even a physician. In this situation, a female nurse is present to assist a male physician.

10. By extending kindness and support to patients' families and friends.

Rights

A *right* is a first claim to anything that is a person's due. Patients and their support persons have become increasingly concerned about their rights. In 1973 the American Hospital Association (AHA) developed and approved a statement of a Patient's Bill of Rights. This statement has served as an impetus to legislation to protect patients and their families in some states and provinces. In 1975 the AHA reprinted the following statement of twelve rights:

A Patient's Bill of Rights*

The American Hospital Association presents a Patient's Bill of Rights with the expectation that observance of these rights will contribute to more effective patient care and greater satisfaction for the patient, his physician, and the hospital organization. Further, the Association presents these rights in the expectation that they will be supported by the hospital on behalf of its patients, as an integral part of the healing process. It is recognized that a personal relationship between the physician and the patient is essential for the provision of proper medical care. The traditional physician–patient relationship takes on a new dimension when care is rendered within an organizational structure. Legal precedent has established that the institution itself also has a responsibility to the patient. It is in recognition of these factors that these rights are affirmed.

1. The patient has the right to considerate and respectful care.

2. The patient has the right to obtain from his physician complete current information concerning his diagnosis, treatment, and prognosis in terms the patient can be reasonably expected to understand. When it is not medically advisable to give such information to the patient, the information should be made available to an appropriate person in his behalf. He has the right to know, by name, the physician responsible for coordinating his care.

3. The patient has the right to receive from his physician information necessary to give informed consent prior to the start of any procedure and/or treatment. Except in emergencies, such information for informed consent should include but not necessarily be limited to the specific procedure and/or treatment, the medically significant risks involved, and the probable duration of incapacitation. Where medically significant alternatives for care or treatment exist, or when the patient requests information concerning medical alternatives, the patient has the right to such information. The patient also has the right to know the name of the person responsible for the procedures and/or treatment.

4. The patient has the right to refuse treatment to the extent permitted by law and to be informed of the medical consequences of his action.

5. The patient has the right to every consideration of his privacy concerning his own medical care program. Case discussion, consultation, examination and treatment are confidential and should be conducted discreetly. Those not directly involved in his care must have the permission of the patient to be present.

6. The patient has the right to expect that all communications and records pertaining to his care should be treated as confidential.

7. The patient has the right to expect that within its capacity a hospital must make reasonable response to the request of a patient for services. The hospital must provide evaluation, service and/or referral as indicated by the urgency of the case. When medically permissible, a patient may be transferred to another facility only after he has received complete information and explanation concerning the needs for and

---

*American Hospital Association: *A Patient's Bill of Rights,* Catalog No. S009, AHA, 1975. Reprinted with the permission of the American Hospital Association, copyright 1975.

alternatives to such a transfer. The institution to which the patient is to be transferred must first have accepted the patient for transfer.

8. The patient has the right to obtain information as to any relationship of his hospital to other health care and educational institutions insofar as his care is concerned. The patient has the right to obtain information as to the existence of any professional relationships among individuals by name, who are treating him.

9. The patient has the right to be advised if the hospital proposes to engage in or perform human experimentation affecting his care or treatment. The patient has the right to refuse to participate in such research projects.

10. The patient has the right to expect reasonable continuity of care. He has the right to know in advance what appointment times and physicians are available and where. The patient has the right to expect that the hospital will provide a mechanism whereby he is informed by his physician or a delegate of the physician of the patient's continuing health care requirements following discharge.

11. The patient has the right to examine and receive an explanation of his bill regardless of source of payment.

12. The patient has the right to know what hospital rules and regulations apply to his conduct as a patient.

No catalog of rights can guarantee for the patient the kind of treatment he has a right to expect. A hospital has many functions to perform, including the prevention and treatment of disease, the education of both health professionals and patients, and the conduct of clinical research. All these activities must be conducted with an overriding concern for the patient, and above all, the recognition of his dignity as a human being. Success in achieving this recognition assures success in the defense of the rights of the patient.

In 1977 the National League for Nursing prepared statements that describe patients' rights and related nursing responsibilities as follows:

Nursing's Role in Patients' Rights*

- People have the right to health care that is accessible and that meets professional standards, regardless of the setting.
- Patients have the right to courteous and individualized health care that is equitable, humane, and given without discrimination as to race, color, creed, sex, national origin, source of payment, or ethical or political beliefs.
- Patients have the right to information about their diagnosis, prognosis, and treatment—including alternatives to care and risks involved—in terms they and their families can readily understand, so that they can give their informed consent.
- Patients have the legal right to informed participation in all decisions concerning their health care.
- Patients have the right to information about the qualifications, names, and titles of personnel responsible for providing their health care.
- Patients have the right to refuse observation by those not directly involved in their care.

- Patients have the right to privacy during interview, examination, and treatment.
- Patients have the right to privacy in communicating and visiting with persons of their choice.
- Patients have the right to refuse treatments, medications, or participation in research and experimentation, without punitive action being taken against them.
- Patients have the right to coordination and continuity of health care.
- Patients have the right to appropriate instruction or education from health care personnel so that they can achieve an optimal level of wellness and an understanding of their basic health needs.
- Patients have the right to confidentiality of all records (except as otherwise provided for by law or third-party payer contracts) and all communications, written or oral, between patients and health care providers.
- Patients have the right of access to all health records pertaining to them, the right to challenge and to have their records corrected for accuracy, and the right to transfer of all such records in the case of continuing care.
- Patients have the right to information on the charges for services, including the right to challenge these.
- Above all, patients have the right to be fully informed as to all their rights in all health care settings.

Guidelines for nursing intervention

1. Be aware of the contents of any bills of rights that have been enacted in your state or province.

2. Respect the dignity of each patient and family.

3. Respect patients' rights to refuse any treatment, procedure, or medication. Report any refusals to the patient's physician and to the responsible nurse.

4. Respect the right of each patient and family to confidentiality of information.

5. Unless otherwise instructed by the physician or responsible nurse, answer patients' questions completely, and provide information normally provided by the health professional responsible.

6. Listen carefully to patients and their support persons, and convey their concerns to the appropriate person in the agency, such as the responsible nurse.

7. As patients are admitted to the agency, inform them and their support persons of agency policies, rules, and regulations.

8. Assist patients to maintain their rights to freedom of movement and freedom to make decisions. The exceptions are mentally incompetent persons, patients who are in the custody of the courts, such as convicted criminals, and persons restricted by their physicians for medical reasons.

Law

Nurses, patients, and support persons have legal rights that protect them. It is necessary for nurses to know some

*National League for Nursing, *Nursing's Role in Patients' Rights,* NLN Pub No. 1–1671 (New York: The League, 1977). Used with permission.

of the basic concepts underlying these laws so that they can protect both patients and themselves.

There are two types of legal actions: civil and criminal. *Civil action* deals with relationships between people, such as an individual's claim that a person has cheated him or her in a sale of goods. *Criminal action* deals with wrongs of individuals against society; for example, a person who stabs another person has violated the law enacted by society prohibiting this behavior. Nurses are more likely to become involved in civil lawsuits than criminal lawsuits. The civil disputes may arise between two people or between a person and an organization such as a hospital. For example, a patient might sue a nurse and a hospital because of a burn the patient received from a hot water bottle.

Contracts

A *contract* is an agreement between two or more competent persons, upon sufficient consideration (remuneration), to do or not to do some lawful act. The agreement may be written or oral. A contract is the basis of the relationship between nurses and their employer. A nurse may be prevented from carrying out the terms of the contract because of illness or death, but personal inconvenience or personal problems are not considered legitimate reasons for failure to fulfill a contract. Employers are also obligated to meet the terms of a contract.

Wills

A *will* is a declaration by a person about how his or her property is to be disposed of after his or her death. For a will to be valid, two conditions are necessary:

1. The person making the will must be of sound mind. This means that the person must be able to understand and retain mentally:
   a. The general nature and extent of the property.
   b. The relationship of the beneficiaries.
   c. The relationship of those not benefiting.
   d. The disposition the person is making of the property.
2. The person making the will must not be unduly influenced by anyone.

Nurses may be asked from time to time to witness a will. In most states and provinces, a will must be signed in the presence of two witnesses, both over the age of 18. In some situations, if the patient cannot sign his or her name, a mark will suffice.

A witness to a will should be someone who is not a beneficiary and should be present at the time the person signs the will. When a nurse serves as a witness, it is wise to note this on the patient's record together with the nurse's opinion of the patient's mental and physical condition.

A nurse who does not wish to act as a witness to a will has a right to refuse. If, for example, the nurse believes that undue influence has been exerted on the patient, the nurse may wish to refuse.

Some hospitals provide a notary public (an individual who certifies written materials) to witness wills and do not expect nurses to do this.

Crimes and torts

A *crime* is an act committed in violation of societal law. It is punishable by a fine and/or imprisonment. A crime does not have to be intentional; for example, accidental administration of a drug that proved lethal is a crime. A *tort* is a wrong committed by a person against another person or the other person's property. *Negligence* is the omission of something a reasonable person would do or the doing of something a reasonable person would not do. *Malpractice* is a part of the law of negligence that applies to professional persons. It is any professional misconduct or unreasonable lack of professional skill. Nurses are responsible for their own nursing actions, even though they are employed by an agency or following a physician's orders. An example of malpractice by omission (neglect) is forgetting to give a medication; an example of malpractice by commission (action carried out) is giving the wrong medication. Common allegations of lawsuits against nurses include charges of negligence and malpractice. Because lawsuits are increasing, nurses in active practice are advised to have malpractice insurance.

Invasion of privacy

Individuals have a right to privacy, that is, a right to withhold themselves and their private lives from public scrutiny. The act of invasion of privacy injures the person's feelings and disregards the effect of the divulged information on the person's standing in the community.

The very fact that a number of people contribute to a patient's diagnosis and treatment may infringe on the patient's right to privacy, but discussions can and should be restricted to the patient's illness and confined to professional persons engaged in the care.

In teaching hospitals it is important to obtain the patient's consent before a demonstration or teaching conference is conducted, to respect the patient's right to privacy. In many agencies, consents are obtained on admission. Patients have a right to refuse to participate in clinical demonstrations for nursing and medical students.

Libel and slander

Libel and slander come under the heading of defamation. *Defamation* is a communication that is false, or made with a careless disregard for the truth, and results in injury to the reputation of a person. *Libel* is defamation by means of print, writing, or pictures. *Slander* is defamation by the spoken word, stating unprivileged (not legally protected) or false words by which a person's reputation is damaged. Nurses can make statements about patients to an attending physician or a member of the patient's health team. These are generally considered *privileged communications* not subject to charges of slander. Unprivileged or false statements may constitute slander, however. It is therefore important for nurses to confine their remarks about patients to the appropriate people and to clinical areas. Statements should never be made in other settings, such as a hospital cafeteria.

Privileged communications

A privileged communication is information given to a professional person such as a physician, nurse, or social worker. Under the law in most states and provinces, physicians generally cannot be made to divulge information about patients in court. Some states, such as New York, New Mexico, and Arkansas, have extended these statutes to include nurses. In Nebraska no physician or person acting as the physician's agent, eg, a nurse, may be required to disclose confidential information (Creighton, 1981, p 216).

When a nurse is given unusual information by a patient, it is prudent to convey this to the physician or the responsible nurse. The law concerning privileged communication is very complex, and it is unwise for nurses to take it upon themselves to keep information from others in the belief that it is privileged.

Assault and battery

Assault can be defined as an attempt to touch another person unjustifiably or the threat to do so. *Battery* is the willful or negligent touching of a person (or the person's clothes or even something the person is carrying), without consent, which may or may not cause harm. Technical assault is assault without the intent to injure the other person. Therefore if patients do not give legal consent to treatment, a nurse or physician could be charged with technical assault.

Informed consent

A patient's consent to treatment is required in most instances. Three groups of persons cannot provide consent:

1. In most areas, for minors to obtain treatment, consent must be given by a parent or guardian. The same is also true of an adult who has the mental capacity of a child.

2. When persons are unconscious or injured in such a way that they are unable to give consent, consent is usually obtained from the closest adult relative. In an emergency, if consent cannot be obtained from the patient or a relative, then the law generally agrees that consent is assumed.

3. Mentally ill persons cannot give consent. States and provinces generally provide in mental health acts or similar statutes definitions of mental illness and the rights of the mentally ill under the law, as well as the rights of the staff caring for such patients.

Guidelines for nursing intervention

1. Be aware of specific legal documents used in the agency, such as consent forms and the patient's chart.

2. Check that a consent form has been signed by the patient before you provide care. If a consent form has not been signed, establish how the physician and/or agency has legally dealt with this problem.

3. Always be considerate of patients. Never threaten a patient with physical force. When you consider restraining a patient, make sure it is for the patient's safety and that you have the appropriate authority.

4. Report patient behavior accurately, and do not make judgmental statements that could be considered libel. For example, report: "Asked 'Where am I?' twice this morning," not "Patient is stupid and does not know where he is."

5. If a patient tells you personal information about his or her condition, consider this a privileged communication and report it only to the responsible nurse or to the attending physician.

Nursing licensure

Licenses are legal documents that entitle practitioners to offer their knowledge and skills to the public in the area of the country covered by the license. Licensing protects the public from unqualified practitioners, and it sets standards for the profession or occupation.

The practical nurse who passes an examination and pays a registration fee becomes licensed under the title *licensed practical nurse* (LPN) or in some jurisdictions *licensed vocational nurse* (LVN). The graduate nurse who passes an examination and pays a registration fee becomes licensed under the title *registered nurse* (RN).

There are two types of licensure: mandatory and permissive. In some areas nurses are legally required to be licensed in order to practice (licensure is mandatory). In other areas nurses need not have a license to practice nursing legally. However, licensure is necessary before a nurse can be called a licensed practical nurse or a registered nurse.

In each jurisdiction there is a nursing body or board that has the authority to grant and revoke (cancel) licenses. Some of the reasons for revoking a license are:

1. Incompetence in nursing practice

2. Conviction of a crime, such as selling drugs

3. Drug addiction

4. Obtaining a license through deception

5. Falsifying school records

Ethics

Ethics are the rules or principles that govern right conduct in a society. A *code of ethics* provides a means by which professional standards of practice are established, maintained, and improved. It is essential to a profession. Codes of ethics are formal guidelines for professional action. They are shared by the persons within the profession and should be generally compatible with a professional member's personal values.

A code of ethics gives the members of the profession a frame of reference for judgments in complex nursing situations. No two situations are identical, and nurses are frequently in situations that require judgment about which course of action to take. A code of ethics serves as a guide in many of these situations.

When people enter the nursing profession, other members of the profession assume that they accept the established nursing codes of ethics. New nurses inherit the trust and the responsibility to carry out ethical practices and to exhibit ethical conduct.

The International Council of Nurses, American Nurses' Association, Canadian Nurses' Association, National Federation of Licensed Practical Nurses, and state and provincial associations have established codes of nursing ethics. If a nurse violates the code, the association may expel the nurse from membership. Increasingly, professional nursing associations are taking an active part in improving and enforcing standards.

The purposes of nursing ethics include:

1. Providing a basis for regulating the relationship between the nurse, the patient, coworkers, society, and the profession.

2. Providing a standard basis for excluding the unscrupulous nursing practitioner and for defending a practitioner who is unjustly accused

3. Providing a basis for professional curricula and for orienting the new graduate to professional nursing practice

4. Assisting the public in understanding professional nursing conduct

Guidelines for nursing intervention

1. Nurses are accountable (answerable) for all their professional activities. They cannot blame others for their own behavior. A nurse who performs a task must be able to explain to others and account for that task and how it was performed. If, for example, the task was carried out unsafely, the nurse must answer for this.

2. Nurses are responsible—that is, their actions are reliable and trustworthy. Nurses report their own actions honestly and accurately.

3. Nurses hold the responsibility to refrain from performing tasks or techniques unfamiliar to them or ones in which they have had no education.

4. All nurses have personal values. Many nurses need to learn new values once they enter nursing. Some of the values they have developed in their homes may be incompatible with nursing practice; other values essential to nursing may not have been emphasized at home. For example, being punctual is a highly held value in nursing but may not be valued in some families.

5. Nurses who hold values that may come into direct conflict with nursing practice need to make this known to their employers. For example, some nurses are strongly opposed to the practice of abortion. These nurses may wish not to be assigned to that area of nursing. It is important that the nurse's values not jeopardize the welfare of any patient.

References

American Hospital Association: *A Patient's Bill of Rights.* Catalog No. S009. AHA, 1975.

Aroskar MA: Anatomy of an ethical dilemma: The theory. *Am J Nurs* (April) 1980; 80:658–660.

Aroskar MA: Anatomy of an ethical dilemma: The practice. *Am J Nurs* (April) 1980; 80:661–663.

Creighton H: *Law Every Nurse Should Know,* 4th ed. Saunders, 1981.

Curtin LL: Is there a right to health care? *Am J Nurs* (March) 1980; 80:462–465.

Davis AJ: To tell or not. *Am J Nurs* (January) 1981; 81:156.

Rabinow J: Patient injury in the hospital: How to protect yourself legally. *Nurs Life* (January/February) 1982; 2:44–48.

Sklar C: Was the patient informed? *Can Nurse* (June) 1980; 76:18, 20, 22.

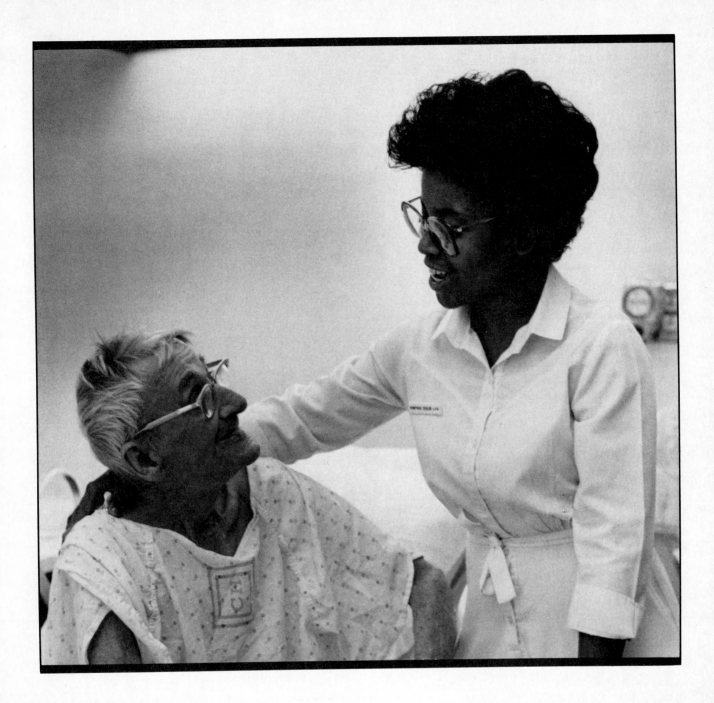

THE NURSING PROCESS

3

The term *nursing process* emerged in the mid-1960s and has become widely accepted to describe the series of steps that a nurse takes when planning and implementing care. It is a systematic method used to assess patients' health problems, to identify nursing diagnoses, to specify plans to solve them, to implement the plans or delegate implementation to others, and, finally, to evaluate the effectiveness of the actions taken in resolving the problems.

The five basic steps of the nursing process are:

1. Collecting data (assessment)
2. Interpreting the data (nursing diagnosis)
3. Planning an intervention
4. Implementing the intervention

5. Evaluating the effectiveness of the other four steps

Implicit in the nursing process is the need to involve the patient and support persons, and the need to tailor the approach to each patient's individual needs.

Chapter Outline

Assessment
    Objective and Subjective Data
    Sources of Data
    Methods of Data Collection

Nursing Diagnosis
    Components
    Format

Planning Nursing Interventions
    Setting Priorities
    Determining Resource Personnel
    Establishing Goals
    Writing a Plan of Action

Nursing Intervention

Evaluation

Objectives

Upon completion of this chapter, the student will:

1. Know essential terms and facts about the nursing process
    1.1 Define selected terms
    1.2 Identify the steps of the nursing process
    1.3 Identify the essential aspects of each phase of the nursing process
    1.4 Identify four major sources of data

    1.5 Identify five methods used to collect data
    1.6 Identify essential aspects of the interview process
    1.7 Identify essential aspects of nursing diagnoses
    1.8 Identify essential aspects of planning nursing interventions
    1.9 Identify essential aspects of formulating patient goals or outcomes

Terms

■ assessment   organized collection of data about a patient; the first step of the nursing process

■ etiology   cause

■ goal (objective)   a hoped-for outcome

■ nursing diagnosis   a problem of a patient that the nurse can treat without a physician's order

■ nursing history   a record compiled by nurses by a systematic method, containing data about a patient's past health and current status

■ nursing process   a systematic method used to assess patients' health problems, identify nursing diagnoses, specify plans to solve them, implement the plans or delegate them to others, and evaluate the effectiveness of the interventions

■ objective data   information about a patient that can be observed or measured by laboratory or other means

■ subjective data   information about a patient that can be offered only by the patient personally, such as thoughts or feelings

ASSESSMENT

Assessment is the first phase in the nursing process, and data collection is the primary tool used during this phase. Data collection is a continuing activity, which can be conducted both formally and informally. An example of formal data collection is the nursing history (nursing assessment); an example of informal data collection is noticing during a handshake that a patient's hand is damp. Assessment is continuous throughout the nursing process. Because the patient is always changing, data are always incomplete.

The purpose of nursing assessment is to gather information about the patient's health so that the nurse can plan individualized care. All other steps in the nursing process depend on the collection of data, which need to be relevant and descriptive. Data must always be factual, not interpretive, and must be reliable and valid. It is a common error to offer opinions, generalizations, and interpretations as data. For example, a nurse may describe a patient as "uncooperative" rather than record specific "uncooperative" behavior—perhaps a refusal to take deep breaths and to cough after surgery. A description of the behavior is more useful than an interpretation, because the causes of specific behavior can be explored. Perhaps the patient refuses to cough because he or she is afraid of rupturing a suture line or has severe pain upon coughing.

Patients sometimes generalize or are not specific. They may describe the reason for their hospitaliztion as a "spell" or "chest pain." It is important that the nurse elicit specifics from the patient. For example, the chest pain needs to be described by its nature and location, its duration, how it was relieved, when it occurred, and whether it was a new experience.

Objective and Subjective Data

Objective data are detectable by an observer or can be tested by using an accepted standard. For example, discoloration of the skin, a blood pressure reading, and the act of crying are objective data. *Subjective data* are apparent only to the person affected and can be described or verified only by that person. Itching, pain, and feeling worried are examples of subjective data. Objective data are sometimes called *signs* or *overt data,* and subjective data are sometimes called *symptoms* or *covert data.*

Data can also be described as *variable* or *constant.* Blood pressure, for example, varies from day to day or even by the hour and needs updating. Constant data are unchanging, for example, a date of birth.

The term *data* has a broader meaning than signs or symptoms. It also includes patient information that is not related to a disease process. In the context of the problem-oriented record, the terms *data base* and *baseline data* are often used. See page 32.

Sources of Data

There are four resources available to the nurse when making an assessment of the patient:

1. The patient
2. Support persons, eg, family members, close friends
3. Health team members
4. Medical and related records

Patients are considered the chief source, since they can provide data that no one else can offer, unless they are very young, confused, or severely ill. Nurses need to recognize, however, that some stoic patients may understate their symptoms, while other patients may exaggerate them.

Family members or friends can often supplement or verify information provided by patients. They may convey information about stresses the patient has undergone prior to illness, the family background in relation to illness and health, and the patient's home environment.

Other members of the health team also can provide information about the patient and the patient's health. The physician may have known the patient before, and a social worker or public health nurse may have already helped the patient. Through consultation, the nurse is often able to supplement data about the patient.

Medical and nursing histories and other clinical records, such as laboratory records, radiologic reports, and vital signs or neurologic records, offer other pertinent data about the patient. The nurse may find from a laboratory record, for example, that a patient's hemoglobin is low, or a radiologic report may indicate that an obstructive lesion exists. The nursing history is discussed in chapter 4.

Methods of Data Collection

Of the five basic methods used by nurses to collect data (observation, physical examination, interviewing, consultation with other health team members, and review of records and reports), the first three are discussed next, while the last two were explored in the previous section.

Observation

To observe is to gather data by use of four senses—sight, smell, hearing, and touch—with an understanding of what has been detected. Nurses not only observe but also realize the significance of their observations and interpret them. For example, when a nurse observes that a patient's face is flushed, it is important to interpret what the flushing means in relation to other data. Related data might be an elevated blood pressure or an elevated body temperature.

Observation is a highly developed skill that uses knowledge from the physical and social sciences as its basis. When nurses have an understanding of normal behavior, they are able to recognize abnormal behavior. Likewise knowledge of normal human physiology is necessary before abnormal physiology can be recognized.

Physical examination

Four methods of assessment commonly used during the physical examination are auscultation, inspection, palpation, and percussion. These are discussed in chapter 10 and in sections on assessment throughout the book. Physical examination of the patient is increasingly a nursing responsibility. It incorporates the methods of observation and interviewing.

Interviewing

More and more nurses are using a nursing history as a tool in initial contact interviews. The patient influences both the time taken for the interview and the assessment itself. With very ill patients, data gathering may be limited to observation and examination. When patients are conscious, however, they are often willing to reveal information other than their immediate health problems; this can facilitate or impede data collection.

During the initial assessment interview, the nurse's objective is to obtain information, and the patient's objective is to convey information. For the nurse, this requires thinking, observing, and verbal and nonverbal activity. At the same time the nurse is initiating a nurse–patient relationship and establishing a climate of trust.

The nurse is largely responsible for the physical arrangements for the assessment interview. It is best carried out in a setting where the patient and the nurse will not be interrupted. Privacy is important so that the patient is more likely to feel comfortable and provide highly personal information. The assessment interview has four parts: the introduction, the body, the recapitulation, and the plans for continuity in patient–nurse planning.

Introduction The introduction should include a number of points:

1. The nurse's name and position in the agency.
2. The kinds of information the nurse requires, and what use is to be made of the data.
3. Where the data will be recorded, and who will be able to see them.
4. How long the interview will take.
5. The patient's right to refuse or consent to provide the data.
6. The patient's right to privileged communication with the nurse. Privileged communication is discussed in chapter 2.

An introduction might run as follows:

Nurse: Hello, Ms. Goodwin, I'm Ms. Fellows. I'm a student nurse, and I'll be assisting with your care here on this unit.

Patient: Hi. Are you a student from the college?

Nurse: Yes, I'm in my final year, and I'd like to sit down with you here for about ten minutes to talk about how I can help you while you're here.

Patient: I'd be glad to talk with you. What do you want to know?

Nurse: Well, in order to plan your care after your operation, I'd like to obtain some information about your normal daily activities and what you expect here in the hospital. I'd like to make notes while we talk, in order to get the important points down and make them available to the other staff members who will be looking after you.

Patient: Okay.... I guess that's all right with me.

Nurse: If there is anything you don't want to say, please feel free to say so, and if there is anything you would rather I didn't write down, just tell me, and it will remain confidential. Shall we start now?

Patient: Sure, now is as good a time as any.

Body of interview In the body of the assessment interview, the patient communicates what she or he thinks, feels, and is experiencing. The information that the nurse requires may be outlined in the nursing history tool. During this part of the interview, the nurse has several responsibilities:

1. To listen carefully
2. To clarify points that the patient does not understand and seek clarification of those the nurse does not understand
3. To be aware of building a relationship of respect, trust, concern, and interest
4. To refocus the patient, if he or she wanders from the subject

There are basically three types of questions that the nurse can use to elicit information: (a) open-ended questions or suggestions, (b) closed questions, and (c) biased or leading questions.

An open-ended question or suggestion is designed to obtain an answer that is longer than one or two words and to allow the patient to divulge information the patient is ready to disclose. It may elicit descriptive or comparative responses or responses that convey to the nurse some attitudes and beliefs held by the patient. The chief disadvantage of the open-ended question is that the patient may spend time conveying irrelevant information. Examples of open-ended questions and suggestions are: "How have you been feeling lately?" "Tell me how you feel about that." "How do you feel about coming to the hospital?"

Closed questions require only one or two words for the answer. The response may be "Yes" or "No," or a specific fact, such as the patient's age or marital status. Highly stressed persons and those who have difficulty communicating usually find closed questions easier to answer than other questions. The amount of information gained is generally limited, however. Examples of closed questions are: "What medication did you take?" "Are you having pain now?" "How long have you lived in the United States?"

Biased or leading questions contain some information about what the questioner expects in the answer. They should not be used. This type of question can provoke the patient to argue with the nurse or not to give accurate information. Examples of biased questions are: "Did you take too many pills because your memory is failing?" "You haven't ever had a venereal disease, have you?"

The use of words about which the patient has many emotions can also bias a question. For example, masturbation and incest have negative connotations to some people, and hence their mention can bias a question.

Recapitulation   The recapitulation phase of the interview follows once the required data have been obtained. It helps the nurse to organize, set priorities for, and verbalize the main points that were identified. It also conveys to the patient what the nurse heard and gives the patient an opportunity to validate or revise the nurse's data.

Plans for continuity   The plans for continuity in patient–nurse planning conclude the interview. At this time the patient should obtain some idea of how he or she will be expected to participate in care planning, which staff members will be seeing the patient in this regard, and when. For example, the nurse might say:

> Ms. Goodwin, I will be responsible for giving you care three days per week while you are here. I will be in to see you each Monday, Tuesday, and Wednesday between 8 o'clock and 12 noon. At those times we can adjust your care if it is needed. When I am not here, Ms. Brown and Mr. Nakamura will be looking after you.

NURSING DIAGNOSIS

In the second step of the nursing process, the patient's problems are outlined. A nursing diagnosis is a problem that the nurse can treat without an order from a physician. In the past decade, considerable attention has been given to the identification, development, and standardization of nursing diagnoses. These diagnoses describe a combination of signs and symptoms indicating actual or potential health problems. Nursing diagnoses differ from medical diagnoses (see Table 3–1).

Components

There are three essential components of a nursing diagnosis; they are referred to as the PES format (Gordon, 1976, p 1299):

1. *The state of the patient or health problem* (P). This component, referred to as the *diagnostic category* label or title, is a description of the patient's condition (actual or potential) for which nursing therapy is given. The state of the patient is described clearly and concisely in a few words. A list of diagnostic categories was adopted by the Fifth National Conference on Classification of Nursing Diagnoses in 1982. Five examples are:

Activity intolerance

Alterations in family processes

TABLE 3–1   ■   Characteristics of Medical and Nursing Diagnoses

Medical diagnosis	Nursing diagnosis
Describes a specific disease process	Describes an individual's response to a disease process, condition, or situation
Is oriented to pathology	Is oriented to the individual
Remains constant throughout the duration of illness	Changes as the patient's responses change
Guides medical management, some of which may be carried out by the nurse	Guides independent nursing care, ie, nursing orders (therapies) and evaluation
Is complementary to the nursing diagnosis	Is complementary to the medical diagnosis
Has a well-developed classification system accepted by the medical profession	Has no universally accepted classification system; such systems are in the process of development

Knowledge deficit (specify)

Impairment of skin integrity

Social isolation (Carpenito, 1983, pp 6–8)

To be clinically useful, category labels need to be specific. Thus, quantifying or qualifying adjectives are sometimes needed to identify areas, stages, or levels of a particular problem. Where the term *specify* follows a category label, the nurse is directed to state the area in which the problem occurs. For example, a knowledge deficit may be in the area of medication prescription, dietary adjustments, or disease process and therapy. Stages may be specified by using qualifying terms such as *acute* or *chronic* (eg, chronic ineffective breathing pattern). Numbered levels are needed to specify a problem such as impaired physical mobility.

2. *The etiology of the problem* (E). This component identifies the probable causes of the patient's state of health and gives direction to the required nursing therapy. Etiology may include behaviors of the patient, environmental factors, or interactions of the two. For example, the probable causes of impaired physical mobility include decreased strength and endurance, pain/discomfort, and musculoskeletal impairment. Differentiating among possible causes in the nursing diagnosis is essential because each may require different nursing therapies.

3. *The defining characteristics or cluster of signs and symptoms* (S). The defining characteristics provide information necessary to arrive at the diagnostic category label (component 1). Each nursing diagnostic category has a set of signs and symptoms that occur as a clinical entity. They are similar to the medical diagnostic categories. For example,

the medical diagnostic category myocardial infarction (heart attack) has a standardized set of signs and symptoms that are universally understood and accepted. Likewise, the nursing diagnostic category impaired physical mobility has a standardized cluster of signs and symptoms.

Format

The nursing diagnostic statement has two parts:

1. Statement of the patient's response
2. Contributing factors or probable causes of the response

The two parts of the nursing diagnosis are joined by the words *related to* or *associated with* rather than *due to*. The phrase *due to* implies a cause-and-effect relationship; one clause causes the other clause. In contrast, the phrases *related to* and *associated with* merely imply a relationship; thus legal hazards are avoided. Examples of nursing diagnoses are:

Potential for injury [*response*] related to poor hearing [*contributing factor*]

Knowledge deficit about diabetes [*response*] related to language difference [*contributing factor*]

Nursing diagnoses are derived from the assessment data. If there are gaps in the nursing diagnoses or if they appear contradictory, the nurse should assess the patient further, consult with other members of the health team, or consult reference sources. The complete assessment data are then divided into normal and abnormal, categorized, and labeled with a nursing diagnosis.

PLANNING NURSING INTERVENTIONS

Planning nursing interventions involves (a) setting priorities, (b) determining resource personnel who can best handle the patient's problems, (c) establishing goals (objectives) for the nursing care, and (d) writing a plan of action.

Setting Priorities

Each of the problems that has been identified in the nursing diagnosis is assigned a priority rating: high, medium, or low priority. This is a nursing judgment, but it must include the patient's views. The hierarchy of needs (see chapter 1) is helpful in setting priorities. In that hierarchy, physiologic needs take precedence, and even within a category some needs are of greater importance than others. Air is essential for the maintenance of life, and people can live longer without water than without air. Once physiologic needs are met, then other needs can

assume a higher priority. The priorities of needs are continually changing, just as the patient's health status changes. Another factor affecting priorities among problems is the patient's view of their urgency.

Determining Resource Personnel

Once priorities have been set among the patient's problems, the nurse assesses whether other personnel may be able to help the patient with one or more problems. Resource personnel may be the patient, support persons, other health team members, and community members such as a family pastor. It is important for nurses to recognize that they cannot help the patient with all problems.

The patient and the nurse can discuss the alternatives and decide whose assistance is required. The particular resources depend on the individual patient and the available personnel. The resources of an urban setting may not be available to people in a rural one.

Establishing Goals

A goal or objective is a hoped-for outcome. It is stated in terms of anticipated patient outcomes, not nursing activities. Goals are of two types: short-term and long-term. A short-term goal is one that the patient could accomplish in the immediate future, ie, an eight-hour shift. For example, "The patient will drink 1,500 mL of fluid in eight hours," or "The patient will raise her right arm to shoulder height once every two hours during the day." A long-term goal in the same context might be, "The patient will demonstrate full range of motion in her right arm during exercise class."

Goals are usually planned by the patient and the nurse. They must be realistic in terms of patient potential and nursing ability. To set a goal that requires the assistance of a nurse when in fact the nurse cannot help is unrealistic.

Goals are worded in a clear, concise manner that can be understood by all health team members. They are written in terms of patient behavior and are exact, rather than general, in wording. Each goal or objective needs to contain three components: the subject, the behavior, and the conditions under which the behavior can be expected to be demonstrated.

Goals must also be stated in measurable terms. For example, if the patient is to understand a technique, the goal must be stated: "The patient will understand the technique, as demonstrated by correct responses to questions after the explanation."

Subject

The subject of a written goal is usually the patient, although it might be a family member or other significant person, or a part of the body such as the ankle or arm.

Behavior

Behavior may be one of four types: psychomotor, affective, cognitive, or physiologic. Psychomotor behavior involves muscle control activities, such as writing or walking. Affective behavior involves feelings and attitudes, such as joy or anger. Cognitive behavior involves the use of intellectual processes such as remembering and understanding. Physiologic behavior is activity of the body processes, such as respiration and elimination.

Conditions

The conditions of a goal are the circumstances in which the behavior is expected to be demonstrated. They are used primarily to make terminal goals more explicit, but they are not necessary for all objectives. In the goals "The patient will walk unassisted," and "The patient will walk using a walker," the conditions are "unassisted" and "using a walker."

Specific criteria of acceptable performance can further clarify a goal. Phrases such as "once an hour" or "the length of the hall" specify minimum conditions of expected behaviors.

Writing a Plan of Action

Once the goals have been determined, the next step is to determine a plan for nursing action. The nursing action or intervention involves assisting patients to meet their goals. It is based on a rationale (an explanation) that includes facts, principles, and knowledge.

At this phase, the nurse may require additional information, from the patient perhaps or from resources such as current literature. This information can add to the rationale for the nursing action.

The plan of action initially involves a decision about each problem. Usually there are three alternatives open to the patient and the nurse:

1. No action is necessary or perhaps possible at this time.
2. The problem needs to be referred to another member of the health team or a member of the family.
3. Nursing intervention is indicated to help the patient resolve the problem.

The problems have already been placed in a hierarchy. It is important to consider each problem now in that sequence. If nursing intervention is indicated, the nurse considers the alternative nursing actions. For most problems, there are a number of alternatives, and the ones selected need to be realistic. This judgment is generally based upon experience, knowledge, and data from other resources. For example, if one nursing diagnosis is "actual impairment of skin integrity related to immobility" the planned nursing interventions (also referred to as *nursing orders, nursing approaches,* or *nursing actions*) may include:

1. Encourage range of motion exercise.

2. Turn the patient every hour using a turning schedule, eg, from right side to back, back to left side, left side to right side, right side to back.
3. Keep the bed as flat as possible.
4. Support the feet with a footboard.
5. Use an egg-crate mattress.
6. With each turning, inspect the skin areas at risk: heels, ischia, and elbows.

In choosing the most desirable nursing actions, a number of criteria should be considered:

1. Will this intervention be effective?
2. Is it realistic for the patient and the nurse?
3. Is it acceptable to the patient and perhaps the support persons?

The nursing interventions chosen are then written in the nursing care plan (discussed in chapter 4) or on specific nursing order sheets.

The degree of detail included in the nursing orders depends to some extent on the health personnel who will carry out the order. It is advisable, however, to be exact. For example, "The patient will force fluids" may have different meanings for different people, whereas "The patient will drink 5,000 mL each 24 hours" provides a precise guide for the patient and all health team personnel.

Nursing orders need to include five components: the date, the precise action verb and possibly a modifier, the content area, the time element, and the signature (Little, Carnevali, 1976, p 213).

Date

Nursing orders are dated when they are written and reviewed regularly at intervals that depend on the individual patient's needs. If a patient is acutely ill—in an intensive care unit, for example—the plan of care is continually monitored and revised. In a community clinic, weekly or biweekly reviews may be indicated.

Action verb

The verb starts the order and is precise in nature. For example, "Explain (to the patient) the actions of his insulin" is a more precise statement than "Teach (the patient) about his insulin." Sometimes a modifier for the verb can make the nursing order more precise. For example, "Apply spiral bandage firmly to left lower leg" is more precise than "Apply spiral bandage to left leg."

Content area

Content is the where and what of the order. In the previous example, "spiral bandage" and "left leg" state the what and the where of the order. The nurse can also clarify whether the foot or toes should be exposed.

Time element

The time element answers when, how long, or how often. Examples are: "Assist patient with tub bath at 0700 daily," "Immerse patient's left arm in sterile saline soak for one hour," "Assist patient to change position q./2h. [every two hours] between 0700 and 2100."

Signature

The signature of the nurse prescribing the order shows the nurse's accountability and has legal significance. See the discussion in chapter 4.

NURSING INTERVENTION

Nursing intervention is the implementation of the nursing plan or the actual assistance provided to the patient and support persons by nursing personnel to help them meet the identified goals. A nurse may carry out the activities, or the actions may be delegated to other nursing personnel.

To delegate is to authorize another as one's representative or to entrust authority to another. Delegating nursing activities is not a simple function; it requires knowledge of the needs and goals of the patient, the support persons, and the nurse and knowledge of the skills of various nursing personnel. It is important that intervention be carried out competently and skillfully. Intervention requires technical, communicative, and intellectual skills.

During the intervention phase, the nurse continually assesses the patient's needs and revises the plan of care accordingly. It is also important to use this phase to help the patient meet learning needs. Often teaching is an important aspect of nursing intervention.

EVALUATION

Evaluation is the process of determining to what extent the goals of nursing care have been attained. It is a crucial step in the nursing process, since, as a result of evaluation, conclusions are drawn and the nursing plan may need to be changed.

If the patient's problem and goals were identified and written in precise terms, then the evaluation process is relatively simple. Did the patient drink 3,000 mL of fluid in 24 hours? Did the patient walk unassisted the specified distance per day?

There are a number of possible outcomes of evaluation:

1. The patient has responded as expected, ie, the outcomes were expected.

2. Short-term goals were achieved, but intermediate and long-term goals have not yet been met.

3. No goals were achieved, ie, the outcomes were unexpected.

4. New problems have arisen.

Evaluation needs to be carried out purposefully and in an organized way. It is an intellectual activity in which the patient is assessed in terms of the identified goals. Both the patient and the nurse participate, whenever this is possible.

During evaluation, the nurse can reflect on a number of questions. What factors affect attainment of the goal? Was the problem correctly identified? Why was the problem not resolved? Was the nursing intervention directed toward the stated goals? What other nursing interventions are more likely to assist the patient to attain the stated goals? If the goal was not attained, the nurse and the patient need to either revise the problem list or restate the goal or adjust the nursing interventions.

References

Abruzzese RS: The nursing process and the problem-oriented system. In: *The Problem-Oriented System—a Multi-Disciplinary Approach.* NLN Pub No. 20–1546. National League for Nursing, 1974.

Bower FL: *The Process of Planning Nursing Care: A Theoretical Model,* 3rd ed. Mosby, 1981.

Carlson JH, Craft CA, McGuire AD (editors): *Nursing Diagnosis.* Saunders, 1982.

Carpenito LJ: *Nursing Diagnosis: Application to Clinical Practice.* Lippincott, 1983.

Edel M: The nature of nursing diagnosis. In: *Nursing Diagnosis.* Carlson JH, Craft CA, McGuire AD (editors). Saunders, 1982.

Gordon M: Nursing diagnosis and the diagnostic process. *Am J Nurs* (August) 1976; 76:1298–1300.

Gordon M: *Nursing Diagnosis: Process and Application.* McGraw-Hill, 1982.

Griffith JW, Christensen PJ: *Nursing Process: Application of Theories, Frameworks, and Models.* Mosby, 1982.

Kim MJ, McFarland GK, McLane AM: *Classification of Nursing Diagnoses: Proceedings of the Fifth National Conference.* Mosby, 1984.

La Monica EL: *The Nursing Process: A Humanistic Approach.* Addison-Wesley, 1979.

Little DE, Carnevali DL: *Nursing Care Planning,* 2nd ed. Lippincott, 1976.

Yura H, Walsh MB (editors): *Human Needs 3 and the Nursing Process.* Appleton-Century-Crofts, 1983.

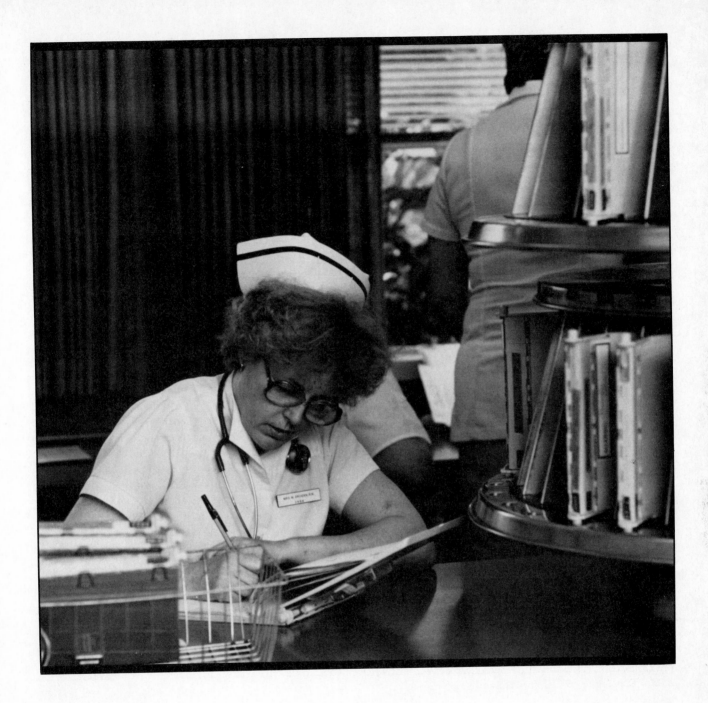

RECORDING

4

A patient's medical record or chart is an account of the patient's health history, current health status, treatment, and progress. It is a highly confidential, legal document by means of which physicians, nurses, social workers, and other health team members communicate about that patient. When a patient goes to a physician's office or enters a hospital, a record is usually started. Records are generally kept in folders, in binders, or on clipboards, and they are updated continually while patients attend the health care facility. When patients are discharged, their records are stored for future reference in the medical records department of the agency.

Records are maintained for a number of reasons other than facilitating communication among health team members, eg, for legal, research, and educational purposes. Although the forms of patient records may vary considerably from place to place, nurses are universally required to make entries of patients' conditions and activities and of all medications, treatments, and nursing techniques offered to patients. The process of making entries on patient records is *charting* or *recording*.

Chapter Outline

Purposes of Patient Records

Types of Records

Types of Progress Records

Computer Records

Guidelines about Recording

Recording on Specific Forms

Objectives

Upon completion of this chapter, the student will:

1. Know essential terms and facts about recording
   1.1 Identify seven purposes of patient records
   1.2 Identify the components of the two types of medical records
   1.3 Identify three types of progress records
   1.4 Identify abbreviations commonly used for charting
   1.5 Identify symbols commonly used for charting
   1.6 Identify medical terms used to describe data about patients
2. Understand facts about recording
   2.1 Identify measures used to maintain the confidentiality of patient records
   2.2 Identify the nurse's role in obtaining consents and releases

2.3 Identify measures used to ensure that recording meets legal standards
3. Record data about patients accurately
   3.1 Record pertinent data about patients
   3.2 Use accepted terms, symbols, and abbreviations
   3.3 Record data on appropriate forms
   3.4 Record information concisely
   3.5 Use terms that are objective and descriptive
   3.6 Record subjective data appropriately
   3.7 Use the format of charting appropriate to the agency (narrative or SOAP)
   3.8 Record the date and time of all entries
   3.9 Correct errors in accordance with agency policy

Terms

■ assessment   organized collection of data about a patient; in the POR, the third step of SOAP, ie, analysis and interpretation of the data and drawing conclusions from them.

■ data base   all information known about a patient; it includes the physician's history and physical examination, the nurse's assessment and history, and material contributed by other members of the health team

■ flow sheet   a record used to record the progress of specific or specialized data such as the vital signs, the fluid balance, or routine medications

■ Kardex   a portable card index file that organizes data about a patient in a concise way and often contains a nursing care plan

■ medical record (chart)   a written account of a patient's health history, current health status, treatment, and progress

■ narrative charting   the writing of all information about a patient in descriptive format as it happens

■ objective data   information about a patient that can be observed or measured by laboratory or other means

■ problem-oriented medical record (POMR; POR)   a patient's record organized according to the patient's problems and recording the reports of several health workers on each problem

■ recording (charting)   the process of making written entries about a patient on the medical record

■ SOAP   the format used in the POR to record the patient's progress; it has four components: S—subjective data, O—objective data, A—assessment, and P—plan

■ source-oriented medical record   a traditional patient's record, organized according to the source of the entries (that is, the person or department reporting); it includes separate records for the doctor, the nurse, the social worker, etc

■ subjective data   information about the patient that

can be offered only by the patient personally, such as thoughts or feelings

---

PURPOSES OF PATIENT RECORDS

Patient records are kept for a number of purposes: communication, legal documentation, research, statistics, education, audit, and planning patient care.

Communication

The record serves as the vehicle by which different members of the health team communicate with each other. Although these members also communicate verbally, the record is an efficient and effective method of sharing information. It also allows health team members on different shifts to convey meaningful data about the patient to one another. An accurate record can prevent errors such as duplication of a medication.

Legal Documentation

The patient's record is a legal document and is admissible in court as evidence. In some jurisdictions the record is considered inadmissible as evidence when the patient objects, because information the patient gives to the physician is confidential.

A record is usually considered the property of the agency, although there is increasing belief that the patient has a right to the information in the record upon request. The National League for Nursing statement on patients' rights supports this view (see chapter 2), and legal decisions have recognized this right (Creighton, 1981, p 329). Some agencies, however, do not permit patients access to their records; thus the nurse needs to be guided by the agency's policy.

Research

The information contained in a record can be a valuable source of data for research. The treatment plans for a number of patients with the same illness can yield information helpful in treating a particular patient.

A record made years earlier may also assist members of the health team with a current problem. A patient's memory of an illness may provide limited data, but a record of that illness will generally reveal additional and accurate data. Records are also very important documents when experimental drugs and treatments are being used.

Statistics

Statistical information from patient records can help an agency anticipate and plan for people's future needs. For example, the number of births or kinds of illnesses can be obtained from records. Some statistics, such as records of births and deaths, are required by law. They are filed with a government agency and become a part of the local, national, and international statistics.

Education

Students in health disciplines can use patient records as educational tools. A record can frequently provide a comprehensive view of the patient, the illness, and the kinds of assistance given. In this context, records are used by nursing students, medical students, dietitians, and other health team members.

Audit

The patient's record is used to monitor the care the patient is receiving and the competence of the people giving that care. A nursing audit, for example, monitors the nursing care and measures it against established standards. Often the audit is a retrospective audit, in that the care has already been given.

When a nursing audit is carried out by other nurses, it is sometimes referred to as a *peer review*. Many agencies have audit committees that monitor the practice of individual nurses. Audits are also carried out by outside groups for approval and accreditation purposes.

Various aspects of care are assessed in nursing audits: the data base, the identification of health problems, the goals of nursing interventions, the choice of nursing interventions, and the level of goal attainment. The nurse's skills, judgment, and knowledge are audited.

Planning Patient Care

The entire health team uses data from the patient's record to plan care for that patient. A physician, for example, may order a specific antibiotic after establishing that the patient's temperature is steadily rising and that laboratory tests reveal the presence of a certain microorganism. Nurses use data from the history they took on the patient's admission to establish an individual nursing care plan. The social worker's data about the patient's home environment can assist the nurse in developing an appropriate discharge teaching plan. Data from the physical therapist help the nurse to implement specific physical exercises for the patient.

TYPES OF RECORDS

There are two types of medical records: the *traditional* or *source-oriented medical record,* and the *problem-oriented medical record* (POMR or POR). The POR is also referred to as the *Weed system,* after its originator, LL Weed.

Source-Oriented Medical Records

In the traditional patient record, each person or department has a record or records for notations. For example, the admission department has an admission sheet; the physician has a doctor's order sheet, a doctor's history sheet, and progress notes; nurses have records that are sometimes called the nurse's notes; and other departments or personnel have their own records. In this type of record, information about a particular problem is distributed throughout the record. For example, if a patient had left hemiplegia (paralysis of the left side of the body) data about this problem might be found in the doctor's history sheet, on the doctor's order sheet, in the nurse's notes, in the physical therapist's record, and in the social service record.

Components

Source-oriented patient records generally have five components:

1. The *admission sheet* is a part of the record in most agencies. It generally contains demographic data about the patient, including an identification number. In hospitals, admission sheets usually set forth the patient's full name, address, date of birth, name of attending physician, sex, marital status, nearest relative, occupation and employer, financial status for hospital payments, religious preference, date and hour of admission to the hospital, hospital unit or agency of admission, previous hospital admission, admitting diagnosis or problem, and identification number. Often this sheet contains a list of allergies presented by the patient.

2. The *physician's order sheet* is a written record of orders. The physician is expected to write the date with the order and sign each order (or sign for several orders written at once). Often agencies have a method of flagging a patient's chart to indicate to the nurse or clerk that there is a new order.

When the doctor phones in orders about a patient, these are written on the physician's sheet by the recipient of the call and signed by that person, indicating a telephone order. Often the physician is expected to countersign the telephone order within 24 or 48 hours of the call.

3. The *history sheet* is a record of the patient's health history, written by the physician. The physician may also use this sheet to record progress notes on the patient and future plans, although some agencies have separate records for progress notes.

4. The *nurse's notes* are a record of the nursing interventions carried out, assessments of the patient, and evaluations of the effectiveness of the interventions. In general, nurses' notes record the following kinds of information:

a. Assessments of the patient by various nursing personnel; eg, pale or flushed skin color or the aroma of urine

b. Dependent nursing interventions, such as medications or treatments ordered by a physician

c. Independent nursing interventions, such as special skin care or health teaching, carried out in the nurses' judgment

d. Evaluation of the effectiveness of each nursing intervention

e. Measures carried out by the physician; for example, shortening a drain in an incision

f. Visits by members of the health team, such as a consulting physician, social worker, or chaplain

5. *Special records* and *reports* also become part of the patient's permanent record. These include roentgenographic reports, laboratory findings, reports of surgery, anesthesia records, physical therapy records, occupational therapy records, and social service records. In addition, special flow sheets are often used to record certain data about the patient. These include graphic records for vital signs, fluid intake and output, and medications. The flow sheets are not to be confused with worksheets used at the patient's bedside. Worksheets are used to collect data that are later transferred to the patient's permanent record. A common example is the daily bedside fluid intake and output worksheet.

Problem-Oriented Medical Records

In a problem-oriented medical record, or POR, data about the patient are recorded and arranged according to the problems the patient has, rather than according to the source of the information. The record integrates all data about a problem, whether gathered by physicians, nurses, or others involved in the patient's care. Then plans for each active problem are drawn up, and progress notes are recorded for each problem. Unlike the traditional record, which separates the medical data on a problem from the nursing data and other data in different sections of the record, the POR coordinates the care given by all health team members and focuses on the patient and the problems.

Components

The POR has four basic components:

1. The defined data base
2. The problem list
3. The initial list of care plans
4. Progress notes

The defined data base The defined data base consists of all information known about the patient when the patient first entered the health care agency. It includes the nursing history and assessment, the physician's history, and the physical examination. To this are added social and family data from other sources, such as the social worker, and baseline laboratory and roentgenographic data. The chief complaint of the patient is an

important piece of data. In most agencies a standardized form is used, to help team members obtain a complete data base.

The problem list The problem list is a carefully drawn list of the problems presented by the patient. Some problems are obvious on initial contact with the patient; others are established as additional data are gathered.

The initial problem list is usually made by the first health care worker to encounter the patient or the person who assumes primary responsibility for the patient's care. Contributions are made subsequently by other members of the health team.

To be complete, the problem list should include socioeconomic, demographic, psychologic, and physiologic problems. The list is attached to the front of the patient's record. Each problem is labeled and numbered so that it can be identified throughout the record. This list has been likened to an index or table of contents. See Figure 4-1. Problems are usually categorized as active or inactive.

FIGURE 4-1 ■ A sample patient's problem list. (Courtesy of the Medical Records Committee of the Medical Board of the University of Maryland Hospital, Baltimore, Maryland.)

If a problem is potential rather than actual, it is generally entered on the progress notes rather than the problem list. Only when a problem actually becomes active is it added to the list.

The initial list of care plans Initial care plans are made with reference to the active problems. Each plan bears the number of the corresponding problem and has three parts:

1. In the *diagnostic workup* the physician indicates what needs to be done first. Setting priorities helps to prevent duplication, may eliminate some distress for the patient, and often saves time and money. Included in the diagnostic workup may be plans to collect further data to establish a medical diagnosis or to assist in therapeutic management of the patient.

2. The *therapy* aspect of the plan presents the physician's orders, often including drug therapy and specific treatments. Each order is numbered to correspond to the problem with which it deals. This organization gives the reader (the nurse) considerable information about the plan, including the reason for each order.

3. The *patient education* aspect of the plan describes the patient's need for skills and information that will assist in the management of the problem.

Progress notes Progress notes in the POR are made by all members of the health team involved in a patient's care: nurse, occupational therapist, dietitian, physician, social worker, and others.

A systematic format for writing progress notes is known as SOAP, an acronym for subjective data, objective data, assessment, and planning.

1. *Subjective data* report what the patient perceives and the way the patient expresses it.

2. *Objective data* include measurements such as the vital signs, observations made by health team members using their senses, laboratory and roentgenographic findings, and patient responses to diagnostic and therapeutic measures such as medications.

3. In the *assessment* stage, the observer makes interpretations and draws conclusions from the subjective and objective data. Again all team members make assessments, using the knowledge in their possession. In the traditional method of recording, nurses are not usually expected to make interpretations and draw conclusions. Thus, for many nurses, assessment is difficult to learn. It entails use of a knowledge base and logical thinking.

4. The *plan* is a revision of the initial care plan. It may describe the need for immediate change or for future change. It should include what the patient has been taught and what the patient has learned. The plan then considers three major aspects of the patient's problem: educational, diagnostic, and therapeutic.

In many agencies only one narrative progress note is made by all health team members, thus encouraging communication and coordination. Each note is signed, with the date and time, by the person writing it.

TYPES OF PROGRESS RECORDS

Three kinds of progress notes are generally recognized: narrative notes, flow sheets, and discharge notes. These are used in both source-oriented and problem-oriented medical records.

Narrative Notes

Narrative notes record the patient's progress descriptively on a day-to-day basis. They are keyed to patient problems and therapy and are filled out by all members of the health team. If there is no additional information to record on a particular day, the nurse need only enter "as above." Narrative notes are discussed further later in this chapter.

Flow Sheets

When specific patient variables such as pulse, blood pressure, medications, or progress in learning a new skill need to be recorded accurately, narrative notes are often too long. Instead the flow sheet, a graphic record, is used, to reflect the patient's condition quickly. A common example is the vital signs graphic sheet.

The time parameters for flow sheets can vary from minutes to months. In a hospital intensive care unit, a patient's blood pressure may be monitored by the minute, whereas in an ambulatory clinic, a patient's blood glucose level may be recorded once a month. Once a problem requiring use of a flow sheet is resolved, a narrative note is written.

Discharge Notes

A discharge note may be written by the physician or another member of the health team, depending upon the health care agency. In a home visiting service or community clinic, it may be written by the nurse. The discharge note refers to the patient problems identified earlier and describes the degree to which each problem has been resolved. If the patient has been referred to another agency, this is also noted.

Some agencies have a nursing discharge profile, a record of information about the patient that is relevant upon discharge.

COMPUTER RECORDS

Since about 1968, a number of health institutions have introduced computers. Early installations were primarily in the business offices of hospitals. However, increasing numbers of computers are being used in health care planning and delivery as well as in laboratories and physicians' clinics.

A nursing unit may use a computer to record and store information about patients. Usually such a computer has a terminal consisting of a keyboard for recording information and a screen for reading the information. Some terminals provide written information (a readout or printout) that becomes part of the patient's record. Some institutions expect nurses to use the computers, while others employ technicians to enter and obtain data from the computer at the request of the professional staff.

Computers used in patient care can:

1. Provide fast communication among professional staff members
2. Offer a greater amount of objective data about patients
3. Notify staff members about problems concerning medications, incompatibilities, allergies, etc
4. Store all material so that it can be retrieved later and adapted for another patient or used for education, research, or audits
5. Reduce the amount of clerical work (such as recording) required of nurses and physicians
6. Reduce errors that are made in copying information

GUIDELINES ABOUT RECORDING

Because the patient's record is a legal document and may be used to provide evidence in court, many factors are considered in recording. Health care personnel not only maintain the confidentiality of the patient's record but also meet legal standards in the process of recording. Some of these factors are described in the sections that follow. They apply to either type of recording system.

Restricted Access

The patient's record is protected legally as a private record of the patient's care. Thus, access to the record is restricted to health workers involved in giving care to the patient. Insurance companies, for example, have no legal right to demand access to medical records, even though they may be determining compensation to the patient. On the other hand, a patient who is making a claim for compensation may ask to have the medical history used as evidence. In this instance, the patient must sign an authorization form for review, copying, or release of information from the record. This form clearly indicates what information is to be released and to whom. In no instance may a nurse allow access to a patient's record by family members or any person other than a caregiver.

For purposes of education and research, most agencies allow student and graduate health workers access to patient records. The records are used in patient conferences, clinics, rounds, and written papers or patient studies. The student or graduate is bound by a strict ethical code to hold all information in confidence. Some agencies code medical records when they are filed, so that the names of patients are removed. This allows records to be used without identifying individuals. When this is not the practice, it is the responsibility of the student or health care worker to protect the patient's privacy by not using a name or any statements in the notations that would identify the patient. Many agencies also require documentation from the student or graduate wishing to use medical records of discharged patients. A permission note from the student's instructor or professor will confirm the person's status as a student at a particular school.

Use of Ink

All entries on the patient's record are made in black or dark blue ink so that the record is permanent and changes can be identified. Dark-colored ink is generally required, since it reproduces well on microfilm and in duplication processes. Entries need to be legible. Hand printing or easily understood handwriting is permissible.

Signature

Each recording on the nursing notes is signed by the nurse making it. The signature consists of the first name, middle initial, legal last name, and the nurse's title or position, abbreviated. For example; "Susan J. Green, RN." The following title abbreviations are often used, but nurses are advised to check the practice in their agencies:

RN   registered nurse
LVN   licensed vocational nurse
LPN   licensed practical nurse
NA   nursing assistant
NS   nursing student
SN   student nurse

Errors

If an error is made, a line is drawn through it, and the word "error" is written above it, with the nurse's initials or name (depending on agency policy). Errors should not be erased or blotted out so that there is no doubt about the nursing care given or the charting error made.

Sample Recording

Date	Time	Notes
12/10/86	0100	error A.J.R. Pulse ~~180 beats/minute~~ 108 beats/minute. ——————— Abby J. Roberts, NS

In the above example, the nature of the error is also clear. When it is not, many attorneys feel it is helpful and legally acceptable to indicate what the error was, in order to protect the patient and the nurse. An example might be, "Charted for wrong patient." The policy of the agency, however, needs to be checked.

Blanks

If a blank appears in a notation, a line is drawn through the blank space and it is signed.

Sample Recording

Date	Time	Notes
11/7/86	0730	Urine appears cloudy, light brown with dark flecks. No odor. ——————— Lin I. Ma, NS C/o burning pain in pubic region prior to voiding. ——————— Lin I. Ma, NS

Accuracy

It is essential that notations on records be accurate and correct. To keep them accurate, notations are written to consist of facts or exact observations, rather than opinions or interpretations of an observation. It is more accurate, for example, to write that the patient "refused medication" (fact) than to write that the patient "was uncooperative" (opinion); to write that a patient "was crying" (observation) is preferable to noting that the patient "was depressed" (interpretation). Opinions or interpretations may or may not be accurate. Similarly, when a patient expresses worry about the diagnosis or problem, this should be quoted directly on the record: "Stated: 'I'm worried about my leg.' " Nurses record what they hear as well as what they observe.

Correct spelling is essential for accuracy in recording. If unsure how to spell a word, the nurse looks it up in a dictionary. Most agency units have one available for this purpose. Two decidedly different medications may have similar spellings—for example, digitoxin and digoxin.

Appropriateness

Only information that pertains to the patient's health problems and care is recorded. Any other personal information that the patient conveys to the nurse is inappropriate for the record. If irrelevant information is recorded, it can be considered an invasion of the patient's privacy and/or libelous. A patient's disclosure that she was a prostitute and has smoked marijuana, for example, would *not* be recorded on the patient's medical record, unless it had a direct bearing on the patient's health problem.

Completeness

Not all data that a nurse obtains about a patient can be recorded. However, the information that is recorded needs to be complete and helpful to the patient, physicians, other nurses, and participating health care workers. Incomplete records could be used as evidence in court to show that the patient did not receive the quality of care considered to meet generally accepted standards. For example, if a diabetic patient's record does not indicate that insulin was given and that the urine was tested, the record could be used as evidence of negligence on the part of the nurse responsible for providing this care. Of course, other examples and evidence would be needed to support a finding of negligence by the nurse. However, the patient's record can be used to indicate the kind of care given. A complete notation for a patient who has vomited, for example, includes the time, the amount, the color, the odor, and any other data about the patient (eg, pain).

Sample Recording

Date	Time	Notes
8/12/86	1410	Vomited approx 500 mL of black liquid with foul fecal odor. C/o cramplike pain in epigastric region immediately prior to vomiting. States feels comfortable following vomiting. ——————— Nancy R. Long, NS

The following guide may assist nurses in selecting essential and complete information to record about patients. Note that the emphasis is on facts that denote a change in the patient's health status or behavior or that indicate a deviation from what is usually expected. Essential information includes:

1. Any behavior changes, for example:

   a. Indications of strong emotions, such as anxiety or fear

   b. Marked changes in mood

   c. A change in level of consciousness, such as stupor

d. Regression in relationships with family or friends

2. Any changes in physical function, such as:

   a. Loss of balance

   b. Loss of strength

   c. Difficulty hearing or seeing

3. Any physical sign or symptom that:

   a. Is severe, such as severe pain

   b. Tends to recur or persist

   c. Is not normal, such as an elevated body temperature

   d. Gets worse, such as gradual weight loss

   e. Indicates a complication, such as inability to void following surgery

   f. Is not relieved by prescribed measures, such as continued failure to defecate or to sleep

   g. Indicates faulty health habits, such as lice on the scalp

   h. Is a known danger signal, such as a lump in the breast

4. Any nursing measures provided, such as:

   a. Medications administered

b. Therapies

c. Activities of daily living, if agency policy dictates

d. Teaching patients self-care

5. Visits by a physician or other members of the health team

Standard Abbreviations, Symbols, and Terms

The nurse needs to use only commonly accepted abbreviations, symbols, and terms that are specified by the agency. Then, if the record is used in court as evidence, other professionals responsible for interpreting the data can do so correctly. Many abbreviations are standard and used universally, while others are confined to certain geographic areas. Some agencies supply a list of the abbreviations they accept. When in doubt about whether to use an abbreviation, the nurse writes the term out in full, until certain about the abbreviation. Table 4–1 lists some commonly used abbreviations (except those used for medications, which are described in chapter 29). Table 4–2 indicates commonly accepted symbols.

TABLE 4–1 ■ Commonly Used Abbreviations *Within an Agency Policies*

Abbrevation	Term	Abbrevation	Term
abd	abdomen	GI	gastrointestinal
ABO	the main blood group system	GP	general practitioner
a.c.	before meals (*ante cibum*)	gtt	drops (*guttae*)
ADL	activities of daily living	h. (hr)	hour (*hora*)
ad lib	as desired (*ad libitum*)	H₂O	water
adm	admitted or admission	h.s.	at bedtime (*hora somni*)
AM	morning (*ante meridiem*)	I & O	intake and output
amb	ambulatory	IV	intravenous
amt	amount	Lab	laboratory
approx	approximately (about)	liq	liquid
b.i.d.	twice daily (*bis in die*)	LMP	last menstrual period
BM (bm)	bowel movment	lt (L)	left
BP	blood pressure	meds	medications
BRP	bathroom privileges	mL	milliliter
c̄ (C)	with	mod	moderate
C	centigrade, celsius	neg	negative
CBC	complete blood count	nil (ō)	none
CBR	complete bed rest	no. (#)	number
c/o	complains of	NPO (NBM)	nothing *per ora*, by mouth
DAT	diet as tolerated	NS (N/S)	normal saline
dc (disc)	discontinue	O₂	oxygen
drsg	dressing	od	daily (*omni die*) qd
Dx	diagnosis	OD	right eye (*oculus dexter*); overdose
ECG (EKG)	electrocardiogram	OOB	out of bed
F	Fahrenheit	os	mouth
fld	fluid	OS	left eye (*oculus sinister*)

TABLE 4–1 ■ continued

Abbrevation	Term	Abbreviation	Term
p.c.	after meals (*post cibum*)	q.i.d.	four times a day (*quater in die*)
PE (PX)	physical examination	req	requisition
per	by or through	Rt (rt, R)	right
PM	afternoon (*post meridiem*)	S (s̄)	without (*sine*)
p.o.	by mouth (*per os*)	SI	seriously ill
postop	postoperative(ly)	spec	specimen
preop	preoperative(ly)	stat	at once, immediately (*statim*)
prep	preparation	t.i.d.	three times a day (*ter in die*)
p.r.n.	when necessary (*pro re nata*)	TL	team leader
pt (Pt)	patient	TLC	tender loving care
q.	every (*quaque*)	TPR	temperature, pulse, respirations
q.d.	every day (*quaque die*)	Tr.	tincture
q.h. (q.1h.)	every hour (*quaque hora*)	VO	verbal order
q.2h., q.3h., etc	every two hours, three hours, etc	VS (vs)	vital signs
q.h.s.	every night at bedtime (*quaque hora somni*)	WNL	within normal limits
		wt	weight

Medical terminology is generally made up of root words, prefixes, and suffixes. A root word may be derived from Latin or Greek. A prefix is a sequence of letters that comes before the word and often describes a variation of the normal. A suffix is a sequence of letters that occurs at the end of the word. It often describes a condition of or act performed upon the root word. Root words, suffixes, and prefixes are provided in Table 4–3. Further terms are given in the glossary at the end of the book.

Dates and Times

Documentation of the date and time of each notation is essential not only for legal reasons but also for safe care.

TABLE 4–2 ■ Commonly Used Symbols

Symbol	Term	Number	Symbol
>	greater than	0	o̅
<	less than	1	ī
=	equal to	2	ii̅
↑	increased	3	iii̅
↓	decreased	4	iv̅
♀	female	5	v̅
♂	male	6	vi̅
°	degree	7	vii̅
#	number; fracture	8	viii̅
ʒ	dram	9	ix̅
℥	ounce	10	x̅
×	times		
@	at		

For example, the time at which a narcotic was administered to a patient needs to be determined before the next one can safely be given. Time can be recorded in the conventional manner, ie, 9 AM or 2:30 PM, or according to the 24-hour clock (military clock), which avoids confusion about whether a time was AM or PM. See Figure 4–2.

FIGURE 4–2 ■ The 24-hour clock.

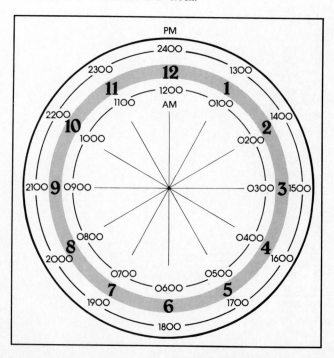

TABLE 4–3 ■ Root Words, Prefixes, and Suffixes

Word element	Meaning	Word element	Meaning
		utero	womb; uterus
Root words		tubo, salpingo	fallopian tube
		ovario, oophoro	ovary
Circulatory system		*Male reproductive system*	
cardio	heart	orchido	testes
angio, vaso	vessel	*Regions of the body*	
hem, hema, hemato	blood	crani, cephalo	head
vena, phlebo	vein	cervico, tracheo	neck
arteria	artery	thoraco	chest
lympho	lymph	abdomino	abdomen
thrombo	clot (of blood)	dorsum	back
embolus	moving clot	*Tissues*	
Digestive system		cutis, dermato	skin
bucca	cheek	lipo	fat
os, stomato	mouth	musculo, myo	muscle
gingiva	gum	osteo	bone
glossa	tongue	myelo	marrow
pharyngo	pharynx	chondro	cartilage
esophago	esophagus	*Miscellaneous*	
gastro	stomach		
hepato	liver	cyto	cell
cholecyst	gallbladder	genetic	formation, origin
pancreas	pancreas	gram	tracing or mark
entero	intestines	graph	writing, description
duodeno	duodenum	kinesis	motion
jejuno	jejunum	meter	measure
ileo	ileum	oligo	small, few
caeco	cecum	phobia	fear
appendeco	appendix	photo	light
colo	colon	pyo	pus
recto	rectum	scope	instrument for visual examination
ano, procto	anus		
Skeletal system		roentgen	x-ray
skeleto	skeleton	lapar	flank; through the abdominal wall
Respiratory system			
naso, rhino	nose	**Prefixes**	
tonsillo	tonsil	a, an, ar	without or not
laryngo	larynx	ab	away from
tracheo	trachea	acro	extremities
bronchus, broncho	bronchus (pl. bronchi)	ad	toward, to
pulmo, pneuma, pneum	lung (sac with air)	adeno	glandular
Nervous system		aero	air
neuro	nerve	ambi	around, on both sides
cerebrum	brain	amyl	starch
oculo, ophthalmo	eye	ante	before, forward
oto	ear	anti	against, counteracting
psych, psycho	mind	bi	double
Urinary system		bili	bile
urethro	urethra	bio	life
cysto	bladder	bis	two
uretero	ureter	brachio	arm
reni, reno, nephro	kidney	brady	slow
pyelo	pelvis of kidney	broncho	bronchus (pl. bronchi)
uro	urine	cardio	heart
Female reproductive system		cervico	neck
vulvo	vulva	chole	gall or bile
perineo	perineum	cholecysto	gallbladder
labio	labium (pl. labia)	circum	around
vagino, colpo	vagina	co	together
cervico	cervix	contra	against, opposite

TABLE 4–3 ■ continued

Word element	Meaning	Word element	Meaning
costo	ribs	macro	large, big
cyto	cell	mal	bad, poor
cysto	bladder	mast	breast
demi	half	medio	middle
derma	skin	mega, megalo	large, great
dis	from	meno	menses
dorso	back	mono	single
dys	abnormal, difficult	multi	many
electro	electric	myelo	bone marrow, spinal cord
en	into, in, within	myo	muscle
encephal	brain	neo	new
entero	intestine	nephro	kidney
equi	equal	neuro	nerve
eryth	red	nitro	nitrogen
ex	out, out of, away from	noct	night
extra	outside of, in addition to	non	not
ferro	iron	ob	against, in front of
fibro	fiber	oculo	eye
fore	before, in front of	odonto	tooth
gastro	stomach	ophthalmo	eye
glosso	tongue	ortho	straight, normal
glyco	sugar	os	mouth, bone
hemi	half	osteo	bone
hemo	blood	oto	ear
hepa, hepato	liver	pan	all
histo	tissue	para	beside, accessory to
homo	same	path	disease
hydro	water	ped	child, foot
hygro	moisture	per	by, through
hyper	too much, high	peri	around
hypo	under, decreased	pharyngo	pharynx
hyster	uterus	phlebo	vein
ileo	ileum	photo	light
in	in, within, into	phren	diaphragm, mind
inter	between	pneumo	air, lungs
intra	within	pod	foot
intro	in, within, into	poly	many, much
juxta	near, close to	post	after
laryngo	larynx	pre	before
latero	side	proct	rectum
lapar	abdomen	pseudo	false
leuk	white	psych	mind

Frequency and Timing of Entries

The frequency of recording depends somewhat on the patient's degree of illness and on the nursing measures and therapy being provided. In most settings recordings are usually made:

1. Immediately after an initial assessment of the patient, for example, on admission to a hospital or directly after returning from the operating room or from a treatment

2. Immediately after administering any medication

3. Before the nurse leaves the nursing unit, for example, to go to lunch, or at the end of the shift

4. Whenever necessary to maintain the currency of the record in relation to the patient's condition

Each recording is made directly *after* carrying out a nursing measure—never before. The present or past tense is therefore used in notations, not the future tense.

Sample Recording: Incorrect

Date	Time	Notes
7/18/86	1400	Will return to bed in 15 min.————— ————————— Morgan F. Smith, NS

TABLE 4–3 ■ continued

Word element	Meaning	Word element	Meaning
pyel	pelvis of the kidney	cule	little
pyo	pus	cyte	cell
pyro	fever, heat	ectasia	dilating, stretching
quadri	four	ectomy	excision, surgical removal of
radio	radiation	emia	blood
re	back, again	esis	action
reno	kidney	form	shaped like
retro	backward	genesis, genetic	formation, origin
rhin	nose	gram	tracing, mark
sacro	sacrum	graph	writing
salpingo	fallopian tube	ism	condition
sarco	flesh	itis	inflammation
sclero	hard, hardening	ize	to treat
semi	half	lith	stone, calculus
sex	six	lithiasis	presence of stones
skeleto	skeleton	lysis	disintegration
steno	narrowing, constriction	megaly	enlargement
sub	under	meter	instrument that measures
super	above, excess	oid	likeness, resemblance
supra	above	oma	tumor
syn	together	opathy	disease of
tachy	fast	orrhaphy	surgical repair
thyro	thyroid, gland	osis	disease, condition of
trache	trachea	ostomy	to form an opening or outlet
trans	across, over	otomy	to incise
tri	three	pexy	fixation
ultra	beyond	phage	ingesting
un	not, back, reversal	phobia	fear
uni	one	plasty	plastic surgery
uretero	ureter	plegia	paralysis
urethro	urethra	rhage	to burst forth
uro	urine, urinary organs	rhea	excessive discharge
vaso	vessel	rhexis	rupture
		scope	lighted instrument for visual examination
Suffixes		scopy	to examine visually
able	able to	stomy	to form an opening
algia	pain	tomy	incision into
cele	tumor, swelling	uria	urine
centesis	surgical puncture to remove fluid		
cide	killing, destructive		

Sources: Courtesy of Margaret Ling, Director of Vocational Nursing, Santa Rosa Junior College, Santa Rosa, Calif.; B Kozier, G Erb: *Fundamentals of Nursing: Concepts and Procedures,* 2nd ed., Addison-Wesley, 1983.

Sample Recording: Correct

Date	Time	Notes
7/18/86	1415	Sat in chair for 15 min.————————— Morgan F. Smith, NS

Brevity

Recordings need to be brief as well as complete, to save time in communication. The patient's name and the word "patient" are omitted, as it is obvious about whom the nurse is charting. Each thought or sentence is terminated with a period.

Sample Recording

Date	Time	Notes
8/21/87	0900	Perspiring profusely. Respirations shallow, wet, 28/min.————————— Julia L. Cardoza, NS

Consents and Releases

Unless the patient gives consent, certain kinds of care could be considered assault or battery and thus cannot be given (see chapter 2). It is important for nurses to ensure that the proper consent forms are signed and made part of the patient's record (see Figure 4–3). A common form gives consent for treatment and operation.

Release of a patient from the hospital without the doctor's consent also necessitates a signed form from the patient, to absolve the physician and the hospital of neglect. The nurse often is the one who obtains the patient's signature in this less frequent situation.

RECORDING ON SPECIFIC FORMS

Patient records on which nurses commonly make notations include:

1. The nursing history
2. Flow sheets such as the clinical record, the medication record, and the fluid intake and output record
3. The nurse's notes (nursing progress notes)
4. The problem list record, in the POR (in source-oriented patient records, the nurse lists the patient's problems on the patient's nursing care plan)
5. The Kardex and/or nursing care plan

Nursing History

Nursing history forms vary considerably among agencies. Even within an agency, forms may differ among nursing units. For example, an adult medical-surgical unit, an obstetric unit, a pediatric unit, and a psychiatric unit may want different nursing histories. Figure 4–4 shows a sample for an infant in a children's hospital.

Histories are usually completed when the patient is admitted to the agency. Most nursing histories include the following information:

LIONS GATE HOSPITAL

CONSENT FOR EXAMINATION AND TREATMENT

I, the undersigned, do hereby certify that the purpose of this visit or admission of me to Lions Gate Hospital has been explained to me by my physician and I agree that any examination and treatment can be administered which the attending physician or physicians and hospital staff may find necessary for my relief.

Dated this 23 day of August, 1986

(1) Signature of Patient: ____________

(2) Signature of Guardian: James Joffery
(or person authorized
to consent for patient)

Father
(Relationship of above)

Margaret Lane
Signature of Witness

Unconscious
(Reason patient unable to sign)

In situations where it is impossible to obtain a signature on line (1) or (2) above, two physicians shall certify by signing the following:

In the opinion of each of the undersigned physicians the treatment to be carried out is necessary and in the best interest of the continued health and well-being of the patient.

Dated this 23 day of August, 1986

R.W. West, M.D. L.C. Spankie, M.D.

Margaret Lane — Signature of Witness
Margaret Lane — Signature of Witness

A.456 Rev. 6/78
10M-S-p

FIGURE 4–3 ■ A sample general consent form for examination and treatment including surgery. (Courtesy of Lions Gate Hospital, North Vancouver, British Columbia.)

THE HOSPITAL FOR SICK CHILDREN

NURSING HISTORY – INFANT

Damian Fields
7 mos.
Persistent Vomiting and
Failure to Thrive

INFORMATION ABOUT INTERVIEW: INFORMANT: Mother

LANGUAGE OF PARENTS English   OF CHILD: —

INTERPRETER?   (NAME & PHONE) —

UNUSUAL CIRCUMSTANCES INFLUENCING INTERVIEW: Admission not planned; sent from Doctor's office

CIRCUMSTANCES LEADING TO THIS HOSPITALIZATION

WHY DID YOU BRING YOUR CHILD TO HOSPITAL? Damian has not been gaining adequate weight and has been vomiting small amounts several times a day.

WHAT HAS THE DOCTOR TOLD YOU ABOUT YOUR CHILD'S ILLNESS?   TESTS, SURGERY, ETC. PLANNED. Damian will have an X-ray of his digestive system and blood and urine tests will be done

HAS THE PATIENT BEEN RECEIVING ANY MEDICATIONS AT HOME?   ALLERGIES:

WHAT?	DOSE & FREQUENCY	WHEN LAST GIVEN?	FOOD	DRUGS	OTHER
—	—	—	orange juice	—	—

PREVIOUS HOSPITALIZATIONS   NO ✓ YES   HOSPITAL:

WHAT WAS THE CHILD ADMITTED FOR:

WHAT WAS HIS AND PARENTS' REACTION TO HOSPITAL?

FAMILY BACKGROUND	OTHER IMPORTANT FAMILY MEMBERS	VISITING PLANS
SIBLINGS (NAMES & AGES) Michael – died at eight months of age of Sudden Infant Death Syndrome (2 years ago)	Grandma and Grampa Fields (maternal grandparents live out west) HOUSEHOLD PETS Cocker Spaniel – "Floppy"	Mother – daily Father – after work WAYS PARENTS WOULD LIKE TO PARTICIPATE IN CARE bath feeding (lunch and supper)

HABITS OF DAILY LIVING	FOOD & FLUIDS:	
LIKES: oatmeal pablum, peaches, pears, carrots, green beans, veal and beef	TYPE OF FORMULA: SMA	TEMPERATURE OF FLUIDS: warm
	AMOUNT/ FEEDING: 4-5 oz.	CONSISTENCY OF SOLIDS strained
	FREQUENCY OF FEEDS: every four hours	(STRAINED, MINCED, CHOPPED)
DISLIKES: peas, apricots	CUP (BOTTLE) 5 bottles each day	# MEALS & SNACKS three meals;
	2 oz. apple juice mid-morning	Breakfast: Supper – Pab: Fruit Lunch: Meat and vegetables

SLEEP: BEDTIME: 8:30pm   SOOTHER OR SPECIAL TOY: Soother

NAPTIMES: afternoon only 1-4pm   BEDCLIMBER? —

SLEEPS THROUGH NIGHT — very rarely   SPECIAL SLEEP HABITS: likes to sleep on tummy

33385

POMR (27)

FIGURE 4-4 ■ A sample nursing history for an infant. (Courtesy of the Hospital for Sick Children, Toronto, Ontario.)

ELIMINATION:	TOILET-TRAINED? —	BLADDER EXPRESSION, ENEMA
USUAL BOWEL HABITS: 3-4 each day	TERMS USED-URINE: —	ROUTINE, LAXATIVE —
FREQUENCY: every day	STOOL: —	
TIMES: usually after feedings	POTTY OR TOILET —	
	DIAPERS AT NIGHT? Yes	

RECREATION AND SOCIABILITY	SPECIAL BELONGINGS: ARE THEY WITH CHILD?
FAVOURITE TOYS & ACTIVITIES musical clown mobile, small blue elephant rattle	Soother and rattle
PLAY WITH OTHERS OR ALONE? likes to watch children play	USED TO BABY SITTERS? Grandparents only
LANAGUAGE SKILLS (SPECIAL WORDS)	PREVIOUS EXPERIENCE AWAY FROM HOME
makes gurgling sounds only	DAY CARE, VISITS, ETC. No

CAPABILITIES OF PHYSICALLY &/OR MENTALLY HANDICAPPED CHILD:	
RESTRICTIONS —	MOBILITY —
	FEEDING —
SELF-HELP —	
	SPEECH

QUESTIONS ASKED BY PARENT &/OR PATIENT: Will the radiation from the x-ray harm Damian? Will the nurses check him often during the night? Do many babies come into hospital because of vomiting?

PERTINENT OBSERVATIONS MADE DURING INTERVIEW: (PARENTS' REACTIONS AND CONCERNS, PARENT-CHILD INTERACTION)

Mother appeared extremely anxious and looked very tired. She was tearful when talking about her first child's death and expressed a fear that Damian may also die. Through out the interview Mrs. Fields held Damian on the edge of her knee and watched him constantly.

NURSING OBSERVATIONS OF PATIENT ON ADMISSION: (PHYSICAL APPEARANCE, ADJUSTMENT TO HOSPITAL)

Damian is a small pale infant who smiles frequently and is alert and interested in his surroundings. He seemed hungry and kept putting his fingers in his mouth. He regurgitated three times during my interview with mother.

PROBLEMS IDENTIFIED FOR THE PATIENT CARE PLAN:

Note frequency, amount and pattern of vomiting.
Observe appetite and response to food.
Observe interaction between mother and child.
Allow for consistency and continuity in assigning nurses to Damian.

DATE: July 27 ___ SIGNATURE J.A. Henderson R.N.

FIGURE 4-4 ■ continued

1. The patient's understanding of the illness

2. The patient's expectations of hospitalization

3. The immediate concerns of the patient or support persons and the circumstances leading to hospitalization

4. The patient's habits of daily living such as food likes and dislikes, elimination patterns, hygienic patterns, and rest and sleep patterns

5. The patient's allergies

6. Medications the patient is currently taking

7. Social and cultural data about the patient's language, family members or other support persons who will visit, education (or developmental data for children), and pertinent beliefs or practices

8. The patient's previous hospitalizations or chronic illnesses

9. The patient's use of aids or prostheses, such as artificial limbs, hearing aids, eyeglasses, or dentures

10. The nurse's observations during the interview

Clinical Record

The clinical record (also called the graphic chart or graphic observation record) indicates:

1. Body temperature

2. Pulse rate

3. Respiratory rate

4. Sugar and acetone present in urine

5. Blood pressure schedule

6. Blood pressure readings

7. Weight

8. Bowel movements

Some agencies also show special medications, such as dicumarol, on the clinical record.

Guidelines for recording on the clinical record

1. Enter the patient's full name (including initials), hospital number, physician's name, and admission date. Some hospitals use Addressographs for this purpose.

2. Date the entry with the month, day, and year.

3. Enter the hospital day number counting from the day of admission as day 1 or day 0 in accordance with agency practice.

4. Enter the patient's temperature on the graph with a dot on the line corresponding to the scale on the left. The dot should be placed in the column for the appropriate time. Draw a line with a ruler joining the dot to the previous dot. If the temperature was taken by any method other than oral, indicate what method.

5. Enter the pulse rate on the line corresponding to the scale on the left. Join the dot to the preceding pulse dot.

Note: Some agencies differentiate between the temperature and the pulse graph by showing the pulse in red or marking the pulse with an X rather than a dot.

6. Enter the respiratory rate in the space allocated. Some agencies also show the respiratory rate on a graph and differentiate it from temperature and pulse by using a small circle (o) instead of a dot or X.

7. Note the other data recorded on the form. See the sample form in Figure 4–6 on the following page.

24-Hour Fluid Balance Record

Before notations are made on a 24-hour fluid balance record, the nurse records the amount of the patient's fluid intake and output on a worksheet kept at the patient's bedside. This worksheet, which does not become part of the patient's record, is discussed in chapter 23. The patient and support persons should be taught to use this record. It documents intake and output for the duration of one shift only (8 or 12 hours). The totals for each shift are then recorded on the 24-hour fluid balance record. In the sample shown in Figure 4–5, the totals for each 8-hour shift (days, evenings, and nights) are recorded, and then the 24-hour totals are calculated.

FIGURE 4–5 ■ A sample 24-hour fluid intake and output record. (Courtesy of Lions Gate Hospital, North Vancouver, British Columbia.)

LIONS GATE HOSPITAL

FLUID BALANCE SHEET

+ Slight
++ Moderate Stool Disphoresis
+++ Profuse

	DATE:				DATE:			
	Nights	Days	Evening	24 Hour Total	Nights	Days	Evening	24 Hour Total
FLUID INTAKE								
Oral	90	180	150	420	170			
Blood								
Intravenous	500	1200	800	2500	300			
Gavage								
TOTAL INTAKE	590	1380	950	2920	470			
FLUID OUTPUT								
Urine: Voided	300	700	550	1550	480			
Catheter								
Ureteral								
Suprapubic								
Emesis:								
Levine								
T-Tube	90	150	100	340	80			
Wound Suction								
Stool								
Diaphoresis								
TOTAL OUTPUT	390	850	650	1890	560			

N.19 REV. 2/75
M-S-p

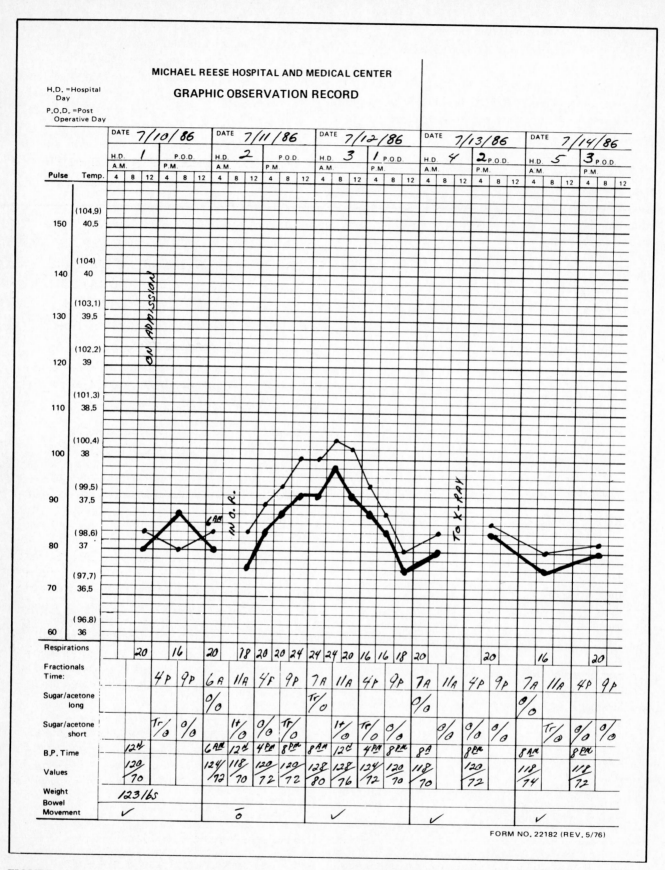

FIGURE 4–6 ■ A sample clinical record (graphic observation sheet). Normally the pulse is shown in red. The pulse line here has been widened to distinguish it from the temperature line. (Courtesy of Michael Reese Hospital and Medical Center, Chicago, Illinois.)

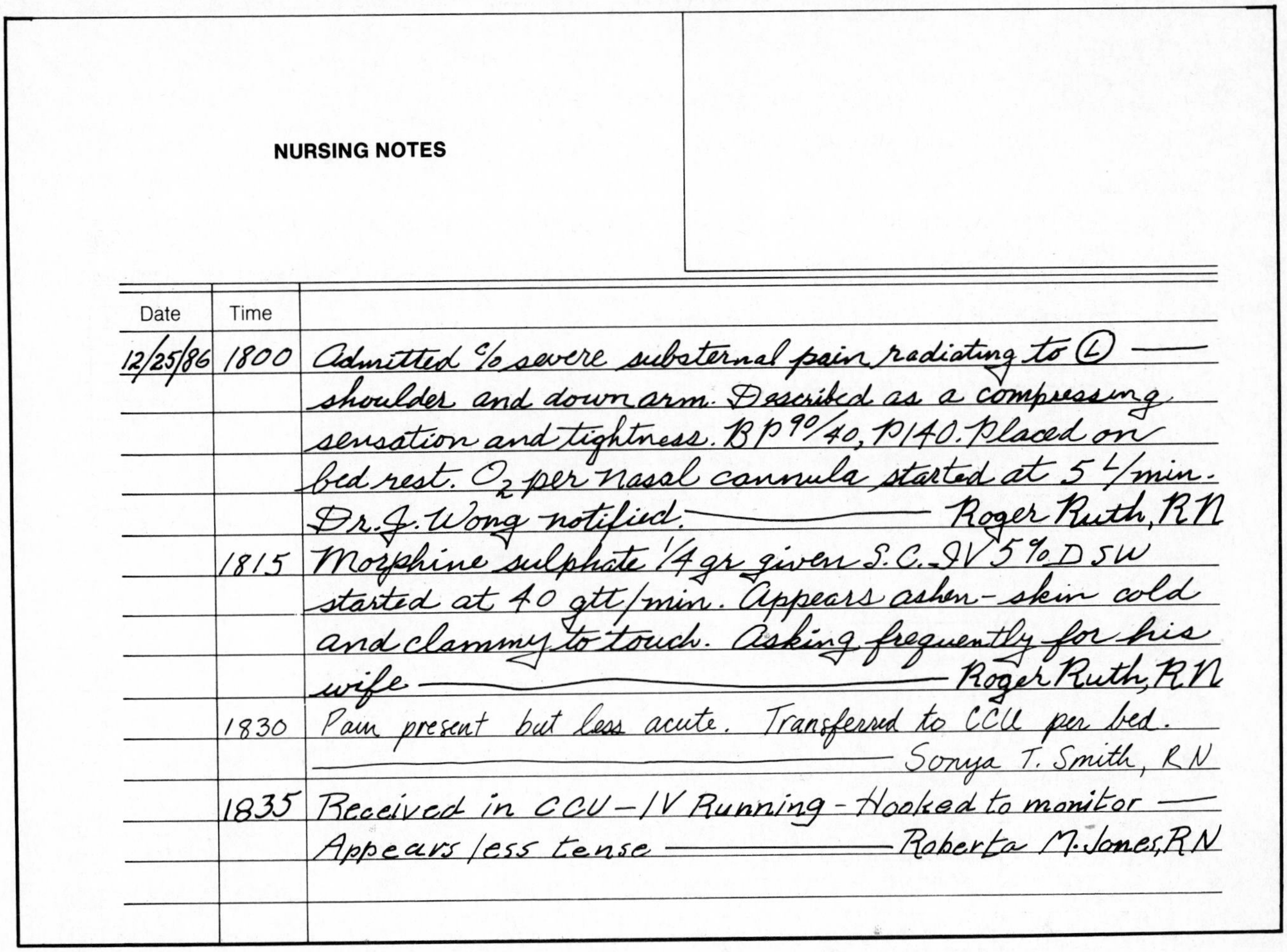

NURSING NOTES

Date	Time	
12/25/86	1800	Admitted ℅ severe substernal pain radiating to Ⓛ — shoulder and down arm. Described as a compressing sensation and tightness. BP 90/40, P140. Placed on bed rest. O₂ per nasal cannula started at 5 L/min. Dr. J. Wong notified. —————— Roger Ruth, RN
	1815	Morphine sulphate ¼ gr given S.C. IV 5% D5W started at 40 gtt/min. Appears ashen – skin cold and clammy to touch. Asking frequently for his wife —————————— Roger Ruth, RN
	1830	Pain present but less acute. Transferred to CCU per bed. —————— Sonya T. Smith, RN
	1835	Received in CCU – IV Running – Hooked to monitor — Appears less tense ———————— Roberta M. Jones, RN

FIGURE 4–7 ■ An example of narrative nurse's notes.

All routes of fluid intake must be measured and recorded: oral, intravenous, and gavage (tube feedings into the stomach). Similarly, all routes of fluid loss or output are measured and recorded: urine, emesis (vomitus), diarrhea, and drainage from any tube, such as a T-tube, Levin (nasogastric) tube, suprapubic drain, wound suction, or bladder or ureteral catheter. When heavy perspiration occurs, this also needs to be estimated. More information about ways to measure and record specific amounts of fluid intake and output are described in chapter 23.

Nurse's Notes

Nurse's notes (also called the *nursing progress notes* or *record*) and the manner of recording vary depending on whether a source-oriented medical record or POR is used.

In source-oriented records, the nursing notes consist of both narrative and chronological charting. *Narrative charting* is a description (narration) of information, and *chronological charting* records data in sequence as time moves forward. The minimum number of words and many abbreviations are used, to keep the information concise. (See the Guidelines about Recording earlier in this chapter.) Figure 4–7 shows a narrative type of nurse's notes. The forms used for the nurse's notes may vary from place to place. Some agencies have separate columns for treatments, nursing observations, and comments.

The major disadvantage of narrative charting is that it is difficult for a reader to find all the data about a specific problem without examining all the information recorded. For this reason, specific flow records are often used for certain information.

In the POR, the nurse's progress notes are written in relation to a specific problem identified on the problem list. Graphic records and flow sheets are used to provide other routine or necessary information. When entering nurse's notes in the POR, the SOAP format is used. See Figure 4–8.

Kardex and Nursing Care Plan

The Kardex (see Figure 4–9) is a widely used concise method of organizing and recording data about a patient, making information quickly accessible to all members of the health team. The system consists of a series of cards kept in a portable index file. The card for a particular patient can be quickly turned up to reveal specific data. Often Kardex data are recorded in pencil so that they can be changed and kept up to date. The information on Kardexes may be organized into sections, for example:

1. Pertinent information about the patient, such as name, room number, age, religion, marital status, admission date, doctor's name, diagnosis, type of surgery and date, occupation, and next of kin

2. List of medications, with the date of order and the times of administration for each

3. List of intravenous fluids, with dates of infusions

4. List of daily treatments and procedures, such as irrigations, dressing changes, postural drainage, or measurement of vital signs

5. List of diagnostic procedures ordered, such as roentgenography or laboratory tests

6. Allergies

7. Specific data on how the patient's physical needs are to be met, such as type of diet, assistance needed with feeding, elimination devices, activity, hygienic needs, and safety precautions (use of side rails etc)

8. A problem list, stated goals, and a list of nursing approaches to meet the goals and relieve the problems

Although much of the information on the Kardex may be recorded by the responsible nurse or a delegate (eg, the ward clerk), any nurse who cares for the patient plays a key role in initiating the record and keeping the data current. When caring for the patient, a nurse has the best opportunity to assess and reassess with the patient the accuracy of the information and the effectiveness of treatment.

FIGURE 4–8 ■ An example of POR nurse's notes using the SOAP format.

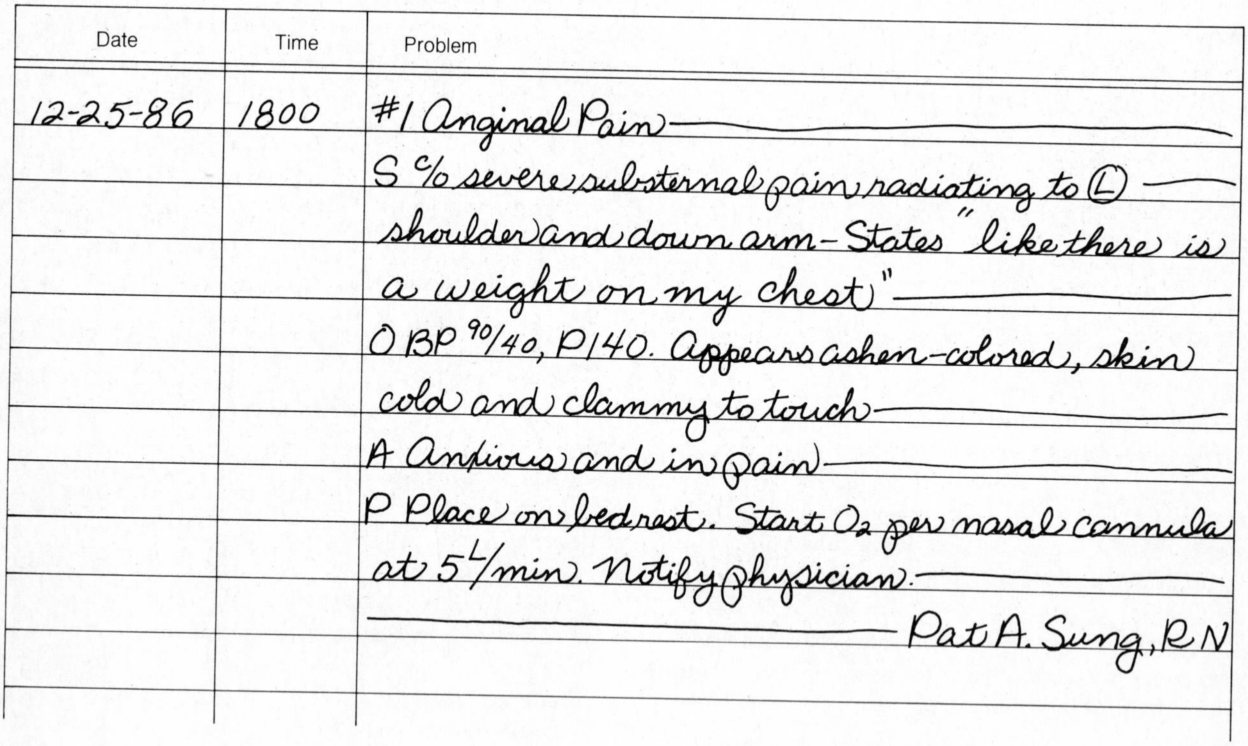

Date	Time	Problem
12-25-86	1800	#1 Anginal Pain
		S c̄ severe substernal pain, radiating to (L) shoulder and down arm—States "like there is a weight on my chest"
		O BP 90/40, P 140. Appears ashen-colored, skin cold and clammy to touch
		A Anxious and in pain
		P Place on bedrest. Start O₂ per nasal cannula at 5 L/min. Notify physician.
		Pat A. Sung, RN

References

Andreoli K, Musser LA: Computers in nursing care: The state of the art. *Nurs Outlook* (January/February) 1985; 33:16–21.

Ball MJ, Hannah KJ: *Using Computers in Nursing.* Reston, 1984.

Creighton H: *Law Every Nurse Should Know,* 4th ed. Saunders, 1981.

Lambert K: Basic principles of the problem-oriented system. In: *The Problem-Oriented System—a Multi-Disciplinary Approach.* NLN Pub No. 20–1546. National League for Nursing, 1974.

Rich PL: With this flow sheet less is more. *Nursing 85* (July 1985; 15:25–29.

Ulisse, GC: *POMR: Application to Nursing Records.* Addison-Wesley, 1978.

Weed LL: *Medical Records, Medical Education and Patient Care: The Problem-Oriented Record as a Basic Tool.* Case Western Reserve University Press, 1971.

DIET
- ☒ Regular *CHINESE*
- ☐ Soft
- ☐ Fluid
- ☐ Clear Fluid
- ☐ N.P.O.
- ☐ Other

FEEDING
- ☒ Self /c *SOME ASSISTANCE*
- ☐ Assist

FLUIDS
- ☐ I. & O.
  .... Am't Daily
- ☐ I.V.
- ☐ Preferred Fluids

ELIMINATION
- ☐ B.R.
- ☒ Commode
- ☐ Ostomy
- ☐ Incontinent
- ☐ Condom
- ☒ Catheter
  Size *#16* Date *JULY 6*
  30cc BALLOON
- ☐ Other Specify:

ACTIVITY
- ☐ Up ad lib
- ☐ B.R.P.
- ☐ Amb c asst
- ☐ Walker
- ☒ Chair *T·I·D 08 - 12 - 16*
- ☐ Dangle
- ☐ Bed rest

HYGIENE
- ☒ Self /c *SOME ASSISTANCE*
- ☐ Partial
- ☐ Bed
- ☐ Tub
- ☐ Shower
- ☐ Mouth Care

SAFETY
Side Rails
- ☒ Constant
- ☐ Night Only
Other

PROSTHESIS
- ☐ Glasses
- ☐ Hearing Aid
- ☐ Dentures
- ☐ Other - Specify

V.S. FREQUENCY
- ☒ B.P. } *O·D*
- ☒ T.P.R. } *@ 0800*
- ☐ Other - Specify

SPECIAL CONSIDERATIONS:
(L)- SIDED WEAKNESS

ALLERGIES

DISCHARGE AND REHAB. PLANS: DATE REVIEWED

DATE	PROBLEM AND SHORT TERM GOAL	APPROACH
JULY 17 #1	PT. WILL BE LESS DEPRESSED, PARTICIPATE MORE IN A·D·L·—↑ HER SELF-ESTEEM	① SHOW CARING BY BEING PATIENT AND UNDERSTANDING. ② BE CONSISTENT IN INVOLVING HER AS MUCH AS POSSIBLE IN A·D·L —AND PRAISE HER WHEN SHE ACCOMPLISHES THEM. ③ MAINTAIN A ROUTINE OF CARE & EXPECT HER TO DO HER SHARE.
JULY 17 #2	PT. WILL BE ABLE TO PARTICIPATE AS MUCH AS POSS· IN A·D·L AND BE AWARE OF POSITIONING OF (L) LIMBS	① ASSIST PT. WHENEVER NECESSARY ② EXPECT PARTICIPATION IN A·D·L. ③ KEEP PT. AWARE OF LEFT LIMB POSITIONS.
JULY 17 #3	PT. WILL UNDERSTAND PROCEDURES ETC.	① GET INTERPRETER WHEN NEC. ② SPEAK SLOWLY

Next of Kin: *HUSBAND - FOO YUNG TOY*   S.I.   Isolation

Occupation: *HOUSEWIFE*   Surgery: *JULY 4 - ESOPHAGOSCOPY*

Age *61*	Religion *NIL*	Mar. Status *M.*	Adm. Date *JUNE 21/86*	Diagnosis ① *ACID INGESTION* ② *DIABETES* ③ *OLD (LT) C·V·A·*

Name: *FOO MUI SENG*	Hosp. No.	Accom. (W) P SP	Doctor *T·Y· TUNG* 016

FIGURE 4-9 ■ A sample nursing Kardex. This is the bottom card; it is folded where the broken line appears. The top card is shown on the following page. (Courtesy of Mount Saint Joseph Hospital, Vancouver, British Columbia.)

X-MATCH

DATE	MEDICATIONS	TIME	DATE	I.V.'s
JULY 4	MYLANTA 15cc q.2.h.	06-08-10 12-14-16		
"	HALDOL 1mgm. T.I.D.	08-14-20		
"	FROSST 292 - CRUSHED FOR PAIN	P.R.N.		
"	BIONETS TO SUCK	P.R.N.		
"	SLIDING SCALE TORONTO INSULIN			
	5% GIVE 12 UNITS.			
	3% " 10 "			
	2% " 8 "			
	2%-0 " 0 "			
JULY 11	AZOGANTRISIN Ī Q.I.D.	06-11 16-22		

TREATMENTS / PROCEDURES

DATE		
JULY 4	CLINITEST T.I.D & H.S -	07-11 17- H.S
JULY 8	IRRIGATE FOLEY CATH. DAILY č N.S	

DATE	MEDICATIONS	TIME
JULY 4	H.S. MED. DALMANE 30 mgm.	H.S.
JULY 14	AMITRIPTYLINE (ELAVIL) 25 mgm	H.S

NAME	ROOM	DOCTOR	015
FOO MUI SENG	306·A	T·Y. TUNG.	

DATE	No.	PROBLEM LIST	RESOLVED	DATE	OTHER RELEVANT DATA (Include x-rays and tests)
JULY 17	#1	PT. STILL VERY DEPRESSED			DATE OF BIRTH
	#2	L-SIDED WEAKNESS		JULY 17	CHEST PHYSIO.
	#3	COMMUNICATION PROBLEMS		JULY 14	BARIUM MEAL ✓
					HEALTH CARE CONSULTANTS
DATE REVIEWED					

FIGURE 4–9 ■ continued

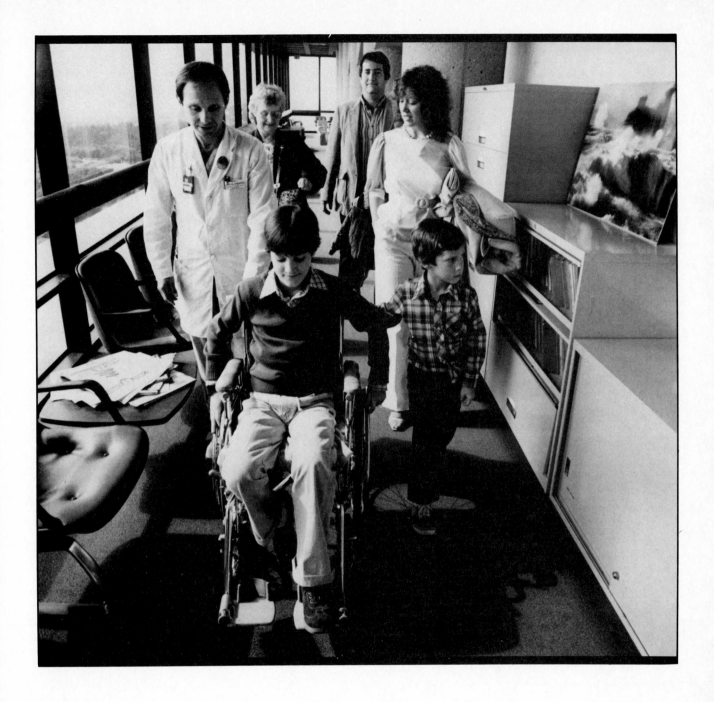

ADMISSION, TRANSFER, AND DISCHARGE

5

Entering a health care facility is a stressful experience for patients. They may or may not be in discomfort, but most, if not all, feel anxious. Relatives and friends are also worried. Thus, the first contact of the patient and the support persons with personnel in the facility is extremely important. Admitting and health care personnel need to convey kindness, concern, and competence in what they do.

Each health care agency has established policies and procedures for the admission of patients, the transfer of patients within the agency and to outside agencies, and the discharge of patients. This chapter focuses on procedures common to many agencies.

Chapter Outline

Preliminary Admission Practices
■ Technique 5–1 Admitting a Patient to a Hospital Unit

■ Technique 5–2 Transferring a Patient
■ Technique 5–3 Discharging a Patient

Objectives

Upon completion of this chapter, the student will:

1. Know essential facts about admission, transfer, and discharge procedures
   1.1 Identify preliminary admission, transfer, and discharge procedures
   1.2 Identify the essential activities in preparing a patient's room prior to admission, transfer, and discharge
   1.3 Identify purposes of the admission, transfer, and discharge procedures
   1.4 Identify information needed to orient a patient to the agency
   1.5 Identify essential data to be recorded on admission
   1.6 Identify the rationale for giving prompt attention to the patient's immediate concerns on admission
   1.7 Identify common reasons for various types of transfers
   1.8 Identify common concerns patients have about transfer
   1.9 Identify essential data to be recorded for a transfer
   1.10 Identify essential aspects of preliminary discharge planning
   1.11 Identify essential data to be recorded when a patient is discharged
   1.12 Identify interventions required to provide safety and comfort for patients during selected techniques
2. Understand facts about techniques used to admit, transfer, and discharge patients

2.1 Identify relevant assessment data
2.2 Identify nursing goals related to the technique
2.3 Explain reasons underlying steps of the technique
2.4 Identify interventions taken to maintain the patient's physical comfort and safety during the technique
2.5 Identify interventions implemented to enhance the patient's psychologic comfort
3. Perform admission, transfer, and discharge techniques effectively
   3.1 Assess the patient adequately
   3.2 Collect additional data from appropriate sources
   3.3 Select pertinent nursing goals for the patient
   3.4 Collect necessary equipment before the technique
   3.5 Implement interventions to enhance the effectiveness of the technique and enhance the patient's comfort and safety
   3.6 Communicate relevant information about the patient to the appropriate persons
4. Evaluate own performance of techniques in a laboratory or clinical setting with the assistance of another individual
   4.1 Use the performance checklists provided
   4.2 Identify areas of strength and weakness
   4.3 Alter performance in response to own evaluation and that of another

PRELIMINARY ADMISSION PRACTICES

The admission of patients to a health care agency involves (a) preliminary routine admission procedures that are usually handled by the admitting office, (b) preparation of the patient's room, and (c) admission procedures conducted by the nurse when the patient arrives at the room.

Patients who are not critically ill generally report first to the admitting office. In some agencies, nurses carry out the initial admission functions. In other agencies, personnel from the business office do. Patients who are critically ill or injured are admitted directly to the emergency unit or, in some agencies, the intensive care unit (ICU).

Preliminary admission procedures generally include:

1. Obtaining essential personal and identifying data for the admission record, such as the patient's full name, age, birth date, physician, religion, and past admissions.

2. Acquiring a signed general consent for care.

3. Putting an identification bracelet (Identaband) on the patient. These are usually made of clear, waterproof plastic and cannot be removed except by cutting. Information on the bracelet may include the patient's name and admission number, the attending physician, and the patient's room number. Bands listing the patient's allergies can also be applied at this time.

4. Notifying the nursing unit that a new patient is being admitted and specifying the room and bed he or she will occupy, what the patient's diagnosis is, who the attending physician is, and other information relevant to the admission (such as "requires continuous oxygen") to alert the nursing staff to make necessary equipment available.

5. Transporting the patient to the room. The patient is always accompanied to the nursing unit by an escort service. Many agencies have volunteer staff or porters for this purpose. Depending upon the patient's condition, a wheelchair or stretcher may be necessary. Most patients, however, can walk to the unit. The unit clerk or nurse there then assists the patient to the room.

TECHNIQUE 5–1 ■ Admitting a Patient to a Hospital Unit

Before admitting a patient it is important to know the following:

1. The agency's policies and practices about admitting patients, in particular in regard to the patient's medications, personal property, and security for valuables

2. The bed and/or room to which the patient will be admitted

3. The patient's general condition and/or medical diagnosis

4. Whether the patient needs any special equipment such as oxygen upon admission

5. Whether the physician has written special orders to be implemented immediately upon the patient's arrival

■ Assessment

Assess the patient for: an initial indication of the patient's physical and emotional status. This assists the nurse to attend to the patient's immediate concerns. Other data include:

1. Information on the patient's record or from health team members.

2. A relevant health history. See Intervention, step 28.

■ Planning

Nursing goals

1. To reduce the anxiety and fear of the patient and support persons and make them feel welcome and as comfortable as possible

2. To provide information that will facilitate the patient's adjustment to the agency environment

3. To assess the patient's physical and emotional status

4. To acquire baseline data for planning care

5. To acquire routine diagnostic specimens

6. To provide immediately needed nursing interventions

Equipment

1. A stethoscope and a sphygmomanometer with a cuff to take the blood pressure. See chapter 8.

2. A watch with a second hand to assess the patient's pulse and respirations.

3. A thermometer, if not provided at the bedside, to assess the patient's temperature.

4. A portable scale to assess the weight, in agencies that require this. In many agencies, the patient's weight and height are recorded as the patient states them.

5. A bedpan or urinal in which to acquire a specimen of urine.

6. A urine specimen container and laboratory urinalysis requisition, both clearly labeled.

7. A hospital gown (and pajama bottoms for males) as necessary. Some agencies, or specific units, permit patients to wear their own night or lounge clothing or daytime dress. Psychiatric nursing units, for example, encourage full dress. Many medical-surgical nursing units, however, require patients to wear hospital gowns.

8. A special envelope to enclose valuables for safekeeping if the admission office has not already provided this.

9. A clothes list or clothing responsibility form. Some agencies have printed checklists of clothing and other personal effects that nurses can use to inventory the patient's articles. A growing trend, however, is to place the clothes in a bedside locker and have

the patient sign a form assuming responsibility for them.

10. Appropriate hospital forms, eg, a responsibility release for personal possessions.

11. Labels to attach to the patient's personal articles at the bedside, eg, a radio.

■ Intervention

Preparing the patient's room

After notification by the head nurse or responsible nurse that a new patient will be admitted to the nursing unit, the nurse assigned prepares the patient's bed unit for the arrival. The bed unit is described in chapter 15.

1. Open a closed bed, for the patient's convenience.

2. Place the bed in a low position, or place a footstool by a bed that is not adjustable, to make it easier and safer for the patient to get into bed. If you know that the patient is being transported by stretcher, place the bed in a high position to facilitate transfer from stretcher to bed.

3. Check that all necessary unit supplies are provided: a full water jug, a bedpan or urinal, a bath basin, a kidney basin, a thermometer container, a call signal, etc.

4. Provide equipment essential to the patient's specific needs, such as an intravenous pole, oxygen equipment, or a footboard.

Meeting the patient

5. Greet the patient in a manner that conveys interest in and concern for him or her. Call the patient by the name he or she desires, introduce yourself, and inquire about any immediate problems that the patient may have. If the patient is feeling distraught or upset, take time to listen and talk, to allay these concerns. If the patient is in acute pain, attend to this at once, contacting the physician for medication orders and/or providing other nursing interventions.

   Rationale By attending to the patient's immediate problems, the nurse indicates a primary concern for the patient's welfare. This makes the patient feel that problems will be attended to, and it does much to initiate a sense of security and a trusting relationship.

Preparing the patient

6. Explain what the admission entails and how the patient can participate.

   Rationale Although the admission procedure often becomes routine for health personnel, it is unfamiliar to patients.

7. Provide privacy when the patient undresses and when she or he gives a urine specimen.

8. Direct support persons to the lounge area unless they can assist the patient to undress. Reassure them that they will be called when it is best for them to return. On pediatric units, the admission procedure is often carried out in the treatment room with the active participation of the support persons.

Orienting the patient to the unit

9. Introduce the patient to the other patients in the room.

10. Introduce the patient to any staff members encountered, even though the patient cannot be expected to remember all of their names.

11. Tell the patient the name of the head nurse or responsible nurse of the unit.

12. Explain equipment in the bedside table and the location of the bedside locker.

13. Explain how the call system works.

14. Show the patient the location of the bathroom.

15. Inform the patient about meal hours and nourishment times.

16. Explain visiting hours and policies.

17. Describe other areas in the hospital that the patient or support persons may use, such as lounges, the cafeteria, the chapel, and the canteen.

18. Explain how the patient may obtain a television or radio.

19. Inform the patient of smoking regulations.

20. Describe expectations of the patient, such as what to wear.

Many agencies provide information pamphlets for patients, covering most of this information. Check what materials are available in your agency.

Admitting the patient

21. Assist the patient to change into the hospital gown, or personal sleeping garments if agency policy allows this. Many patients do not require assistance undressing but need to be informed which way to put on a hospital gown, ie, with the ties at the back.

22. Assist the patient as needed to a comfortable position in bed.

23. Hang the clothes in the bedside locker and either list the clothes or have the patient sign a form assuming responsibility for them, following the policy of the agency. Some agencies have support persons take the patient's clothing home.

24. Inform the patient of agency policy about valuables. Special envelopes are usually provided by the agency to store valuables such as money, jewelry, and keys in a locked safe in the business office. Supply an envelope, if this is agency policy. Assure the patient that the valuables will be safely handled and

returned at discharge. Have the patient sign a statement absolving the hospital of responsibility for valuables kept at the bedside, if this is agency policy. Agency policies generally state the amount of money the patient should keep at the bedside. Patients undergoing prolonged hospitalization sign special release forms to be able to withdraw small amounts of money from safekeeping as needs arise. Label large items, such as radios, with the patient's full name. Some agencies require that personal electronic equipment be checked by the engineering department before it is used.

25. Ask whether the patient has brought medications. If so, request that they be taken home, or send them to the hospital pharmacy or designated area for safekeeping. It is usual for only certain medications, such as nitroglycerin, to be kept at the bedside. Check agency policy.

    Rationale   While the patient is in the hospital, medications must be carefully regulated, to be therapeutic and to avoid incompatibilities.

26. Take the patient's temperature, pulse, respirations, blood pressure, and weight. In some agencies, the blood pressure is not taken for children under 6, however. See chapter 8.

    Rationale   These vital signs provide baseline data for subsequent assessments during hospitalization. They are indicators of the patient's general condition.

27. Obtain a urine specimen. Explain to the patient that this is a routine procedure for all patients on admission. Direct ambulatory patients to the bathroom to provide a specimen. Provide a bedpan or urinal for bed patients to use. Apply a urine collector to children who are not toilet trained.

    Rationale   Urine specimens are taken routinely at admission as a precautionary measure to screen for diabetes or infections of the urinary tract. See chapter 27.

28. Obtain a nursing history. If forms are not available:
    a. Ask for the patient's perceptions of his or her illness.
    b. Ask about the chief discomforts and complaints.
    c. Ascertain any allergies.
    d. Determine what medications have been taken routinely or recently.
    e. Observe the patient's general appearance.
    f. Note any objective signs of illness, such as a rash or a cough.

    Rationale   The nursing history provides baseline data for subsequent care planning.

29. Inform the patient that a blood specimen and chest x-ray film will be taken by a technician, if applicable.

Rationale   A blood specimen is routinely taken from many or all patients, to do a hemoglobin assessment, blood typing, and cross-matching for patients having surgery. Chest x-ray films are taken to ascertain the presence of any lung disease such as tuberculosis.

30. Inform the patient of any treatments to be administered in the near future, eg, during the next shift or day. Patients who are having surgery, for example, need to know what preoperative preparations (such as a surgical shave) are required. See chapter 31.

31. Place the call signal within easy reach of the patient, and explain how it works.

32. Provide a container for dentures if the patient requires one.

33. Inform support persons when they can return, and inform them about visiting hours.

34. Send specimens to the laboratory with appropriate labels and requisitions.

35. Place allergy alerts, if necessary, on the patient and the chart, according to agency policy. Record allergies in red ink both on the front of the patient's chart and on the nursing Kardex. A sign indicating specific allergies may also be placed on the foot of the patient's bed or on the wall above the head of the bed. If the patient has food allergies, notify the dietary department.

36. Record assessment data on the appropriate forms of the patient's record, in accordance with agency procedure. Some agencies, for example, record the vital signs on both the nurse's notes and the graphic record. Selected data from the nursing history form are generally transferred to the nurse's notes as well as the patient's Kardex. Record on the nurse's notes and on the valuables envelope the disposition of the valuables.

Sample Recording

Date	Time	Notes
12/5/86	1140	Admitted walking. T 97, P 82, R 14, BP 130/70. Appears alert. States is in to have gallbladder removed, has no discomfort at present. States has no known allergies. States takes thyroid pills twice a day before breakfast and at bedtime. Urine specimen sent to lab. Gave watch and ring to wife to take home. $50.00 cash placed in valuables envelope and given to hospital Business Office to place in safe. Oriented to hospital routines and equipment. Given information pamphlet about preop prep.——— Sheila S. Murphy, NS
	1150	Dr. L. Stein notified of admission.——— Sheila S. Murphy, NS
	1230	Blood sample taken by lab technician.——— Sheila S. Murphy, NS

TECHNIQUE 5–2 ■ Transferring a Patient

Patients may be transferred (moved) to another nursing unit within the hospital, to another bed within the nursing unit, or to another agency. Some transfers are requested by the physician, some are occasioned by hospital policy. Examples of reasons for transferring patients are:

1. To obtain special care, eg, in an intensive care unit
2. To obtain a different type of accommodation, such as a single room rather than a four-bed room
3. To obtain another type of medical service, such as surgery instead of rehabilitation

In-unit transfers

Transfers may be made within a nursing unit. The patient changes rooms on the same unit, often for one of the following reasons:

1. To obtain a different type of accommodation, such as a private room
2. To be nearer to the nurses' station if frequent observations and care are required, eg, for a seriously ill or confused patient
3. To obtain compatible roommates, eg, other non-smokers

This type of move is not considered a usual transfer, since the only change is the room number. The new number is recorded on the patient's chart and other documents (the medication record, the nursing care plan or Kardex, etc). It is also important to notify the business office, the information desk, the dietary department, etc, to assure continuity of services. All the patient's personal belongings and equipment should be moved with the patient.

Interhospital transfers

In some regions patients are transferred from one hospital to another, when necessary. For example, a patient may move from an acute hospital to a long-term care facility. In these transfers, the patient's records, medications, etc, often go with the patient, accompanied by a form containing pertinent information about the patient. The transferring agency will usually have guidelines for nursing personnel to follow in making the transfer.

■ Assessment

The nurse in the current unit assesses the patient for: current health status reflecting nursing and medical problems, eg, respirations, pulse, condition of skin.

Other data include: information about the transfer, eg, the name of the unit to which the patient is moving.

■ Planning

Nursing goals

1. To move the patient with the least amount of discomfort
2. To assist the patient in adjustment to the new unit

■ Intervention

Nurse in current unit

1. Explain to the patient about the transfer. Be sure to tell the patient that the hospital's information desk will be given the new room number so that visitors can be told.

   Rationale Many patients worry about change and are reassured by knowing the reason for the transfer, what the other nursing unit is like, when the move will take place, and any arrangements that are being made.

2. Gather all the patient's personal belongings and place them in the patient's suitcase or in bags provided by the agency:
   a. Clothes in locker
   b. Slippers
   c. Clothes in drawers
   d. Dentures, cosmetics, etc, usually in the bedside table or the bathroom
   e. Magazines, books, flowers, etc

3. Collect the equipment used at the bedside:
   a. Bedpan, urinal
   b. Washbasin, towels, etc
   c. Emesis basin
   d. Denture cup

   Some agencies leave this equipment at the bedside and provide another set at the new bed. Check agency policy.

4. Collect the patient's record and related supplies, such as:
   a. Medication cards
   b. The nursing care plan
   c. Medications

5. If agency policy indicates, write a discharge

summary similar to that discussed in Technique 5–3 and shown in Figure 5–2 on page 59. Many agencies require the nurse to write a discharge summary when the patient is transferred to another nursing unit.

6. Establish the method by which the patient can move, such as wheelchair or stretcher. This may be indicated in the patient's record or by the responsible nurse. Patients normally are transferred by wheelchair unless they are too ill to sit up.

7. Lock the wheels on the stretcher or wheelchair when the patient moves on and off it.
   Rationale   Locking prevents the wheels from moving and thus endangering the patient's safety.

8. Assist the patient to the wheelchair or stretcher. Provide warm coverings for the patient.
   Rationale   Assistance prevents undue exertion. Coverings prevent chilling and maintain the patient's sense of modesty.

9. Record in the patient's chart the time of the transfer, the unit to which the patient is moving, the mode of transport, eg, by wheelchair, and any significant assessments. This is an exception to the rule that charting is done after the technique. This recording is done just prior to moving the patient (see the Sample Recording following the technique).

10. Take the patient and the supplies to the other unit, or arrange for transport service.

11. Call at the nurses' station upon arrival at the receiving unit, and introduce the nurse in charge to the patient. Review the patient's chart or discharge summary with a nursing staff member (receiving nurse) on this unit.

12. Leave the chart, medications, and nursing care plan at the nurses' station.

13. Take the patient to the new room and assist him or her into bed. The receiving nurse may go with you.

14. Return to your nursing unit with the stretcher or wheelchair.

15. Notify the information desk and other departments (such as the dietary department and pharmacy) of the transfer. Most agencies indicate which departments need to be notified when a patient is transferred.

16. At the patient's former bed unit, strip the bed and arrange for terminal cleaning. In some agencies, housekeeping personnel carry out this cleaning; in others, nursing personnel do it.

Nurse in receiving unit

17. With the transferring nurse, review the patient's chart, or discharge summary if written, and the patient care required.

18. Assess the patient's immediate condition, and provide any interventions immediately needed.

19. Welcome the patient and any accompanying support persons. Introduce other patients in the room. Orient the patient to any practices that are different on this unit from those of the previous unit.

20. Confirm that other departments, such as the dietary department, know the new location of the patient.

21. Record on the patient's chart the time of arrival, method of transport, and assessment data.

Sample Recording: Transferring Nurse

Date	Time	Notes
6/12/86	1100	Transferred by wheelchair to A6. P 96, BP 160/120/90. All personal items including dentures moved with pt. Meds given to L. Jones, HN.———— Eliza L. Begbie, NS

Sample Recording: Receiving Nurse

Date	Time	Notes
6/12/86	1115	Received by wheelchair. Color pale. P 106, BP 165/90. C/o fatigue. Oriented to unit practices. Dr. Bedow notified.———— Karen S. Stockley, NS

TECHNIQUE 5–3   ■   Discharging a Patient

When patients leave a hospital they are normally discharged with the physician's authorization (a written order by the physician, eg, "May go home tomorrow," on the patient's chart). Occasionally, patients leave an agency without the permission of the physician. These are *unauthorized discharges,* and the patient is asked to sign a special form releasing the hospital from any responsibility after the patient's departure. See the sample release in Figure 5–1.

Usually patients plan and look forward to their

(NAME OF HOSPITAL)

RESPONSIBILITY RELEASE

This is to certify that I, the undersigned, am this day leaving the (Name of Hospital) contrary to the expressed wishes of my Medical Advisor, Dr. _____ and the Hospital Authorities, and I hereby relieve the said Doctor and the Hospital Authorities of all responsibility as to my future welfare and progress.

_____
(Signature of Patient)

_____
(Signature of Witness)

Dated at (name of city, town) this ____ day of _____ 19 ____

RE: _____ Patient # _____
(Name of Patient)

FIGURE 5–1 ■ An example of a form for a patient release without authorization.

discharge from the hospital. Several members of the health team, such as a dietitian, a social worker, and a community nurse may be working with the patient and support persons to make discharge plans.

■ Assessment

Assess the patient for:

1. Readiness to be discharged, eg, physical and emotional readiness. Some agencies have discharge profiles to use for final assessment purposes. See Figure 5–2.
2. Acquisition of skills required for follow-up care.

Prior to the discharge, also make sure that the patient and support persons have received and understood written information about follow-up care.

■ Planning

Plans for the patient's discharge generally include plans for continued care after discharge, teaching specific skills and knowledge to the patient and support persons, and plans for physical arrangements that need to be made in the patient's home. Some agencies have special departments to deal solely with discharge planning.

Nursing goals

1. To help the patient and support persons feel secure and comfortable about leaving the health care agency
2. To instruct the patient and support persons in care required at home

3. To help the patient and support persons plan support services and make necessary home adjustments

Planning follow-up care

After a stay in the hospital, patients may require follow-up care. Some hospitals and community health agencies provide aftercare for patients in the home. The care may vary from dressing changes to exercises for a partially paralyzed limb. It is important to notify the agency involved as early as possible. Another common part of aftercare is a visit to the physician's office at a specified time after discharge.

It is wise for the nurse to provide written data about any follow-up care and arrangements that have been made for the patient. Patients excited about going home often forget verbal information given at departure. A written list of directions can be reviewed and followed later.

Teaching specific skills and knowledge

Often a patient and/or support persons need to learn specific skills and knowledge as a consequence of an illness. The skills might be how to administer medications, change dressings, or give certain treatments. The knowledge might be about activity, diet, or exercises. Learning is absorbed best if taught over a period of time, not just before the patient is discharged. Unfortunately, this is not always possible, and last minute teaching is unavoidable at times.

Planning physical arrangements in the home

Physical arrangements must often be made in a home to accommodate the hospitalized patient after discharge. This is particularly true for the elderly, who tend to require longer than younger people to regain their strength. Some communities provide nursing service to assist support persons with these arrangements, while others rely on the hospital nurses to help patients and their support persons plan to meet these needs.

■ Intervention

1. Determine whether and at what time the patient has made arrangements for transportation. If an ambulance is required, at many hospitals the nurse telephones to make the arrangements.
2. If the patient has valuables in safekeeping, obtain his or her signature on the release form, and return the valuables to the patient. Assist the patient to dress.
3. Confirm that the business office has completed its procedures for the patient. If it has not, make arrangements for the patient to visit the office or for an office representative to visit the patient. The

THE MONTREAL GENERAL HOSPITAL

NURSING DISCHARGE PROFILE
RESUME DU DOSSIER SOINS INFIRMIERS

Smith, Mrs. Jane

PATIENT'S LEVEL OF SELF CARE
HABITUDES QUOTIDIENNES DU PATIENT

	INDEP.	ASSIST(E)	DEPEND.	COMMENTS (COMMENTAIRES/PREFERENCES)		
				☐ BED BATH BAIN AU LIT	☑ TUB BATH BAIN: BAIGNOIRE	☑ SHOWER DOUCHE
BATH/BAIN	✓					
DRESSING/HABILLEMENT	✓					
FEEDING/ALIMENTATION	✓					
AMBULATION/DEPLACEMENT	✓					
STAIRS/ESCALIERS	✓					

NUTRITION/DIETE	BLADDER/VESICALE	BOWELS/INTESTINALE	VISION/VUE
☑ Regular/Régulière	☑ Normal	☑ Normal	☑ Adequate/Suffisante
☐ Diabetic/Diabétique	☐ Incontinent/Incontinence	☐ Incontinent/Incontinence	☐ Impaired/Déficiente
☐ Low Salt/Sel↓	☐ Frequency/Frequence	☐ Diarrhea/Diarrhée	☐ (R) Eye/Oeil droit
☐ Other/Autre	☐ Catheter/Sonde	☐ Constipation	☐ (L) Eye/Oeil gauche
AS TOLERATED	☐ Ostomy/Ostomie	☐ Aids/Moyens	☐ Glasses/Lunettes
			☐ Contact Lens/Verres de contact

HEARING/OUIE	SPEECH/EXPRESSION	LANGUAGE/LANGUE	
☑ Adequate/Suffisante			
☐ Impaired/Déficiente	Difficulty/Difficultés	☑ Eng./Anglais ☑ Fr./Français	
☐ Aid/Appareil	☐ Yes/Oui ☑ No/Non	☐ Other/Autre	

NURSING CONCERNS/PROBLEMES SOINS INFIRMIERS	NURSING APPROACH/APPROCHE SOINS INFIRMIERS
1) WOUND CARE (DRAIN SITE OOZING SMALL AMOUNT SEROUS FLUID)	CLEANSE WITH NORMAL SALINE DAILY. APPLY DRY DRESSING.
2) FATIGUE (TIRES EASILY, HAS FOUR YOUNG CHILDREN TO CARE FOR)	HOMEMAKER × 5 DAYS

ATTITUDES TO PLAN OF CARE/ATTITUDES ENVERS LE PLAN DE SOINS (PATIENT & FAMILY/MALADE & FAMILLE) ANXIOUS TO GO HOME. AWARE THAT SHE WILL NEED LOTS OF REST

TEACHING DONE/ENSEIGNEMENT FAIT UNDERSTANDS & HAS DEMONSTRATED WOUND CARE. KNOWS THAT SHE CAN CALL SOCIAL WORKER FOR EXTENSION OF HOMEMAKER SERVICES

RESOURCES/RESSOURCES (FAMILY/FAMILLE, COMMUNITY/COMMUNAUTE) HOMEMAKER × 5 DAYS. PARENTS LIVE NEARBY - CAN HELP WITH CHILDREN

DISCHARGE DIAGNOSIS/DIAGNOSTIC AU RENVOI DU MALADE CHOLECYSTECTOMY

MEDICATION RECEIVED DAY OF DISCHARGE/MEDICAMENTS RECUS LE JOUR DE RENVOI —

DATE OF DISCHARGE/JOUR DE RENVOI JULY 11/86   TIME/HEURE 10.30   TO/A Home

FOLLOW-UP APPOINTMENTS/RENDEZ-VOUS JULY 26, 1986 - SURGICAL CLINIC

SIGNATURE (NURSE/INFIRMIER(E)) a. Carpenter, RN   DATE July 11, 1986

NURSING DISCHARGE PROFILE

FIGURE 5–2 ■ A sample nursing discharge profile. (Courtesy of the Department of Nursing, Montreal General Hospital, Montreal, Quebec.)

patient's support persons may be able to attend to this. Arrangements for paying are usually made at the time of admission.

4. If the physician has left a prescription for the patient, make sure that the patient has this and understands directions for taking the medication. The hospital may have facilities to make up the prescription for the patient.

5. Assess the patient's health, eg, check the surgical dressing, assess the pulse and blood pressure if indicated.

6. Contact the transport service or obtain a wheelchair if required for the patient, unless an ambulance will be taking the patient. Obtain a utility cart to transport the patient's personal effects, if the patient cannot hold them.

   Rationale Some hospitals require that the patient use a wheelchair even though he or she feels able to walk, because of the danger of overexertion. The ambulance crew will have a stretcher for the patient.

7. Lock the wheels of the chair. Then assist the patient onto the wheelchair.

   Rationale Locking the wheels prevents the chair from moving and endangering the patient's safety.

8. Take the patient and the personal effects to meet the arranged transportation.

9. Lock the wheels of the chair before assisting the patient to move.

10. Assist the patient to the automobile and place the personal effects inside it.

11. Report to the responsible nurse and/or the unit clerk that the patient has been discharged.

12. Record in the patient's chart the discharge, the time, the method of transport to the agency door, and assessment data. Some agencies also suggest that the patient's destination, eg, a nursing home, be included in the discharge notes.

Sample Recording

Date	Time	Notes
12/5/86	1400	Discharged by wheelchair to Sunnyvale Lodge. Meds taken by wife. Written instructions provided about leg exercises.—————————— Maria L. Chavez, NS

13. Write a discharge profile. Some agencies require a discharge summary of nursing care given. Check agency practice.

14. Check that the record for discharge has been completed. If not, leave it in the appropriate place for the physician. Once it is completed, send the record to the records office.

15. Return to the patient's room, strip the bed, and arrange for terminal cleaning.

References

DeYoung M: Planning for discharge. *Geriatr Nurs* (November/December) 1982; 3:396–399.

Johnston M, Salazar M: Preadmission program for rehospitalized children. *Am J Nurs* (August) 1979; 79:1420–1422.

Lore A: Supporting the hospitalized elderly person. *Am J Nurs* (March) 1979; 79:496–499.

Weinstein SM: Special teams in home care. *Am J Nurs* (March) 1984; 84:342–345.

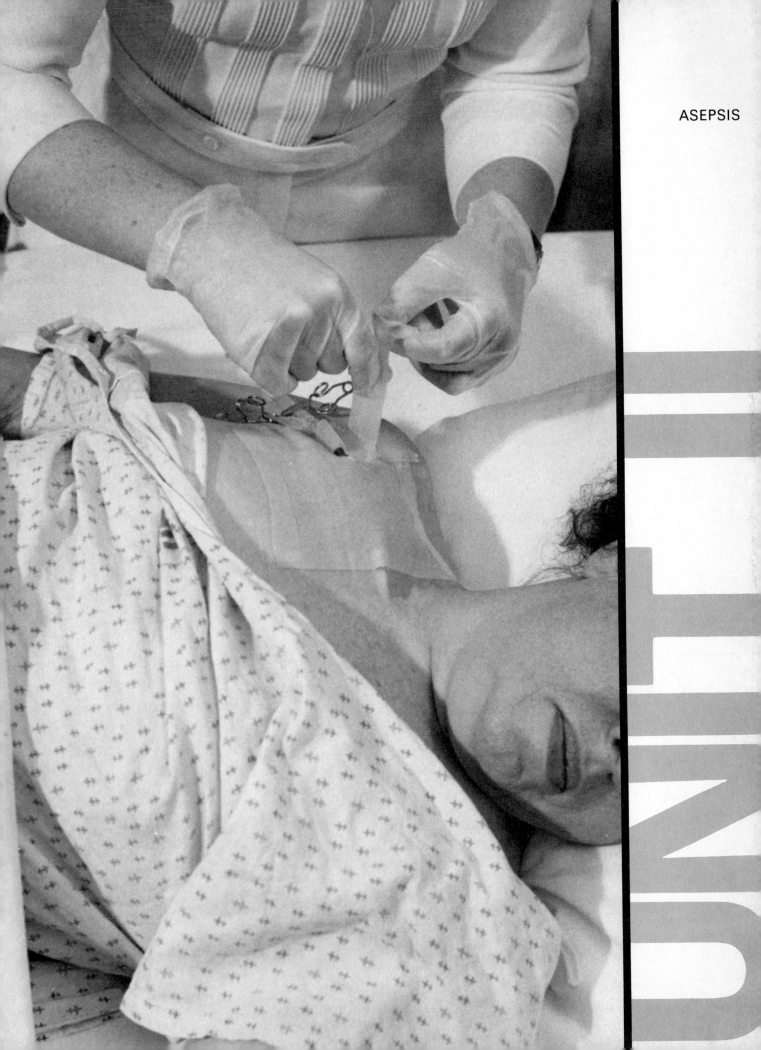

UNIT II

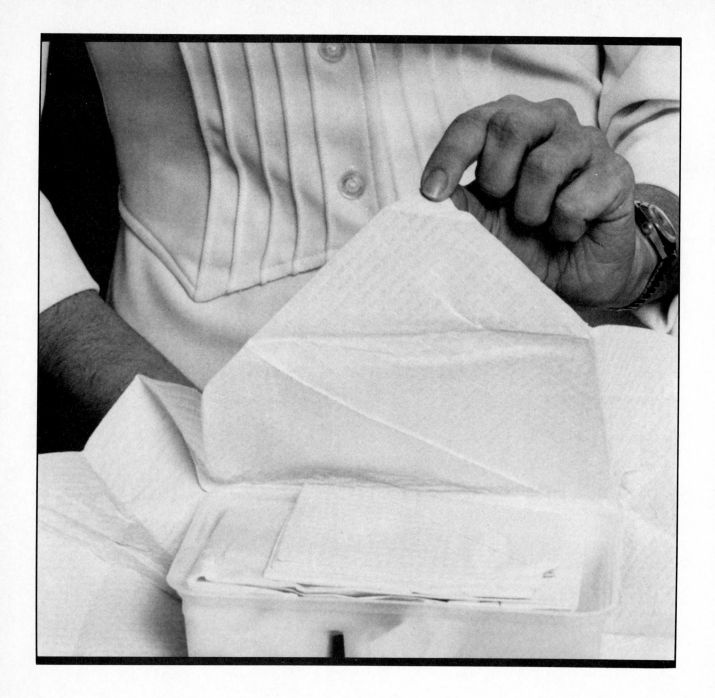

MEDICAL ASEPSIS AND INFECTION CONTROL

6

Asepsis is the absence of disease-producing microorganisms (germs). Microorganisms are always present in the environment. Some live on the skin, in the nose, in the mouth, and in the bowel; others are found in the air, in the soil, on clothes, and elsewhere. Most microorganisms do not produce disease in ordinary circumstances (they are nonpathogenic). Those that do produce disease are called *pathogens* or *pathogenic microorganisms.* The disease process caused by the pathogens is *infection.*

Controlling the transmission of microorganisms and protecting

...fections are major concerns in hospitals ...mes. Several risk factors make a patient ...le to acquiring an infection. Some ...ly have and are being treated for an ...are more susceptible to secondary infections. Other patients do not have an infection but because of the severity of their illness have lowered resistance to infectious agents. In addition, many medical therapies are risk factors. For example, surgery, intravenous therapy, and injected medications break the body's protective skin barrier to invading micro-organisms. The risk of introducing an infection is a constant threat for patients receiving such therapies. Infections acquired in a hospital or similar institution are referred to as *nosocomial* infections. When nurses work with patients who have infections, they need to

understand the infectious disease process and how infectious agents are transmitted, so that they can prevent the spread of microorganisms among patients, personnel, and visitors.

Agencies employ special practices when personnel or equipment becomes contaminated—that is, comes in direct contact with pathogenic microorganisms. These practices, referred to as *protective aseptic precautions* or *isolation precautions,* are designed to interrupt the chain of infection primarily at the transmission stage. Such practices include hand washing before and after patient contact and correct cleaning, disinfecting, and disposal of equipment and supplies.

Hand washing is often described as the single most important means of preventing the spread of infection.

Chapter Outline

The Chain of Infection

Medical Aseptic Practices

Protective Asepsis (Isolation Precautions)

Guidelines for Protective Aseptic Practices

Psychologic Problems of Protective Asepsis

■ Technique 6–1 Hand Washing

■ Technique 6–2 Initiating Protective Aseptic Practices

■ Technique 6–3 Donning and Removing a Face Mask

■ Technique 6–4 Gowning for Protective Asepsis
■ Technique 6–5 Donning and Removing Disposable Gloves
■ Technique 6–6 Double-Bagging
■ Technique 6–7 Assessing the Vital Signs of a Patient on Protective Asepsis
■ Technique 6-8 Reverse Protective Asepsis (Barrier Technique; Reverse Isolation)

Objectives

Upon completion of this chapter, the student will:

1. Know essential terms and facts about medical asepsis
   1.1 Define terms associated with medical asepsis
   1.2 Identify the six components of the chain of infection
   1.3 Identify major vehicles that transport microorganisms
   1.4 Identify exit methods of microorganisms from six parts of the body
   1.5 Identify major barriers of the body that prevent the entrance of microorganisms
   1.6 Identify the seven types of protective asepsis
   1.7 Identify precautions for each type of protective asepsis
   1.8 Identify psychologic problems associated with protective asepsis
   1.9 Identify general guidelines for protective aseptic techniques
   1.10 List equipment essential for protective aseptic techniques

   1.11 Identify the order in which certain protective aseptic techniques are carried out
2. Understand the protective aseptic practices used to prevent the spread of microorganisms
   2.1 Explain the hand-washing technique used in medical asepsis
   2.2 Give reasons for certain dress standards
   2.3 Explain the essential steps for cleaning articles that are soiled with organic material
   2.4 Compare two types of chemical decontamination
   2.5 Identify four methods for sterilizing objects
   2.6 Identify measures to strengthen the body's barriers against infection
   2.7 Give examples of effective ways to handle body secretions
   2.8 Explain why air currents and dust are kept to a minimum
3. Understand facts about protective aseptic techniques
   3.1 Identify relevant assessment data
   3.2 Identify nursing goals related to the technique

3.3 Identify reasons underlying selected steps of the technique

4. Perform protective aseptic techniques safely
   4.1 Assess the patient adequately
   4.2 Collect additional data from appropriate sources
   4.3 Select pertinent nursing goals for the patient
   4.4 Establish relevant outcome criteria for the patient, if indicated, following the technique
   4.5 Collect necessary equipment before the technique
   4.6 Implement interventions to enhance the effectiveness of the technique and enhance the patient's comfort and safety
   4.7 Communicate relevant information about the patient to the appropriate persons
   4.8 Determine the evaluative outcomes of the technique, if indicated

5. Evaluate own performance of protective aseptic techniques in a laboratory or clinical setting with the assistance of another
   5.1 Use the performance checklists provided
   5.2 Identify areas of strength and weakness
   5.3 Alter performance in response to own evaluation and that of another

Terms

■ **aerobe** an organism that requires oxygen to live

■ **anaerobe** an organism that does not require oxygen to live or requires the absence of oxygen

■ **antiseptic** an agent that inhibits the growth of some microorganisms on skin or tissue

■ **asepsis** the absence of disease-producing microorganisms

■ **autoclave** an apparatus that sterilizes, using steam under pressure

■ **bactericide** an agent capable of destroying some microorganisms

■ **bacteriostatic agent** an agent that prevents the growth and reproduction of some microorganisms

■ **carrier** a person who carries pathogens but is not ill

■ **clean** free of pathogenic organisms

■ **contaminated** possessing pathogenic organisms

■ **disinfectant** an agent that inhibits the growth or reproduction of microorganisms on inanimate environmental surfaces

■ **enteric** referring to the gastrointestinal system or the organisms that inhabit the system

■ **environmental stimulus** anything in the environment that arouses or incites action by a receptor (the terminus of a sensory nerve)

■ **fomite** an inanimate object that can harbor pathogenic microorganisms

■ **germicide** an agent that kills some pathogens

■ **hallucination** a distortion of sensory perceptions; hearing voices or seeing things that do not exist

■ **infection** the disease process produced by microorganisms or the toxins they produce

■ **medical asepsis** practices that limit the transmission of microorganisms; also called *clean technique*

■ **microorganism** a small (minute) living body visible under a microscope

■ **nonpathogen** a microorganism that does not produce disease under usual conditions

■ **nosocomial** associated with or originating in a hospital or similar institution, eg, a nosocomial infection

■ **pathogen** a microorganism that produces disease in most circumstances

■ **phagocyte** a cell, eg, a white blood cell, that ingests microorganisms, other cells, and foreign particles

■ **phagocytosis** the process by which cells engulf microorganisms, other cells, or foreign particles

■ **protective asepsis (isolation)** practices setting someone or something apart from others or separating it; practices used to prevent the spread of infections and communicable diseases

■ **reverse protective asepsis (barrier technique; reverse isolation)** practices used to prevent an individual from coming in contact with microorganisms, eg, when a patient has severe burns

■ **sensory deprivation** lack of sensory stimulation

■ **spore** a round or oval structure resistant to destruction that is formed by some bacterial cells as part of the reproductive process

■ **sterilization** a process that destroys all microorganisms, including spores

■ **surgical asepsis** measures that render and maintain objects free from microorganisms, ie, that produce sterility

■ **thought disorganization** a condition in which a person has difficulty remembering what he or she is saying, is confused about time (eg, time of day or the day of the week), gives inappropriate verbal responses, and has sensory distortions

■ **virulence** ability to produce disease

THE CHAIN OF INFECTION

The chain of infection or infectious cycle (see Figure 6–1) is the process through which a microorganism produces infection in a person. This chain has six components: the microorganism, the source or reservoir, the exit or escape, the method of transmission, the portal of entry, and the susceptible host. It is important for nurses to understand this chain, so that they can prevent microorganisms from causing infections.

The Microorganism

Whether a particular microorganism will cause disease depends on a number of factors related to the microorganism:

1. The number of microorganisms. An attack by many microorganisms is more likely to cause disease than an invasion by a few.

2. The potency or virulence of the microorganism. Microorganisms vary in ability to produce disease. Some, such as the smallpox virus, are highly virulent; others, such as streptococci, are less so.

3. The ability of the microorganism to establish itself within the body, in light of environmental conditions for growth.

FIGURE 6–1 ■ The chain of infection.

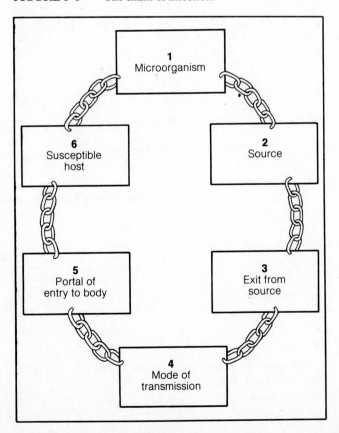

4. The ability of the microorganisms to enter the body. Pathogenic organisms on intact skin rarely cause an infection unless they can enter the body, eg, through a cut in the skin, contact with mucous membranes, or with food entering the digestive tract.

The Source or Reservoir

The source of pathogenic microorganisms can be an animal, a person, or any aspect of the environment, including water and food. All humans and animals carry microorganisms within them and may be sources of infectious agents to others, yet they themselves may not become ill. They are sometimes referred to as *carriers*.

The Exit from the Source

The means by which microorganisms leave the source are varied. In humans, methods of exit depend on the site of the microorganisms within the body and the particular pathogen. There are six primary exits, which are detailed in Table 6–1.

The Method of Transmission

After a microorganism leaves its source or reservoir, it requires a means of transmission to reach another person or host. There are five common methods:

1. *Direct contact.* When a person touches an infected person, microorganisms can transfer to the uninfected person.

2. *Air.* A few microorganisms can attach to dust particles in the air and then can be inhaled directly from the air.

3. *Food or water.* When food or water becomes contaminated, agents such as hepatitis A can infect whole communities.

TABLE 6–1 ■ **Portals of Exit and Transport Vehicles for Microorganisms**

Exit	Transport vehicle	Example of microorganism
1. Respiratory tract	Droplets expelled while sneezing, coughing, breathing	*Streptococcus pneumoniae*
2. Gastrointestinal tract	Emesis, feces, drainage (such as from the gallbladder), saliva	*Salmonella enteritidis*
3. Urinary tract	Urine	*Escherichia coli*
4. Reproductive tract	Discharge from the vagina or penis	*Neisseria gonorrhoeae*
5. Blood	Blood sample	Hepatitis B virus
6. Tissue	Drainage from a cut or wound	*Staphylococcus aureus*

4. *Fomites.* Articles soiled with body substances such as feces, blood, or wound drainage can transmit microorganisms to others.

5. *Animals or insects.* Domestic animals harbor microorganisms such as *Salmonella* that can cause gastrointestinal infections when transmitted to humans. Flies and fleas can also transmit pathogens.

The Portal of Entry

The portals by which microorganisms enter the body of a person may be the same as the exits from the body. All portals have barriers to the entry of microorganisms. Normally these barriers are effective, but if they are damaged or have been compromised by invasive medical devices, they will permit microorganisms to pass. Table 6–2 lists the portals and major barriers.

The Susceptible Host

A susceptible host is a person who is likely to develop an infection when pathogens enter the body. A number of factors make a person more susceptible than others at a particular time:

TABLE 6–2 ■ **Portals of Entry and Major Barriers to Microorganisms**

Portal of entry	Major barriers*
1. Respiratory tract	Cilia (microscopic, hairlike process of the nose, larynx, pharynx, and trachea), mucous membrane, mucus, sneezing and coughing
2. Gastrointestinal tract	Mucous membrane, mucus, cilia of the pharynx
3. Urinary tract	Mucous membrane, mucus, acid medium of the urine
4. Reproductive tract	**Males** Mucous membrane, mucus
	Females Mucous membrane, mucus, vaginal secretion (which is normally slightly acid)
5. Blood	Skin, mucous membrane, mucus, blood vessels
6. Tissue	Skin, mucous membrane, mucus

*The immune system (antibodies etc) is a major barrier that protects the entire body from infection.

1. High-level or prolonged stress
2. Poor nutrition
3. Fatigue
4. Age (the very young are susceptible to certain infections, the very old to others, etc)
5. Medical treatments (eg, chemotherapy for leukemia depletes the white blood cells needed to combat infection)

MEDICAL ASEPTIC PRACTICES

Medical aseptic practices are designed to weaken or destroy the links in the chain of infection. Following are some of the specific methods used.

Hand Washing

Washing hands is the medical aseptic practice nurses do most frequently. It is an important, simple, and effective method of reducing to a minimum the number of microorganisms on the hands and thus limiting transmission. Some antiseptic agents that do not require hand washing with running water are gaining acceptance in situations where the hands are not physically soiled.

Standards of Dress

Uniforms are kept clean. Some agencies supply and launder staff uniforms to ensure cleanliness, especially in high-risk areas such as the nursery or operating room. Rings, other than plain bands, and other jewelry are not worn in some agencies because it is thought that microorganisms can lodge in grooved areas and stone settings and be carried from patient to patient. Rings other than plain bands are also a safety hazard.

Cleaning

Dirt, food, and organic material provide sources and means of transport for bacteria. Many general cleaning procedures are carried out by the housekeeping department; however, nurses assume responsibility for cleaning various pieces of equipment and supplies in some agencies.

An article is considered clean or *decontaminated* when it is free of pathogenic organisms; an article that has pathogens on it is considered *dirty* or *contaminated*. The steps for cleaning most articles in a hospital or home where pathogens are present are:

1. Wearing gloves, rinse the article with cold water to remove organic material, such as blood or pus. Hot water coagulates the protein of organic material and tends to make it stick to the article.

2. Wash the article in hot water and soap. Soap has an emulsifying action and reduces surface tension, facilitating the removal of dirt. Water assists in rinsing the dirt away.

3. Use an abrasive such as a stiff-bristled brush to clean articles that have grooves and corners.

4. Rinse the article well with hot water.

5. Dry the article; it is now clean.

6. Disinfect or sterilize the article, if indicated.

Floors are always considered heavily contaminated. This is because microorganisms have an affinity for dust particles, which are heavier than air and eventually settle on the floor. The microorganisms may originate from any source—the skin, clothing, a dressing, or body discharge. Thus, an item that falls to the floor is discarded or cleaned with a disinfectant before use.

Chemical Decontamination (Disinfectants and Antiseptics)

Both antiseptics and disinfectants are said to have *bactericidal* or *bacteriostatic* actions. Whether a chemical agent destroys microorganisms or inhibits their growth depends upon its mechanism of action, the length of time it is used, the number of microorganisms present, the concentration of the agent, the temperature, and the presence and amount of organic matter (such as blood, mucus, or some other body discharge).

Chemical disinfection is achieved by the use of compounds such as phenolics or iodophors that destroy most microorganisms except some spore-forming bacteria. Although heat or steam can also destroy pathogens, the term *disinfectant* is generally used for chemical substances, such as phenol and iodine compounds. Disinfectants are usually caustic or toxic substances. They therefore are used to decontaminate equipment, floors, walls, and furniture rather than living tissue.

An *antiseptic,* which may be bacteriostatic or bactericidal, is used on skin or tissue. Examples of antiseptics are alcohol and iodophors.

Sterilization

In contrast to disinfecting, sterilization is a process that destroys *all* microorganisms, including spores. Various methods are used to sterilize objects, since not all objects can withstand certain types of sterilization without damage. Methods and uses include:

1. *Hot-air oven.* Dry heat at a temperature of 180 °C (350 °F) for two hours will sterilize glassware and some metal objects. Dry heat is especially useful for sterilizing dressings for home use. The package should be no thicker than 15 cm (6 in) and should be baked for one hour at 180 °C (350 °F). The oven door should be left slightly ajar to prevent scorching.

2. *Boiling.* Boiling is useful for sterilizing metal instruments, eg, forceps, or glass items for home use. It is believed that boiling for 10 minutes will destroy all microorganisms except spores and the virus of infectious hepatitis. Spores are destroyed after 20 minutes of boiling. The article to be sterilized must be completely submerged in water during the entire time. The boiling time is counted after the water comes to a full boil.

3. *Steam.* Steam under pressure requires an *autoclave,* a special self-locking apparatus fitted with a gauge that automatically regulates the degree of heat and steam pressure on the contents. The amount of time and degree of temperature needed for effective sterilization vary with the article being sterilized. Articles wrapped in paper or cloth need more time for the steam to penetrate than unwrapped articles that are directly exposed to the steam. Commonly, steam at 121 °C (250 °F) and at 17 lb pressure is used for 30 minutes. Autoclaving is used to sterilize surgical dressings, surgical linens, intravenous solutions, metal, glass, and some rubber objects. Small items can be sterilized in the home in a pressure cooker for 15 minutes.

4. *Ethylene oxide gas (ETO).* Sterilization without extreme heat, using ethylene oxide gas instead, is employed in some agencies. Because exposure to ETO is more costly and time consuming than steam autoclaving, it is recommended for equipment that cannot tolerate the high temperatures of autoclaving, such as plastic or rubber articles. Objects sterilized by ETO are subjected to a temperature of about 43 °C (110 °F) in a concentration of ethylene oxide 440 mg/L. Examples of articles that can be sterilized by gas are oxygen and suction gauges, blood pressure apparatus, stethoscopes, sheepskins, plastic drinking glasses, and catheters.

Handling of Body Secretions

Common body discharges come from the nose, throat, urinary bladder, vagina, penis, and rectum. Discharges are always present from open wounds, which may be or become infected. Measures taken to handle body secretions relate largely to the exit of microorganisms from their reservoir and the next link in the chain of infection, transmission. Measures for handling body secretions effectively include:

1. Covering the mouth and nose with a protective tissue when coughing, sneezing, or blowing the nose. This measure applies to both patients and nurses. It prevents droplets and microorganisms from spraying into the air where someone else may breathe them or dropping on surfaces where they may be touched. The tissue is discarded in an appropriate container, preferably a plastic-

lined receptacle. The hands are then washed before picking up objects or touching others.

2. Wearing gloves and washing hands thoroughly after handling any excretions in bedpans or from wound drainage. Bedpans are emptied promptly, handled carefully, and cleaned appropriately. Patients are given the opportunity to wash their hands following elimination. Wet dressings from wounds are discarded in plastic-lined refuse containers.

3. Avoiding talking, coughing, or sneezing over open wounds. Agencies have policies restricting work when nurses have upper respiratory tract infections. Such policies are usually followed strictly around patients who are less resistant to infection, such as newborns, patients with open wounds, the very ill, patients with limited immune responses, and patients in the operating room.

4. Teaching patients to avoid direct contact with others and to handle their own discharges effectively. Paper tissues and plastic or waxed waterproof disposal bags are generally provided at every bedside for disposal of nose and mouth secretions. Special containers are usually available for patients to dispose of excessive sputum (mucus from the lungs). Each patient uses his or her own personal items, such as linens, hairbrush, and comb. To prevent cross-contamination, patients are instructed *not* to sit on another patient's bed.

5. Avoiding direct contact by nurses with infective secretions. For example, nurses wear gloves when removing soiled dressings. The gloves are discarded in a plastic-lined container, to prevent contamination of the garbage handlers.

6. Preventing cross-contamination of patient linens. Nurses avoid placing linens for one patient on the bed of another. Linens may be soiled with urine, feces, blood, or wound drainage.

Minimizing Air Currents and Dust

Since bacteria are found in dust particles, measures are taken to keep dust to a minimum. For example, wet vacuum pickup machines are used rather than dry mops and damp dusting of furniture. Nurses need to be constantly aware of minimizing air currents. The shaking and handling of linens produce lint, dust, and air currents, and these increase the bacteria count in the air. Thus, excessive shaking of linens is avoided.

PROTECTIVE ASEPSIS (ISOLATION PRECAUTIONS)

Protective aseptic practices are indicated when a patient has an infection that can be transmitted to others. In 1983, the Centers for Disease Control (CDC) published recommendations regarding protective asepsis practices in hospitals. Seven categories for isolation were described: strict isolation, contact isolation, respiratory isolation, tuberculosis isolation, enteric precautions, drainage/secretion precautions, and blood/body fluid precautions (see Table 6–3).

The CDC recommendations also presented an alternative system to the categories of isolation, referred to as *disease-specific isolation precautions.* Many diseases are listed, and for each the CDC specifies the category in which the disease falls, the type of infective material present, and the length of time that precautions need to be employed. In addition, it recommends that modified isolation precautions be employed in intensive care units, in newborn and infant nurseries, and for care of the severely compromised and patients with burns. Agencies may also develop their own systems and not use either CDC system.

The CDC guidelines are designed (a) to establish a balance between ideal and practical isolation precautions, (b) to eliminate practices that are not based on scientific data, and (c) to establish effective precautions that isolate the disease but not the patient.

GUIDELINES FOR PROTECTIVE ASEPTIC PRACTICES

1. A private room reduces the spread of microorganisms by separating the infected patient from susceptible patients. Visitors and personnel are reminded to wash their hands before leaving the room. The private room should have hand-washing and toilet facilities. In some instances, eg, tuberculosis isolation, the room also needs special ventilation—the air pressure in the room is kept lower than the air pressure in the connecting room or hall so that the air will not move readily out of the room; instead, it is discharged outdoors or into vents equipped to filter out any microorganisms.

2. Masks prevent the transmission of microorganisms through the air. Masks should be used only once and discarded in the appropriate receptacle when they become moist.

3. Gowns are worn when it is possible that clothes will become contaminated. Gowns should be worn only once and then discarded. Contaminated gowns must not be worn outside the room because they may contaminate other people or objects.

4. Gloves are used for several purposes: to protect the nurse from microorganisms; to reduce the likelihood that the nurse may transmit microorganisms to the patient; to reduce the possibility that the nurse may acquire microorganisms that can be transmitted to others. Disposable

TABLE 6–3 ■ Category-Specific Protective Asepsis (Isolation)

Isolation category	Purpose	Private room	Gowns	Masks	Gloves	Hand washing	Disposal of contaminated articles
Strict isolation (for, eg, diphtheria pneumonic plague, smallpox, varicella [chickenpox], zoster)	To prevent transmission of pathogens spread both by contact and by airborne sources	Necessary; door must be kept closed	Must be worn by all persons entering room; for smallpox, coverings for cap and shoes are also recommended	Must be worn by all persons entering room	Must be worn by all persons entering room	Necessary after touching patient or potentially contaminated articles and before caring for another patient	Discard in plastic-lined container or bag and label before sending for decontamination and reprocessing
Contact isolation (for, eg, acute respiratory infections and influenza in children, pediculosis, wound infections, herpes simplex, impetigo, rubella, scabies)	To prevent transmission of highly transmissible infections not requiring strict isolation but spread by close or direct contact	Necessary	Must be worn if soiling is likely	Must be worn if person comes near patient	Worn if touching infective material	Same as for strict isolation	Same as for strict isolation
Respiratory isolation (for, eg, epiglottitis, measles, meningitis, mumps, pertussis, pneumonia in children)	To prevent transmission of infection by airborne sources and contaminated articles (eg, tissues) from respiratory droplets that are coughed, sneezed, or exhaled	Necessary	Not necessary	Must be worn by all persons in close contact	Not necessary	Same as for strict isolation	Same as for strict isolation
Tuberculosis isolation (AFB isolation) (for pulmonary tuberculosis when patients have positive sputum smear or suggestive chest x-ray film)	To prevent spread of acid-fast bacilli (AFB)	Necessary, with special ventilation	Necessary only if clothing may become contaminated	Necessary if patient is coughing and does not always cover mouth	Not necessary	Same as for strict isolation	Clean and disinfect (although these articles rarely transmit disease)
Enteric precautions (for, eg, hepatitis A, some gastroenteritis, typhoid fever, cholera, diarrhea with suspected infectious etiology, encephalitis, meningitis)	To prevent infections spread through direct or indirect contact with feces	Necessary if patient hygiene is poor, eg, patient is incontinent and soils enviroment	Same as for tuberculosis isolation	Not necessary	Necessary if touching infective material	Same as for strict isolation	Same as for strict isolation
Drainage/secretion precautions (for, eg, any draining lesion, abscess, infected burn, infected skin, decubitus ulcer, conjunctivitis)	To prevent infections through direct or indirect contact with material or drainage from body site	Not necessary unless patient hygiene is poor	Same as for tuberculosis isolation	Not necessary	Same as for enteric precautions	Same as for strict isolation	Same as for strict isolation

TABLE 6–3 ■ continued

Isolation category	Purpose	Private room	Gowns	Masks	Gloves	Hand washing	Disposal of contaminated articles
Blood/body fluid precautions (for, eg, hepatitis B, syphilis, AIDS [acquired immuno-deficiency syndrome], malaria)	To prevent infections spread through direct or indirect contact with infected blood or body fluids	Necessary if patient hygiene is poor	Same as for tuberculosis isolation	Not necessary	Necessary if touching infective blood or body fluid	Necessary if hands can become contaminated and before caring for another patient	Same as for strict isolation; used needles must be placed in puncture-proof container for disposal

Source: Adapted from JS Garner, BP Simmons: CDC guidelines for isolation precautions in hospitals, *Infect Control* (July/August) 1983; 4(4):258–260.

gloves should be used only once and then discarded in the appropriate receptacle.

5. Soiled articles are bagged and labeled before being removed from the room. A single bag that is impervious and sturdy can be used, as long as the outside of the bag is unsoiled.

6. Use of disposable equipment reduces the possibility of transferring microorganisms if the equipment is discarded correctly.

7. Contaminated reusable equipment is bagged, labeled, and decontaminated and/or sterilized.

8. Used needles are not recapped but placed in labeled, puncture-proof containers for disposal. Reusable syringes are bagged and labeled for decontamination and reprocessing.

9. Soiled linen is handled minimally. It is bagged and labeled before being sent for decontamination. Handling is reduced when contaminated linen is placed in hot-water-soluble laundry bags, which can be put directly into the washing machine. Hot-water-soluble bags may need to be double-bagged, however, because they are more easily torn than standard laundry bags and dissolve when wet.

10. Dishes normally do not require special precautions unless they are visibly contaminated. Disposable contaminated drinking cups or glasses are discarded the same way as disposable contaminated equipment. Reusable contaminated dishes may be bagged, labeled, and sent to the hospital kitchen for decontamination. Fluid containers and glasses are handled the same way as dishes.

11. Dressings, paper tissues, and contaminated disposable items are bagged, labeled, and discarded according to the agency's policy for disposal of contaminated wastes.

12. Urine and feces are normally flushed down the toilet. Urinals and bedpans are decontaminated or sterilized before use by another patient.

13. When nurses collect specimens, care is taken to keep the outside of the container uncontaminated. If it comes in contact with infective material it is disinfected, placed in an impervious bag, and labeled for transport to the laboratory.

14. Visitors are given information about the precautions they need to take when visiting a patient on medical aseptic precautions. They may need help with gowns, masks, etc, depending on the patient's illness.

15. When patients are transported out of their rooms, barriers are set up to prevent the transmission of microorganisms to others. For example, a patient on respiratory isolation and transport personnel should wear masks; a patient with an infected draining wound requires a moisture-proof dressing.

16. The patient's chart is not allowed to come into contact with infective objects or material.

17. Books and toys that become visibly contaminated with infective material are disinfected or destroyed.

18. In terminal cleaning, all items that have come in direct contact with the patient or infective secretions are decontaminated.

19. Nurses caring for a patient on medical aseptic precautions are constantly aware of their hands. Once contaminated, the hands do not touch any clean objects, eg, the nurse's hair or watch or the medication tray.

20. Any cut or scratch on the nurse's hands is covered with an occlusive bandage impervious to moisture, because the abrasion can become the portal of entry for microorganisms. The nurse may need to wear gloves while giving care.

PSYCHOLOGIC PROBLEMS OF PROTECTIVE ASEPSIS

Patients who are placed on protective aseptic precautions can develop several problems as a result of the separation from others and the special precautions. Two of the most common are sensory deprivation and feelings of inferiority. Sensory deprivation occurs when the environment lacks normal stimuli for the patient, eg, frequent communications with others. Because the patient is usually in a private room, contact with other patients is lacking. Because a gown may have to be put on before entering the room, support persons may not visit as often as usual. Visits by other patients are usually discouraged. Nurses should therefore be alert to common clinical signs of sensory deprivation: boredom, inactivity, slowness of thought, daydreaming, increased sleeping, thought disorganization, anxiety, panic, and hallucinations.

A patient's feeling of inferiority can occur because of the infection itself and because of the precautions. In North America, many people place a high value on cleanliness, and the idea of being "contaminated" or "dirty" can give patients the feeling that they are at fault and substandard. While this is obviously not true, the infected person may feel "not as good" as others and inflict self-blame for the situation.

Nurses need to provide care that prevents these two problems and/or deals with them positively. Nursing interventions include:

1. Assessment of the individual's need for stimulation.

2. Measures to help meet the need, including regular communication with the patient; diversionary activities, eg, toys for a child and books, television, or radio for an adult; stimulation of the sense of taste with a variety of foods; stimulation of the visual sense by providing a view or an activity to watch.

3. Explanation of the infection and the associated procedures, to help patients and their support persons understand and accept the situation.

4. Warm, accepting behavior. This is particularly important for patients on protective asepsis. The nurse needs to make efforts not to convey to the patient any sense of annoyance about the precautions or any feelings of revulsion about the infection.

TECHNIQUE 6–1 ■ Hand Washing

Hand washing is important in every setting where people are ill, including hospitals. It is considered one of the most effective infection control measures. The goal of hand washing is to remove microorganisms that might be transmitted to patients, visitors, or other health care personnel.

Any patient may harbor microorganisms that are currently harmless to the patient yet could be harmful to another person or to the same patient if they find a portal of entry. It is important that hands be washed at the following times to prevent the spread of these microorganisms.

For patients
1. Before eating
2. After using the bedpan or toilet
3. After the hands have come in contact with any known infective material, such as sputum or drainage from a wound

For visitors
1. After contact with a patient's excreta or secretions
2. After contact with any contaminated equipment
3. Before handling food

For nurses
1. Before and after touching a patient
2. After contact with any excreta, secretions, or contaminated equipment, such as a bedpan

3. Before handling any sterile equipment, such as a syringe (see chapter 7)
4. Before leaving the nursing unit

When a patient is suspected or known to have an infection, hand washing is extremely important. The CDC recommends that personnel wash their hands:

1. After taking care of an infected patient, even when gloves are used
2. After touching excretions (urine, feces, or material soiled by them) or secretions (from wounds, skin infections, etc), before touching another patient
3. Before performing invasive procedures, touching wounds, or touching patients who are particularly susceptible to infection
4. Between all patient contacts in intensive care units and newborn nurseries

It is also recommended that nurses use antiseptics for hand washing, rather than soap and water, when taking care of patients who are infected with virulent or epidemiologically important microorganisms, eg, the varicella (chicken pox) virus, especially in intensive care units. Antiseptics should not be used as a substitute for thorough hand washing, however (Garner, Simmons, 1983.) The recommended duration of hand washing for nurses is:

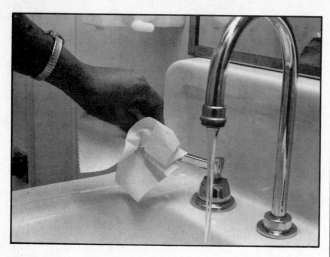

FIGURE 6–2

1. Two minutes at the start and end of nursing duty
2. One minute after contact with contaminated equipment, before leaving for a break or a meal, and before charting or preparing medications
3. Ten to fifteen seconds between patients

■ Planning

Nursing goals

1. To remove pathogenic microorganisms from the hands
2. To prevent the transfer of microorganisms to other patients, personnel, family members, and articles
3. To prevent microorganisms from entering the nurse's body, eg, through a scratch or with food

FIGURE 6–3

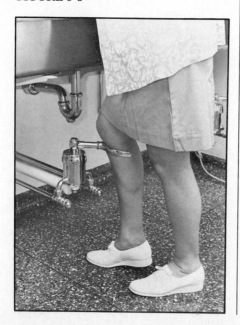

Equipment

1. Soap. Most hospitals supply soaps that contain a germicide. Liquid soaps are frequently supplied in dispensers at the sink.
2. Warm running water.
3. Towels. Nurses usually dry their hands with paper towels; they discard the towels in the appropriate container immediately after use.

■ Intervention

1. File the nails short.

   Rationale Short nails are less likely to harbor microorganisms or scratch a patient. Long nails are hard to clean.

2. Remove jewelry, except a plain band, from the hands and arms. Some nurses slide their watches up above their elbows. Others pin the watch to the uniform so that it can still be used.

   Rationale Microorganisms can lodge in the settings of jewelry. Removal facilitates proper cleaning of the hands and arms.

3. Check hands for breaks in the skin, such as hangnails or cuts. Report cuts to the instructor or responsible nurse before beginning work, or check agency policy about cuts. Use lotions to prevent hangnails and cracked, dry skin. A nurse who has open sores may have to change work assignments or wear gloves to avoid contact with patients' body substances.

4. Stand in front of the sink. Do not lean on the sink or splash water on your uniform. Flex your knees slightly if the sink is low.

   Rationale Microorganisms thrive in moisture. Dampness can contribute to contamination of the uniform. Flexing the knees keeps the nurse's waist below the level of the sink.

5. Turn on the water. There are four types of faucet controls:

   a. Hand-operated handles. Use paper towels to turn these. Some agencies use paper towels only to turn the faucets on, others to turn faucets off, others at both times, and some in neither instance. See Figure 6–2.

      Rationale Towels protect the hands from possible contamination.

   b. Knee levers. Move these with the knee to regulate flow and temperature. See Figure 6–3.

   c. Foot pedals. Press these with the foot to regulate flow and temperature. See Figure 6–4.

   d. Elbow controls. Move these with the elbows, instead of the hands. This type of handle is most frequently used for surgical asepsis. See chapter 7.

6. Adjust the flow so that the water is warm.

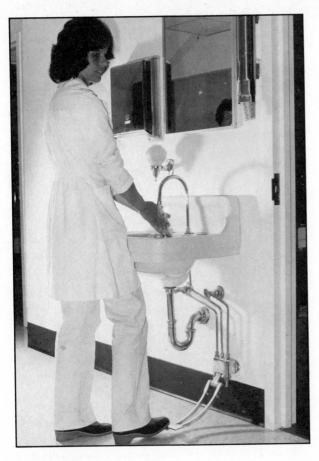

FIGURE 6–4

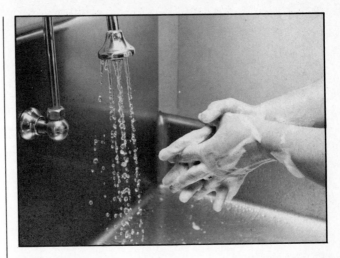

FIGURE 6–5

between the hands, and rinse the bar before returning it to the dish.

Rationale Rinsing the bar removes microorganisms.

9. Use firm, rubbing, circular movements to wash the palm, back, and wrist of each hand. Interlace the fingers and thumbs, and move the hands back and forth. See Figure 6–5. Continue this motion for 10 to 15 seconds.

Rationale The circular action helps remove microorganisms. Interlacing the fingers and thumbs cleans the interdigital spaces.

10. For a one-minute hand wash, repeat steps 7 through 9. For two- and three-minute hand washes, repeat steps 7 through 9 but extend the washing time. See the durations recommended on pages 71–72.

11. Dry the hands and arms thoroughly with the paper towel. Discard it in the appropriate container.

Rationale Moist skin becomes chapped readily; chapping produces lesions.

12. Turn off the water. Use paper towels to grasp hand-operated control.

Rationale This prevents picking up microorganisms from the faucet knobs.

Rationale Warm water removes less of the protective oil of the skin than hot water.

7. Wet the hands and lower arms thoroughly by holding them under the running water. Hold the hands lower than the elbows so that the water flows from the arms to the fingertips.

Rationale The water should flow from the least contaminated to the most contaminated area, and the hands are more contaminated than the lower arms.

8. Apply soap to the hands. If the soap is liquid, apply 2 to 4 mL (1 tsp). If it is bar soap, rub it firmly

✳ *Rinse w/fingertips up, Dry same*

TECHNIQUE 6–2 ▪ Initiating Protective Aseptic Practices ⌂

The nurse first confirms the precautions that are appropriate for the patient and determines the type of protective asepsis required and the reason. At some hospitals precautions must be ordered by the physician; in other agencies it may be a nursing decision or specified by agency policy.

The equipment required depends primarily on the type of protection and the physical arrangement of the agency. Practices vary, and thus the necessary equipment and supplies also vary. For example, masks are advised for nurses caring for patients on respiratory protective asepsis, but they are not required when caring for patients on enteric precautions. Some patients are able to cooperate with the precautions, whereas others, eg, a confused adult, cannot. Nurses may not need to gown when measuring the blood pressure of a rational, cooperative patient, while gowning would be essential with a confused patient who is likely to contaminate the nurse's uniform.

Physical arrangements also affect the equipment and supplies required. Some hospitals have specially designed rooms for protective asepsis with an anteroom on the nursing unit. These rooms have most of the equipment in place, so very little setting up is required. Generally a private room is highly desirable to prevent the transmission of microorganisms.

■ Assessment

The assessment practices described below are not always carried out before a unit is set up; some practices may be appropriate at that time, and others while protective asepsis is being implemented.

1. Assess the ability of the patient to understand and to cooperate with the practices.
2. Assess the patient's understanding of the procedures and need for information.
3. Continually assess the patient's need for stimulation. Be aware of the clinical signs of sensory deprivation: boredom, inactivity, slowness of thought, daydreaming, increased sleeping, thought disorganization, anxiety, panic, and hallucinations.
4. Assess the amount, color, consistency, and odor of body drainage, excreta, or secretions pertinent to the patient's condition.

■ Planning

Nursing goals

1. To provide the equipment to implement the required protective aseptic practices
2. To arrange the equipment and supplies for the patient's safety and comfort and for effective practice
3. To facilitate the patient's adjustment to protective aseptic practices

Equipment

The equipment required depends upon the type of protective asepsis. The following equipment is usually needed:

1. A sink with liquid germicidal soap for washing hands and cleaning used articles.
2. Paper towels near the sink.
3. At least one waste container with a moisture-proof liner.

4. A laundry hamper to collect used linen. Some agencies use hampers specially marked with red or "isolation."
5. A table on which to place supplies, eg, a stethoscope and thermometer.
6. A toilet for the disposal of excreta. Some agencies also dispose of waste food in the toilet. Others provide a hopper in addition to a toilet for the disposal of waste products.
7. A tub or shower for the patient.
8. Bedside supplies for the patient, eg, tissues, drinking water, and a cup.
9. Clean supplies such as gowns, plastic bags, isolation tags, disinfectant solutions, masks, plastic disposal bags, plastic gloves, moisture-proof bags, as needed by the specific patient.
10. A sign to place on the outside of the door, indicating the type of precautions and saying "Visitors inquire at the desk."

■ Intervention

1. Arrange the equipment and supplies for the patient's safety and comfort and for effective practice.
2. Explain the practices and the reasons for them to the patient. If appropriate, provide explanations and demonstrations after the patient is moved to the unit or after the equipment has been set up. Explain in clear simple language what substances are presumed to have the infectious agent and what precautions are necessary. Reassure and support the patient. If the patient is being moved to a private room, assist him or her to gather clothing and personal effects.
3. Explain to support persons the practices that they need to carry out, eg, gowning. Demonstrating procedures is often helpful.
4. Assess the patient's response to the practices.
5. Arrange diversionary activities for the patient, as appropriate.
6. Arrange a teaching plan as needed for the patient and support persons.
7. Report to the responsible nurse when the protective aseptic practices have been implemented.
8. Record on the patient's chart that protective asepsis has been implemented, the type, the time, and the patient's response.

Sample Recording

Date	Time	Notes
8/16/86	1800	Enteric precautions implemented. Cooperative and aware of precautions. No discomfort. No further stools passed.————————————Sheri A. Miranda, SN

■ Evaluation

Expected outcome

The patient and/or support persons carry out the practices as taught.

Unexpected outcome

The patient and/or support persons are unable to carry out the practices as taught. Upon obtaining an unexpected outcome:

1. Reassess the patient's and/or support persons' needs and capacities to understand and cooperate with the practices.
2. Reassess your own teaching methods.
3. Report your findings to the responsible nurse.

TECHNIQUE 6–3 ■ Donning and Removing a Face Mask

Masks are worn to prevent the transmission of microorganisms through the air. They protect the wearer from inhaling microorganisms and from transmitting microorganisms to others by exhaled air. The CDC recommends that masks be worn:

1. Only by those close to the patient if the infection is transmitted by large-particle aerosols (droplets), eg, acute respiratory diseases in children, measles, and mumps. Large-particle aerosols are transmitted by close contact and generally travel short distances (about 1 m, or 3 ft).
2. By all persons entering the room if the infection is transmitted by small-particle aerosols (droplet nuclei), eg, diphtheria. Small-particle aerosols remain suspended in the air and thus travel greater distances by air.

Masks are worn by nurses when they are in close contact with patients who require (a) contact isolation, (b) respiratory isolation, and (c) tuberculosis isolation when the patient is coughing and does not cover her or his mouth. They are worn by all persons entering the rooms of patients who require strict isolation. They are also worn during certain techniques requiring surgical asepsis (see chapter 7).

■ Planning

Nursing goals

1. To prevent the inhalation of pathogenic microorganisms
2. To prevent the spread of microorganisms to patients at risk, eg, a patient who has an exposed open wound

Equipment

A clean mask. High-efficiency disposable masks are more effective than cotton gauze or paper tissue masks (Garner, Simmons, 1983, p 254).

■ Intervention

Donning a face mask

1. Wash hands if they are not clean.
   Rationale   The hands will touch the nurse's hair and ears while the nurse is donning the mask.
2. Place the upper edge of the mask over the bridge of the nose and tie the upper ties at the back of the head or secure the loops around the ears. If glasses are worn, fit the upper edge of the mask under the glasses.
   Rationale   With the edge of the mask under the glasses, clouding of the glasses is less likely to be a problem.
3. Secure the lower edge of the mask under the chin, and tie the lower ties at the nape of the neck. See Figure 6–6.
   Rationale   To be effective, a mask must cover both the nose and the mouth, because air moves in and out of both.

FIGURE 6–6

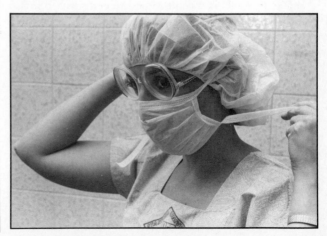

4. If the mask has a metal strip, adjust this firmly over the bridge of the nose.

   Rationale A secure fit prevents both the escape and the inhalation of microorganisms around the edges of the mask and the fogging of eyeglasses.

5. Avoid talking, sneezing, or coughing when caring for an at-risk patient, eg, when exposing an open wound.

Removing a face mask

6. Remove gloves if used, or wash hands if they have been in contact with a patient.

Rationale Microorganisms on the hands can be transmitted to the nurse's hair upon contact.

7. Remove and discard a disposable mask in the waste container.

   Rationale A mask should be used only once because it becomes ineffective when moist (Garner, Simmons, 1983, p 254).

8. Wash hands if they have become contaminated by accidentally touching the soiled part of the mask.

TECHNIQUE 6–4 ■ Gowning for Protective Asepsis

Clean or disposable gowns are worn for protective asepsis when the nurse's uniform is likely to become contaminated, ie, when a patient has infected excreta or secretions that may come in contact with the nurse's clothes. Gowns are also required when persons enter the room of a patient who has an infection that could cause serious illness if spread to others, even though soiling of the clothing is not likely (Garner, Simmons, 1983, p 254). Sterile gowns may be indicated when changing the dressings of a patient who has extensive wounds, eg, burns.

■ Planning

Nursing goals

1. To prevent contamination of the nurse's clothing
2. To prevent transmission of microorganisms from the nurse to the patient at risk (barrier technique)

Equipment

A clean gown. It is recommended that a gown be used only once and then discarded in the receptacle designated for the purpose. Gowns may be disposable or reusable after laundering.

■ Intervention

1. Wash hands thoroughly to prevent the transmission of microorganisms to the patient.

   Rationale Infected patients may have a lowered resistance to microorganisms that do not usually cause infection.

2. Don a face mask if required.

Donning a clean gown

3. Pick up a clean gown, and allow it to unfold without touching the floor or any known area of contamination.

4. Slide your arms and hands through the sleeves. See Figure 6–7.

FIGURE 6–7

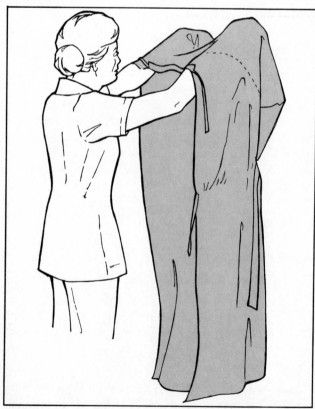

5. Fasten the ties at the neck. See Figure 6–8.

6. Overlap the gown at the back as much as possible, and fasten the waist ties or belt. See Figure 6–9.

    Rationale   Overlapping securely covers the uniform at the back.

7. Don disposable gloves if required. See Technique 6–5.

FIGURE 6–8

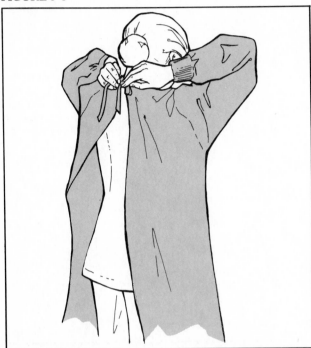

FIGURE 6–9

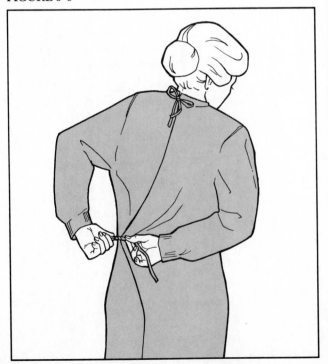

Removing a contaminated gown

No special precautions are necessary when removing a gown unless the gown is soiled with infectious materials. The most important action is to wash hands thoroughly after the gown is removed. Following are steps that have traditionally been followed to remove a contaminated gown so that it does not contaminate your uniform.

8. Remove disposable gloves if worn, and dispose of them in the appropriate container. See Technique 6–5.

    Rationale   The gloves are likely to be more contaminated than the waist ties and are therefore removed first.

9. Untie the waist belt or ties, and let the ends hang freely at the sides.

10. Untie the neck ties, and bring them forward until the gown is partially off your shoulders. Avoid touching soiled parts on the outside of the gown if possible. The top part of the gown may be soiled if you have been holding an infant with a respiratory infection.

11. Slide the gown down your arms and over your hands working from the inside of the gown. See Figure 6–10.

FIGURE 6–10

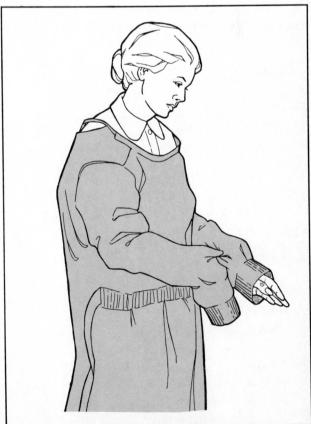

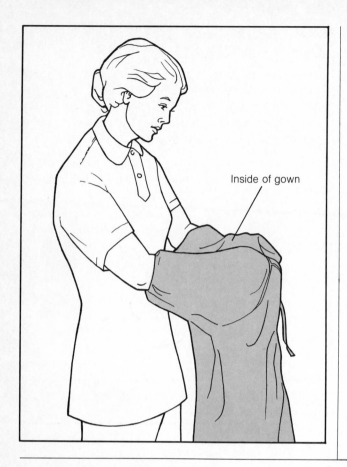

Inside of gown

FIGURE 6-11

12. Holding the gown away from your body, grasp the gown with both hands inside the shoulders at the shoulder seams. Bring your hands together. See Figure 6–11. Invert one shoulder over the other so that the clean part (inside) is outermost.

13. Roll the gown up inside out, and discard it in the appropriate container.

14. Wash your hands if they are soiled with infectious material.

15. Remove and discard the mask in the appropriate container.

16. Wash your hands.

TECHNIQUE 6–5 ■ Donning and Removing Disposable Gloves

Disposable gloves are used to protect the hands from soiling. Clean gloves are worn for protective aseptic precautions. Sterile gloves are used when the hands will come in contact with an open wound or mucous membrane or when the hands might transmit microorganisms into a body orifice.

Gloves are therefore indicated when the nurse will be touching infective materials such as excretions, secretions, blood, or body fluids. Gloves are otherwise not usually necessary when infected material will not be touched. Gloves are also indicated when caring for patients who require strict isolation: eg, patients who have diphtheria (Garner, Simmons, 1983, p 258).

■ Planning

Nursing goals

1. To reduce the possibility that the nurse will become infected, eg, when cleaning the mouth of a patient with an oral herpes simplex infection.

2. To prevent the transfer of microorganisms present on the nurse's hands to the patient (sterile gloves), eg, when changing a surgery patient's dressing.

3. To reduce the possibility of acquiring microorganisms on the hands that could be transmitted to other patients. While adequate hand washing prevents this transmission, gloves are also a practical means of prevention.

Equipment

A pair of disposable gloves.

■ Intervention

Donning gloves

1. Don a mask if required, wash and dry the hands, and don a gown.

2. Don disposable gloves carefully so as not to tear them. No special technique is required because dis-

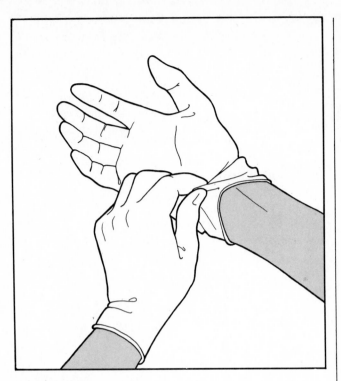

FIGURE 6–12

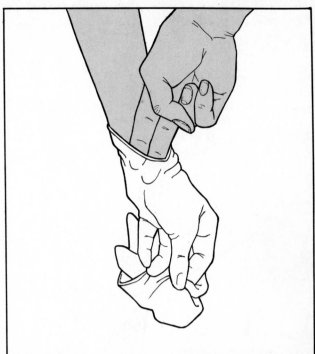

FIGURE 6–13

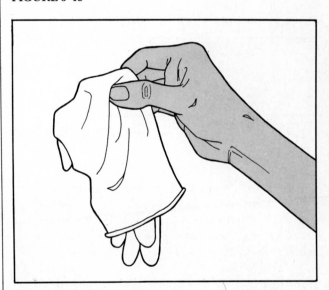

FIGURE 6–14

posable gloves are relatively shapeless and designed to fit either hand.

3. If you are wearing a gown, pull the gloves up to cover the cuffs of the gown. If you are not wearing a gown, pull the gloves up to cover your wrists.

Removing gloves

4. Grasp the first glove to be removed on its palmar surface just below the cuff, taking care to touch only glove to glove. See Figure 6–12.

    Rationale   The outsides of the used gloves are contaminated and should not touch the skin of the wrist or hand, which is considered clean.

5. Pull the first glove completely off by inverting or rolling the glove inside out.

6. Continue to hold the inverted removed glove by the fingers of the remaining gloved hand.

7. Place the first two fingers of your bare hand inside the cuff of the second glove. See Figure 6–13.

    Rationale   The bare hand is considered clean and should therefore not touch the outside of the second glove, which is contaminated.

8. Pull the second glove off to the fingers by turning it inside out. This pulls the first glove inside the second glove.

    Rationale   The contaminated part of the glove is folded to the inside to reduce the chance of transferring microorganisms by direct contact.

9. Using your bare hand, continue to remove the gloves, which are now inside out, and dispose of them in the refuse container. See Figure 6–14.

    Rationale   The bare hands, which are considered clean, touch only the insides of the gloves, which are also considered clean.

10. Wash your hands well.

    Rationale   Even though gloves were worn, it is considered safe practice to wash the hands following a contaminated procedure.

TECHNIQUE 6–6 ■ Double-Bagging

Articles contaminated with infective material must be bagged before they are removed from the room or unit of a patient on protective aseptic precautions. Only articles that are contaminated or likely to be contaminated with infective material need to be bagged. The 1983 CDC guidelines recommend the following methods:

1. A single bag, if it is sturdy and impervious to microorganisms, and if the contaminated articles can be placed in the bag without contaminating its outside.
2. Double-bagging if the above conditions are not met.
3. Labeling of all bags or use of color-coded bags or markers to alert all staff members that the bags contain contaminated articles.

Double-bagging consists of placing contaminated items into bags inside the patient's room and in turn placing those bags inside clean bags held outside the room. Two

FIGURE 6–15

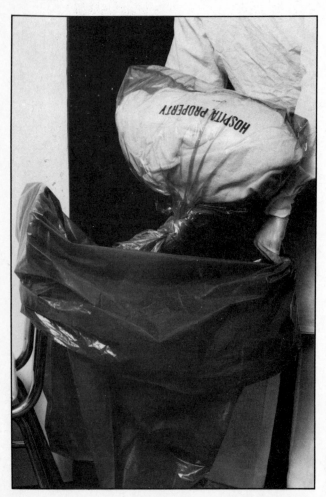

nurses are required to carry out this procedure. One nurse, who may be gowned, works inside the patient's room. The second nurse may be inside or outside the patient's room and acts as a "clean receiving nurse." This nurse holds the outside bag, maintaining the cleanliness of its outside surface, and does not become contaminated.

The nurse who cares for the patient is responsible for ensuring that all items are placed in the appropriate containers inside the patient's room. This nurse determines what the agency's practices are first. Some general guidelines are:

1. Handle soiled linen as little as possible and with the least agitation possible, to prevent gross microbial contamination of the air and/or persons handling the linen. Place soiled linen in the linen hamper in the infected patient's room or unit. Some agencies use hot-water-soluble bags, which can be placed directly into the washing machine and eliminate sorting of the linen by laundry personnel before it is laundered. Such bags may require double-bagging, however, because they are generally easily torn or punctured and dissolve when wet.
2. Place garbage and contaminated disposable equipment in the plastic bag that lines the waste container. Some agencies separate dry and wet waste material and send dry items, eg, paper towels and disposable items, to the incinerator for burning. They place other waste materials in a central garbage chute or storage area.
3. Place glass bottles or jars in separate plastic or paper containers.
4. Place leftover food in the wet garbage container or flush it down the toilet.
5. Food trays and dishes do not require special precautions unless they are visibly contaminated with infective material. If the patient's hygienic practices are unsafe, use disposable dishes and discard them in the appropriate waste receptacle in the patient's unit. Bag and label contaminated nondisposable (reusable) dishes, utensils, and trays before sending them to the food service department.
6. Place dressings in either the wet or the dry waste container depending on how soiled they are.
7. Place special nondisposable equipment in a separate bag to be sent to the central supply area. Place glass and metal equipment in separate bags from rubber and plastic items. Glass and metal can be sterilized in an autoclave, but rubber and plastic are damaged by this process and must be cleaned by other methods, eg, gas sterilization.

■ Planning

Nursing goals

1. To prevent inadvertent exposure of health personnel and others to articles contaminated with infective material
2. To prevent contamination of the environment

Equipment

1. A gown for the nurse inside the room if the type of isolation requires it
2. A mask for the nurse inside the room if the type of isolation requires it
3. Sufficient bags, color-coded or with coded markers

■ Intervention

First nurse

1. Seal all bags securely. Check agency practice, because equipment and practices vary.

Rationale Sealing the bags ensures that microorganisms are confined to the bag.

2. Place the bag or bags in an appropriate clean bag opened by the nurse at the room entrance.
3. Remove your gown, mask, and gloves if required, and wash your hands.

Second nurse

4. Make a cuff on the bag and hold the bag wide open or place it on a frame for the first nurse to place the sealed bag into it. See Figure 6–15.

Rationale A cuff on the bag protects the nurse's hands from contamination by the articles placed inside.

5. Seal the bag securely in accordance with agency practice so that the contaminated inner part of the cuff is inside the bag.
6. Label the bag with a protective asepsis (isolation) tag, and mark its contents as required.
7. Take the bag to the appropriate disposal area.

TECHNIQUE 6–7 ■ Assessing the Vital Signs of a Patient on Protective Asepsis

Most agencies arrange for a thermometer, stethoscope, and sphygmomanometer (including cuff) to be kept at the bedside. The thermometer may be kept in a tube of disinfectant solution that is changed daily. Many agencies use disposable or electronic thermometers to measure a patient's temperature. If there is no sphygmomanometer or stethoscope for the patient's use only, no special precautions are indicated unless the equipment is contaminated or is likely to be contaminated with infective material. When the equipment is contaminated, it must be bagged, labeled, and/or disinfected in accordance with agency practice.

The nurse's watch, stethoscope, vital signs notebook or worksheet, and pencil also require no special precautions unless they are contaminated with infected material. Although microorganisms may be present on table tops, walls, and floors in protective asepsis rooms, such environmental surfaces, unless visibly contaminated, are rarely associated with transmission of infections to others. If the nurse's watch, notebook, or stethoscope does become contaminated with infectious material, alcohol swabs or spray disinfectants are often used to decontaminate it. The nurse should check agency practice.

TECHNIQUE 6–8 ■ Reverse Protective Asepsis (Barrier Technique; Reverse Isolation)

In barrier technique, the patient must be protected from microorganisms transmitted by health care personnel and the environment. Patients who are severely compromised and highly susceptible to infection require barrier technique. Included are those who:

1. Have certain diseases, such as leukemia
2. Have extensive skin impairments such as severe dermatitis or major burns that cannot be effectively covered with dressings

3. Are receiving therapeutic regimes such as steroid or antimetabolite therapy or total body irradiation

The 1983 CDC guidelines state that barrier technique "does not appear to reduce the risk of infection for severely compromised patients any more than strong emphasis on appropriate handwashing during patient care" (Garner, Simmons, 1983, p 325). Compromised patients are often infected (a) by their own microorganisms, (b) by microorganisms transmitted by inadequately washed hands of health personnel, and (c) by nonsterile items (food, water, air, and patient care equipment).

The 1983 CDC guidelines recommend the following for severely compromised patients (Garner, Simmons, 1983, p 254):

1. Frequent and appropriate hand washing by all personnel before, during, and after patient care
2. Private rooms whenever possible
3. Use of sterile gloves, sterile gowns, and masks when caring for patients with major wounds or burns that cannot be enclosed by dressings

Although the effectiveness of barrier technique is questionable for many compromised patients, such as oncology patients, the technique may be required for other patients.

■ Planning

Nursing goal

To protect patients who have impaired resistance against microorganisms in the environment and microorganisms carried by nurses and others.

Equipment

The exact equipment required depends upon agency practices and facilities. The following equipment is often needed:

1. A table upon which to place supplies.
2. Caps.
3. Masks.
4. Sterile gowns.
5. Sterile gloves.
6. A laundry hamper to collect used linens.
7. Bed linen. Some agencies advocate the use of sterile linen.
8. Personal hygiene equipment. Some agencies advocate the use of sterile equipment.
9. A sink with liquid germicidal soap and paper towels.
10. At least one waste container with a moisture-proof liner.
11. Bedside supplies for the patient, eg, tissues, drinking water, and a cup.

12. Signs to place on the outside of the door indicating the type of precautions and "Visitors inquire at the desk."

■ Intervention

1. Before entering the room, check that all supplies required for care, eg, linen and dressing materials, are available.
2. Don a cap and a mask. Caps and face masks are usually worn for patients with extensive open skin wounds.
   Rationale The cap and mask prevent the transmission of microorganisms from the nurse's hair, mouth, and nose.
3. Do a surgical hand wash. See Technique 7–1 on page 87.
   Rationale This hand washing removes contaminants before the nurse handles sterile supplies.
4. Open the sterile gown package and the sterile glove package.
5. Open the sterile packages of supplies and equipment that are needed in the room.
   Rationale These supplies are opened in readiness for the nurse to handle after gowning and gloving.
6. Pick up the sterile gown from the sterile package by grasping it at the inside of the neck.
   Rationale This ensures that the outside of the gown remains sterile.
7. Move away from the supply cart, hold the gown up and away from your body, and allow the gown to unroll, or gently shake the gown to open it. Take care that the gown does not touch anything.
   Rationale This prevents contamination of the gown through contact with unsterile objects.
8. Put on the sterile gown, grasping it by the inside only. Place both arms in the sleeves and work the arms down the sleeves and the hands out through the cuffs.
   Rationale Touching only the inside of the gown maintains the sterility of the outside.
9. Tie the neck ties.
   Rationale The neck ties and neck area of the gown are subsequently considered unsterile and may be touched with bare (unsterile) hands.
10. Put on the sterile gloves (see Technique 7–6 on page 96). Extend the gloves well over the gown cuffs.
    Rationale This ensures that the cuffs and gloves do not separate and create a break in the continuity of the sterile area.
11. Grasp the waist ties of the gown, pull them around, and tie them in front. Keep your sterile gloved hands in sight.

Rationale Sterile items, such as gloved hands, can become contaminated without the nurse realizing it. If they are out of vision and below waist level, they should be considered contaminated.

12. After providing patient care, remove the gloves, gown, mask, and cap, and dispose of them appropriately.
13. Wash hands.

References

Axnick KJ, Yarbrough M (editors): *Infection Control: An Integrated Approach.* Mosby, 1984.

Carroll M: Infection control in long-term care. *Geriatr Nurs* (March/April) 1984; 5:100–103.

Fox MK, Langner SB, Wells RW: How good are hand washing practices? *Am J Nurs* (September) 1974; 74:1676–1678.

Garner JS, Simmons BP: CDC guidelines for isolation precautions in hospitals. *Infect Control* (July/August) 1983; 4:254–325.

Hardy CS: Infection control: What can one nurse do? *Nursing 73* (August) 1973; 3:18–21.

Jackson MM: From ritual to reason—with a rationale approach for the future: An epidemiologic perspective. Fifth Annual Carole DeMille Lecture. *Am J Infect Control* (August) 1984; 12(4):213–220.

Jenny J: What you should be doing about infection control. *Nursing 76* (November) 1976; 6:78–79.

Kolff CA, Sánchez R: *Handbook for Infectious Disease Management.* Addison-Wesley, 1979.

Kozier B, Erb G: *Fundamentals of Nursing: Concepts and Procedures,* 2nd ed. Addison-Wesley, 1983.

Larson E: Bringing the new isolation guideline into focus. *Am J Infect Control* (December) 1984; 12(6):312–316.

Nottebart HC: The CDC guidelines for prevention and control of nosocomial infections: View from the trenches. (Commentary.) *Am J Infect Control* (February) 1985; 13(1):40–44.

Williams P, Bierer B: Wash your hands! *Geriatr Nurs* (March/April) 1984; 5:103–104.

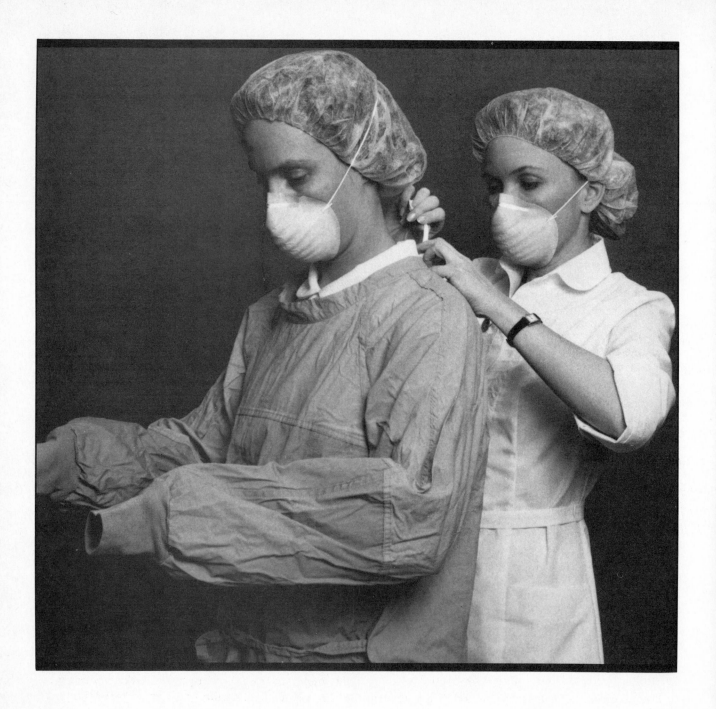

SURGICAL ASEPSIS

7

Sterile technique or surgical asepsis is an essential practice carried out by nurses, not only in operating rooms and delivery rooms but also in most patient care areas. Surgical asepsis goes one step beyond medical asepsis in that it controls the transmission of all microorga-nisms including spores. In other words, surgical asepsis means freedom from both types of microor-ganisms.

Surgical asepsis is indicated in the following instances:

1. Whenever the patient's skin is in-

tentionally perforated for therapeutic reasons, such as by a hypodermic injection or a surgical incision

2. Whenever the skin is unintentionally diseased or injured, for example, by a burn or ulceration

3. Whenever a body cavity that is considered sterile, such as the urinary bladder, is entered by a catheter or surgical instrument

Nurses need to understand the basic principles and practices of surgical asepsis to provide care that protects patients from infection. Many techniques detailed in subsequent chapters require surgical asepsis. This chapter provides basic principles and practices of surgical asepsis that are common to all sterile techniques.

Chapter Outline

Principles and Practices of Surgical Asepsis
■ Technique 7–1 Hand Washing for Surgical Asepsis
■ Technique 7–2 Opening and Closing Sterile Packages
■ Technique 7–3 Establishing a Sterile Field
■ Technique 7–4 Handling Sterile Forceps
■ Technique 7–5 Removing Sterile Supplies from a Container

■ Technique 7–6 Donning and Removing Sterile Gloves (Open Method)
■ Technique 7–7 Donning a Sterile Gown and Sterile Gloves (Closed Method)

Objectives

Upon completion of this chapter, the student will:

1. Understand principles and practices of surgical asepsis
   1.1 Define relevant terms
   1.2 Differentiate surgical asepsis from medical asepsis
   1.3 Give three instances in which sterile technique is indicated
   1.4 Identify nine principles of surgical asepsis
   1.5 Identify basic practices of surgical asepsis
   1.6 Relate the practices to the principles of surgical asepsis
   1.7 Explain the reasons for selected steps of basic sterile techniques

2. Perform sterile techniques safely and accurately
   2.1 Maintain surgical aseptic technique
   2.2 Maintain medical aseptic technique
3. Evaluate own performance of sterile techniques in a laboratory or clinical setting with the assistance of another individual
   3.1 Use the performance checklists provided
   3.2 Identify areas of strength and weakness
   3.3 Alter performance in response to own evaluation and that of another

Terms

■ spore a round or oval structure, highly resistant to destruction, that is formed in some bacterial cells
■ sterile free from microorganisms and their pathogenic by-products

■ sterile field a specified area that is considered sterile
■ surgical asepsis (sterile technique) those practices that maintain the sterility of designated objects
■ unsterile (contaminated) containing microorganisms

PRINCIPLES AND PRACTICES OF SURGICAL ASEPSIS

The nine basic principles of surgical asepsis, and practices that relate to each of them, are:

1. All objects used in a sterile procedure are sterile, and their sterility is maintained.
   a. All articles are sterilized appropriately by dry or moist heat, chemicals, or radiation before use.
   b. Sterile articles are stored in double-thickness cloth

wrappers or special paper for only prescribed periods of time.

c. Storage areas are kept clean and dry.

d. The sterilization dates and periods labeled on wrapped items are always checked before using the items.

e. Chemical indicators of sterilization are always checked before packages are used. Such an indicator may be tape used to fasten the package or contained within the package. The indicator changes color during the sterilization process, indicating that the contents are appropriately sterilized. If the color change is not evident, the package is considered unsterile. Commercially prepared sterile packages may not have indicators but will be marked "sterile." They are considered sterile unless there is any evidence that they have been opened.

2. Sterile objects become contaminated when touched by unsterile objects.

a. Sterile objects are handled only by sterile forceps or by hands encased in sterile gloves or in sterile drapes.

b. Sterile objects that become contaminated by unsterile objects are discarded or resterilized.

c. Whenever the sterility of an object is questionable, the article is considered unsterile.

3. Sterile items that are out of vision or below the waist level of the nurse are considered contaminated.

a. A sterile field is never left unattended; a field that is left unattended is considered contaminated.

b. Sterile objects are always kept in view and above the waist level of the nurse. Nurses do not turn their backs on a sterile field.

c. Only the front part of a sterile gown from the waist to the shoulder level and the front part of the sleeves are considered sterile.

d. Sterile gloved hands are always kept in sight above waist level and touch only objects that are sterile.

e. Once a sterile field becomes contaminated it must be set up again before proceeding.

4. Sterile objects can be contaminated by airborne microorganisms.

a. Areas in which sterile technique is carried out are kept as clean as possible by frequent damp cleaning with detergent germicides.

b. The health care worker's uniform is kept clean and dry.

c. The health care worker's hair is kept clean and is short or enclosed in a net to prevent the hair from falling on sterile objects.

d. Surgical caps are worn in operating rooms and delivery rooms.

e. Masks are worn to cover the mouth and the nose whenever working over a sterile field or an open wound.

f. The health care worker who has a mild upper respiratory infection refrains from carrying out sterile techniques or wears a mask.

g. Talking is kept to a minimum whenever working over a sterile field.

h. The health care worker refrains from reaching over a sterile field and from moving unsterile objects over a sterile field.

i. Sterile objects are moved as little as possible within the sterile field.

j. Doors are closed and traffic is kept to a minimum in areas where sterile technique is performed.

k. Sterile draped tables in the operating room or elsewhere are considered sterile only at the table level.

l. Any article that falls outside the edges of a sterile field is considered unsterile.

m. Sterile packages are opened by grasping only the outer edges or corners of the coverings.

n. When transfer forceps are removed from a container of antiseptic solution, the edge of the container is not touched.

5. Fluids flow in the direction of gravity.

a. Wet forceps are always held with the tips below the handles. When the tips are held higher than the handles, fluid flows to the handle and becomes contaminated by the hands. When the forceps are again pointed downward, the fluid flows back down and contaminates the tips.

b. During a surgical hand wash, the hands are held higher than the elbows to prevent contaminants from the forearms from reaching the hands.

6. Moisture that penetrates through a sterile object draws microorganisms from unclean surfaces above or below to the sterile surface by capillary action.

a. Sterile metal trays or nonabsorbent materials are used beneath sterile objects. Liquids (sterile saline or antiseptics) are frequently poured into containers on a sterile field. If they are spilled within the sterile field, the nonabsorbent tray prevents penetration of the liquid beneath the sterile field.

b. The sterile covers on sterile equipment are kept dry.

c. When pouring sterile solutions into sterile containers, care is taken to avoid dampening the sterile covers.

d. Sterile drapes that become moist are replaced.

7. The edges of a sterile field are considered contaminated.

a. A 2.5 cm (1 in) margin at each edge of an opened drape is considered contaminated, since the edges are in contact with unsterile surfaces.

b. All sterile objects are placed more than 2.5 cm (1 in) inside the edges of a sterile field.

8. The skin cannot be sterilized and is considered contaminated.

   a. Sterile gloves are worn and/or sterile forceps are used to handle sterile items.

   b. Prior to surgical aseptic practice, hands are washed to reduce the number of microorganisms on them.

9. Conscientiousness, alertness, and honesty are essential qualities in maintaining surgical asepsis.

   a. When a sterile object becomes contaminated, it does not necessarily change in appearance.

   b. The person who sees a sterile object become contaminated must correct the situation.

TECHNIQUE 7-1 ■ Hand Washing for Surgical Asepsis

Surgical aseptic hand washing differs from medical aseptic practice in that the hands are held higher than the elbows. The elbows are considered more contaminated than the hands, and the washing and rinsing water runs from the cleanest to the least clean area (from the hands to the elbows).

Surgical aseptic hand washes for hospital clinical areas, in contrast to operating rooms, are usually one minute long—a wash and rinse of 25 to 30 seconds repeated once. Some agencies require a three-minute scrub using a brush when hand washing in a surgical clinical area. The scrub in an operating room depends on agency practice; it may be as long as ten minutes for the first scrub of the day.

■ Planning

Nursing goal

To render the hands and forearms as free as possible of microorganisms.

Equipment

1. A germicidal soap or detergent. Most agencies supply liquid detergent beside the sink. The container of detergent is often operated by a foot pedal.

2. A deep sink with foot, knee, or elbow controls for the water and a faucet high enough so that the hands and forearms can be positioned under it. See Figure 7-1. For a description of the types of faucet controls, see Technique 6-1 on page 71.

3. Towels for drying the hands. Many agencies supply paper towels, which are discarded after use.

4. A nail cleaning tool, such as a file or orange stick.

■ Intervention

1. Remove your wristwatch and rings, and make sure your sleeves are above the elbows. Ensure that your fingernails are trimmed.

Rationale A wristwatch and rings can harbor microorganisms and be damaged by water. The sleeves should be above the elbows because the forearms need to be washed.

2. Turn on the water and adjust the temperature to lukewarm.

   Rationale Warm water removes less protective oil from the skin than hot water. Soap irritates the skin more when hot water is used.

FIGURE 7-1

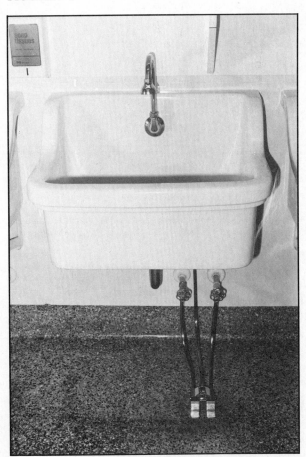

3. Wet the hands and forearms under running water, holding the hands above the level of the elbows so that the water runs from the fingertips to the elbows. See Figure 7–2.

   Rationale The hands will become cleaner than the elbows. The water should run from the least contaminated to the most contaminated area.

4. Apply 2 to 4 mL (1 tsp) soap to the hands.

5. Use firm, rubbing, circular movements to wash the palms and backs of the hands, the wrists, and the forearms. Interlace the fingers and thumbs, and move the hands back and forth. Continue washing for 20 to 25 seconds. Some agencies require scrubbing with a brush.

FIGURE 7–2

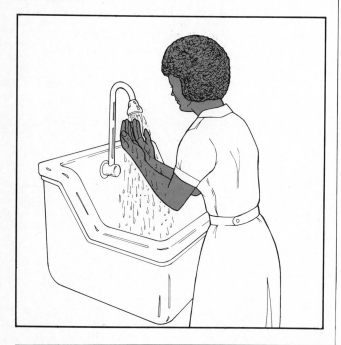

Rationale Circular strokes clean most effectively and rubbing ensures a thorough mechanical cleaning action. The areas between the fingers need to be cleaned.

6. Hold the hands and arms under the running water to rinse thoroughly, keeping the hands higher than the elbows.

   Rationale Soap remaining on the skin is irritating. The nurse rinses from the cleanest to the least clean area.

7. Check the nails, and clean them with a file or orange stick if necessary. Rinse the nail tool after each nail is cleaned.

   Rationale Sediment under the nails is removed more readily when the hands are moist. Rinsing the nail tool prevents the transmission of sediment from one nail to another.

8. Repeat steps 4 through 6.

9. Use a towel to dry one hand thoroughly from the fingers to the elbow. Use a rotating motion. Use a new, clean towel to dry the second hand in the same manner.

   Rationale Moist skin readily becomes chapped and subject to open sores. Thorough drying also makes it easier to don sterile gloves. The nurse dries the hands from the cleanest to the least clean area.

10. Discard each towel in the waste container.

11. Turn off the water. If the faucet has hand controls, use the elbows, if possible; otherwise use a dry paper towel when touching the handle.

    Rationale Touching the handle directly contaminates the hands.

12. Keep the hands in front of you and above your waist.

    Rationale This position maintains their cleanliness and prevents accidental contamination.

TECHNIQUE 7–2 ■ Opening and Closing Sterile Packages

Sterile packages of such items as dressing gauzes, catheterization trays, or dressing sets are commercially prepared in paper or plastic containers. In hospitals, sets are prepared in a double-thickness linen, or special paper may be used to wrap nondisposable items. Sterile equipment is stored in clean, dry areas to preserve its sterility. If the equipment is moist, it is considered contaminated and should not be used. The sterilization date is checked to ensure that the wrapped item has not been kept beyond its sterilized period. Frequently, chemical indicators are checked to be sure the package has been sterilized. If the proper color change is not evident, the package is considered unsterile. Commercially prepared sterile packages are marked "sterile." They should be checked to be sure they have not been opened previously.

Sterile packages may be opened by (a) placing them on a clean, dry surface and unwrapping them in such a way that the sterility of the contents, including the inside of the wrapper, is maintained, or (b) holding the outside of the package with one hand and opening it with

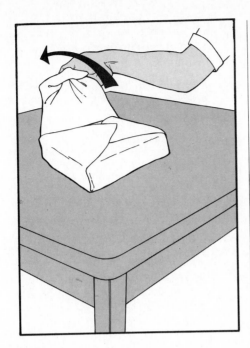

FIGURE 7-3

the other hand. The nurse's hands must be thoroughly washed before opening any sterile item.

Sterile items are packaged so that the package can be opened without contaminating the contents. A large, clean working area above the waist must be used if the package is to be opened on a surface. The area should also be away from contaminated supplies and protected from air currents, which could carry microorganisms.

■ Planning

Nursing goals

1. To maintain the sterility of the contents of the package
2. To maintain the sterility of the inner aspect of the wrapper, if the package is to be rewrapped or if it is to be used as a sterile field on which supplies will be placed

Equipment

1. A sterile package. The package must be clean and dry; if moist, it is considered contaminated and discarded. Check the sterilization dates on the package, and look for any indications that it has been previously opened. Follow agency practice about the disposal of possibly contaminated packages.
2. Other supplies needed for the particular procedure, such as antiseptic solutions.
3. A mask as required by the agency.

■ Intervention

Opening a wrapped package on a surface

1. Place the package in the center of the work area so that the top flap opens away from you.

   Rationale This position prevents subsequent reaching directly over the exposed sterile contents, which could contaminate them.

2. Reaching around the package (not over it) pinch the first flap on the outside of the wrapper between your thumb and index finger. See Figure 7-3. With some folded packages, it may be necessary to grasp the uppermost flap at each corner. See Figure 7-4. Pull the flap open, laying it flat on the far surface.

   Rationale Touching only the outside of the wrapper maintains the sterility of the inside of the wrapper.

3. Repeat for the side flaps, opening the top one first. Use the right hand for the right flap, and the left hand for the left flap. See Figure 7-5.

   Rationale Both hands are used to avoid reaching over the sterile contents.

4. Pull the fourth flap toward you by grasping the corner that is turned down. See Figure 7-6.

5. Lay the last flap on the near surface, making sure it does not touch your uniform.

   Rationale If the inner surface touches any unsterile article, it is contaminated.

FIGURE 7-4

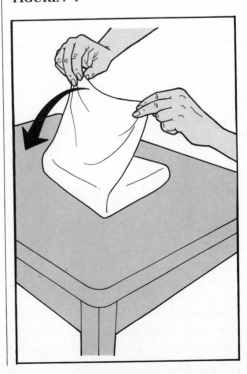

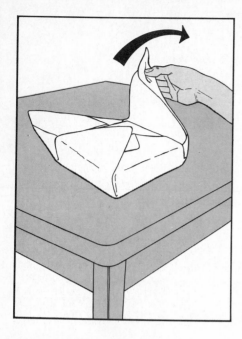

FIGURE 7–5

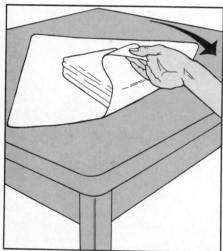

FIGURE 7–6

FIGURE 7–7

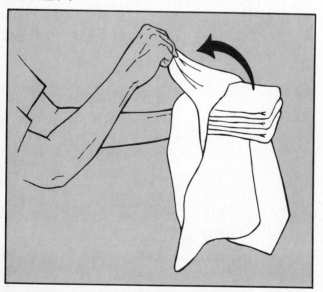

Opening a wrapped package while holding it

6. Hold the package in one hand with the top flap opening away from you.

7. Using the other hand, open the package as described in steps 2–4, pulling the corners of the flaps well back. See Figure 7–7.

   Rationale The hands are considered contaminated, and at no time should they touch the contents of the package.

Closing a wrapped package

Occasionally it is necessary to cover up items in a sterile wrapper, to maintain their sterility for a few minutes, for example, when taking the package to a patient's bedside.

8. Pick up the flap closest to you, handling it at the corner (see Figure 7–8), and lay it over the contents. Make sure the corner is folded toward you, as it was before this flap was opened.

   Rationale This corner is contaminated because it was touched, so it should not touch the package contents.

9. Select the side you opened third. Pinch the side flap from the underside (see Figure 7–9), and lay it over the contents. Use the right hand for the right flap and the left hand for the left flap.

   Rationale By this method the nurse avoids touching the inner sterile surface of the wrapper and avoids reaching over the sterile contents and thereby contaminating them.

10. Repeat for the other side.

11. Pinch the far flap from the underside by reaching around the package, and bring the flap over the contents. Tuck it in loosely. See Figure 7–10.

12. Use the rewrapped package immediately.

    Rationale Although the contents are covered, they will not remain sterile for any length of time, because the package is loosely wrapped.

13. Reopen the package using the method described in steps 1–5.

    Rationale Using the same sequence of steps should keep the contents sterile.

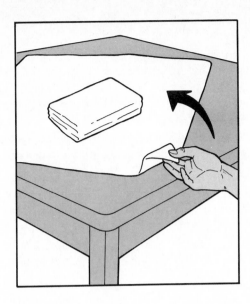

FIGURE 7–8

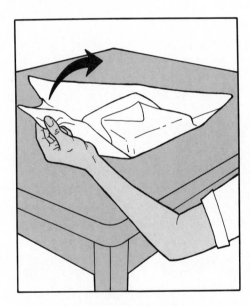

FIGURE 7–9

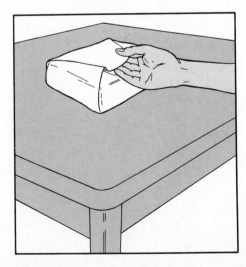

FIGURE 7–10

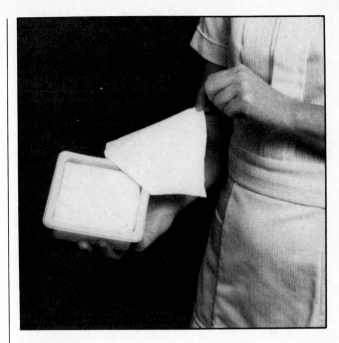

FIGURE 7–11

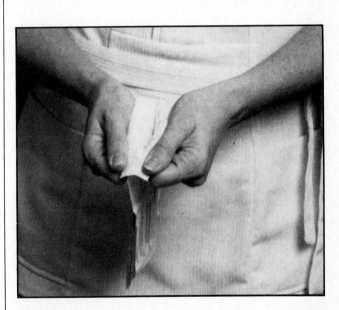

FIGURE 7–12

Opening commercially prepared packages

Commercially prepared sterile packages and containers usually have manufacturers' directions for opening.

14. If the flap of the package has an unsealed corner, hold the container in one hand, and pull back on the flap with the other hand. See Figure 7–11.

15. If the package has a partially sealed edge, grasp both sides of the edge, one with each hand, and pull apart gently. See Figure 7–12.

TECHNIQUE 7–3 ■ Establishing a Sterile Field 🏠

A sterile field is often established by using the innermost side of a sterile wrapper (see Technique 7–2) or by using a wrapped sterile drape.

■ Planning

Nursing goal

To establish an area free of microorganisms to receive sterile supplies.

Equipment

1. A package containing a sterile drape
2. Sterile equipment as needed, eg, wrapped sterile gauze, a wrapped sterile bowl, antiseptic solution

■ Intervention

Preparing the field

1. Open the package containing a sterile drape as described in Technique 7–2, checking the sterility of the contents.

FIGURE 7–13

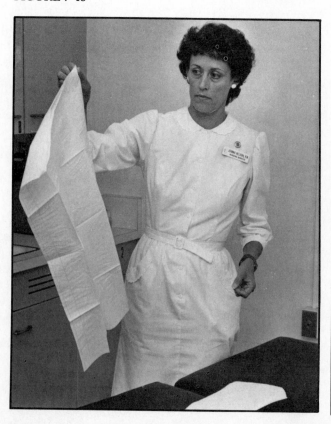

2. With one hand, pluck the corner of the drape that is folded back on the top.
3. Lift the drape out of the cover, and permit it to open freely without touching any articles. See Figure 7–13.

   Rationale If the drape touches the outside of the package, the nurse's uniform, or any unsterile surface, it is considered contaminated.

4. Discard the cover.
5. With the other hand, carefully pick up another corner of the drape holding it well away from yourself.
6. Lay the drape on a clean, dry surface, placing the bottom, freely hanging side farthest from you. See Figure 7–14.

   Rationale By placing the lowermost side farthest away, the nurse avoids leaning over the sterile field and contaminating it.

FIGURE 7–14

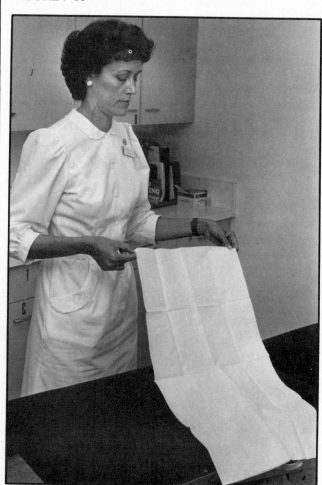

Adding wrapped supplies to a sterile field

7. Open each wrapped package as described in Technique 7–2, steps 6–7.

8. With your free hand, grasp the corners of the wrapper and hold them against the wrist of the hand holding the package. See Figure 7–15.

    Rationale The hand is now covered by the sterile wrapper and rendered sterile.

9. Place the sterile bowl, drape, etc, on the sterile field approaching from an angle rather than holding your arm over the field.

10. Discard the wrapper.

Adding commercially packaged supplies to a sterile field

11. Open each package, eg, gauze, as described in Technique 7–2, step 14 or 15.

12. Hold the package 15 cm (6 in) above the field, and permit the contents to drop on the field. See Figure 7–16. Keep in mind that 2.5 cm (1 in) around the edge of the field is considered contaminated.

    Rationale At a height of 15 cm (6 in), the outside of the package is not likely to touch and contaminate the sterile field.

Adding sterile solution to a sterile bowl

Sterile liquids (eg, normal saline) frequently need to be poured into metal or nonabsorbent containers within a sterile field. Bottles or flasks that contain sterile solutions are considered sterile on the inside and contaminated on the outside, since the bottle may have been handled. Bottles used in an operating room may be sterilized on the outside as well as the inside, however, and these are handled with sterile gloves.

Before pouring any liquid, read the label three times. See chapter 29, item 6, on page 696.

13. Obtain the exact amount of solution, if possible.

    Rationale Once a sterile container has been opened, its sterility cannot be assured for a future use unless it is used again immediately.

14. From the label, confirm the name of solution and its strength.

15. Remove the lid or cap from the bottle and invert the lid before placing it on a surface that is not sterile.

    Rationale Inverting the lid maintains the sterility of the inside surface, because it is not allowed to touch an unsterile surface.

16. Hold the bottle with the label uppermost.

    Rationale Any solution that flows down the outside of the bottle during pouring will then not damage or obliterate the label.

17. Hold the bottle of fluid at a height of 10 to 15 cm

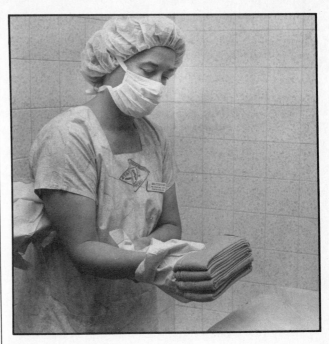

FIGURE 7–15

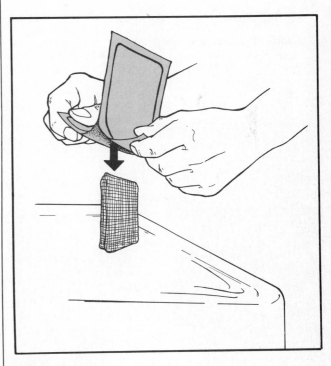

FIGURE 7–16

(4 to 6 in) over the bowl and to the side of the sterile field so that as little of the bottle as possible is over the field.

Rationale At this height there is less likelihood of contaminating the sterile field by touching the field or by reaching an arm over it.

18. Pour the solution gently so as not to splash the liquid.

    Rationale If the sterile drape is on an unsterile surface any moisture will contaminate the field.

19. Replace the lid securely on the bottle if you plan to use it again. In many agencies, a sterile container of solution that is opened is used only once and then discarded.

    Rationale Replacing the lid immediately maintains the sterility of the inner aspect of the lid.

TECHNIQUE 7–4 ■ Handling Sterile Forceps

Sterile forceps are used in many situations for handling sterile supplies. Hemostat and tissue forceps are commonly used for such techniques as changing a sterile dressing and shortening a drain. Sponge forceps are usually used to transfer a sterile article from one place to another, such as taking sterile gauze from a package and moving it to a sterile dressing tray. Forceps are usually packaged, and once used they are discarded or resterilized. In some places, lifting forceps are kept in solution. It is important that the forceps and the container be sterilized and the solution changed regularly.

Commonly used forceps are:

1. Hemostats or artery forceps. See Figure 7–17.
2. Tissue forceps. See Figure 7–18.
3. Sponge or transfer (lifting) forceps. (These are shown in Figure 7–20 later.)

■ Planning

Nursing goals

1. To maintain the sterility of the tips of the forceps
2. To maintain the sterility of the sterile supplies

Equipment

Sterile forceps. Determine that the forceps are sterile before using them.

■ Intervention

1. Keep the tips of the forceps, which are wet, lower than the wrist at all times. See Figure 7–19.

   Rationale Gravity then prevents liquids on the forcep tips from flowing to the handles and later back to the tips, which would contaminate the forceps. The handles are contaminated once they are held by the bare hand.

FIGURE 7–17 ■ Hemostat forceps (straight and curved).

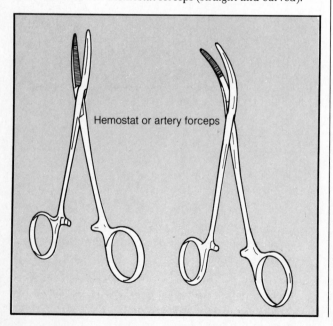

FIGURE 7–18 ■ Tissue forceps (toothed and plain).

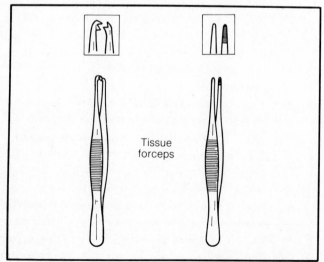

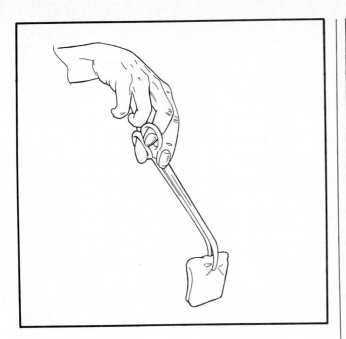

FIGURE 7-19

2.   Hold sterile forceps above waist level.

     Rationale   There is less danger of contamination if the forceps are held nearer to eye level.

3.   Hold sterile forceps within sight.

     Rationale   Forceps that are out of sight may inadvertently become contaminated and therefore should be considered contaminated.

4.   Remove transfer forceps from a solution container by lifting the forceps directly upward. See Figure 7-20. Make sure that the forceps do not touch the edge or inside of the container.

     Rationale   The edge and inside of the container above the solution are exposed to the air and are considered contaminated.

5.   When using forceps to lift sterile supplies out of a commercially prepared package, be sure that the forceps do not touch the edges or outside of the package.

     Rationale   The edges and outside of the package are exposed to the air and handled and are thus contaminated.

6.   When placing used forceps on a sterile field, position the handles outside the sterile area. See Figure 7-21.

     Rationale   The handles of used forceps are contaminated, unless the nurse is wearing sterile gloves.

7.   Deposit a sterile item on a sterile field without permitting moist forceps to touch the sterile field when the surface under the absorbent sterile cover is unsterile.

     Rationale   Dampness facilitates the movement of microorganisms through the sterile cover from the

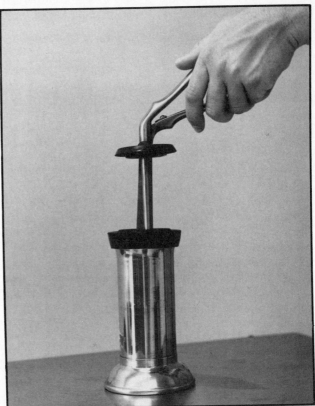

FIGURE 7-20

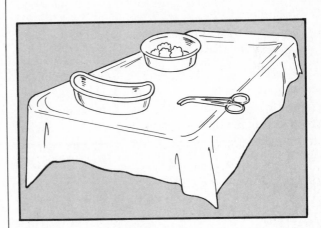

FIGURE 7-21

unsterile surface, contaminating the sterile field. If the underlying surface is sterile (eg, a plastic container) the field will not become contaminated when moist.

8.   Replace transfer forceps in the solution container, making sure that they do not touch the edge or inside of the container.

     Rationale   If the forceps have become contaminated, they will contaminate the edge and inside of the container above the solution.

9. If the transfer forceps were contaminated, indicate on the container the time by which they will be sterilized by the solution.

Rationale Others will consider the forceps sterile unless notified. The length of time they will remain unsterile depends upon the type of solution.

TECHNIQUE 7–5 ■ Removing Sterile Supplies from a Container

Although commercially packed one-use supplies are generally used in health agencies, sterile containers of various shapes and sizes may still be used in some settings to store sterile supplies. The sterility of these containers is always a concern, because they are opened many times. Sterile containers and their contents must be resterilized at regular intervals and whenever they become contaminated. Most agencies have regular schedules for resterilization.

■ Planning

Nursing goals

1. To maintain the sterility of the inside of a container and the supplies in it
2. To remove sterile supplies without contaminating them

Equipment

1. A pair of forceps to transfer the supplies from the container. Check agency practice on the use of sterile packaged forceps or forceps soaking in solution.
2. A sterile container holding the sterile articles or supplies. Check that the supplies are sterile.

■ Intervention

1. Open the sterile container for as short a period as possible.
   Rationale The longer a sterile container is open, the greater the opportunity for microorganisms in the air to contaminate it.
2. Do not talk, cough, or sneeze while the sterile container is open. Some agencies require masking before handling sterile supplies.
   Rationale Microorganisms on droplets from the nurse's respiratory tract could contaminate the container.
3. Remove the lid, and hold it above your waist with the innermost side facing downward. Hold the lid still; do not move it around.
   Rationale Fewer microorganisms will come in contact with the lid in this position. Moving it around brings it in contact with more microorganisms in the air.
4. Remove the sterile articles without touching the rim of the container.
   Rationale The rim of the container and the edge of the lid are in contact with the air and are considered contaminated.
5. If it is necessary to put the lid down, invert it first, so that the innermost side is facing upward.
   Rationale The inner sterile surface of the lid will not come in contact with the unsterile surface beneath it.
6. Remove the sterile articles using sterile forceps as described in Technique 7–4.
7. Once sterile supplies have been removed from the container, do not return them to it even if they are unused.
   Rationale The sterility of the supplies is questionable because of exposure to the air and possible contact with unsterile objects. Most agencies have a place to put these supplies for resterilization later.
8. Replace the lid on the container without contaminating its inner surface.

TECHNIQUE 7–6 ■ Donning and Removing Sterile Gloves (Open Method)

Sterile gloves may be donned by the open method or the closed method. The open method is most frequently used outside the operating room, since the closed method requires that the nurse wear a sterile gown.

Gloves are worn for many sterile techniques, to maintain the sterility of equipment and protect a patient's open wound. Gloves may or may not be used with sterile forceps. For example, to catheterize a patient the nurse generally wears gloves and uses sterile forceps, but to change a patient's dressing the nurse may not wear gloves while using sterile forceps.

■ Planning

Before donning sterile gloves the nurse follows agency practices about enclosing hair in a cap and donning a face mask.

Nursing goals

1. To don sterile gloves maintaining the sterility of the outside surfaces
2. To maintain the cleanliness of the hands while removing the gloves

Equipment

A package of sterile gloves. Gloves are packaged with a cuff often about 5 cm (2 in) and with the palms facing upward when the package is opened. The package usually indicates the size of the gloves (eg, size 6 or 7½), so that the nurse can select the appropriate size.

■ Intervention

Donning sterile gloves

1. Place the package of gloves on a clean dry surface.
   Rationale Any moisture on the surface could contaminate the gloves.
2. Some gloves are packed in an inner as well as an outer package. Open the outer package without contaminating the gloves or the inner package. See Technique 7–2. Remove the inner package from the outer package.
3. Open the inner package as described in Technique 7–2 or according to the manufacturer's directions. Some manufacturers provide a numbered sequence for opening the flaps and folded tabs to grasp for opening the flaps. If no tabs are provided, pluck the flap so that your fingers do not touch the inner surfaces.
   Rationale The inner surfaces, which are next to the sterile gloves, will remain sterile.
4. If the gloves are packaged so they lie side by side, grasp the glove for your dominant hand by its cuff (on the palmar side) with the thumb and first finger of the nondominant hand. Touch only the inside of the cuff. See Figure 7–22.
   or

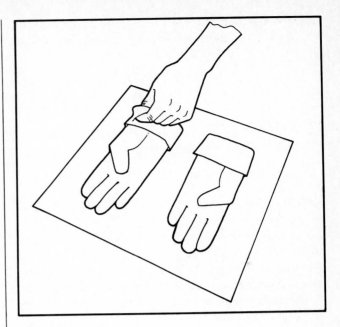

FIGURE 7–22

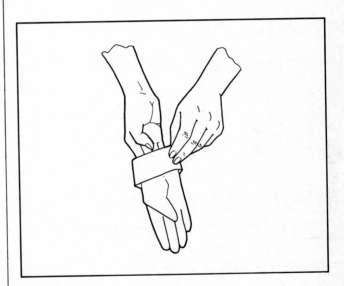

FIGURE 7–23

If the gloves are packaged one on top of the other, grasp the cuff of the top glove as above, using the opposite hand.

Rationale The hands are not sterile. By touching only the inside of the glove, the nurse avoids contaminating the outside.

5. Insert the dominant hand into the glove and pull the glove on. Keep the thumb of the inserted hand against the palm of the hand during insertion. See Figure 7–23. Leave the cuff turned down.

Rationale If the thumb is kept against the palm, it is less likely to contaminate the outside of the glove.

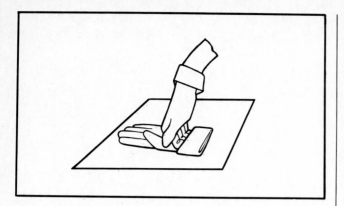

FIGURE 7-24

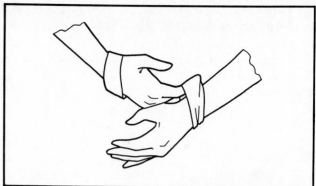

FIGURE 7-25

6. Pick up the other sterile glove with the sterile gloved hand, inserting the gloved fingers under the cuff and holding the gloved thumb outermost to the gloved palm. See Figure 7-24.

   Rationale This helps prevent accidental contamination of the glove by the bare hand.

7. Pull on the second glove carefully. Hold the thumb of the gloved first hand outermost. See Figure 7-25.

   Rationale In this position the thumb is less likely to touch the arm and become contaminated.

8. Adjust each glove so that it fits smoothly, and carefully pull the cuffs up by sliding the fingers under the cuffs.

Removing used gloves

9. Pluck either glove near the cuff end and pull the glove over the hand so that the glove inverts itself with the contaminated surface inside.

   Rationale Sterile gloves are considered contaminated once they have been used.

10. Slide two fingers of the bare hand against the wrist under the cuff of the other glove and slide the second glove off, inverting it over itself and the first glove. Discard the gloves in the designated container.

TECHNIQUE 7-7 ■ Donning a Sterile Gown and Sterile Gloves (Closed Method)

Sterile gowning and closed gloving are chiefly carried out in the operating room or delivery room where surgical asepsis is necessary. Prior to these techniques, the nurse dons a hair cover and a mask.

■ Planning

Nursing goal

To don a sterile gown and gloves maintaining their sterility.

Equipment

A sterile pack containing a sterile gown and sterile gloves. In some agencies the gloves are provided in a separate package.

■ Intervention

Donning a sterile gown

1. Open the sterile pack. See Technique 7-2, steps 1-5.

2. Remove the outer wrap from the sterile gloves, and drop the gloves in their inner sterile wrap on the sterile field established by the sterile outer wrapper. See Technique 7-3, steps 7-10.

3. Carry out a surgical hand wash for the length of time required by the agency. See Technique 7-1. For areas such as the operating room, the time required is commonly longer than for clinical areas, eg, ten minutes, and includes scrubbing with a stiff-bristled brush.

4. Grasp the sterile gown at the crease near the neck, and permit it to unfold freely without touching anything, including your uniform.

Rationale   The gown will be unsterile if the outside of it touches any unsterile articles.

5. Put your hands inside the shoulders of the gown and work your arms part way into the sleeves without touching the outside of the gown. See Figure 7–26.

6. Work your hands down the sleeves only to the proximal edge of the cuff, if donning sterile gloves using the closed method (see steps 8–16 below).

   or

   Work your hands down the sleeves and through the cuffs if donning sterile gloves using the open method (see Technique 7–6).

7. A coworker wearing a hair cover and mask grasps the neck ties without touching the outside of the gown and pulls the gown upward to cover the neckline of your uniform in front and back. The coworker ties the neck ties. Gowning continues at step 17.

Donning sterile gloves (closed method)

8. Open the inner sterile wrapper containing the sterile gloves using your hands covered by the sleeves. See Figure 7–27.

FIGURE 7–26

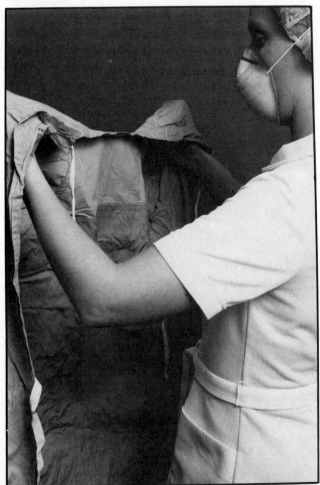

9. With your dominant hand, pick up the opposite glove with your thumb and index finger, handling it through the sleeve.

10. Lay the glove on the opposite gown cuff, thumb side down, with the glove opening pointed toward the fingers. See Figure 7–28. Position your nondominant hand palm upward inside the sleeve.

11. With the nondominant hand, grasp the cuff of the glove through the gown cuff and firmly anchor it.

FIGURE 7–27

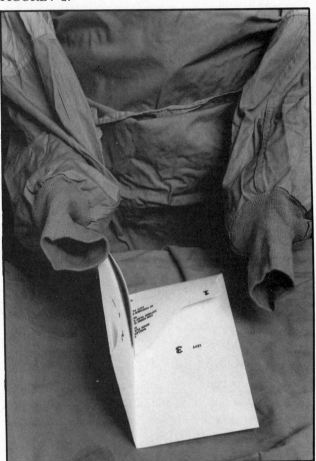

FIGURE 7–28

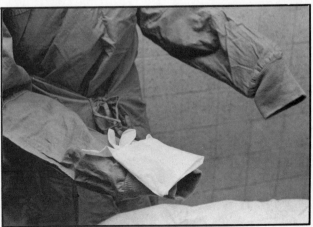

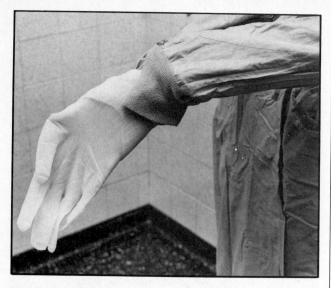

FIGURE 7–29

12. With your dominant hand working through its sleeve, grasp the upper side of the glove's cuff and stretch it over the cuff of the gown.

13. Pull the sleeve up to draw the cuff over the wrist as you extend the fingers of the nondominant hand into the glove's fingers. See Figure 7–29.

14. To don the second glove, place the fingers of the gloved hand under the cuff of the remaining glove. See Figure 7–30.

15. Place the glove over the cuff of the second sleeve.

16. Extend the fingers into the glove as you pull the glove up over the cuff. See Figure 7–31.

Completion of gowning

17. A coworker who is masked and whose hair is covered holds the waist tie of your gown, using sterile gloves or a sterile wrapper or drape.

    Rationale   The tie remains sterile.

18. Make a three-quarter turn, then take the tie, and secure it in front of the gown.

    or

19. A coworker wearing sterile gloves takes the two ties at each side of the gown and ties them at the back of the gown making sure that your uniform is completely covered.

    Rationale   In both methods the back of the gown remains sterile.

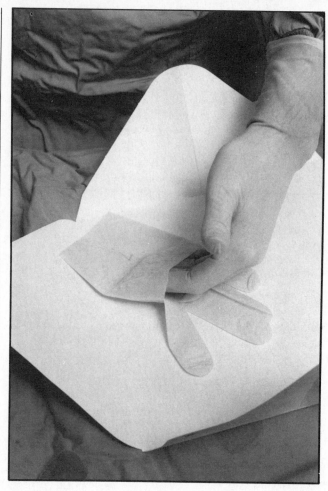

FIGURE 7–30

FIGURE 7–31

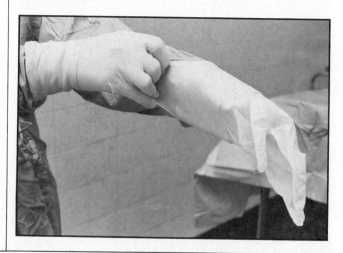

References

Kozier B, Erb G: *Fundamentals of Nursing: Concepts and Procedures,* 2nd ed. Addison-Wesley, 1983.

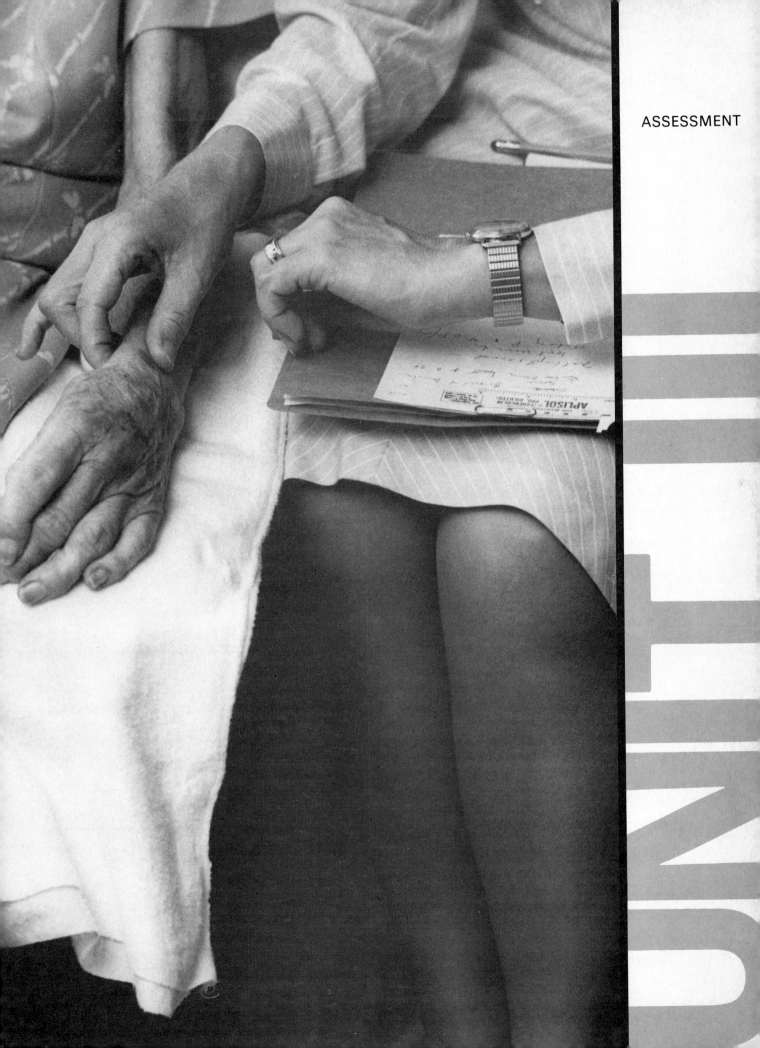

ASSESSMENT

UNIT

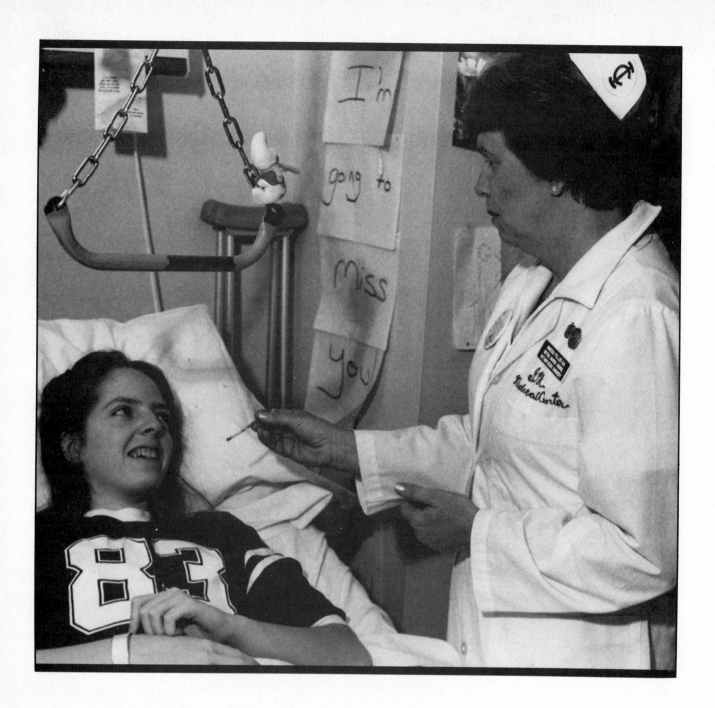

VITAL SIGNS

8

The vital signs (VS), also referred to as the *cardinal signs,* are body temperature, pulse, respirations, and blood pressure. TPR stands for temperature, pulse, and respirations; BP stands for blood pressure. These signs are valuable indicators of the internal functions of the body.

Changes in any of them may indicate changes in the patient's condition and therefore need to be reported accurately and immediately.

Within the range of normalcy there are variations in an individual's vital signs, due to such factors as the time of day and the person's age, emotional status, amount of exercise, and food intake. Because of these differences, vital signs are usually measured when a patient first enters the hospital. The initial readings then provide a reference point for assessing any later changes. Accurate assessment of the vital signs is an important and frequently used nursing skill.

Chapter Outline

Objectives

Upon completion of this chapter, the student will:

1. Know essential terms and facts related to body temperature, pulse, respirations, and blood pressure
   1.1 Define relevant terms and abbreviations
   1.2 Identify factors that affect the vital signs
   1.3 Identify the normal ranges for each vital sign
   1.4 Convert to a centigrade temperature reading from a Fahrenheit reading and vice versa
   1.5 Identify qualitative data (other than rates) needed to assess pulse and respirations
   1.6 Identify the variations in normal body temperature, pulse, respirations, and blood pressure that occur from infancy to old age
   1.7 Identify common problems associated with each vital sign
2. Understand facts about techniques for assessing vital signs
   2.1 Identify relevant assessment data
   2.2 Identify nursing diagnoses for which the technique may be implemented
   2.3 Identify nursing goals related to the technique
   2.4 Identify expected and unexpected outcomes from assessment data
   2.5 Identify reasons underlying selected steps of the technique
3. Perform techniques for assessing vital signs safely
   3.1 Assess the patient adequately
   3.2 Collect additional data from appropriate sources
   3.3 Select pertinent nursing goals for the patient
   3.4 Establish relevant outcome criteria for the patient following the technique
   3.5 Collect necessary equipment before the technique
   3.6 Implement interventions to enhance the effectiveness of the technique and enhance the patient's comfort and safety
   3.7 Communicate relevant information about the patient to the appropriate persons
   3.8 Determine the evaluative outcomes of the technique
4. Evaluate own performance assesssing specific vital signs in a laboratory or clinical setting with the assistance of another
   4.1 Use the performance checklists provided
   4.2 Identify areas of strength and weakness
   4.3 Alter performance in response to own evaluation and that of another

Terms

■ **apnea** a complete absence of respirations
■ **arrhythmia** a pulse that has an abnormal rhythm
■ **axilla** armpit
■ **basal metabolic rate** the heat produced through the metabolism (burning) of food
■ **bradycardia** a very slow pulse rate

■ **bradypnea** abnormally slow respirations, usually fewer than 10 respirations per minute
■ **cardiac output** the amount of blood ejected by the heart with each ventricular contraction
■ **centigrade (Celsius)** a thermometer scale used to measure heat; the freezing point of water is 0 °C and the boiling point is 100 °C

- conduction   the transfer of heat from one molecule to another
- convection   the transfer of heat through the air
- cyanosis   bluish discoloration of the skin and mucous membranes, due to reduced oxygen in the blood
- defervescence   the stage of abatement of a fever
- diaphoresis   profuse sweating
- diaphragm   the structure separating the abdominal and thoracic cavities
- diastolic pressure   the pressure of the blood against the arterial walls when the ventricles of the heart are at rest
- dyspnea   difficult respirations
- eupnea   normal, quiet breathing
- evaporation   conversion of a liquid or solid into a vapor
- exhalation (expiration)   the act of breathing out
- Fahrenheit   a thermometer scale used to measure heat; the freezing point of water is 32 °F and the boiling point is 212 °F
- febrile   pertaining to a fever; feverish
- hemorrhage   bleeding
- hyperpyrexia   an extremely elevated body temperature
- hypertension   an abnormally high blood pressure
- hypotension   an abnormally low blood pressure
- hypothermia   an abnormally low body temperature
- inhalation (inspiration)   the act of breathing in
- oral   referring to the mouth
- orthopnea   ability to breathe only when in an upright position (sitting or standing)
- pulmonary   referring to the lungs
- pulse   the wave of blood within an artery that is created by contraction of the left ventricle of the heart
- pulse pressure   the difference between the systolic and the diastolic pressures

- pulse rate   the number of pulse beats per minute
- pyrexia   an elevated body temperature; fever
- radiation   the transfer of heat from the surface of one body to the surface of another without contact between the two
- rales   bubbling or rattling sounds, audible by ear or stethoscope on inhalation; they are a result of fluid in the lungs
- rectum   the distal portion of the large intestine
- respiration   the act of breathing
- rhonchi   dry, wheezy sounds, audible by ear or stethoscope chiefly on exhalation; they are a result of a constricted airway
- rhythm   the pattern of pulse beats and of the intervals between beats
- sphygmomanometer   an instrument used to measure the pressure of the blood within the arteries
- stethoscope   an instrument used to listen to various sounds inside the body such as the heartbeats
- stridor   a harsh, crowing sound made on inhalation due to constriction of the upper airway
- systolic pressure   the pressure of the blood against the arterial walls when the ventricles of the heart contract
- tachycardia   a very fast pulse rate
- tachypnea   abnormally fast respirations, usually more than 24 respirations per minute
- tension   the elasticity of the arteries
- thermometer   an instrument used to determine body temperature
- thorax   the chest cavity
- vaporization   evaporation
- volume   the force of the blood with each beat produced by contraction of the left ventricle
- wheezing   a rasping or whistling sound in breathing due to constrictions in the upper airway

---

BODY TEMPERATURE

The body temperature is the balance between the heat produced by the body and the heat lost from the body to the environment. Heat is produced in the body by:

1. Metabolism of food
2. Exercise
3. Shivering or the unconscious tensing of the muscles
4. Increased production of certain hormones
5. Certain disease processes

Heat produced through the metabolism of food is called the *basal metabolic rate.* Exercise and shivering (contraction of the arrector pili muscles in the skin) add to this heat. The basal metabolic rate itself is increased by the increased production of certain body hormones, such as thyroxine, epinephrine, and norepinephrine. The stimulated metabolism increases the heat produced in the

TABLE 8-1   ■   Variations of Vital Signs by Age

Age	Average temperature	Pulse rate at rest/min Average	Pulse rate at rest/min Range	Respiratory rate/min	Mean blood pressure
Newborn	36.1–37.7 °C 97.0–100.0 °F (axilla)	125	70–190	30–80	78 systolic, 42 diastolic; by flush technique: 30–60
1 year	37.7 °C 99.7 °F	120	80–160	20–40	96 systolic, 65 diastolic
2 years	37.2 °C 98.9 °F	110	80–130	20–30	100 systolic 63 diastolic
4 years		100	80–120	20–30	97 systolic 64 diastolic
6 years	37.0 °C 98.6 °F (oral)	100	75–115	20–25	98 systolic 65 diastolic
8 years		90	70–110		106 systolic 70 diastolic
10 years		90	70–110	17–22	110 systolic 72 diastolic
12 years		Male: 85 Female: 90	65–105 70–110	17–22	116 systolic 74 diastolic
14 years		Male: 80 Female: 85	60–100 65–105		120 systolic 76 diastolic
16 years		Male: 75 Female: 80	55–95 60–100	15–20	123 systolic 76 diastolic
18 years		Male: 70 Female: 75	50–90 55–95	15–20	126 systolic 79 diastolic
Adult		Same as 18 years		15–20	120 systolic 80 diastolic
Elderly (over 70 years)	36.0 °C 96.8 °F	Same as 18 years		15–20	Same as adult

Sources: Pulse rates: RE Behrman, VC Vaughan III (editors): *Nelson Textbook of Pediatrics,* 12th ed, Saunders, 1983, p 1100. Respiratory rates and blood pressures: SR Mott, NF Fazekas, SR James: *Nursing Care of Children and Families,* Addison-Wesley, 1985, p 1745; for newborn and 1 year ages, National Heart, Lung, and Blood Institute, Task Force on Blood Pressure Control in Children: Report of the Task Force on Blood Pressure Control in Children, *Pediatrics* (May) 1977; 59 (Suppl):819–820.

body. Certain disease processes, such as infections, also increase heat production. For this reason body temperature is one important measure of a patient's condition.

The body loses heat by four major methods:

1. Radiation
2. Conduction
3. Convection
4. Vaporization

Heat is lost through *radiation* in the form of infrared rays. An example of radiation loss is the loss of body heat a person experiences when standing in front of an open freezer.

For *conduction* to transfer heat, two objects must come in contact. An example occurs when an arm is immersed in ice, thus lowering the temperature of the arm.

Convection occurs as the air near the body becomes warmed and is replaced by cooler air. Use of a fan or the

breeze from an open window to cool the body illustrates convection.

Vaporization is the method of transfer when sweating decreases body heat. The air must be dry enough to absorb the moisture for this method to cause heat loss.

Developmental Variables

Age affects body temperature to some degree. See Table 8–1. A newborn's body temperature mechanism is imperfect. As a result, the baby is greatly influenced by the temperature of the environment and must be protected from extreme changes. In the newborn, the normal body temperature fluctuates between 36.1 and 37.7 °C (97 and 100 °F). In fact, a child's temperature continues to be more labile than an adult's until puberty. A 2-year-old's body temperature is about 37.2 °C (98.9 °F); a 12-year-old's, an average of 37 °C (98.6 °F), the same as an adult's.

In elderly adults, body temperature drops to an average of 36 °C (96.8 °F). Thus, elderly people have less heat to lose than younger adults before reaching *hypothermia* (very low temperature) levels.

Common Problems

Pyrexia, hyperpyrexia, and *hypothermia* are three common problems of body temperature. Elevated temperatures are considered to have three stages: onset, course, and defervescence. Onset and defervescence may be gradual (taking place over a number of days) or sudden (occurring within hours).

Types of Thermometers

Traditionally, body temperatures have been measured using glass thermometers. Oral thermometers may have long slender tips, short rounded tips, or pear-shaped tips. See Figure 8–1. The rounded thermometer can be used at the rectal as well as other sites. In some agencies thermometers may be color coded; for example, blue-colored thermometers may be used for rectal temperatures and silver-colored ones for oral and axillary temperatures. Disposable thermometers are also manufactured; these are used only once.

Electronic thermometers offer another method of assessing body temperatures. They can provide a reading in only 2 to 60 seconds, depending on the model. The equipment consists of a battery-operated portable electronic unit, a probe that the nurse attaches to the unit, and a probe cover, which is usually disposable. See Figure 8–2. Some models have a different circuit for each method of measurement, and the nurse needs to make sure that the correct circuit is switched on before taking the temperature.

Chemical disposable thermometers are also used to measure body temperatures. They come in individual cases and are discarded after use. One type has small chemical dots at one end that respond to body heat by changing color, thereby providing a reading of the body temperature. The thermometer comes in a plastic case. To activate the chemicals, the nurse holds the thermometer with the handle toward herself or himself, moves the handle up and down, and then pulls the plastic straight off the thermometer.

The thermometer is inserted under the patient's tongue, the same as a glass thermometer, and left in place for the time recommended by the manufacturer (eg, 45 seconds). After it is removed, the dots are observed for a change in color. The dot that has changed in color and represents the highest reading indicates the temperature measurement. See Figure 8–3. The chemical thermometer is then discarded.

FIGURE 8–2 ■ An electronic thermometer. Note the probe and the probe cover beside it.

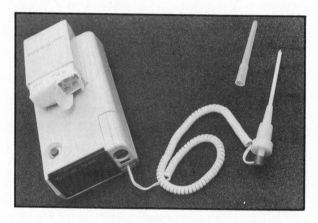

FIGURE 8–3 ■ A chemical thermometer showing a 99.2 °F reading.

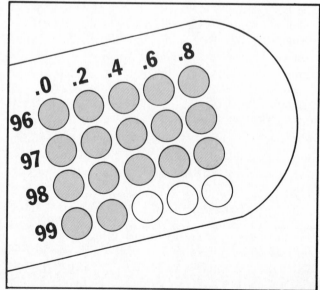

FIGURE 8–1 ■ Three types of thermometer tips.

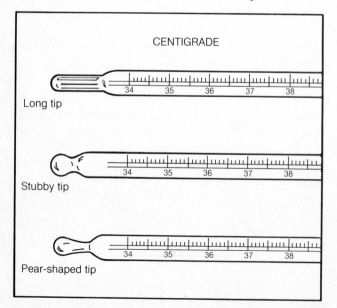

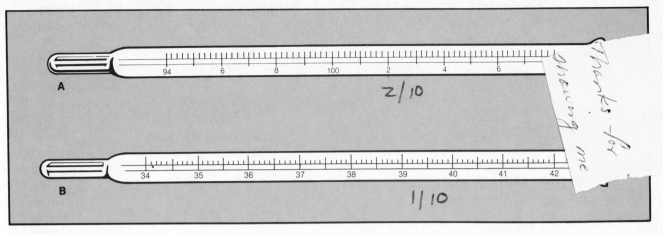

FIGURE 8-4 ■ Thermometers: The upper one shows the Fahrenheit scale; the lower one the centigrade scale.

Temperature-sensitive tape is used to obtain a general indication of body temperature. When applied to the skin, usually of the forehead or abdomen, the tape responds by changing color. The skin area should be dry. After the length of time specified by the manufacturer (eg, 15 seconds), a color appears on the tape. On one brand, a green N indicates a normal temperature, a brownish NF indicates a transition phase, and a blue-green F indicates an elevated temperature. The transition phase reflects the onset of a high temperature in the area where the tape was placed—for example, a sunburn on the forehead. Because infants under 2 years of age generally have an immature temperature-regulating system, any variation from the normal in an infant should be confirmed by a regular thermometer. The tape is removed and discarded after the color has been noted. This method is particularly useful at home and for infants whose temperatures are to be monitored for any reason.

Temperature Scales

The body temperature is measured in degrees on two scales: centigrade and Fahrenheit. The thermometer is the tool generally used to measure body temperature. The most common type is a glass tube with a column of mercury inside it. Heat expands the mercury, thus extending the column along the tube, where it can be measured against marked calibrations. The centigrade scale normally extends from 34.0 to 42.0 °C. The Fahrenheit scale usually extends from 94 to 108 °F. See

Figure 8-4. Body temperatures rarely extend beyond these scales.

Sometimes a nurse needs to convert a centigrade reading to Fahrenheit or vice versa. To convert from Fahrenheit to centigrade, deduct 32 from the Fahrenheit reading and then multiply by the fraction 5/9. That is:

$$C = (Fahrenheit\ temperature - 32) \times 5/9$$

For example, when the Fahrenheit reading is 100:

$$\begin{aligned} C &= (100 - 32) \times 5/9 \\ &= (68) \times 5/9 \\ &= 37.7\ °C \end{aligned}$$

To convert from centigrade to Fahrenheit, multiply the centigrade reading by the fraction 9/5 and then add 32. That is:

$$F = (centigrade\ temperature \times 9/5) + 32$$

For example, when the centigrade reading is 40:

$$\begin{aligned} F &= (40 \times 9/5) + 32 \\ &= 72 + 32 \\ &= 104\ °F \end{aligned}$$

A body temperature is normally measured with a thermometer at one of three sites: mouth, rectum, or axilla. The oral temperature is the one most frequently taken. Measures from these three sites vary somewhat. A rectal temperature will measure about 0.4 °C (0.7 °F) higher than an oral temperature. An axillary temperature will, on the average, be 0.6 °C (1 °F) lower than an oral temperature.

TECHNIQUE 8-1   ■   Assessing Body Temperature by Mouth

The body temperature is most frequently measured by mouth (per os, abbreviated po). This method is conve-

nient, is usually the least disruptive to the patient, and is considered to reflect changing temperature more quickly than the rectal method (Blainey, 1974, p 1861). It is generally used for all patients *except*:

1. Children under the age of 6, because of the possibility that they will bite and break the thermometer.

2. Irrational or unconscious persons, because of the danger that they may bite and break the thermometer.

3. Patients who are receiving oxygen or are breathing through their mouths, since the accuracy of such an oral temperature measurement is questionable. Recent evidence, however, supports the oral route for patients receiving oxygen by nasal cannula, aerosol mask, Venturi mask, and nasal prongs (Graas, 1974, p 1863; Hasler, Cohen, 1982, p 265).

4. Patients who have a wired jaw, have oral inflammation, or have had oral surgery.

Nurses assess a patient's body temperature:

1. For baseline data, eg, upon admission to a hospital

2. When there are clinical signs of hyperthermia or hypothermia

3. At specific times for hospitalized patients, eg, 0700 hours (7 AM) and 1500 hours (3 PM)

4. When monitoring a patient's response to specific therapies, eg, every four hours following surgery

■ Assessment

Assess the patient for:

1. The clinical signs of a fever, which vary depending on the stage of the fever (Davis-Sharts, 1978, pp 1875–1877).

   Onset (cold or chill stage)
   a. Increased heart rate
   b. Increased respiratory rate and depth
   c. Shivering, due to increased skeletal muscle tension and contractions
   d. Pallid, cold skin, due to vasoconstriction
   e. Cyanotic nail beds, due to vasoconstriction
   f. Complaints of feeling cold
   g. "Gooseflesh" appearance of the skin, due to contraction of the arrector pili muscles
   h. Cessation of sweating
   i. Rise in body temperature

   Course
   a. Skin that feels warm and appears flushed, due to vasodilation
   b. Complaints of feeling hot or warm
   c. Increased pulse and respiratory rates
   d. Increased thirst
   e. Mild to severe dehydration

   f. Simple drowsiness, restlessness, or delirium and convulsions, due to irritation of the nerve cells
   g. Herpetic lesions of the mouth
   h. Loss of appetite with prolonged fever
   i. Malaise, weakness, and aching muscles, due to protein catabolism

   Defervescence (fever abatement)
   a. Skin that appears flushed and feels warm
   b. Sweating
   c. Decreased shivering
   d. Possible dehydration

2. The clinical signs of an abnormally low body temperature:
   a. Pallor
   b. Shivering and/or a "gooseflesh" appearance of the skin
   c. Bradycardia
   d. Skin that feels cold to the touch
   e. Complaints of feeling cold
   f. Irritability

3. The time the patient last took hot or cold food or fluids and the time he or she last smoked. To obtain an accurate oral temperature reading it is recommended that nurses allow at least 15 minutes to elapse between a patient's intake or smoking and the measurement (Blainey, 1974, p 1861).

Other data include:

1. Baseline data regarding body temperature
2. The most recent previous assessments
3. Any nursing or medical orders to be implemented as a result of the assessment

■ Nursing Diagnosis

Nursing diagnoses that may indicate the need to assess a patient's body temperature include:

1. Actual or potential fluid volume deficit related to:
   a. Decreased fluid intake
   b. Abnormal fluid loss

2. Alterations in respiratory function related to:
   a. Excessive or thick secretions
   b. Infection
   c. Neuromuscular impairment
   d. Loss of lung elasticity
   e. Anesthesia
   f. Smoking
   g. Suppressed cough reflex
   h. Immobility

3. Alterations in patterns of urinary elimination related to:

a. Dysuria

b. Incontinence

■ Planning

Nursing goals

1. To acquire a baseline measurement against which future readings can be compared

2. To assess an abnormally high or low body temperature

3. To evaluate a patient's temperature response and progress following special procedures, such as a tepid sponge bath

Equipment

1. An oral thermometer

2. Soft tissues to wipe the thermometer, if clean plastic sheaths are not used

3. A pencil or pen to record the temperature

4. A book, record, or worksheet on which to record the temperature

■ Intervention

1. Explain to the patient what you plan to do. Adjust the explanation to the patient's need.

   Rationale By explaining, the nurse reassures the patient by giving knowledge of what will happen and ascertains that this method of taking the temperature is appropriate.

2. a. If using a mercury thermometer: Remove the thermometer from its container. If the thermometer is stored in disinfectant, wipe the solution from the thermometer with a soft tissue or rinse it under cold water. Wipe from the bulb end to fingers in a rotating fashion. Discard the tissue.

   Rationale Disinfectant can irritate the mucous membrane and taste unpleasant. Cold water is used because hot water causes the mercury to expand and can break the thermometer. The thermometer is wiped from the cleanest to the least clean area. Rotating ensures that all sides are wiped.

   b. If using an electronic thermometer: Gather the kit and disposable probe covers. Attach the probe to the unit, being sure to attach it to the appropriate circuit (oral, rectal, or axillary) in models that have separate circuits for each. Place a cover on the probe. Warm up the machine by switching it on, if not kept on.

3. Check the temperature reading on the thermometer. If necessary, shake down a mercury thermometer by holding it between the thumb and forefinger at the end farthest from the bulb. See Figure 8–5. Sharply

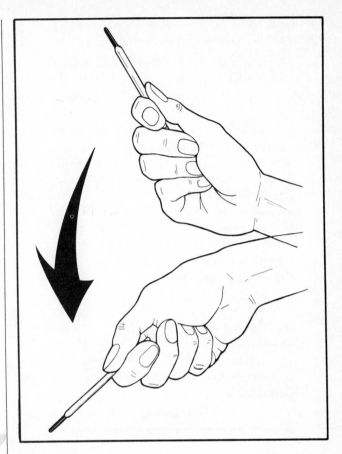

FIGURE 8–5

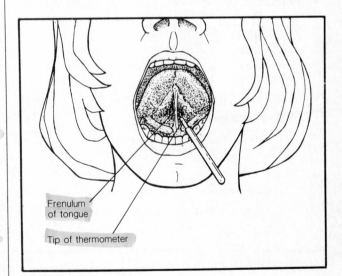

Frenulum of tongue

Tip of thermometer

FIGURE 8–6

snap the wrist downward. Repeat until the mercury is below 34 °C (95 °F).

4. Ask the patient to open his or her mouth, and place the thermometer or probe at the base of the tongue to the right or left of the frenulum (posterior sublingual pocket). See Figure 8–6.

   Rationale The thermometer needs to reflect the core

temperature of the blood in the larger blood vessels of the posterior pocket.

5. Ask the patient to close the lips, not the teeth, around the thermometer.

   Rationale A patient who bites the thermometer can break it.

6. Leave the thermometer in place according to agency policy.

   Rationale The nurse must allow sufficient time for the temperature to register. The recommended time is two minutes (Baker et al, 1984, p 111) or three minutes (Graves, Markarian, 1980, p 323). If an electronic oral thermometer is used, the patient holds the thermometer under the tongue 10 to 20 seconds or until it completes registering.

7. If using an electronic thermometer, read the temperature on the dial or readout.

8. Remove the thermometer. Remove the plastic sheath or wipe the thermometer with a tissue. Start at the end held by you, and wipe in a rotating manner toward the bulb. Discard the tissue. If using an electronic thermometer, remove and discard the probe cover.

   Rationale The thermometer is wiped from the area of least contamination to that of greatest contamination.

9. Read the temperature, if using a mercury thermometer. Hold it at eye level, and rotate it until the mercury column is clearly visible. The upper end of the mercury column registers the patient's body temperature. On the Fahrenheit thermometer, each long line reflects 1 degree and each short line 0.2 degree. On the centigrade thermometer, each long line reflects 0.5 degree and each short line 0.1 degree.

10. Wash the mercury thermometer in tepid soapy water, rinse it in cold water, dry it, and disinfect it.

    Rationale Organic material such as mucus must be removed before the thermometer is placed in disinfectant. Organic materials on the thermometer can inhibit the action of the disinfectant solution. Effective disinfectants are ethyl alcohol 70%, benzalkonium chloride (Zephiran chloride) 1:1000, and synthetic phenols.

11. Shake down the thermometer and return it to its container. Many agencies store the thermometer in a small container of disinfectant at the bedside; others place it in a large container in the utility area. Some agencies also have special equipment for spinning down the mercury levels.

12. Record the temperature to the nearest indicated tenth (eg, 98.4 °F, 37.1 °C) on the book, record, or worksheet.

    Rationale Recording the temperature immediately ensures it is not forgotten.

■ Evaluation

Expected outcome

A body temperature within the normal range for the patient.

Unexpected outcome

A body temperature above or below the normal range for the patient. Upon obtaining an unexpected outcome:

1. Reassess the patient's temperature in one half to one hour, or sooner depending upon the patient's condition, using another thermometer to verify the results.

2. Assess the patient for other signs of an abnormally high or abnormally low body temperature. See Assessment earlier in this technique.

3. Assess the patient's pulse and respirations.

4. Report your findings to the responsible nurse and/or physician.

TECHNIQUE 8–2 ■ Assessing Body Temperature by Axilla

Measurement of the body temperature by axilla is a safe, easily accessible method that is less distressing psychologically than the rectal method. Although the axillary temperature was considered less accurate than the rectal or oral method, studies now indicate that there is no clinically important difference in accuracy between axillary and rectal temperatures (Eoff, Joyce, 1981, p 1011:

Axillary temps safer, 1978, p 1081; Schiffman, 1982, p 274). The axilla is therefore the preferred site for temperature measurements in children, not only because it is easily accessible but also because there is less likelihood of (a) spreading infection, and (b) rectal perforation and subsequent peritonitis (Eoff, Joyce, 1981, p 1010; Axillary temps safer, 1978, p 1081).

Patients requiring this method of assessment include:

1. Newborns and infants
2. Toddlers and preschoolers
3. Patients who have oral inflammation, oral surgery, or wired jaws
4. Patients who are breathing through their mouths, eg, following nasal surgery
5. Irrational patients
6. Patients for whom oral and rectal temperatures are contraindicated

■ **Assessment**   See Technique 8–1 on page 108.

■ **Nursing Diagnosis**   See Technique 8–1 on page 108.

■ **Planning**

Nursing goals   See Technique 8–1 on page 109.

Equipment

1. An axillary thermometer. Oral thermometers are usually used in most agencies.
2. Soft tissues to wipe the thermometer.
3. A towel to remove perspiration from the axilla.
4. A pencil or pen to record the temperature.
5. A book, record, or worksheet on which to record the temperature.

■ **Intervention**

1. Follow steps 1–3 in Technique 8–1 on page 109.
2. Expose the patient's axilla. If the axilla is moist, dry it with the towel, using a patting motion.
   Rationale   Friction created by rubbing can raise the temperature of the axilla.

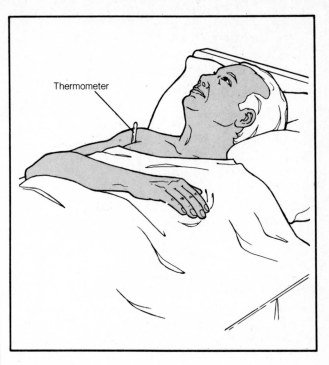

Thermometer

FIGURE 8–7

3. Place the thermometer in the patient's axilla.
4. Assist the patient to place the arm tightly across the chest. See Figure 8–7.
   Rationale   This position keeps the thermometer in place.
5. Leave the thermometer in place for nine minutes (Nichols et al, 1966, p 310). Remain with the patient, and hold the thermometer in place, if the patient is irrational or very young. For infants and children, leave the thermometer in place five minutes (Eoff, Joyce, 1981, p 1011).
6. Follow steps 7–12 in Technique 8–1.

■ **Evaluation**   See Technique 8–1 on page 110.

TECHNIQUE 8–3   ■   Assessing Body Temperature by Rectum

In the past, a rectal body temperature has generally been considered more accurate than an oral or axillary temperature, as it reflects the temperature of the blood inside the large blood vessels of the rectum—the superior, inferior, and middle arteries and veins. This belief is thought to have arisen from the fact that the rectum was less influenced by external factors than the axillae or mouth.

Blainey (1974, pp 1860–1861) points out several disadvantages of rectal temperatures:

1. Placement of the rectal thermometer at different sites within the rectum yields different temperatures, yet placement at the same site each time is difficult.
2. A rectal temperature does not respond to changes in arterial temperatures as quickly as an oral

temperature, a fact that may be potentially dangerous for febrile patients, since misleading information may be acquired.

3. The presence of stool may interfere with thermometer placement. If the stool is soft, the thermometer may be embedded in stool rather than against the wall of the rectum. If the stool is impacted, the depth of thermometer insertion may be insufficient.

4. In newborns and infants, insertion of the rectal thermometer has resulted in tragic ulcerations and rectal perforations. Many agencies advise against using rectal thermometers on neonates until the first meconium stool has been passed, and the rectum is known to be patent.

The rectal site may nevertheless be indicated for patients who cannot have an oral or axillary temperature measurement. Rectal temperatures are generally contraindicated for patients who have rectal pathologic conditions, have had rectal surgery, and have convulsive disorders. If a patient were to have a convulsion while a rectal temperature was being taken, there is danger the thermometer would break and injure the patient. In some agencies rectal temperatures are also contraindicated for patients with myocardial infarction. It is believed that rectal temperature measurement produces vagal stimulation, which in turn can increase myocardial damage. Recent research, however, indicates that the rectal method produces no deleterious effects on the heart (Creative Care Unit, 1977, p 997).

■ **Assessment**   See Technique 8–1 on page 108.

■ **Nursing Diagnosis**   See Technique 8–1 on page 108.

■ **Planning**

Nursing goals   See Technique 8–1 on page 109.

Equipment

1. A rectal thermometer
2. Soft tissues to wipe the thermometer
3. Lubricant to apply to the thermometer to ease insertion into the rectum
4. A pencil or pen to record temperature

5. A book, record, or worksheet on which to record the temperature

■ **Intervention**

1. Follow steps 1–3 in Technique 8–1 on page 109.
2. Assist the patient to assume a lateral position. A newborn may be placed in a lateral or prone position (Axillary temps safer, 1978, p 1081). Provide privacy before folding the bedclothes back to expose the buttocks.

   Rationale   Privacy is essential since exposure of the buttocks embarrasses most patients.
3. Place some lubricant on a piece of tissue. Then apply lubricant to the thermometer. For an adult, lubricate 2.5 to 4 cm (1 to 1.5 in) of the bulb end of the thermometer. For an infant, lubricate 1.5 to 2.5 cm (0.5 to 1 in).

   Rationale   The lubricant facilitates insertion of the thermometer without irritating the mucous membrane.
4. With one hand, raise the patient's upper buttock to expose the anus.
5. Ask the patient to take a deep breath, and insert the thermometer into the anus anywhere from 1.5 to 4 cm (0.5 to 1.5 in), depending on the age and size of the patient (for example, 1.5 cm for an infant, 4 cm for a large adult). *Do not force insertion of the thermometer.*

   Rationale   Having the patient take a deep breath relaxes the external sphincter muscle, thus easing insertion. Inability to insert the thermometer into a newborn could indicate the rectum is not patent. The end of the thermometer should not be embedded in feces or the temperature measurement will not be accurate.
6. Hold the thermometer in place for two minutes (Nichols, 1972) or for the length of time recommended by the agency. For neonates hold the thermometer in place for five minutes (Schiffman, 1982, p 276). Hold an electronic thermometer in place for 10 to 20 seconds.
7. Follow steps 7–12 in Technique 8–1.

■ **Evaluation**   See Technique 8–1 on page 110.

PULSE

The pulse is the wave of blood within an artery created by contraction of the left ventricle of the heart. It can be palpated (felt with the fingers) at sites where an artery passes alongside or over a bone, by placing slight pressure on the artery.

Nine of the sites where a pulse is commonly taken (see Figure 8–8) are:

FIGURE 8–8 ■ Nine sites commonly used for assessing a pulse.

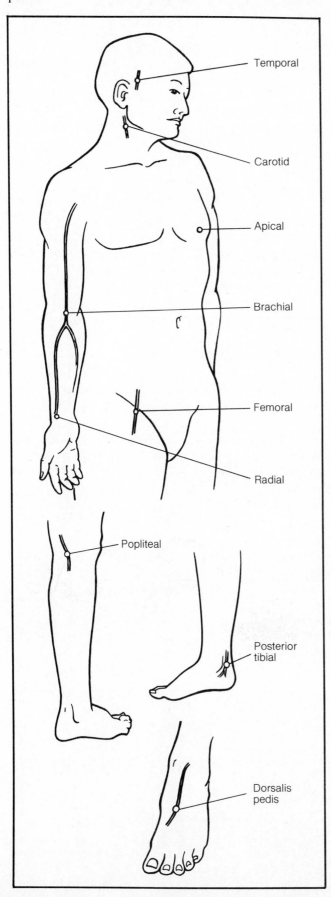

1. *Temporal:* where the temporal artery passes over the temporal bone of the head. The site is superior (above) and lateral (away from the midline) to the eye.

2. *Carotid:* at the side of the neck below the lobe of the ear where the carotid artery runs between the trachea and the sternocleidomastoid muscle.

3. *Apical:* at the apex of the heart. In an adult this is located on the left side of the chest, no more than 8 cm (3 in) to the left of the sternum (breastbone) and under the fourth, fifth, or sixth intercostal space (area between the ribs). Another way to locate the apex is to find the midclavicular line (MCL), an imaginary line dropping straight down from the center of the clavicle (collarbone). See Figure 8–9. Normally the apex lies inside or on the MCL at the fourth, fifth, or sixth intercostal space. In men, the MCL will usually pass through the nipple area. To locate the center of the clavicle, first feel for the medial end of this bone where it joins the sternum. This joint can be felt more readily by having the patient move the shoulder forward. Next, locate the lateral end of the clavicle, where it joins the shoulder, by feeling along the front edge of the clavicle until a bony prominence or notch is felt at the shoulder. Midway between these identified points at the sternum and the shoulder is the center of the clavicle.

For a child 7 to 9 years of age, the apical pulse is located between the fourth and fifth intercostal spaces. Before 4 years of age it is left of the MCL, between 4 and 6 years it is at the MCL. See Figure 8–9.

4. *Brachial:* at the inner aspect of the biceps muscle of the arm or medially in the antecubital space (elbow crease).

5. *Radial:* where the radial artery runs along the radial bone, on the thumb side of the inner aspect of the wrist.

FIGURE 8–9 ■ Location of the apical pulse for a child under 4 years, a child 4 to 6 years, and an adult.

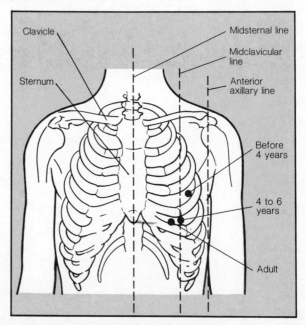

6. *Femoral:* where the femoral artery passes alongside the inguinal ligament.

7. *Popliteal:* where the popliteal artery passes behind the knee. This point is difficult to find, but it can be palpated if the patient flexes the knee slightly.

8. *Posterior tibial:* on the medial surface of the ankle where the posterior tibial artery passes behind the medial malleolus.

9. *Pedal (dorsalis pedis):* where the dorsalis pedis artery passes over the bones of the foot. This artery can be palpated by feeling the dorsum (upper surface) of the foot on an imaginary line drawn from the middle of the ankle to the space between the big and second toes.

The reasons for use of each site are given in Table 8-2. The radial site is most commonly used. It is readily found in most people and accessible.

The *rate* of a pulse is expressed in beats per minute. It varies according to the patient's age, sex, level of exercise, and emotions. Age is discussed under Developmental Variables, next. Boys and men tend to have a slightly slower rate than girls and women. Exercise and emotions normally increase the pulse rate. Heat, including fever, and prolonged assumption of a horizontal position in bed also increase the rate.

The *rhythm* of the pulse is the pattern of the beats and the intervals between the beats. A normal pulse has a regular rhythm and equal time periods between beats. See Figure 8-10.

Pulse *volume* is the force of the blood with each beat. A normal pulse can be felt with moderate pressure of the fingers. In contrast, a weak pulse can be obliterated easily with finger pressure, while a full or bounding pulse is obliterated only with difficulty. See Figure 8-11.

The *tension* of the pulse is a measure of the elasticity of the arteries. Normal arteries are smooth and straight. The arteries of elderly people are often hard or inelastic and may feel irregular or twisted.

Developmental Variables

The pulse rate varies according to age. See Table 8-1 earlier. In the newborn, the normal rate may be as high as 190 beats per minute. It slows with age until at 18 years it has reached the normal adult level, between 50 and 90 beats per minute for males. The rate for females is 5 beats higher in childhood and adulthood. The rate for older adults tends to be similar to the adult rate, and rhythm and volume are normally regular.

Common Problems

The three common problems related to the pulse rate are: *tachycardia,* a rate over 100 beats per minute for an adult; *bradycardia,* a rate usually below 50 beats per minute; and

TABLE 8-2 ■ Reasons for Using Specific Pulse Sites

Pulse site	Reasons for use
Radial	Readily accessible and routinely used
Temporal	Used when radial pulse is not accessible
Carotid	Used for infants
	Used in cases of cardiac arrest
	Used to determine circulation to the brain
Apical	Routinely used for infants and children up to 3 years of age
	Used to determine discrepancies with radial pulse
	Used in conjunction with some medications
Brachial	Used to measure blood pressure
	Used during cardiac arrest for infants
Femoral	Used in cases of cardiac arrest
	Used for infants and children
	Used to determine circulation to a leg
Popliteal	Used to determine circulation to the lower leg
	Used to determine leg blood pressure
Posterior tibial	Used to determine circulation to the foot
Pedal	Used to determine circulation to the foot

FIGURE 8-10 ■ Two comparative electrocardiographs, one illustrating regular cardiac rhythm and one irregular cardiac rhythm.

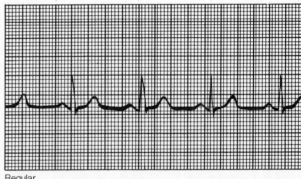
Regular

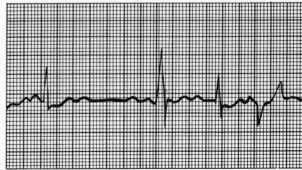
Irregular

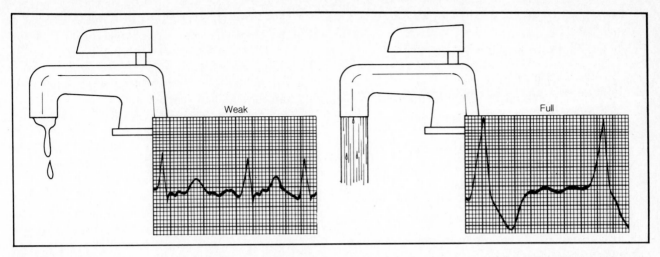

FIGURE 8-11 ■ Two comparative electrocardiographs, one illustrating a weak pulse volume and one a full pulse volume.

arrhythmia. In terms of volume, a pulse that is weak and easily obliterated is described as *weak, feeble,* or *thready;* an abnormally strong pulse is referred to as *full* or *bounding.*

Abnormalities of pulse tension are an arterial wall that feels *rough* or *beady* (uneven) and an artery that lacks elasticity and feels *hard* or *gritty* to the touch.

TECHNIQUE 8-4   ■   Assessing a Peripheral Pulse   🏠

A pulse is commonly measured by palpation (feeling) or auscultation (hearing). The middle three fingertips are used for palpating all pulse sites except the apex of the heart. A stethoscope is used for assessing apical pulses and fetal heart tones. Increasingly ultrasound (Doppler) equipment is being used to assess pulses that are difficult to assess. See Intervention, step 3b.

Occasionally a radial pulse and an apical pulse are taken simultaneously by two persons (see Technique 8-6). This is called an apical–radial pulse. Differences between the two rates can indicate cardiovascular disorders.

The cardiac monitoring machine is another device for assessing the pulse rate. It indicates the rate on a screen or readout graph. However, this method is beyond the scope of this chapter.

A peripheral pulse, usually the radial pulse, is assessed for all individuals *except:*

1. Newborns and children up to 2 or 3 years. Apical pulses are assessed in these patients.
2. Very obese or elderly patients, whose radial pulse may be difficult to palpate. Doppler equipment may be used for these patients or the apical pulse is assessed.
3. Individuals with a heart disease, who require apical pulse assessment.

4. Individuals in whom the circulation to a specific body part must be assessed, eg, following leg surgery the pedal (dorsalis pedis) pulse is assessed.

■ Assessment

Assess the patient for:

1. Skin color and warmth, eg, assess the color and warmth of the foot when taking a pedal pulse
2. Facial pallor and cyanosis of the lips and nail beds

Additional data include:

1. Baseline data about the peripheral pulse rate, volume, and rhythm and the arterial wall
2. Most recent pulse assessments
3. Nursing or medical orders to be implemented as a result of the assessment

■ Nursing Diagnosis

Nursing diagnoses that may indicate the need to assess a patient's peripheral pulse include:

1. Potential or actual activity intolerance related to:
   a. Alterations in the oxygen transport system (cardiac, respiratory, or circulatory)

b. Chronic disease

c. Malnourishment

d. Prolonged bed rest

e. Sedentary life-style

2. Alterations in cardiac output (decreased) related to:

a. Cardiac factors

b. Pulmonary disorders

c. Endocrine disorders

d. Hematologic disorders

e. Fluid and electrolyte imbalances

f. Stress

g. Surgery

h. Medications (diuretics, antihypertensives, vaso-constrictors, vasodilators)

i. Allergic response

j. Sepsis

3. Alterations in respiratory function related to:

a. Excessive or thick secretions

b. Infection

c. Neuromuscular impairment

d. Loss of lung elasticity

e. Anesthesia

f. Smoking

g. Suppressed cough reflex

h. Immobility

4. Actual or potential fluid volume deficit related to:

a. Decreased fluid intake

b. Abnormal fluid loss

■ Planning

Nursing goals

1. To acquire baseline data against which future assessments can be compared

2. To evaluate a patient's pulse following special therapy, such as digitalis medication

3. To assess an abnormal pulse

Equipment

1. A watch with a second hand or indicator to count the pulse rate

2. A pencil or pen to record pulse data

3. A book, record, or worksheet on which to record pulse data

4. If a Doppler ultrasound stethoscope (DUS) will be used, the transducer in the DUS probe (a device resembling a small transistor radio), a stethoscope headset, and transmission gel. See Figure 8–12. Do not use K-Y jelly, which contains probe-damaging

salts. The DUS headset has earpieces similar to standard stethoscope earpieces but it has a long cord attached to a volume-controlled audio unit and an ultrasound transducer. The DUS detects *movement* of red blood cells through a blood vessel. In contrast, the conventional stethoscope amplifies only *sound*, not movement. The DUS can detect blood flow if the blood cells are moving faster than 6 cm per second and at a depth of about 5 cm (Hudson, 1983, p 55). It cannot detect blood flow in deep vessels or in those underlying bone, such as the vessels in the abdomen, thorax, or skull. The DUS is battery operated, and batteries need replacement about every 6 months. Many agencies write the date of battery installation on a small adhesive label and attach it to the case as a reminder to replace the battery.

■ Intervention

1. Select the pulse point. Normally, the radial pulse is taken, unless it cannot be exposed or circulation to another body area is to be assessed.

2. Assist the patient to a comfortable resting position. When the radial pulse is assessed the arm can rest alongside the patient with the palm facing downward or the forearm can rest at a 90° angle across the chest with the palm downward. For the patient who can sit, the forearm can rest across the thigh with the palm of the hand facing downward or inward.

3. a. When palpating the pulse, place three middle fingertips lightly and squarely over the pulse point. See Figure 8–13.

   Rationale Using the thumb is contraindicated because the thumb has a pulse that the nurse could mistake for the patient's pulse.

   b. For using a Doppler ultrasound device, Hudson (1983, p 56) outlines the following steps:

FIGURE 8–12 ■ An ultrasound (Doppler) stethoscope.

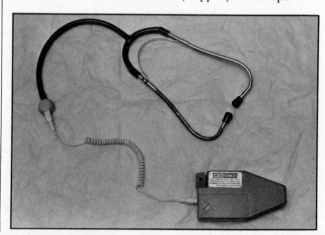

- Plug the stethoscope headset into one of the two output jacks located next to the volume control. DUS units have jacks for two headpieces and accessory loudspeakers so that another person can listen to the signals.

- Apply transmission gel either to the probe, at the narrowed end of the plastic case housing the transducer, or to the patient's skin.

  Rationale Ultrasound beams do not travel well through air. The gel makes an airtight seal, which promotes optimal ultrasound wave transmission.

- Press the "on" button.

- Hold the probe at a 45° angle against the skin over the pulse site. Use a light pressure, and keep the probe in contact with the skin.

  Rationale Too much pressure can stop the blood flow and obliterate the signal.

- Distinguish between artery and vein sounds. The artery sound (signal) is distinctively pulsating and has a pumping quality. The venous sound is like the wind, is intermittent, and varies with respirations.

  Rationale Both artery and vein sounds are heard simultaneously through the DUS, since major arteries and veins are situated close together throughout the body.

- If you have difficulty hearing arterial sounds, reposition the probe.

4.   Count the pulse for 30 seconds and multiply by 2

FIGURE 8–13

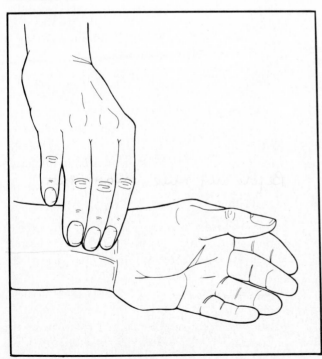

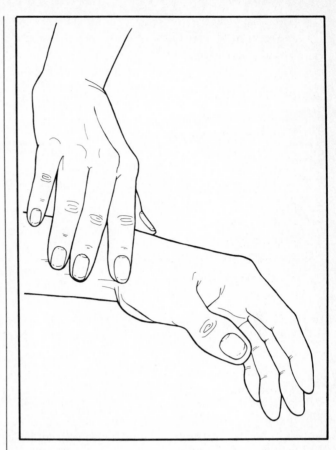

FIGURE 8–14

if the pulse is regular. If it is irregular, count for one full minute.

Rationale An irregular pulse requires a full minute's count for a correct assessment.

5.   Assess the pulse rhythm by noting the pattern of intervals between the beats. A normal pulse has equal time periods between beats. If this is an initial assessment, assess for one full minute.

6.   Assess the pulse volume. A normal pulse can be felt with moderate pressure, and the pressure is equal with each beat. A forceful pulse volume is full; an easily obliterated pulse is weak.

7.   To assess the arterial wall, compress the artery firmly and run a finger distal to the heart along the artery. See Figure 8–14. A normal arterial wall is smooth and straight.

8.   Record the pulse rate, rhythm, and volume, and the condition of the arterial wall.

Sample Recording

Date	Time	Notes
5/8/86	0900	Pale and listless. Pulse 116, weak and threadly. Reported above to Ms. N. McNamara. ———— Sally M. Sahara, NS

9. After using the DUS, remove all the gel from the probe to prevent damage to its surface. Clean the transducer with aqueous solutions.

Rationale Alcohol or other disinfectants may damage the face of the transducer.

■ Evaluation

Expected outcomes

1. A pulse rate within the normal range for the patient
2. A normal pulse volume for the patient
3. A regular pulse rhythm
4. An arterial wall that is smooth and straight

Unexpected outcomes

1. A pulse rate faster or slower than normal for the patient
2. A full, bounding or weak pulse volume
3. An irregular pulse rhythm
4. A tortuous arterial wall

Upon obtaining an unexpected outcome:

1. Reassess the patient's pulse immediately.
2. Assess the patient's respirations and blood pressure.
3. Report your findings to the responsible nurse and/or physician.

TECHNIQUE 8–5 ■ Assessing an Apical Pulse

An apical pulse, at the apex of the heart, is commonly assessed for newborns, infants, and children up to 2 or 3 years. It may also be indicated for patients with cardiac arrhythmias and those receiving medications to improve heart action.

■ Assessment

Assess the patient for:

1. Skin pallor and/or cyanosis of the lips or nail beds
2. Shortness of breath or restlessness
3. The emotional state, since emotions can increase the pulse rate

Other data include:

1. Baseline data about the apical pulse and recent previous assessments
2. The frequency and times at which the apical pulse has been assessed
3. Nursing and/or medical orders to be implemented as a result of the assessment

■ Nursing Diagnosis   See Technique 8–4 on page 115.

■ Planning

Nursing goals

1. To establish a baseline in the initial assessment of the patient

2. To determine a change from prior measurements
3. To determine the rate, rhythm, and volume of the apical pulse

Equipment

1. A watch with a second hand to time the rate of the apical pulse.
2. A stethoscope with a bell-shaped or a flat-disc diaphragm to listen to the heartbeats. See Figure 8–15.
3. Antiseptic wipes to clean the earpieces and diaphragm of the stethoscope if their cleanliness is in doubt. Only the diaphragm needs to be cleaned if the nurse's own stethoscope is used.
4. If using ultrasound, a Doppler ultrasound stethoscope, probe (transducer), and transmission gel.
5. A pencil or pen to record pulse data.
6. A book, record, or worksheet on which to record pulse data.
7. A pacifier if necessary to quiet a newborn or infant.

Before any other treatment

■ Intervention

1. Assist an adult or young child to a comfortable supine position with the head of the bed elevated or to a sitting position on a chair, the edge of the bed, or the examination table. Place a baby on his or her back, and offer a pacifier if the baby is crying or restless.

Rationale Crying and physical activity increase the pulse rate. For this reason, the nurse also takes the apical pulse rate of infants and small children before assessing body temperature.

2. Expose the area of the chest over the apex of the heart. If the patient is in bed, fold the top bedding down to the bottom of the patient's rib cage, and roll the gown up toward the neck. If the patient is sitting, remove the upper clothing. Untie a hospital gown at the back, and draw it down in front just enough to expose the apical area, or lift the gown up from the bottom and drape it over the patient's shoulder.

3. Warm the diaphragm of the stethoscope by holding it in the palm of the hand for a moment.

   Rationale   The metal of the diaphragm is usually cold and can startle the patient when placed immediately on the chest.

4. Insert the earpieces of the stethoscope into your ears. The earpieces may be straight or bent. If they are bent, place them in the direction of the ear canals, slightly forward, to facilitate hearing.

5. Place the diaphragm of the stethoscope over the apex of the patient's heart or over the point where the beats are most clearly heard. For the location of the apex of the heart in a child under 4 years, a child 4 to 6 years, and an adult, see Figure 8–9 earlier.

   Rationale   The heartbeat is normally loudest over the apex of the heart.

6. Count the heartbeats for 30 seconds and multiply by 2 if the rhythm is regular; count the beats for 60 seconds if the rhythm is irregular.

   Rationale   A 60-second count provides a more accurate assessment of an irregular pulse.

7. Assess the rhythm of the heartbeat by noting the pattern of intervals between the beats. A normal pulse has equal time periods between beats. See Figure 8–10 earlier for comparative electrocardiograms illustrating regular and irregular rhythm.

8. Assess the strength (volume) of the heartbeat. Normally the heartbeats are equal in strength and can be described as strong or weak. See Figure 8–11 earlier.

9. Record the pulse on the book, record, or worksheet, noting that it is an apical pulse rate.

Sample Recording

Date	Time	Notes
1/26/87	0900	Apical pulse 56. Beats strong and equal. Digitoxin withheld. Notified Ms. S. Santos, responsible nurse. — Thomas A. Jones, NS

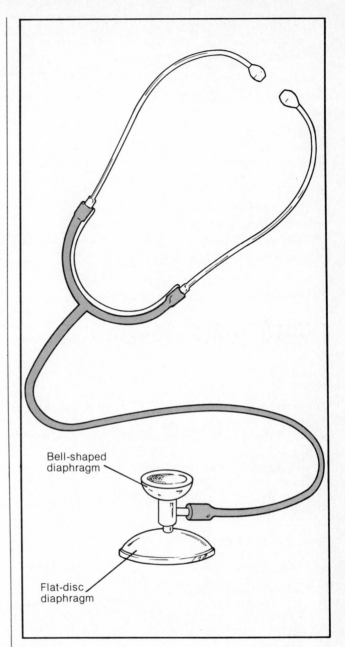

Bell-shaped diaphragm

Flat-disc diaphragm

FIGURE 8–15

■ **Evaluation**

Expected outcomes   See Technique 8–4, outcomes 1–3, on page 118.

Unexpected outcomes   See Technique 8–4, outcomes 1–3, on page 118.

TECHNIQUE 8–6 ■ Assessing an Apical–Radial Pulse

An apical–radial pulse may be required for patients who have certain cardiovascular disorders. Normally the apical and radial rates are identical. An apical pulse rate greater than the radial pulse rate can indicate that the thrust of the blood from the heart is too feeble for the wave to be felt at the peripheral pulse site, or it can indicate that vascular disease is preventing impulses from being transmitted. Any discrepancy between the two pulse rates needs to be reported promptly. In no instance will the radial pulse be greater than the apical pulse. One or two nurses can carry out this technique.

■ **Assessment**   See Technique 8–4 on page 115.

■ **Nursing Diagnosis**   See Technique 8–4 on page 115.

■ **Planning**

Nursing goals

1.   To establish a baseline in the initial assessment of the patient
2.   To determine any change from previous measurements
3.   To determine the rate, rhythm, and volume of the radial and apical pulses
4.   To determine any pulse deficit (difference between the two pulse rates)

Equipment

1.   A watch with a second hand or indicator shared by the two nurses while counting the pulse rates
2.   A stethoscope used by one nurse to listen to the apical pulse
3.   Antiseptic wipes to clean the earpieces and diaphragm of the stethoscope
4.   A pencil to record pulse data
5.   A book, record, or worksheet on which to record the pulse data

■ **Intervention**

1.   Assist the patient to assume the position described for taking the apical pulse. See Technique 8–5, step 1. If previous measurements were taken, determine what position the patient assumed, and use the same position, to ensure an accurate comparative measurement.

Two nurses

2.   Place the watch where both nurses can see it. The nurse who is taking the radial pulse may hold the watch. See Figure 8–16.
3.   One nurse locates the apical pulse site with the stethoscope while the other nurse palpates the radial pulse site. See Techniques 8–4 and 8–5.
4.   Decide on a time to begin counting while watching the second hand of the watch. A time when the second hand is on 12, 3, 6, or 9 is usually selected. The nurse taking the radial pulse says "Start" at the designated time.
     Rationale   This ensures that simultaneous counts are taken.
5.   Each nurse counts the pulse rate for 60 seconds. Both nurses end the count when the nurse taking the radial pulse says "Stop."
     Rationale   A full minute's count is necessary for accurate assessment of any discrepancies between the two pulse sites.
6.   The nurse assessing the apical rate also assesses the apical pulse rhythm and volume, ie, whether the heartbeat is strong or weak. If the pulse is irregular, note whether the irregular beats come at random or at predictable times creating a regular irregularity.
7.   The nurse assessing the radial pulse rate also assesses the radial pulse rhythm (see step 6 above) and volume, ie, whether the pulse can be readily obliterated with pressure or can be obliterated only with difficulty.
8.   Record the apical and radial pulse rates, rhythm, volume, and any pulse deficit on the book, record, or worksheet.
9.   Promptly report to the responsible nurse any notable changes from previous measurements or any discrepancy between the two pulses.
10.   Record the apical and radial (AR) pulse rates on the patient's record in accordance with agency policy.
11.   Record any other pertinent observations, such as pallor, cyanosis, dyspnea, or anxiety.
12.   Check the physician's orders for any directions related to a discrepancy in the apical and radial pulse rates.

One nurse

One-nurse technique may not be as accurate as two-nurse technique.

13. Assess the apical pulse for 60 seconds. See Technique 8–5.

14. Assess the radial pulse for 60 seconds. See Technique 8–4.

15. Complete the technique as in steps 8–12 above.

Sample Recording

Date	Time	Notes
12/2/87	1000	AR pulse 88/88. Apical and radial impulses regular and strong. —— Inez R. Ortega, RN

■ **Evaluation**   See Technique 8–4 on page 118.

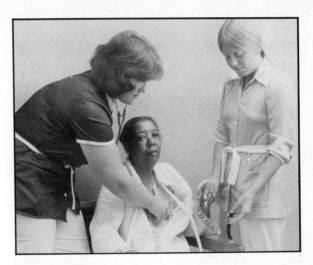

FIGURE 8–16

TECHNIQUE 8–7   ■   Assessing a Fetal Heartbeat

The fetal heart rate (FHR) is audible as early as the tenth week of pregnancy, using the Doppler stethoscope with ultrasound. At about 18 to 20 weeks, the FHR can be heard by fetoscope or other stethoscope.

The FHR is usually between 120 and 160 beats per minute. It can be detected during the early months of pregnancy at the midline of the abdomen over the mother's symphysis pubis (above the pubic hairline); later in the pregnancy, the location varies with the position of the fetus. See Figure 8–17. The nurse first determines the position of the fetus either by palpating the mother's abdomen or from the mother's record.

■ **Assessment**

Assessment varies according to the stage of the pregnancy. Consult a maternal–child nursing textbook for assessment information. Other data from the patient's record include:

1. The frequency and times of assessment. Often FHRs are taken:
   a. If there is any concern about the health of the fetus
   b. On the patient's admission
   c. Every hour during the onset of regular contractions of the uterus
   d. Every 30 minutes during cervical dilation
   e. Every five minutes or continually during the second stage of labor
   f. Immediately after the rupture of the uterine membranes

2. The location on the patient's abdomen where the FHR is most clearly heard. The best location for auscultating the fetal heart may be recorded on the patient's chart and/or marked on the patient's abdomen. The location of maximum intensity will depend on the position of the fetus, because the beats are most clearly transmitted through the back or chest of the fetus. See Figure 8–18.

3. A previous FHR and maternal pulse rate as baseline data.

■ **Planning**

Nursing goals

1. To establish a baseline in the initial assessment of the patient

2. To determine any change from previous measurements

3. To determine the rate, rhythm, and strength of the fetal heartbeat

Equipment

1. One of the following kinds of stethoscopes:
   a. A fetal heart stethoscope (fetoscope) with a large

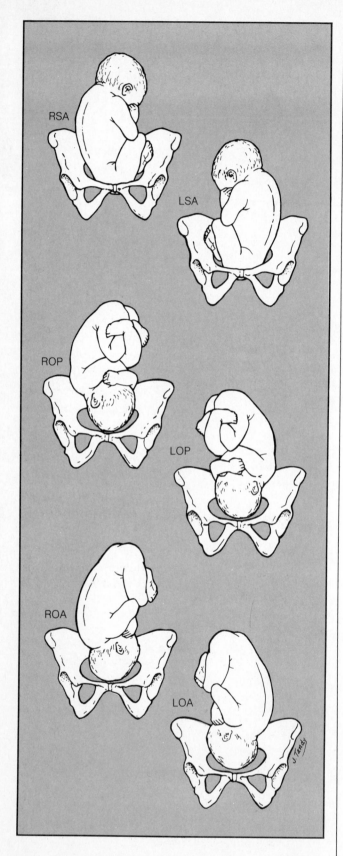

FIGURE 8–17 ■ Six positions of the fetus are: right sacrum anterior (RSA), right occiput posterior (ROP), right occiput anterior (ROA), left sacrum anterior (LSA), left occiput posterior (LOP), and left occiput anterior (LOA).

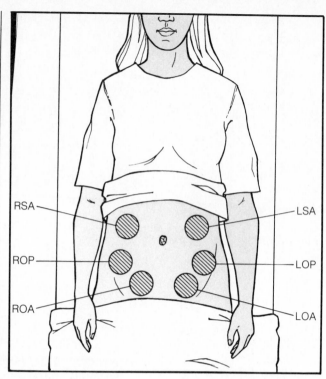

FIGURE 8–18 ■ Locations of maximum FHR intensity according to the position of the fetus.

weighted bell designed specifically for fetal heart auscultation. The weighted bell negates the need to hold the stethoscope in place, thus avoiding the noise of finger movement, which can interfere with auscultation. Some fetal heart stethoscopes can be adapted to monitor the mother's heart rate and blood pressure by substituting a smaller bell.

b. A head stethoscope, which augments the fetal heart sounds, since sounds are transmitted not only to the nurse's eardrums but also by bone conduction through the headpiece the nurse wears.

c. A regular bell stethoscope held by rubber bands.

d. A Doppler ultrasound stethoscope with probe (transducer) and transmission gel. See Figure 8–12 earlier. The Doppler stethoscope is a more sensitive and reliable instrument than other fetoscopes. The transducer is applied to the woman's abdomen in lieu of the bell of other fetoscopes.

2. a. Antiseptic wipes to clean the stethoscope if the cleanliness of earpieces or diaphragm is in doubt. Only the diaphragm needs to be cleaned if the nurse's own stethoscope is used.

b. Soft tissues and aqueous solution if Doppler equipment is used.

3. A watch with a second hand or indicator to time the fetal heart rate.

4. A pencil or pen to record the data.

5. A book, record, or worksheet on which to record the data.

■ Intervention

Using a fetoscope or stethoscope

1. Verify the woman's radial pulse rate to avoid mistaking the uterine souffle for the fetal heart. A uterine souffle has the same rate as the woman's heart rate. For information about the uterine souffle, see step 5 below.

2. Assist the patient to a supine position and expose the abdomen.

3. Locate the point on the abdomen where the fetal heartbeat is most clearly heard.

4. Place the bell of the fetoscope, head stethoscope, or regular stethoscope held by elastic bands firmly on the maternal abdomen over the area of maximum intensity of the FHR in accordance with the identified fetal position: right sacrum anterior (RSA), right occiput posterior (ROP), right occiput anterior (ROA), left sacrum anterior (LSA), left occiput posterior (LOP), and left occiput anterior (LOA). See Figure 8-18.

   Rationale   The FHR is best heard when sounds are transmitted through the fetus's back or chest.

5. Listen to and identify the fetal heart tone, differentiating it from the uterine souffle by simultaneously taking the maternal radial pulse. See Figure 8-19. The *uterine souffle* is the soft blowing sound made when the maternal heart propels the blood through the large blood vessels of the uterus. It synchronizes with the maternal heart rate and can be heard distinctly upon auscultation of the lower portion of the uterus.

   Another blowing or whizzing sound may be heard during fetal heart auscultation. This *funic* (umbilical cord) *souffle* is a sharp hissing sound caused by blood rushing through the umbilical cord and is equivalent to the fetal heart rate, that is, about 140 beats per minute.

6. Count the fetal heart rate for at least 15 seconds whenever it is monitored during the gestation period before labor. During labor, count the fetal heart rate for 60 seconds during the relaxation period between contractions to determine the baseline FHR. Then count the FHR for 60 seconds during a contraction and for 30 seconds immediately following a contraction.

   Rationale   Signs of fetal distress may occur during a contraction but most often occur immediately after it. The normal fetal heart rate is 120 to 160 beats per minute. More than 160 or fewer than 120 beats per minute may indicate fetal distress.

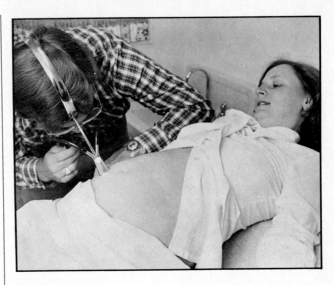

FIGURE 8-19

7. Assess the FHR rhythm. A normal fetal heart rate has equal time periods between beats.

8. Assess the fetal heartbeat strength (volume). Normally the pressure of blood with each beat is equal.

9. Assist the woman to listen to the FHR if she wishes.

10. Record the FHR, including rhythm and strength, on the appropriate record.

Sample Recording

Date	Time	Notes
9/14/87	1300	FHR 136 over right lower quadrant. Beats regular and strong. —Eva L. Mendez, SN

11. If the fetal heart rate or strength is abnormal, report this immediately to the responsible nurse or physician, and initiate electronic fetal monitoring if appropriate.

Using a Doppler stethoscope

12. Follow the manufacturer's instructions about attaching the headset to the audio unit and transducer.

13. Apply transmission gel to the woman's abdomen over the area on which the transducer is to be placed.

    Rationale   Gel creates an airtight seal between the skin and the transducer and promotes optimal ultrasound wave transmission. In the early months of pregnancy, having the patient drink plenty of fluids before the procedure, to fill the bladder, will also improve ultrasound transmission. Later in the pregnancy this may cause discomfort to the patient (Nursing Photobook Series, 1982, p 97).

14. Place the earpieces of the headset in your ears, adjust the volume of the audio unit, hold that unit in one hand, and place the transducer on the mother's abdomen.

15. After you have determined the FHR, remove the excess gel from the mother's abdomen and from the transducer with soft tissues.

16. Clean the transducer with aqueous solutions.

    Rationale Alcohol or other disinfectants may damage the face of the transducer.

■ Evaluation

Expected outcome

A regular, strong FHR between 120 and 160 beats per minute.

Unexpected outcomes

1. An irregular FHR
2. A weak FHR
3. An FHR below 120 beats per minute or above 160 beats per minute

Upon obtaining an unexpected outcome:

1. Reassess the fetal heart in 30 minutes.
2. Assess any discomfort or other complaints experienced by the woman.
3. Reassess the fetal position.
4. Report your findings to the responsible nurse and/or physician.

RESPIRATIONS

Respiration includes the intake of oxygen and the output of carbon dioxide. Respirations are generally described as deep or shallow. In deep respirations a large volume of air is inhaled and exhaled. In shallow respirations the volume of air moved is small.

In inhalation the following processes normally occur (see Figure 8–20):

1. The diaphragm contracts (flattens).
2. The ribs move upward and outward.
3. The sternum moves outward.
4. The thorax enlarges, and thus the lungs expand.

In exhalation (see Figure 8–21):

1. The diaphragm relaxes (its curvature increases).
2. The ribs move inward and downward.
3. The sternum moves inward.
4. The thorax decreases in size, and thus the lungs are compressed.

Respirations are assessed for rate, depth, rhythm, and character. They are measured by observing the patient's chest during the breathing process. The patient needs to be resting and unaware that the nurse is observing the respirations; otherwise the patient may voluntarily control their rate, depth, or rhythm.

The *rate* is measured in breaths per minute; the normal adult rate is 16 to 20, varying with such factors as age (see Developmental Variables, next), emotional intensity, activity, and certain disease processes. The latter three factors tend to increase the respiratory rate, reflecting the body's need for increased oxygen.

Respiration *depth* is generally described as normal, shallow, or deep. Depth can also be measured accurately by pulmonary equipment, usually operated by a physician or a respiratory technologist.

The *rhythm* of respirations refers to the regularity of inhalations and exhalations. Normally respirations are evenly spaced. Certain disease processes, eg, pneumonia, and other circumstances, eg, varying blood carbon dioxide levels, produce irregular respirations.

The *character* of respirations primarily denotes deviations from eupnea. These deviations are discussed under Common Problems.

Developmental Variables

The respiratory rate normally varies with age. See Table 8–1 earlier. Newborns range from 30 to 80 respirations per minute. By 2 years of age, the rate slows to between 20 and 30 breaths per minute, and by 12 years it further slows to between 17 and 22 respirations per minute. The adult rate is normally between 15 and 20 breaths per minute. In the elderly, respiratory rates above 20 breaths per minute are not unusual.

Common Problems

Respiration problems may relate to rate, depth, rhythm, or character. An adult respiratory rate higher than 24 breaths per minute is called *tachypnea*. A rate below 10 respirations per minute is described as *bradypnea*. The complete absence of respirations is called *apnea*.

Abnormally shallow respirations move a small volume of air into and out of the lungs in relation to the normal lung capacity; abnormally deep respirations exchange a large volume of air in relation to the normal capacity. Either abnormality can lead to disturbances of the acid–base balance in the body.

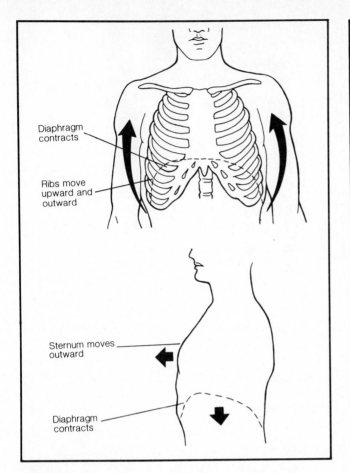

FIGURE 8–20   ■   Respiratory inhalation: anterior and lateral views.

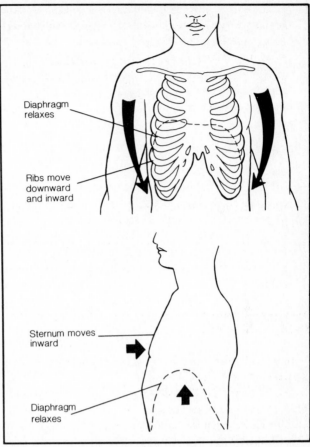

FIGURE 8–21   ■   Respiratory exhalation: anterior and lateral views.

A problem of rhythm is irregular breathing—uneven time periods between respirations. Cheyne-Stokes respirations, often associated with cardiac failure or brain damage, are an example of an irregular breathing pattern. They are characterized by rhythmic waxing and waning from very deep to very shallow respirations, including periods of apnea.

Respirations abnormal in character include dyspnea, orthopnea, wheezing, stridor, and rales or rhonchi.

TECHNIQUE 8–8   ■   Assessing Respirations

Respirations are usually counted and observed at the same time that the body temperature and pulse are taken. Breathing is essential to life, and assessing respirations can be critical to determining a patient's condition. People can adjust their respirations consciously to a large degree; therefore, respirations are usually counted directly after counting the pulse, so that the patient is unaware that breaths are being counted. The nurse's hand usually remains on the patient's wrist with the same amount of pressure (as if counting the pulse) while the respirations are assessed.

■ Assessment

Assess the patient for:

1. The color of the skin and mucous membranes, eg, for cyanosis and/or pallor
2. The rate, depth, rhythm, and character of the breathing
3. The position that the patient assumes for breathing, eg, whether the patient is orthopneic
4. Any complaints of dyspnea by the patient

5. Any change that might indicate cerebral anoxia (decreased oxygen to the brain), eg, anxious behavior, irritability, restlessness, drowsiness, or loss of consciousness

6. If severe respiratory disease is present, specific chest movements, such as intercostal retractions (indrawing between the ribs) and substernal or suprasternal retractions (indrawing below or above the sternum)

Other data from the patient's record include:

1. The patient's activity schedule, to determine a suitable time to assess respirations. A patient who has been exercising will need to rest for a few minutes to permit the accelerated respiratory rate to return to normal. An infant or child who is crying will have an abnormal respiratory rate and will need quieting before an accurate assessment of the respirations can be made.

2. Baseline data about the patient's respirations and recent respiratory assessment.

3. The frequency and times at which the respirations need to be assessed.

4. Any nursing or medical orders to be implemented as a result of the assessment.

■ Nursing Diagnosis

Nursing diagnoses that may indicate the need to assess a patient's respirations include:

1. Potential or actual activity intolerance related to:
   a. Alterations in the oxygen transport system (cardiac, respiratory, or circulatory)
   b. Chronic diseases
   c. Malnourishment
   d. Prolonged bed rest
   e. Sedentary life-style

2. Alterations in cardiac output (decreased) related to:
   a. Cardiac factors
   b. Pulmonary disorders
   c. Endocrine disorders
   d. Hematologic disorders
   e. Fluid and electrolyte imbalances
   f. Stress
   g. Surgery
   h. Medications (diuretics, antihypertensives, vasoconstrictors, vasodilators)
   i. Allergic response
   j. Sepsis

3. Alterations in respiratory function related to:
   a. Excessive or thick secretions
   b. Infection
   c. Neuromuscular impairment
   d. Loss of lung elasticity
   e. Anesthesia
   f. Smoking
   g. Suppressed cough reflex
   h. Immobility

4. Fluid volume excess (edema) related to:
   a. Renal failure
   b. Decreased cardiac output
   c. Liver disorder
   d. Excessive sodium intake

5. Anxiety related to:
   a. Actual or perceived threat to self-concept
   b. Actual or perceived loss of significant others
   c. Actual or perceived threat to biologic integrity
   d. Actual or perceived change in environment
   e. Actual or perceived change in socioeconomic status

■ Planning

Nursing goals

1. To acquire baseline data against which future measurements can be compared.

2. To determine the rate, rhythm, depth, and character of the patient's respirations.

3. To monitor abnormal respirations, for example, for patients with chest or heart disease.

4. To assess a patient's respirations prior to the administration of a medication such as morphine. (An abnormally slow respiratory rate may warrant withholding the medication.)

5. To assess respirations following the administration of a general anesthetic or any medication that influences respirations.

Equipment

1. A watch with a second hand or indicator to time the respiratory rate

2. A pencil or pen to record the data

3. A book, record, or worksheet on which to record the data

■ Intervention

1. Inform the patient about measuring his or her temperature, pulse, and blood pressure, but do not mention respirations.

   Rationale An explanation about assessing respirations could cause the patient to alter his or her respiratory pattern.

2. Place a hand against the patient's chest to feel the patient's chest movements or place the patient's arm across his or her chest and/or observe the chest movements while supposedly taking the radial pulse.

3. Count the respiratory rate for 30 seconds if the respirations are regular. Count for 60 seconds if they are irregular. An inhalation and an exhalation count as one respiration.

4. Observe the respirations for depth by watching the movement of the chest. During deep respirations a large volume of air is exchanged; during shallow respirations a small volume is exchanged.

5. Observe the respirations for regular or irregular rhythm. Normally respirations are evenly spaced.

6. Observe the character of respirations—the sound they produce and the effort they require. Normally respirations are silent and effortless.

7. Record the respiratory rate, depth, rhythm, and character on the appropriate record.

Sample Recording

Date	Time	Notes
6/20/86	0900	R 38 and shallow. Dyspneic when talking. Dr. Woo notified.—— John P. Brown, NS

■ Evaluation

Expected outcomes

1. A respiratory rate within the normal range for the patient

2. Regular respiratory rhythm

3. Adequate respiratory depth

4. Quiet, effortless breathing

Unexpected outcomes

1. A respiratory rate significantly above or below the normal range

2. An irregular respiratory rhythm

3. An inadequate respiratory depth

4. An abnormal character of breathing, eg, dyspnea, orthopnea, wheezing, stridor, rales, or rhonchi

Upon obtaining an unexpected outcome:

1. Reassess the patient's respirations for rate, depth, rhythm, and character in 30 minutes or sooner depending upon the patient's condition.

2. Assess the temperature, blood pressure, and pulse rate, since tachypnea may accompany a fever, low blood pressure, and rapid pulse rate.

3. Assess the patient's emotional status, since anxiety, fear, or stress can produce an increase in respiratory rate.

4. Assess the patient for pallor or cyanosis, especially at the lips and nail beds.

5. Report your findings to the responsible nurse and/or physician.

BLOOD PRESSURE

Blood pressure is the measure of the pressure of the blood as it circulates in the arteries. Because the blood moves in waves, there are two blood pressures: *systolic pressure,* or the pressure of the blood at the height of the wave when the heart muscle contracts; and *diastolic pressure,* or the pressure of the blood at the low point in the wave when the heart muscle relaxes. The diastolic pressure is the lowest pressure, and it is present at all times within the arteries. The difference between the systolic pressure and the diastolic pressure is called the *pulse pressure.*

Blood pressure is measured in millimeters of mercury (mm Hg). It varies with a number of factors, including the patient's age (see Developmental Variables), cardiac output, blood volume, the elasticity and size of arteries, and the size of the capillaries.

Cardiac output is normally 70 mL of blood for each contraction. Exercise and fever cause this output to increase. Blood volume also affects the blood pressure. Normally an adult has about 6 L of circulating blood. Loss of blood due to hemorrhage or a reduced blood volume due to dehydration can lower the blood pressure.

The size of the arteries and the capillaries creates greater or less resistance to the circulating blood. The smaller the lumen (channel) of the blood vessel, the greater the resistance. Elasticity of the artery walls also affects resistance to the blood. In elderly people, elasticity is decreased; the arteries are more rigid and less yielding to the pressure of the blood. This produces an elevated systolic pressure. Because the walls no longer retract as flexibly with decreased pressure, there is also a lower diastolic pressure.

Blood pressure is also increased by exercise, emotions, and physical stress. It is therefore important that the patient be resting and not under excessive stress (free of pain, for example) when the blood pressure is measured.

Korotkoff's Sounds

When taking a blood pressure using a stethoscope, the nurse identifies five phases in the series of sounds, called *Korotkoff's sounds*. First the nurse pumps the cuff up to about 30 mm Hg above the point where the last sound is heard; that is the point when the blood flow in the artery is stopped. Then the pressure is released slowly (2 to 3 mm Hg per second), while the nurse observes the pressure readings on the manometer and relates them to the sounds heard through the stethoscope. Five phases occur (American Heart Association, 1980, p 11):

Phase 1. The period initiated by the first faint clear tapping sounds. These sounds gradually become more intense. To ensure that they are not extraneous sounds, the nurse should identify at least two consecutive tapping sounds.

Phase 2. The period during which the sounds have a swishing quality.

Phase 3. The period during which the sounds are crisper and more intense.

Phase 4. The period during which the sounds become muffled and have a soft, blowing quality.

Phase 5. The point where the sounds disappear.

The American Heart Association (AHA) recommends that the systolic pressure be considered the point where the first tapping sound is heard (Phase 1). In adults the diastolic pressure is the point where the sounds become

FIGURE 8–22 ■ **A,** A blood pressure cuff and bulb; **B,** the bladder inside the cuff.

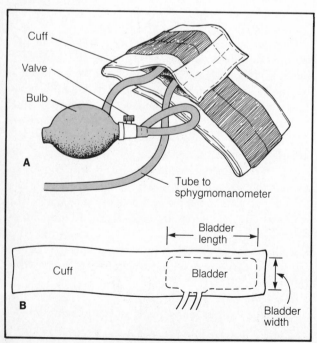

inaudible (Phase 5). In children, however, the AHA recommends that diastolic pressure be considered to be the onset of Phase 4, where the sounds become muffled. In agencies where the fourth phase is considered the diastolic pressure of adults, three measures are recommended (systolic pressure, diastolic pressure, and Phase 5). These may be referred to as systolic, first diastolic, and second diastolic pressures. The Phase 5 (second diastolic pressure) reading may be zero; that is, the muffled sounds are heard even when there is no air pressure in the blood pressure cuff. In some instances, muffled sounds may never be heard, in which case a dash is inserted where the reading would normally be recorded.

Developmental Variables

Normal blood pressures vary with age. See Table 8–1 earlier, for average rates. Newborns have a mean systolic pressure of 78 mm Hg. The pressure rises with age, reaching a peak at the onset of puberty, and then tends to decline somewhat. One quick way to determine the normal systolic blood pressure of a child is to use the following formula (Evans, 1983, p 61):

Normal systolic BP = 80 + (2 × child's age in years)

Elderly people show very little increase in systolic pressure from the adult level. However, exercise and stress tend to raise the blood pressure more in elderly people than in younger people, and it takes longer to return to normal.

Common Problems

Two common problems of blood pressure are exceptionally high pressure and exceptionally low pressure. An adult pressure above 140 mm Hg systolic and/or 90 mm Hg diastolic constitutes hypertension when these pressures are confirmed at a minimum of two subsequent visits (National Heart, Lung, and Blood Institute, 1984, p 1045). An adult pressure below 100 mm Hg systolic constitutes hypotension.

Blood Pressure Equipment

Blood pressure is measured with a *blood pressure cuff,* a *sphygmomanometer,* and a *stethoscope.* The blood pressure cuff consists of a rubber bag that can be inflated with air. It is called the *bladder.* See Figure 8–22. It is usually covered with cloth and has two tubes attached to it. One tube connects to a rubber bulb that inflates the bladder. A small valve on the side of this bulb releases the air in the bladder when turned counterclockwise. When the valve is tightened (turned clockwise), air pumped into the bladder is held there. The other tube is attached to a sphygmomanometer.

The sphygmomanometer is an instrument that indicates the pressure of the air within the bladder. There are two types of sphygmomanometers: *aneroid* and *mercury.*

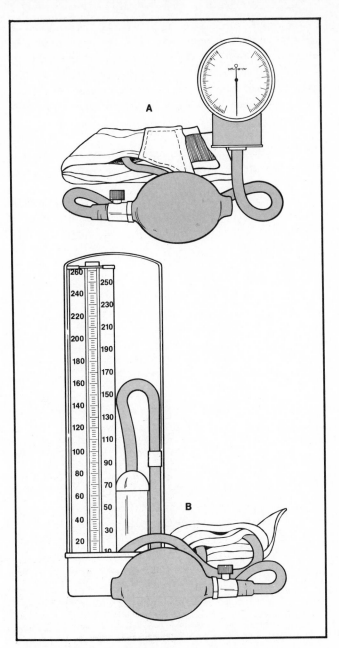

FIGURE 8-23   ■   Blood pressure equipment: **A,** an aneroid manometer and cuff; **B,** a mercury manometer and cuff.

See Figure 8-23. The aneroid sphygmomanometer is a calibrated dial with a needle that points to the calibrations. The mercury sphygmomanometer is a calibrated cylinder filled with mercury. The pressure is indicated at the point to which the meniscus of the mercury (the crescent-shaped surface of the column) rises. It is important to examine the meniscus at eye level to avoid distortions in the reading from viewing it at an angle.

Some agencies use electronic sphygmomanometers, which eliminate the need to listen to the sounds of the patient's systolic and diastolic blood pressures through a stethoscope. On some models, as the pressure in the cuff is lowered, a light flashes to indicate the systolic and diastolic pressures.

Ultrasound (Doppler) stethoscopes are also used to assess blood pressure. See Figure 8-12 earlier. These are of particular value when Korotkoff's sounds are difficult to hear, eg, in infants, obese patients, and patients in shock. Transmission gel is applied to a transducer probe, which is placed over the pulse point, and the blood pressure is measured. A systolic blood pressure assessed using a Doppler stethoscope is recorded with a large D, eg, 85D. Systolic pressure may be the only blood pressure obtained by some ultrasound models.

Blood pressure cuffs come in various sizes, since the bladder must be the correct width and length for the patient's arm. If the bladder width is too narrow, the blood pressure reading will be erroneously elevated; if it is too wide, the reading will be erroneously low. The width should be 40% of the circumference or 20% wider than the diameter of the midpoint of the limb on which it is used (American Heart Association, 1980, p 4). To determine whether the width of a blood pressure cuff is appropriate, lay the cuff lengthwise at the midpoint of the upper arm. Hold the outermost side of the bladder edge laterally on the arm. With the other hand wrap the width of the cuff around the arm and determine whether the width is 40% of the arm circumference. See Figure 8-24.

FIGURE 8-24   ■   Determining if a blood pressure cuff is the correct width.

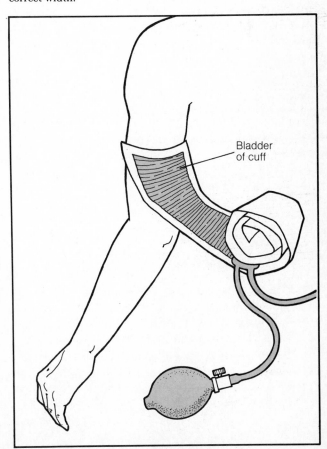

Bladder of cuff

TABLE 8-3 ■ Recommended Blood Pressure Cuff Bladder Dimensions by Arm Circumference

Arm circumference at midpoint* (cm)	Cuff name	Bladder width (cm)	Bladder length (cm)
5–7.5	Newborn	3	5
7.5–13	Infant	5	8
13–20	Child	8	13
17–26	Small adult	11	17
24–32	Adult	13	24
32–42	Large adult	17	32
42–50†	Thigh	20	42

Source: American Heart Association: *Recommendations for Human Blood Pressure Determination by Sphygmomanometers,* Pub No. 70–019–B, 80–100M, 9–81–100M, American Heart Association, 1980, p 5. Reprinted by permission of the American Heart Association, Inc.

*The midpoint of the arm is defined as half the distance from the acromion to the olecranon.

†In persons with very large limbs, the indirect blood pressure should be measured in the leg or forearm.

The length of the bladder also affects the accuracy of measurement. The length should almost encircle the limb and cover from 60% to 100% of its circumference, preferably 80%, ie, twice the recommended width (ibid, pp 4, 5). The bladder dimensions of various cuff sizes, which are given age group names, are shown in Table 8–3; the arm circumference, not the age of the patient, should always determine bladder size.

Blood pressure cuffs are made of nondistensible material so that an even pressure is exerted around the limb. Most cuffs are held in place by hooks, snaps, or Velcro. Others have a cloth bandage that is long enough to encircle the limb several times; this type is closed by tucking the end of the bandage into one of the bandage folds.

TECHNIQUE 8–9 ■ Assessing Blood Pressure 🏠

The blood pressure is usually assessed in the patient's arm using the brachial artery and a standard stethoscope. If the arm is very large or grossly misshapen and the conventional cuff cannot be properly applied, leg or forearm measurements can be taken. To obtain a leg blood pressure, a standard-sized cuff is applied over the lower leg with the distal border of the cuff at the malleoli. Korotkoff's sounds are auscultated over the posterior tibial or dorsalis pedis arteries. To obtain a forearm blood pressure an appropriate-sized cuff is applied to the forearm 13 cm (5 in) from the elbow. Korotkoff's sounds are heard over the radial artery (American Heart Association, 1980, p 13).

■ Assessment

Assess the patient for:

1. Clinical signs of hypertension. Although early hypertension does not usually have associated signs or symptoms, late or untreated hypertension may be accompanied by frequent nosebleeds, periodic facial flushing, irritability, and a ringing sound in the ears.

2. Clinical signs of hypotension, such as an increased pulse rate, cold clammy skin, mental confusion, and dizziness.

3. Calm physical and emotional status. The patient should be resting before the blood pressure is measured. Exercise increases blood pressure; thus, a measure taken directly after exercise may provide an unreliable reading. Crying and anxiety also raise the blood pressure.

Other data include:

1. The patient's baseline blood pressure and/or recent assessments.

2. Baseline data about other vital signs and recent assessments.

3. The patient's age and size, since these affect the cuff size required. An emaciated adult patient, for example, may need a small cuff.

4. The time the patient last ate, smoked, or performed exercise. Measurement should not be taken within 30 minutes of eating, smoking, or exertion (eg, climbing two flights of stairs) (American Heart Association, 1980, p 10).

5. Any particular problems about taking the blood pressure. For example, the patient's chart or nursing care plan might indicate that the blood pressure is difficult to detect in the right arm.

6. The position the patient assumed for the previous blood pressure measurement, eg, sitting, lying, or standing.

7. Whether the patient's arm should not be used to assess blood pressure. When neither arm can be used, the popliteal artery of the leg is usually the site of choice. See Technique 8–10. The blood pressure is *not* measured on a particular arm where:

   a. The patient has a cast.

   b. The shoulder, arm, or hand is injured or diseased.

   c. The patient has had breast or axilla surgery on that side.

   d. The patient has an intravenous infusion or a blood transfusion running.

   e. The patient has a shunt (a surgical opening that joins a vein or an artery). Shunts are used, for example, for renal dialysis and for the administration of heparin.

■ Nursing Diagnosis

Nursing diagnoses that may indicate the need to assess the patient's blood pressure include:

1. Alteration in cardiac output related to:

   a. Cardiac factors

   b. Pulmonary disorders

   c. Endocrine disorders

   d. Hematologic disorders

   e. Fluid and electrolyte imbalances

   f. Stress

   g. Surgery

   h. Medications (diuretics, antihypertensives, vasoconstrictors, vasodilators)

   i. Allergic response

   j. Sepsis

2. Potential or actual fluid volume deficit related to:

   a. Decreased fluid intake

   b. Abnormal fluid loss

3. Alteration in tissue perfusion related to:

   a. Cardiovascular disorders

   b. Hypotension

   c. Blood dyscrasias

   d. Renal failure

   e. Edema or inflammation

   f. Cancer or tumor

   g. Prolonged immobility or bed rest

■ Planning

Nursing goals

1. To establish a baseline in the initial assessment of the patient

2. To assess any change from previous measurements

Equipment

1. A stethoscope. Clean the ear attachments with disinfectant, if others have worn it.

   or

   An ultrasound (Doppler) stethoscope (see Figure 8–12 earlier).

2. A blood pressure cuff of the appropriate size (newborn, infant, child, small adult, adult, large adult, thigh).

3. A sphygmomanometer.

■ Intervention

1. Help the patient to assume the appropriate position. A sitting position is normally used unless otherwise specified. The arm should be slightly flexed with the palm of the hand facing up and the forearm supported at heart level. Readings in any other position should be specified.

   Rationale The blood pressure is normally similar in sitting, standing, and lying positions, but it can vary significantly by position in certain persons. There is an increase in the blood pressure when the arm is below heart level and a decrease when it is above heart level (American Heart Association, 1980, p 12).

2. Expose the upper arm.

3. Wrap the deflated cuff evenly around the upper arm so that the center of the bladder is applied directly over the medial aspect of the arm. To take an adult's blood pressure, place the lower border of the cuff about 2.5 cm (1 in) above the antecubital space. The lower edge can be nearer the antecubital space of an infant.

   Rationale The bladder inside the cuff must be directly over the artery to be compressed if the reading is to be accurate.

4. If this is the patient's initial examination, perform a preliminary palpatory determination of systolic pressure.

   Rationale The initial estimate tells the nurse the maximal pressure to which the manometer needs to be elevated in subsequent determinations. It also prevents underestimation of the systolic pressure or overestimation of the diastolic pressure should an auscultatory gap occur. An auscultatory gap, which occurs particularly in hypertensive patients, is the temporary disappearance of sounds normally heard over the brachial artery when the cuff pressure is high and then the reappearance of the sounds at a lower level. This temporary disappearance of sounds occurs in the latter part of Phase 1 and Phase 2 and may cover a range of 40 mm Hg (American Heart Association, 1980, p 11).

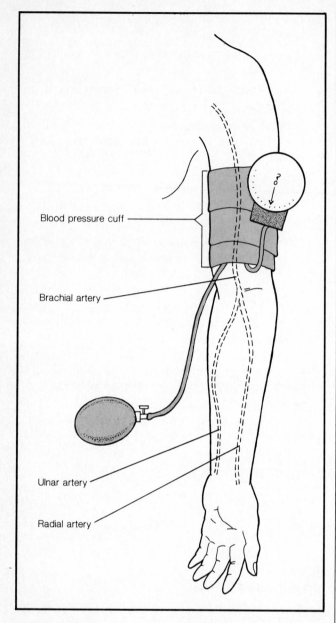

FIGURE 8-25

a. Palpate the brachial artery with the fingertips. The brachial artery is normally found medially in the antecubital space. See Figure 8-25.

b. Close the valve on the pump by turning the knob clockwise.

c. Pump up the cuff until you no longer feel the brachial pulse.

Rationale At that pressure the blood cannot flow through the artery.

d. Note the pressure on the sphygmomanometer at which the pulse is no longer felt.

Rationale This gives an estimate of the maximum pressure required to measure the systolic pressure.

e. Release the pressure completely in the cuff and wait one to two minutes before further measurements are made.

Rationale A waiting period gives the blood trapped in the veins time to be released.

5. Insert the ear attachments of the stethoscope in your ears so that they tilt slightly forward.

Rationale Sounds are sharper when the ear attachments follow the direction of the ear canal.

6. Ensure that the stethoscope hangs freely from the ears to the diaphragm.

Rationale Rubbing the stethoscope against an object can obliterate the sounds of the blood within an artery.

7. Place the diaphragm of the stethoscope over the brachial pulse. Use the bell-shaped diaphragm of the stethoscope (see Figure 8-15 earlier) (American Heart Association, 1980, p 7). Hold the diaphragm with the thumb and index finger.

8. Pump up the cuff until the sphygmomanometer registers about 30 mm Hg above the point where the brachial pulse disappears.

9. Release the valve on the cuff carefully so that the pressure decreases at the rate of 2 to 3 mm Hg per second.

Rationale If the rate is faster or slower, an error in measurement may occur (American Heart Association, 1980, p 11).

10. As the pressure falls, identify the manometer reading at each of the five phases.

11. Deflate the cuff rapidly and completely and wait one to two minutes before repeating.

Rationale This permits blood trapped in the veins to be released.

12. Repeat steps 8-11 once or twice as necessary to confirm the accuracy of the reading.

13. Remove the cuff from the patient's arm.

14. If this is the patient's initial examination, repeat the procedure on his or her other arm. The arm found to have the higher pressure should be used for subsequent examinations (American Heart Association, 1980, p 10).

15. Record the blood pressure according to agency policy. Record two pressures in the form "130/80" where "130" is the systolic (Phase 1) and "80" is the diastolic (Phase 5) pressure. Record three pressures in the form "130/110/90" where "130" is the systolic, 110 is the first diastolic (Phase 4), and "90" is the second diastolic (Phase 5) pressure. Use abbreviations RA for right arm and LA for left arm.

16. Report any significant change in the patient's blood pressure to the responsible nurse.

Sample Recording

Date	Time	Notes
8/14/87	1300	BP 130/90 in RA in bed-sitting position. Color pale. ——— Ruth P. O'Shea, SN

■ Evaluation

Expected outcomes

1. Systolic blood pressure within the normal range for the patient
2. Diastolic blood pressure within the normal range for the patient

Unexpected outcomes

1. Systolic blood pressure (of an adult) above 140 mm Hg
2. Diastolic blood pressure (of an adult) above 90 mm Hg
3. Systolic blood pressure (of an adult) below 100 mm Hg
4. A significant change in the systolic and/or diastolic pressures from the baseline data

Upon obtaining an unexpected outcome:

1. Reassess the patient's blood pressure in the other arm immediately.
2. Assess the patient's pulse and respirations.
3. Assess for clinical signs of hemorrhage if appropriate, eg, in a postsurgical patient.
4. Report your findings to the responsible nurse and/or physician.

TECHNIQUE 8–10   ■   Assessing Thigh Blood Pressure

Assessing the blood pressure on a patient's thigh is usually indicated:

1. When the blood pressure cannot be measured on either arm, eg, because of burns or casts
2. When the blood pressure in one thigh is to be compared with the blood pressure in the other thigh or in the arm, eg, when there is disease of the aorta

■ **Assessment**   See Technique 8–9 on page 130.

■ **Nursing Diagnosis**   See Technique 8–9 on page 131.

■ **Planning**

Nursing goals

1. To establish a baseline in the initial assessment of the patient
2. To assess any change from previous measurements

Equipment

1. A stethoscope. Clean the ear attachments with a disinfectant, if others have used it. Only the diaphragm needs to be cleaned if your own stethoscope is used.
2. A thigh blood pressure cuff of the appropriate size. The cuff width and length should be greater than that normally used for an arm blood pressure, eg, for an adult 20 cm (7.8 in) wide and 42 cm (16.5 in) long (American Heart Association, 1980, p 5).
3. A sphygmomanometer.

■ **Intervention**

1. Help the patient to assume a prone position. If the patient cannot assume this position, measure the blood pressure while the patient is in a supine position with the knee slightly flexed.
   Rationale   Slight flexing of the knee will facilitate placing the stethoscope over the popliteal space.
2. Expose the thigh, taking care not to expose the patient unduly.
3. Wrap the cuff evenly around the midthigh with the compression bladder over the posterior aspect of the thigh.
   Rationale   The bladder must be directly over the artery if the reading is to be accurate.
4. If this is the patient's initial examination, perform a preliminary palpatory determination of systolic pressure.
   Rationale   This is done to estimate the maximal

pressure to which the manometer needs to be elevated in subsequent determinations and to prevent underestimation of systolic pressure or overestimation of the diastolic pressure in hypertensive patients should an auscultatory gap occur.

a. Palpate the popliteal artery with the fingertips. The popliteal artery is found behind the knee. See Figure 8–26.

b. Close the valve on the pump by turning the knob clockwise.

FIGURE 8–26

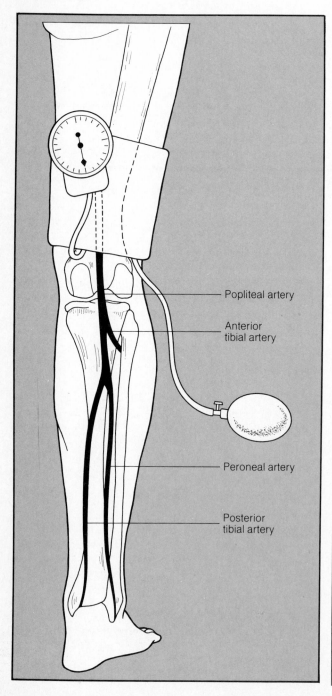

- Popliteal artery
- Anterior tibial artery
- Peroneal artery
- Posterior tibial artery

c. Pump up the cuff until you no longer feel the popliteal pulse.

Rationale At that pressure the blood cannot flow through the artery.

d. Note the pressure on the sphygmomanometer at which the pulse is no longer felt.

Rationale This will give an estimate of the maximum pressure required to measure the systolic pressure and will help to prevent an error in measurement.

e. Release the pressure completely in the cuff and wait one to two minutes.

Rationale A waiting period gives the blood trapped in the veins time to be released.

5. Insert the ear attachments of the stethoscope in your ears so that they point slightly forward.

Rationale Sounds are heard more clearly when the ear attachments follow the direction of the ear canals.

6. Make sure that the stethoscope hangs freely from the earpieces to the diaphragm.

Rationale Rubbing the stethoscope against any object can obliterate the sounds of the blood in the artery.

7. Place the diaphragm of the stethoscope over the popliteal artery.

8. Pump up the cuff until the pressure is about 30 mm Hg above the point where the popliteal pulse disappears.

9. Release the valve on the cuff so that the pressure falls at a rate of 2 to 3 mm Hg per second.

Rationale If the rate is faster or slower, the measurement may be inaccurate (American Heart Association, 1980, p 11).

10. As the pressure falls, identify the manometer reading at each of the five phases.

11. Deflate the cuff completely and rapidly and wait one to two minutes before making further determinations.

Rationale This permits blood trapped in the veins to be released.

12. Repeat steps 8–11 once or twice as necessary.

Rationale It may be necessary to establish the accuracy of the readings.

13. Remove the cuff from the patient's thigh.

14. Record the systolic and diastolic pressures. The systolic pressure in the popliteal artery is usually 10 to 40 mm Hg higher than that in the brachial artery due to use of a larger bladder (American Heart Association, 1980, p 13); the diastolic pressure is usually the same.

15. Record an adult's pressure readings in the form "RT

130/80" where "RT" is right thigh, "130" is systolic pressure (Phase 1), and "80" is diastolic pressure (Phase 5). Record a child's pressure readings in the form "LT 140/90" where "LT" is left thigh, "140" is systolic pressure (Phase 1), and "90" is diastolic pressure (Phase 4). In agencies where the onset of

the fourth phase is considered the diastolic pressure of adults, take three readings: Phase 1, Phase 4, and Phase 5. Record the readings in the form "RT 130/100/80."

■ **Evaluation**   See Technique 8–9 on page 133.

TECHNIQUE 8–11   ■   Assessing an Infant's Blood Pressure

The blood pressure of an infant can be measured by auscultation, palpation, ultrasound, or flush technique. Auscultation is often difficult on infants under age 3, because Korotkoff's sounds are relatively inaudible, but it is the method of choice for children over 3 years of age. When the blood pressure cannot be auscultated, it can be palpated or measured by the flush technique. Both of these methods reveal only a mean pressure between the systolic and diastolic pressures when the blood returns to the limb. The flush technique is largely being replaced by use of an ultrasound device. Some ultrasound models measure only systolic pressures; others measure both systolic and diastolic pressures.

The procedure for measuring an infant's blood pressure differs from that used for an adult. The systolic pressure (Phase 1) is noted when the first two or three tapping sounds are heard. Phase 4 (muffling of sounds) is used as the diastolic pressure and Phase 5 (disappearance of sounds) may or may not be identifiable. If Phases 1, 4, and 5 are measured, they are recorded in the form "118/78/68." If only Phases 1 and 4 could be identified, they are recorded "118/78/0." This indicates that sounds were heard to the 0 point on the manometer.

■ **Assessment**   See Technique 8–9 on page 130.

■ **Nursing Diagnosis**   See Technique 8–9 on page 131.

■ **Planning**

Nursing goals

1. To establish a baseline in the initial assessment of the patient
2. To determine any change from previous measurements
3. To determine the adequacy of the arterial blood pressure

Equipment

1. A blood pressure cuff of a suitable size. The inflatable bladder within the cuff should completely or nearly encircle the limb. The bladder width should be 40% of the circumference of the limb (American Heart Association, 1980, p 17).
2. A sphygmomanometer (auscultatory method).
3. A stethoscope (auscultatory method).
4. An elastic bandage of a suitable width to cover the limb distal to the cuff (flush method).

■ **Intervention**

1. Be sure the environment in which the blood pressure measurement is to take place is quiet and reassuring to the infant. Frightening sounds or sights can contribute to error in measurement, since anxiety and restlessness increase the blood pressure.
2. Allow time for the infant to recover from any activity or apprehension.
3. Assist the child to a comfortable position. Infants and children up to 5 years should assume a supine position; children over 5 years should assume a sitting position. Expose the arm fully and support it comfortably at the child's heart level.

Auscultation

The auscultatory method is essentially the same for children as for adults.

1. Place the cuff around the limb so that the lower edge is about 1 cm (0.4 in) above the antecubital space. See Figure 8–27.
2. Follow steps 4–9 in Technique 8–9 on page 131.
3. Identify the manometer reading at Phases 1, 4, and 5 of Korotkoff's sounds. Phase 1 is the systolic pressure and Phase 4 the diastolic pressure.
4. Follow steps 11–16 in Technique 8–9.

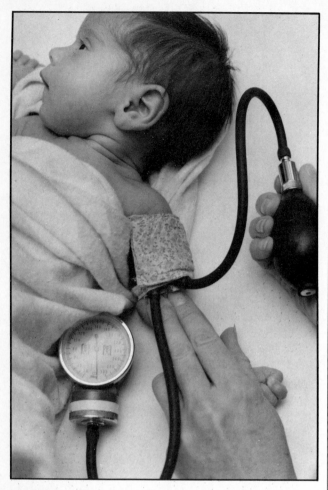

FIGURE 8-27

Palpation

5. Place the cuff around the limb so that the lower edge is about 1 cm (0.4 in) above the antecubital space. See Figure 8-27.

6. Palpate the brachial pulse.

7. Inflate the cuff to about 30 mm Hg beyond the point where the brachial pulse disappears.

8. Release the cuff at the rate of 2 to 3 mm Hg per second and identify the manometer reading at the point where the pulse returns in the brachial artery. This pressure is a mean pressure between the systolic and diastolic pressures.

Flush technique

This procedure (American Heart Association, 1980, p 18) requires two people and a well-lighted room, so that the pressure at which the flush appears can be accurately determined.

9. Place the cuff on the infant's wrist or ankle.

10. Elevate the limb.

   Rationale This promotes venous blood flow to the heart.

11. Wrap the limb distal to the cuff with an elastic bandage. Wrap firmly starting at the fingers or toes and working up to the blood pressure cuff.

   Rationale The bandage will force venous blood into the upper part of the limb and restrict arterial blood flow into the lower part of the limb.

12. Lower the extremity to heart level.

13. Inflate the bladder of the cuff rapidly to about 200 mm Hg.

   Rationale This stops arterial blood flow to the limb.

14. Remove the bandage. The limb should appear pale due to the absence of blood.

15. Gradually release the pressure at no more than 5 mm Hg per second.

16. Record the pressure at the appearance of a flush as the blood returns in the extremity distal to the cuff. This pressure is a mean blood pressure between the systolic and diastolic pressures.

■ **Evaluation**   See Technique 8-9 on page 133.

References

Abbey JC et al: How long is that thermometer accurate? *Am J Nurs* (August) 1978; 78:1375-1376.

Adelman EM: When the patient's blood pressure falls . . . . What does it mean? What should you do? *Nursing 80* (February) 1980; 10:26-33.

American Heart Association. *Recommendations for Human Blood Pressure Determination by Sphygmomanometers.* Pub No. 70-019-B, 80-100M, 9-81-100M. American Heart Association, 1980.

Axillary temps safer in infants. (Medical Highlights.) *Am J Nurs* (June) 1978; 78:1081.

Baker NC et al: The effect of type of thermometer and length of time inserted on oral temperature measurements of afebrile subjects. *Nurs Res* (March/April) 1984; 33:109-111.

Behrman RE, Vaughan VC III (editors): *Nelson Textbook of Pediatrics,* 12th ed. Saunders, 1983.

Blainey CG: Site selection in taking body temperature. *Am J Nurs* (October) 1974; 74:1859-1861.

Canetto V: T.P.R. q.4h. ad infinitum? *Am J Nurs* (November) 1964; 64:132.

Carpenito LJ: *Nursing Diagnosis: Application to Clinical Practice.* Lippincott, 1983.

Castle M, Watkins J: Fever: Understanding a sinister sign. *Nursing 79* (February) 1979; 9:26–33.

Correcting common errors in blood pressure measurement, programmed instruction. *Am J Nurs* (October) 1965; 65: 133–164.

Creative Care Unit: Turnabout: Rectal temperatures for postcoronary patients. *Am J Nurs* (June) 1977; 77:997.

Davis-Sharts J: Mechanisms and manifestations of fever. *Am J Nurs* (November) 1978; 78:1874–1877.

Eoff MJ, Joyce B: Temperature measurement in children. *Am J Nurs* (May) 1981; 81:1010–1011.

Eoff MJ, Meier RS, Miller C: Temperature measurement in infants. *Nurs Res* (November/December) 1974; 23:457–460.

Erickson R: Oral temperature differences in relation to thermometer and technique. *Nurs Res* (May/June) 1980; 29: 157–164.

Evans MJ: Tips for taking a child's blood pressure quickly. *Nursing 83* (March) 1983; 13:61.

Felton G: Effect of time cycle change on blood pressure and temperature in young women. *Nurs Res* (January/February) 1970; 19:48–58.

Graas S: Thermometer sites and oxygen. *Am J Nurs* (October) 1974; 74:1862–1863.

Graves RD, Markarian MF: Three-minute time intervals when using an oral mercury-in-glass thermometer without J-temperature sheaths. *Nurs Res* (September/October) 1980; 29; 323–324.

Hasler ME, Cohen JA: The effect of oxygen administration on temperature assessment. *Nurs Res* (September/October) 1982; 31:265–268.

Hill MN: Hypertension: What can go wrong when you measure blood pressure. *Am J Nurs* (May) 1980; 80:942–945.

Hudson B: Sharpen your vascular skills with the Doppler ultrasound stethoscope. *Nursing 83* (May) 1983; 13:55–57.

Jarvis CM: Vital signs: How to take them more accurately and understand them more fully. *Nursing 76* (April) 1976; 6: 31–37.

Kolanowski A, Gunter L: Hypothermia in the elderly. *Geriatr Nurs* (September/October) 1981; 2:362–365.

Lim-Levy F: The effect of oxygen inhalation on oral temperature. *Nurs Res* (May/June) 1982; 31:150–152.

National Heart, Lung, and Blood Institute. *The 1984 Report of the Joint National Committee on Detection, Evaluation, and Treatment of High Blood Pressure,* US Department of Health and Human Services, Public Health Service, National Institutes of Health, 1984. Reprinted from *Arch Intern Med* (May) 1984; 144:1045–1057.

National Heart, Lung, and Blood Institute, Task Force on Blood Pressure Control in Children: Report of the Task Force on Blood Pressure Control in Children. *Pediatrics* (May) 1977; 59 (Suppl):819–820.

Nichols GA: Taking adult temperatures: Rectal measurement. *Am J Nurs* (June) 1972; 72:1092–1093.

Nichols GA, Kucha DH: Taking adult temperatures: Oral measurement. *Am J Nurs* (June) 1972; 72:1090–1093.

Nichols GA, Verhonick PJ: Time and temperature. *Am J Nurs* (November) 1967; 67:2304–2306.

Nichols GA et al: Oral, axillary, and rectal temperature determinations and relationships. *Nurs Res* (Fall) 1966; 15:307–310.

Nursing Photobook Series: *Attending Ob/Gyn Patients.* Intermed Communications, 1982.

Patient assessment: Pulses, programmed instruction. *Am J Nurs* (January) 1979; 79:115–132.

Perfecting your blood pressure technique. *Nursing 84* (Canadian ed) (June) 1984; 14:17.

Purintun LR, Bishop BE: How accurate are clinical thermometers? *Am J Nurs* (January) 1969; 69:99–100.

Scharping EM: Physiologic measurements of the neonate. *Maternal Child Nurs* (January/February) 1983; 8:70–73.

Schiffman RF: Temperature monitoring in the neonate: A comparison of axillary and rectal temperatures. *Nurs Res* (September/October) 1982; 31:274–277.

Takacs KM, Valenti WM: For the research record: Perforation of the plastic thermometer sheaths. *Am J Nurs* (June) 1981; 81:1198.

Takacs KM, Valenti WM: Temperature measurement in a clinical setting. *Nurs Res* (November/December) 1982; 31:368–370.

Tate GV et al: Correct use of electric thermometers. *Am J Nurs* (September) 1970; 70:1898–1899.

Thompson LR: Thermometer disinfection. *Am J Nurs* (February) 1963; 63:113–115.

Warren FM: Blood pressure readings: Getting them quickly on an infant. *Nursing 75* (April) 1975; 5:13.

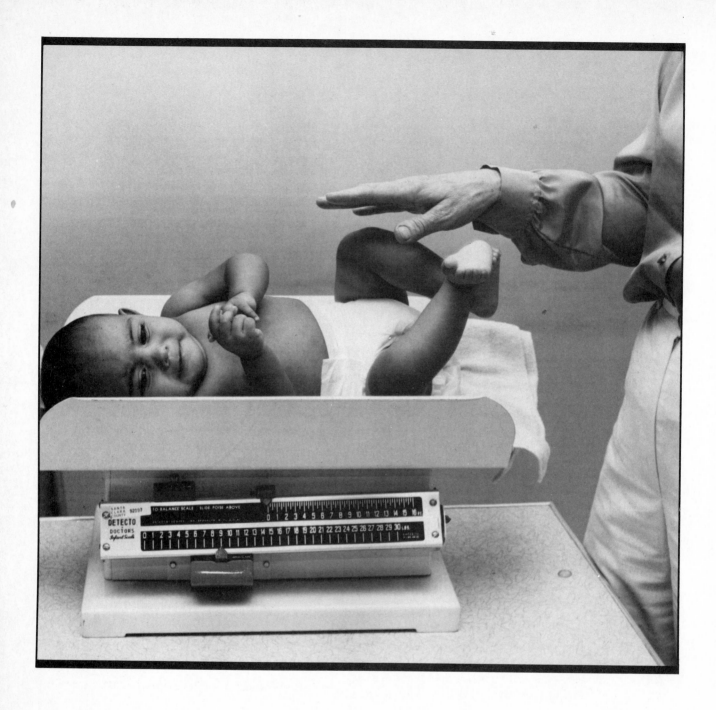

HEIGHT, WEIGHT, AND CIRCUMFERENCES

9

Height, weight, and head and chest circumferences are standard measurements that are frequently taken in health care agencies, schools, and homes. Recording the height and head and chest circumferences of an infant or growing child provides an index of normal or abnormal growth, while weight provides a general measure of health. However, these measurements vary considerably among individuals.

Adults have their weight and height measured at various times. Often an individual's stated height and weight are accepted as baseline data upon admission to a health agency. However, ill adults who have fluid and electrolyte problems and those who are obese are usually weighed initially and daily. Infants are generally weighed daily to assess their growth.

Height is measured less frequently, although this measurement is also extremely important in assessing the growth of infants and children. It is an essential

measurement, along with weight, to determine safe dosages of medications to give to infants and children. See chapters 29 and 30.

Head and chest circumferences of infants are evaluated at each health assessment visit to physicians or nurse practitioners to determine appropriate growth proportions between the two.

Chapter Outline

Height or Length
- Technique 9–1 Measuring the Height of a Child or Adult
- Technique 9–2 Measuring the Recumbent Length of an Infant

Weight
- Technique 9–3 Measuring the Weight of a Child or Adult

- Technique 9–4 Measuring the Weight of an Infant

Head and Chest Circumferences
- Technique 9–5 Measuring Head and Chest Circumferences

Objectives

Upon completion of this chapter, the student will:

1. Know essential terms and facts related to height, weight, and head and chest circumferences
   1.1 Define relevant terms and abbreviations
   1.2 Identify average heights of individuals of selected ages
   1.3 Identify average weights of individuals of selected ages
   1.4 Identify average head and chest circumferences of infants
   1.5 Identify causes of impaired growth and excessive growth
   1.6 Identify reasons for weight loss and weight gain
2. Understand facts about techniques used to measure body height, weight, and circumferences
   2.1 Identify relevant assessment data
   2.2 Identify nursing diagnoses for which the technique may be implemented
   2.3 Identify nursing goals related to the technique
   2.4 Identify expected and unexpected outcomes from assessment data
   2.5 Explain reasons underlying selected steps of the technique

3. Perform techniques for assessing body height, weight, and circumferences safely and accurately
   3.1 Assess the patient adequately
   3.2 Collect additional data from appropriate sources
   3.3 Select pertinent nursing goals for the patient
   3.4 Establish relevant outcome criteria for the patient following the technique
   3.5 Collect necessary equipment before the technique
   3.6 Implement interventions to enhance the effectiveness of the technique and enhance the patient's comfort and safety
   3.7 Communicate relevant information about the patient to the appropriate persons
   3.8 Determine the evaluative outcomes of the technique
4. Evaluate own performance of specific techniques in a laboratory or clinical setting with the assistance of another
   4.1 Use the performance checklists provided
   4.2 Identify areas of strength and weakness
   4.3 Alter performance in response to own evaluation and that of another

Terms

- habitus   the body build or body type; it can vary from the slender, wiry body to the heavy, soft body
- height   a vertical measurement extending from the highest point of the head to the surface on which the

individual is standing, normally measured in centimeters or inches

- hydrocephalus   Abnormal accumulation of fluid within the ventricular system of the brain; head enlargement

- microcephalus   very small head size
- recumbent length   the measurement from the soles of the feet to the vertex of the head while the individual is supine; it is often measured in centimeters for accuracy, although inches can also be used
- stature   the height or tallness of a person when standing

- vertex   the top of the head
- weight   the heaviness of a body or object, normally measured in kilograms or pounds

HEIGHT OR LENGTH

Developmental Variables

The average length of newborns in the United States is approximately 50 cm (20 in), with a range of 45 to 55 cm (18 to 22 in) (Behrman, Vaughan, 1983, p 13). The first growth spurt takes place between birth and 1 year of age. During the first six months of life, infants grow rapidly, adding about 15 cm (6 in); during the second six months, their length increases another 20 cm (8 in) or so. Between the first and second year, the average increase in height is 10 to 12 cm (4 to 5 in). After 2 years of age, the rate of growth slows. Preschool children grow on the average about 7.5 cm (3 in) per year. At 4 years of age the average height is 102 cm (40 in), double the birth length. At 6 years of age, both boys and girls are about 115 cm (46 in) tall. School-age children grow about 5 cm (2 in) per year until reaching an average height of 150 cm (59 in) by age 12. See Tables 9–1 and 9–2.

The second growth spurt occurs during adolescence. For boys, the maximum rate of growth takes place at about 14 years and the maximum height is reached at about 18 or 19 years. In their 20s some men add another 1 to 2 cm (0.3 to 0.8 in) to their height as the spinal column slowly continues to grow. Girls, on the other hand, have their fastest growth rate at about 12 years and reach their maximum height at about 15 or 16 years. This sex difference is the reason some adolescent girls are taller than boys of the same age, which is awkward socially for some.

Many factors influence physical growth:

1. Age (infant versus adult)
2. Sex (female versus male)

TABLE 9–1 ■ Length and Weight by Sex and Age, Birth to 24 Months

Sex	Age (mo)	Length Median Cm	Length Median In	Length 5th–95th percentiles Cm	Length 5th–95th percentiles In	Weight Median Kg	Weight Median Lb	Weight 5th–95th percentiles Kg	Weight 5th–95th percentiles Lb
Boys	Birth	50.5	20	46.4–54.4	18¼–21½	3.3	7¼	2.5–4.1	5½–9¼
	1	54.6	21½	50.4–58.6	19¾–23	4.3	9½	3.2–5.4	7–11¾
	3	61.1	24	56.7–65.4	22¼–25¾	5.9	13¼	4.4–7.4	9¾–16¼
	6	67.8	26¾	63.4–72.3	25–28½	7.8	17¼	6.2–9.5	13¾–20¾
	9	72.3	28½	68–77.1	26¾–30¼	9.2	20¼	7.5–10.9	16½–24
	12	76.1	30	71.7–81.2	28¼–32	10.1	22½	8.4–11.9	18½–26½
	18	82.4	32½	77.5–88.1	30½–34¾	11.5	25¼	9.6–13.4	21¼–29½
	24	87.6	34½	82.3–93.8	32½–37	12.6	27¾	10.5–14.7	23¼–32½
Girls	Birth	49.9	19¾	45.4–52.9	17¾–20¾	3.2	7	2.4–3.8	5¼–8½
	1	53.5	21	49.2–56.9	19¼–22½	3.9	8¾	2.9–4.9	6½–10¾
	3	59.5	23½	55.4–63.4	21¾–25	5.4	12	4.2–6.7	9¼–14¾
	6	65.9	26	61.8–70.2	24¼–27¾	7.2	16	5.8–8.7	12¾–19¼
	9	70.4	27¾	66.1–75	26–29½	8.6	18¾	7–10.2	15½–22½
	12	74.3	29¼	69.8–79.1	27½–31¼	9.5	21	7.8–11.2	17¼–24¾
	18	80.9	31¾	76.0–86.1	30–34	10.8	23¾	8.9–12.8	19¾–28¼
	24	86.5	34	81.3–92.0	32–36¼	11.9	26¼	9.9–14.1	21¾–31

Source: Adapted from RE Behrman, VC Vaughan III (editors): *Nelson Textbook of Pediatrics,* 12th ed, Saunders, 1983, p 27.

TABLE 9-2 ■ Height and Weight by Sex and Age, 3 to 18 Years

Sex	Age (yr)	Height Median Cm	Median In	5th–95th percentiles Cm	5th–95th percentiles In	Weight Median Kg	Median Lb	5th–95th percentiles Kg	5th–95th percentiles Lb
Boys	3	94.9	37¼	89–102	35–40½	14.6	32¼	12.1–17.8	26½–39¼
	4	102.9	40½	95.8–109.9	37¾–43¼	16.7	36¾	13.6–20.3	30–44¾
	5	109.9	43¼	102–117	40¼-46	18.7	41¼	15.3–23.1	33¾–51
	6	116.1	45¾	107.7–123.5	42½–48½	20.7	45½	16.9–26.3	37¼–58
	7	121.7	48	113–129.7	44½–51	22.8	50¼	18.6–30.1	41–66½
	8	127	50	118.1–135.7	46½–53½	25.3	55¾	20.4–34.5	45–76
	9	132.2	52	122.9–141.8	48½–55¾	28.1	62	22.2–39.6	49–87¾
	10	137.5	54¼	127.7–148.1	50¼–58¼	31.4	69¼	24.3–45.3	53¾–99¾
	11	143.3	56½	132.6–154.9	52¼–61	35.3	77¾	26.8–51.5	59–113½
	12	149.7	59	137.6–162.3	54¼–64	39.8	87¾	29.8–58.1	65¾–128
	13	156.5	61½	142.9–169.8	56¼–66¾	44.9	99	33.6–65	74¼–143¼
	14	163.1	64¼	148.8–176.7	58½–69½	50.8	112	38.2–72.1	84¼–159
	15	169	66½	155.2–181.9	61–71½	56.7	125	43.1–79.1	95–174½
	16	173.5	68¼	161.1–185.4	63½–73	62.1	137	47.7–85.6	105¼–188¾
	17	176.2	69¼	164.9–187.3	65–73¾	66.3	146¼	51.5–91.3	113½–201¼
	18	176.8	69½	165.7–187.6	65¼–73¾	68.8	151¾	53.9–95.8	119–211
Girls	3	94.1	37	88.3–100.6	34¾–39½	14.1	31	11.6–17.2	25½–38
	4	101.6	40	95–108.3	37½–42¾	15.9	35¼	13.1–19.9	29–44
	5	108.4	42¾	101.1–115.6	39¾–45½	17.7	39	14.5–22.6	32–49¾
	6	114.6	45	106.6–122.7	42–48¼	19.5	43	16.1–25.7	35½–56¾
	7	120.6	47½	111.8–129.5	44–51	21.8	48¼	17.7–29.7	39–65½
	8	126.4	49¾	116.9–136.2	46–53½	24.8	49¾	19.6–34.7	43¼–76½
	9	132.2	52	122.1–142.9	48–56¼	28.5	62¾	21.8–40.6	48–89½
	10	138.3	54½	127.5–149.5	50¼–58¾	32.5	71¾	24.4–47.2	53¾–104
	11	144.8	57	133.5–156.2	52½–61½	36.9	81½	27.2–54	60–119
	12	151.5	59¾	139.8–162.7	55–64	41.5	91½	30.5–60.8	67¼–134
	13	157.1	61¾	145.2–168.1	57¼–66¼	46.1	101¾	34.1–67.3	75¼–148¼
	14	160.4	63¼	148.7–171.3	58½–67½	50.3	110¾	37.8–73.1	83¼–161
	15	161.8	63¾	150.5–172.8	59¼–68	53.7	118¼	40.9–77.8	90¼–171½
	16	162.4	64	151.6–173.3	59¾–68¼	55.9	123¼	43.4–80.9	95¾–178½
	17	163.1	64¼	152.7–173.5	60–68¼	56.7	125	44.7–82.5	98¾–181¾
	18	163.7	64½	153.6–173.6	60½–68¼	56.6	124¾	45.3–82.5	99¾–181¾

Source: Adapted from RE Behrman, VC Vaughan III (editors): *Nelson Textbook of Pediatrics,* 12th ed, Saunders, 1983, pp 30, 31.

3. Race (Oriental, Caucasian, etc)

4. Heredity (short parents, tall parents)

5. Nutrition

6. Illness

7. Medical care

8. Physical and emotional environments

Generally, the average heights of people in the United States and Canada have increased in recent years. This is thought to be due largely to nutrition.

Common Problems

Impaired growth

Shortness of stature and dwarfism occur for a variety of reasons. Functionally, failure to grow can be classified according to four major causes:

1. Abnormal regulation of the endocrine glands

2. Genetic defects

3. Nutritional factors

4. Chronic inflammation

The three major endocrine glands that affect growth are the pituitary gland, which produces growth hormone, the thyroid gland, and the adrenal gland. Growth failures occur if the pituitary gland produces insufficient growth hormone, if the thyroid gland produces insufficient amounts of its hormone thyroxine (hypothyroidism), and if the adrenal glands produce excessive amounts of corticosteroids (hyperadrenocorticism). Large amounts of corticosteroids block the release of growth hormone by the pituitary gland. In addition, conditions that affect the hypothalamus can retard growth since the hypothalamus produces a growth hormone releasing factor that is essential for stimulating the pituitary gland to produce its growth hormone. Because the hypothalamus is readily influenced by emotions, it is thought that very disturbed children who are deprived of affection may exhibit impaired growth. When these children are moved to more secure and loving surroundings they undergo a "catch-up" growth spurt.

Persons with Down's syndrome (mongolism) and the pygmies of Africa manifest two common genetic conditions that produce impaired growth. These people have normal amounts of the growth hormones but specific genes in their cells prevent the normal response of growth.

Severe dietary deficiencies of calories, essential proteins, vitamins, or minerals can also impair growth.

In infants and children who have congenital heart disease and suffer from inadequate oxygen to the tissues, growth failure is also evident until the problem is corrected. Some chronic diseases, eg, juvenile rheumatoid arthritis and chronic kidney disease, are another cause of growth failure.

Excessive growth

Most cases of excessive tallness are the result of augmented nutrition and an increased response of tissue cells to growth hormones. Gigantism due to excessive growth hormones is very rare.

TECHNIQUE 9–1 ■ Measuring the Height of a Child or Adult

Height is measured starting at the age when children can stand. It is measured in centimeters or in feet and inches, depending on the agency's practice.

■ Assessment

Assess the patient for appropriateness of stature. This includes:

1. The midpoint of the stature. For the newborn it is approximately at the umbilicus; for the adult it is at the symphysis pubis.
2. The ratio of sitting height to total body height. This decreases with age until the extremities stop growing. In the newborn, sitting height is about 70% of body length; in the 3-year-old, about 57%; in girls at the time of menarche, and in boys at age 15, about 52%. The sitting height then increases a few percentage points, since the trunk continues to grow slightly after the extremities have completed growth.

Additional data include:

1. Whether the patient's height can be measured in a standing position and/or whether assistance is required.
2. The preferred time for taking this measurement, eg, after an analgesic has taken effect.
3. The normal standing height. See Tables 9–2 (earlier) and 9–3.

■ Nursing Diagnosis

Nursing diagnoses that may indicate the need to assess a patient's height include:

1. Alteration in nutrition: less than body requirements, related to lack of knowledge of adequate nutrition

2. Potential disturbance in self-concept related to inadequate body size

■ Planning

Nursing goals

1. To ascertain whether normal growth has taken place.
2. To relate an individual's height to his or her weight. See Tables 9–1 to 9–3 for average heights and weights from birth to adulthood.
3. To ascertain the size of orthopedic appliances required for patients.
4. To acquire baseline data against which future measurements can be compared.

Equipment

1. A measuring stick. Some weight scales have a built-in measuring stick. There are also measuring sticks that can be placed against or attached to a wall.
2. A protector on which the patient stands, to prevent the spread of microorganisms.
3. A ruler, book, or measuring square.

■ Intervention

1. Assist the patient to the appropriate place for measurement, and help the patient to remove shoes or slippers.
2. Assist the patient to stand on the clean protector with her or his back against the measuring stick. The patient stands erect with heels together, with heels, buttocks, and occiput (back of the head) against the

measuring stick, and with eyes looking straight ahead.

3. Place the ruler, book, or measuring square on top of the patient's head at a right angle to the measuring stick. See Figure 9-1.

4. Determine the point on the measuring stick to which the bottom side of the ruler or book comes.

5. Assist the patient to put on shoes or slippers and to resume activity or to assume a comfortable position in bed.

6. Discard the protector in the waste container.

   Rationale The protector will possess microorganisms from the patient that could be transmitted to others.

7. Record the patient's height in the appropriate place. Heights are often recorded on the graphic sheet.

■ Evaluation

Expected outcome

A height appropriate for the patient's age, nutritional status, health, and therapy.

Unexpected outcome

A height greater or less than the anticipated height for the patient. Upon obtaining an unexpected outcome:

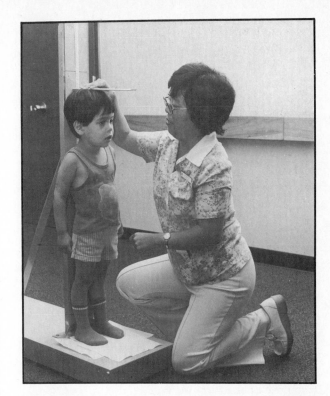

FIGURE 9-1

1. Remeasure the patient's height to verify the results.
2. Report your findings to the responsible nurse.

TABLE 9-3 ■ 1983 Metropolitan Height and Weight Tables, Men and Women, Ages 25 to 59

Men				Women			
	Weight (lb)				Weight (lb)		
Height	Small frame	Medium frame	Large frame	Height	Small frame	Medium frame	Large frame
5' 2"	128–134	131–141	138–150	4'10"	102–111	109–121	118–131
5' 3"	130–136	133–143	140–153	4'11"	103–113	111–123	120–134
5' 4"	132–138	135–145	142–156	5' 0"	104–115	113–126	122–137
5' 5"	134–140	137–148	144–160	5' 1"	106–118	115–129	125–140
5' 6"	136–142	139–151	146–164	5' 2"	108–121	118–132	128–143
5' 7"	138–145	142–154	149–168	5' 3"	111–124	121–135	131–147
5' 8"	140–148	145–157	152–172	5' 4"	114–127	124–138	134–151
5' 9"	142–151	148–160	155–176	5' 5"	117–130	127–141	137–155
5'10"	144–154	151–163	158–180	5' 6"	120–133	130–144	140–159
5'11"	146–157	154–166	161–184	5' 7"	123–136	133–147	143–163
6' 0"	149–160	157–170	164–188	5' 8"	126–139	136–150	146–167
6' 1"	152–164	160–174	168–192	5' 9"	129–142	139–153	149–170
6' 2"	155–168	164–178	172–197	5'10"	132–145	142–156	152–173
6' 3"	158–172	167–182	176–202	5'11"	135–148	145–159	155–176
6' 4"	162–176	171–187	181–207	6' 0"	138–151	148–162	158–179

Source of basic data: *1979 Build Study,* Society of Actuaries and Association of Life Insurance Medical Directors of America, 1980. Courtesy Metropolitan Life Insurance Company.

Weights at ages 25–59 based on lowest mortality.

Weight in indoor clothing weighing 5 lb for men, 3 lb for women; height in shoes with 1" heels.

TECHNIQUE 9-2 ■ Measuring the Recumbent Length of an Infant

Until an infant can stand alone, the recumbent length of the child is measured.

■ Assessment

1. See Technique 9-1 on page 142.
2. Assess the symmetry of body development, eg, the length of each leg.
3. Determine whether the infant's legs can straighten for the measurement.

■ Nursing Diagnosis   See Technique 9-1 on page 142.

■ Planning

Nursing goals

1. To ascertain whether normal growth has taken place.
2. To relate the infant's length to his or her weight. See Table 9-1 earlier.
3. To ascertain the child's length, which is used with the weight to calculate the body surface area and thus some medication dosages.

Equipment

1. A measuring board or a measure, usually calibrated in centimeters. The centimeter measure facilitates accuracy.
2. A brace for the feet, eg, a box, if a measuring board is not available.
3. A ruler or measuring square.
4. A clean protector for the scale.

■ Intervention

1. Explain the procedure to the accompanying adults.
   Rationale By explaining, the nurse reassures the adults.
2. Remove the infant's shoes. It is unnecessary to undress the infant, but remove any bulky outdoor clothing so that the infant can lie horizontally with the knees extended.
3. Reassure the infant with a soothing voice and gentle, sure movements.
4. Place a clean protector on the measuring surface.

Rationale This protects the infant from microorganisms present on the measuring board.

5. Place the infant supine on the measuring surface parallel to the measuring rule. Do not leave the infant, because he or she may roll off. The measuring surface must be firm to make an accurate measurement.
6. Hold the infant's head facing the ceiling, and press the top of the head against an upright structure that is at point zero on the measuring rule.
7. Make sure that the infant's knees are extended.
8. Place the ruler or measuring square against the soles of the feet at a right angle to the measuring board. See Figure 9-2.
9. Determine the point on the measuring board to which the ruler or measuring square comes.
10. Take the infant off the measuring surface.
11. Put shoes and any clothes removed back on the infant, and put him or her in a safe place.
12. Discard the protector in the waste container.
13. Record the infant's length in the appropriate place.

■ Evaluation   See Technique 9-1 on page 143.

FIGURE 9-2

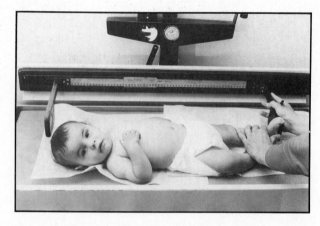

WEIGHT

Developmental Variables

At birth, most babies weigh 2.5 to 4.6 kg (5½ to 10 lb) (Behrman, Vaughan, 1983, p 13). The average birth weight of White American male babies is 3.4 kg (7½ lb) and of female babies is 3.2 kg (7 lb). The weights of newborns of Black, Oriental, and Native American origin are on the average lower. During the first few days of life, newborns normally lose about 10% of their birth weight due to fluid loss. However, after the first week a steady weight gain ensues.

By 6 months of age, the birth weight has doubled; by 12 months it has tripled; and by 2 years it has quadrupled. At 3 years of age, toddlers weigh about 15 kg (33 lb), and, by 5 years, children weigh 18 to 20 kg (40 to 45 lb). The average gain per year by preschoolers is about 2.2 kg (5 lb). During the school years, children add an average of 2.7 to 3.2 kg (6 to 7 lb) per year, until at age 12 they weigh approximately 40 kg (90 lb). See Table 9–2 on page 141. During the adolescent growth spurt between ages 12 and 18, boys increase their weight about 25 kg (55 lb), while girls gain about 15 kg (35 lb). At the end of adolescence, weight generally stabilizes until the middle years of life, when weight tends to increase. Table 9–3 indicates suggested adult weights for health (weights of the lowest mortality) according to height and body frame.

Common Problems

Weight deficit

Weight deficit results from insufficient intake of one or more nutrients required to meet metabolic needs (eg, protein, vitamins, iron). The following signs may indicate insufficient nutrient intake and weight:

1. Weight 20% or more under the ideal for the patient's height and frame
2. Loss of weight with adequate food intake
3. Food intake less than that recommended by food guides, or evidence of lack of food
4. Eating difficulties
5. Gastrointestinal signs, such as abdominal pain, cramping, diarrhea, and hyperactive bowel sounds
6. Muscle weakness and reduced energy level
7. Excessive loss of hair
8. Pallor of skin, mucous membranes, and conjunctiva

A very severe protein deficit results in kwashiorkor, a disease seen in many Eastern undernourished populations. It is characterized by retarded growth and development; mental apathy; extreme muscular wasting, which may be masked by edema; depigmentation of the hair and skin; and scaly changes in skin texture.

Obesity

Obesity is the result of calorie intake that exceeds metabolic need. It is evidenced by weight 20% greater than the ideal for the patient's height and frame and by triceps skin folds greater than 15 mm in men and 25 mm in women (Kim, Moritz, 1982, p 300). *Overweight* refers to weight 10% greater than the ideal for the patient's height and frame (White, Schroeder, 1981, p 550). Obesity is currently one of the most prevalent health problems in North America. It is associated with hypertension, cardiovascular diseases, and diabetes. Factors contributing to obesity include:

1. Sedentary habits (low activity level)
2. Inappropriate eating patterns (eg, eating large amounts of carbohydrates and saturated fats)
3. Depression or anxiety (often accompanied by stressors such as a death in the family or a change in marital or work status)
4. Eating the largest meal at the end of the day

Factors placing a person at risk for obesity may include sedentary habits, genetic predisposition, obesity in one or both parents, and a pattern of excessive food intake in early infancy and childhood.

Types of Scales

The following types of scales are used to weigh adults and children:

1. *Standing scale.* This requires the patient to stand on a small platform. It may have wheels to facilitate moving the scale. The standing upright balance scale (gravity) has two calibrated arms: the lower one has the larger weight demarcations, eg, 50, 100, 150, 200 lb, or 25, 50, 75, 100 kg. The upper arm measures smaller weight variations, eg, eighths of a pound, or tenths of a kilogram. When the scale is balanced, the patient's weight is the sum of the weights on both arms.

Another type of standing scale uses multiple weights. Weights are added to a balance arm until it falls. The main arm is then adjusted using smaller weights, until it balances. The weight of the patient is the sum of the weight on the main arm and the smaller weights.

A third type of standing scale has a digital display panel. On some types a button is pressed before the patient stands on the scale. The weight is reflected on a panel in either pounds or kilograms.

2. *Bed scale.* There are several types of bed scales for patients who cannot stand. Figure 9–3 shows one. These scales have either canvas straps or a stretcherlike apparatus. A machine lifts the patient 5 cm (2 in) above the

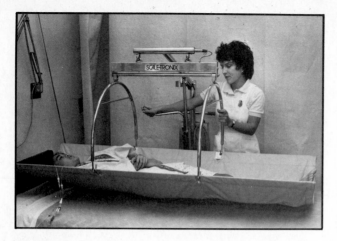

FIGURE 9–3 ■ A bed scale.

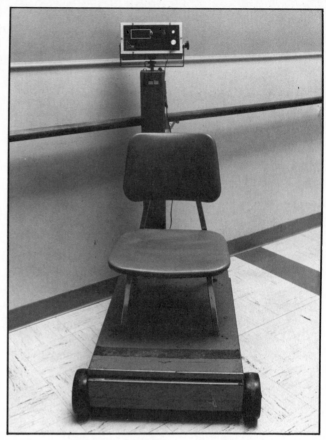

FIGURE 9–4 ■ A chair scale.

surface of the bed, and the weight is reflected either on a digital display panel or on a balance arm like that on a standing scale.

3. *Chair scale.* In this device the patient sits on a chair attached to a scale. See Figure 9–4. The scale may have a balance arm or a digital display panel to indicate the patient's weight.

4. *Tray scale.* A number of types of tray scales are available. Hospitals frequently use balanced weight scales with a tray or basket container for weighing infants. Some scales are portable and easily taken by community nurses to the home.

TECHNIQUE 9–3 ■ Measuring the Weight of a Child or Adult

Weight is often measured on a patient's admission to a health agency. The weight of some patients is measured regularly, eg, each morning before breakfast. This regular weighing is usually done for obese patients on reducing diets or for patients who retain excess fluid (edema).

Weight is measured in kilograms or pounds. A person who weighs 100 lb is calculated to weigh 45.45 kg, as follows:

$$2.2 \text{ lb} = 1 \text{ kg}$$
$$100 \text{ lb} = \frac{100 \text{ kg}}{2.2}$$
$$100 \text{ lb} = 45.45 \text{ kg}$$

A person who weighs 80 kg is calculated to weigh 176 lb, as follows:

$$2.2 \text{ lb} = 1 \text{ kg}$$
$$x \text{ lb} = 80 \text{ kg}$$
$$x = 80 \times 2.2$$
$$x = 176 \text{ lb}$$

■ **Assessment**

Assess the patient for:

1. Appearance of being overweight or underweight
2. Presence of edema

Additional data include:

1. The time to weigh the patient, if the patient is being weighed regularly. It is important that regular weighings be done at the same time each day so that the weights can be reliably compared. The weight of some people varies considerably during the 24-hour period. In some hospitals weights are measured in the early morning, before the patient has breakfast and dresses.

2. The type of scale the patient requires, whether the patient can stand on a scale, and the amount of assistance he or she requires.

3. Baseline data for weight and/or recent weight measurements.

■ Nursing Diagnosis

Nursing diagnoses that may indicate the need to assess a patient's weight include:

1. Alteration in nutrition (more than body requirements) related to:
    a. Stress
    b. Depression
    c. Sedentary life-style
    d. Decreased activity patterns
    e. Decreased metabolic needs
2. Alteration in nutrition (less than body requirements) related to:
    a. Absorptive disorder
    b. Anorexia
    c. Inability to procure food
    d. Crash or fad diet
    e. Chewing or swallowing difficulty
3. Actual or potential fluid volume excess related to:
    a. Decreased cardiac output
    b. Liver disease
    c. Steroid therapy
    d. Excessive sodium intake
4. Activity intolerance related to:
    a. Lack of motivation
    b. Sedentary life-style
    c. Malnourishment
    d. Congestive heart failure
5. Alteration in cardiac output (decreased) related to:
    a. Congestive heart failure
    b. Chronic obstructive pulmonary disease

■ Planning

Nursing goals

1. To assess the growth and development of children
2. To determine whether a patient is overweight or underweight
3. To assess the effectiveness of a diet or a medication such as a diuretic
4. To determine baseline data essential for calculating medication dosages

Equipment

1. A suitable scale (see Types of Scales, earlier).

2. A protector for the scale, eg, for a standing scale a clean paper towel on which the patient can stand. When a canvas sling or chair is used, it should be protected by a plastic cover that can be readily cleaned after use.

■ Intervention

1. Place the scale next to the patient's bed or assist the patient to the location of the scale.
2. Lock the wheels of the scale to prevent it from slipping.
3. Provide privacy as necessary for the patient. Patients do not usually undress, but, if repeated weighings are done, the patient should wear a similar amount of clothing each time. In a hospital, patients usually wear their hospital gowns or pajamas. Patients usually remove shoes or slippers before being weighed.
4. Place a paper protector on the platform of a standing scale.
    Rationale   The protector prevents the transfer of microorganisms from the scale to the feet, when several people are using the same scale.
5. Check that the scale registers zero. Adjust it, if necessary.

For a standing scale

6. Assist the patient onto the scale. Make sure the patient is not leaning on the bed or holding a chair. If the patient is unsteady, remain nearby to assist. Be sure the patient stands on the center of the platform.
    Rationale   Standing in the center is necessary both for accurate measurement and for safety.
7. Read the weight on the dial or adjust the counterbalance to obtain the patient's weight. Determine whether the scale is in pounds or kilograms.
8. Assist the patient off the scale. Dispose of the paper protector in the waste container.
9. Record the patient's weight on the chart.

For a bed scale

10. Check the manufacturer's instructions.
11. Adjust the scale stretcher to a horizontal position, and lock it in place.
12. Turn the patient to a lateral position, with her or his back toward the scale.
13. Roll the base of the scale under the bed; widen the base (if adjustable).
    Rationale   The wider base provides maximum stability.

14. Lock the wheels.

15. Lower the stretcher onto the bed so that it is centered on the bed.

16. Roll the patient onto the stretcher.

17. Move the weighing arms over the patient and attach them securely to the stretcher.

18. Gradually pump the handle to raise the patient 5 cm (2 in) above the bed surface. Pump slowly and evenly to avoid jerking the patient.

19. Ensure that the stretcher is not touching any part of the bed or its attachments.
    Rationale Touching any equipment will affect the reading of the weight.

20. Press the button (on a digital scale) to display the weight. Adjust the counterbalance on a balance scale or refer to the dial on a dial scale.

21. After observing the weight registered, lower the patient gradually to the bed using the pump handle.

22. Detach the stretcher from the arms.

23. Roll the patient off the stretcher.

24. Remove the stretcher, and assist the patient to a comfortable position.

25. Release the lock on the wheels. Clean the scale and return it to storage with the stretcher in the vertical position.

26. Record the weight on the patient's chart.

For a chair scale

27. Check the manufacturer's instructions.

28. Position the chair scale beside the patient, and lock the wheels.

29. If the side arm nearest the patient moves, unlock it, and move it away from the chair.
    Rationale This can facilitate the patient's transfer.

30. Transfer the patient onto the chair of the scale.

31. Return the arm, and lock it in place.
    Rationale The arm provides additional security for the patient.

32. Adjust the counterbalances or read the digital display.

33. Unlock the chair arm, and transfer the patient back to the bed or a wheelchair.

34. Unlock the wheels, lock the balance arm, clean the scale, and return it to storage.
    Rationale An unlocked balance arm can be damaged during movement.

35. Record the weight on the patient's chart.

■ Evaluation

Expected outcome

A weight appropriate for the patient's age, nutritional status, health, and therapy.

Unexpected outcome

A weight greater or less than the anticipated weight for the patient. Upon obtaining an unexpected outcome:

1. Determine that the scale was balanced and in good working order.

2. Reassess the patient's weight to verify the results.

3. If the weight was greater than anticipated, assess the patient for edema.

4. If the weight was greater than anticipated, determine the balance between fluid intake and output.

5. Report your findings to the responsible nurse and/or physician.

TECHNIQUE 9–4 ■ Measuring the Weight of an Infant

■ Assessment

Assess the infant for:

1. General nutritional status, eg, thin, obese
2. Any skin abnormalities, such as irritations, rashes, or bruises

For additional data, see Technique 9–3, items 1 and 3, on pages 146 and 147.

■ Nursing Diagnosis See Technique 9–3 on page 147.

■ Planning

Nursing goals

1. To determine the weight of an infant for baseline data.

2. To assess an infant's growth, health, and nutritional needs. See Table 9–1 earlier.

3. To ascertain the weight, to use with the length to calculate the body surface area, for some medication dosages.

Equipment

1. A scale with a tray. See Figure 9–5.

2. A paper protector to cover the tray before placing the infant on it. Some agencies use a special sterile paper that does not allow fluids such as urine to seep through and contaminate the scale.

■ Intervention

1. Remove the infant's clothing. In most instances the infant's naked weight is taken. Often the infant's weight is measured in association with hygienic care. If for some reason an infant cannot be unclothed at the time, the clothes are later weighed separately, and that weight is deducted from the earlier weight to determine the infant's naked weight.

2. Reassure the infant with a soothing voice and gentle, sure movements.

3. Drape the scale tray with the paper protector.
   Rationale   The protector prevents the transfer of microorganisms from one infant to another using the same scale.

4. Check that the scale registers zero, and adjust it if necessary.

5. Gently lift and place the infant on the tray.

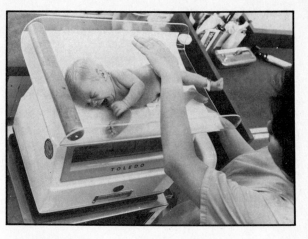

FIGURE 9–5

6. Hold one hand about an inch above but not touching the baby. See Figure 9–5. Use the other hand to adjust the scale. Never leave an infant unattended.
   Rationale   The nurse holds one hand over the baby for safety reasons but avoids touching the baby because this would distort the weight measurement.

7. Determine the weight.

8. Clothe the infant and return her or him to the crib.

9. Discard the paper protector in the waste container.

10. Record the infant's weight on the appropriate record. In most agencies the weight is recorded on a special flow sheet.

■ **Evaluation**   See Technique 9–3 on page 148.

HEAD AND CHEST CIRCUMFERENCES

The head circumference of the newborn is about 34 to 35 cm (13 to 14 in) (Behrman, Vaughan, 1983, p 16). It is normally 1 to 2 cm larger than the chest until after the first year of life. One exception occurs during the first 24 hours of life, when head molding from delivery may create a slightly smaller head circumference than that of the chest. A molded head contour returns to normal within 48 to 72 hours.

By 6 months of age, head circumference increases to about 44 cm (17 in) and by 1 year to about 46 cm (18 in). See Table 9–4. By 1 year of age, the head and chest circumferences are approximately equal. In comparison to the sizable 12 cm (4 in) increase in head circumference in the first year, the second year increase is minimal— about 2.3 cm (0.9 in)—since brain growth decelerates. By the end of the first year, the brain has reached about two thirds of its adult size and, by the end of the second year, four fifths. Chest growth begins to exceed head size during early childhood, until the head is 5 to 7 cm (2 to 2.75 in) smaller than the chest.

Common Problems

When head growth is greater than normal, hydrocephalus, intracranial bleeding, or a brain tumor may be suspected. *Hydrocephalus* is the abnormal accumulation of fluid in the ventricular system of the brain. It is also known as *water on the brain*. Enlargement occurs as a result of an imbalance between production and absorption of cerebrospinal fluid (CSF). This condition is characterized by enlargement of the head, prominence of the forehead, elevated CSF pressure, atrophy of the brain, mental deterioration, and convulsions. It may be acquired or congenital, and slowly progressive or sudden in onset. Infants with a rapid, progressive hydrocephalus have a

TABLE 9-4 ■ Median Head Circumferences, by Sex, Birth to 36 Months

Age (mo)	Boys				Girls			
	Median		5th–95th percentiles		Median		5th–95th percentiles	
	Cm	In	Cm	In	Cm	In	Cm	In
Birth	34.8	13.7	32.6–37.2	12.8–14.7	34.3	13.5	32.1–35.9	12.6–14.1
1	37.2	14.7	34.9–39.6	13.7–15.6	36.4	14.3	34.2–38.3	13.5–15.1
3	40.6	16.0	38.4–43.1	15.1–17.0	39.5	15.6	37.3–41.7	14.7–16.4
6	43.8	17.2	41.5–46.2	16.3–18.2	42.4	16.7	40.3–44.6	15.9–17.6
9	45.8	18.0	43.5–48.1	17.1–18.9	44.3	17.4	42.3–46.4	16.7–18.3
12	47.0	18.5	44.8–49.3	17.6–19.4	45.6	18.0	43.5–47.6	17.1–18.7
18	48.4	19.1	46.3–50.6	18.2–19.9	47.1	18.5	45.0–49.1	17.7–19.3
24	49.2	19.4	47.3–51.4	18.6–20.2	48.1	18.9	46.1–50.1	18.2–19.7
30	49.9	19.7	48.0–52.2	18.9–20.6	48.8	19.2	47.0–50.8	18.5–20.0
36	50.5	19.9	48.6–52.8	19.1–20.8	49.3	19.4	47.6–51.4	18.8–20.2

Source: Adapted from RE Behrman, VC Vaughan III (editors): *Nelson Textbook of Pediatrics,* 12th ed, Saunders, 1983, p 17. Data from Health Survey of National Center for Health Statistics, 1976.

large, bulging frontal (anterior) fontanelle and palpable separation of cranial sutures. See Figure 9–6 for the location of skull sutures and fontanelles.

When head growth is less than normal, microcephalus or premature closure of the sutures may be suspected. *Microcephalus,* less common than hydrocephalus, is a very small head size in relation to the rest of the body and is usually associated with mental retardation. Micro-cephalus is a defect in the growth of the brain as a whole. *Premature closure* of one or more sutures of the skull results in deformities of the head. For example, with premature closure of the sagittal suture, the head becomes long and narrow; with closure of the coronal sutures, the top of the head becomes pointed (steeple head), and facial deformities occur. Depending on which skull suture is involved, damage to the brain and the eyes may result.

FIGURE 9–6 ■ The bones of the skull, showing the fontanelles and suture lines.

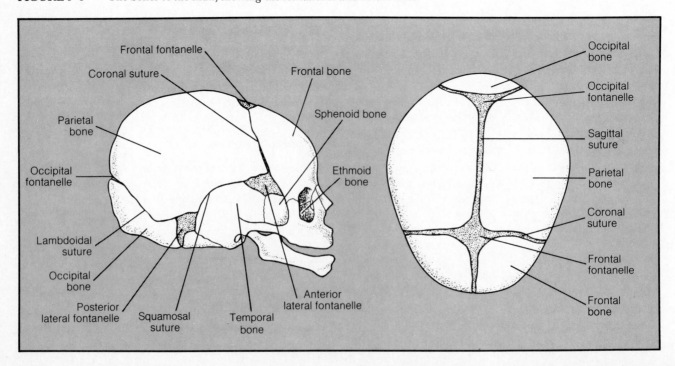

TECHNIQUE 9–5   ■   Measuring Head and Chest Circumferences

Head and chest circumferences are measured regularly during health care visits for the first 2 years of life and then at least twice a year up to 3 years of age or at any initial physical examination for children at any age, if indicated.

■ Assessment

Assess the infant for:

1. Smaller or larger head circumference than expected for the age of the infant.
2. Head circumference disproportionate to chest circumference.
3. Skull symmetry and any bulges on the scalp or skull.
4. Closure of fontanelles earlier or later than scheduled. Generally the frontal (anterior) fontanelle closes between 9 and 18 months; the occipital (posterior) fontanelle by 4 months (Behrman, Vaughan, 1983, p 16). The fontanelles are felt as soft concavities.
5. Fontanelles with diameters larger than 5 or 6 cm (2 or 2.4 in). At birth, the frontal fontanelle measures 4 to 6 cm (1.6 to 2.4 in) in its largest diameter; the occipital fontanelle is 1 to 2 cm (0.4 to 0.8 in).
6. Palpable overriding suture lines or widely separated suture lines. Sutures are normally felt as slightly depressed ridges. These usually flatten so that they are not palpable by 6 months of age.

Additional data include: baseline head and chest circumferences and/or recent measurements.

■ Planning

Nursing goal

To ascertain whether normal growth has taken place.

Equipment

A measuring tape. A steel or disposable paper tape is preferred, since cloth tape stretches with age. When a cloth tape is used, check it against a wooden or steel standard first.

■ Intervention

Head circumference

1. Reassure the infant with a soothing voice and gentle, sure movements.
2. Place the infant in a recumbent position.
3. Place the tape under the infant's head.
4. Apply the tape snugly around the greatest circumference of the head:
   a. Posteriorly at the level of the occipital protuberances.
   b. Anteriorly at the midforehead level just above the eyebrows.
5. If the head has an abnormal shape, as in hydrocephalus, position the tape over whatever points on the forehead or occiput give the greatest circumference.
6. Record the head circumference on the appropriate record.

Chest circumference

7. Place the infant in a recumbent position on a firm surface, eg, a crib or examining table.
8. Place the tape under the infant's back.
9. Apply the tape snugly around the chest at the level of the xiphoid cartilage (at the nipple line) and at right angles to the spinal column. Make sure the tape is at the same level in the front and back.
10. Record the chest circumference on the appropriate record.

■ Evaluation

Anticipated outcome

Head and chest circumferences appropriate for the patient's age and in appropriate proportion to each other

Unanticipated outcomes

1. A head circumference too small or too large for the patient's age
2. Head circumference disproportionate to chest circumference

Upon obtaining an unanticipated outcome:

1. Remeasure the patient's head and chest circumferences to verify the results.
2. Report your findings to the responsible nurse and/or physician.

References

Behrman RE, Vaughan VC III: *Nelson Textbook of Pediatrics,* 12th ed. Saunders, 1983.

Bowers AC, Thompson JM: *Clinical Manual of Health Assessment,* 2nd ed. Mosby, 1984.

Kim MJ, Moritz DA (editors): *Classification of Nursing Diagnoses: Proceedings of the Third and Fourth National Conferences.* McGraw-Hill, 1982.

White JH, Schroeder MA: When your client has a weight problem: Nursing assessment. *Am J Nurs* (March) 1981; 81:550–552.

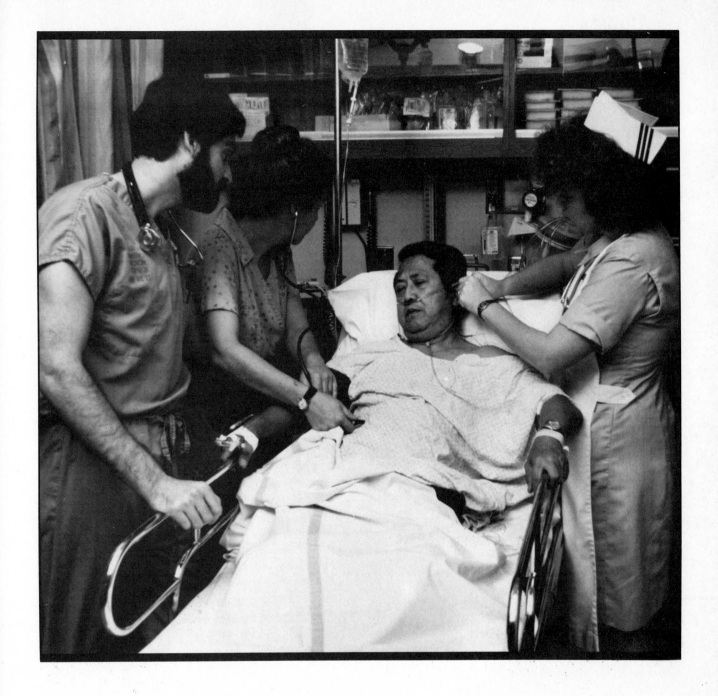

HEALTH ASSESSMENT OF THE ADULT

10

An assessment of a patient's health encompasses both physical and psychosocial aspects. It is also adjusted to the patient's needs. A health assessment may be (a) a complete assessment, eg, on admission to a health agency; (b) an assessment of a body system, eg, the cardiovascular system; (c) an assessment of a body part, eg, the lungs when difficulty breathing is observed. This chapter discusses health assessment techniques applied only to adults.

A complete health assessment is generally conducted from the head to the toes; however, the procedure can vary in many ways according to the age of the individual, the severity of the illness, the preferences of the nurse, and the agency's priorities and procedures. Regardless of what procedure is used, the patient's energy and time need to be considered. The health assessment is therefore conducted in a systematic and efficient manner that requires the fewest position changes for the patient.

Because assessment is an integral part of the nursing process, aspects of specific assessment techniques should be used in all nursing interventions. The assessment required by an individual at a given time is a nursing judgment based upon knowledge and the patient's needs.

Chapter Outline

Methods of Physical Assessment

Positions and Draping

- Technique 10–1 Assessing General Appearance and Mental Function
- Technique 10–2 Assessing the Skin
- Technique 10–3 Assessing the Hair
- Technique 10–4 Assessing the Nails
- Technique 10–5 Assessing the Head, Face, and Neck
- Technique 10–6 Assessing the Mouth
- Technique 10–7 Assessing the Nose and Sinuses
- Technique 10–8 Assessing the Eyes and Vision
- Technique 10–9 Assessing the Ears and Hearing
- Technique 10–10 Assessing the Thorax, Lungs, and Breasts
- Technique 10–11 Assessing the Heart
- Technique 10–12 Assessing the Peripheral Vascular System
- Technique 10–13 Assessing the Abdomen
- Technique 10–14 Assessing the Rectum and Anus
- Technique 10–15 Assessing the Female Genitals
- Technique 10–16 Assessing the Male Genitals
- Technique 10–17 Assessing the Musculoskeletal System
- Technique 10–18 Assessing the Neurologic System

Objectives

Upon completion of this chapter, the student will:

1. Know essential terms and facts related to health assessment
   1.1 Define terms associated with health assessment
   1.2 Describe specific positions patients assume during assessment
   1.3 Identify various ways patients are draped during assessment
   1.4 Identify essential aspects of the four basic methods of physical assessment
2. Demonstrate skills in assessment of various body systems
   2.1 Establish relevant nursing goals
   2.2 Identify equipment and supplies required during the assessment
   2.3 Identify the various steps in selected assessment techniques
   2.4 Give reasons for selected steps in the assessment techniques
   2.5 Identify expected and unexpected outcomes of health assessment
3. Evaluate own performance of health assessments in a laboratory or clinical setting with the assistance of another
   3.1 Use the performance checklists provided
   3.2 Identify areas of strength and weakness
   3.3 Alter performance in response to own evaluation and that of another

Terms

- acne   an inflammatory disease of the sebaceous glands
- acromegaly   a disorder caused by excessive growth hormone; it is characterized by excessive skeletal growth of the hands, feet, nose, jaw, and forehead
- adventitious sounds   sounds not normally heard over the lung fields
- affect   the emotional state of a person as it appears to others
- alopecia   abnormal loss of hair
- aneurysm   localized dilation of the wall of an artery at a weak point in the wall
- angle of Louis   the angle between the manubrium and the body of the sternum

■ **annulus**   a ringlike structure, eg, around the tympanic membrane

■ **anterior chamber (of the eye)**   the area immediately behind the cornea and in front of the iris

■ **anthelix**   the anterior curve on the upper aspect of the auricle of the ear

■ **arrector pili muscle**   the erector muscle attached to the hair follicle

■ **arteriosclerosis**   a condition in which the walls of the arteries become hardened and thickened

■ **ascites**   the accumulation of fluid in the abdominal cavity

■ **astigmatism**   a visual refractive error due to differences in curvature of the cornea and the lens

■ **ataxia**   impairment of position sense

■ **atelectasis**   collapse of a lung or a portion of it

■ **atrophy**   a wasting away or decrease in the size of a cell, tissue, body organ, or muscle

■ **auricle (pinna)**   the visible part of the ear

■ **auscultation**   the process of listening to sounds produced within the body

■ **Bass method**   *see* sulcular technique

■ **Beau's line**   a transverse white line or groove on the nail associated with an acute and severe illness

■ **Bell's palsy**   paralysis of the seventh cranial (facial) nerve

■ **borborygmi**   gurgling, splashing sounds heard over the large intestine

■ **bradycardia**   an abnormally slow heart rate (below 60 beats per minute)

■ **bruit**   a blowing or swishing sound created by turbulent blood flow

■ **buccal mucosa**   the mucous membrane lining the inner surface of the cheeks

■ **bulbar conjunctiva**   the mucous membrane over the eyeball

■ **callus**   a thickened portion of the skin

■ **canthus**   the angular junction of the eyelids at each corner of the eyes

■ **carotid sinus**   a dilated portion of the internal carotid artery that contains pressoreceptors that are stimulated by changes in blood pressure

■ **caruncle (of the eye)**   the red fleshy emminence at the inner canthus of the eye

■ **cataract**   an opacity of the lens of the eye

■ **cementum**   calcified tissue covering the root of a tooth

■ **cerumen**   the waxlike substance secreted by glands in the external ear canal

■ **clubbing (of a nail)**   elevation of the proximal aspect of the nail and softening of the nail bed due to a long-term lack of oxygen

■ **cochlea**   a seashell-shaped structure located in the inner ear; it has numerous apertures for passage of the cochlear division of the auditory nerve

■ **comedo**   a blackhead

■ **conjunctiva**   the membrane covering the eyelids and eyeball

■ **conjunctivitis**   inflammation of the membrane covering the eyelids and eyeball

■ **contracture**   permanent shortening of a muscle and subsequent shortening of tendons and ligaments

■ **contusion**   a bruise; an injury to soft tissue, produced by a blunt force

■ **convergence**   a moving together toward a common point

■ **cornea**   a transparent convex avascular structure forming the anterior surface of the eyeball

■ **crown (of a tooth)**   the exposed part of a tooth outside the gum

■ **Cushing's syndrome**   increased production of adrenal hormones

■ **cuticle**   the flat, thin rim of skin surrounding the nail

■ **cyanosis**   a bluish tinge to the skin and mucous membranes manifested when there is excessive reduced hemoglobin in the blood

■ **cystocele**   protrusion of the urinary bladder through the vaginal wall

■ **cytology**   the study of the origin, structure, function, and pathology of cells

■ **dacryocystitis**   inflammation of the lacrimal sac

■ **dandruff**   a dry or greasy scaly material shed from the scalp

■ **delusion**   a false belief

■ **dentin**   the chief substance of teeth, forming the body, neck, and roots; it is covered by enamel

■ **dentures**   a natural or artificial set of teeth; usually the term designates artificial teeth

■ **dermis (corium)**   true skin, containing blood vessels, nerves, hair follicles, and glands

■ **diaphoresis**   profuse perspiration

■ **diastasis rectus abdominus**   separation of the rectus abdominis muscles, often due to pregnancy or obesity

■ **diastole**   the period when the ventricles of the heart are relaxed

■ **dullness**   a thudlike percussion sound produced from underlying dense tissue

■ **duration (of a sound)**   the length of a sound heard during auscultation and percussion

■ **dyspnea**   difficult and labored breathing, in which the patient has a persistent unsatisfied need for air and feels distressed

■ **ecchymosis**   a bruise; bleeding into the tissues larger than 1 cm in diameter

■ ectropion   eversion; outward turning of the eyelid

■ emmetropia   normal refraction, in which the eyes focus objects on the retina

■ emphysema   a chronic obstructive lung disorder in which the terminal bronchioles become distended and plugged with mucus

■ enamel (of a tooth)   the covering over the crown of the tooth

■ enterocele   any hernia of the intestine through the intact vaginal mucosa

■ entropion   inversion; inward turning of the eyelid

■ epidermis   the outermost, nonvascular layer of skin

■ erythema   redness that is associated with a variety of rashes

■ eustachian tube   a channel lined with mucous membrane that connects the middle ear and the nasopharynx; it acts as an air pressure stabilizer

■ excoriation   loss of superficial layers of the skin

■ excursion   movement of a part in the performance of a function

■ exophthalmus   protrusion of the eyeballs with elevation of the upper lids; a staring, startled expression

■ external auditory meatus   the entrance to the ear canal

■ extinction   failure to perceive touch on one side of the body when two symmetric areas are touched simultaneously

■ fasciculation   abnormal contraction of a bundle of muscle fibers

■ fenestrated drape   a drape with an opening in its center

■ fissure   a cleft or groove; a crack line

■ flatness (of a sound)   an extremely dull sound heard on percussion from very dense tissue

■ fovea centralis   a tiny pit in the center of the macula of the eye

■ fremitus (tactile, vocal)   the vibration felt through the chest wall when a person speaks

■ frenulum   a midline fold connecting the undersurface of the tongue to the floor of the mouth

■ fundus   the larger part, base, or body of a hollow organ; in the eye, the back portion of the interior of the eyeball, visible only through an ophthalmoscope

■ genupectoral (knee–chest) position   a position in which the weight is borne by the patient's knees and chest and the body is at a 90° angle to the hips

■ gingiva   the gum

■ gingivitis   acute or chronic inflammation of the gums

■ glaucoma   an eye disease characterized by increased intraocular pressure, which causes damage to the retina and optic nerve and blindness if left untreated

■ glossitis   inflammation of the tongue

■ goiter   an enlargement of the thyroid gland, causing a swelling in the front part of the neck

■ graphesthesia   the act of recognizing a number or letter when it is drawn on the palm of the hand

■ hair follicle   a pouchlike depression in the skin enclosing the root of a hair

■ hair shaft   the visible part of the hair

■ halitosis   an unpleasant odor of the breath

■ hallucination   a false perception of a stimulus

■ hangnail   a shred of epidermal tissue at either side of the nail

■ helix   the posterior curve of the upper aspect of the auricle of the ear

■ hemangioma   a large, persistent, bright red or dark purple vascular area of the skin

■ hematoma   a collection of blood in a tissue or cavity

■ hemoptysis   the presence of blood in the sputum

■ hemorrhoids   distended veins in the rectum

■ hordeolum (sty)   an inflammation of one or more sebaceous glands of the eyelid

■ hyperopia   farsightedness; abnormal refraction in which light rays focus behind the retina

■ hyperresonance   a booming sound not normally produced by percussion, eg, from emphysematous lung tissue

■ hypertrophy   an increase in the size of a cell, tissue, or body organ such as a muscle

■ hypodermis (subcutaneous tissue)   the connective tissue beneath the skin

■ hypoesthesia   abnormally decreased sensitivity to stimulation

■ hypotonia   diminished tone of skeletal muscles

■ incus   an anvil-shaped ossicle of the middle ear; it communicates sound waves from the malleus to the stapes

■ inspection (observation)   assessment that uses the sense of sight; visual examination

■ intensity (of a sound)   the loudness or softness of a sound as heard during auscultation and percussion

■ iris   the colored part of the eye perforated by the pupil

■ iritis   inflammation of the iris

■ ischemia   deficiency of blood in a part due to constriction or obstruction of a blood vessel

■ jaundice   a yellowish tinge to the skin and mucous membrane

■ keratin   the type of protein found in epidermis, hair, and nails

■ keratotic spots   horny growths, such as warts or calluses

■ labia   the fleshy edges of a structure, usually the female genitals

- lacrimal canal   a passageway from the innermost corner of the eye to the lacrimal sac
- lacrimal duct   a small passageway from the lacrimal gland draining the tears into the conjunctiva at the upper outer corner of the eye
- lacrimal gland   the organ that lies over the upper outer corner of the eye and secretes tears
- lacrimal sac   a pouchlike structure located in a groove in the lacrimal bone between the inner corner of the eye and the bridge of the nose
- lithotomy position   a back-lying position in which the feet are supported in stirrups
- lobule   small lobe; the earlobe
- macula lutea   an irregular, yellowish depression on the retina, lateral to and slightly below the optic disc
- malleus   a hammer-shaped ossicle of the middle ear; it is connected to the tympanic membrane and transmits sound waves to the incus
- manubrium   a general term for a handlelike structure or part; in relation to the sternum it is the superior portion that joins with the clavicles
- mastication   the act of chewing
- mastoid   breast-shaped; the bony prominence of the temporal bone behind the ear
- melanin   the dark pigment of the skin
- miosis   constriction of the pupil
- mood   the emotional state of a person as he or she describes it
- multiparous   having had two or more pregnancies that resulted in viable fetuses
- mydriasis   enlargement of the pupil
- myopia   nearsightedness; abnormal refraction in which light rays focus in front of the retina
- myxedema   hypothyroidism
- nasolabial folds   creases extending from the angle of the nose to the corner of the mouth
- nasolacrimal duct   the channel between the lacrimal sac and the nose
- normocephalic   normal head circumference
- nulliparous   having never given birth to a viable fetus
- nystagmus   involuntary rhythmic movements of the eyeball
- ophthalmoscope   the instrument used to examine the interior of the eye
- orthopnea   the ability to breathe only in the upright position, ie, sitting or standing
- ossicles   the bones of sound transmission in the middle ear
- osteitis deformans (Paget's disease)   a disorder in which bony thickness increases
- otitis externa   inflammation of the external ear canal

- otitis media   inflammation of the middle ear
- otoscope   the instrument used to examine the eardrum and external ear canal
- Paget's disease   see osteitis deformans
- palate   the roof of the mouth
- pallor   the absence of normal skin color
- palpation   the act of feeling with the hands, usually the fingers; examination of the body using the sense of touch
- palpebral conjunctiva   the mucous membrane lining the eyelids
- palpebral fissure   the opening between the eyelids
- palpitation   a subjective sensation of an irregular or unduly rapid heartbeat
- paralytic ileus   obstruction of the intestines resulting from inhibition of nerve impulses, which leads to decreased bowel motility
- paresthesia   abnormal sensation such as burning, pricking, or numbness
- Parkinson's disease   a neurologic disorder characterized by muscle tremor and muscular rigidity
- paronychia   infection of the tissue surrounding the nail
- parotitis   inflammation of the parotid salivary gland
- parous   having borne one or more viable fetuses
- pediculosis capitis   infestation with head lice
- percussion   an assessment method in which the body surface is struck to elicit sounds or vibrations
- percussion hammer   an instrument shaped like a hammer with a head often made of plastic
- perfusion   the act of pouring over or through; the passage of a fluid through the vessels of a specific organ, eg, passage of blood constituents through blood vessels
- periodontal disease   a general term for a number of inflammatory and degenerative diseases that affect the supporting structures of the mouth
- peritonitis   inflammation of the peritoneum
- petechiae   pinpoint red areas in the skin
- phlebitis   inflammation of a vein
- photophobia   abnormal intolerance of light
- pinna   see auricle
- pitch (of a sound)   the frequency of the vibrations; the high or low quality of a sound as heard during auscultation and percussion
- pleximeter   the finger that is struck during percussion
- plexor   the finger that strikes during percussion
- pneumothorax   accumulation of air or gas in the pleural cavity
- point of maximal impulse (PMI)   the point where the apex of the left ventricle touches the anterior chest wall;

the point where the apical beat is most clearly palpated or auscultated

■ precordium   the area of the chest overlying the heart

■ presbyopia   impaired vision, usually farsightedness, as a result of loss of elasticity of the lens with aging

■ proctocele   *see* rectocele

■ proprioceptor   a sensory nerve terminal in a muscle, a tendon, a joint, or the internal ear that gives information about movements and the position of the body

■ ptosis   drooping of the eyelid so that one or both lids lie at or below the pupil margin

■ punctum   an extremely small point or spot; the opening into the lacrimal canal

■ pyorrhea   purulent periodontal disease

■ quality (of sound)   the subjective description of a sound as heard during percussion and auscultation

■ rectocele (proctocele)   a protrusion of part of the rectum into the vagina

■ reflex   involuntary activity in response to a stimulus

■ resonance   a hollow sound produced on percussion from tissue filled with air

■ retina   the innermost of three coverings of the eyeball

■ S₁   the first heart sound that occurs, when the atrioventricular valves close; it is a dull, low-pitched sound

■ S₂   the second heart sound that occurs, when the semilunar (aortic and pulmonary) valves close; it is a high-pitched, snappy sound

■ sclera   a tough white covering over about 75% of the eye; it is continuous with the cornea anteriorly and with the external sheath of the optic nerve posteriorly

■ sebaceous gland   a gland of the dermis that secretes sebum

■ seborrheic dermatitis   a chronic disease of the skin, characterized by scaling and crusted patches on various body areas, including the scalp

■ sebum   the oily, lubricating secretion of sebaceous glands in the skin

■ semicircular canals   passages shaped like half-circles in the inner ear that control the sense of balance by the effect of fluid moving against hairlike nerves

■ serous otitis   inflammation of the eustachian tube

■ smegma   a thick, white, cheeselike secretion that accumulates between the labia and under the foreskin

■ sordes   the accumulation of foul matter (food, microorganisms, and epithelial elements) on the teeth and gums

■ spasticity   sudden, prolonged involuntary muscle contraction

■ speculum   a funnel-shaped instrument used to widen and examine canals of the body, eg, the vagina or nasal canal

■ spoon nail   a thin nail with a concave profile

■ stapes   a stirrup-shaped ossicle of the middle ear; it transmits sound waves from the incus to the internal ear

■ stenosis   constriction or narrowing of a body canal or opening

■ stereognosis   the act of recognizing objects by touching and manipulating them

■ sternal angle (suprasternal notch)   the point where the clavicles meet

■ sternum   the breastbone

■ stomatitis   inflammation of the entire mouth

■ strabismus   crossed eyes; squint

■ striae   stretch marks

■ sty   *see* hordeolum

■ subcutaneous tissue   *see* hypodermis

■ sudoriferous gland   a gland of the dermis that secretes sweat

■ sulcular technique (Bass method)   a technique of brushing the teeth under the gingival margins

■ sulcus   the groove between the surface of the tooth and the gum

■ suprasternal notch   *see* sternal angle

■ syncope   fainting or temporary loss of consciousness

■ systole   the period when the ventricles of the heart are contracted

■ thecal whitlow   acute inflammation of the tissue surrounding the nail

■ thrill   a vibrating sensation

■ thrombus   a solid mass of blood constituents in the circulatory system; a clot (plural: thrombi)

■ thyroid isthmus   the portion connecting the two lobes of the thyroid gland; it lies across the trachea below the cricoid cartilage

■ tonicity   the normal condition of tension or tone, eg, of a muscle

■ tortuous   twisted

■ tragus   a cartilaginous protrusion at the entrance to the ear canal

■ tremor   involuntary trembling of a limb or part

■ turgor   the normal fullness and elasticity of the skin

■ tympanic membrane   the eardrum

■ tympany   a musical, drumlike sound produced on percussion from the least dense tissue

■ umbo   a round projection; eg, the umbo of the tympanic membrane is a slight projection on its external surface

■ uvula   a fleshy mass suspended at the midline and back of the palate

■ varicose veins   swollen, distended, and knotted veins

- vellus   fine, nonpigmented body hair
- vertigo   dizziness
- vestibule (of the ear)   a cavity at the entrance to the ear

- visual acuity   the degree of detail that the eye can discern in an image
- visual field   the area an individual can see when looking straight ahead

METHODS OF PHYSICAL ASSESSMENT

There are four commonly used methods of asessment: inspection, auscultation, palpation, and percussion.

Inspection

Inspection is visual examination, that is, assessment using the sense of sight. It includes looking with the naked eye and using instruments such as an otoscope or ophthalmoscope. The otoscope assists with visual examination of the ear and the ophthalmoscope with visual examination of the inside of the eye.

Inspection is an active not passive process, in which the nurse must know what to look for and where. Nurses use inspection frequently to assess color, rashes, scars, body shape, facial expressions that may reflect emotions, as well as body structures, eg, the inner eye. Inspection should be systematic, so that no area is missed. Inspection using lighted instruments, such as the otoscope, is discussed under the body area or system examined.

Auscultation

Auscultation is the process of listening to sounds produced within the body. Auscultation may be direct or indirect. Direct auscultation uses the unaided ear, eg, to listen to a respiration wheeze or the grating of a moving joint. Indirect auscultation uses a stethoscope, which amplifies the sounds and conveys them to the nurse's ears A stethoscope is used primarily to listen to sounds from within the body, eg, bowel sounds in the abdomen or valve sounds of the heart.

The stethoscope should be 30 to 35 cm (12 to 14 in) long, with an internal diameter of about 0.3 cm (⅛ in). It should have both a flat-disc and a bell-shaped diaphragm. See Figure 8–15 on page 119. The flat-disc diaphragm best transmits high-pitched sounds, eg. bronchial sounds, and the bell-shaped diaphragm low-pitched sounds, such as some heart sounds.

The earpieces of the stethoscope should fit comfortably into the nurse's ears. The diaphragm of the stethoscope is placed firmly but lightly against the patient's skin. If a patient has a very hairy skin, it may be necessary to dampen the hairs with a cloth so that they will lie smoothly against the skin and not cause scratching sounds.

Auscultated sounds are described according to their pitch, intensity, duration, and quality. The *pitch* is the frequency of the vibrations (the number of vibrations per second). Low-pitched sounds, eg, some heart sounds, have fewer vibrations per second than high-pitched sounds, such as bronchial sounds. The *intensity* (amplitude) refers to the loudness or softness of a sound. Some body sounds are loud, eg, bronchial sounds heard over the trachea, while others are soft, eg, normal breath sounds heard in the lungs. The *duration* of a sound is its length (long or short). The *quality* of sound refers to the subjective description of a sound, eg, whistling, gurgling, or snapping.

Palpation

Palpation is the examination of the body using the sense of touch. The pads of the fingers are used because their concentration of nerve endings makes them highly sensitive to tactile discrimination.

Palpation is used to determine:

1. Texture, eg, of the hair
2. Temperature, eg, of a skin area
3. Vibration, eg, of a joint
4. Position, size, consistency, and mobility of organs or masses
5. Distention, eg, of the urinary bladder
6. Presence and rate of peripheral pulses
7. Tenderness or pain

There are two types of palpation: light and deep. Light (superficial) palpation should always precede deep palpation, because heavy pressure on the fingertips can dull the sense of touch. For light palpation, the nurse extends dominant hand fingers parallel to the skin surface and presses gently downward while moving the hand in a circular fashion. If it is necessary to determine the details of a mass, the nurse presses lightly several times rather than holding the pressure.

Deep palpation is done with two hands (bimanually) or one hand. In deep bimanual palpation, the nurse extends the dominant hand as for light palpation, then places the fingerpads of the nondominant hand on the dorsal surfaces of the distal interphalangeal joint of the middle three fingers of the dominant hand. See Figure 10–1. Pressure is applied by the top hand while the lower hand remains relaxed to perceive the tactile sensations. For deep palpation using one hand, the fingerpads of the dominant hand press over the area to be palpated. Often the other hand is used to support a mass or organ from below. See Figure 10–2.

The effectiveness of palpation depends largely on the patient's relaxation. Nurses can assist a patient to relax by: (a) gowning and/or draping the patient appropriately; (b) positioning the patient comfortably; (c) ensuring that their own hands are warm before beginning, eg, running them under warm water if they are cold; and (d) commencing palpation with areas that are not painful. During palpation, the nurse should be sensitive to the patient's verbal and facial expressions indicating discomfort.

Percussion

Percussion is an assessment method in which the body surface is struck to elicit sounds that can be heard or vibrations that can be felt. A commonly used percussion technique is to place the middle finger of the nondominant hand, referred to as the *pleximeter*, on the patient's skin. Only the distal phalanx of this finger should be in contact with the skin. Using the tip of the flexed middle finger of the other hand, called the *plexor*, the nurse strikes the pleximeter between the nail and the distal interphalangeal joint. See Figure 10–3. The striking motion should come from the wrist; the forearm remains stationary. The angle between the plexor and the

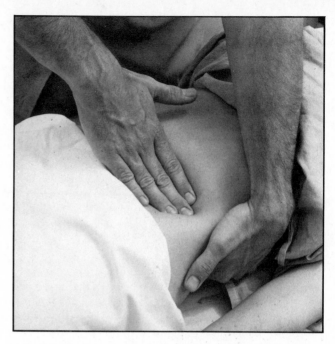

FIGURE 10–2 ■ Deep palpation using one hand below to support while the hand above palpates the organ.

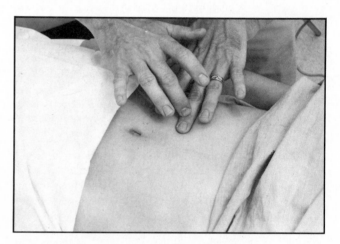

FIGURE 10–3 ■ The position of the fingers for percussion. Only the middle finger of the nondominant hand is in contact with the skin.

FIGURE 10–1 ■ The position of the hands for deep bimanual palpation.

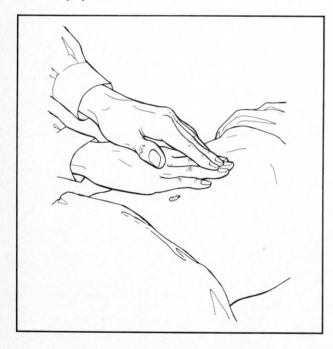

pleximeter should be 90°, and the blows must be firm, rapid, and short to obtain a clear sound.

Percussion is used to determine the size and shape of internal organs by establishing their borders. It indicates whether tissue is fluid-filled, air-filled, or solid. Percussion elicits five types of sound: flatness, dullness, resonance, hyperresonance, and tympany. *Flatness* is an extremely dull sound produced by very dense tissue such as muscle or bone. *Dullness* is a thudlike sound produced by dense tissue such as the liver, spleen, or heart. *Resonance* is a hollow sound such as that produced by lungs filled with air. *Hyperresonance* is not produced in the normal body. It is described as booming and can be heard over an emphysematous lung. *Tympany* is a musical or drumlike sound produced from an air-filled stomach. On a continuum, flatness reflects the most dense tissue (least amount of air) and tympany the least dense tissue (the most amount of air).

A percussion sound, such as resonance, is described according to its intensity, pitch, duration, and quality. See Table 10–1 and the discussion of auscultation earlier.

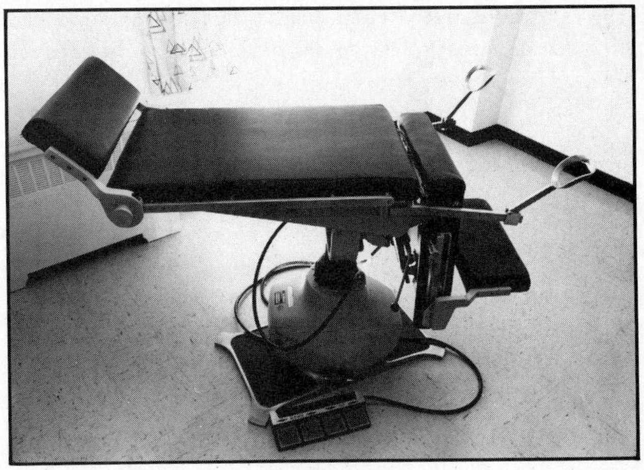

FIGURE 10–4 ■ An electrically operated examination table.

POSITIONS AND DRAPING

Patients frequently need to assume one or more positions during a physical examination. Some of these may be uncomfortable. The nurse indicates specific positions for the patient at the time needed. Patients who are assessed while in bed or on a stretcher can assume only some of the positions. Many hospitals, offices, and clinics have special examination tables, usually with extendable leaves for the supine and Sims's positions, stirrups for the lithotomy position (see Figure 10–4), and a platform for the genupectoral position.

Patients need to be draped appropriately during an examination to prevent unnecessary exposure, chilling, and embarrassment. An embarrassed or chilled patient is usually tense, which can limit the effectiveness of some aspects of the examination.

Drapes are made of cloth or paper. Bedding (bath blankets, sheets, and drawsheets) can also be used for draping. Some drapes are specially made, eg, circumcision drapes or special socks to cover the patient's feet and legs. A drape with one or more round or rectangular openings is referred to as a *fenestrated* (window) drape.

Dorsal Recumbent (Supine) Position

For physical assessments, the dorsal recumbent position is frequently used. Some agencies differentiate between the horizontal recumbent position and the dorsal recumbent position. The horizontal recumbent position is a flat back-lying position, while in the dorsal recumbent position the knees are flexed and the hips are externally rotated.

The appropriate drapes for a patient in this position usually include:

1. A hospital gown or bath towel for the chest
2. A bath blanket or sheet to cover the remainder of the body from the waist to the toes

The bath towel is placed across the chest, and the bath blanket or sheet is placed diagonally over the patient. See Figure 10–5, *A*. If the patient's perineal area is to be examined, opposite corners of the sheet are wrapped around the feet to cover the legs. See Figure 10–5, *B*.

TABLE 10–1   Percussion Sounds

Sound	Intensity	Pitch	Duration	Quality	Example of location
Flatness	Soft	High	Short	Extremely dull	Muscle, bone
Dullness	Medium	Medium	Moderate	Thudlike	Liver, heart
Resonance	Loud	Low	Long	Hollow	Lung
Hyperresonance	Very loud	Very low	Very long	Booming	Emphysematous lung
Tympany	Loud	High (distinguished mainly by musical timbre)	Moderate	Musical	Stomach filled with gas (air)

The corner between the patient's legs can be raised to expose the perineum at the appropriate time. See Figure 10–5, C.

Knee–Chest (Genupectoral) Position

This position is used to view the rectal and sometimes the vaginal areas. The patient kneels, using knees and chest to bear the body's weight. The back is straight and the body is at a 90° angle to the hips. The head is turned to one side and the arms are held above the head. Some agencies provide a special table, which supports the patient in this position.

The drapes often used for a patient in this position are:

1. A hospital gown to cover the upper body.

2. A fenestrated drape to cover the patient's back, buttocks, and thighs. The hole in the drape exposes only the area to be examined. See Figure 10–6, A. If a fenestrated drape is not available, a rectangular drape can be used. The two lateral corners are tucked around the patient's thighs. See Figure 10–6, B. The corner between the thighs can then be lifted up to expose the area to be examined, eg, the anus. See Figure 10–6, C.

3. Socks to cover the feet and lower legs (optional).

Lithotomy Position

The lithotomy position is frequently used for examinations of the vagina, and sometimes for urinary catheterizations in women. The patient assumes a back-lying

FIGURE 10–5 ■ Draping for the dorsal recumbent position.

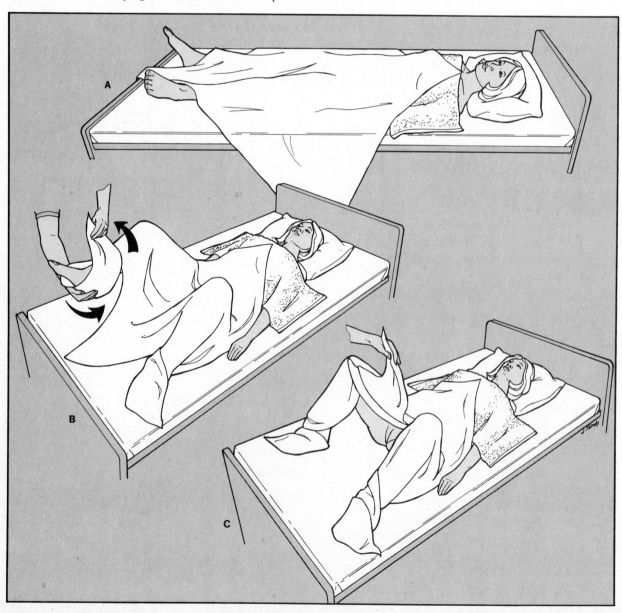

For the lithotomy position, the drapes usually used are:

1. A hospital gown for the upper body (optional)
2. A rectangular sheet or a fenestrated sheet
3. Socks for the patient's feet (optional)

The socks are put on the patient before the feet are placed in the stirrups. The sheet is placed diagonally on the patient so that the top part covers the patient's chest and abdomen. See Figure 10–7, *A*. The side corners are wrapped around the patient's legs and feet. If the patient is wearing socks, the drape need not cover the feet, but it should overlap the socks. See Figure 10–7, *B*. The corner between the patient's legs is lifted to expose the

FIGURE 10–7 ■ Draping for the lithotomy position.

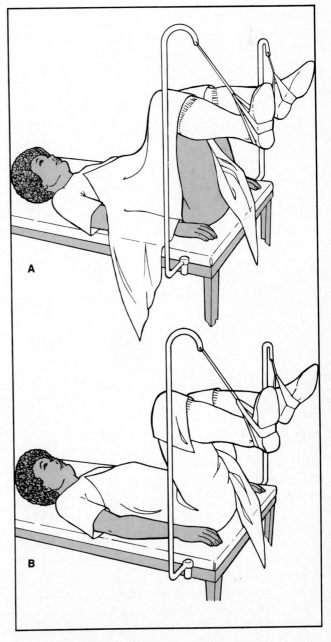

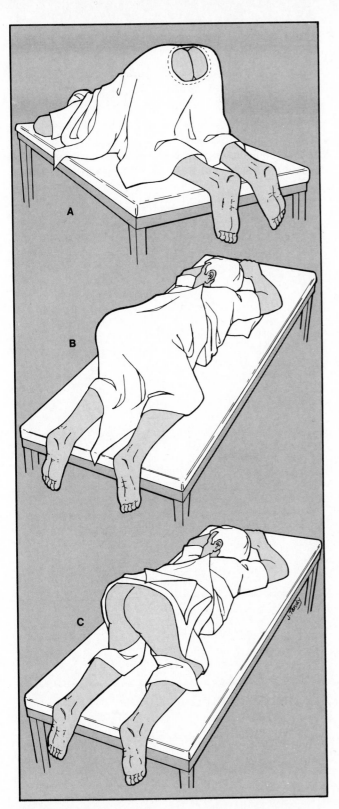

FIGURE 10–6 ■ Draping for the genupectoral position.

position, and the feet are held in supports called *stirrups*. The knees are flexed, and the hips are externally rotated. The patient's hips are usually brought down to the bottom edge of the examining table, to expose the perineal area.

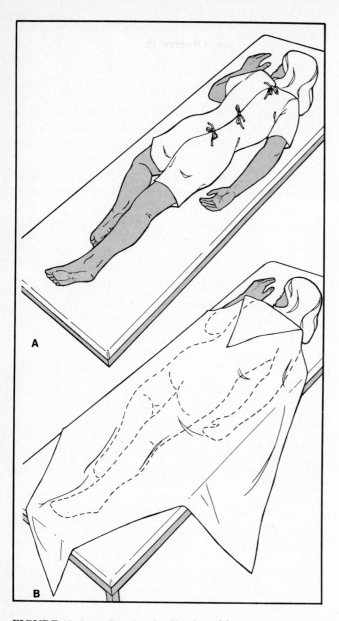

FIGURE 10-8 ■ Draping for Sims's position.

perineal area. A fenestrated drape is placed the same way as a rectangular sheet but with the opening directly over the area to be examined.

Sims's Position

Sims's position (see Figure 10–8, *A*) is usually assumed for examinations of the rectum and/or vagina. The drape is usually one rectangular sheet, placed diagonally on the patient. See Figure 10–8, *B*. At the time of examination, the corner is folded back to expose the area. Because this position can be difficult for some patients to assume, particularly the elderly and the obese, it is normally not assumed until immediately before the examination.

TECHNIQUE 10-1 ■ Assessing General Appearance and Mental Function

The general appearance and mental function of an individual must be assessed in terms of culture, educational level, socioeconomic status, and current circumstances. An individual who has recently experienced a personal loss may naturally appear depressed. An individual who has had an accident while working may be dressed in work clothes that she or he would not normally wear when seeing a nurse or physician.

Assessment should be carried out systematically so as not to miss portions of the patient.

■ Planning

Nursing goals

1. To determine baseline data about a patient's general appearance and mental status
2. To screen for mental problems

■ Intervention

See Table 10–2 for normal and abnormal findings and associated conditions.

General appearance

1. *Sex, race, and culture.* Observe the patient's sex and race. Assessment findings should be considered in light of these.

   Rationale The patient's sex, race, and cultural beliefs can affect the meaning of specific assessment data.

2. *Body build.* Observe body build, height, and weight in relation to the patient's age, life-style, and health.

3. *Posture and gait.* Observe the patient's posture and gait, standing, sitting, and walking. See Table 19–5 on page 451.

4. *Hygiene and grooming.* Observe the patient's overall hygiene and grooming; then assess these factors from head to toe. Include cleanliness of the hair and nails. Relate this to the person's activities prior to the assessment.

5. *Dress.* Observe the patient's dress in relation to his or her age, life-style, climate, socioeconomic staus, and culture.

6. *Body odor.* Using your sense of smell, assess the

TABLE 10–2 ■ General Appearance and Mental Function

Nursing history: Determine chronologic age, race, cultural background, and general health status; achievement of developmental tasks; body image concerns; self-esteem; educational level, thought processes; general health history; stressors (past and present); changes in personality, behavior, or memory; lifelong problems, eg, poor job history, alcoholism, drug abuse, discipline.

Test, structure, or process	Normal findings	Abnormal findings	Some associated conditions
General appearance			
Body build, height, weight, muscularity, shapeliness	Varies with life-style	Excessively thin	Anorexia nervosa
		Obese	Hypothyroidism
Posture, gait	Relaxed, erect posture; coordinated movement	Tense, slouched, bent posture; uncoordinated movement; tremors	Parkinsonism
Hygiene	Clean, neat	Dirty, unkempt	Chronic brain syndrome
Body odor	None or some relative to work or exercise	Foul odor	Poor hygiene
		Ammonia odor	Renal failure
	No breath odor	Acetone breath odor	Diabetes
		Foul breath	Poor oral hygiene
Dress	Appropriate for age, life-style, culture, socioeconomic status, climate	Inappropriate	Depression, cerebral disorder
Signs of distress	None	Distress	
Signs of health	Healthy	Weakness, obvious illness	
Mental status			
Attitude	Cooperative	Negative, hostile, withdrawn	
Affect/mood	Appropriate to circumstances	Inappropriate to situation	Depression
Speech	Understandable, moderate pace, exhibits thought association	Rapid or slow, uses generalizations, lacks association, exhibits confabulation	Manic psychosis (rapid pace)
Memory	Recall: recalls 7 digits readily	Lack of or impaired memory	Pathology of cerebral cortex
	Recent memory: can relate events of day		
	Past memory: can relate previous illnesses		

TABLE 10–2 ■ continued

Test, structure, or process	Normal findings	Abnormal findings	Some associated conditions
Thought processes	Logical sequence, makes sense, sense of reality	Illogical sequence, flight of ideas, confusion	Neuroses, psychoses
Self-concept	Healthy self-concept, body image conforms to reality, high self-esteem	Anxiety, guilt, anger, power-lessness, low self-esteem	
Knowledge	Appropriate for education and culture	Inadequate in light of education and culture	Amnesia, brain lesions
Judgment	Appropriate for culture	Inappropriate	Brain lesions
Orientation	Oriented to time, place, and person	Confused as to time, place, and/or person	Cerebral disorder, sensory deprivation
Concentration and calculation	Can recall 5 to 8 digits forward, 4 to 6 backward; appropriate for education and language or cultural level	Unable to recall 5 to 8 digits	Cerebral disorder, severe anxiety
	Can subtract 4 from 100 progressively	Unable to subtract 4 progressively	
Consciousness	Oriented and alert	Not alert (see Table 10–3)	Brain tumor, cerebrovascular accident

patient's body and breath odor. Relate these to the patient's activity.

Rationale People who have been exercising may have a normal body odor.

7. *Distress.* Observe for signs of distress in posture, facial expression, etc, such as wincing or labored breathing. Question the patient about any pain.

Rationale A person may hold or rub a painful limb in a protective manner, bend over because of abdominal pain, hold a painful side, etc.

8. *Health.* Observe for obvious signs of health or illness, eg, in color or breathing.

Mental status

9. *Attitude.* Observe the patient's attitude through appearance, speech, and behavior.

10. *Affect/mood. Affect* is the emotional state as it appears to others. *Mood* is the emotional state as described by the individual. Observe affect through appearance and behavior. Assess mood from the patient's speech. Assess for appropriateness, swings, and harmony. Affect and mood are considered to be in disharmony when, eg, the person laughs but says he or she is sad.

11. *Speech.* Listen to the patient's speech for quantity,

quality, and organization. Quantity refers to the amount of speech and the pace of talking (slow or rapid). Quality refers to loudness, clarity, and inflection. Organization includes coherence of thought, overgeneralizations, tendency to use global pronouns such as "they," and vagueness.

12. *Memory.* Listen for lapses in recall, recent memory, or remote memory.

a. To assess recall, ask the patient to repeat a series of digits spoken slowly.

b. To assess recent memory, ask the patient to recall the events of the day.

c. To assess remote memory, ask the patient to recall a previous illness, eg, five years ago, or a birthday or anniversary.

13. *Thought processes.* Listen to the patient's health history for relevance and organization of the thoughts. Does the thought flow logically? Is there contact with reality, or is the patient experiencing delusions or hallucinations? A *delusion* is a false belief, one not based upon fact. A *hallucination* is the false perception of a stimulus, eg, a shadow that the patient believes to be a large ant is a visual hallucination.

14. *Self-concept.*

a. Ask the patient, "What do you like or dislike about yourself?" "How would you describe yourself?"

b. Ask the patient to describe his or her physical self, eg, personal perceptions of his or her shape, size, and appearance.

c. Note whether the patient establishes eye contact.

15. *Knowledge.* Ask questions you would expect the patient to be able to answer, eg, "What are the seasons of the year?"

16. *Judgment.* Ask simple questions requiring judgment, such as "What would you do if you broke your neighbor's shovel?" "What would you do if you were stopped by the police?"

17. *Orientation.* Ask questions about time, place, and person: "What is the day of the week?" "Where are you?" "What is your name?"

18. *Concentration and calculation.*

a. Recite eight digits, eg, 6–8–9–4–3–8–7–2. Ask the patient to recall them in the same order, and then backwards.

b. Ask the patient to calculate by subtracting 4 progressively from 100.

19. *Consciousness.* See Table 10–3.

a. Inspect the patient for level of consciousness.

b. Speak to the patient to arouse her or him if necessary.

c. Press your fingernail to the patient's nail to arouse the patient.

d. Determine the status of the patient's reflexes as described in Table 10–3, if indicated.

20. Record your findings on the appropriate records.

21. Report abnormal findings to the responsible nurse and/or physician.

TABLE 10–3 ■ Levels of Consciousness

Level	Behavior
Alert	Awake and aware of environment without stimulation
	Oriented to time, place, and person
	Responds briskly and appropriately to minimal visual, auditory, and tactile stimuli
Lethargic	Sleeps much of the time when not stimulated
	Is easily aroused, and when aroused is oriented
	Speech may be slow or hesitant
Obtunded	Difficult to arouse from sleep (eg, must be shaken or given a painful stimulus)
	Responds verbally when awakened, but the response is confined to a few words that do not make sense
	Quickly returns to a sleeping state when stimulation is removed
Stuporous	Aroused only by painful stimuli (eg, when the nurse presses a fingernail into the patient's nailbed or pinches the patient's Achilles tendon)
	No verbal response to painful stimuli
	Is never fully wakened
Semicomatose	Reflex movement is elicited by painful stimuli
	Gag reflex is present (checked by holding tongue down with tongue blade and touching oropharynx with cotton-tipped applicator)
	Corneal (blink) reflex is present (checked by lightly touching the cornea with a wisp of cotton
	Decorticate or decerebrate posturing may be present*
Comatose	No response to maximal painful stimuli
	Reflexes absent
	Absence of muscle tone in extremities

Source: Adapted from A Ladyshewsky: Increased intracranial pressure: When assessment counts, *Can Nurse* (October) 1980; 76:34.

Decerebrate posturing (indicating midbrain damage) is recognized by extension, adduction, and internal rotation of the arms; extension of the legs with feet in plantar flexion; and arching of the back. *Decorticate posturing* (indicating damage to the internal capsule and corticospinal tracts above the brain stem) is recognized by flexion and adduction of fingers, wrists, and shoulders; extension and internal rotation of legs and feet; and rigidity of all extremities.

TECHNIQUE 10-2 ■ Assessing the Skin

Assessment of an individual's skin includes the entire body skin including skin folds. For information about developmental variables and skin lesions, see chapter 14.

■ Nursing Diagnosis

Nursing diagnoses that may indicate a need to assess a patient's skin include:

1. Actual impairment of skin integrity related to:
   a. Shearing forces
   b. Pressure
   c. Altered nutritional state: emaciation
   d. Altered circulation
2. Potential impairment of skin integrity related to:
   a. Radiation therapy
   b. Physical immobilization
   c. Altered sensation
   d. Immunologic deficit
   e. Urinary incontinence

■ Planning

Nursing goals

1. To determine baseline data about the patient's skin
2. To determine the patient's skin hygiene practices
3. To develop an appropriate plan of skin care

■ Intervention

See Table 10–4 for normal and abnormal findings and associated conditions.

1. With adequate light, inspect the skin surface for color and uniformity of color. This is best determined on areas not exposed to the sun and in an environment that is neither hot nor cold.
   Rationale Sun-darkened areas may hide pigmentation changes. A hot or cold environment can cause flushing of the skin or skin pallor.
2. Inspect the skin and skin folds for moisture. The environment should not be hot.
   Rationale A hot enviroment can cause excessive perspiration.
3. Using the backs of your fingers, palpate the skin surface for temperature, including the extremities. Compare the two feet and the two hands.

Rationale Comparison can indicate vascular abnormalities, eg, excessive coolness of left foot compared to the right foot.

4. With the pads of the fingers, stroke the inner aspects of the patient's arms to determine skin texture. Normal skin texture in this area is soft and smooth.
5. Inspect skin surfaces for variations in thickness, particularly on areas where there is pressure or rubbing. Thickened skin areas, eg, calluses, may be present on the soles of the feet and palms of the hands.
6. Inspect the skin for hygiene. Normally, clean skin is free from odor, crusts, and dirt.
7. Pinch the skin to determine tissue turgor and mobility. Note how quickly the skin returns to place (to assess turgor) and how easily it is moved (to assess mobility). Usually this is done inferior to the clavicle and on the lower extremities.
   Rationale Under the clavicle there is usually no excessive skin.
8. Inspect all skin surfaces for abnormalities. See Table 10–4.
9. Inspect all skin pressure points of patients at risk for skin breakdown, eg, persons who are immobilized or restrained.
   a. Determine that skin surface is intact.
   b. Determine that the surface temperature is the same as that of the surrounding skin.
   c. Apply pressure, and determine that the skin quickly becomes red (reactive hyperemia), then returns to normal color.
10. Record your findings on the patient's record.

■ Evaluation

Expected outcomes

1. Skin color is light to dark brown, whitish pink to deep pink, yellow in overtones, or olive.
2. Skin texture is smooth and soft.
3. Skin integrity is uninterrupted.

See also Table 10–4.

Unexpected outcomes

See Table 10–4. Upon obtaining an unexpected outcome: Report your findings to the responsible nurse and/or physician.

TABLE 10-4   ■   Skin

Nursing history: Determine presence of pain or itching; presence and spread of any lesions, bruises, abrasions, pigmented spots; previous experience with skin problems; associated clinical signs; family history; presence of problems in other family members; related systemic conditions; use of medications, lotions, home remedies; whether skin feels dry or very moist; whether patient bruises easily; whether problem is associated with season of year, stress, occupation, medications, recent travel, housing, personal contact, etc; any recent contact with allergens, eg, metal paint.

Assessment data	Normal findings	Abnormal findings
General color tone, best assessed on areas not exposed to sun	Light to deep brown; ruddy pink to light pink; yellow overtones to olive	Cyanosis, paleness, jaundice
Uniformity of color	Generally uniform; dark-skinned people have areas of lighter pigmentation (palms, lips, nail beds); areas are darkened by sun	Areas of hyperpigmentation or hypopigmentation
Hydration	Dampness in axilla and skin folds	Excessive oiliness or dryness
Vascularity and edema	No edema or vascular abnormalities	Petechiae, telangiectasias, bruises, erythema, edema
Pigmented spots	Freckles, some birthmarks, some flat and raised nevi	Various other lesions
Abrasions and excoriations	None	Various interruptions in skin integrity
Turgor and elasticity	When pinched, springs back to previous state	Stays pinched, moves back slowly
Mobility	Moves freely	Moves with difficulty, eg, edema
Texture and thickness	Smooth, soft, even; thickness is widely variable	Rough, coarse, or velvety smooth; excessive thickness
Surface temperature	Uniform, within normal range	Excessive coolness of some areas, eg, one extremity
Lesions (see Table 14–3)	No lesions present	Lesions, macules, papules, etc

TECHNIQUE 10-3   ■   Assessing the Hair

Scalp hair is inspected routinely during a complete physical examination, for distribution, texture, condition of the scalp, and infestations. For information about the anatomy of hair and developmental variables, see chapter 12. The condition of the hair is also a useful indicator of the patient's personal hygiene, emotional status, and social group identification.

■ Nursing Diagnosis

Nursing diagnoses that may indicate the need to assess a person's hair include:

1. Alterations in health maintenance related to:
   a. Inadequate health practices
   b. Substance abuse

■ Planning

Nursing goals

1. To determine baseline data about the patient's hair
2. To determine the patient's hair hygienic practices
3. To develop an appropriate plan of hair and/or scalp care

TABLE 10–5 ■ Hair

Nursing history: Determine recent use of hair dyes, rinses, or curling or straightening preparations; recent chemotherapy (if alopecia is present); presence of disease, such as hypothyroidism, which can be associated with dry, brittle hair.

Assessment method	Data	Normal findings	Abnormal findings	Some associated conditions
Inspection				
Ensure that lighting is appropriate	Hair growth and distribution	Evenly distributed hair	Patchy losses of hair (alopecia)	Chemotherapy, radiation therapy
	Hair texture and oiliness	Silky, resilient hair	Brittle hair	Hypothyroidism
			Excessively oily or dry hair	
	Condition of scalp	Smooth, intact skin	Dandruff	
			Sores	
			Itching	
	Infestations	None	Lice	
			Ticks	
			Nits	

■ Intervention

See Table 10–5 for normal and abnormal findings. Taking into account the many individual variations in hair, assess:

1. The evenness of hair growth over the scalp and, in particular, any patchy loss of hair. Normal scalp hair is evenly distributed.

2. Texture, ie, whether the hair is coarse or silky. Normal hair has resilience. Brittle hair may be associated with hypothyroidism.

3. Oiliness, ie, whether the hair is dry or greasy.

4. Thickness or thinness. Some therapies for cancer cause thinning and loss of the hair (alopecia). With hyperthyroidism, the hair often becomes very thin.

5. Any reddened areas, sores, or flaking on the scalp or infestations of lice, nits, or ticks. To assess for these, part the hair in several areas.

6. Personal hygienic practices and learning needs. See chapter 12, page 278.

■ Evaluation

See Table 10–5 for expected and unexpected outcomes. Upon obtaining an unexpected outcome: Report your findings to the responsible nurse and/or physician.

TECHNIQUE 10–4 ■ Assessing the Nails

The nails and surrounding tissues are inspected for shape, texture, and color, and palpated for capillary refill. For information about nail structure, developmental variables, and common problems, see chapter 12. For normal nail contour and angle, clubbing, spoon-shaped nails, and Beau's line, see Figures 12–13, 12–14, and 12–15.

■ Planning

Nursing goals

1. To determine baseline data about the patient's nails
2. To determine the patient's nail hygienic practices
3. To develop an appropriate plan of nail care

TABLE 10–6 ■ Nails

Nursing history: Determine presence of diabetes mellitus or peripheral circulatory disease.

Assessment method	Data	Normal findings	Abnormal findings	Some associated conditions
Inspection				
Inspect nail profile to determine its curvature and angle	Nail plate shape	Convex curvature	Spoon shape Claw nails	Prolonged iron-deficiency anemia
	Angle between nail and nail bed	About 160° angle	Clubbing (180° or greater angle)	Long-term lack of oxygen
Use adequate lighting to determine nail texture, color, and capillary refill	Nail texture	Smooth	Excessively thick nails	Aging
			Excessively thin nails Presence of grooves or furrows	Prolonged iron-deficiency anemia
	Nail bed color	In Caucasians, pink; in Blacks, brown or black pigmentation in longitudinal streaks or along edge of nail	Pallor	Poor arterial circulation
			Cyanotic	Lack of oxygenated hemoglobin
	Tissues surrounding nails	Intact epidermis	Hangnails	
			Inflammation	Paronychia, ingrown toenails
Palpation				
Blanch test: Press two or more nails between thumb and index fingers; look for blanching and return of pink color to nail bed	Capillary refill	Prompt return of pink color	Delayed return of pink color	Circulatory impairment, anemia

---

■ **Intervention**

See Table 10–6 for normal and abnormal findings. Assess:

1. The shape, thickness, smoothness, color, and length of the nails. The normal nail is smooth to the touch, has a convex shape, and has a pink nail bed (the tissue under the nail).

2. The tissues around the nails, for dryness, hangnails, and paronychia.

3. The rate of return of nail bed color after the *blanch test:* Normal nail bed capillaries blanch when pressed but quickly turn pink (in Caucasians) or their usual color when pressure is released. In dark-skinned people, the nail may be pigmented along the edges or in lines along the nail, and the rate of return of nail bed color may be more significant than the color. A slow rate of capillary refill may indicate circulatory problems.

4. The patient's personal hygienic practices and learning needs. See chapter 12, page 278.

■ **Evaluation**

See Table 10–6 for expected and unexpected outcomes. Upon obtaining an unexpected outcome: Report your findings to the responsible nurse and/or physician.

TECHNIQUE 10–5 ■ Assessing the Head, Face, and Neck

Assessment of the head, face, and neck involves inspection and palpation, often used simultaneously, and auscultation. This technique excludes the hair, mouth, eyes, ears, nose, and nasopharynx, which are discussed in separate techniques.

The head is examined for skull size, shape, and contour. Size is of utmost importance in infants and toddlers. On measuring head circumference, see Technique 9–5. The face is examined for status of the facial skin, symmetry, shape changes, and movements. The neck is examined for range of motion and symmetry. Neck examination includes the trachea, thyroid gland, and lymph nodes; other structures are discussed in cardiovascular and respiratory assessment; see Techniques 10–10 and 10–11 later in this chapter.

■ Planning

Nursing goal

To identify problems of the head, face, and neck.

Equipment

1. A good light source
2. A glass of water
3. A stethoscope

■ Intervention

See Table 10–7 for normal and abnormal findings.

TABLE 10–7 ■ Head, Face, and Neck

Nursing history: Determine any past problems with lumps or bumps, neck pain, stiffness, itching, scaling, or dandruff; any history of loss of consciousness, dizziness, seizures, headache, facial pain, or injury; when and how any lumps occurred; length of time any other problem existed; any known cause of problem; associated symptoms, treatment, and recurrences; any previous diagnosis of thyroid problem, whether thyroid was over- or underfunctioning, what tests were taken, test results, whether and what medications were ordered, amounts taken, whether still being taken, and whether other treatments were provided (eg, surgery, radiation).

Structure	Normal findings	Abnormal findings	Some associated conditions
Head	Rounded (normocephalic and symmetrical, with frontal, parietal, and occipital prominences)	Increased size with prominent nose and forehead, longer mandible	Acromegaly
		Increased size with prominent superficial veins	Osteitis deformans
	Smooth skull contour	Lumps, depressions, or nodules	Trauma, sebaceous cysts
Face	Consistent pink or other natural skin color	Bluish or cyanotic lips, nose, cheeks, or earlobes	Cardiac or pulmonary disease or local stasis of circulation
		Pallor	Anemia, shock
		Yellow color (jaundice)	Increase in bilirubin
		Localized color change	Acne; moles; scar tissue
		Reddened discoloration bridging cheeks and nose	Lupus erythematosus
		Increased facial hair	Increased production of adrenal hormones
		Thinning of eyebrows	Myxedema
	Facial features symmetric or slightly asymmetric	Features asymmetric	Trauma; masses
	Palpebral fissures equal in size	Edema of eyelids	Cardiovascular or kidney disease

TABLE 10–7   ■   Continued

Structure	Normal findings	Abnormal findings	Some associated conditions
	Nasolabial folds are symmetrical	Exophthalmus	Hyperthyroidism
		"Myxedema face"	Hypothyroidism
		"Moon face"	Cushing's syndrome; intake of synthetic adrenal hormones
		Sunken eyes, cheeks, and temples	Dehydration; prolonged illness; starvation
	Facial movements symmetric	Facial movements asymmetric, eg, eye on affected side cannot close completely, lower eyelid and mouth droop	Facial nerve lesions; Bell's palsy
Neck muscles	Muscles equal in size; head position centered	Unilaterial neck swelling; head tilted to one side	Masses; injury; muscle weakness; shortening of sterno-cleidomastoid muscle; scars
	Movements coordinated, smooth, without discomfort	Muscle tremor, spasm, or stiffness	
	Head flexes 45°	Painful movement	Irritation of meninges, neck injury
	Head hyperextends 60°	Limited range of motion	Cervical arthritis
	Head laterally flexes 40°	Up and down nodding movement	Parkinson's disease
	Head laterally rotates 70°		
	Strength among muscles equal	Unequal strength	Muscle injury
Trachea	Central placement	Deviation to one side	Neck tumor; thyroid enlargement; enlarged lymph nodes; tension pneumothorax; unilateral emphysema; atelectasis
Thyroid gland	Not visible on inspection	Visible diffuse or local enlargement	Hyperthyroidism; goiter
	Lobes may not be palpated	Solitary nodules	Carcinoma
	If palpated, lobes are small, smooth, centrally located, painless, and rise freely with swallowing	Gland not fully movable with swallowing	
Lymph nodes	Not palpable	Enlarged, palpable, and possibly tender	Infection; metastatic carcinoma
		Enlargement of submental and submaxillary nodes	Infection of the tongue
		Enlargement of preauricular, mastoid, and deep cervical nodes	Infection of the ear
		Enlargement of deep cervical nodes	Rubella; infectious mononucleosis; hepatitis

Head and face

1. Although there is a large range of normal shapes of skulls, inspect the head at all angles for size, shape, and symmetry. Areas of the head are named from underlying bones: frontal, parietal, occipital, mastoid process, mandible, maxilla, and zygomatic. See Figure 10–9. Note particularly areas of local trauma, lumps or bumps, and overall size. In adults, a large head may result from osteitis deformans or acromegaly. *Osteitis deformans* (Paget's disease) is a disorder in which bony thickness increases. The skull, spine, pelvis, and femur are the usual sites of involvement. When the skull is involved, it appears enlarged, with prominent superficial veins, and often there is hearing impairment. *Acromegaly* is a disorder caused by excessive growth hormone secretion. The

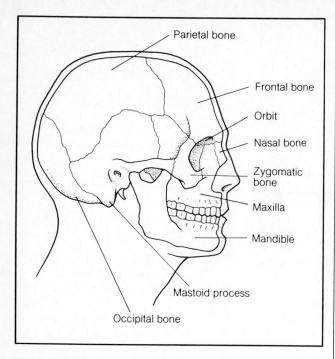

Parietal bone

Frontal bone

Orbit

Nasal bone

Zygomatic bone

Maxilla

Mandible

Mastoid process

Occipital bone

FIGURE 10–9

skull becomes thickened and enlarged, mandible length increases, the nose and forehead become more prominent, and the facial features look coarsened. Associated signs include changes in the skin, which becomes thickened, coarse, leathery, and oily and develops thick folds, and similar bone and skin changes in the hands and feet.

2. Palpate the skull for nodules or masses. Use a gentle rotating motion with the fingertips. Begin at the front and palpate down the midline; then palpate each side of the head. In the occipital region, palpate the occipital lymph nodes. See step 17 below.

   Rationale Palpation may detect sebaceous cysts, local deformities resulting from trauma, or enlarged lymph nodes. Sebaceous cysts result from occlusion of the sebaceous gland ducts; they feel smooth, rounded, and nodular.

3. Auscultate over the occipital, temporal, and orbital regions for bruits. See Figure 10–10. Bruits are discussed in carotid artery assessment in Technique 10–12 on page 212.

Face

4. Inspect the facial skin for color, the hair distribution and condition, and the facial structures (eyebrows, eyes, nose, mouth, and ears) for size and symmetry. Many disorders cause a change in facial shape or condition. Kidney or cardiac disease can cause edema of the eyelids. Thyroid overactivity (hyperthyroidism) can cause protrusion of the eyeballs with elevation of the upper eyelids, resulting in a startled

or staring expression. Thyroid underactivity (hypothyroidism or myxedema) can cause a dry, puffy face with dry skin and coarse features, referred to as *myxedema facies,* and thinning of scalp hair and eyebrows. *Cushing's syndrome,* a disorder in which there is increased adrenal hormone production, can cause a round face with reddened cheeks, referred to as *"moon face,"* and excessive hair growth on the upper lips, chin, and sideburn areas. Intake of synthetic adrenal hormones also produces these changes. Prolonged illness, starvation, and dehydration can result in sunken eyes, cheeks, and temples.

5. Ask the patient to elevate the eyebrows, frown or lower the eyebrows, close the eyes tightly, puff the cheeks, and smile and show the teeth.

   Rationale These movements determine the function of the muscles of facial expression and the seventh cranial (facial) nerve. (Sensation of the face, supplied by the fifth cranial [trigeminal] nerve, is tested as part of the neurologic examination. See Technique 10–18.)

6. Palpate the facial sinuses. See Technique 10–7, step 3.

Neck

7. Have the patient hold his or her head erect, and inspect the neck muscles (sternocleidomastoid and trapezius) for abnormal swellings or masses. Each sternocleidomastoid muscle extends from the upper sternum and the medial third of the clavicle to the mastoid process of the temporal bone behind the ear.

FIGURE 10–10

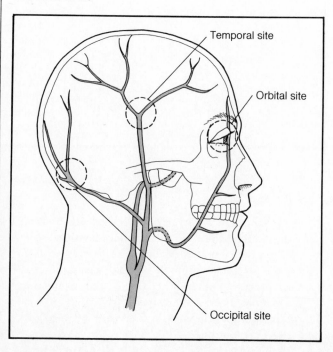

Temporal site

Orbital site

Occipital site

See Figure 10–11. These muscles turn and laterally flex the head. Each trapezius muscle extends from the occipital bone of the skull to the lateral third of the clavicle. These muscles draw the head to the side and back, elevate the chin, and elevate the shoulders to shrug them. Areas of the neck are defined by the sternocleidomastoid muscles, which divide each side of the neck into two triangles: the anterior and posterior triangles. See Figure 10–11. The trachea, thyroid gland, anterior cervical nodes, and carotid artery lie with the anterior triangle (the carotid artery runs parallel and anterior to the sternocleidomastoid muscle); the posterior lymph nodes lie within the posterior triangle. See Figure 10–12.

8. Instruct the patient to:

a. Move the chin to the chest (head flexion).

Rationale   This determines function of the sternocleidomastoid muscle.

b. Move the head back so that the chin points upward (head hyperextension).

Rationale   This determines function of the trapezius muscle.

c. Move the head so that the ear is moved toward the shoulder (lateral flexion) on each side.

FIGURE 10–11

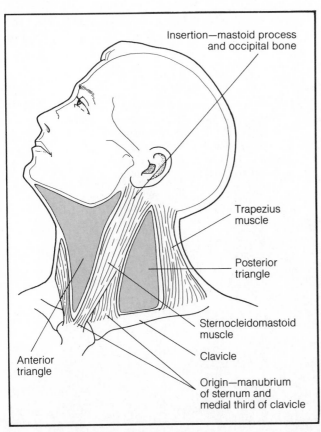

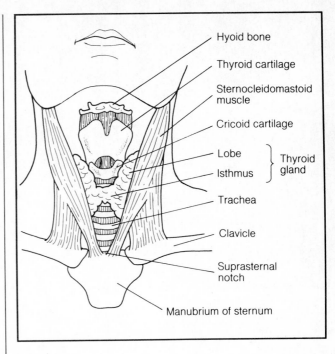

FIGURE 10–12

Rationale   This determines function of the sternocleidomastoid muscle.

d. Turn the head to the right and to the left (lateral rotation).

Rationale   This determines function of the sternocleidomastoid muscle.

9. Have the patient turn the head to one side against the resistance of your hand. Repeat with the other side.

Rationale   This determines the strength of the sternocleidomastoid muscle.

10. Have the patient shrug his or her shoulders against the resistance of your hands.

Rationale   This determines the strength of the trapezius muscles.

Trachea

11. Palpate the trachea for lateral deviation. Place a fingertip or a fingertip and thumb on the trachea in the suprasternal notch (see Figure 10–12) and then move the finger(s) laterally to the left and the right in the spaces bordered by the clavicle, the anterior aspect of the sternocleidomastoid muscle, and the trachea. See Figure 10–13. These spaces are normally equal on both sides, and the trachea is centrally placed.

Thyroid gland

12. Inspect the thyroid gland:

a. Stand in front of the patient.

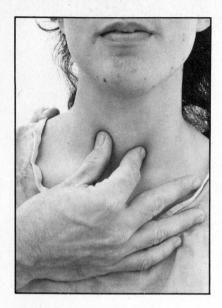

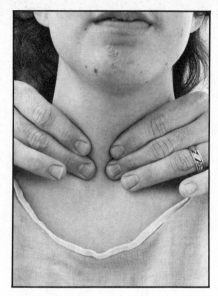

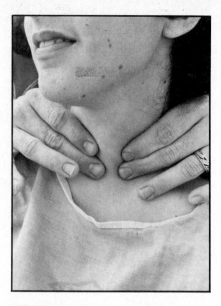

FIGURE 10–13

FIGURE 10–14

FIGURE 10–15

b. Observe the lower half of the neck overlying the thyroid gland for symmetry and visible masses.

c. Have the patient hyperextend the head and swallow. If necessary offer a glass of water to make it easier for the patient to swallow.

Rationale This determines movement of the thyroid and cricoid cartilages (see Figure 10–12) and whether swallowing causes a bulging of the gland. Normally the thyroid gland ascends during swallowing and is not visible.

13. To palpate the thyroid gland, stand either in front of or behind the patient and have the patient lower the chin slightly.

Rationale Lowering the chin relaxes the neck muscles, facilitating palpation.

14. For the posterior approach:

a. Place your hands around the patient's neck with your fingertips on the lower half of the neck over the trachea. See Figure 10–14.

b. Have the patient swallow (using a sip of water, if necessary), and feel for any enlargement of the *thyroid isthmus,* as it rises. The isthmus lies across the trachea below the cricoid cartilage. See Figure 10–12 earlier.

c. To examine the right thyroid lobe, have the patient lower the chin slightly and turn his or her head slightly to the right (the side being examined). With your left fingers displace the trachea slightly to the right. With your right fingers palpate the right thyroid lobe for any enlargement, masses, or nodules. See Figure 10–15. Have the patient swallow while you are palpating.

d. Repeat step c in reverse to examine the left thyroid lobe.

15. For the anterior approach:

a. Place the tips of your index and middle fingers over the trachea, and palpate the thyroid isthmus as the patient swallows.

b. To examine the right thyroid lobe, have the patient lower the chin slightly and turn his or her head slightly to the right. With your right fingers, displace the trachea slightly to the patient's right (your left). With your left fingers, palpate the right thyroid lobe. See Figure 10–16.

FIGURE 10–16

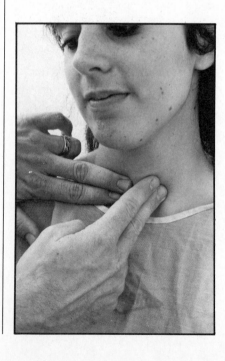

TABLE 10–8 ▪ Lymph Nodes of the Head and Neck

Node center	Location	Area drained
Head		
Occipital	At the posterior base of the skull	The occipital region of the scalp and the deep structures of the back of the neck
Postauricular (mastoid)	Behind the auricle of the ear over or in front of the mastoid process	The parietal region of the head and part of the ear
Preauricular	In front of the tragus of the ear	The forehead and upper face
Floor of mouth		
Submandibular (submaxillary)	Along the medial border of the lower jaw, halfway between the angle of the jaw and the chin	The chin, upper lip, cheek, nose, teeth, eyelids, part of the tongue and of the floor of the mouth
Submental	Behind the tip of the mandible, in the midline, under the chin	The anterior third of the tongue, gums, and floor of the mouth
Neck		
Superficial (anterior) cervical chain	Along and anterior to the sterno-cleidomastoid muscle	The skin and neck
Posterior cervical chain	Along the anterior aspect of the trapezius muscle	The posterior and lateral regions of the neck, occiput, and mastoid
Deep cervical chain	Under the sternocleidomastoid muscle	The larynx, thyroid gland, trachea, and upper part of the esophagus
Supraclavicular	Above the clavicle, in the angle between the clavicle and the sternocleido-mastoid muscle	The lateral regions of the neck and lungs

c. To examine the left thyroid lobe, repeat step c in reverse.

16. If enlargement of the gland is suspected, auscultate over the thyroid area for a bruit. Use the bell-shaped diaphragm of the stethoscope.

    Rationale In an enlarged hyperactive thyroid gland, blood flow through the thyroid arteries is increased and produces vibrations that may be heard as a soft rushing sound (bruit). See Technique 10–12 for further discussion of bruits.

Lymph nodes

Several lymph nodes or centers in the head collect lymph from the head, ears, nose, cheeks, and lips. Nodes in the neck that collect lymph from the head and neck structures are grouped serially and referred to as *chains*. See Figure 10–17 and Table 10–8. The deep cervical chain is not shown in Figure 10–17, since it lies beneath the sterno-cleidomastoid muscle.

17. Palpate the entire neck for enlarged lymph nodes, using the following guidelines:

    a. Face the patient to palpate all nodes.

    b. Bend the patient's head forward slightly or toward the side being examined to relax the soft tissue and muscles.

FIGURE 10–17

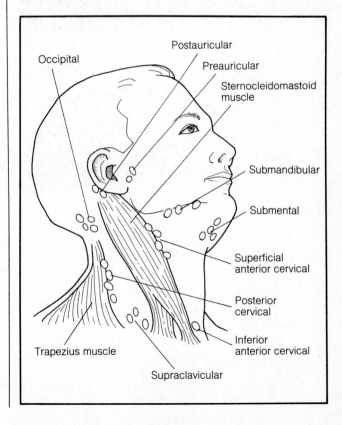

c. Palpate the nodes using the tips of the fingers. Move the fingertips in a gentle rotating motion.

d. When examining the submental and submandibular nodes, place the fingertips under the mandible on the side nearest the palpating hand, and pull the skin and subcutaneous tissue laterally over the mandibular surface so that it rolls over the nodes.

e. When palpating the supraclavicular nodes, have the patient bend her or his head forward to relax the tissues of the anterior neck and to relax the shoulders so that the clavicles are dropped. Use your hand nearest the side to be examined when facing the patient, ie, your left hand for the patient's right nodes. Use your free hand to flex the patient's head forward if necessary. Hook your index and third fingers over the clavicle lateral to the sternocleidomastoid muscle. See Figure 10–18.

f. When palpating the anterior cervical nodes and posterior cervical nodes, move your fingertips slowly in a forward circular motion against the sternocleidomastoid and trapezius muscles respectively.

g. To palpate the deep cervical nodes, bend or hook your fingers around the sternocleidomastoid muscle.

■ Evaluation

For expected and unexpected outcomes, see Table 10–7. Upon obtaining an unexpected outcome: Report your findings to the responsible nurse and/or physician.

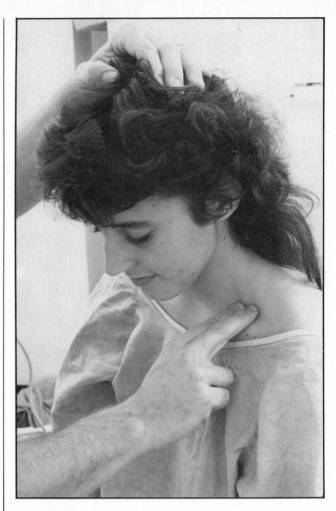

FIGURE 10–18

TECHNIQUE 10–6 ■ Assessing the Mouth

Assessment of an individual's mouth includes examination of its physical characteristics, consideration of developmental changes, and determination of the person's hygienic practices. Oral assessment should be carried out as part of the patient's initial assessment. Periodic reassessments need to be made for long-term care patients. Physical examination of the mouth includes inspection and palpation techniques. The status of the lips, mucous membranes, teeth, gingiva (gums), tongue, palates, and uvula is assessed.

■ Nursing Diagnosis

Nursing diagnoses that may indicate the need to assess a patient's mouth include:

1. Self-care deficit (oral hygiene) related to:
   a. Neuromuscular impairment
   b. Musculoskeletal disorder
   c. Visual disorder
   d. Surgical procedure
2. Alteration in health maintenance related to:
   a. Loss of independence
   b. Lack of knowledge
   c. Inadequate health practices
   d. Lack of supervision (children, the elderly)

■ Planning

Nursing goals

1. To determine baseline data regarding the patient's oral health
2. To determine the patient's oral hygienic practices
3. To develop an appropriate plan of oral care for the patient

Equipment

1. A tongue blade
2. Some 2 × 2 gauze squares
3. A fingercot or disposable glove
4. A penlight or flashlight

■ Intervention

See Table 10–9 for normal and abnormal findings and associated conditions.

Lips

1. Inspect the *outer lips.* Have the patient open his or her mouth. Observe the lips for symmetry of contour, color, and texture. See Figure 10–19.

   Rationale   Opening the mouth aids visual examination of these aspects.

2. Inspect *lip movement.* Have the patient purse the lips as if to whistle.

   Rationale   Inability to purse the lips can indicate damage to the facial (seventh cranial) nerve.

Inner lips and buccal mucosa

3. Inspect and palpate the inner lips and buccal mucosa for color, moisture, and texture.

   a. To inspect the *inner lip mucosa* of the bottom and top lips, have the patient relax the mouth and pull the lip outward away from the teeth. Grasp the lip on each side between the thumb and index finger. See Figure 10–20. Gloves may be worn.

      Rationale   Spreading the lips away from the teeth enables better vision of any abnormalities.

   b. To inspect the *buccal mucosa* (inner cheeks), have the patient close the teeth and relax the mouth. Retract the cheeks with a tongue blade or an index finger covered with a piece of gauze. See Figure 10–21. Use a penlight if needed to ensure adequate vision.

   c. To palpate the buccal mucosa, have the patient open the mouth. Using a fingercot (or gloves) and a penlight (optional), move a finger along the inside cheek. Another finger may be moved outside the cheek.

      Rationale   Palpation can determine the presence of nodules, ulcerations, or cysts.

Teeth and gums

4. Inspect the teeth and gums while examining the inner lips and buccal mucosa.

   a. Examine the *back teeth* while examining the buccal mucosa. Use the index fingers of both hands to retract the cheek if necessary. See Figure 10–22. Have the patient relax the lips and first close the teeth, then open them. Observe the number of

FIGURE 10–19

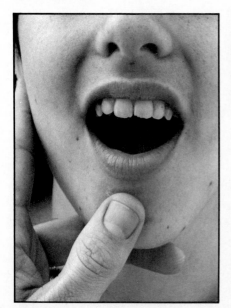

FIGURE 10–20

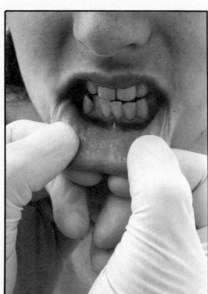

FIGURE 10–21

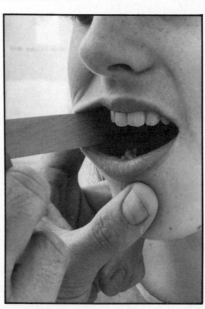

TABLE 10–9 ■ Mouth

Nursing history: Determine patient's routine pattern of dental care, when patient last visited dentist; length of time ulcers or other lesions have been present; whether any dentures produce discomfort; any medications patient is receiving.

Structure	Normal findings	Abnormal findings	Some associated conditions
Lips	Uniform pink color (darker in Mediterranean groups and Blacks, eg, bluish hue)	Pallor	Anemia
		Bluish discoloration	Cyanosis
		Blisters	Herpes simplex
	Soft, moist, smooth texture	Generalized swelling	Allergic reaction
	Symmetry of contour	Localized swelling	Trauma
	Ability to purse lips	Fissures, crusts, scales	Excessive moisture; nutritional deficiency; fluid deficit
		Inability to purse lips	Facial nerve damage
Inner lips and buccal mucosa	Uniform pink color (brown freckled pigmentation in Blacks)	Pallor	Anemia
		White patches (leukoplakia)	Early oral cancer; heavy smoking and drinking
	Moist, smooth, soft and elastic texture (drier oral mucosa in elderly due to decreased salivation)	Excessive dryness	Dehydration
		Mucosal cysts	Glandular irritation
		Irritations	Infections; ill-fitting dentures
		Abrasions	Trauma
		Ulcerations, nodules	Possible carcinoma
Teeth	32 adult teeth (see Figure 13–3; for eruption of temporary teeth, see Figure 13–2)	Missing teeth, bridges, full or partial dentures	Trauma; dental disease
		Dental caries	Poor oral hygiene
	Smooth, white tooth enamel	Discoloration of enamel	Excessive use of tobacco; certain medications (eg, iron)
Gums	Pink color (bluish or dark patches in Blacks)	Excessive redness	Ill-fitting dentures; periodontal disease
	Moist, firm texture	Spongy texture, bleeding, tenderness	Periodontal disease
	No retraction (pulling away from the teeth)	Receding atrophied gums	Normal aging process
		Swelling that partially covers the teeth	Dilantin therapy; leukemia
Tongue	Central position	Deviated from center	Damage to hypoglossal (12th cranial) nerve
	Pink color (some brown pigmentation on tongue borders in Blacks), moist, slightly rough, thin whitish coating	Dry, furry	Fluid deficit
		Smooth and red	Iron, vitamin B_{12}, or Vitamin B_3 deficiency
		Nodes, ulcerations, discolorations, restricted mobility	Possible carcinoma
	Moves freely		
	Smooth tongue base with prominent veins	Varicosities (tiny bluish-black or purple swollen areas)	Normal aging process
Palates	Light pink, smooth, soft palate	Discolorations	Jaundice
	Lighter pink hard palate, more irregular texture	Palates the same color	Anemia
		Irritations	Ill-fitting dentures
Uvula	Positioned in midline of soft palate	Deviation to one side	Tumor; trauma
		Immobility	Damage to trigeminal (fifth cranial) nerve or vagus (tenth cranial) nerve
Oropharynx and tonsils	Pink and smooth posterior wall	Reddened, lesions, plaques	Pharyngitis
	Tonsils pink and normal size	Tonsillar crypts inflamed, filled with exudate, swollen	Tonsillitis

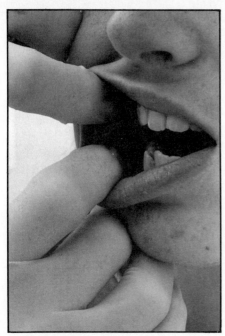

FIGURE 10–22

teeth, tooth color, the state of fillings, the presence of partial or complete dentures, and how they fit. By age 25, most people have 32 permanent teeth. See Figure 13–3 on page 298.

Rationale Adequate retraction of the cheeks is necessary for proper vision of the molars. Closed teeth assist in observation of the tooth alignment and loss of teeth; opened teeth assist in observation of dental fillings and caries.

b. Assess the *gums around the molars* while examining the buccal mucosa. Observe the color and moisture of the gums. Assess the texture of the gums by gently pressing the gum tissue with a tongue blade.

c. Inspect the *front teeth and gums* while examining the inner lip mucosa. Have the patient "grit" the teeth and retract the lips, or follow step 3a on page 179.

d. If the patient has complete or partial dentures, ask him or her to remove them. Inspect the condition of the dentures, eg, broken parts.

Tongue

5.   Inspect and palpate the *tongue* for color, texture, position, and mobility.

a. To inspect the *surface of the tongue,* have the patient protrude the tongue. Observe it for position, color, and texture.

b. To inspect *tongue movement,* have the patient roll the tongue upward and move it from side to side.

c. To inspect the *base of the tongue,* the *mouth floor,* and the *frenulum,* have the patient place the tip of the tongue against the roof of the mouth.

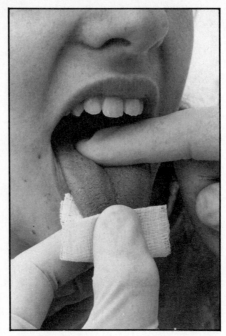

FIGURE 10–23

d. To palpate the tongue, grasp its tip, using a piece of gauze, and with the index finger of the other hand, palpate the back of it, its borders, and its base. See Figure 10–23.

Rationale Grasping the tongue stabilizes it for proper palpation.

Palate and uvula

6.   Inspect the *hard and soft palate* for color and texture. Have the patient tilt back the head and open the mouth widely. Depress the tongue with a tongue blade. Use a penlight for better vision.

7.   Inspect the *uvula* for position and mobility, while examining the palates.

Oropharynx and tonsils

8.   Inspect the *oropharynx* one side at a time to avoid eliciting the gag reflex. The oropharynx is that area of the pharynx behind the mouth and tongue.

a. With a tongue depressor, press the tongue to one side while the patient is sticking the tongue out. Use a penlight to view the oropharynx, if needed.

b. Repeat for the other side of the oropharynx.

9.   Inspect the *tonsils* behind the fauces for color and size. The tonsils are oval-shaped lymphoid tissues situated on each side of the fauces. The fauces is the passage from the mouth to the oropharynx. See Figure 10–24. The tonsils may be normally enlarged in the young child.

10.   Elicit the *gag reflex* by pressing the posterior tongue with the tongue depressor.

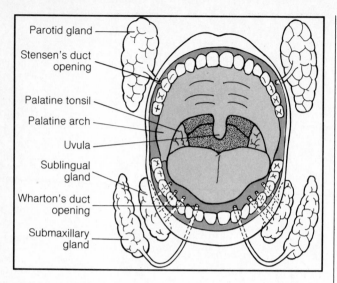

Parotid gland
Stensen's duct opening
Palatine tonsil
Palatine arch
Uvula
Sublingual gland
Wharton's duct opening
Submaxillary gland

FIGURE 10–24

Rationale Lack of the gag reflex can indicate problems with the glossopharyngeal or vagus nerves.

11. Record your findings on the appropriate records.

Sample Recording

Date	Time	Notes
4/7/87	1500	C/o discomfort from ill-fitting upper dentures and difficulty chewing. Refuses to wear dentures. Oral cavity assessed. Left superior buccal mucosa reddened. Hard palate swollen and reddened, is tender to touch. Dr. Woo notified.———————— ———————— Susan M. Maraket, SN

TECHNIQUE 10–7 ■ Assessing the Nose and Sinuses

Assessment of the nose and sinuses includes inspection and palpation.

■ Planning

Nursing goals

1. To determine the effectiveness of nasal or sinus therapies
2. To screen for nasal or sinus problems

Equipment

1. A nasal speculum (a lighted instrument to examine the nares)
2. A small flashlight or penlight to inspect the sinuses

■ Intervention

See Table 10–10 for normal and abnormal findings and associated conditions.

Nose

1. Palpate the external nose lightly for tenderness.
2. Inspect both nares (nasal chambers) using a lighted nasal speculum. The nares open externally via the anterior nares and internally through the posterior nares into the nasopharynx. See Figure 10–25.

   a. Inspect the lining of the nares (mucosa) and the coarse hairs that filter the air. Note the presence of redness, swelling, growths, and discharge.

   b. Inspect the position of the nasal septum between the nasal chambers, in particular any deviation to right or left.

   c. Inspect the inferior and middle turbinates. The superior turbinate is difficult to inspect because of its position. See Figure 10–25. These bones increase the mucous membrane surface in the

FIGURE 10–25

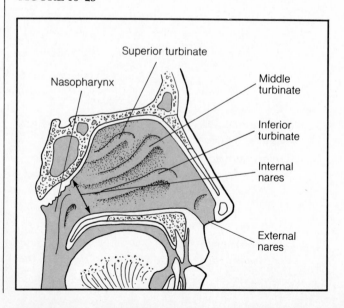

Superior turbinate
Nasopharynx
Middle turbinate
Inferior turbinate
Internal nares
External nares

TABLE 10-10   ■   Nose and Sinuses

Nursing history: Determine whether patient has history of allergies, difficulty breathing through the nose, sinus infections, injuries to nose or face, nosebleeds; whether patient takes any medications; any changes in sense of smell.

Structure	Normal findings	Abnormal findings	Some associated conditions
Nose (external)	Nares patent	Decreased air movement through one or both nares	Allergies
	External nose symmetrical and straight; no discharge	Discharge from nares	Upper respiratory infection
	Not tender; no lesions	Tenderness upon palpation; lesions	
Nose (internal)	Nasal septum intact and in midline	Septum deviated	Injury to nose
	Mucosa pink with clear watery discharge	Mucosa red, edema Abnormal (eg, purulent) discharge	Upper respiratory infection
	No lesions	Lesions, eg, polyps	
Sinuses	Not tender	Tenderness	Infection
	Sinuses contain air and light up equally	Fluid in sinus appears darker upon transillumination	

nares. The mucous membranes warm and moisten the inspired air. The clefts between the turbinates are called meati. Each meatus is named for the adjacent turbinate, eg, the inferior meatus is near the inferior turbinate.

d. Inspect the mucous membranes for purulent drainage and nasal polyps.

Sinuses

3. Palpate the maxillary and frontal sinuses. See Figure 10-26.

   Rationale   Palpation can reveal tenderness.

4. Transilluminate the frontal sinuses by placing a penlight against the inner aspect of the supraorbital ridge of the frontal bone (see Figure 10-26). This is best done in a darkened room. Normally the light shines through the bone and outlines the sinus.

   Rationale   Transillumination can reveal the presence of air or fluid in the sinuses. The sinuses will appear darker when fluid is present.

5. Transilluminate the maxillary sinuses by placing a penlight in the patient's mouth and shining it to the left and to the right.

6. Record your assessments on the appropriate record.

FIGURE 10-26

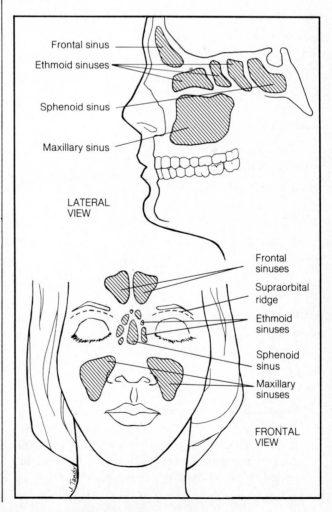

■ **Evaluation**

Expected outcomes

1. Mucous membranes of the nose are smooth and have a small amount of clear drainage.
2. Nares are patent.
3. Nasal septum is intact and in the midline.

4. Sinuses are clear.

Unexpected outcomes

See Table 10–10. Upon obtaining an unexpected outcome: Report your findings to the responsible nurse and/or physician.

TECHNIQUE 10–8 ■ Assessing the Eyes and Vision

Vision is considered by many people the most important sense, since it allows them to interact freely with their environment and enjoy the beauty of life around them. To maintain optimum vision, the eyes need to be examined throughout the life cycle. It is recommended that people under age 40 have their eyes tested every three to five years, or more frequently if there is a family history of diabetes, hypertension, blood dyscrasia, or eye disease (eg, glaucoma). After age 40, an eye examination is recommended every two years, to rule out the possibility of glaucoma.

An eye assessment should be carried out as part of the patient's initial physical examination; periodic reassessments need to be made for long-term care patients. Examination of the eyes includes assessment of visual acuity, ocular movement, visual fields, external structures, and the fundus. Most eye assessment procedures involve inspection. Consideration is also given to developmental changes and to individual hygienic practices, if the patient wears contact lenses or an artificial eye.

For the anatomic structures of the eye, see Figures 13–13 and 13–14 on pages 306 and 307.

■ **Planning**

Nursing goals

1. To obtain baseline data on the patient's vision, eye mobility, and health status of the external and internal eye structures
2. To screen for specific eye problems

Equipment

1. Newsprint for testing near vision.
2. A Snellen eye chart; for a person unable to read, a Snellen E chart; for a child of 3 years, a chart with identifiable pictures. See Figure 10–27.

3. A penlight.
4. An eye cover or opaque index card.
5. A cotton-tipped applicator stick (optional) for examining the palpebral conjunctiva.
6. A cotton wisp.
7. An ophthalmoscope. See Figure 10–28.

■ **Intervention**

See Table 10–11 for normal and abnormal findings and associated conditions.

Visual acuity

1. *Near vision.* Provide adequate lighting and have the patient read from a magazine or newspaper held at a distance of 36 cm (14 in). If the patient normally wears corrective lenses, the glasses or lenses should be worn as she or he reads.

FIGURE 10–27 ■ Three types of eye charts: the preschool children's chart (left), Snellen standard chart (center), and Snellen E chart for patients unable to read (right).

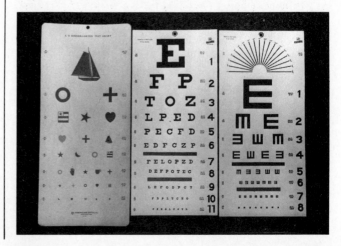

2. *Distance vision.* Have the patient wear her or his corrective lenses, unless they are used for reading only, ie, for distances of only 30 to 36 cm (12 to 14 in). Have the patient stand or sit 6 m (20 ft) from a Snellen chart. Take three readings as follows:

   a. Have the patient cover the eye not being tested (left eye) and identify the letters on the Snellen chart, starting at the line he or she can most comfortably read and continuing to lower lines. If the patient is unable to read, use the Snellen E chart, and ask him or her to say in which direction the E is pointing.

   Rationale   The right eye is usually tested first. It is wise to get in the habit of starting with the right eye, to prevent inadvertent errors in documenting data about each eye.

   b. Have the patient cover the right eye, and identify the letters with the left eye.

   c. Have the patient read the Snellen chart with both eyes *uncovered.*

   d. Record the readings of each eye and both eyes, ie, the smallest line from which the patient is able to read one half or more of the letters. The Snellen chart has standardized numbers (fractions) at the end of each line of the chart. For the top line it is 20/200. The numerator (top number) is always 20, the distance the patient stands from the chart. The denominator (bottom number) is the distance from which the normal eye can read the chart. Therefore, if a patient has 20/40 vision, he or she can see at 20 feet from the chart what a normal-sighted person can see at 40 feet from the chart. Normal 20/20 vision is acquired by 6 years of age. Visual acuity is recorded as s̄c (without correction), or c̄c (with correction). You can also indicate how many letters were misread in the line, eg, "visual acuity 20/40 – 2 c̄c" indicates that two letters were misread in the 20/40 line by a patient wearing corrective lenses.

3. *Functional vision.* If the patient is unable to see the top line (20/200) of the Snellen chart, perform functional vision tests (Boyd-Monk, 1980, p 63):

   a. *Light perception* (LP). Shine a penlight into the patient's eye from a lateral position and then turn the light off. Ask the patient to tell you when the light is on or off. If the patient knows when the light is on and off, he or she has light perception, and the vision is recorded as LP.

   b. *Hand movements* (H/M). Hold your hand 30 cm (1 ft) from the patient's face and move it slowly back and forth, stopping it periodically. Ask the patient to tell you when your hand stops moving. If the patient knows when your hand stops moving, record the vision as H/M 1 ft.

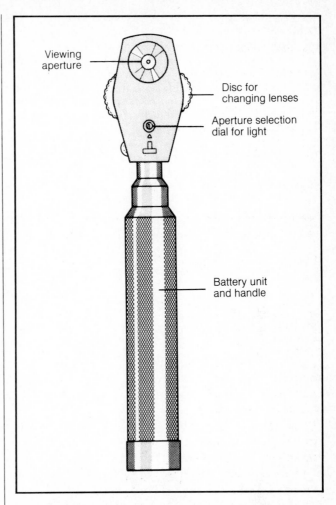

FIGURE 10–28 ■ The ophthalmoscope used to examine the interior of the eye through the pupil.

   c. *Counting fingers* (C/F). Hold up some of your fingers 30 cm (1 ft) from the patient's face, and ask him or her to count your fingers. If the patient can do so, note on the vision record C/F 1 ft.

   Rationale   Patients who can pass these three functional tests are able to manage fairly well independently. If the person is unable to perform them in either eye, he or she is blind. Legal blindness is a visual acuity of 20/200 or less in both eyes with corrective lenses.

Extraocular movements (EOM)

Three tests can be performed on patients over 6 months of age.

4. *Six cardinal fields of gaze* (determines eye coordination and alignment).

   a. Stand directly in front of the patient and hold the penlight at a comfortable distance, eg, 30 cm (1 ft) in front of the patient's eyes.

   b. Ask the patient to hold his or her head in a fixed

TABLE 10–11 ■ Eyes and Vision

Nursing history: Determine family history of diabetes, hypertension, blood dyscrasia, or eye disease, injury, or surgery; when patient last visited an ophthalmologist; whether patient is currently taking eye medications; whether patient wears contact lenses or eyeglasses; hygienic practices for corrective lenses; current symptoms of eye problems, such as changes in visual acuity, blurring of vision, tearing, spots, photophobia, itching, or pain.

Test or structure	Normal findings	Abnormal findings	Some associated conditions
Visual acuity			
Near vision	Able to read newsprint	Difficulty reading newsprint	Aging
Distance vision	20/20 vision on Snellen chart from age 6 onward	Denominator of 40 or more on Snellen chart with corrective lenses	Refractive errors
Functional vision		Functional vision only (eg, light perception, hand movements, counting fingers at 1 ft)	
Extraocular movement			
Positions of gaze	Both eyes coordinated, move in unison, with parallel alignment	Eye movements not coordinated or parallel; one or both eyes fail to follow penlight in specific directions	Strabismus
	End-point nystagmus	Nystagmus other than end-point	Neurologic impairments, eg, cerebrovascular accident, multiple sclerosis; Dilantin toxicity
Cover-uncover patch test	Uncovered eye does not move when index card is placed over other eye	Uncovered eye moves to focus on fixed point	
	Newly uncovered eye does not move when index card is removed	Newly uncovered eye moves to focus on fixed point	
Corneal light reflex text	Light reflection appears at symmetric spots in both eyes	Light reflection appears at different spots in each eye (asymmetric)	
Visual fields	Temporal field, 90° Upward field, 50° Downward field, 70° Nasal field, 50–60°	Visual field smaller than normal	Glaucoma
		One-half vision in one or both eyes	Nerve damage
External structures			
Eyebrows	Hair evenly distributed	Loss of hair	
	Skin intact	Scaling and flakiness of skin	
	Eyebrows symmetrically aligned; movement is equal	Unequal alignment and movement	
Eyelashes	Equally distributed		
	Curled slightly outward	Turned inward (see inversion of eyelid below)	
Eyelids	Skin intact; no discharge; no discoloration	Redness, swelling, flaking, crusting, plaques, discharge, nodules, lesions	Infections; sebaceous gland blockages; carcinoma
	Lids close symmetrically	Asymmetric lid closure; incomplete or painful closure	
	Approximately 15 to 20 involuntary blinks per minute; blinking bilateral	Blinking rapid, monocular, absent, or infrequent	

TABLE 10–11   ■   continued

Test or structure	Normal findings	Abnormal findings	Some associated conditions
Eyelids (continued)	When lids open, no visible sclera above corneas, and upper and lower borders of cornea are slightly covered	Lid lies at or below the pupil margin (ptosis)	Aging; edema from drug allergy or systemic disease (eg, kidney disease); congenital lid muscle dysfunction; neuromuscular disease (eg, myasthenia gravis); third cranial nerve impairment
		Eversion (outturning of lid) (ectropion)	Aging; scarring injury
		Inversion of lid (entropion)	Aging; scarring injury
		Rim of sclera shows between lid and iris	Hyperthyroidism
Lacrimal apparatus	No edema over lacrimal gland or sac	Swelling over lacrimal gland and/or sac; evidence of increased tearing; regurgitation of fluid on palpation of lacrimal sac	
Bulbar conjunctiva	Transparent; capillaries sometimes evident; sclera appears white (yellowish in Blacks)	Jaundiced sclera	Liver disease
		Excessively pale sclera	Anemia
		Reddened sclera; lesions or nodules	Damage by mechanical, chemical, allergenic, or bacterial agents
Palpebral conjunctiva	Pink and smooth	Extremely pale	Anemia
		Red	Inflammation
Corneal sensitivity (reflex) test	Patient blinks when cornea is touched	One or both eyelids fail to respond	Fifth (trigeminal) cranial nerve impairment
Cornea	Transparent, shiny, and smooth; details of iris visible	Opaque; surface not smooth	Trauma; abrasion
	Thin, grayish-white ring around margin in elderly people (arcus senilis)	Arcus senilis in patient under age 40	
Anterior chamber	Transparent	Cloudy	
	No shadows of light on iris	Crescent-shaped shadow on far side of iris	
	Depth of about 3 mm	Shallow chamber	Glaucoma
Pupil and iris	Black in color; equal in size; normally 3 to 7 mm in diameter; round, smooth border	Cloudy	Cataract
		Enlarged (mydriasis)	Injury, glaucoma, drugs (atropine)
		Constricted (miosis)	Drugs (morphine, pilocarpine); inflammation of iris
		Unequal pupils (anisocoria)	Central nervous system disorder
	Iris flat and round	Bulging toward cornea	Increased intraocular pressure
Pupillary reflexes Direct and consensual reaction to light	Illuminated pupil constricts (direct response) Nonilluminated pupil constricts (consensual response)	Neither pupil constricts Unequal responses Absent responses	Blind eye in monocular blindness
Accommodation	Pupils constrict when looking at near object Pupils dilate when looking at far object Pupils converge when near object is moved toward nose	One or both pupils fail to constrict, dilate, or converge	

TABLE 10–11 ■ continued

Test or structure	Normal findings	Abnormal findings	Some associated conditions
Internal structures			
Red reflex	Bright, round, red-orange glow through pupil	Decreased redness or roundness	
		Opacities	Cataracts
Optic disc and cup	Yellowish or creamy pink, almost round disc; lighter than retina	Pale disc	Optic atrophy; glaucoma
	Distinct regular outline (nasal edge less distinct than temporal edge)	Blurred disc margins and reddened disc	Papilledema
	About 1.5 mm in diameter but appears larger with magnification × 15	Discs unequal size and shape	
	Physiologic cup occupies one third to one half of disc area	Cup extends to disc border, is asymmetric	Glaucoma
	Cups equal in size	Cups unequal in size	
	Cup paler than disc (yellow-white)		
Retinal vessels	Arteries		
	Light red color	Copper or silver color	Arteriosclerosis
		Pale or white vessel	Previous vascular event
	Narrow band of light in center (arteriolar light reflex) about one-fourth diameter of blood column Arteries two-thirds to four-fifths diameter of veins	Narrowed light reflex	Hypertension
	Regular calibre, decreasing in size toward periphery	Irregularities in calibre (dilations or constrictions)	
	Veins		
	Larger than arteries	Dilated and tortuous veins	
	Darker color than arteries		
	No prominent light reflex		
	Arteriovenous crossings		
	Calibre of underlying vessel; not indented, pinched, or displaced		
Retinal background (periphery)	Uniform orange-pink color; lighter in fair people, darker in Black people	Pallor	
		Linear, or large or small dark or red patches	Hemorrhage
		Discrete tiny red dots	Microaneurysms
		Fuzzy white patches	Exudates
Macula and fovea	Slightly darker than retina	Same as for retinal background, above	
	Tiny capillaries may be evident on surface		
	Fovea seen as tiny bright light in center		

position facing you and to follow the movements of the penlight with the *eyes only*.

c. Move the penlight in a slow, orderly manner through the six cardinal fields of gaze: from the center of the eye along the lines of the arrows in Figure 10–29 and back to the center.

Rationale   These six positions are used because six muscles guide the movement of each eye. Four *rectus* muscles (superior, inferior, lateral, and medial) move the eye in the directions indicated. Two *oblique* muscles (superior and inferior) rotate the eyeball on its axis. Cranial nerves III (oculomotor), IV (trochlear), and VI (abducens) innervate these muscles. The six positions can identify a nonfunctioning muscle or associated cranial nerve.

d. Stop the movement of the penlight periodically.

Rationale   This enables the nurse to detect *nystagmus* (an involuntary rapid movement of the eyeball). Slight nystagmus on the extreme lateral gaze (end-point nystagmus) occurs normally in many people. Other nystagmus is abnormal.

5. *Cover-uncover patch test* (determines eye alignment).

a. Ask the patient to stare straight ahead at a fixed point, eg, at a penlight held 15 cm (6 in) in front of the eyes.

FIGURE 10–29

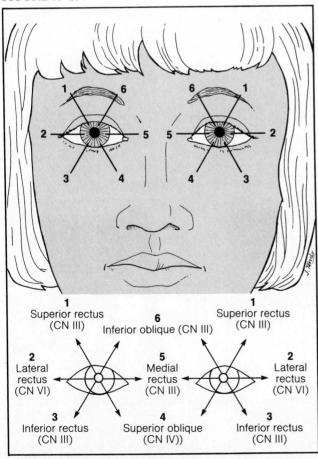

1
Superior rectus
(CN III)

6
Inferior oblique (CN III)

1
Superior rectus
(CN III)

2
Lateral rectus
(CN VI)

5
Medial rectus
(CN III)

2
Lateral rectus
(CN VI)

3
Inferior rectus
(CN III)

4
Superior oblique
(CN IV))

3
Inferior rectus
(CN III)

b. Cover one of the patient's eyes with an eye cover or index card while observing the uncovered eye. If well aligned, the uncovered eye should not move from the fixed point when the other eye is covered. If it does move, to focus on the fixed point, it was *not* well aligned before the other eye was covered; it is shifting from a lateral to central gaze.

c. Remove the eye cover, and observe the newly uncovered eye for movement. The newly uncovered eye, if well aligned, should not move. If it does move to focus on the fixed point when uncovered, it was *not* well aligned when covered. Muscle weakness is apparent when the eye turns outward while covered. As the eye is uncovered, a quick inward movement occurs to bring it back to alignment.

d. Repeat steps a–c for the other eye.

e. Test each eye several times to confirm your findings.

6. *Corneal light reflex test* (determines eye alignment).

a. Darken the room.

b. Ask the patient to stare straight ahead.

c. Shine a penlight on the bridge of the nose.

d. Observe the light reflection in both corneas. Light reflection is normally situated in the same spot on both eyes.

Visual fields

7. *Peripheral visual field: confrontation method* (determines function of retina, neuronal visual pathways to the brain, and second (optic) cranial nerve function.

a. Have the patient sit directly facing you at a distance of 60 to 90 cm (2 to 3 ft).

b. Ask the patient to cover the left eye with a card and to look directly at your nose.

Rationale   It is wise to get in the habit of testing the right eye first. The patient must always look straight ahead in order to test what he or she can see in all areas away from the centralmost point of vision.

c. Cover or close your eye directly opposite the patient's covered eye (ie, your right eye), and look directly at the patient's nose.

Rationale   The nurse acts as a control. It is assumed that she or he has good visual fields.

d. Hold an object (eg, a penlight or pencil) in your fingers, extend your arm, and move the object into the visual field from various points in the periphery. See Figure 10–30. The object should be an equal distance from the patient and yourself. Ask the patient to tell you when he or she first sees the moving object.

Rationale   The object is placed equidistant from

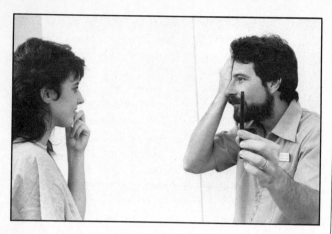

FIGURE 10-30

the nurse and the patient so that both can see it at the same time.

- To test the *temporal* field of the right eye, extend and move your left arm in from the patient's right periphery. Temporally, peripheral objects can be seen at right angles (90°) to the central point of vision.

- To test the *upward* field of the right eye, extend and move the left arm down from the upward periphery. The upward field of vision is normally 50°.

  Rationale The orbital ridge is in the way.

- To test the *downward* field of the right eye, extend and move the left arm up from the lower periphery. The downward field of vision is normally 70°.

  Rationale The cheekbone is in the way.

- To test the *nasal* field of the right eye, extend and move your right arm in from the periphery. The nasal field of vision is normally 50° away from the central point of vision.

Rationale The nose is in the way.

e. Repeat the above steps for the left eye, reversing the process.

External eye structures

Have the patient sit at eye level directly in front of you. Inspect the external ocular structures in the order described. See Table 10-11 for normal and abnormal findings.

8. *Eyebrows.* Inspect the eyebrows for hair distribution and alignment, skin quality, and movement. Ask the patient to raise and lower the eyebrows.

9. *Eyelashes.* Inspect the eyelashes for evenness of distribution and direction of curl.

10. *Eyelids.* Inspect the eyelids for surface characteristics, (eg, skin quality and texture), position, ability to close, ability to blink, and frequency of blinking.

  a. To inspect the *upper* lids, have the patient close the eyes. Elevate the eyebrows with your thumb and index finger. See Figure 10-31. Note skin color, skin texture, and eyelid closure.

  Rationale Elevating the eyebrows stretches the skin folds for proper visual examination.

  b. To inspect the *lower* lids, have the patient open the eyes. Note the characteristics listed for the upper lids, ability to blink, frequency of blinking, and the position of the eyelids in relation to the cornea.

11. *Lacrimal apparatus.* See Figure 13-13 on page 306.

  a. Inspect and palpate the lacrimal gland. See Figure 10-32. Note any edema or tenderness.

  b. Inspect and palpate the lacrimal sac and nasolacrimal duct. See Figure 10-33. Observe for edema between the lower lid and the nose and for

FIGURE 10-31

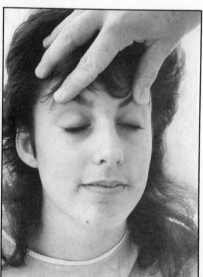

FIGURE 10-32

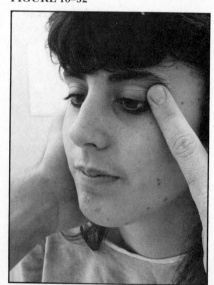

FIGURE 10-33

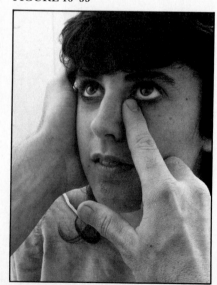

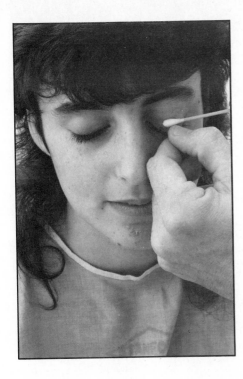

FIGURE 10–34

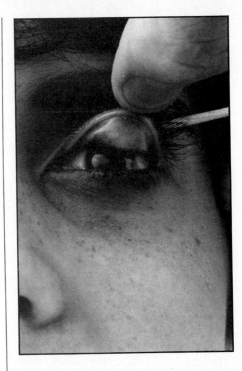

FIGURE 10–35

evidence of increased tearing. Using the tip of your index finger, palpate inside the lower orbital rim near the inner canthus, not on the side of the nose.

12. *Bulbar conjunctiva.*

   a. Retract the patient's eyelids with your thumb and index finger, exerting pressure over the upper and lower bony orbits.

   b. Ask the patient to look up, down, and from side to side.

   c. Inspect the conjunctiva for color, texture, and presence of lesions.

13. *Palpebral conjunctiva.* Assessment requires eversion of the eyelids.

   a. Evert both *lower* lids. Ask the patient to look up, and gently retract the lower lids with your index fingers. Inspect the conjunctiva for color, texture, and presence of lesions.

   b. Evert the *upper* lids only if a problem is suspected.

   ■ Ask the patient to look down and to keep the eyes slightly open.

   Rationale   Closing the eyelids contracts the orbicular muscle, which prevents lid eversion.

   ■ Gently grasp the eyelashes with your thumb and index finger. Pull the lashes gently downward.

   Rationale   Upward or outward pulling on the eyelashes causes muscle contraction.

   ■ Place a cotton-tipped applicator stick about 1 cm above the lid margin, and push it gently downward while still holding the eyelashes. See Figure 10–34. These actions evert the lid, ie, flip the lower part of the lid over on top of itself.

   ■ Hold the margin of the everted lid or the eyelashes against the ridge of the upper bony orbit with the applicator stick or your thumb. See Figure 10–35.

   ■ Inspect the conjunctiva for color, texture, lesions, and foreign bodies.

   ■ Gently pull the lashes forward, and ask the patient to look up and to blink.

   Rationale   This returns the lid to its normal position.

14. *Corneal sensitivity test* (determines the function of the fifth [trigeminal] cranial nerve).

   a. Ask the patient to keep both eyes open and look straight ahead.

   b. With a wisp of cotton, approach from behind and beside the patient and lightly touch the cornea with the cotton wisp. The blink response normally occurs when the cornea is touched, indicating that the trigeminal nerve is intact.

15. *Cornea.*

   a. Ask the patient to look straight ahead.

   b. Hold a penlight at an oblique angle to the eye, and move the light slowly across the corneal surface.

   c. Inspect the cornea for clarity and texture.

16. *Anterior chamber.*

   a. Use the same oblique lighting as used to test the cornea.

   b. Inspect the anterior chamber for transparency and depth. Normally no shadows of light appear on the iris. If a crescent-shaped shadow appears on

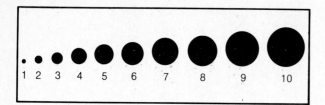

FIGURE 10–36

the far side of the iris, it indicates a bulging iris, a shallow anterior chamber, and a predisposition to glaucoma.

17. *Pupil.*

a. Ask the patient to look straight ahead.

b. Inspect the pupils for color, shape, and symmetry of size. The pupil is normally 2 to 5 mm in diameter. Pupil charts are available in some agencies. See Figure 10–36 for variations in pupil diameters in millimeters.

c. Assess each pupil's direct and consensual reaction to light to determine the function of the second (oculomotor) and third (trochlear) cranial nerves.
   - Partially darken the room.
   - Ask the patient to look straight ahead.
   - Using a penlight and approaching from the side, shine a light on the pupil.
   - Observe the response of the illuminated pupil. It should constrict (direct response).
   - Again shine the light on the pupil, and observe the response of the other pupil. It should also constrict (consensual response).

d. Assess each pupil's reaction to accommodation.
   - Hold an object (a penlight or pencil) about 10 cm (4 in) from the bridge of the patient's nose.
   - Ask the patient to look first at the top of the object and then at a distant object (eg, the far wall) behind the penlight. Alternate the gaze from the near to the far object.
   - Observe the pupil response. The pupils should constrict when looking at the near object and dilate when looking at the far object.
   - Next move the penlight or pencil toward the patient's nose. The pupils should converge.

e. To record normal assessment of the pupils, use the abbreviation PERRLA (pupils equally round and react to light and accommodation).

Internal eye structures

The internal part of the eye posterior to the lens, visible through the pupil by an ophthalmoscope, is called the *fundus* of the eye. Structures of the fundus include the retina, choroid, fovea, macula, disc, and retinal vessels. Ophthalmic or fundic examination of the eye requires practice and skill.

18. *Red reflex through pupil.*

a. Assemble the ophthalmoscope. See Figure 10–28 on page 185. Align the base of the head with lugs on the top of the handle. Push the head down and rotate it, until you hear it click into place.

b. Darken the room to dilate the pupils.

c. Have the patient remove his or her eyeglasses. Contact lenses may be left in, although removal can decrease light reflection.

d. Have the patient sit or stand in front of you.

e. Adjust the aperture selection dial on the back of the ophthalmoscope head, to regulate the amount of light. Use the largest round light at first.

f. Select the appropriate lens by adjusting the lens selection wheel on the side of the ophthalmoscope head. To begin, you may set the lens wheel at the 0 setting.

g. To examine the right eye, hold the ophthalmoscope comfortably against your right eye with your right hand. Reverse the position to examine the left eye.

h. Hold the ophthalmoscope at least 30 cm (1 ft) from the patient's pupil and at an angle of about 25° lateral to the patient's line of central vision.

i. Ask the patient to keep both eyes open and to focus on a distant object.

j. Shine the light on the patient's pupil.

k. Observe the bright orange glow through the pupil (the red reflex). In dark-skinned persons, the fundus may appear brown or purplish.

19. *Optic disc and cup.*

a. Keeping the red reflex in sight, slowly move the ophthalmoscope close to the patient's pupil.

   Rationale Slow movement promotes dilation of the pupil and prevents eye movement.

b. Locate some retinal structure, such as a blood vessel, and focus the image. Adjust the lens until the margins of the structure appear sharp.

c. Locate the optic disc by following the blood vessels toward the midline. See Figure 10–37.

d. Note the color, size, and shape of the disc, the distinctness of its margins, and its physiologic cup (the depressed central area of the disc).

20. *Retinal blood vessels.*

a. Follow the blood vessels peripherally in each of four quadrants: superior temporal, inferior temporal, superior nasal, and inferior nasal.

   Rationale The central retinal artery arises from the depth of the optic disc and divides into four main branches, which supply each retinal quadrant. The central retinal vein leaves the disc in company with the central artery and has similar branches in each quadrant. The four quadrants

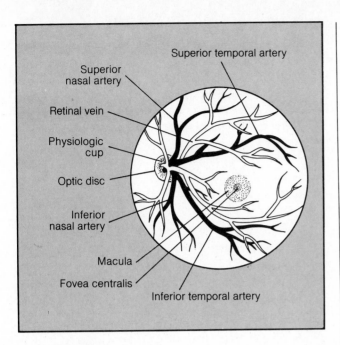

Superior temporal artery

Superior nasal artery

Retinal vein

Physiologic cup

Optic disc

Inferior nasal artery

Macula

Fovea centralis

Inferior temporal artery

FIGURE 10-37

are scanned, since blood vessel abnormalities are not evenly distributed.

b. Inspect the vessels for size, color, pattern, and arteriovenous crossings. See Table 10–11 earlier for normal and abnormal findings.

21. *Retinal background (periphery).*

a. Ask the patient to look upward, downward, and from side to side.

b. Inspect the retinal background of the four quadrants.

c. Note color and surface characteristics.

22. *Macula and fovea centralis.*

a. Avoid directing light on the macula for long periods.

   Rationale   The macula is the center of most acute vision and is sensitive. Prolonged light on it can be uncomfortable for the patient.

b. Locate the macula by first locating the optic disc and then looking two disc diameters (DD) away toward the patient's temple. It is a small circular structure 1 DD in size.

   or

c. Ask the patient to look directly at the light.

d. Inspect the macula for color and surface characteristics. Note the tiny glistening spot of reflected light in the center of the macula. This is the *fovea centralis.*

23. Record your findings on the appropriate records. Identify the right eye as OD (oculus dexter), the left as OS (oculus sinister), and both eyes as OU (oculus uterque).

Sample Recording

Date	Time	Notes
5/7/87	0900	C/o "sore" left eye and tearing. Near vision 14/14 OU c̄c. Distant vision 20/40 – 2 s̄c OD, 20/30 – 1 s̄c OS. EOM intact. Visual fields intact (confrontation method). Eyebrows, eyelashes, eyelids intact; no evidence of inflammation, lesions, or position abnormalities. Lacrimal apparatus intact; no evidence of swelling or regurgitation of fluid on palpation of lacrimal sac. Right conjunctiva/sclera white. Left conjunctiva/sclera red; no apparent lesions or purulent discharge. Corneas clear and smooth. Irises brown, flat, and round. PERRLA. Ophthalmic exam: Discs round and creamy pink; cups equal in size and color. Retinal vessels even caliber and intact. Retinal background has uniform orange-pink color. Maculae 2 DD from discs; no lesions apparent. ———— Simone L. White, RN

■ **Evaluation**

For normal and abnormal findings, see Table 10–11. Upon obtaining an unexpected outcome: Report your findings to the responsible nurse and/or physician.

TECHNIQUE 10–9   ■   Assessing the Ears and Hearing

Assessment of the ear includes direct inspection and palpation of the external ear, inspection of the remaining parts of the ear by an otoscope, and determination of auditory acuity. The ear is usually assessed during an initial physical examination; periodic reassessments may be necessary for long-term patients or those who have hearing problems.

■ **Planning**

Nursing goals

1. To determine baseline data on the patient's hearing

2. To detect ear or hearing problems

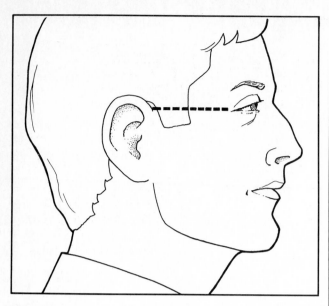

FIGURE 10-38

Equipment

1. An otoscope with several sizes of ear specula and an air insufflator
2. A tuning fork
3. A ticking watch

■ Intervention

See Table 10-12 for normal and abnormal findings.

Auricles

The auricles are inspected and palpated.

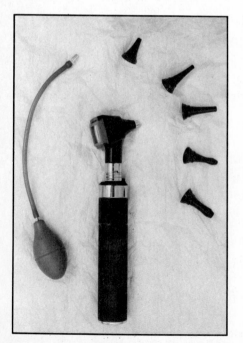

FIGURE 10-39

1. Assist the patient to a comfortable sitting position.
2. Inspect the auricles for color, texture, and symmetry of size and position. To inspect position, note the level at which the superior aspect of the auricle attaches to the head in relation to the eye. There should be a straight line from the lateral angle of the eye to the point where the superior aspect of the auricle joins the head. See Figure 10-38.
3. Palpate the auricle for texture, elasticity, and areas of tenderness.
   a. Pull the auricle upward, downward, and backward.
   b. Fold the pinna forward (it should recoil).
   c. Push in on the tragus.
   d. Apply pressure to the mastoid process.

External ear canal

Use the otoscope to inspect the remaining parts of the ear. See Figure 10-39. The air insufflator (at the left) may be used to test tympanic membrane movement.

4. Attach a speculum to the otoscope. Use the largest diameter that will fit the ear canal without causing discomfort.
   Rationale Maximum vision of the tympanic membrane is achieved.
5. Hold the otoscope either:
   a. Right side up with your fingers between the otoscope handle and the patient's head.
      or
   b. Upside down with your fingers and the ulnar surface of your hand against the patient's head. See Figure 10-40.

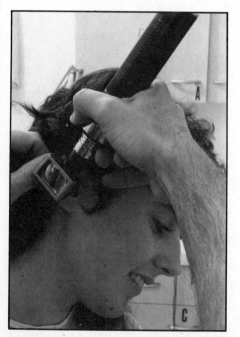

FIGURE 10-40

TABLE 10–12 ■ Ears and Hearing

Nursing history: Determine family history of hearing problems or loss; whether patient has had any ear problems; medication history, especially if there are complaints of ringing in ears; any hearing difficulty, its onset, factors contributing to it, and how it interferes with activities of daily living; whether a corrective hearing device is used, when, and from whom it was obtained.

Test or structure	Normal findings	Abnormal findings	Some associated conditions
Auricle	Color same as facial skin	Bluish color of earlobes	Cyanosis
		Pallor	Frostbite
		Excessive redness	Febrile condition
	Symmetric position		
	Line drawn from lateral angle of eye to point where top part of auricle joins head is horizontal	Low-set ears	Mongolism; renal disease
	Smooth texture	Lesions such as cysts or moles	
		Flaky, scaly skin	Seborrhea
	No tenderness on palpation; mobile and firm	Tenderness when moved or slight pressure is applied	Inflammatory process
	Pinna recoils after it is folded	Pinna is rigid	Frostbite
External ear canal	Distal third contains hair follicles and glands	Redness and discharge Scaling	Inflammation, infection
	Dry cerumen, grayish-tan in color; or wet cerumen, sticky and various shades of brown	Excessive cerumen obstructing canal	
Tympanic membrane	Pearly gray color, semitransparent	Pink to red, some opacity	Inflammation
		Yellow-amber	Serum in middle ear
		White	Pus
		Blue or deep red	Blood in middle ear
		Dull surface	Fibrosis
	Superior aspect is more anterior than lower rim; dimension is slightly conical	Loss of conical dimension and convex bulging	Inflammation, serum, pus, or blood in middle ear
	Fluctuates (vibrates) slightly when patient swallows	Membrane fixed, does not fluctuate	Inflammation, serum, pus, or blood in middle ear; obstructed eustachian tube; perforation of eardrum
	Light reflex (cone of light) bright to dim	Light reflex dimmed or absent	Inflammation; infection in middle ear
	Malleus is dense whitish streak	Malleus poorly defined or not visible	Inflammation; infection
	Umbo appears regressed	Umbo not visible	Inflammation; infection
	Annulus is defined and whitish-gray	Annulus poorly defined or not visible	Inflammation; infection
Hearing acuity Weber test	Sound heard in both ears, indicating proper bone conduction	Sound heard better in impaired ear	Bone conductive hearing loss (obstruction of ossicles)
		Sound heard better in ear without problem	Sensorineural disturbance (nerve or inner ear damage)
Rinne test	Positive, AC > BC	Negative, BC > AC or BC = AC	Conductive loss

Rationale Holding the fingers and/or ulnar surface of the hand between the otoscope and the patient's head stabilizes the head and protects the eardrum and canal from injury if a quick head movement occurs.

6. Tip the patient's head away from you and straighten the ear canal.

a. For an adult, straighten the ear canal by pulling the pinna up and back. See Figure 10–41.

b. For a child under 3 years of age, pull the pinna down and back. See Figure 10–42.

Rationale Both of these actions facilitate vision of the tympanic membrane.

7. Gently insert the tip of the otoscope into the ear canal.

Rationale The inner two thirds of the ear canal is bony; if the speculum is pressed against either side, the patient will experience pain.

8. Inspect the ear canal for cerumen, inflammation, scaling, foreign bodies, or other lesions.

9. If there is excessive cerumen in the canal, remove it. Dry cerumen is best removed by an irrigation. Wet and waxy cerumen can be removed with a curette (cerumen spoon) or a cotton-tipped applicator.

Rationale Removal of cerumen is essential for proper vision of the canal and tympanic membrane.

Tympanic membrane

10. Locate the tympanic membrane. If you have difficulty seeing it, try repositioning the patient's head and pulling the pinna in a slightly different direction.

FIGURE 10–41

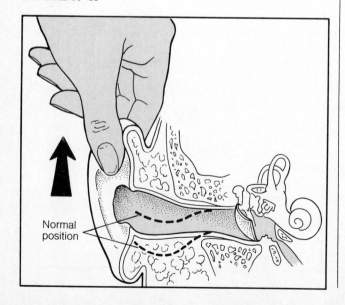

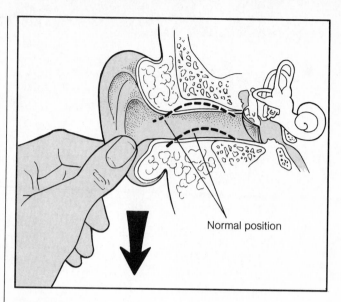

FIGURE 10–42

11. Inspect it for color and gloss, position, movement, and appearance of specific landmarks: the umbo, the annulus, the malleus, and the light reflex (cone of light). The membrane is systematically inspected in terms of four quadrants: anterior superior, anterior inferior, posterior superior, and posterior inferior. The anterior–posterior division is a hypothetical straight line running through the handle of the malleus. See Figure 10–43. The tympanic membrane is nearly oval in shape, measuring about 9 to 10 mm in its downward and forward diameter, and 8 to 9 mm in its shorter diameter. The greater part of its circumference is thickened, forming a fibrocartilaginous ring (*tympanic ring* or *annulus*). Inside the ring, a triangular part of the tympanic membrane, located at the top between two folds (anterior and posterior malleolar folds), is lax and thin; it is referred to as the *pars flaccida*. The remainder of the membrane is taut and is referred to as the *pars tensa*. The *malleus* (hammer) originates in the anterior superior quadrant of the membrane and extends approximately to its center. The handle of the malleus is firmly attached to the inner surface of the tympanic membrane as far as its center, which projects inward toward the tympanic cavity, making the inner surface of the membrane convex. The point of greatest convexity is called the *umbo*. The *light reflex* (a cone of light) is seen in the anterior inferior quadrant. Its point is directed toward the umbo and its broad base is at the periphery of the tympanic annulus. See Table 10–12 for normal and abnormal findings.

Hearing acuity: gross hearing

12. *Normal voice.* Note generally how well the patient

hears your voice. If the patient has difficulty, proceed with steps 13–14.

13. *Whispered voice.*

    a. Stand 30 to 60 cm (1 to 2 ft) from the patient in a position where the patient cannot read your lips. Ask the patient to occlude one ear by putting his or her finger in it.

    b. Whisper some nonconsecutive numbers and have the patient tell you what he or she heard. Increase the loudness of the whisper until the patient can identify at least 50% of the numbers. Repeat the process with the other ear.

    Rationale   Nonconsecutive numbers are used so that the patient cannot anticipate what number will follow. This test is used for screening purposes only, since it is difficult to maintain consistency in the whispered voice.

14. *Watch tick.* The ticking of a watch has a higher pitch than the human voice.

    a. Have the patient occlude one ear. Out of the patient's sight, place a ticking watch 2 to 5 cm (1 to 2 in) from the unoccluded ear.

    b. Ask the patient whether he or she can hear it. Repeat with the other ear.

Hearing acuity: tuning fork

15. *Weber test.* This test assesses bone conduction by testing the lateralization (sideward transmission) of sounds.

    a. Hold the tuning fork at its base. Activate it by tapping the fork gently against the back of your hand near the knuckles or by stroking the fork between your thumb and index fingers. It should be made to ring softly.

    Rationale   If the tone is too loud it takes a long while for it to quiet. A quiet tone is all that is needed.

    b. Place the base of the vibrating fork on top of the patient's head (see Figure 10–44) and ask the patient where she or he hears the noise. Normally the sound will be heard in both ears or localized at the center of the head (Weber negative). With a conductive hearing loss, the sound is heard better in the poor or damaged ear. With a sensorineural loss, the sound is heard better in the ear without a problem. Record positive findings as Weber right or Weber left.

16. *Rinne test.* This test compares air conduction to bone conduction.

    a. Have the patient intermittently block the hearing in one ear by moving a fingertip in and out of the ear canal.

    b. Hold the *handle* of the activated tuning fork on the mastoid process of one ear (see Figure 10–45)

until the patient tells you he or she can no longer hear the vibrations.

    c. Then immediately hold the still vibrating fork *prongs* in front of the patient's ear canal. Push aside the patient's hair if necessary. See Figure 10–46. Ask whether the patient now hears it again.

    Rationale   Air conduction is more sensitive than bone conduction. The tuning fork vibrations are therefore heard longer by air conduction.

    d. Repeat the procedure with the other ear. When air-conducted hearing is greater than bone-conducted hearing, the Rinne test is normal and is said to be positive, ie, AC > BC. When there is a conductive loss, the bone conduction time is equal to or longer than the air conduction time, ie, negative Rinne test, BC = AC or BC > AC.

17. Record your findings on the appropriate records.

Sample Recording

Date	Time	Notes
7/12/86	1300	C/o difficulty hearing in left ear. Ear: position bilateral and symmetric. Auricles: smooth, without lesions. External canal: small amount tan cerumen. Tympanic membrane: intact, all landmarks visible. Auditory: Hears low whisper at 30 cm. Weber: lateralization to left ear. Rinne: negative (BC>AC) in left ear; positive (AC>BC) in right ear. ——— Mark L. James, RN

FIGURE 10–43

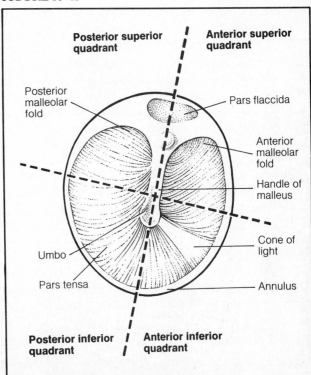

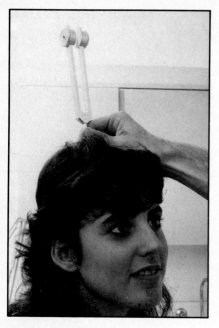

FIGURE 10-44

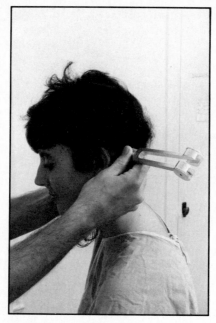

FIGURE 10-45

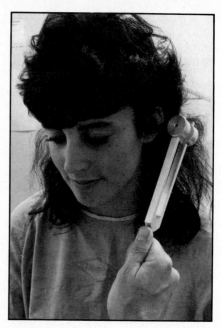

FIGURE 10-46

■ Evaluation

See normal and abnormal findings in Table 10–12. Upon obtaining an unexpected outcome: Report your findings to the responsible nurse and/or physician.

TECHNIQUE 10–10 ■ Assessing the Thorax, Lungs, and Breasts

Assessing the thorax and lungs is frequently critical to an assessment of the patient's aeration status. Two of the chief functions of the respiratory system are to maintain the exchange of oxygen and carbon dioxide in the lungs and the tissues and to maintain acid–base balance in the body. Changes in the respiratory system can come about slowly or quickly. For patients who have chronic obstructive pulmonary disease (COPD) changes are frequently gradual; however, for patients who are acutely ill, eg, those who have a pneumothorax (accumulation of gas or fluid in the pleural cavity), changes occur quickly, and if immediate action is not taken, death can result.

The breasts are frequently examined as part of the female reproductive system. Patients should examine their own breasts regularly, eg, once a month, to detect signs of breast cancer early. Breast self-examination (BSE) can be conducted using a procedure similar to that described in this technique.

■ Nursing Diagnosis

Nursing diagnoses that may indicate the need for respiratory assessment include:

1. Alteration in respiratory function related to:
   a. Ineffective ventilation
   b. Chronic obstructive pulmonary disease (COPD)
   c. Immobility
2. Alteration in tissue perfusion related to aging
3. Ineffective breathing patterns related to pulmonary disease

■ Planning

Nursing goals

1. To determine baseline data regarding a patient's thorax, lungs, and breasts
2. To assess respiratory function

Equipment

1. A stethoscope
2. A plumb line (a line or string with a weight at one end)
3. A marking pencil

■ **Intervention**

See Table 10–13 for normal and abnormal findings and some associated conditions.

Thorax

1. Inspect the body posture.
    a. Ask the patient to remove all clothing above the waist.
    b. Observe the posture of the patient in a standing, sitting, or lying position. Check whether the back is straight or bent.

2. Observe the shape of the thorax from posterior, anterior, and lateral views. Compare the anterioposterior diameter to the lateral diameter. These are normally 1:2 in the adult.

3. Inspect the spinal alignment for deformities. From a lateral position observe the curvatures of the spine. The spine has three normal curvatures: cervical, thoracic, and lumbar. From the posterior, drop a plumb line from the occiput of the skull to the gluteal cleft. The spine is normally aligned in a vertical line when the patient stands.

4. Palpate the anterior and posterior chest muscles, ribs, and skin.
    Rationale Palpation can reveal areas of tenderness and the presence of masses.

Lungs

Have the patient assume a sitting position for lung examination.

5. Examine the rate, depth, and type of respirations. See chapter 8, page 124.

6. Palpate the posterior chest for respiratory excursion (expansion). Place the palms of both hands over the lower thorax with the thumbs adjacent to the spine and the fingers stretched laterally. See Figure 10–47. Ask the patient to take a deep breath while you observe the movement of your hands and any lag in movement.
    Rationale When the patient takes a deep breath, the nurse's thumbs should move apart an equal distance and at the same time, reflecting chest expansion.

7. Palpate the anterior chest as in step 6, placing the palms of both hands on the lower thorax with the fingers laterally along the lower rib cage and the thumbs along the costal margins. See Figure 10–48.

8. Palpate the lungs for vocal (tactile) *fremitus,* the vibration felt through the chest wall when the patient speaks.
    a. Place the palms of your hands on the posterior chest near the apex of the lungs, position *A* in Figure 10–49.

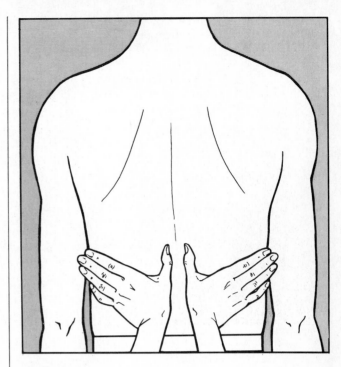

FIGURE 10–47

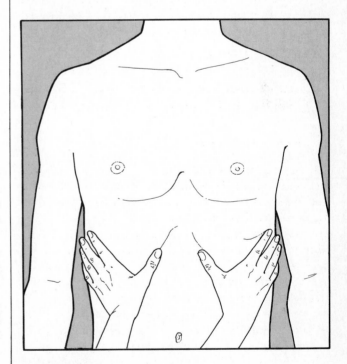

FIGURE 10–48

b. Ask the patient to repeat words such as "blue moon" or "one, two, three."

c. Repeat steps a and b with the hands moving sequentially to the base of the lungs, through positions *B–E* in Figure 10–49.

d. Compare the fremitus on both lungs and between the apex and the base of each lung.

TABLE 10–13 ■ Thorax, Lungs, and Breasts

Nursing history: Determine family history of illness, including cancer, allergies, tuberculosis; life-style, including smoking, occupational hazards, eg, inhaling fumes; whether patient is taking any medications; current problems, eg, swellings, cough, wheezing, pain; onset of menstruation for females, last menstrual period (LMP) for females.

Structure	Normal findings	Abnormal findings	Some associated conditions
Thorax	No lesions on skin		
	Adult chest configuration anterioposterior to lateral diameter of 1:2	Barrel chest, funnel chest, pigeon chest (increased anterioposterior to lateral diameter)	Kyphosis; osteoporosis; emphysema
	Chest symmetric	Chest asymmetric	Scoliosis
	Muscles, ribs not tender	Tenderness	Fractured ribs
Lungs	Respiratory rate 16–20/min and regular (adult)	Increased or decreased rate	Pneumonia
		Irregular pattern	
		Retraction or bulging of intercostal muscles	
	Respiratory excursion is full and symmetric	Impairment in movement	Emphysema
	Vocal fremitus is symmetric bilaterally	Decreased or increased fremitus	Obstruction of bronchi
	Percussion notes resonant except over liver, heart, sternum, scapula, and stomach	Asymmetry in percussion	
		Areas of dullness	Tumors; atelectasis; pleural fluid
		Areas of hyperresonance	Emphysema
	Auscultated vesicular breath sounds (see Table 10–14)	Auscultated adventitious breath sounds (see Table 10–15)	
		Rales	Pulmonary edema
		Rhonchi	Bronchi filled with fluid
		Wheeze	Chronic bronchitis
		Friction rub	Pleurisy
Breasts	Rounded shape; small, medium, or large size	Change in breast size, swellings	Inflammation
	Symmetric	Marked asymmetry	
	Skin smooth, intact	Dimpling, redness, vascularities, edema	
		Retraction	Scarring, carcinoma
	Nipples everted, no discharge or lesions	Nipples inverted, crusting, ulcers, cracks, discharge	Inflammation; abscess; malignancy
	No swelling in axilla	Swelling, tenderness in axilla	Malignancy
	No tenderness, masses, or nodules on palpation	Tenderness, masses, or nodules (note location, patient's position, size, mobility, consistency, surface, tenderness, and shape)	Tumor; abscess

Rationale The vibrations from speaking are normally transmitted through the chest wall. They are felt most clearly at the apex of the lungs. Low-pitched voices of males are more readily palpated than the higher pitches of females.

Increased fremitus occurs with consolidated lung tissue as in pneumonia, and decreased or absent fremitus occurs in pneumothorax.

9. Repeat steps 8a–d for the anterior chest. See Figure 10–50, positions *A–E*.

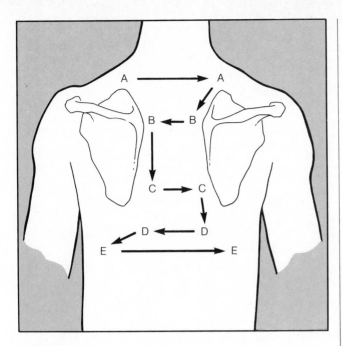

FIGURE 10-49

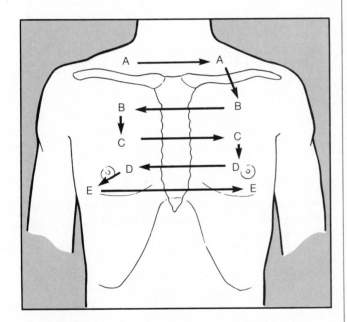

FIGURE 10-50

10. Percuss the anterior surface of the chest. See the description of percussion earlier in this chapter.

   a. Percuss in the intercostal spaces in a systematic sequence, beginning above the clavicles in the supraclavicular space, and proceeding downward to the diaphragm. See Figure 10-51.

   Rationale   Percussion on a rib will normally elicit dullness. The lowest point where resonance can normally be detected is at the diaphragm, ie, at the level of the eighth to tenth rib.

   b. Compare one side of the chest with the other. For each percussion, note the intensity, pitch, and duration. See Table 10-1 earlier in this chapter.

11. Percuss the lateral chest wall, starting at the axilla and working down to the tenth rib. Percuss every few inches. Repeat for the other side.

12. Percuss the posterior chest wall while the patient leans forward, neck flexed. Start at the apex of each lung and proceed downward to the diaphragm. See Figure 10-52. Compare one side of the chest to the other.

FIGURE 10-51

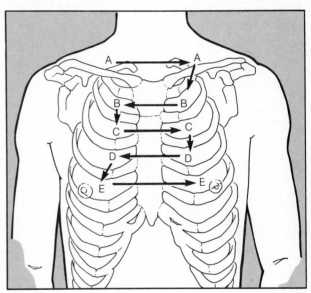

FIGURE 10-52

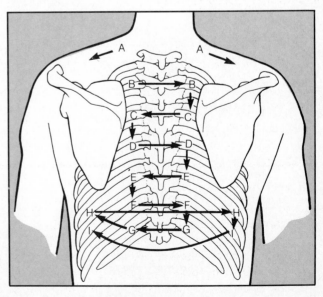

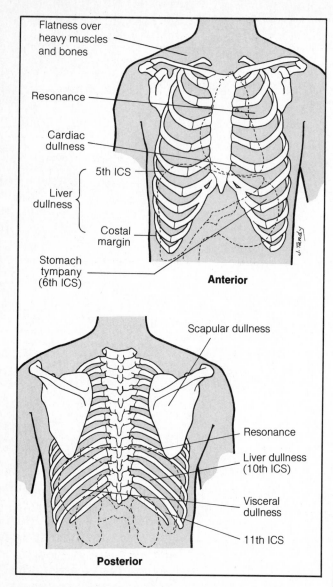

Flatness over heavy muscles and bones

Resonance

Cardiac dullness

5th ICS

Liver dullness

Costal margin

Stomach tympany (6th ICS)

Anterior

Scapular dullness

Resonance

Liver dullness (10th ICS)

Visceral dullness

11th ICS

Posterior

FIGURE 10–53

FIGURE 10–54

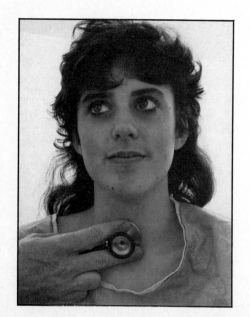

Rationale Percussion sounds are loudest where the chest wall is thinnest. For normal percussion sounds, see Figure 10–53.

13. Determine the excursion (movement) of the diaphragm.

a. Ask the patient to take a deep breath and hold it.

Rationale On inspiration, the diaphragm normally moves downward.

b. Percuss downward on one side of the posterior chest until dullness is produced.

Rationale The dullness indicates the level of the diaphragm.

c. With a pencil place a mark on the skin at the level of dullness.

d. Ask the patient to completely expel the breath and hold it.

Rationale Upon expiration, the diaphragm normally moves upward.

e. Percuss as in step b for the level of dullness.

Rationale The level normally is above the inspiratory level, because the lungs have deflated.

f. Mark the level of dullness on the skin.

g. Measure the distance between the two marks.

Rationale Normal excursion is 3 to 5 cm (1 to 2 in) in females and 5 to 6 cm (2 to 2.3 in) in males.

h. Repeat steps a–g on the other side of the posterior chest.

14. To auscultate the lungs, use the flat-disc diaphragm of the stethoscope.

Rationale The flat diaphragm best transmits high-pitched sounds, eg, breath sounds.

a. Facing the patient, place the diaphragm firmly against the skin starting over the trachea. See Figure 10–54.

b. Ask the patient to breathe normally.

c. Proceed in the sequence shown in Figure 10–51, earlier, first auscultating over the bronchi between the sternum and the clavicles, then following the sequence for percussion in Figure 10–51.

d. Listen for normal and adventitious breath sounds at each point on the chest. See Tables 10–14 and 10–15.

Rationale Breath sounds occur as a result of the movement of the air through the trachea, bronchi, and alveoli.

e. Repeat for the lateral chest and the posterior chest. Follow the percussion sequence described in steps 11–12 and shown in Figure 10–52.

15. When abnormal breath or percussion sounds are discovered, carry out further investigation: bronchophony, whispered pectoriloquy (exaggerated bronchophony), and egophony.

TABLE 10-14 ■ Normal Breath Sounds

Type	Description	Location	Characteristics
Vesicular	Soft, low-pitched, "gentle sighing"	Over bronchioles and alveoli; best heard at base of lungs	Best heard on inspiration
Bronchial (tracheal)	Moderately high-pitched, "harsh"	Over trachea; not normally heard over lung tissue	Louder than vesicular sounds; long inspiratory phase and short expiratory phase
Bronchovesicular	Moderate intensity	Over bronchioles lateral to the sternum at the first and second intercostal spaces and between the scapulae	Equal inspiratory and expiratory phases

Rationale   Fluid or consolidated tissue will transmit vibrations of the spoken or whispered voice through the chest wall.

a. *Bronchophony and whispered pectoriloquy.* Using a stethoscope, listen to the chest, using the sequence described for assessing vocal fremitus. See Figures 10–49 and 10–50, earlier. Have the patient softly repeat "one, two, three."

Rationale   With tissue consolidation, the words may be clearly heard in the periphery of the lung.

b. *Egophony.* Listen to the chest while the patient repeats the sound of a long *e,* as in "she."

Rationale   Fluid in the lungs will alter the sound from an *e* to an *ay,* as in "say," when heard through the stethoscope.

Breasts

16. Ask the female patient to assume a sitting position, and assess the breasts.

a. Inspect the size, shape, and symmetry of the breasts. Breasts are normally round and fairly symmetric, and may be described as small, medium, or large.

b. Inspect the skin for lesions, increased vascular patterns, edema, and "pig skin" or a pitted appearance.

Rationale   Pitting of the skin can be the result of lymphatic edema.

c. Inspect the color of the areola. It is normally darker in brunettes and pregnant women than in fair-haired women.

d. Inspect the breast and nipples for any dimpling or retraction, which can be the result of scar tissue formation or can be caused by the presence of a lesion. See Figure 10–55. In front of a mirror, show the patient how to accentuate any retraction by raising her arms above her head, pushing her hands together with elbows flexed (see Figure 10–56), or pressing her hands down on her hips (see Figure 10–57).

e. Inspect the nipples for any discharge, ulceration, inversion, crusting, or scaling. Note the position

TABLE 10-15 ■ Adventitious Breath Sounds

Name	Description	Characteristics
Rales	Fine crackling sounds; alveolar rales are high-pitched; bronchial rales are lower-pitched	Best heard on inspiration
Rhonchi	Coarse, gurgling, harsh, louder sounds as air passes through bronchi filled with fluid	Best heard on expiration
Wheeze	Squeaky musical sounds often indicative of bronchial constriction	Best heard on expiration
Friction (pleural rub)	Rubbing of the pulmonary and visceral pleura; grating sound	Best heard over the lower anterior and lateral chest

of the nipples. Both nipples normally point in the same direction.

17. Inspect the axilla and clavicular areas for any swelling or redness.

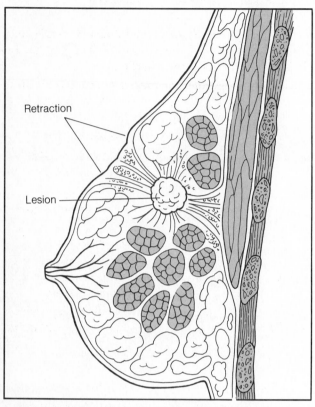

FIGURE 10-55

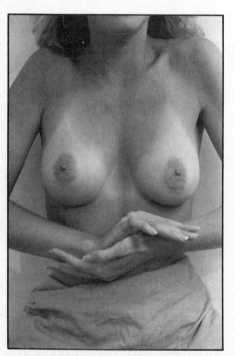

FIGURE 10-56

18. Palpate around the nipple to check for discharge. If discharge is present, strip the breast by compressing the breast tissue between the thumb and index finger while moving the fingers toward the nipple. Strip one lobe at a time to identify the source of the discharge.

    a. Observe any discharge for amount, color, consistency, and odor.

    b. Note any tenderness upon palpation.

19. Palpate the clavicular and axillary regions while the patient is sitting, arms at her sides.

    Rationale These areas contain lymph nodes that drain the breasts. See Figure 10-58.

20. Lightly palpate each breast. A bimanual technique is often preferred, particularly for large breasts. The nondominant hand is placed under the breast, and the dominant hand palpates the breast.

    Rationale A bimanual technique can be most effective in detecting small deep masses.

    a. Press the palmar surfaces of the middle three fingers on the skin surface starting in the upper lateral quadrant.

    b. Use a gentle rotary motion pressing the breast tissue against the other hand (bimanual) or against the chest wall.

    c. Palpate from the periphery to the areola.

    d. Move your peripheral starting point around the breast clockwise. See Figure 10-59.

21. Record the following data about any masses:

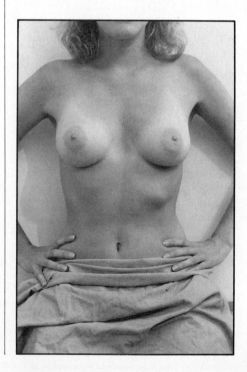

FIGURE 10-57

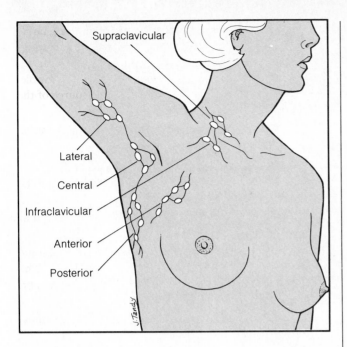

FIGURE 10–58

FIGURE 10–59

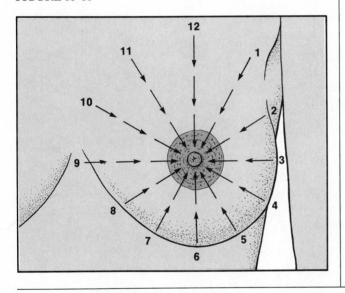

a. *Location:* the exact location relative to the clock (as in Figure 10–59) and the distance from the nipple in centimeters.

b. *Patient's position:* whether the arms were raised or lowered, the patient was sitting or supine.

   Rationale   The position can change the perceived location of the mass.

c. *Size:* the length, width, and thickness of the mass in centimeters. If you are unable to determine the discrete edges, record this fact.

d. *Mobility:* whether the mass is movable or fixed. If it is fixed, determine whether it is firmly or moderately fixed, if possible.

e. *Consistency:* whether the mass is hard or soft.

f. *Surface:* whether the surface is smooth or irregular.

g. *Tenderness:* whether palpation is painful to the patient.

h. *Shape:* whether the mass is round, discoid, regular, or irregular.

22. Repeat steps 20–21 for the other breast.

23. Assist the patient to a supine position, with a small pillow or towel under the shoulder of the side to be palpated. Repeat steps 20–21 for each breast.

   Rationale   Slightly raising the shoulder helps spread the breast tissue over the chest wall, facilitating palpation.

■ Evaluation

See Tables 10–13, 10–14, and 10–15. Upon obtaining an unexpected outcome: Report your findings to the responsible nurse and/or physician.

TECHNIQUE 10–11   ■   Assessing the Heart

Heart function can be assessed to a large degree by findings in the history, by symptoms such as shortness of breath, by the patient's general appearance (eg, cyanosis and edema of the legs suggest impaired function), and by pulse rate, rhythm, and quality. Direct examination of the heart, however, offers more specific information, including the heart sounds, the heart size, and findings such as lifts, heaves, or murmurs. Nurses assess heart function through observation (inspection), palpation, and auscultation, in that sequence. Auscultation is more meaningful when other data are obtained first. The heart is usually assessed during an initial physical examination; periodic reassessments may be necessary for long-term or at-risk patients or those who have cardiac problems.

A nursing history taken in conjunction with physical assessment needs to include:

1. Pertinent family health history.

2. Past history of heart problems.
3. Presence of symptoms indicative of heart disease.
4. Presence of diseases that affect the heart.
5. Habits and life-style data that indicate potential risk factors. See Table 10–16.

TABLE 10–16 ■ Heart

Nursing history: Determine family history of incidence and age of heart disease, high cholesterol levels, high blood pressure, stroke, obesity, congenital heart disease, and rheumatic fever; patient's past history of rheumatic fever, heart murmur, heart attack, or heart failure; present symptoms indicative of heart disease, eg, fatigue, dyspnea, orthopnea, edema, cough, chest pain, palpitations, syncope, hypertension, wheezing, hemoptysis; presence of diseases that affect heart, eg, obesity, diabetes, lung disease, endocrine disorders; life-style habits that are risk factors for cardiac disease, eg, smoking, alcohol intake, eating and exercise patterns, areas and degree of stress perceived.

Assessment method, area, or stage	Normal findings	Abnormal findings	Some associated conditions
Precordial inspection and palpation			
Aortic area	Possible pulsations	Pulsations	
Pulmonic area	No pulsations	Pulsations	
Tricuspid area	No pulsations	Pulsations	
	No lift or heave	Diffuse lift or heave	Enlargement or overactivity of right ventricle
Apical area	Pulsations visible in 50% of adults and palpable in most		
	PMI in fifth LICS at or medial to MCL	PMI displaced laterally or lower	Enlarged heart
	Diameter of 1 to 2 cm (⅓ to ½ in)	Diameter over 2 cm	Enlarged heart or aneurysm
	No lift or heave	Diffuse lift or heave lateral to apex	Enlargement or overactivity of left ventricle
Epigastric area	Aortic pulsations	Bounding pulsations	Aortic aneurysm
Auscultation			
S_1	Usually heard at all sites	Increased or decreased intensity	
	Usually louder at apical area	Varying intensity with different beats	Complete heart block
S_2	Usually heard at all sites	Increased intensity at aortic area	Arterial hypertension
	Usually louder at base of heart	Increased intensity at pulmonic area	Pulmonary hypertension
Systole	Silent interval	Sharp-sounding ejection clicks	Valvular deformities
	Slightly shorter duration than diastole at normal heart rate (60 to 90 beats/min)		
Diastole	Silent interval	S_3 in older adults	Heart failure
	Slightly longer duration than systole at normal heart rates		
	S_3 in children and young adults		
	S_4 in older adults		

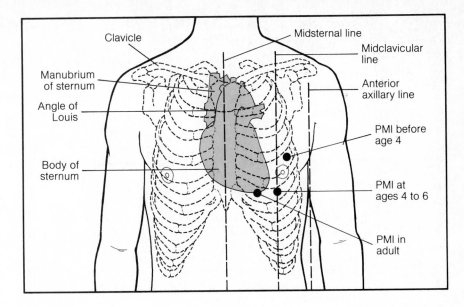

FIGURE 10-60 ■ The location of the apical pulse of a child under 4 years, a child 4 to 6 years, and an adult.

To perform cardiac assessment, the nurse must first know the exact location of the heart. In the average adult, most of the heart lies behind and to the left of the sternum. A small portion (the right atrium) extends to the right of the sternum. The upper portion of the heart (both atria), referred to as its base, lies toward the back. The lower portion (the ventricles), referred to as its apex, points forward. The apex of the left ventricle actually touches the anterior chest wall at or medial to the left midclavicular line (MCL) and at or near the fifth left intercostal space (LICS), which is slightly below the left nipple. See Figure 10-60. This point where the apex touches the anterior chest wall is known as the *point of maximal impulse* (PMI). In infants and small children, because their hearts are positioned more horizontally, the PMI is located at the third or fourth LICS just to the left of the MCL. By the age of 7, however, a child's PMI is found in the same location as the adult's.

■ Planning

Nursing goals

1. To determine baseline data about the patient's cardiac function
2. To detect cardiac problems
3. To identify potential risk factors for cardiac disease

Equipment

A stethoscope with a bell-shaped and flat-disc diaphragm.

■ Intervention

See Table 10-16 for normal and abnormal findings and associated conditions.

Inspection and palpation

The *precordium*, the area of the chest overlying the heart, is inspected and palpated simultaneously for the presence of abnormal pulsations or lifts or heaves. It is inspected in a systematic manner at the following anatomic sites: aortic area, pulmonic area, tricuspid (or ventricular) area, apical (or mitral) area, and epigastric area. See Figure 10-61. All pulsations are described by their location in an intercostal space and their distance from the midsternal, midclavicular, or axillary line.

1. Assist the patient to a supine position, and stand at the patient's right side.
   Rationale This position facilitates palpation of the cardiac area and allows for optimal inspection.
2. Locate the angle of Louis, the angle between the manubrium and the body of the sternum. It is felt as a prominence on the sternum.

FIGURE 10-61

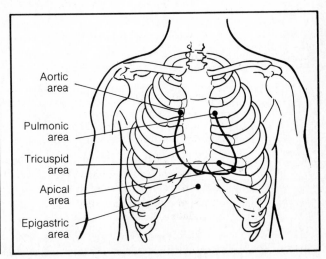

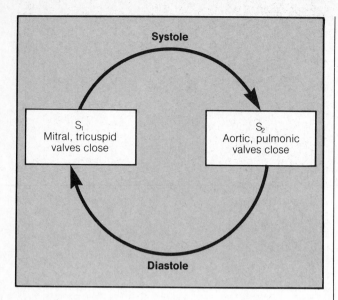

FIGURE 10-62

3. Move your fingertips down each side of the angle until you can feel the second intercostal spaces. The patient's *right* second intercostal space is the aortic area, and the *left* second intercostal space is the pulmonic area.

4. Inspect and palpate the aortic and pulmonic areas, observing them at an angle and to the side, to note the presence or absence of pulsations.

   Rationale Observing these areas at an angle increases the likelihood of seeing pulsations.

5. From the pulmonic area, move your fingertips down three left intercostal spaces along the side of the sternum. The left fifth intercostal space close to the sternum is the tricuspid or ventricular area. Inspect and palpate the tricuspid area for pulsations and heaves or lifts. The terms *lift* and *heave,* often used interchangeably, refer to a rising along the sternal border with each heartbeat. A lift occurs when cardiac action is very forceful (overactive). It should be confirmed by palpation with the palm of the hand. Enlargement or overactivity of the left ventricle produces a heave lateral to the apex, while enlargement of the right ventricle produces a heave at or near the sternum.

6. From the tricuspid area, move your fingertips laterally 5 to 7 cm (2 to 3 in) to the left midclavicular line (LMCL). This is the apical or mitral area, or PMI.

7. Inspect and palpate the apical area for pulsation, noting its specific location (it may be displaced laterally or lower) and diameter. An apical impulse can be seen in about 50% of the adult population. The apical impulse is a good index of cardiac size. If the heart is enlarged, this impulse is lateral to the MCL. Record the distance between the apex and the MCL in centimeters. If the apical beat cannot

be observed, the apex may be located by palpation, but not always. If you have difficulty locating the PMI, have the patient roll onto the left side.

   Rationale Moving the patient onto his or her left side moves the apex closer to the chest wall.

8. Inspect and palpate the epigastric area at the base of the sternum for aortic pulsations.

Auscultation

Several heart sounds can be heard by auscultation. Only the first and second heart sounds (S_1 and S_2) will be emphasized in this technique. The normal first two heart sounds are produced by closure of the valves of the heart. The first heart sound (S_1) occurs when the atrioventricular (A-V) valves close. These valves close when the ventricles have been sufficiently filled. Although the right and left A-V valves do not close simultaneously, the closures occur closely enough to be heard as one sound (S_1), a dull, low-pitched sound described as "lub." After the ventricles empty their blood into the aorta and pulmonary arteries, the semilunar valves close, producing the second heart sound (S_2), described as "dub." S_2 has a higher pitch than S_1 and is also shorter. These two sounds, S_1 and S_2 ("lub-dub"), occur within 1 second or less, depending on the heart rate.

Auscultation is performed systematically, starting at the aortic area, then moving to the pulmonic, the tricuspid, and the apical. See Figure 10–61, earlier. Auscultation need not be limited to these areas, however. First locate these areas, and then move the stethoscope to find the most audible sounds for each particular patient. The two heart sounds are audible anywhere on the precordial area, but they are best heard over these areas. Each area is associated with the closure of heart valves: the aortic area with the aortic valve (inside the aorta as it arises from the left ventricle); the pulmonic area with the pulmonic valve (inside the pulmonary artery as it arises from the right ventricle); the tricuspid area with the tricuspid valve (between the right atrium and ventricle); and the apical (mitral) area with the mitral valve (between the left atrium and ventricle).

Associated with these sounds are *systole* and *diastole.* Systole is the period in which the ventricles are contracted. It begins with the first heart sound and ends at the second heart sound. Systole is usually shorter than diastole. Diastole is the period in which the ventricles are relaxed. It starts with the second sound and ends at the subsequent first sound. Normally no sounds are audible during these periods. See Figure 10–62. The experienced examiner, however, may perceive extra heart sounds (S_3 and S_4) during diastole. Both sounds are low in pitch and heard best at the apical site, with the bell of the stethoscope, and with the patient lying on the left side. S_3 occurs early in diastole right after S_2 and sounds like "lub-dub-*ee*" (S_1, S_2, S_3) or "Ken-tuc-*ky*." It often disappears when the patient sits up. S_3 is normal in

TABLE 10–17   ■   Normal Heart Sounds

Sound or phase	Description	Area			
		Aortic	Pulmonic	Tricuspid	Apical
S_1	Dull, low-pitched, and longer than S_2; sounds like "lub"	Less intensity than S_2	Less intensity than S_2	Louder than or equal to S_2	Louder than or equal to S_2
S_2	High-pitched, snappy, and shorter than S_1; creates sound of "dub"	Louder than S_1	Louder than S_1; abnormal if louder than the aortic S_2 in adults over 40	Less intensity than or equal to S_1	Less intensity than or equal to S_1
Systole	Normally silent interval between S_1 and S_2				
Diastole	Normally silent interval between S_2 and next S_1				

children and young adults. In older adults it may indicate heart failure. S_4 is rarely heard in normal patients. It occurs near the very end of diastole just before S_1 and creates the sound of "*dee*-lub-dub" (S_4, S_1, S_2) or "*Ten*-nes-see." S_4 may be heard in many elderly patients and can be a sign of hypertension.

For heart auscultation a stethoscope with a bell-shaped and a flat-disc diaphragm is needed. The bell transmits lower-pitched sounds best, while the flat disc transmits higher-pitched sounds best. The bell should be used for the tricuspid and mitral valve areas.

9. Eliminate all sources of room noise.

   Rationale   Heart sounds are of low intensity, and other noise lowers the nurse's receptivity to them.

10. Assist the patient to a supine position, and stand at the patient's right side. Later reexamine the heart while the patient is in the upright sitting position.

    Rationale   Certain sounds are more audible in certain positions.

11. Auscultate the heart in the following manner using both the flat-disc diaphragm and the bell to listen to all areas. See Table 10–17 for descriptions of normal heart sounds. See Table 10–16, earlier, for normal and abnormal findings. In every area of auscultation, both S_1 and S_2 need to be distinguished. When auscultating, concentrate on one particular sound at a time in each area; the first heart sound, followed by systole, then the second heart sound, then diastole. Systole and diastole are normally silent intervals.

    a. Locate and auscultate the aortic area using the flat diaphragm and bell attachment of the stethoscope. Listen for both sounds and for systole and diastole. S_2 is loudest in this area, louder than S_1.

    Rationale   The higher-pitched sounds of S_1 and S_2 are transmitted better through the flat diaphragm of the stethoscope. The lower-pitched sounds of S_3 and S_4 are best transmitted through the bell of the stethoscope.

    b. Locate and auscultate the pulmonic area as in step a. S_2 is normally louder than S_1 in this area.

    c. Compare the loudness of S_2 between the aortic and pulmonic areas.

    Rationale   The loudness of S_2 in the pulmonic area relates to the blood pressure in the pulmonary artery, while the loudness of S_2 in the aortic area relates to the arterial blood pressure in the systemic circulation. Thus when the pulmonary artery pressure increases, eg, in patients with some chronic obstructive lung diseases, the loudness of pulmonic S_2 also increases. In contrast, the aortic S_2 is louder than normal in patients with hypertensive disease. When the pulmonic S_2 is louder than the aortic S_2 in adults over age 40, the finding is abnormal.

    d. Locate and auscultate the tricuspid area as in step a. S_2 is normally louder than or equal to S_1 in this area.

    e. Locate and auscultate the apical (mitral) area as in step a. S_2 is normally louder than or equal to S_1 in this area.

    f. Assess the heart rate and rhythm at the apical area as described in Technique 8–5 on page 118. Note irregularities in rhythm, and note murmurs. *Murmurs* result when blood flow becomes turbulent within the heart due to valve defects or abnormal openings between the compartments of the heart. Not all murmurs indicate cardiac disease. Murmurs are described in terms of their location of maximum intensity, quality (eg, loud, harsh, rumbling), and timing in relation to the phases of the cardiac cycle. Diastolic murmurs are usually considered abnormal. Murmurs relating to the valves are usually heard over the valvular areas. To increase your ability to hear an S_3 sound or a mitral murmur, have the patient lie on the left side. Using the bell of your stethoscope, listen carefully in and around the apical area.

g. Record your assessment findings. Describe the *intensity* or *loudness* of the sounds as normal, absent, diminished, or accentuated, and the *quality* of sounds as sharp, full, booming, or snapping.

■ Evaluation

See Table 10–16. Upon obtaining an unexpected outcome: Report your findings to the responsible nurse and/or physician.

TECHNIQUE 10–12 ■ Assessing the Peripheral Vascular System

Assessment of the peripheral vascular system includes measurement of the blood pressure; palpation of peripheral pulses; inspection, palpation, and auscultation of the carotid pulse; inspection of the jugular and peripheral veins; and inspection of the skin and tissues to determine perfusion to the extremities.

■ Planning

Nursing goals

1. To determine baseline data about the patient's peripheral vascular function
2. To detect vascular problems

3. To identify potential risk factors for vascular disease

Equipment

1. A blood pressure cuff
2. A sphygmomanometer
3. A stethoscope
4. A watch with a second hand or indicator

■ Intervention

See Table 10–18 for normal and abnormal findings and some associated conditions.

TABLE 10–18 ■ Peripheral Vascular System

Nursing history: Determine past history of heart disorders, varicosities, arterial disease, and hypertension; life-style, specifically exercise patterns, activity patterns and tolerance, smoking habits, and use of alcohol.

Structure	Normal findings	Abnormal findings	Some associated conditions
Peripheral arteries	Symmetric pulse volumes	Asymmetric volumes	Arterial disease
	Full pulsations	Absent pulsation	Arterial stenosis; occlusion
		Decreased, weak, thready pulsations	Decreased cardiac output from failure of left side of heart, hemorrhage, shock, or endocardial, myocardial, or pericardial disease
		Increased, bounding pulsations	Increased cardiac output from excessive exercise, anxiety, fear, fever, or disease
Carotid arteries	Symmetric pulse volumes	Asymmetric volumes	Stenosis or thrombosis
	Full pulsations, thrusting quality	Decreased pulsations	Failure of left side of heart; severe shock; aortic stenosis

TABLE 10-18   ■   continued

Structure	Normal findings	Abnormal findings	Some associated conditions
Carotid arteries (continued)	Quality remains same when patient breathes, turns head, and changes from sitting to supine position	Increased pulsations	Hypertension; complete heart block; hyperthyroidism; anemia; extreme bradycardia
	Elastic arterial wall	Thickened, hard, rigid, beaded, inelastic wall	Arteriosclerosis
	No sound heard on auscultation	Presence of bruit in one or both arteries	Occlusive artery disease
Jugular veins	Distended and visible in supine position; not visible in upright position	Distended veins; JVP exceeds 3 cm above the sternal angle	Failure of right side of heart is most common cause
Peripheral veins	In dependent position, distention and nodular bulges at calves When limbs elevated, veins collapse (veins may appear tortuous or distended in older people)	Distended veins in the anteromedial part of thigh and/or lower leg or on posterolateral part of calf from knee to ankle Pitting edema	Varicose veins
	Limbs not tender, symmetric in size	Tenderness on palpation or positive Homans' sign Warmth and redness over vein Swelling of one calf or leg	Phlebitis
Peripheral perfusion	Skin color pink	Skin cyanotic	Venous insufficiency
		Pallor that increases with limb elevation	Arterial insufficiency
		Dusky red color when limb lowered	Arterial insufficiency
		Brown pigmentation around ankles	Arterial insufficiency
	Skin not excessively warm or cold	Skin cool Marked swelling or edema	Arterial insufficiency Venous insufficiency
	Skin resilient, moist	Skin thin and shiny or thick, waxy, shiny, and fragile, with reduced hair and ulceration	Venous or arterial insufficiency
	After arterial adequacy test, original color returns in 10 seconds; veins in feet or hands fill in about 15 seconds	Delayed color return or mottled appearance; delayed venous filling; marked redness of arms or legs	Arterial insufficiency
	After capillary refill test, immediate return of color	Delayed return of color	Arterial insufficiency

Blood pressure

1. Measure the patient's blood pressure. See Technique 8-9 on page 130.

   Rationale The blood pressure reflects the overall status of the arterial system. Inelastic, narrowed arterioles cause an abnormal elevation in the blood pressure.

Peripheral pulses

2. Palpate the peripheral pulses (except the carotid pulse) on both sides of the patient's body simultaneously and systematically. (Pulse sites and assessing pulses are described in chapter 8.)

   Rationale This determines the symmetry of pulse volume. Inequality may indicate arterial disease.

   a. Start at the head, and assess the temporal and facial pulses.

   b. Move to the arms, and assess the brachial, radial, and ulnar pulses.

   c. Move to the legs, and assess the femoral, popliteal, posterior tibial, and pedal pulses.

d. For all pulse volumes, note whether they are absent; weak, thready, or decreased; normal; or increased and bounding.

3. If you have difficulty palpating some peripheral pulses, use a Doppler ultrasound probe, if available. See the discussion of this device in chapter 8.

   a. Lubricate the transducer with transmission gel.

   b. Position the earpieces (if present) in your ears.

   c. Place the probe over the pulse site. See Figure 10–63, which shows the probe over the patient's brachial pulse site.

   d. Listen for wavelike "whooshing" sounds, which indicate blood flow.

   e. Record either the presence or absence of pulsations, their rate, and their intensity.

Carotid arteries

The carotid arteries supply oxygenated blood to the head and neck. See Figure 10–64. Since they are the only source of blood to the brain, prolonged occlusion of one of these arteries can result in serious brain damage. The carotid pulses correlate with central aortic pressure, thus reflecting cardiac function better than the peripheral arteries. When cardiac output is diminished, the peripheral pulses may be difficult or impossible to feel, but the carotid pulse should be felt easily.

4. With the patient in a sitting position, inspect the carotid arteries for obvious pulsations; sometimes a wave can be seen.

5. To palpate the carotid arteries, have the patient turn

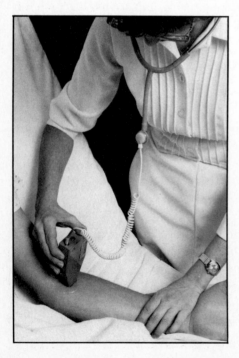

FIGURE 10–63

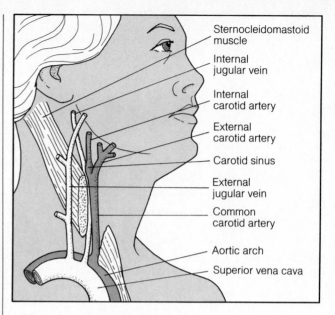

FIGURE 10–64

her or his head slightly toward the side being examined.

Rationale This makes the artery more accessible.

a. Palpate *one* carotid artery at a time.

   Rationale This ensures adequate cerebral blood flow through the other and prevents possible cerebral ischemia.

b. Avoid exerting too much pressure and massaging the area.

   Rationale Pressure can occlude the artery. Carotid sinus massage can precipitate bradycardia. The carotid sinus is a small dilation at the beginning of the internal carotid artery just above the bifurcation of the common carotid artery, in the upper third of the neck.

c. Note the rate, rhythm, and volume of each carotid pulse and the condition of the artery wall. Compare their equality.

6. To auscultate the carotid artery, turn the patient's head slightly away from the side being examined. Auscultate the carotid artery on one side and then the other.

   Rationale Turning the head facilitates placement of the stethoscope.

a. Listen for the presence of a *bruit* (a blowing or swishing sound) created by turbulence of blood flow due to a narrowed arterial lumen (a common development in older people) or a high cardiac output condition, such as anemia or hyperthyroidism. Normally no sound is heard by auscultation.

b. If you hear a bruit, gently palpate the artery to determine the presence of a thrill, which frequently accompanies a bruit. A *thrill* is a vibrating sensation like the purring of a cat or water running through a hose. It too is caused by turbulent blood flow from arterial obstruction.

Jugular veins

The jugular veins drain blood from the head and neck directly into the superior vena cava and right side of the heart. See Figure 10–64. The external jugular veins are superficial and may be visible above the clavicle. The internal jugular veins lie deeper along the carotid artery and may transmit pulsations onto the skin of the neck. Normally, external neck veins are distended and visible when a person lies down; they are flat and not as visible when a person stands up, since gravity encourages venous drainage. By inspecting the jugular veins for pulsations and distention, you can assess the adequacy of function of the right side of the heart and venous pressure.

7. Remove clothing around the patient's neck and thorax, and assist the patient to a semi-Fowler's position with the head supported on a small pillow.

   Rationale Clothing is removed to prevent constriction. Semi-Fowler's position is used, since at a 30° to 45° angle neck veins should not be prominent if the right side of the patient's heart is functioning normally. A small pillow aligns the head sufficiently to prevent neck hyperextension; a large pillow would create neck flexion.

8. If jugular distention is present, assess the jugular venous pressure (JVP) as follows:

   a. Locate the highest visible point of distention of the internal jugular vein.

      Rationale Although either the internal or the external jugular vein can be used, the internal jugular vein is more reliable. The external jugular vein is more easily affected by obstruction or kinking at the base of the neck.

   b. Measure the vertical height of this point in centimeters from the sternal angle or suprasternal notch (the point at which the clavicles meet). See Figure 10–65.

   c. Repeat steps a–b on the other side. Bilateral measurements above 3 cm are considered elevated and may indicate right-sided heart failure. Unilateral distention may be caused by local obstruction.

   d. Note whether other veins in the neck, shoulder, and upper chest are distended.

Peripheral veins

9. Inspect the arms and legs for presence and/or appearance of superficial veins in the dependent position and when the limbs are elevated.

10. Assess the peripheral leg veins for signs of phlebitis.

    a. Inspect the calves for redness and swelling over vein sites. These may be indicative of phlebitis.

    b. Palpate the calves for firmness or tension of the muscles, the presence of edema over the dorsum of the foot, and areas of localized warmth.

       Rationale Palpation augments inspection findings particularly in highly pigmented people in whom redness may not be visible.

    c. Push the calves from side to side to test for tenderness.

    d. Firmly dorsiflex the foot while supporting the entire leg in extension (Homans' test) or have the person stand or walk.

       Rationale Forceful dorsiflexion of the foot produces pain in the calf muscles if a deep phlebitis of the leg is present. This is called a *positive Homans' sign.*

Peripheral perfusion

11. Inspect the skin of the hands and feet for color, temperature, edema, and skin changes.

12. Assess the adequacy of arterial flow if arterial insufficiency is suspected.

    a. Assist the patient to a supine position. Have him or her raise one leg or one arm about 30 cm (1 ft) above heart level, move the foot or hand briskly up and down for about 1 minute, and then sit up and dangle the leg or arm. This procedure is called *Buerger's test.*

    b. Observe the time of return of original color and vein filling. Original color normally returns in 10 seconds, and the veins fill in about 15 seconds. Delayed color return indicates arterial insufficiency.

FIGURE 10–65

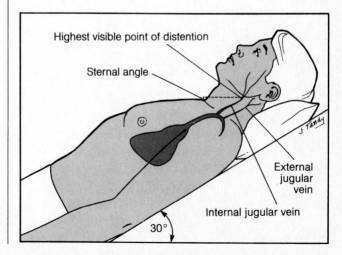

Highest visible point of distention

Sternal angle

External jugular vein

Internal jugular vein

30°

13. Test capillary refill:
    a. Squeeze a fingernail and a toenail between your fingers sufficiently to cause blanching.
    b. Release the pressure and observe how quickly normal color returns. Color normally returns immediately.
14. Inspect the fingernails for changes indicative of circulatory impairment. See Technique 10–4.

15. Record your findings on the patient's record.

■ Evaluation

See Table 10–18. Upon obtaining an unexpected outcome: Report your findings to the responsible nurse and/or physician.

TECHNIQUE 10–13 ■ Assessing the Abdomen

Assessment of the abdomen involves all four methods of examination (inspection, palpation, auscultation, and percussion). Several body organs are assessed during the abdominal examination: the stomach, intestines, liver, spleen, kidneys, and, if distended or enlarged, bladder. More revealing data can be obtained from the nursing history. See Table 10–21 later in this chapter.

Abdominal subdivisions and landmarks

Description of abdominal findings is facilitated by two commonly used methods of subdivision: quadrants and nine regions. To divide the abdomen into quadrants, a vertical line is made from the xiphoid process to the pubic symphysis, and a horizontal line is drawn across the umbilicus. See Figure 10–66. These quadrants are labeled upper right quadrant (1), upper left quadrant (2), lower right quadrant (3), and lower left quadrant (4). The

second method, division into nine regions, uses two vertical lines that extend superiorly from the midpoints of the inguinal ligaments and two horizontal lines, one at the level of the edge of the lower ribs and the other at the level of the iliac crests. See Figure 10–67. Specific organs or parts of organs lie in each abdominal region. See Tables 10–19 and 10–20.

In addition, certain landmarks are often used to facilitate the location of abdominal signs and symptoms. These are the xiphoid process of the sternum, the costal margins, the midline (a line drawn from the tip of the sternum through the umbilicus to the pubic symphysis), the anterosuperior iliac spine, the inguinal ligaments (Poupart's ligaments), and the superior margin of the pubic symphysis. See Figure 10–68.

FIGURE 10–66 ■ The four abdominal quadrants and the underlying organs: 1, upper right quadrant; 2, upper left quadrant; 3, lower right quadrant; 4, lower left quadrant.

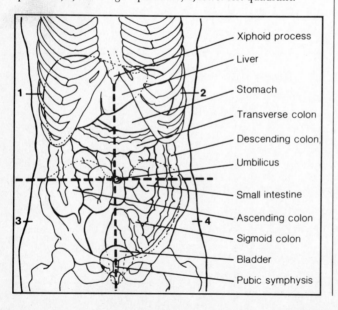

FIGURE 10–67 ■ The nine abdominal regions: 1, epigastric; 2, 3, left and right hypochondriac; 4, umbilical; 5, 6, left and right lumbar; 7, suprapubic or hypogastric; 8, 9, left and right inguinal or iliac.

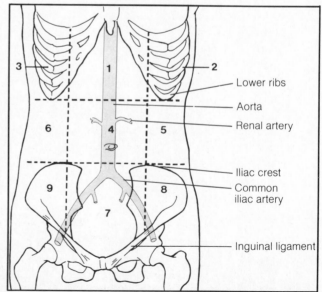

TABLE 10–19   ■   Organs in the Four Abdominal Quadrants

Upper right quadrant	Upper left quadrant
Liver	Left lobe of liver
Gallbladder	Stomach
Duodenum	Spleen
Head of pancreas	Upper lobe of left kidney
Right adrenal gland	Pancreas
Upper lobe of right kidney	Left adrenal gland
Hepatic flexure of colon	Splenic flexure of colon
Section of ascending colon	Section of transverse colon
Section of transverse colon	Section of descending colon

Lower right quadrant	Lower left quadrant
Lower lobe of right kidney	Lower lobe of left kidney
Cecum	Sigmoid colon
Appendix	Section of descending colon
Section of ascending colon	Left ovary
Right ovary	Left fallopian tube
Right fallopian tube	Left ureter
Right ureter	Left spermatic cord
Right spermatic cord	Part of uterus (if enlarged)
Part of uterus (if enlarged)	

Midline

Uterus
Bladder

TABLE 10–20   ■   Organs in the Nine Abdominal Regions

Right hypochondriac	Epigastric	Left hypochondriac
Right lobe of liver	Aorta	Stomach
Gallbladder	Pyloric end of stomach	Spleen
Part of duodenum	Part of duodenum	Tail of pancreas
Hepatic flexure of colon	Pancreas	Splenic flexure of colon
Upper half of right kidney	Part of liver	Upper half of left kidney
Suprarenal gland		Suprarenal gland
Right lumbar	**Umbilical**	**Left lumbar**
Ascending colon	Omentum	Descending colon
Lower half of right kidney	Mesentery	Lower half of left kidney
Part of duodenum and jejunum	Lower part of duodenum	Part of jejunum and ileum
	Part of jejunum and ileum	
Right inguinal	**Hypogastric (pubic)**	**Left inguinal**
Cecum	Ileum	Sigmoid colon
Appendix	Bladder (if enlarged)	Left ureter
Lower end of ileum	Uterus (if enlarged)	Left spermatic cord
Right ureter		Left ovary
Right spermatic cord		
Right ovary		

■ Planning

Nursing goals

1. To establish baseline data about the patient's abdomen, liver, spleen, kidneys, and bladder
2. To detect problems of the abdomen, liver, spleen, kidneys, and bladder

Equipment

1. A stethoscope
2. A tape measure (metal or unstretchable cloth)
3. A skin-marking pencil
4. An examining light

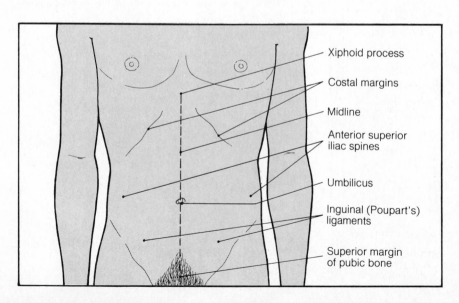

FIGURE 10–68   ■   Landmarks commonly used to identify abdominal areas.

Xiphoid process
Costal margins
Midline
Anterior superior iliac spines
Umbilicus
Inguinal (Poupart's) ligaments
Superior margin of pubic bone

■ Intervention

See Table 10-21 for normal and abnormal findings and some associated conditions. When assessing the abdomen, inspection is done first, followed by auscultation, palpation, and/or percussion. Auscultation is done before palpation and percussion since movement or stimulation of the bowel caused by palpation and percussion can increase bowel motility and thus heighten bowel sounds, creating false results.

1. Ensure that the patient's bladder has been recently emptied. Assist the patient to a supine position with the arms placed comfortably at the sides. Place small pillows beneath the knees and the head.

   Rationale This position and an empty bladder prevent tension in the abdominal muscles, compared to a sitting position or a supine position with knees extended and arms extended upward with hands clasped behind the head.

2. Ensure that the room is warm, and expose only the patient's abdomen from chest line to the pubic area.

   Rationale Chilling and shivering can tense the abdominal muscles.

Inspection

3. Direct the examining light over the abdomen, and inspect the abdominal surface, with your head only slightly higher than the patient's abdomen. Note surface characteristics, distention, masses, visible peristaltic waves or pulsations, movements with respiration, abdominal and umbilical contours, and presence of scars or rashes. Abdominal contour is the profile line from the rib margin to the pubic bone viewed by the examiner at a right angle to the umbilicus when the patient is supine. Abdominal contour is described as flat, rounded, or scaphoid. The flat contour lies in an approximately horizontal plane from the rib cage to the pubic area; the rounded contour is convex to the horizontal plane; and the scaphoid is concave to the horizontal plane.

4. Instruct the patient to take a deep breath and to hold it. Inspect the abdominal contour.

   Rationale A deep breath forces the diaphragm downward, thus decreasing the size of the abdominal cavity and making masses such as an enlarged liver or spleen more obvious.

5. Instruct the patient to raise his or her head and shoulders without using the arms for support. Again inspect the abdominal contour, and observe the rectus abdominus muscles for separation (diastasis recti abdominis). See Figure 10-69.

   Rationale Separation of the rectus abdominis muscles can be observed as a ridge or bulge between the muscles when intraabdominal pressure is increased by raising the head and shoulders. This

defect does not seriously affect the functions of abdominal organs.

6. Move to the foot of the bed or examining table, and inspect the contour of the abdomen for symmetry.

   Rationale Asymmetry of the abdominal contour is more readily assessed from this position.

Auscultation

Listen for two abdominal sounds: bowel or peristaltic sounds caused by gas and food moving along the intestines, and vascular sounds. In the pregnant woman, fetal heart sounds are also assessed. See chapter 8.

7. Warm your hands and the stethoscope diaphragms.

   Rationale Cold hands and a cold stethoscope may cause the patient to contract the abdominal muscles, and these contractions may be heard during auscultation.

8. Applying only light pressure with the stethoscope, use the flat-disc diaphragm to listen to the abdominal intestinal sounds, and use the bell-shaped diaphragm to detect arterial and venous sounds.

   Rationale Light pressure is adequate to detect the sounds. Intestinal sounds are relatively high-pitched and best accentuated by the flat diaphragm; arterial and venous sounds are lower-pitched and best accentuated by the bell.

9. Ask when the patient last ate.

   Rationale Shortly after or long after eating, bowel sounds may be normally increased. They are loudest when a meal is long overdue. Four to seven hours after a meal, bowel sounds may be heard continuously over the ileocecal valve area, while the digestive contents from the small intestine empty through the valve into the large intestine.

10. Place the flat diaphragm of the stethoscope in each of the four quadrants of the abdomen, and listen for active bowel sounds—irregular gurgling noises occur-

FIGURE 10-69

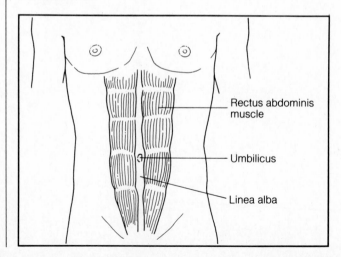

Rectus abdominis muscle

Umbilicus

Linea alba

TABLE 10–21   Abdomen

Nursing history: Determine incidence of abdominal pain, its location, onset, sequence, and chronology; its quality (description); its frequency; associated symptoms, eg, nausea, vomiting, diarrhea; bowel habits; incidence of constipation or diarrhea (have patient describe what he or she means by these terms); change in appetite, food intolerances, and foods ingested in last 24 hours; specific signs and symptoms such as heartburn, flatulence and/or belching, difficulty swallowing, hematemesis, blood or mucus in stools, and aggravating and alleviating factors; previous problems and treatment, eg, stomach ulcer, gallbladder surgery, history of jaundice.

Method and structure	Normal findings	Abnormal findings	Some associated conditions
Inspection			
Abdomen	Smooth, soft; flat, rounded, or scaphoid contour	Tense, glistening skin	Ascites; edema
		Distention	Ascites; intestinal obstruction
		Visible peristalsis	Bowel obstruction
		Visible midline pulsations	Aortic aneurysm
	Symmetric contour	Asymmetric contour, eg, localized protrusions around umbilicus, around inguinal ligaments, or near scars	Tumor; hernia
	Silver-white striae or surgical scars	Purple striae	Cushing's disease
	Unblemished skin	Rash or other skin lesions	Allergy; skin disorder
	After deep breath, smooth, even, symmetric movements	After deep breath, bulges or masses appear	Enlarged liver or spleen
		After deep breath, abdominal movement is restricted	Peritonitis; abdominal infection
	After raising head and shoulders, little or no midline bulge	After raising head and shoulders, marked ridge or bulge	Separation of rectus abdominis muscles (diastasis recti abdominis)
Auscultation			
Abdomen	Audible bowel sounds	Absent or hypoactive bowel sounds	Decreased motility due to post-operative paralytic ileus, electrolyte disorders (eg, low potassium), or late bowel obstruction
		Hyperactive bowel sounds	Laxative ingestion; gastro-enteritis; early bowel obstruction
	Absence of arterial bruits	Loud bruit over aortic area	Aortic aneurysm
		Bruit over renal or iliac arteries	Renal or iliac arterial stenosis
	Absence of venous hum	Medium-pitched hum in peri-umbilical region	Obstructed portal circulation
		Friction rub	Splenic infection, abscess, or tumor; metastatic liver disease or liver abscess
Percussion			
Abdomen	Predominantly tympanic percussion sound; suprapubic dullness over distended bladder	Dullness in localized area	Fluid or solid mass
Liver	Span of 6–12 cm at midclavicular line and 4–8 cm at midsternal line	Span exceeding 12 cm at midclavicular line and 8 cm at midsternal line	Hepatomegaly
		Midsternal line span is equal to midclavicular line span	Cirrhosis of liver
		Lower liver border displaced inferiorly	Pulmonary edema
		Lower liver border displaced superiorly	Pregnancy; ascites

TABLE 10–21 ■ continued

Method and structure	Normal findings	Abnormal findings	Some associated conditions
Spleen	Span of about 7 cm at left midaxillary line between sixth and tenth ribs	Span exceeds 7 cm	Mononucleosis
Shifting dullness test		Change in first and second demarcation lines (between tympany and dullness)	Ascites
Fist percussion	No tenderness of liver or kidney	Tenderness of liver Tenderness of kidney	Hepatitis; cholecystitis Kidney inflammation
Palpation			
Light abdominal	No tenderness; relaxed abdomen with smooth, consistent tension	Tenderness and hypersensitivity Superficial masses Localized areas of increased tension	
Deep abdominal	Tenderness may be present near xiphoid process, over cecum, and over sigmoid colon	Generalized or localized areas of tenderness Mobile or fixed masses	
Liver	May not be palpable Border feels smooth	Enlarged but smooth and not tender Smooth but tender Nodular Hard	Portal obstruction and cirrhosis; congestion of liver Acute hepatitis Metastatic carcinoma Carcinoma
Spleen	Not palpable	Palpated	Splenic enlargement (inflammation or mass)
Kidney	Neither kidney palpable Pole of right kidney palpable, feels smooth and firm	Either or both kidneys palpable Enlarged, hard, tender, or nodular	Kidney enlargement (inflammation or mass)
Bladder	Not palpable	Distended and palpable as smooth, round, tense mass	Urinary retention

ring about every 5 to 20 seconds. The duration of a single sound may range from less than a second to more than several seconds. The frequency of sounds relates to the state of digestion or the presence of food in the gastrointestinal tract. Normal bowel sounds are described as audible. Alterations in sounds are described as (a) absent or hypoactive, ie, extremely soft and at a slow rate (eg, one per minute), and (b) hyperactive or increased (borborygmi), ie, high-pitched, loud, rushing sounds at a faster rate (eg, every 3 seconds).

11. If bowel sounds appear to be absent, listen for three to five minutes before concluding that they are absent. Listen over all the auscultatory sites shown in Figure 10–70.

    Rationale Because bowel sounds are so irregular, a longer time and more sites are used to confirm absence of sounds.

12. Place the bell of the stethoscope over the aorta, renal arteries, and iliac arteries, and listen for arterial sounds (bruits).

    a. Auscultate the aorta superior to the umbilicus.

    b. Auscultate the renal arteries at or to the left and right of the upper abdominal midline or further toward the flank.

    c. Auscultate the iliac arteries to the left and right of the abdominal midline below the umbilicus. See Figure 10–67, earlier, to locate these areas.

13. Place the bell of the stethoscope over the periumbilical (around the umbilicus) region and listen for a venous hum, rarely heard in the abdomen.

14. At the various auscultating sites, especially the liver and splenic sites, listen for peritoneal friction rubs that sound like two pieces of leather rubbing together.

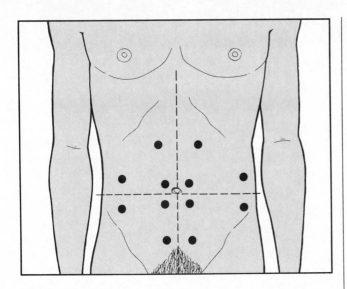

FIGURE 10–70

Rationale The liver and spleen have large surface areas in contact with the peritoneum; thus they are most frequently the beginning sites for friction rubs.

a. To auscultate the splenic site, place the stethoscope over the left lower rib cage in the anterior axillary line and have the patient take a deep breath.

Rationale A deep breath may accentuate the sound of a friction rub area.

b. To auscultate the liver site, place the stethoscope over the lower right rib cage.

Percussion

Percussion is used to detect gas, fluid, and/or masses within the abdomen as well as the position and size of the liver and spleen.

15. Lightly percuss the entire abdomen in a systematic manner:

a. Move from the right upper quadrant in a clockwise direction from the patient's perspective (counterclockwise from your perspective). See Figure 10–71.

b. If the patient is experiencing pain or tenderness in a specific area, percuss that area last.

Rationale Evoking pain early in the percussion sequence might cause the patient to tense the abdominal muscles, making evaluation of percussion sounds more difficult.

c. Percuss for areas of tympany and dullness, noting specifically areas of dullness. *Tympany* is a bell-like, musical percussion sound of somewhat higher pitch than resonance. It is characteristic of a gas-filled cavity or organ. Tympanic sounds pre-

dominate in the abdomen due to the presence of gas in the stomach and intestines. *Dullness* is a decrease, absence, or flatness of resonance. Dullness is heard over solid masses such as ascites, a distended bladder, a sigmoid colon filled with stool, enlarged organs such as the liver or spleen, and tumors.

16. *Liver size and position.*

a. Begin percussion in the right midclavicular line at or below the level of the umbilicus, and percuss upward over tympanic areas until a dull percussion sound indicates the lower liver border. Mark this site with a skin-marking pencil. See Figure 10–72.

b. Then percuss downward at the right midclavicular line beginning from an area of lung resonance and progressing downward until a dull percussion sound indicates the upper liver border. Mark this site.

c. Measure the distance between the two marks (upper and lower liver border) in centimeters, to establish the liver span or size. Normally the range of liver span in the midclavicular line is 6 to 12 cm, and the lower liver border is at or just below the rib cage.

d. Repeat steps a–c at the midsternal line. Normally the range of liver span at the midsternal line is 4 to 8 cm.

17. *Liver descent.*

a. Have the patient take a deep breath and hold it.

b. Again percuss upward in the midclavicular line.

c. Estimate liver descent in centimeters.

Rationale On inspiration the diaphragm moves

FIGURE 10–71

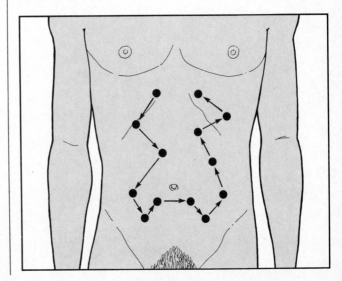

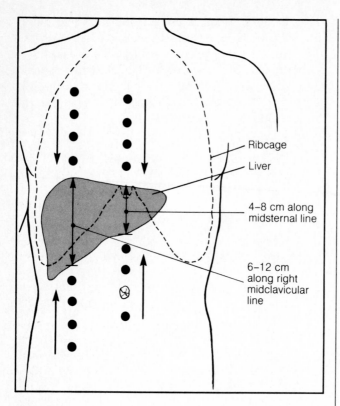

FIGURE 10-72

downward and shifts the span of liver dullness downward 2 to 3 cm.

18. *Spleen size and position.* The spleen is most easily percussed when it is enlarged. Percuss upward and downward along the left midaxillary line and note where a dull tone is heard. Normally a dullness is heard between the sixth and tenth ribs for a span of about 7 cm.

19. *Shifting dullness test.* This test is used to detect free-floating intraabdominal fluid (ascites) in the peritoneal cavity.

a. While the patient is supine, percuss the abdomen, progressing laterally from the umbilicus toward the flank. Mark the point where dullness is first percussed.

   Rationale From the umbilical area, tympanic sounds will be elicited over gas-filled structures until the area of fluid is reached; at this point, dullness will be heard. When the patient is supine, free-floating fluid in the abdomen moves to the flank areas because of gravity. The level of the fluid-filled area is determined by percussing the height of dullness.

b. Have the patient turn on her or his side facing you, and again percuss the abdomen as in step a. Mark the new line between the areas of tympany and dullness.

   Rationale When the patient lies on one side, ascitic fluid that rested in the opposite flank area

flows by gravity to the dependent flank and shifts the line of dullness closer to the umbilicus. If the area of dullness does not shift significantly, the fluid is not free-floating and may be confined within the bowel, cysts, or the abdominal wall. This technique also helps the nurse to make a rough estimate of fluid volume.

20. *Fist percussion.* Fist percussion is used to detect areas of tenderness over regions of dullness of the liver and kidney. Two methods are used to apply fist percussion: direct and indirect. In the indirect method, the palm of the nondominant hand is placed over the specific region, eg, the liver, and is then struck with a light blow by the fisted dominant hand. In the direct method, the side of the fisted hand is applied directly to the specific region, eg, the kidney. Do not apply fist percussion until the end of the examination, since it may produce discomfort and tenderness. You will assess the tenderness by the patient's reaction. Always alert the patient before fist percussion. Otherwise, although the patient's reaction may simply indicate surprise, you may interpret it as an indication of tenderness.

a. For the liver, apply only indirect fist percussion. Place the palm of your nondominant hand parallel to and below the right costal margin and strike it with the back of the fist of the other hand. See Figure 10-73. Note if tenderness occurs.

b. For the kidney, apply either direct or indirect fist percussion while the patient is sitting upright or lying on his or her side. Place the palm of your nondominant hand or the back of your clenched fist over the costovertebral angle between the spine and the 12th rib. See Figure 10-74.

Palpation

Palpation is used to detect tenderness, the outline and position of abdominal organs (eg, the liver, spleen, and

FIGURE 10-73

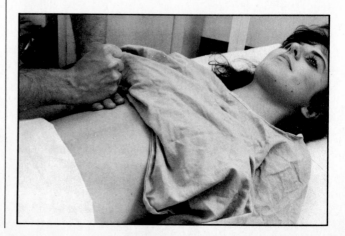

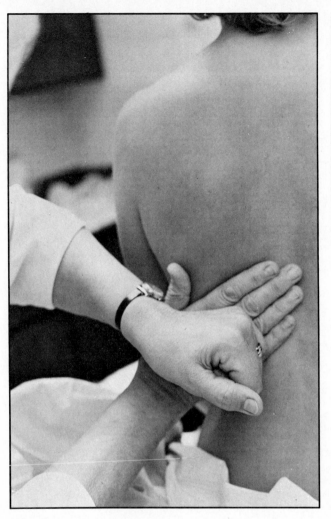

FIGURE 10–74

kidneys), and the presence of masses or distention. Two types of palpation are used: light and deep.

21. Warm your hands.

Rationale   Cold hands can elicit muscle tension that impedes palpatory evaluation.

22. *Light palpation.* Perform light palpation first, and systematically explore all four abdominal quadrants.

Rationale   Light palpation alerts the nurse to areas of tenderness and/or muscle guarding (stiffening) before more vigorous palpation is performed.

a. Hold the palm of your hand slightly above the patient's abdomen with your fingers parallel to the abdomen.

b. Depress the abdominal wall lightly, about 1 cm or to the depth of the subcutaneous tissue, with the pads of the fingers. See Figure 10–75.

c. Move the finger pads in a slight circular motion.

d. If the patient is extremely ticklish, place his or her hand under or over your own hand.

Rationale   This decreases the degree of ticklishness and resulting muscle tenseness.

e. Note areas of slight tenderness or superficial pain, large masses, and muscle guarding. To determine areas of tenderness, have the patient tell you about them, watch for changes in the patient's facial expressions, and note areas of muscle guarding.

23. *Deep palpation.* Perform deep palpation systematically over all four quadrants.

a. Palpate sensitive areas last.

b. Press the distal half of the palmar surface of the fingers of one hand into the abdominal wall.

or

Use the bimanual method of palpation discussed earlier in this chapter, on page 159.

c. Depress the abdominal wall about 4 to 5 cm or an appropriate distance beyond subcutaneous tissue. See Figure 10–76.

d. Note masses and the structure of underlying contents. If a mass is present, determine its size, location, mobility, contour, consistency, and tenderness. Normal abdominal structures that may be mistaken for masses include: the lateral borders of the rectus abdominis muscles; the feces-filled

FIGURE 10–75

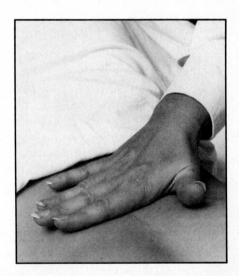

FIGURE 10–76

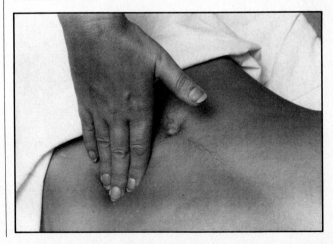

ascending, descending, or sigmoid colon; the aorta; the uterus; the common iliac artery; and the sacral promontory.

24. *Liver palpation.* The liver is palpated to detect enlargement and tenderness. Two bimanual approaches are used.

a. Stand on the patient's right side.

b. Place your left hand on the posterior thorax at about the 11th or 12th rib.

c. Push upward with the left hand.

   Rationale This hand braces the subsequent anterior palpation.

d. Place your right hand along the rib cage at about a 45° angle to the right of the rectus abdominis muscle or parallel to the rectus muscle with the fingers pointing toward the rib cage. See Figure 10–77.

e. While the patient exhales, exert a gradual and gentle downward and forward pressure beneath the costal margin until a depth of 4 to 5 cm is reached.

   Rationale During expiration, the abdominal wall is relaxed and facilitates deep palpation.

f. Maintain your hand position, and ask the patient to inhale deeply.

   Rationale This makes the liver border descend and moves the liver into a palpable position.

g. While the patient inhales, feel the liver border move against your hand. It should feel firm and have a regular contour. If the liver is not palpated initially, have the patient take two or three more deep breaths, while you maintain or apply slightly more palpation pressure. Livers are harder to palpate in obese, tense, or very physically fit people.

h. If the liver is enlarged, ie, palpable below the costal margin, measure the number of centimeters it extends below the costal region.

The second method is the bimanual palpation method discussed on page 159, in which one hand is superimposed on the other. It uses the same techniques and principles as steps d–h.

25. *Spleen palpation.* Although the spleen is not palpable in the normal adult, the splenic area is palpated in the same manner as the liver.

a. Have the patient turn onto his or her right side.

   Rationale This brings the spleen forward and down by gravity and closer to the abdominal wall.

b. Palpate at the left costal margin.

26. *Kidney palpation.* The upper lobes of both kidneys touch the diaphragm, and the kidneys descend upon inhalation. The right kidney is normally more easily palpated than the left, because the right one lies a little lower than the left. The right kidney lies in line with the 12th rib and the left kidney with the 11th rib. See Figure 10–78, *A,* for the anterior view, and

FIGURE 10–77

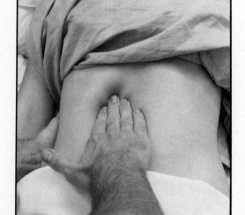

FIGURE 10–78

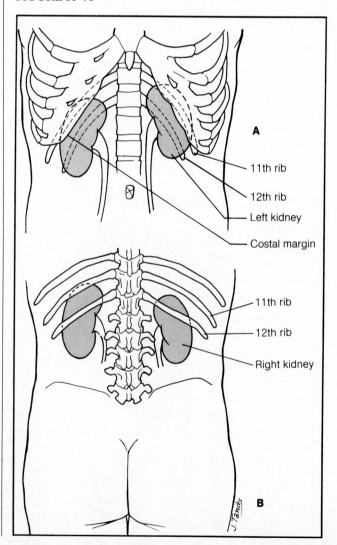

10–78, *B,* for the posterior view. The adult kidney is normally smooth, solid, firm, and shaped like a lima bean. It is generally about 11 cm (4.5 in) long, 5 to 7 cm (2 to 3 in) wide, and 2.5 cm (1 in) thick. To palpate the kidneys, have the patient in a supine position, and stand at his or her right side while assessing either kidney.

a. To palpate the right kidney, place your left hand under the patient's flank to elevate the kidney anteriorly.

b. Place your right hand on the anterior abdominal wall at the midclavicular line and at the inferior edge of the costal margin.

c. Press directly upward beneath the costal margin while the patient takes a deep breath. See Figure 10–79.

   Rationale   Inhaling moves the diaphragm and the inferior aspect of the kidney downward, so that the kidney may be felt. Normally the kidneys of the adult are not palpable, but in very thin people the lower part of the right kidney may be felt.

d. If the kidney is palpable, check it for contour (shape), size, tenderness, and lumps.

e. To palpate the left kidney, reach across the patient, and place your left hand under the patient's flank. See Figure 10–80.

f. Follow steps b–d.

27. *Bladder palpation.* With one or two hands, palpate the area above the symphysis pubis. See Figure 10–81. The bladder is palpable only when distended with

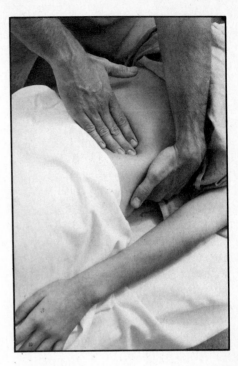

FIGURE 10–80

urine. If it is distended, percuss the area for level of dullness.

■ Evaluation

See Table 10–21 for expected and unexpected outcomes. Upon obtaining an unexpected outcome: Report your findings to the responsible nurse and/or physician.

FIGURE 10–79

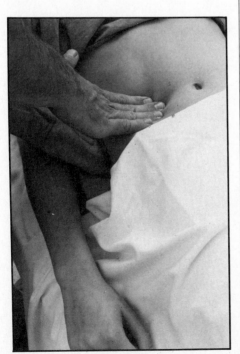

FIGURE 10–81

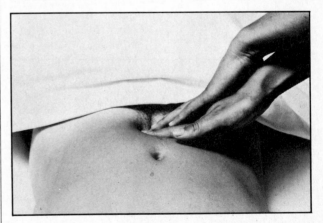

TECHNIQUE 10-14 ▪ Assessing the Rectum and Anus

The anal canal is the most distal portion of the gastrointestinal tract. At the point where it joins the rectum, the skin lining the anal canal changes to mucous membrane lining the rectum. In an adult, the anal canal is about 4 cm (1.5 in) long, and the rectum is about 12 cm (8 in) long. On its proximal end, the rectum joins the sigmoid colon. Distally it opens onto the body surface; the orifice is called the *anus*. The anus has many somatic nerve endings and thus is highly sensitive to discomfort. The rectum is innervated by the vagus nerve; care must be taken not to overstimulate this nerve, because of the danger of causing a decreased heart rate, since the vagus nerve also innervates the heart.

The lumen of the rectum has three folds, called *Houston's valves*, which help hold feces in the rectum. The most inferior fold, which projects posteriorly, can sometimes be felt digitally.

▪ Planning

Nursing goals

1. To determine baseline data regarding the patient's anus, rectum, and (in males) prostate gland
2. To determine the presence of fecal impaction

Equipment

1. Drapes so as to expose the patient only minimally
2. A disposable examining glove
3. Lubricant

FIGURE 10-82

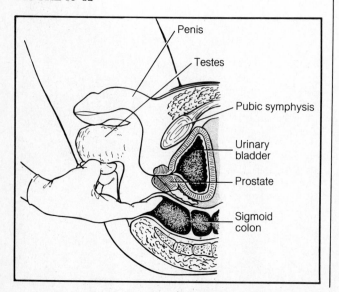

Penis

Testes

Pubic symphysis

Urinary bladder

Prostate

Sigmoid colon

▪ Intervention

1. Assist the patient to a dorsal recumbent position with hips externally rotated and knees flexed, or to Sims's position. Drape the patient appropriately. See pages 161-162 or 164.

2. Spread the buttocks, and ask the patient to bear down.

   Rationale Bearing down normally causes the anal sphincter to contract, so that this tests whether the nerves to the area are intact.

3. Inspect the anus for protruding hemorrhoids (distended veins that appear as red bodies), fissures, cracks, and redness. Normally the skin is intact, and there are no hemorrhoids, lesions, or reddened areas.

4. Don a glove, and lubricate the index finger. Slowly insert the finger into the anus and into the rectum.

   Rationale If the finger is inserted slowly, the anal sphincter muscles will relax, permitting the finger to extend into the rectum.

5. Palpate the rectal walls with the pad of the index finger, feeling for nodules, masses, and tenderness. Normally the wall will be smooth and not tender. If you palpate a mass, note the location on the rectum, eg, anterior wall, 2 cm proximal to the internal anal sphincter.

6. In the male, palpate the prostate gland through the anterior wall of the rectum. See Figure 10-82. You should be able to feel the median sulcus, which divides the gland into two lobes. The prostate should be about 4 cm (1.5 in) in diameter, firm and rubbery, with discrete edges. Tenderness is not normally experienced by the patient.

7. In the female, palpate the cervix of the uterus through the anterior rectal wall. See Figure 10-83. The cervix normally feels smooth, round, firm, and movable. It is not normally tender.

8. Upon withdrawing your finger from the rectum and anus, observe it for feces. Feces are normally brown. Note any mucus or blood.

9. Record the color of the feces, and send a sample to the laboratory to test for occult blood.

10. Record your findings on the appropriate record.

▪ Evaluation

Expected outcomes

1. Anal sphincter intact

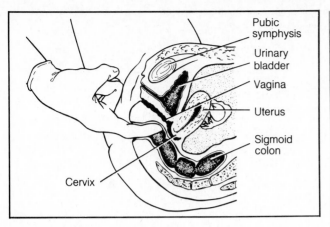

FIGURE 10–83

2. Absence of lesions, fissures, external hemorrhoids
3. No visible mucus or blood in feces

4. No tenderness, masses, or internal hemorrhoids
5. Prostate firm, smooth, mobile, normal size, and not tender
6. Cervix smooth, round, firm, and movable

Unexpected outcomes

1. Presence of external hemorrhoids
2. Mucus visible with feces
3. Mass palpated on posterior rectal wall
4. Prostate enlarged (5–6 cm) and tender, with nodular surface
5. Cervix tender

Upon obtaining an unexpected outcome: Report your findings to the responsible nurse and/or physician.

TECHNIQUE 10–15   ■   Assessing the Female Genitals

The female genitourinary system includes three main parts: the inguinal lymph nodes; the genitals and orifices, eg, labia majora; the internal genitals, eg, the cervix.

■ Planning

Nursing goals

1. To obtain baseline data on the patient's genitourinary system and lymph nodes
2. To obtain a specimen, eg, a cervical smear for diagnostic purposes

Equipment

1. Good lighting. A flashlight may be necessary to view the cervix.
2. Drapes to avoid undue exposure of the patient.
3. An examining table on which the patient can assume the lithotomy position.
4. Disposable gloves.
5. A vaginal speculum of the correct size. A virgin or an elderly woman will probably require a small speculum. The size of speculum required otherwise depends on the individual's sexual and obstetric history. See Figure 10–84.
6. Warm water to lubricate the speculum.
7. Lubricant.

8. Supplies for cytology studies: cotton applicators, normal saline solution, an Ayre spatula (for a cervical scrape), slides, and fixative spray or solution for the specimen.

■ Intervention

See Table 10–22 for normal and abnormal findings and associated conditions.

FIGURE 10–84

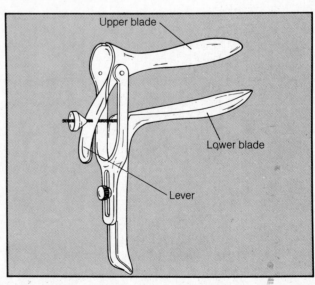

TABLE 10-22 ■ Female Reproductive System

Nursing history: Determine age of onset of menstruation, last menstrual period (LMP), regularity of cycle, duration, amount of daily flow, and whether menstruation is painful; incidence of pain during intercourse; vaginal discharge; number of pregnancies, number of live births, labor or delivery complications; frequency, urgency, frequency of urination at night, blood in urine, painful urination, incontinence; history of sexually transmitted disease, past and present.

Structure	Normal findings	Abnormal findings	Some associated conditions
External genitals	Normal pubic hair pattern and amount	Scant pubic hair	Aging
	Labia majora and minora intact		
	Absence of lesions, scars, fissures, swelling, or erythema		
	No urethral discharge	Urethral discharge	Urethritis
	Skene's and Bartholin's glands not tender or inflamed	Inflamed Bartholin's glands	
Vagina	Walls intact	Cystocele, rectocele, enterocele	Prolapse of vaginal wall
	Pelvic musculature has good tone		
	Mucosa pink, no discharge	Vaginal discharge, mucosa inflamed	Vaginitis, malignancy
Cervix	Positioned posteriorly		
	Smooth, mobile, not tender	Nodular, tender	Cervical cancer
	Size 2-3 cm (0.7-1 in) in diamater	Lacerations, erosions, masses, discharge, polyps, cysts	Chronic cervicitis; cervical cancer
	Nulliparous os is round or oval		
	Parous os is slitlike		
Uterus	About fist size		
	Freely movable	Not movable, tender	Malignancy
	Positioned anteriorly, firm, smooth surface		
Ovaries	Slightly tender	Acute discomfort	
	Less than 4 cm (1.5 in)		
	Smooth, mobile	Nodular surface, fixed	Inflammation
Rectovaginal wall	Smooth, thin, and pliable	Bulging, inflamed	Tumor
	Posterior surface of uterus smooth	Surface nodular	

Inguinal lymph nodes

There are two groups of superficial lymph nodes in the inguinal area: the superior (horizontal) group, and the inferior (vertical) group. See Figure 10-85. The superior group drain the skin of the abdominal wall, below the external genitals, anal canal, and lower vagina. The inferior group receives lymph from the medial aspect of the leg and foot.

1. Assist the patient to a back-lying position and drape her appropriately (see pages 161–162).
2. Palpate the groin area for the lymph nodes indicated in Figure 10-85, using the pads of your fingers in a rotary motion.
3. Assess the lymph nodes for enlargement and tenderness.

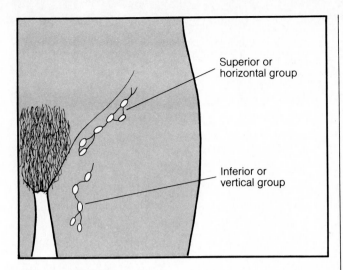

FIGURE 10–85

External genitals

4. Ask the patient to empty her bladder before the pelvic examination. A urine specimen may or may not be sent for urinalysis.

   Rationale   The patient will feel more comfortable during the examination. Relaxation of the abdominal muscles is important for successful assessment.

5. Assist the patient to a lithotomy position, and drape her appropriately.

6. Inspect the distribution and amount of pubic hair. There are wide variations. Generally in the adult, during menstruating years, it may be kinky; after menopause, it is thinner and straighter.

7. Inspect the skin in the pubic area for lice, lesions, erythema, leukoplakia, fissures, and excoriations.

8. Separate the labia majora, and inspect the interior of the labia majora and the labia minora for the problems noted in step 7.

9. Inspect the clitoris for size and lesions. The normal clitoris is about 0.5 cm (0.2 in) in diameter.

10. Inspect the urethral meatus for signs of inflammation.

11. Palpate the Skene's (paraurethral) glands at the urethral meatus. These are located on either side of the urethral orifice. They are not normally palpable. See Figure 10–86.

    a. Insert a gloved index finger, palm uppermost, into the entrance of the vagina about 2.5 cm (1 in).

    b. While pressing gently upward, palpate for the Skene's glands, then draw the finger outward.

       Rationale   This action will milk the urethra of any discharge.

    c. Observe for any discharge.

12. Palpate the Bartholin's glands, which are normally

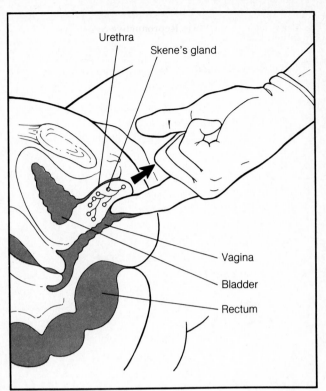

FIGURE 10–86

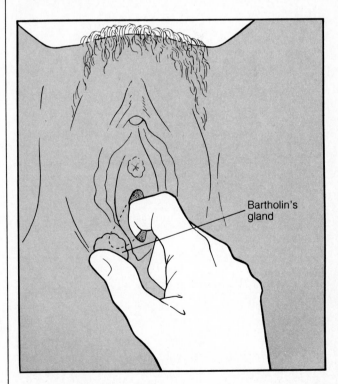

FIGURE 10–87

located on the posterior aspect of the vaginal orifice. See Figure 10–87.

a. Insert a gloved finger into the entrance of the vagina.

b. Move the finger to the side and posterior aspect of the vagina.

c. Palpate against the thumb at the posterior aspect of the labia majora.

d. Repeat for the other side.

Rationale The Bartholin's glands are not normally tender or palpable.

13. While the gloved finger is in the vaginal orifice, assess the pelvic musculature.

a. Ask the patient to constrict her vaginal orifice. A nulliparous female will probably have a high degree of muscle tone, while a multiparous female will have less tone.

b. Ask the patient to bear down while the fingers spread the vaginal wall laterally. Observe the vaginal wall for bulges. A *cystocele* is a bulging of the anterior vaginal wall as a result of a prolapse of the anterior wall and the bladder. A *rectocele* is a bulging of the posterior vaginal wall as a result of a prolapse of the posterior wall and the rectum. An

FIGURE 10–88

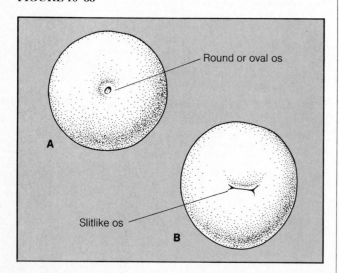

FIGURE 10–89

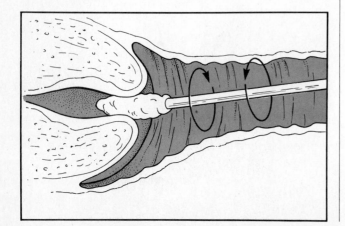

enterocele is a bulging from the posterior fornix as a result of prolapse of the pouch of Douglas into the vagina.

Vagina and cervix

14. Lubricate the vaginal speculum. Use warm water rather than lubricating jelly if a specimen is to be taken.

Rationale Lubricants can interfere with cytologic studies.

15. With two fingers just inside the vaginal entrance, press gently down on the posterior wall.

16. Make sure that there is no pubic hair at the vaginal entrance.

Rationale The hair can get caught in the speculum and be pulled, causing discomfort.

17. Insert the speculum at a 45° angle with slight pressure toward the posterior wall.

Rationale The vagina slants toward the sacrum.

18. Once the speculum is in the vagina, turn it so the handle is down, ie, the blades are in a horizontal position.

19. Open the blades, locate the cervix, and lock the blades open.

20. Inspect the cervix and os for size, lacerations, erosions, nodules, masses, discharge, and color. The normal nulliparous cervical os is round or oval (see Figure 10–88, *A*); the normal parous os is slitlike (see Figure 10–88, *B*).

21. Acquire a specimen for cytology, if indicated.

Endocervical smear

a. Insert the end of a cotton-tipped applicator into the cervical os. See Figure 10–89. The applicator may or may not be dipped first in normal saline, depending on agency practice.

b. Rotate the applicator clockwise and counterclockwise in the os.

c. Remove the applicator, and roll it on a glass slide (numbered 1).

d. Fix the specimen with a fixative spray or solution.

Cervical scrape

e. Insert an Ayre spatula with the longer end extending into the cervical os. See Figure 10–90.

f. Rotate the spatula a full circle.

g. Place the scrapings on a glass slide (numbered 2).

h. Fix the specimen with a fixative.

Vaginal smear

i. Insert a cotton-tipped applicator to a position below the cervix. See Figure 10–91. The applicator may be dipped in normal saline, particularly if the vaginal mucosa is dry.

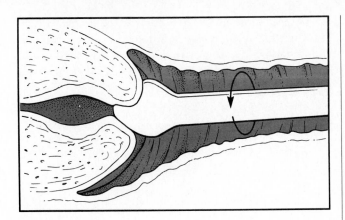

FIGURE 10-90

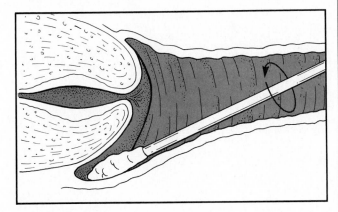

FIGURE 10-91

j. Roll the applicator on the vaginal wall below the cervix.

k. Place the smear on a glass slide (numbered 3).

l. Fix the specimen with a fixative.

22. Withdraw the speculum slowly while observing the vagina.

23. When the speculum is clear of the cervix, release the screws, and close the speculum as it is withdrawn from the vaginal entrance.

24. Insert your index and middle fingers or just your index finger, gloved and lubricated, into the vagina. Abduct your thumb, and flex your other fingers into the palm of the hand. See Figure 10-92.

    Rationale   The number of fingers inserted will depend on the size of the vagina.

25. Press the other hand downward about halfway between the umbilicus and the symphysis pubis.

    Rationale   The second hand stabilizes the uterus.

26. Palpate the cervix for smoothness, size, mobility, and tenderness.

Uterus

27. Place the fingers of the vaginal hand on either side of the cervix, palm facing upward.

Rationale   This helps to stabilize the uterus.

28. Press down with the hand on the abdomen and identify the uterus between the two hands.

29. Palpate the uterus for size, shape, consistency, and mobility. Determine if there are any masses or areas of tenderness.

Ovaries

30. Place the vaginal fingers in the right lateral fornix (to the right of the cervix). See Figure 10-93.

31. Press the abdominal hand down firmly but gently in the lower right quadrant.

FIGURE 10-92

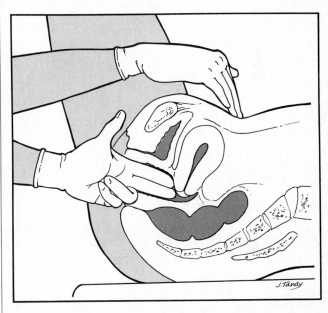

FIGURE 10-93

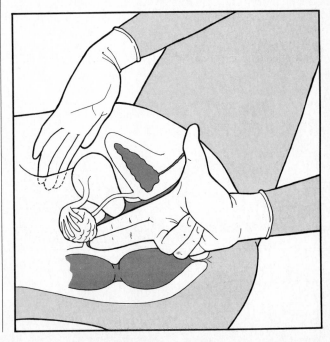

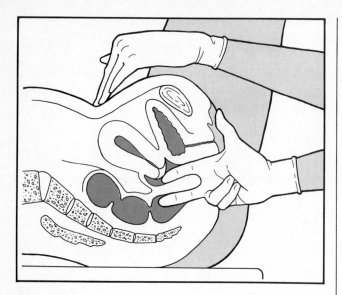

FIGURE 10-94

32. Palpate the right ovary between the two hands. The fallopian tube is not normally palpated.

33. Palpate the ovary for size, mobility, shape, consistency, and tenderness. Normally, five years after menopause the ovaries cannot be palpated because of atrophy.

34. Repeat steps 30–33 for the left ovary, with the vaginal hand in the left lateral fornix and the abdominal hand pressed downward in the left lower quadrant.

Rectovaginal–abdominal palpation

35. Don clean gloves, and lubricate the index and middle fingers.

    Rationale Clean gloves will prevent cross-contamination between the vagina and the rectum.

36. Insert the index finger into the vagina and the middle finger into the rectum. See Figure 10–94. The patient may feel that her bowels will move.

37. Apply pressure with the abdominal hand to move the uterus. The posterior surface of the uterus can then be palpated by the finger in the rectum.

38. Palpate carefully behind the cervix for masses and areas of tenderness.

39. Record your assessments on the appropriate record.

■ Evaluation

See Table 10–22. Upon obtaining an unexpected outcome: Report your findings to the responsible nurse and/or physician.

TECHNIQUE 10–16 ■ Assessing the Male Genitals

The male reproductive and urinary systems share the urethra, which is the passageway for both urine and semen. Therefore, in physical assssessment of the male these two systems are frequently assessed together.

■ Planning

Nursing goals

1. To establish baseline data regarding a patient's genitourinary system
2. To detect genitourinary problems

Equipment

1. A flashlight
2. A disposable glove
3. Lubricant

■ Intervention

See Table 10–23 for normal and abnormal findings and associated conditions.

External genitals

See Figure 10–95.

1. Inspect the amount and pattern of the pubic hair. There are wide variations among people, and only

FIGURE 10-95

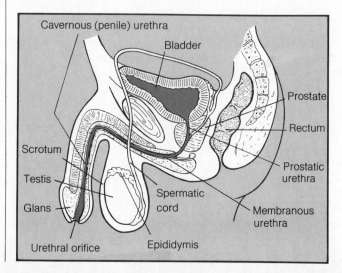

Cavernous (penile) urethra

Bladder

Prostate

Rectum

Prostatic urethra

Membranous urethra

Scrotum

Testis

Glans

Spermatic cord

Epididymis

Urethral orifice

TABLE 10-23 ▪ Male Genitourinary System

Nursing history: Determine usual fluid intake and output, voiding patterns and any changes, bladder control, urinary incontinence, frequency, urgency, abdominal pain; any symptoms of sexually transmitted disease; any swellings that could indicate presence of hernia; family history of nephritis, malignancy of the prostate, or malignancy of the kidney.

Structure	Normal findings	Abnormal findings	Some associated conditions
Pubic hair	Usually triangular pattern	Scant amount	
Skin over penis and scrotum	Intact	Excoriations, ulcers, lesions	
Penis	Normal size	Extremely large or small	
	Foreskin retracts Absence of tenderness, thickening, or nodules	Foreskin does not retract	Phimosis
	Urethral meatus at tip	Meatus on underside of penis	Hypospadius
		Meatus on upper side of penis	Epispadius
	Urethral meatus has no discharge, swelling, ulcers, scars, nodules, or inflammation	Discharge	Gonorrhea; urethritis
	No discomfort voiding, good urinary stream	Dysuria, poor or recently changed urinary stream	Prostatic hyperplasia
Scrotum	Skin intact, no inflammation	Ulcers, swellings, excoriations, nodules	
	Testicles rubbery, smooth, free of nodules and masses	Testicles enlarged, uneven surface	Tumor
	Testis about 2 × 4 cm (0.7 × 1.5 in)	Testis has swelling that transilluminates	Hydrocele
Epididymis	Tender, softer than the spermatic cord		
Spermatic cord	Firm		
Inguinal and femoral areas	No swellings or bulges	Swelling or bulge	Inguinal hernia; femoral hernia
Prostate gland	Size 4 cm (1.5 in) in diameter, firm, rubbery, smooth, movable, with discrete borders	Enlarged, not movable, nodular surface, tender	Prostatitis; prostatic hyperplasia; tumor

very thin hair or absence of hair should be reported. The normal pattern is triangular, often spreading up the abdomen.

2. Inspect the skin covering the penis and scrotum for excoriations, ulcers, and lesions.

3. Inspect the size of the penis. Variations are normal, and only an extreme variation is probably significant.

4. Retract the foreskin or have the patient do this. The foreskin should retract readily. A small amount of thick white smegma will normally be seen between the glans and the foreskin.

5. Palpate the penile shaft for tenderness, thickening, and nodules.

6. Locate the site of the urethral meatus, which is normally at the tip of the penis. Variations in its location are: *hypospadius,* on the underside of the penile shaft, and *epispadius,* on the upper side of the penile shaft.

7. Inspect the urethral meatus and the glans for ulcers, scars, nodules, inflammation, and discharge. Compress the glans slightly to open the urethral meatus to inspect it for discharge. If the patient has pain on voiding (dysuria) or a poor urinary stream, assess for a urethral stricture or prostatic hyperplasia.

8. Inspect the scrotum for redness, swelling, ulcers, excoriations, or nodules. Lift the scrotum to inspect the posterior aspect.

FIGURE 10–96

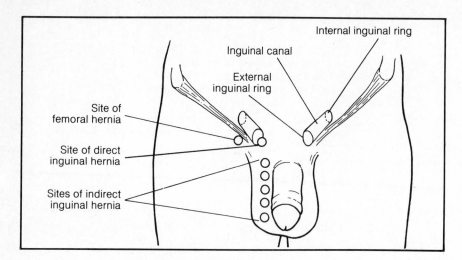

9. Palpate the scrotum and testicles. Using your index finger and thumb, palpate each testis for size, consistency, shape, smoothness, and masses. The testicle normally feels rubbery, smooth, and free from nodules or masses. Each testis is normally about 2×4 cm (0.7×1.5 in).

10. Palpate the epididymis between your thumb and index finger. It is located at the top of the testis and extends behind it. The epididymis is normally tender.

11. Palpate the spermatic cord between thumb and index finger. It is usually found at the top lateral portion of the scrotum and will feel harder than the epididymis.

12. Inspect any swelling of the scrotum by transillumination.

    a. Darken the room.

    b. Shine the flashlight from behind the scrotum through the mass. Serous fluid will cause the light to show with a red glow; tissue or blood will not transilluminate.

Hernias

13. Inspect the inguinal and femoral areas for swellings. See Figure 10–96.

14. Palpate for an inguinal hernia.

    a. Ask the patient to stand, with the leg on the side to be examined slightly flexed.

    b. Using your right hand for the patient's right side or left hand for the patient's left side, insert your index finger into the loose scrotal skin.

    c. Advance your finger up to the external inguinal ring. See Figure 10–97.

    d. If the ring is enlarged, extend your finger through the ring.

    e. Ask the patient to "bear down" or cough; an inguinal hernia may touch your finger.

15. Palpate the anterior thigh in the area of the femoral canal for a femoral hernia.

    a. Ask the patient to cough or strain during palpation.

    b. Note any bulging, swelling, or tenderness in the area.

    c. Ask the patient to lie down. Often a hernia will return to the abdomen.

Prostate gland

16. Assist the patient to a lateral or Sims's position, and drape him appropriately (see page 164), or have the patient stand leaning over a table or bed.

17. Don a disposable glove, and lubricate the index finger.

FIGURE 10–97

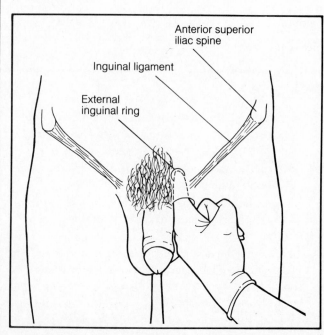

18. Insert the index finger slowly through the anal canal into the rectum. See Technique 10–14.
19. Palpate the prostate gland through the anterior rectal wall.
    a. Identify the median sulcus, which divides the gland into two lobes.
    b. Palpate the prostate for size, consistency, smoothness, mobility, and discrete borders. The prostate is normally firm and rubbery, about 4 cm (1.5 in) in diameter, smooth, with discrete borders, movable, and not tender.
20. Record your findings on the appropriate record.

■ Evaluation

See normal and abnormal findings in Table 10–23. Upon obtaining an unexpected outcome: Report your findings to the responsible nurse and/or physician.

TECHNIQUE 10–17   ■   Assessing the Musculoskeletal System

The musculoskeletal system encompasses the muscles, bones, and joints. The completeness of an assessment of this system will depend largely upon the needs of the individual patient, ie, their health problems.

The assessment of the muscles includes muscle strength, tone, and size, and symmetry of muscle development. Bones are assessed as to the normalcy of their form. Joints are assessed for tenderness, swelling, thickening, crepitation, presence of nodules, and range of motion. Range of motion is discussed in detail in chapter 19.

■ Planning

Nursing goals

1. To determine baseline data about the muscles, bones, and joints
2. To determine changes in mobility, strength, and/or endurance of specific body parts

Equipment

Measuring tape.

■ Intervention

Muscles

1. Inspect the muscle for size, eg, arm, thigh, calf muscles. Compare the muscle on one side of the body with the same one on the other side. Determine if there is any atrophy or hypertrophy.
2. If there appears to be a discrepancy between the sides, measure the muscles with a tape.
3. Observe muscles and tendons for contractures. These can be indicated by malposition of a body part, eg, a foot fixed in dorsiflexion.
4. Observe muscles for fasciculations and tremors. A *fasciculation* is an abnormal contraction (shortening) of a bundle of muscle fibers. A *tremor* is an involuntary trembling of a limb or body part. Tremors may involve large groups of muscle fibers or small bundles of muscle fibers. An *intention tremor* is a tremor that becomes more apparent when an individual attempts a voluntary movement, eg, holding a cup of coffee. A *resting tremor* is more apparent at rest and diminishes with activity.
5. Inspect any tremors of the hands and arms by having the patient hold his or her arms out in front.
6. Palpate muscles at rest to determine muscle tonicity. Muscle *tonicity* is the normal condition of tension (tone) of a muscle at rest. Muscles are normally firm.
7. Palpate muscles while the patient is active and passive (see chapter 19) for flaccidity, spasticity, and smoothness of movement. *Flaccidity* is weakness or laxness. *Spasticity* is a sudden involuntary muscle contraction.
8. Test muscle strength by having the patient squeeze or push against each of your hands. Compare the right side with the left side.
9. To test muscle strength, ask the patient to move various body parts, eg, head, arms. The patient should be able to move body parts horizontally in spite of gravity.
10. Apply resistance to the body movements. See Figure 10–98. An individual normally has equal strength on each body side. Muscle strength is graded from zero (complete paralysis) to five (normal). See Table 10–24.

Bones

11. Inspect the skeleton for normal structure and deformities. See chapter 16 for information about body alignment.
12. Palpate the bones to locate any areas of edema or tenderness.

Rationale Tenderness can reflect conditions such as fractures, neoplasms, and osteoporosis.

13. Inspect bones for bruising and swelling.

Rationale Bruises and swelling can indicate fractures.

Joints

14. Inspect each joint for swelling.

Rationale Swelling could indicate arthritis.

15. Palpate each joint for tenderness, smoothness of movement, swelling, crepitation (a crackling, grating sound), and the presence of nodules. Normally joints are not tender, move smoothly, and have no swelling, crepitation, or nodules.

16. Assess the patient's range of motion. See chapter 19.

17. Record your findings on the appropriate record.

■ Evaluation

Expected outcomes

1. Muscles symmetrical and normal size
2. Normal positions of body parts: no contractures
3. Absence of fasciculations and tremors
4. Good muscle tone and consistency
5. Normal muscle strength
6. Absence of swelling of joints
7. Normal joint range of motion

Unexpected outcomes

1. Flaccid or spastic muscles
2. Bones not in normal alignment
3. Presence of fasciculations and tremors
4. Joints swollen
5. Limited range of motion of joints

Upon obtaining an unexpected outcome: Report your findings to the responsible nurse and/or physician.

FIGURE 10-98

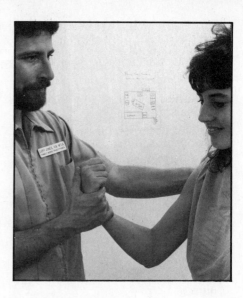

TABLE 10-24 ■ Grading Muscle Strength

Scale	Percentage of normal strength	Characteristics
0	0	Complete paralysis
1	10	No movement
		Contraction of muscle is palpable or visible
2	25	Full muscle movement against gravity, with support
3	50	Normal movement against gravity
4	75	Normal full movement against gravity and against minimal resistance
5	100	Normal strength
		Normal full movement against gravity and against full resistance

TECHNIQUE 10–18 ■ Assessing the Neurologic System

The nervous system integrates all other body systems, but it is also dependent upon the appropriate functioning of peripheral organs from which it receives internal and external environmental stimuli. A thorough neurologic examination may take one to three hours; however, routine screening tests are usually done first, and if the results of these tests are questionable, then more extensive evaluations are made. Three major considerations determine the extent of a neurologic exam: (a) the patient's chief complaints, (b) the patient's physical condition (ie, level of consciousness and ability to ambulate), since many parts of the exam require movement and coordination of the extremities, and (c) the patient's willingness to participate and cooperate.

Examination of the neurologic system includes assessment of the cranial nerves, the proprioception and cerebellar function, the motor system, the sensory system, reflexes, and mental status. Mental status and levels of consciousness are discussed in Technique 10–1 on page 164.

■ Planning

Nursing goals

1. To acquire baseline data about the patient's neurologic status
2. To detect specific neurologic problems

Equipment

1. Vials of coffee, tobacco, vanilla, and oil of cloves for olfactory assessment
2. Applicator sticks and vials of salt solution, sugar solution, vinegar or lemon juice, and quinine for taste assessment
3. Test tubes of hot and cold water for temperature assessment
4. Sterile safety pin or sterile hypodermic needle for pain sensation
5. Wisps of cotton for corneal and facial sensation assessment
6. Snellen chart for visual acuity
7. Large tuning fork
8. Tongue blade
9. Reflex hammer

■ Intervention

Cranial nerves

Assessment of the functions of the twelve pairs of cranial nerves is included to a large degree in an examination of the head and neck. A neurologist usually conducts specific examinations of these nerves, if needed; however, the routine neurologic assessment of a basic physical examination includes assessment of some of them. For the specific functions and assessment methods of each cranial nerve, see Table 10–25. The nurse needs to be aware of these functions to detect abnormalities. (The names and order of the cranial nerves can be recalled by remembering this sentence: "On old Olympus's treeless top, a Finn and German viewed a hop." The first letter of each word in the phrase is the same as the first letter of the names of the cranial nerves.)

The sense of smell (cranial nerve I) and the sense of taste (cranial nerves VII and IX) are not routinely tested. Vision and eye movements have been previously discussed in Technique 10–8; these activities involve cranial nerves II, III, IV, and VI. The cranial nerves V (trigeminal) and VII (facial) are not routinely tested other than by observing facial expression and the symmetry of the face, both moving and at rest. Any facial weakness

TABLE 10–25 ■ Cranial Nerve Functions and Assessment Methods

Cranial nerve	Name	Type	Function	Assessment methods
I	Olfactory	Sensory	Smell	Ask patient to close eyes and identify different mild aromas, such as coffee, tobacco, vanilla, oil of cloves, peanut butter, orange, lemon, lime, chocolate
II	Optic	Sensory	Vision and visual fields	Ask patient to read Snellen chart; check visual fields by confrontation; and conduct an ophthalmoscopic examination (see Technique 10–8)
III	Oculomotor	Motor	Extraocular eye movement (EOM); movement of sphincter of pupil; movement of ciliary muscles of lens	Assess directions of gaze and pupil reaction (see Technique 10–8)
IV	Trochlear	Motor	EOM, specifically moves eyeball downward and laterally	Assess directions of gaze

TABLE 10–25 ■ continued

Cranial Nerve	Name	Type	Function	Assessment methods
V	Trigeminal			
	Ophthalmic branch	Sensory	Sensation of cornea, skin of face, and nasal mucosa	While patient looks upward, lightly touch lateral sclera of eye to elicit blink reflex; to test light sensation, have patient close eyes, wipe a wisp of cotton over patient's forehead and paranasal sinuses; to test deep sensation, use alternating blunt and sharp ends of a safety pin over same areas
	Maxillary branch	Sensory	Sensation of skin of face and anterior oral cavity (tongue and teeth)	Assess skin sensation as for ophthalmic branch above
	Mandibular branch	Motor and sensory	Muscles of mastication; sensation of skin of face	Ask patient to clench teeth
VI	Abducent	Motor	EOM; moves eyeball laterally	Assess directions of gaze
VII	Facial	Motor and sensory	Facial expression; taste (anterior two thirds of tongue)	Ask patient to smile, raise the eyebrows, frown, puff out cheeks, close eyes tightly; ask patient to identify various tastes placed on tip and sides of tongue: sugar (sweet), salt, lemon juice (sour), and quinine (bitter); identify areas of taste
VIII	Auditory			
	Vestibular branch	Sensory	Equilibrium	Assessment methods are discussed with cerebellar functions (in next section)
	Cochlear branch	Sensory	Hearing	Assess patient's ability to hear spoken word and vibrations of tuning fork (see Technique 10–9)
IX	Glossopharyngeal	Motor and sensory	Swallowing ability and gag reflex, tongue movement, taste (posterior tongue)	Use tongue blade on posterior tongue while patient says "ah" to elicit gag reflex; apply tastes on posterior tongue for identification; ask patient to move tongue from side to side and up and down
X	Vagus	Motor and sensory	Sensation of pharynx and larynx; swallowing; vocal cord movement	Assessed with cranial nerve IX; assess patient's speech for hoarseness
XI	Accessory	Motor	Head movement; shrugging of shoulders	Ask patient to shrug shoulders against resistance from your hands and turn head to side against resistance from your hand (repeat for other side)
XII	Hypoglossal	Motor	Protrusion of tongue	Ask patient to protrude tongue at midline, then move it side to side

may be made more obvious by having the patient close the eyes tightly, wrinkle the forehead, and show the teeth. Only the cochlear branch of nerve VIII (vestibulocochlear) is routinely tested, that is, hearing ability. The vestibular branch of nerve VIII is concerned with balance and is tested with cerebellar functions. Swallowing, the gag reflex, tongue movement, and phonation, which involve cranial nerves IX, X, and XII, are routinely tested in the examination of the mouth. Nerves IX and X are tested together. Each side of the pharynx is touched with a tongue blade, which normally elicits the gag reflex (contraction of the pharyngeal muscles). Another test is to have the patient say "ah." The soft palate normally moves; imperfect movement suggests difficulty with nerves IX and X. Nerve XII (hypoglossal) can be readily examined by having the patient protrude the tongue as far as possible. Deviation of the tongue toward either side suggests paralysis. Cranial nerve XI (accessory), which is the motor nerve of the sternocleidomastoid muscle, can be tested by having the patient attempt to shrug the shoulders while the nurse presses down on them with the hands. Any weakness is noted.

Proprioception and Cerebellar Function

Examination of proprioception and cerebellar function includes assessment of the proprioceptive system. Structures involved in proprioception are the proprioceptors, the posterior columns of the spinal cord, the cerebellum, and the vestibular apparatus (which is innervated by cranial nerve VIII) in the labyrinth of the internal ear.

Proprioceptors are sensory nerve terminals, occurring chiefly in the muscles, tendons, joints, and the internal ear, that give information about movements and position of the body. Stimuli from the proprioceptors travel through the posterior columns of the spinal cord. Deficits of function of the posterior columns of the spinal cord result in impairment of muscle and position sense. A patient with such an impairment often must watch his or her own arm and leg movements to ascertain the position of the limbs. The posterior columns also carry nerve fibers for tactile discrimination.

The cerebellum performs three general functions below the level of consciousness:

1. It helps to control posture.
2. It acts with the cerebral cortex to produce skilled movements by coordinating the activities of groups of muscles. It therefore makes body movements smooth, steady, efficient, and coordinated instead of jerky, trembling, ineffective, awkward, and uncoordinated.
3. It controls skeletal muscles to maintain equilibrium. Afferent (sensory) impulses from the vestibular apparatus of the labyrinth of the ear travel to the cerebellum, where connections are made with the proper efferent (motor) fibers for contraction of the neces-

sary muscles to maintain bodily equilibrium. Vestibular dysfunction is characterized by vertigo, nausea, and vomiting.

Cerebellar disorders cause certain characteristic and common symptoms: *ataxia,* impairment of position sense, muscle incoordination, hypotonia, tremors, disturbance of equilibrium, disturbance in the timing of movements, and disturbance of gait. An example of ataxia is overshooting a mark or stopping before reaching it when trying to touch a given point on the body. Tremors are especially pronounced toward the end of movements. Patients with cerebellar disease also have difficulty performing rapid skilled movements, alternating movements such as supinating and pronating the arms or hands, and starting and stopping motions and replacing them with a movement in the opposite direction. The cerebellar gait, although it may vary, is commonly characterized by a wide base of support; a rigid head, trunk, and arms; lurching or staggering; legs bending at the hips; arm movements not coordinated with stride; a clumsy manner of raising the foot too high and bringing it down with a clap; and frequent falling. Paralysis does not occur with cerebellar disorders.

1. *Gross motor and balance tests.* See Table 10–26 for normal and abnormal findings. Use only two of the following tests to screen for gross motor function and balance.

   a. Have the patient walk across the room and back, and assess his or her gait.

   b. Romberg test: Ask the patient to stand with feet together and arms resting at the sides, first with eyes open, then closed. Stand close during this test to prevent the patient from falling. A positive Romberg's sign is indicated by excessive swaying or an inability to maintain the stance without widening the foot base (with eyes open or shut). If the patient has trouble maintaining his or her balance with the eyes shut, he or she has a loss of position sense referred to as *sensory ataxia.* If balance cannot be maintained whether the eyes are open or shut, the condition is referred to as *cerebellar ataxia.*

   c. Have the patient close his or her eyes and stand on one foot and then the other.

   d. Ask the patient to walk a straight line, placing the heel of one foot directly in front of the toes of the other foot.

   e. Have the patient walk several steps on the toes and then on the heels.

   f. Instruct the patient to hop in place on one foot and then the other. A certain amount of muscle strength is required for this test and is not indicated for a frail or elderly patient.

   g. Ask the patient to stretch the arms forward (in

TABLE 10–26 ■ Proprioception and Cerebellar Function

Test	Normal findings	Abnormal findings
Gross motor function and balance		
Walking gait	Has upright posture and steady gait with opposing arm swing; walks unaided maintaining balance	Has poor posture and unsteady, irregular, staggering gait with wide stance; bends legs only from hips; has rigid or no arm movements
Romberg test	May sway slightly but is able to maintain upright posture and foot stance	Cannot maintain foot stance; moves the feet apart to maintain stance
Standing on one foot with eyes closed	Maintains stance for at least 5 seconds	Cannot maintain stance for 5 seconds
Heel–toe walking	Maintains heel–toe walking along a straight line	Assumes a wider foot gait to stay upright
Toe or heel walking	Able to walk several steps on toes or heels	Cannot maintain balance on toes or heels
Hopping in place	Has adequate muscle strength to hop on one foot	Cannot hop or maintain single leg balance
Knee bends	Has adequate balance and muscle strength to perform knee bends	Does not have adequate balance or muscle strength to perform knee bends
Fine motor function: upper extremities		
Finger-to-nose test	Repeatedly and rhythmically touches the nose	Misses the nose or gives lazy response
Alternating supination and pronation of hands on knees	Can alternately supinate and pronate hands at rapid pace	Performs with slow, clumsy movements and irregular timing, has difficulty alternating from supination to pronation
Finger to nose and to examiner's finger	Performs with coordination and rapidity	Misses the finger and moves slowly
Fingers to fingers	As above	Moves slowly and is unable to touch fingers consistently
Fingers to thumb (same hand)	Rapidly touches each finger to thumb with each hand	Cannot coordinate this fine discrete movement with either one or both hands
Patting and polishing the examiner's hand	Performs these maneuvers smoothly and rapidly	Performs with clumsy movements and irregular timing
Fine motor function: lower extremities		
Heel down opposite shin	Demonstrates bilateral equal coordination	Has tremors, is awkward, heel moves off shin
Toe or ball of foot to examiner's finger	Moves smoothly, with coordination	Misses the examiner's finger, is unable to coordinate movement
Figure-eight	Can perform this test	Unable to perform the test

front of the body at shoulder level) and then do several knee bends. This test also requires muscle strength and is not indicated for weak patients.

2. *Fine motor tests for the upper extremities.* Use only two of the following tests to screen for fine motor function of the upper extremities. The patient may be seated for these tests. Have the patient:

a. Abduct and extend the arms at shoulder height and rapidly touch the nose alternately with one index finger and then the other. The patient repeats the test with the eyes closed if the test is performed easily. In abnormal responses, the patient misses the nose and may bring the finger beyond the nose (past-pointing). See Figure 10–99.

b. Alternately pat both knees with the palms of both hands and then with the backs of the hands at an ever-increasing rate. See Figure 10–100.

c. Touch his or her nose and then the examiner's index finger, held at a distance of about 45 cm (18 in), at a rapid and increasing rate.

d. Spread the arms broadly at shoulder height and

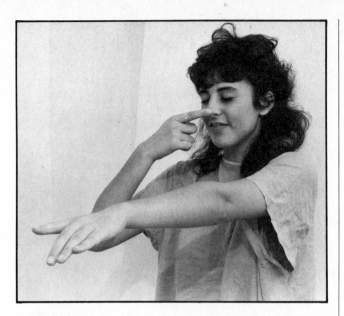

FIGURE 10-99

FIGURE 10-100

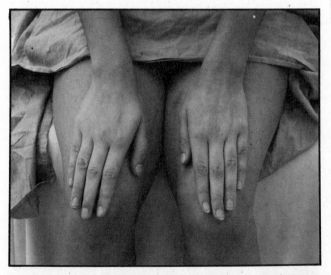

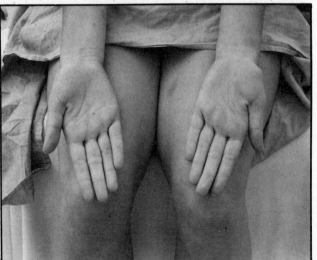

then bring the fingers together at the midline, first with the eyes open and then closed, first slowly and then rapidly.

e. Touch each finger of one hand to the thumb of the same hand as rapidly as possible. See Figure 10–101.

f. Pat the back of the examiner's hand with increasing speed; then use a circular motion on the back of the examiner's hand with increasing speed.

3. *Fine motor tests for the lower extremities.* Use only two of the following tests to screen for fine motor function of the lower extremities. Have the patient lie supine and:

a. Place the heel of one foot just below the opposite knee and run the heel down the shin to the foot. Repeat with the other foot. See Figure 10–102. (The patient may also use a sitting position for this test.)

c. Touch the examiner's finger with the large toe of each foot. See Figure 10–103.

d. Touch the examiner's finger with the ball of each foot.

e. Draw a figure-eight in the air.

Motor function

Assessment of muscle size, strength, and tone and of involuntary movements are discussed in Technique 10–17 on page 233.

Sensory function

Sensory functions include touch, pain, vibration, position, temperature, and discrimination. The first three are routinely tested in a few locations. Vibration is tested at the wrists, elbows, knees, and ankles. Generally the face, arms, legs, hands, and feet are tested for touch and pain, although all parts of the body can be tested. If the patient complains of numbness, peculiar sensations, or paralysis,

FIGURE 10-101

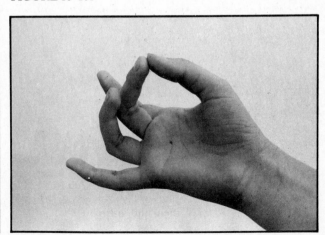

sensation should be checked more carefully over flexor and extensor surfaces of limbs. Abnormality of touch or pain should then be mapped out clearly by examining responses in the area about every 2 cm (1 in). This is a lengthy procedure. A more detailed neurologic examination includes position sense, temperature sense, and discrimination.

Sensory function of neurologically impaired patients can be evaluated by the use of dermatome zones, or segmented skin bands, that compare anatomically to the innervation by a dorsal root cutaneous nerve. See Figure 10–104. These nerves deliver the sensations of pain, temperature, touch, and vibration to the spinal cord and, ultimately, to the brain. The *spinothalmic tract* transmits the sensations of pain, temperature, and crude touch; the *dorsal column tract* transmits the perceptions of light touch and vibrations. Even though there is usually a great deal of overlap in nerve distribution, a knowledge of the dermatome zones can help you locate the approximate level of the neurologic lesion or injury. For example, a diminished or heightened response at the client's thumb can alert you to a potential disorder at level C-6 of the spinal cord.

FIGURE 10–102

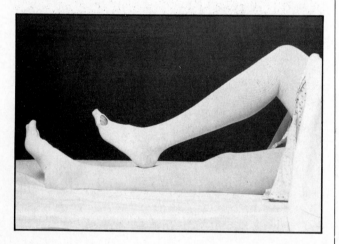

FIGURE 10–103

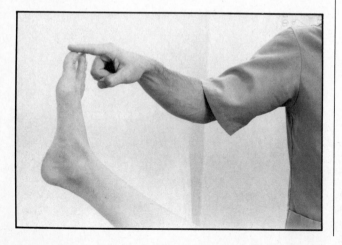

1. *Light touch sensation.*
   a. Ask the patient to close the eyes and to respond by saying "yes" or "now" whenever he or she feels the cotton wisp touching the skin.
   b. With a wisp of cotton, lightly touch one specific spot and then the same spot on the other side of the body. See Figure 10–105. Normally, a light tickling or touch sensation occurs.
      Rationale Sensitivity to touch varies with different skin areas, so it is important to compare the sensation of symmetrical areas of the body.
   c. Test areas on the forehead, cheek, hand, lower arm, abdomen, foot, and lower leg. A specific area of the limb is checked first (ie, the hand before the arm and the foot before the leg), since the sensory nerve may be assumed to be intact if sensation is felt at its most peripheral part.
      Rationale This ensures assessment of the major dermatome zones and peripheral nerves.
   d. Have the patient point to the spot where the touch was felt.
      Rationale This demonstrates whether the patient is able to determine tactile location (point localization), ie, can accurately perceive where he or she was touched.
   e. If areas of sensory dysfunction are found, determine the boundaries of sensation by testing responses about every 2.5 cm (1 in) in the area. Make a sketch of the sensory loss area for recording purposes. Note if the response is loss of sensation to touch stimuli (anesthesia); more than normal sensation (hyperesthesia); less than normal sensation (hypoesthesia); or an abnormal sensation such as burning, pain, or the feel of an electric shock (paresthesia).

2. *Pain.*
   a. Ask the patient to close his or her eyes and to say "sharp," "dull," or "don't know" when the sharp or dull end of the safety pin or needle is felt.
   b. Alternately use the sharp and dull end of the sterile pin or needle to lightly prick designated anatomic areas at random, eg, hand, forearm, foot, lower leg, abdomen. The face is not tested in this manner. See Figure 10–106.
      Rationale Alternating the sharp and dull ends of the instrument more accurately evaluates the patient's response. A sterile safety pin or needle is used to avoid the risk of infection.
   c. Allow at least 2 seconds between each test.
      Rationale This prevents summation effects of stimuli, ie, several successive stimuli perceived as one stimulus.
   d. Note areas of reduced, heightened, or absent

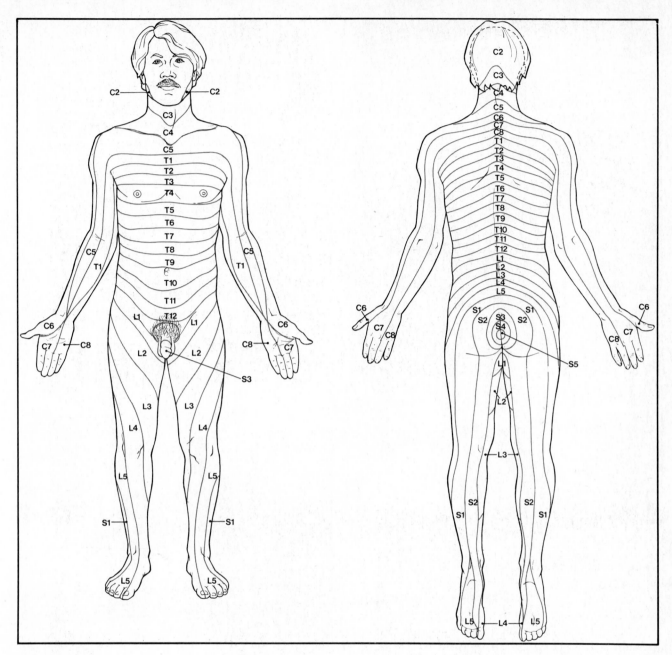

FIGURE 10–104

sensation, and map them out for recording purposes.

e. If pain sensation is dulled or lost, assess temperature sensation in these areas.

   Rationale When sensations of pain are dulled, temperature sense is usually also impaired because distribution of these nerves over the body is similar.

3. *Temperature sensation.* Temperature sensation is not routinely tested if pain sensation is found to be within normal limits. If pain sensation is not normal or is absent, testing sensitivity to temperature may prove more reliable.

a. Touch skin areas with test tubes filled with hot or cold water.

b. Have the patient respond by saying "hot" or "cold" or "don't know."

4. *Vibration.* The vibratory sense is tested with a vibrating tuning fork held firmly against a bone. Bones commonly used are in the ankle, the knee, the thumb side of the wrist, and the outside of the elbow. Routinely, the distal bones of an extremity are tested first. If some impairment is noted, the more proximal bones are also tested. The nurse may test other bones, such as fingers, toes, the sternum, the clavicle, the spinous processes, and the iliac crests. A person

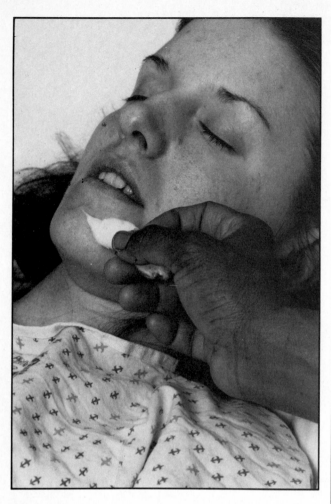

FIGURE 10–105

normally perceives the vibration as a buzzing or tingling sensation. In older persons (over 65 years of age), vibratory sensation may be diminished, particularly in the extremities. A large tuning fork is recommended because vibration cycles decline more slowly in a larger instrument.

a. Ask the patient to close his or her eyes and to tell you (a) when vibrations are first felt by indicating "yes" or "now" and (b) when vibrations stop by indicating "not now" or "gone."

b. Apply the vibrating tuning fork to the designated area. See Figure 10–107.

c. Stop the vibrations between successive tests to facilitate more rapid assessment.

d. Compare the patient's response to your own to confirm a normal response.

e. Compare the vibratory sensations felt on symmetrical sides of the body.

f. If you believe the patient is confusing the pressure of the fork against the skin with its vibrations, strike the tuning fork but place it on the patient

only after the vibrations stop; the patient then should not report vibrations.

5. *Position or kinesthetic sensation.* Commonly the middle fingers and the large toes are tested for the sense of position.

a. To test the fingers, support the patient's arm with one hand and hold the patient's palm in the other; to test the toes, place the patient's heels on the examining table.

b. Have the patient close his or her eyes.

c. Grasp a middle finger or big toe firmly between your thumb and index finger and exert the same pressure on both sides of the finger or toe while moving it.

d. Move the finger or toe until it is up, down, or straight out, and ask the patient to identify the position.

e. Use a series of brisk up-and-down movements before coming to rest suddenly in one of the three positions. Normal persons can readily determine the position of their fingers and toes.

6. *Tactile discrimination.* Three types of tactile discrimina-

FIGURE 10–106

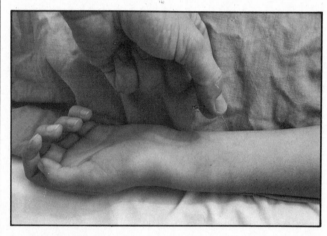

FIGURE 10–107

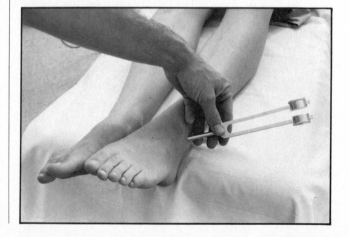

TABLE 10–27 ■ Grading Reflex Responses

Scale	Response
0	No reflex response
+1	Minimal activity (hypoactive)
+2	Normal response
+3	More active than normal
+4	Maximum activity (hyperactive)

tion are generally tested: *one- and two-point discrimination,* the ability to sense whether one or two areas of the skin are being stimulated by pressure; *stereognosis,* the act of recognizing objects by touching and manipulating them; and *extinction,* the failure to perceive touch on one side of the body when two symmetrical areas of the body are touched simultaneously. For all tests the patient's eyes need to be closed.

a. To assess one- and two-point discrimination, alternately stimulate the skin with two pins simultaneously and then with one pin. Ask the patient if he or she feels one or two pinpricks. Wide perceptual variability occurs in adults over different parts of the body. Normally a person can distinguish between a one- and two-point stimulus within the following minimum distances:

- Fingertips, 2.8 mm
- Palms of hands, 8 to 12 mm
- Chest, forearm, 40 mm
- Back, 50 to 70 mm
- Upper arm, thigh, 75 mm
- Toes, 3 to 8 mm

b. To assess stereognosis, place familiar objects, such as a key, paper clip, or coin, in the patient's hand and ask her or him to identify them. If the patient has a motor impairment of the hand and is unable to voluntarily manipulate an object, write a number or letter on the patient's palm, using a blunt instrument, and ask the patient to identify it. Recognition of a figure drawn on the hand is called *graphesthesia.*

c. To assess the extinction phenomenon, simultaneously stimulate two symmetrical areas of the body, such as the thighs, the cheeks, or the hands. Normally, both points of stimulus are felt. Failure to perceive the stimulus on one side is called extinction and is frequently noted in lesions of the sensory cortex.

Deep tendon reflexes

A *reflex* is an automatic response of the body to a stimulus. It is not voluntarily learned or conscious. The deep tendon reflex (DTR) is activated when a tendon is stimulated (tapped) and its associated muscle contracts. The quality of a reflex response varies among individuals and by age. As a person ages and the nervous system gradually deteriorates, reflex responses become less intense.

Reflexes are tested using a percussion hammer. The response is described on a scale of 0 to +4 (+ + + +). See Table 10–27. Experience is necessary to determine appropriate scoring for an individual. It is important to compare one side of the body with the other when assessing reflexes to evaluate the response in terms of symmetry.

Several reflexes are normally tested during a physical examination. These are (a) the biceps reflex, (b) the triceps reflex, (c) the bradioradialis reflex, (d) the patellar reflex, (e) the Achilles reflex, and (f) the plantar reflex.

7. *Biceps reflex.* This reflex tests the spinal cord level C-5, C-6.

   a. Partially flex the patient's arm at the elbow, and rest the forearm over his or her thighs placing the palm of the hand down.

   b. Place the thumb of your nondominant hand horizontally over the biceps tendon.

   c. With your other hand, hold the percussion hammer between thumb and index finger.

   d. Deliver a blow (slight downward thrust) with the percussion hammer to your thumb.

   e. Observe the normal slight flexion of the elbow and feel the bicep's contraction through your thumb. See Figure 10–108.

8. *Triceps reflex.* This reflex tests the spinal cord level C-7, C-8.

   a. Flex the patient's arm at the elbow and support it in the palm of your nondominant hand.

   b. Palpate the triceps tendon about 2 to 5 cm (1 to 2 in) above the elbow.

FIGURE 10–108

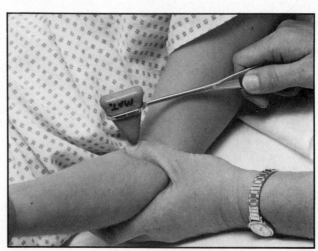

c. Deliver a blow with the percussion hammer directly to the tendon. See Figure 10–109.

d. Observe the normal slight extension of the elbow.

9. *Brachioradialis reflex*. This reflex tests the spinal cord level C-3, C-6.

a. Rest the patient's arm in a relaxed position on your forearm or on the patient's own leg.

b. Deliver a blow with the percussion hammer directly on the radius 2 to 5 cm (1 to 2 in) above the wrist or the styloid process (bony prominence on the thumb side of the wrist). See Figure 10–110.

c. Observe the normal flexion and supination of the forearm. The fingers of the hand may also extend slightly.

FIGURE 10–109

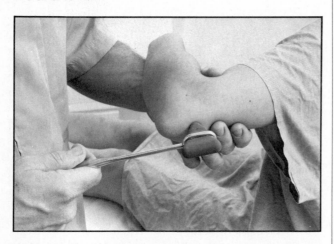

FIGURE 10–110

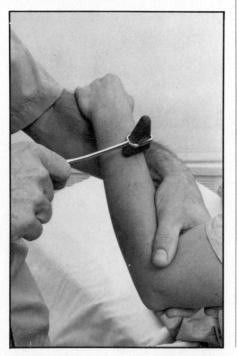

10. *Patellar reflex*. This reflex tests the spinal cord level L-2, L-3, L-4.

a. Have the patient sit on the edge of the examining table so that the legs hang freely.

b. Locate the patellar tendon directly below the patella (kneecap).

c. Deliver a blow with the percussion hammer directly to the tendon. See Figure 10–111.

d. Observe the normal extension or kicking out of the leg as the quadriceps muscle contracts.

e. If no response is obtained and you suspect the patient is not relaxed, ask him or her to interlock his or her fingers and pull. This action often enhances relaxation so that a more accurate response is obtained.

11. *Achilles reflex*. This reflex tests the spinal cord level S-1, S-2.

a. With the patient in the same position as for the patellar reflex, slightly dorsiflex the patient's ankle by grasping the toes in the palm of your hand.

b. Deliver a blow with the percussion hammer directly to the Achilles tendon just above the heel. See Figure 10–112.

c. Observe and feel the normal plantar flexion (downward jerk) of the foot.

12. *Plantar (Babinski) reflex*. This reflex is a superficial reflex.

a. Use a moderately sharp object such as the handle

FIGURE 10–111

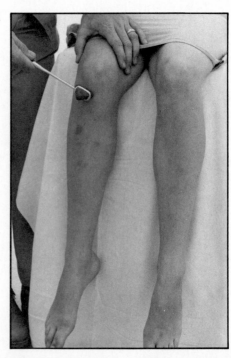

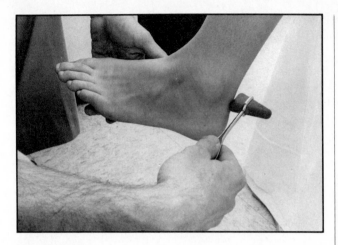

FIGURE 10-112

of the percussion hammer, a key, or the dull end of a pin or applicator stick.

b. Stroke the lateral border of the sole of the patient's foot, starting at the heel, continuing to the ball of the foot, and then proceeding across the ball of the foot toward the big toe. See Figure 10-113.

c. Observe the response. Normally, all five toes bend downward; this reaction is negative Babinski. In an abnormal response, positive Babinski, the toes spread outward and the big toe moves upward. Positive Babinski is abnormal after age 1.

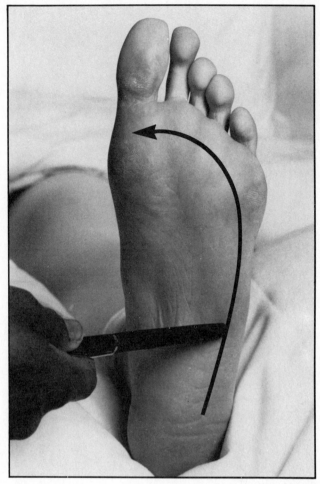

FIGURE 10-113

REFERENCES

Bates B: *A Guide to Physical Examination,* 3rd ed. Lippincott, 1983.

Bellack JP, Bamford PA: *Nursing Assessment: A Multidimensional Approach.* Wadsworth Health Sciences Division, 1984.

Block GJ, Nolan JW, Dempsey MK: *Health Assessment for Professional Nursing: A Developmental Approach.* Appleton-Century-Crofts, 1981.

Bowers AC, Thompson JM: *Clinical Manual of Health Assessment,* 2nd ed. Mosby, 1984.

Boyd-Monk H: Examining the external eye, part I. *Nursing 80* (May) 1980; 10:58–63.

Burns KR, Johnson PJ: *Health Assessment in Clinical Practice.* Prentice-Hall, 1980.

Carpenito LJ: *Nursing Diagnosis: Application to Clinical Practice.* Lippincott, 1983.

Grimes J, Iannopollo E: *Health Assessment in Nursing Practice.* Wadsworth Health Sciences Division, 1982.

Hagerty BK: *Psychiatric-Mental Health Assessment.* Mosby, 1984.

Malasanos L et al: *Health Assessment.* Mosby, 1981.

Nurses Reference Library Series: *Assessment.* Intermed Communications, 1982.

Nursing 80 Photobook Series: *Assessing Your Patients.* Intermed Communications, 1980.

Swearingen PL: *The Addison-Wesley Photo-Atlas of Nursing Procedures.* Addison-Wesley, 1984.

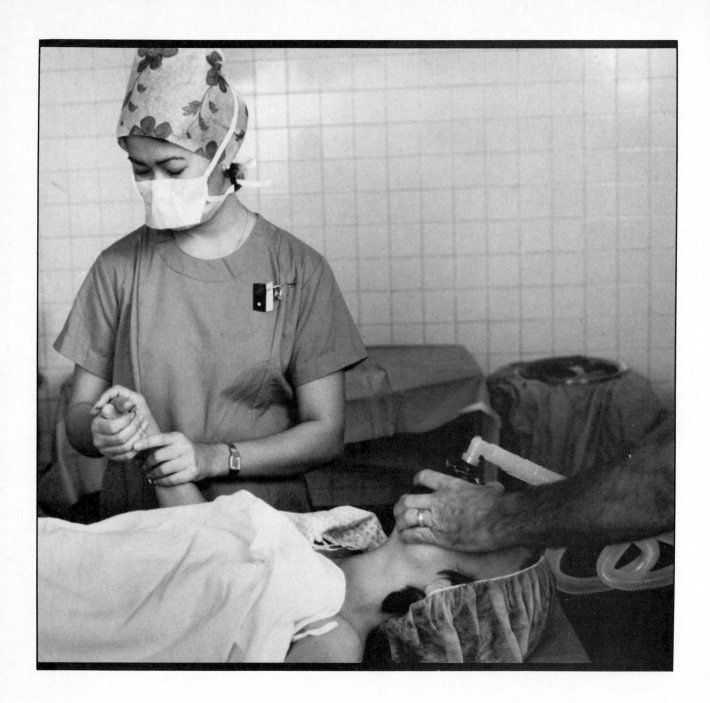

SPECIAL PROCEDURES

11

Many patients undergo special diagnostic and/or therapeutic procedures. The results of a *diagnostic procedure* help the physician to determine the patient's pathology. For example, an electrocardiogram (ECG or EKG) provides information about the heart's functioning and diseases of the heart. A *therapeutic procedure* treats the patient. For example, a thoracentesis removes fluid from the pleural cavity, which can ease the patient's breathing.

In special procedures, the nurse has two chief concerns: the patient and his or her support persons and the procedure itself. The nurse's function can be divided into three areas: preparing the patient and/or the support persons, assisting the physician with the procedure, and caring for the patient during and after the procedure.

Tests and treatments are frightening to many patients. People may fear pain, the results of tests, or their reactions to either the pain or the findings. Fear of the unknown increases these misgivings. It is important for the nurse to be aware of the needs of patients and families and to help them meet these needs.

The nurse is often responsible for certain aspects of tests or treatments. For example, it is frequently a nursing function to assemble the equipment before tests or treatments performed in a clinical nursing unit or a physician's office. The nurse is also responsible for assessing the patient during and after the procedure. Many tests and treatments require special nursing intervention afterward. The nurse is responsible for certain pretest interventions that help assure success. A well-prepared patient is likely to experience the least possible discomfort during tests.

Diagnosis after tests often requires the services of specialists in laboratory tests, radiologic (roentgenographic) techniques, cardiac testing, etc. The nurse helps coordinate the services of these personnel, assists in scheduling, and helps the patient meet schedules.

Chapter Outline

Removal of Body Fluids and Tissues
- Technique 11–1 Assisting with a Lumbar Puncture
- Technique 11–2 Assisting with an Abdominal Paracentesis
- Technique 11–3 Assisting with a Thoracentesis
- Technique 11–4 Assisting with a Bone Marrow Biopsy
- Technique 11–5 Assisting with a Liver Biopsy

Visual Inspection Procedures
- Technique 11–6 Assisting with a Proctoscopy

Measurement of Electric Impulses
- Technique 11–7 Assisting with an Electrocardiogram

Roentgenography (X-Ray), Ultrasound, and Nuclear Medicine Procedures
- Technique 11–8 Assisting with Roentgenography

Objectives

Upon completion of this chapter, the student will:

1. Know essential terms and facts related to assisting patients undergoing special procedures
   1.1 Define selected terms
   1.2 Identify various procedures
   1.3 Identify purposes of specific procedures
   1.4 Identify essential assessment data for specific procedures
   1.5 Identify essential instructions required by the patient for specific procedures
   1.6 Outline interventions that physically prepare the patient for specific procedures
   1.7 Identify interventions implemented to maintain the patient's physical comfort and safety
   1.8 Identify interventions implemented to enhance the patient's psychologic comfort
   1.9 Give reasons for essential aspects of specific procedures
   1.10 Explain the outcomes of the procedures
2. Demonstrate ability to assist patients undergoing special procedures effectively
   2.1 Assess the patient adequately
   2.2 Collect additional data from appropriate sources
   2.3 Select pertinent nursing goals for the patient
   2.4 Establish relevant outcome criteria for the patient following the technique
   2.5 Collect necessary equipment before the technique
   2.6 Implement interventions to enhance the effectiveness of the technique and enhance the patient's comfort and safety
   2.7 Communicate relevant information
   2.8 Evaluate the patient's responses to the technique
3. Demonstrate skills to assist the person conducting the procedure effectively
   3.1 Provide essential equipment and supplies in advance
   3.2 Open sterile packages correctly
   3.3 Pour antiseptic solutions using surgical aseptic technique
   3.4 Provide assistance as necessary
4. Evaluate own performance of assisting patients with special procedures in a laboratory or clinical setting with the assistance of another
   4.1 Use the performance checklists provided
   4.2 Identify areas of strength and weakness
   4.3 Alter performance in response to own evaluation and that of another

Terms

■ **abdominal paracentesis** removal of fluids from the peritoneal cavity

■ **angiography** a diagnostic procedure enabling x-ray visual examination of the vascular system after injection of a radiopaque dye

■ **anoscopy** visual examination of the anal canal using an anoscope (a lighted instrument)

■ **ascites** the accumulation of fluid in the abdominal cavity

■ **aspirate** to remove gases or fluids from a cavity by using suction

■ **atrioventricular (AV) node** the neuromuscular tissue of the heart at the base of the atrial septum that conveys impulses to the ventricles

■ **barium enema** x-ray filming of the large intestine using a contrast medium; also called a *lower gastrointestinal series*

■ **barium swallow** x-ray filming of the esophagus, stomach, and duodenum; also referred to as an *upper gastrointestinal series*

■ **bronchogram** an x-ray film of the bronchial tree taken after injection of an iodized oil dye, used as a contrast medium

■ **bronchoscopy** visual examination of the bronchi using a bronchoscope

■ **cannula** a tube with a lumen (channel) that is inserted into a cavity or duct and is often fitted with a trocar during insertion

■ **CAT scan** *see* tomography

■ **cholecystogram (oral cholecystography)** an x-ray film of the gallbladder after the ingestion of a contrast dye

■ **cisterna** a space that is enclosed and serves as a reservoir for body fluid

■ **cisternal puncture** insertion of a needle into the subarachnoid space of the cisterna magna

■ **colonoscopy** visual examination of the interior of the colon with a colonoscope

■ **computerized axial tomography** *see* tomography

■ **cystoscopy** visual examination of the urinary bladder with a cystoscope

■ **depolarize (cardiac muscle)** to reduce toward a nonpolarized state; to cause loss of charge

■ **electrocardiogram (ECG, EKG)** a graph of the electric activity of the heart

■ **electrocardiograph** a machine that measures and records the impulses from the heart on an electrocardiogram

■ **electroencephalogram (EEG)** a graph of the electric activity of the brain

■ **electroencephalograph** a machine that measures and records impulses from the brain on an electroencephalogram

■ **electromyogram (EMG)** a record of the electric potential created by the contraction of a muscle

■ **electromyograph** a machine that measures and records impulses from the muscles on an electromyogram

■ **endoscope** an instrument used for examining the interior of a hollow organ, eg, the bladder, rectum, stomach, or bronchi

■ **esophagoscopy** visual examination of the interior of the esophagus with a lighted instrument

■ **fasciculation** abnormal contraction of a muscle involving the whole motor unit of the muscle

■ **gastroscopy** visual examination of the stomach with a lighted instrument (gastroscope)

■ **hematoma** a collection of blood in a tissue, organ, or space due to a break in the wall of a blood vessel

■ **hemoptysis** the presence of blood in the sputum

■ **hypovolemic shock** a state of shock due to a sudden redirection of the blood flow

■ **insufflator** an instrument used to blow air into a part of the body, eg, the rectum

■ **intrapleural** within the pleural cavity

■ **intravenous cholangiogram** an x-ray film of the bile ducts after intravenous injection of a contrast dye

■ **intravenous pyelogram** an x-ray film of the kidney taken after intravenous injection of a radiopaque dye

■ **intravenous pyelography (IVP); intravenous urography (IVU)** x-ray filming of the kidney and ureters after intravenous injection of a radiopaque material

■ **laryngoscopy** visual examination of the larynx with a laryngoscope

■ **lumbar puncture (LP, spinal tap)** insertion of a needle into the subarachnoid space at the lumbar region

■ **manometer** an instrument used to measure the pressure of fluids or gases

■ **mediastinal shift** a lateral movement of the organs in the mediastinum, ie, the heart and major blood vessels

■ **myelogram** an x-ray film of the spinal cord, nerve roots, and vertebrae after injection of a contrast medium into the subarachnoid space

■ **pericardium** a fibrous sac that surrounds the heart

■ **peritoneal cavity** the area between the layers of the peritoneum in the abdomen; a potential space

■ **pleural cavity** a potential space between the two layers of the pleura

■ pneumoventriculogram   an x-ray film of the ventricles of the brain after the introduction of oxygen

■ polarized (cardiac muscle)   electrically charged

■ proctoscopy   visual examination of the interior of the rectum with a proctoscope

■ proctosigmoidoscopy   visual examination of the rectum and sigmoid colon with a proctosigmoidoscope

■ Purkinje's fibers   a network of modified cardiac muscle fibers concerned with the conduction of impulses in the heart; dense networks of these fibers form the sinoatrial and atrioventricular nodes

■ repolarized (cardiac muscle)   reacquiring an electric charge

■ retrograde pyelogram   an x-ray film taken after a contrast medium is injected through ureteral catheters into the kidneys

■ scan   a noninvasive type of x-ray procedure capable of distinguishing minor differences in the radiodensity of soft tissues

■ sigmoidoscopy   visual examination of the interior of the sigmoid colon with a sigmoidoscope

■ sinoatrial (SA) node   the pacemaker of the heart; the collection of the Purkinje's fibers in the right atrium of the heart where the rhythm of contraction is initiated

■ stopcock   a valve that controls the flow of fluid or air through a tube

■ stupor   a condition of partial or nearly complete unconsciousness characterized by lethargy and reduced response to stimulation

■ stylet   a metal or plastic probe inserted into a needle or cannula to render it stiff and to prevent occlusion of the needle by particles of tissue

■ subarachnoid space   the area between the arachnoid membrane and the pia mater

■ subcostal   below the ribs

■ thoracentesis (thoracocentesis)   insertion of a needle into the pleural cavity for diagnostic or therapeutic purposes

■ tomogram   an image acquired from a CAT scan

■ tomography   a scanning procedure during which a narrow x-ray beam passes through the body part from different angles; *see also* scan

■ trocar   a sharp pointed instrument that fits inside a cannula and is used to pierce body tissues

■ ventriculogram   an x-ray film of the ventricles of the brain after the introduction of an opaque medium

■ ultrasound   a noninvasive diagnostic technique that uses sound waves to measure the acoustic density of tissues

REMOVAL OF BODY FLUIDS AND TISSUES

A number of body fluids and tissues may be removed for diagnostic purposes. Table 11–1 lists common procedures. The procedure is normally performed by a physician, at the bedside, in an examining room, or sometimes in the emergency department of a hospital. All the procedures described here involve inserting an instrument, often a needle, through the skin and withdrawing some fluid or tissue. The fluid or tissue is usually placed in a special container and sent to the hospital laboratory for examination. Although the techniques for taking specimens are considered safe, there can be complications with each of them. Some agencies require that a patient sign a special consent form prior to the procedure. In other agencies the general consent form signed by the patient on admission suffices.

TABLE 11–1   ■   Common Diagnostic or Therapeutic Procedures

Name	Type of specimen	Source	Common tests
Lumbar puncture	Spinal fluid	Subarachnoid space of the spinal canal	Pressure, appearance, sugar, protein, cell count, bacteria, Queckenstedt-Stookey test
Abdominal paracentesis	Ascitic fluid	Peritoneal cavity	Cell count, cells, specific gravity, protein
Thoracentesis	Pleural fluid	Pleural cavity	Cell count, protein
Bone marrow biopsy	Bone marrow	Iliac crest, posterior superior iliac spine, or sternum	Cells, iron
Liver biopsy	Liver tissue (needle biopsy specimen)	Liver	Carcinoma, cells

TECHNIQUE 11-1 ■ Assisting with a Lumbar Puncture

In a lumbar puncture (LP, or spinal tap), cerebrospinal fluid (CSF) is withdrawn by inserting a needle into the subarachnoid space of the spinal canal between the third and fourth lumbar vertebrae or between the fourth and fifth lumbar vertebrae. At this level the needle avoids damaging the spinal cord and major nerve roots. See Figure 11-1. A spinal tap is carried out by a physician.

FIGURE 11-1 ■ A diagram of the vertebral column, indicating a site for insertion of the lumbar puncture needle into the subarachnoid space of the spinal canal.

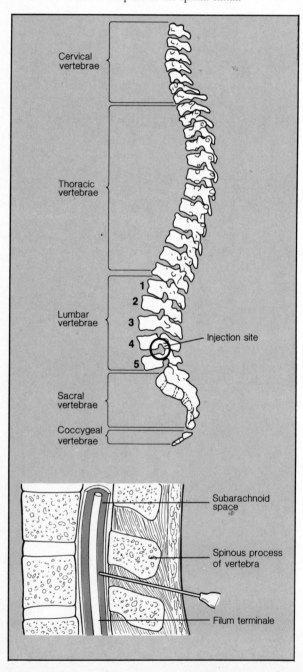

The nurse may have to obtain a signed consent to the procedure from the patient in some agencies. Strict sterile technique is essential to prevent the introduction of microorganisms into the spinal canal. Lumbar punctures are carried out for a variety of reasons:

1. To analyze the constituents of a specimen of fluid for diagnostic purposes
2. To test the pressure of the CSF for diagnostic purposes
3. To relieve pressure by removing CSF
4. To inject a spinal anesthetic, dye, or air into the spinal canal

The physician locates the appropriate intervertebral space, disinfects the site, drapes the area with sterile drapes, and administers a local anesthetic. After the area is numbed, the physician inserts the spinal needle with the stylet and removes the stylet. When the flow of CSF is ascertained, the stopcock and manometer are attached, and an initial CSF pressure reading is taken at the point where the CSF stops rising in the manometer tube. Normal opening pressures are 60–180 mm of water. Pressures above 200 mm are considered abnormal.

A Queckenstedt-Stookey test may also be done while the manometer is in place. If the nurse is not supporting the patient in position, she or he may be asked to exert digital (finger) pressure on one or both of the internal jugular veins. See Figure 11-2. The normal response is an increase in CSF pressure.

The physician usually takes specimens of CSF and hands the specimen tubes to the nurse, who numbers them in the sequence taken. A total of 10 mL of fluid is generally collected, with 2 to 3 mL of fluid in each

FIGURE 11-2 ■ Location of the internal jugular vein for the Queckenstedt-Stookey test.

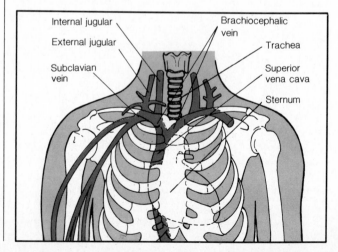

specimen tube. Specimens of CSF are often tested in the laboratory for the presence of certain elements (eg, protein, sugar, cell count, bacteria). See Table 11–1.

After collecting the specimens, the physician may take a final or closing CSF pressure reading before removing the spinal needle.

■ Assessment

Assess the patient for:

1. Vital signs, health status, and neurological status prior to the procedure to obtain baseline data for comparison following the procedure
2. Drug allergies, particularly allergies to the medications contained in local anesthetics and skin antiseptics

■ Planning

Nursing goals

1. To minimize the patient's discomfort
2. To help the physician perform the lumbar puncture safely and expediently

Equipment

1. A sterile lumbar puncture set. See Figure 11–3. The set contains:
   a. Sterile sponges or gauze squares with an antiseptic solution to apply to the site of the puncture. If the skin antiseptic is not included in the set, a container of it must be obtained.
   b. Drapes. One may be fenestrated.
   c. A syringe and needle to administer the local anesthetic. A 2-mL syringe and #24 and #22 needles are often provided.
   d. A spinal needle 5 to 12.5 cm (2 to 5 in) long, with

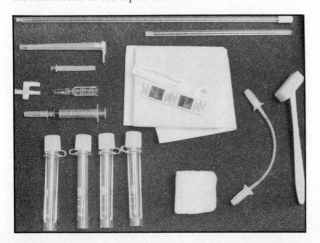

FIGURE 11–3 ■ A preassembled lumbar puncture set. Note the manometer at the top of the set.

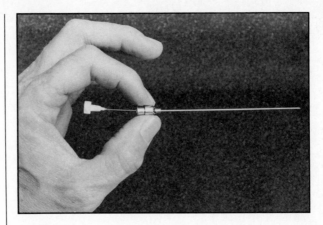

FIGURE 11–4 ■ A spinal needle with the stylet protruding from the hub.

a stylet, to insert into the spinal canal. See Figure 11–4. The shorter needles are used for infants.
   e. A manometer (a glass or plastic tube calibrated in millimeters) to measure the pressure of CSF.
   f. A three-way stopcock (a valve between the spinal needle and the manometer that regulates the flow of CSF by shutting off the CSF drainage, allowing the CSF to flow either into the manometer or out into a receptacle).
   g. Specimen containers (test tubes).
   h. A local anesthetic, eg, 1% procaine, to anesthetize the lumbar site. This may or may not be included in the preassembled set. If included, it will be supplied in a small glass ampule. If not included, a vial or ampule must be obtained.
   i. A small dressing to apply over the puncture site.
2. Face masks for the physician and the nurse (optional).
3. Sterile gloves for the physician to put on after scrubbing.
4. A completed laboratory requisition and specimen labels.
5. A gooseneck lamp if the light in the room is inadequate.

Arrange the equipment so that it is readily accessible to the physician.

■ Intervention

1. Even though a patient may appear confused or stuporous, explain:
   a. That the physician will be taking a small sample of spinal fluid from the lower spine.
   b. That a local anesthetic will be given so that the patient will feel no pain.
   c. When and where the procedure will occur, eg, at the bedside or in the treatment room.

d. Who will be present, ie, the physician and the nurse.

e. The time involved, eg, about 15 minutes.

In addition, tell the patient what to expect during the procedure. The patient may feel slight discomfort (like a pinprick) when the local anesthetic is injected and a sensation of pressure when the spinal needle is being inserted. Remind the patient that it is important to remain still and in one position throughout the procedure. A restless patient or a child will need to be held to prevent movement.

2. Have the patient empty his or her bladder and bowels prior to the procedure to prevent unnecessary discomfort.

3. Position the patient laterally with the head bent toward the chest, the knees flexed onto the abdomen, and the back at the edge of the bed or examining table. Place a very small pillow under the patient's head to maintain the horizontal alignment of the spine. In this position the back is arched, increasing the spaces between the vertebrae so that the spinal needle can be inserted readily. Drape the patient to expose only the lumbar spine.

4. Open the lumbar puncture set, and supply the physician with the sterile gloves and antiseptic, in a container or poured onto sterile gauze squares, if necessary.

5. Stand in front of the patient, and support the back of the patient's neck and knees if the patient needs help to remain still. See Figure 11–5. Reassure the patient throughout the procedure by explaining what is happening. Encourage him or her to breathe normally and relax as much as possible.

Rationale Excessive muscle tension, coughing, or changes in breathing can increase CSF pressure, giving a false reading.

FIGURE 11–5

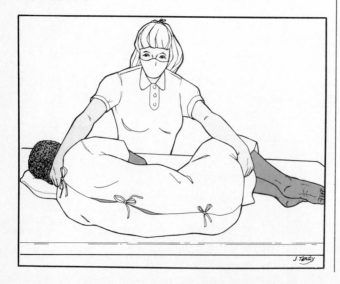

6. If the Queckenstedt-Stookey test is being done, place digital pressure on the patient's jugular veins. See Figure 11–2, earlier.

7. Label the specimen tubes in sequence if they are not already labeled. While handling the tubes, take care to prevent contamination of the physician's sterile gloves, the sterile field, and yourself, since the CSF may contain virulent microorganisms, eg, organisms that cause meningitis.

8. Place a small sterile dressing over the site of the puncture to help prevent infection after the needle is removed.

9. Assist the patient to a dorsal recumbent position with only one head pillow. The patient remains lying down for 8 to 24 hours, until the spinal fluid is replaced. Check agency practice about the length of time recommended for this position. Some patients experience a headache following a lumbar puncture, and the dorsal recumbent position tends to prevent or alleviate it. Often analgesics are ordered and can be given for headaches.

10. Assess the patient's response to the procedure, ie, pallor, feeling of faintness, changes in pulse rate and other vital signs, changes in neurological status, headache, swelling or bleeding at the puncture site, and numbness, tingling, or pain radiating down the legs, which may be due to nerve irritation.

11. Ensure that the CSF specimens are correctly labeled and send them immediately to the laboratory, with the completed requisition.

12. Record the procedure on the patient's chart, including the date and time it was performed; the name of the physician; the color, character (clear, cloudy, etc), and amount of CSF obtained; the pressure readings; the number of specimens obtained; and the response of the patient.

Sample Recording

Date	Time	Notes
5/24/87	1500	Lumbar puncture performed by Dr. Guido. 4 2-mL specimens of cloudy serous CSF sent to lab. Initial pressure 130 mm. Closing pressure 100 mm. No apparent discomfort. Resting. ————Sarah D. Nicols, NS

13. Adjust the nursing care plan to include the patient's positioning and assessment needs following the procedure.

■ **Evaluation**

Expected outcomes

1. No significant change in vital signs

2. If the LP was done to relieve pressure, an improvement in neurologic status

Unexpected outcomes

1. Significant changes in vital signs
2. Alterations in neurologic status such as numbness, tingling, or pain radiating down the legs

3. Headache
4. Swelling or bleeding at the puncture site
5. Feeling of faintness

Upon observing an unexpected outcome: Report your findings to the responsible nurse and/or physician.

TECHNIQUE 11–2 ■ Assisting with an Abdominal Paracentesis

Normally the peritoneum creates just enough peritoneal fluid for lubrication. The fluid is continuously formed and absorbed into the lymphatic system. However, in some disease processes, a large amount of fluid accumulates in the cavity; this condition is called *ascites*. Normal ascitic fluid is serous, clear, and light yellow in color. An abdominal paracentesis is carried out to obtain a fluid specimen for laboratory study and to relieve pressure on the abdominal organs due to the presence of excess fluid. See Table 11–1 on page 249.

The procedure is carried out by a physician with the assistance of a nurse. Strict sterile technique is followed. A common site for abdominal paracentesis is midway between the umbilicus and the symphysis pubis on the midline. See Figure 11–6. The physician disinfects the site of the incision, drapes the area with sterile drapes, and administers a local anesthetic. After the area is numbed, the physician makes a small incision with a scalpel, inserts the trocar and cannula (the trocar inside the cannula), and then withdraws the trocar. Tubing is attached to the cannula and the fluid flows through the tubing into a receptacle. Normally about 1,500 mL is the maximum amount of fluid drained at one time, to avoid hypovolemic shock. The fluid is drained very slowly for the same reason. Some fluid is placed in the specimen container before the cannula is withdrawn. The small incision may or may not be sutured; in either case, it is covered with a small sterile bandage.

This procedure may require a signed consent from the patient. The nurse must determine agency policy and obtain the consent if necessary.

■ **Assessment**

Assess the patient for:

1. Vital signs (body temperature, pulse, respirations, and blood pressure) to obtain baseline data.
2. Degree of ascites in the abdomen, general appear-

ance, and health status. Measure the patient's abdominal girth at the level of the umbilicus. See Figure 11–7. Record the measurement exactly so that a comparative measurement can be done after the procedure.
3. Drug allergies, particularly allergies to the drugs contained in local anesthetics and antiseptics.

■ **Planning**

Nursing goals

1. To minimize the patient's discomfort
2. To assist the physician to perform the paracentesis safely and expediently

Equipment

1. A sterile set containing:
   a. Sterile sponges or gauze squares with an antiseptic solution to apply to the puncture site. If the skin

FIGURE 11–6 ■ A common site for an abdominal paracentesis.

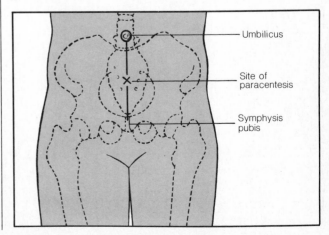

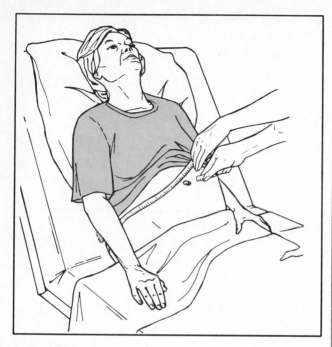

FIGURE 11-7

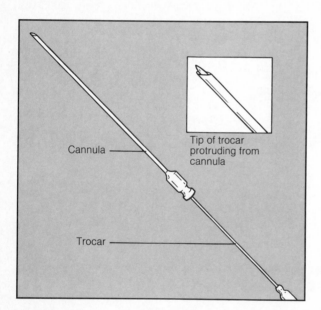

Cannula

Tip of trocar protruding from cannula

Trocar

FIGURE 11-8

antiseptic is not included with the set, it is necessary to acquire a container of it.

b. A drape (or drapes) to place over the patient's abdomen. The drape is often fenestrated, and the opening is placed at the site where the fluid will be removed.

c. A 2-mL syringe and #24 and #22 needles to administer the anesthetic. These may already be in the set, or the nurse may need to obtain them.

d. A small scalpel to make an incision in the abdomen and a needle holder and sutures to sew

up the incision after withdrawing the fluid. Suturing is done at the physician's discretion.

e. A receptacle for the fluid.

f. A trocar and cannula. The trocar is a sharp pointed instrument that fits inside the cannula. The cannula is a tube through which plastic tubing can be threaded to drain the fluid. See Figure 11-8. If the purpose of the paracentesis is to obtain a specimen, the physician may use an aspirating needle attached to a syringe rather than making an incision and using a trocar and cannula.

g. Plastic tubing or a special catheter.

h. A specimen container.

i. A local anesthetic, which is often packaged in an ampule.

2. Masks for the nurse and the physician (optional). Determine agency policy.

3. Sterile gloves for the physician.

4. A completed laboratory requisition and a label for the specimen.

Arrange the equipment so that it is easily accessible when the physician sits beside the patient.

■ Intervention

1. Explain the procedure to the patient. Normally an abdominal paracentesis is not painful, and, when a patient has considerable ascites, the procedure can relieve discomfort caused by the fluid. The procedure to remove ascitic fluid usually takes 30 to 60 minutes. Obtaining a specimen usually takes about 15 minutes. Emphasize the importance of remaining still during the procedure. Include in your explanation when and where the procedure will occur and who will be present.

2. Have the patient void just before the paracentesis to lessen the possibility of puncturing the urinary bladder. Notify the physician if the patient cannot void prior to the procedure.

3. Help the patient assume a sitting position in bed so that the fluid accumulates in the lower abdominal cavity, and the force of gravity and the pressure of the abdominal organs will help the flow of the fluid from the cavity. Some patients may be able to sit on the edge of the bed with pillows to support the back. Cover the patient to expose only the necessary area. See Figure 11-7 earlier.

4. Open the paracentesis set, and supply the physician with the sterile gloves and antiseptic in a container or poured onto sterile gauze squares.

5. Open and hold the ampule or vial of local anesthetic, if it is not part of the sterile set.

6. Support the patient verbally, and describe the steps of the procedure if the physician does not do so. Observe the patient closely for signs of distress. A major concern is hypovolemic shock induced by the loss of fluid. See step 8.

7. Place a small sterile dressing over the site of the incision after the cannula is withdrawn.

8. Assess the patient's response in terms of pulse rate, skin color, and blood pressure. Hypovolemic shock can occur when the fluid in the circulatory system is redirected to the abdominal area as a result of reduced pressure from the removal of the ascitic fluid. Shock is evidenced by pallor, dyspnea, diaphoresis, and a drop in blood pressure.

9. Measure the abdominal girth with a tape measure in the same place as before the procedure.

10. Arrange for the specimen with the completed requisition and label to be transported to the laboratory.

11. Record the procedure on the patient's chart, including the date and time; the name of the physician; the girth of the patient's abdomen before and after the procedure; the color, clarity, and amount of drained fluid; and the response of the patient.

Sample Recording

Date	Time	Notes
7/18/86	1400	Paracentesis performed by Dr. Johnson. 300 mL clear serosanguinous fluid obtained. Abdominal girth at umbilical level 114 cm before, 109 cm after. Specimen sent to laboratory. P 72, BP 120/85. Slight pallor. Resting comfortably. ———————————————— Roxanne J. Tuttle, NS

12. Adjust the nursing care plan to include continuing assessment for hypovolemic shock; signs of infection (peritonitis), such as elevated body temperature; and signs of internal hemorrhage, such as lowered blood pressure and accelerated pulse.

■ **Evaluation**

Expected outcomes

1. No significant change in vital signs
2. Reduction in abdominal girth measurement

Unexpected outcomes

1. Signs of hypovolemic shock (a drop in blood pressure, accelerated pulse rate, pallor, dyspnea, diaphoresis)
2. Signs of infection (elevated body temperature)
3. Bleeding at the paracentesis site

Upon observing an unanticipated outcome: Report your findings to the responsible nurse and/or physician.

TECHNIQUE 11-3   ■   Assisting with a Thoracentesis

Normally only sufficient fluid to lubricate the pleura is present in the pleural cavity. However, excessive fluid can accumulate as a result of injury, infection, or other pathology. In such a case, or in a case of pneumothorax, a physician may perform a thoracentesis to remove the excess fluid or air. Thoracentesis is also performed to introduce chemotherapeutic drugs intrapleurally.

The physician and the assisting nurse follow strict sterile technique. The physician dons sterile gloves, cleans the site with an antiseptic solution, and administers a local anesthetic. The physician attaches a syringe and/or stopcock to the aspirating needle. The stopcock must be in the closed position so that no air will enter the pleural space. The physician inserts the needle through the intercostal space to the pleural cavity. In some instances, a small plastic tube is threaded through the needle and the needle is then withdrawn. (The tubing is less likely to puncture the pleura.) If a syringe is used, the plunger is pulled out to draw out the pleural fluid as the stopcock is opened. If a large container is used to receive the fluid, the tubing is attached from the stopcock to the adapter on the receiving bottle. When the adapter and stopcock are opened, negative pressure in the container will draw the fluid from the pleural cavity. After the fluid has been withdrawn, the physician removes the needle or plastic tubing.

This procedure may require a signed consent from the patient. The nurse must determine agency policy and obtain the consent if necessary.

■ Assessment

Assess the patient for:

1. Vital signs (body temperature, pulse, respirations, and blood pressure) to obtain baseline data, if these are not already available
2. Respiratory depth and the movement of both sides of the chest during inspiration, to note differences between the two sides
3. Chest pain
4. Breath sounds
5. Dyspnea
6. Type and frequency of cough, if present, and character and amount of sputum
7. Drug allergies, particularly allergies to the medications contained in local anesthetics and skin antiseptics

■ Planning

Nursing goals

1. To minimize the patient's discomfort
2. To assist the physician to perform the thoracentesis safely and expediently

Equipment

1. A sterile set containing:
   a. Sterile sponges or gauze squares with an antiseptic solution to apply to the site of the thoracentesis. If the skin antiseptic is not included in the set, it is necessary to obtain a container of it.
   b. A drape or drapes to place over the patient's chest. The drape is often fenestrated, and the opening is placed at the site of the thoracentesis.
   c. A 2-mL syringe and #24 and #22 needles to administer the anesthetic. If these are not in the set, they need to be obtained.
   d. A receptacle for the fluid. This may be a syringe (50 mL) and #16 needle or an airtight container with negative pressure created by a pump or a suction machine. The negative pressure in the container must be greater than that of the pleural space. Negative pressure also prevents air from entering the pleural space and causing a pneumothorax (air in the pleural cavity).

   e. A three-way stopcock to prevent air from entering the pleural space.
   f. A two-way stopcock with connecting tubing to maintain the negative pressure in the receptacle and to direct the flow of pleural fluid into the container.
   g. A thoracentesis needle, usually a #15 needle about 5 to 7.5 cm (2 to 3 in) long.
   h. A specimen container.
   i. A local anesthetic. The anesthetic is usually packaged in an ampule.
2. Sterile gloves for the physician.
3. Masks for the nurse and the physician (optional). Determine agency policy.
4. A completed laboratory requisition and label for the specimen.

Arrange the equipment at the bedside so that it is readily accessible to the physician.

■ Intervention

1. From the patient's chart, note the physician's orders, eg, to give the patient a cough medicine to suppress coughing 30 minutes before the thoracentesis.
2. Explain the procedure to the patient. Normally a thoracentesis is not painful, although the patient may experience a feeling of pressure when the needle is inserted. The patient may experience considerable relief if breathing has been difficult. The procedure takes only a few minutes, depending primarily on the time it takes for the fluid to drain from the pleural cavity. It is important for the patient not to cough while the needle is inserted, to avoid puncturing the lungs. Include in your explanation when and where the procedure will occur and who will be present.
3. Help the patient assume a comfortable position. This is usually a sitting position with the arms above the head, which spreads the ribs and enlarges the intercostal space. Two positions commonly used are: arm elevated and stretched forward (see Figure 11–9, A), and leaning forward over a pillow (see Figure 11–9, B). To make sure that the needle is inserted below the fluid level when fluid is to be removed (or above any fluid if air is to be removed), the physician will palpate the chest and select the exact site for insertion of the needle. A site on the lower posterior chest is often used to remove fluid, and a site on the upper anterior chest is used to remove air.
4. Open the thoracentesis set, and supply the sterile gloves to the physician. Pour antiseptic solution into a container or onto sterile gauze squares if necessary.

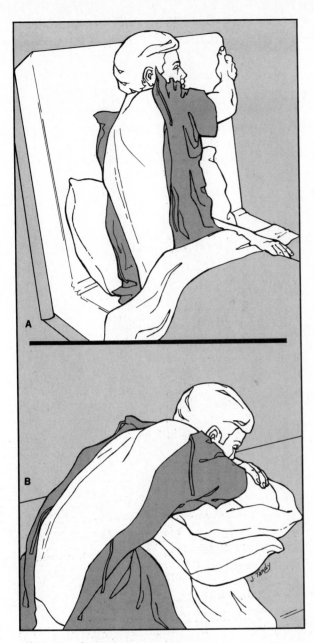

FIGURE 11-9

shift in the mediastinum (heart and large blood vessels) can occur with removal of large amounts of fluid. Also note changes in the patient's cough, sputum, respiration depth, breath sounds, and chest pain.

9. Arrange for the specimen and the completed requisition to be transported to the laboratory.

10. Record the procedure on the patient's chart, including the date and time; the name of the physician; the amount, color, and clarity of fluid drained; and any other significant data, such as the patient's respiration rate.

Sample Recording

Date	Time	Notes
4/18/86	1500	Thoracentesis performed by Dr. Sargent. 275 mL of cloudy serosanguinous fluid removed. Specimen sent to laboratory. R 32, shallow and wet. P 76. Skin pale. Coughing occasionally. Small amount of thick white sputum. Resting more comfortably. ——————————— Ron L. Landry, NS

11. Adjust the nursing care plan to include special assessment of respirations,

■ Evaluation

Expected outcomes

1. No significant change in temperature, pulse rate, blood pressure, and skin color
2. Return of normal chest movement on affected side
3. Normal breath sounds on affected side
4. Relief of dyspnea
5. Relief of chest pain

Unexpected outcomes

1. Signs of mediastinal shift (pallor, accelerated pulse rate, dyspnea, accelerated respiration rate, dizziness)
2. Hemoptysis
3. Severe dyspnea, restlessness
4. Sudden pain

Upon observing an unexpected outcome: Report your findings to the responsible nurse and/or physician.

5. Open and hold the ampule or vial of local anesthetic if it is not part of the sterile set.

6. Support the patient verbally, and describe the steps of the procedure if the physician does not do so. Observe the patient closely for signs of distress, such as dyspnea, pallor, and coughing. If the patient becomes distressed or has to cough, the procedure is halted briefly. The physician may withdraw the needle slightly to avoid puncturing the pleura.

7. Following the procedure, place a small sterile dressing over the site of the puncture.

8. Assess the patient's response in terms of changes in pulse and respiration rate or skin color, because a

TECHNIQUE 11–4 ■ Assisting with a Bone Marrow Biopsy

A bone marrow biopsy is the removal of a specimen of bone marrow for laboratory study. The biopsy is used to detect specific diseases of the blood, eg, pernicious anemia and leukemia, by studying a sample of the bone marrow for abnormal blood cell development. The bones of the body commonly used for a bone marrow biopsy are the sternum and the iliac crests. See Figure 11–10.

The physician dons sterile gloves, applies a drape, and cleans the skin with antiseptic. The physician administers a local anesthetic into the skin and the periosteum of the bone. See Figure 11–11. Then the physician introduces a bone marrow needle with stylet through the skin and bone into the red marrow of the spongy bone. Once the needle is in the marrow space, the physician removes the stylet, attaches a 10-mL syringe to the needle, and draws the plunger back until 1 or 2 mL of marrow has been withdrawn. The physician replaces the stylet in the needle, withdraws the needle, and places the specimen in test tubes and/or on glass slides.

FIGURE 11–10 ■ The sternum and the iliac crests are common sites for a bone marrow biopsy.

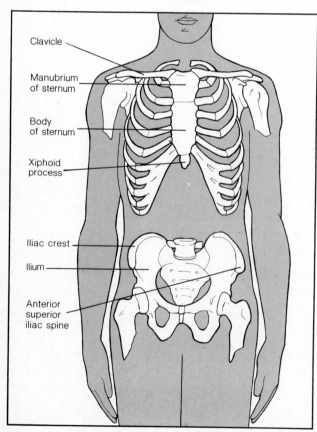

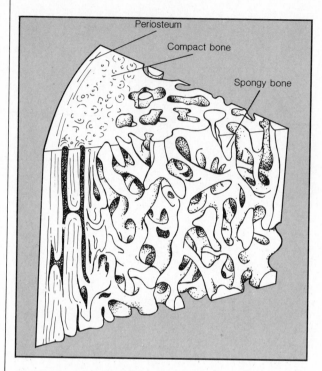

FIGURE 11–11 ■ A cross section of a bone.

This procedure may require a signed consent from the patient. The nurse must determine agency policy and obtain the consent if necessary.

■ Assessment

Assess the patient for:

1. Vital signs (body temperature, pulse, respirations, and blood pressure) for baseline data, if these are not already available
2. Drug allergies, particularly allergies to the drugs contained in the local anesthetics and skin antiseptics

■ Planning

Nursing goals

1. To minimize the patient's discomfort
2. To help the physician perform the bone marrow biopsy safely and expediently

Equipment

1. A sterile set containing:

a. A drape or drapes. One drape is often fenestrated, and the opening is placed over the aspiration site.

b. Antiseptic to clean the skin.

c. A local anesthetic.

d. A 2-mL syringe and #25 needle to administer the local anesthetic.

e. A 10-mL syringe to withdraw the bone marrow.

f. A bone marrow needle with stylet.

g. Sterile gauze squares to apply the antiseptic and cover the wound.

h. Test tubes and/or glass slides for the specimen.

2. Masks for the nurse and physician (optional). Determine agency policy.

3. Sterile gloves for the physician.

4. A completed laboratory requisition and labels for the specimen.

Arrange the equipment so that it is within easy reach of the physician.

■ **Intervention**

1. Explain the procedure to the patient. The patient may experience pain when the marrow is aspirated. There may be a crunching sound when the needle is pushed through the cortex of the bone. The entire procedure usually takes 15 to 30 minutes. Include in your explanation when and where the procedure will occur and who will be present.

2. Help the patient assume a supine position (with one pillow if desired) for a biopsy of the sternum (sternal puncture) or a prone position for a biopsy of either iliac crest. Fold the bedclothes back to expose the area.

3. Open the bone marrow set, and supply the sterile gloves to the physician. Pour the antiseptic into a container in the set or over sterile gauze squares.

4. Open and hold the ampule or vial of local anesthetic, if it is not in the set.

5. Describe the steps of the procedure to the patient, and provide verbal support. Observe the patient for pallor, diaphoresis, and faintness.

6. Place a small dressing over the site of the puncture after the needle is withdrawn.

7. Assess the patient's response in terms of discomfort and bleeding from the site. The patient may experience some tenderness in the area. Bleeding and hematoma formation need to be assessed for several days.

8. Provide an analgesic if required by the patient and ordered by the physician.

9. Arrange for the specimen with the completed requisition and label to be transported to the laboratory.

10. Record the procedure on the patient's chart, including the date and time of the procedure, the name of the physician, and the response of the patient.

Sample Recording

Date	Time	Notes
8/19/86	0900	Bone marrow biopsy from right iliac crest performed by Dr. Rosenthal. Site dry, no apparent bleeding. No complaints of discomfort. Specimen sent to laboratory.——————————— Donna S. Lambert, NS

11. Adjust the nursing care plan to include regular assessment for discomfort and bleeding.

■ **Evaluation**

Expected outcomes

1. No significant change in vital signs
2. Tenderness at the puncture site

Unexpected outcome

Bleeding and hematoma formation at the puncture site. Upon observing an unexpected outcome: Report your findings to the responsible nurse and/or physician.

TECHNIQUE 11–5 ■ Assisting with a Liver Biopsy

A liver biopsy is a short, sterile procedure, generally performed at the patient's bedside. A physician inserts a needle in the intercostal space between two of the right lower ribs and into the liver (see Figure 11–12) or through the abdomen below the right rib cage (subcostally) to aspirate a sample of liver tissue. Liver biopsies are usually conducted to obtain data about the nature of liver disease, to facilitate diagnosis, and to gain information about specific changes in the liver tissue.

The physician puts on sterile gloves, applies an antisep-

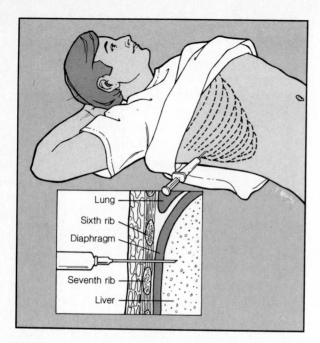

Lung
Sixth rib
Diaphragm
Seventh rib
Liver

FIGURE 11-12 ■ A common site for a liver biopsy.

tic to the biopsy site, drapes the area with sterile drapes, and injects the local anesthetic. When the area feels numb, the patient holds his or her breath, and the physician inserts the biopsy needle, injects a small amount of sterile normal saline to clear the needle of blood or particles of tissue picked up during insertion, and aspirates liver tissue by drawing back on the plunger of the syringe. After the needle is withdrawn, the nurse applies pressure to the site to prevent bleeding.

This procedure may require a signed consent from the patient. The nurse must determine agency policy and obtain the consent if necessary.

■ **Assessment**

Assess the patient for:

1. Vital signs (body temperature, pulse, respirations, and blood pressure) for baseline data if these are not already available.
2. Drug allergies, particularly allergies to medications contained in the local anesthetics and skin antiseptics.
3. Ability to hold his or her breath for up to 10 seconds. It is vitally important that the patient do so and remain still while the biopsy needle is inserted.

Additional data from the patient's record include:

1. The patient's prothrombin time and platelet count. Ensure that these are normal. Because many patients with liver disease have blood clotting defects and are prone to bleeding, prothrombin time and platelet

count are normally taken well in advance of the test. If the test results are abnormal, the biopsy may be contraindicated.

2. Preprocedural medications. Ensure that ordered medications have been given. Several days before the test, vitamin K may be administered intramuscularly to reduce the risk of hemorrhage. Vitamin K may be lacking in some patients with liver disease. It is essential for the production of prothrombin, which is a requisite for blood clotting.

■ **Planning**

Nursing goals

1. To minimize the patient's discomfort
2. To help the physician perform the liver biopsy safely and expediently

Equipment

1. A sterile liver biopsy set containing:
   a. Sterile sponges or gauze squares with an antiseptic solution to apply to the skin site.
   b. A 2-mL syringe and #22 and #25 needles (¾ in) to inject the local anesthetic.
   c. A large biopsy syringe and needle.
   d. Drapes.
   e. A local anesthetic.
   f. Sterile normal saline to clean the biopsy needle after insertion.
   g. A specimen container with formalin to preserve the liver tissue.
2. Face masks for the physician and the nurse (optional). Determine agency policy.
3. Sterile gloves for the physician to don after scrubbing.
4. A laboratory requisition and a specimen label.

■ **Intervention**

1. Explain the procedure to the patient, including:
   a. What the physician will do, ie, take a small sample of liver tissue by putting a needle into the patient's side or abdomen.
   b. That a sedative and local anesthetic will be given, so the patient will feel no pain.
   c. When and where the procedure will occur.
   d. Who will be present.
   e. The time required.
   f. What to expect as the procedure is being performed, eg, the patient may experience mild dis-

comfort when the local anesthetic is injected and slight pressure when the biopsy needle is inserted.

2. Ensure that the patient fasts for at least two hours before the procedure.

3. Administer the appropriate sedative about 30 minutes beforehand or at the specified time.

4. Help the patient assume a supine position, with the upper right quadrant of the abdomen exposed. Cover the patient with the bedclothes so that only the abdominal area is exposed.

5. Open the sterile set and provide the sterile gloves for the physician. Pour antiseptic over the sterile sponges or gauze, or into a container, as requested.

6. Support the patient in a supine position.

7. Instruct the patient to take a few deep inhalations and exhalations and to hold his or her breath after the final exhalation for up to 10 seconds as the needle is inserted, the biopsy obtained, and the needle withdrawn.

   Rationale Holding the breath after exhalation immobilizes the chest wall and liver and keeps the diaphragm in its highest position, avoiding injury to the diaphragm and laceration of the liver.

8. Instruct the patient to resume breathing when the needle is withdrawn.

9. Apply pressure to the site of the puncture.

   Rationale   Pressure will help stop any bleeding.

10. Apply a small dressing to the site of the puncture.

11. Assist the patient to a right side-lying position with a small pillow or folded towel under the biopsy site. See Figure 11–13. Instruct him or her to remain in this position for several hours.

    Rationale   The right lateral position compresses the biopsy site of the liver against the chest wall and minimizes the escape of blood or bile through the puncture site.

12. Send the labeled specimen immediately to the laboratory along with the completed requisition.

13. Record the procedure on the patient's chart, including the date and time it was performed, the name of the physician, and the patient's response.

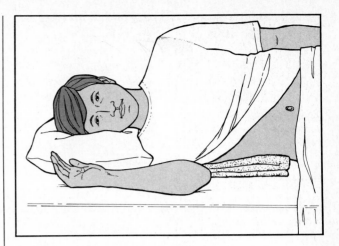

FIGURE 11–13

14. Assess the patient's response to the procedure in terms of pulse, respirations, and blood pressure every 15 minutes for the first hour following the test or until they are stable. Complications of a liver biopsy are rare, but hemorrhage from a perforated blood vessel can occur.

15. Determine whether the patient is experiencing abdominal pain. Severe abdominal pain may indicate bile peritonitis (an inflammation of the peritoneal lining of the abdomen caused by bile leaking from a perforated bile duct).

16. Check the biopsy site for localized bleeding. Pressure dressings may be required if bleeding occurs.

■ Evaluation

Expected outcome

No significant change in vital signs.

Unexpected outcomes

1. Abdominal pain

2. Internal bleeding and shock, indicated by falling blood pressure, accelerated pulse rate, and pallor

3. Bleeding at the biopsy site

Upon observing an unexpected outcome: Report your findings to the responsible nurse and/or physician.

Sample Recording

Date	Time	Notes
2/13/87	1000	Liver biopsy performed by Dr. Martinez. Specimen sent to laboratory. P 86, R 16 and regular, BP 110/76/70. Small amount bleeding at site (0.3 cm diameter). Resting comfortably in right lateral position. ——————————— Theresa A. Milligan, NS

VISUAL INSPECTION PROCEDURES

Visual inspection or direct visualization procedures use special instruments called *endoscopes,* by which interior parts of the body can be seen. Three of the most common procedures are *proctoscopy* or *sigmoidoscopy, bronchoscopy* or *laryngoscopy,* and *cystoscopy.*

A proctoscopy is carried out at the bedside or in a special treatment room. A nurse assists the patient and the examiner. Bronchoscopies (laryngoscopies) and cystoscopies require general or local anesthetics and are usually carried out in the operating room. The nurse prepares the patient and provides aftercare. These procedures are beyond the scope of this book. Assisting with a proctoscopy is discussed here because of the nurse's assisting function.

TECHNIQUE 11-6 ■ Assisting with a Proctoscopy

A proctoscopy is an examination of the rectum using a lighted instrument. During a proctoscopy it is not unusual for the physician to obtain a specimen of tissue. The nurse serves similar functions for a proctoscopy, proctosigmoidoscopy, and anoscopy.

The physician usually examines the rectum digitally (with the fingers) as well as visually, to ascertain that there is no obstruction and to dilate the anal sphincter. See Figure 11–14 for a cross-section of the rectum and anal canal, including the anal sphincters. The physician lubricates the proctoscope and inserts it as far as the patient can tolerate it. It is withdrawn gradually, and

FIGURE 11–14 ■ A cross section of the rectum and the anal canal, including the anal sphincters.

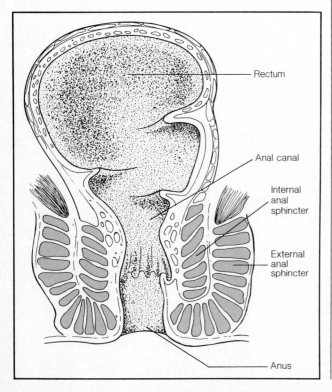

Rectum

Anal canal

Internal anal sphincter

External anal sphincter

Anus

suction and air may be used alternately. The suction removes fecal material and blood if bleeding occurs. The air from an insufflator expands the bowel, thus improving visual examination.

This procedure may require a signed consent from the patient. The nurse must determine agency policy and obtain the consent if necessary.

■ Assessment

Assess the patient for:

1. Vital signs for baseline data if not already available.
2. Color, odor, and consistency of feces and any abnormal constituents, eg, visible blood.
3. Abdominal discomfort, including abdominal distention, type of pain, location, and time of onset.
4. Ability to assume a genupectoral (knee–chest) position for the length of time required (about 30 minutes). See Figure 11–15.

■ Planning

Nursing goals

1. To minimize the patient's discomfort
2. To help the physician perform the proctoscopy safely and expediently

Equipment

1. A sterile proctoscopy set. A proctoscopy is not a sterile procedure, but the set will probably be sterilized as a safety precaution to avoid transmitting microorganisms into the rectum. Sterile technique is usually practiced if a tissue biopsy is to be taken. The following equipment is included in the set:

   a. A drape to cover the patient. A fenestrated drape

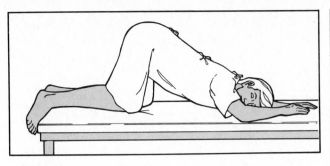

FIGURE 11–15 ■ The genupectoral (knee–chest) position.

is often used, with the opening placed over the anus.

   b. An endoscope and biopsy forceps. Special types of endoscopes used are: a proctoscope for a proctoscopy, a sigmoidoscope for a sigmoidoscopy, and an anoscope for an anoscopy. Proctoscopes are shorter than sigmoidoscopes, and anoscopes are shorter than proctoscopes. Some models have a mechanism that permits alternate suctioning and insufflation.

   c. Gauze squares.

   d. Lubricant for the endoscope.

2. Sterile gloves.

3. Suction to remove fecal matter. Suction is frequently provided through wall outlets. Make sure it is functioning.

4. An insufflator to force air into the colon to separate the mucosal folds. Check that it is functioning.

5. A specimen container, a label, and a completed laboratory requisition.

Arrange the equipment within easy reach of the physician.

■ **Intervention**

1. Note the preparation required of the patient from the chart, and confirm that this was done. The physician usually orders an enema, a laxative, a suppository, or a combination administered to the patient the day before or the morning of the examination, to clear the large intestine of fecal material.

2. Explain the procedure to the patient. A proctoscopy can be uncomfortable because of the position the patient must assume and because the instrument is inserted into the rectum. The patient will need to assume and maintain a knee–chest position for perhaps 30 minutes. Special tables called *Ritter tables,* which break at the level of the hips and provide a platform on which the patient can kneel,

provide more support for the patient than the knee–chest position on a bed.

3. Drape the patient appropriately so that he or she is well covered except for the anal area.

4. Open the proctoscopy set, and supply the gloves to the physician.

5. Explain the steps of the procedure to the patient, and verbally support the patient. Assess the patient for pallor, diaphoresis, and faintness.

   Rationale   The patient may feel faint because of the knee–chest position, from the discomfort caused by the proctoscope, or when a biopsy is obtained.

6. After the proctoscope is removed, wipe the patient's anus with gauze.

7. Assist the patient from the knee–chest position to a comfortable position.

8. Assess the response of the patient in terms of pulse rate, color, and rectal discomfort. Note any sanguinous discharge from the anus, which could result from the biopsy or inadvertent tissue injury.

9. Send the labeled specimen and completed requisition to the laboratory.

10. Record the procedure on the patient's chart, including the date and time, the name of the physician, the specimen taken if any, and the response of the patient.

Sample Recording

Date	Time	Notes
1/14/87	0900	Proctoscopy performed by Dr. Simpson. Two biopsy specimens sent to laboratory. C/o sharp pain in rectal area; color pale; pulse 125.——— Roger S. Sandusky, NS

11. Adjust the nursing care plan to include regular assessment for bleeding etc.

■ **Evaluation**

Expected outcome

No significant change in vital signs.

Unexpected outcomes

1. Rectal discomfort
2. Rectal bleeding

Upon observing an unexpected outcome: Report your findings to the responsible nurse and/or physician.

MEASUREMENT OF ELECTRIC IMPULSES

A number of machines measure and record electric impulses. The *electrocardiograph* receives impulses from the heart, the *electroencephalograph* from the brain, and the *electromyograph* from muscles. All these machines have electrodes that attach to body parts. The electrodes are sensitive to electric activity, which is recorded graphically. The graphic reading can also be shown on an oscilloscope screen.

Electrocardiography

An *electrocardiogram* (ECG or EKG) is a graph of electric impulses from the heart. The heart muscle is said to be *polarized* or charged when it is at rest. When the muscle cells of the ventricles and the atria contract, they *depolarize* or lose their charge. During a resting stage, they regain their electric charge or *repolarize*. Cardiac depolarization and repolarization are recorded on an electrocardiogram.

The heartbeat is normally initiated at the *sinoatrial (SA) node*, which is located in the upper aspect of the right atrium. The SA node is often referred to as the pacemaker of the heart. The impulse it initiates radiates over the atria, causing them to contract. It is then picked up by the *atrioventricular (AV) node*, situated at the base of the atrial septum. The impulse travels from the AV node down two bundle branches throughout the ventricles of the heart. The SA and AV nodes and the bundle branches have dense networks of *Purkinje's fibers*, modified cardiac tissue that helps conduct the impulse. As the impulse travels throughout this system, the ventricles contract or depolarize. Figure 11–16 shows a normal electrocardiogram and indicates the intervals of depolarization and repolarization. The P wave arises when the impulse from the SA node causes the atria to contract or depolarize. The QRS wave occurs with contraction and depolarization of the ventricles. The T wave represents the resting or repolarization of the ventricles. Repolarization of the atria occurs during the QRS segment of the graph; it is normally not seen on an ECG. The ECG is produced on finely lined paper. The horizontal lines represent the voltage of the electric

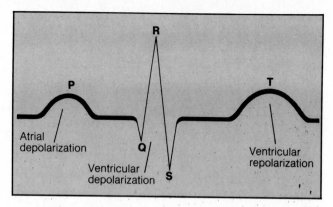

FIGURE 11–16 ■ Schematic of a normal electrocardiogram.

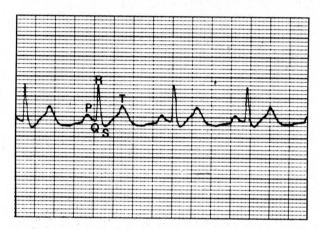

FIGURE 11–17 ■ A normal electrocardiogram.

impulse, and the vertical lines represent time. See Figure 11–17. The graph waves can be abnormal in size, position, and form when cardiac pathology exists.

Patients who require ECGs may go to a special department of a hospital or laboratory. If the patient is very ill, a portable ECG machine can be brought to the bedside in a home or hospital. If the patient is critically ill, the heart may be monitored continually. For such patients, a *cardiac monitor* is used. This machine shows cardiac waves on an oscilloscope.

Electrocardiography is painless and usually takes about 10 minutes. Some physicians order an electrocardiogram as part of routine physical examinations of patients over age 40. No special preparation is required before the test.

TECHNIQUE 11–7 ■ Assisting with an Electrocardiogram

An electrocardiogram is usually taken by a specially trained technician or by a physician. Electrodes are attached by leads to the electrocardiograph. The elec-

trodes are attached to the patient's body by paste, suction cups, or tape. One electrode is attached to the lower part of each limb, and a fifth electrode is moved to six different positions on the chest. The first position is on the right sternal border; subsequent positions follow the general outline of the heart around to the left sternal border and laterally as far as the midaxillary line. See Figure 11–18. The heart's electric impulses register on a graph that the machine produces during the procedure. A physician interprets the graph after the test.

■ Assessment

Assess the patient's vital signs (body temperature, pulse, respirations, and blood pressure) for baseline data, if not already available.

■ Planning

Nursing goal

To minimize discomfort to the patient.

Equipment

A portable ECG unit can be brought to or kept on the nursing unit. The physician usually decides whether to take the ECG at the central laboratory or at the bedside, depending on the patient's condition.

■ Intervention

The nurse assists in this procedure as requested by the physician or technician. Nursing assistance may not be required.

1. Determine whether the patient has had an electrocardiogram before, and explain the procedure as the patient requires. The patient may be anxious, not about the test, which is painless and takes only 10 to 15 minutes, but about the results, which might indicate a problem with the heart.
2. No special preparation is required unless the physician specifies, eg, "exercise strenuously for five minutes just prior to ECG."
3. Provide privacy, because the patient's limbs and chest will be exposed.

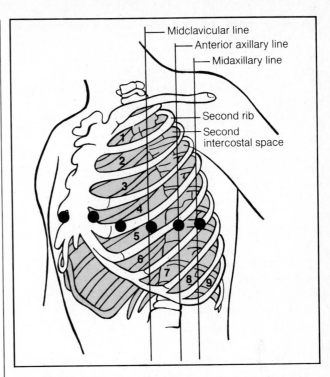

FIGURE 11–18 ■ The placement of electrodes on the chest of an adult for electrocardiography.

4. Following the test, assess the patient's response to the test, including discomfort, pulse, respirations, and blood pressure.
5. If the patient is particularly anxious about the test, notify the physician so that the results can be explained as soon as possible.
6. Record on the patient's chart that an ECG was carried out, by whom, and the patient's response.

Sample Recording

Date	Time	Notes
4/24/87	1500	ECG taken by Dr. Tekawa. C/o sharp chest pains following. R 20 and shallow, P 108 and irregular, BP 180/90/80. Dr. Tekawa notified. ————Amanda V. Arguello, SN

Electroencephalography

Electroencephalograms (EEGs) are recordings of electric activity in the brain. Electroencephalographs have leads to electrodes that attach to the patient's scalp with paste or small needles. The patient lies in a dorsal recumbent position in a darkened room. The patient may be asked to hyperventilate, and readings may also be taken while the patient sleeps. If performed on a sleeping patient, the test may take two hours; otherwise it lasts no more than one hour. The test is normally painless, although the patient may feel occasional pinpricks if needle electrodes are used in the scalp.

Preparation for an EEG varies. Some agencies advise that, on the day of the test, the patient not take stimulants such as coffee or depressants such as alcohol. Usually the patient takes no medications prior to the test, and the nurse shampoos the patient's hair, which should be free of hair spray, hair creams, and the like.

Electromyography

An *electromyogram* (EMG) is a record of the electric potential created by the contraction of a muscle. Two electrodes are attached with paste or small needles to the skin over the muscle. This test is used to discern muscle abnormalities such as *fasciculation* (abnormal contraction involving the whole motor unit). No special preparation is necessary for this procedure. The patient may experience some discomfort when the needle electrodes are inserted and some residual discomfort if many muscles are tested.

Often a *nerve conduction study* is done in conjunction with the EMG. This procedure determines the excitability and conduction velocities of motor and sensory nerves and the presence of disease of the peripheral nerves. A stimulating electrode and a recording electrode are placed over specific sites to test a specific nerve. The distance between the electrodes and the time required for a nerve impulse to pass from the point of stimulation to the point of recording are precisely measured. Conduction velocity is then calculated. The patient will experience the discomfort of mild electric shock during this procedure, but there should be no residual discomfort.

ROENTGENOGRAPHY (X-RAY), ULTRASOUND, AND NUCLEAR MEDICINE PROCEDURES

Roentgenography

Roentgen rays are part of the spectrum of electromagnetic radiation. They travel at the speed of light and have considerably shorter wavelengths than light or radio waves. This distinctive property enables radiation to penetrate organs and tissues according to their thickness and density. High-voltage x rays have shorter wavelengths and produce a more penetrating (harder) radiation; low-voltage x rays have longer wavelengths and produce a more easily absorbable (softer) radiation. X rays that are not absorbed pass through the tissue to form an image on the photographic film (a plain, or static, radiograph) or on a fluorescent screen (fluoroscopy).

It is the differential absorption of x rays by the various tissues that makes roentgenography diagnostically useful.

Bones, which are dense, permit fewer x rays to pass through to the film, so they appear as light areas; the soft tissues surrounding bone are less dense, so they appear darker on the film. Natural contrasts in density also occur between blood-filled cardiovascular structures and air-filled lung areas. Such natural contrasts, however, do not occur in the abdomen or between the soft tissue structures of the extremities. Thus contrast agents must be introduced for certain body parts, eg, the digestive tract and blood vessels, to show on the film.

Contrast materials (solids, liquids, or gaseous substances) must absorb either more or fewer x rays than the surrounding tissues. Commonly used contrast agents are compounds of iodine, barium, air, and carbon dioxide. Iodine and barium absorb more x rays than soft tissues; air and carbon dioxide absorb fewer.

Contrast materials are introduced into the body in four ways to view specific organs:

1. Orally or rectally for the digestive tract (esophagus, stomach, intestines) and gallbladder. See Figure 11-19.

2. Intravenously for the blood vessels, bile ducts, and kidneys.

3. Into the subarachnoid space for the spine and the ventricles of the brain.

4. Through a nasotracheal tube or bronchoscope for the bronchial tree. This method is used infrequently now, since the advent of fiberoptic bronchoscopy, which has increased the area available to direct visual examination.

FIGURE 11-19 ■ An x-ray film of the small and large intestines using a contrast medium.

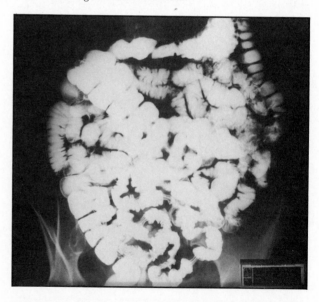

TECHNIQUE 11–8 ■ Assisting with Roentgenography

The nurse's role in assisting with an x-ray procedure is largely preparation of the patient for the examination and provision of follow-up care. The reasons for roentgenography are:

1. To determine abnormalities in the structure or appearance of body organs, eg, ulcerations in the stomach, tumors, bone fractures, or consolidated infectious material in the lungs

2. To determine disruptions in the function of body organs, eg, decreased function of the gallbladder or thyroid gland

3. To determine the presence of obstructions to body ducts or vessels, eg, stones in the bile ducts or urinary system, or blood clots in the arteries

4. To determine the extent or spread of malignant tumors

■ Assessment

Assess the patient for:

1. Vital signs to provide baseline data for comparison following the procedure.

2. Allergies, particularly to iodine. The oral contrast agents (eg, Telepaque tablets) used for gallbladder x-ray films are iodine compounds. Most of the intravenous contrast agents used for angiograms and intravenous urography also contain iodine compounds. See Table 11–2.

■ Planning

Nursing goals

1. To prepare the patient before the procedure, so that the roentgenography will be successful

2. To provide follow-up care that minimizes the patient's discomfort and maintains the patient's safety

■ Intervention

1. Check the physician's order sheet to determine the specific examination ordered. For example, a cholecystogram and a cholangiogram may appear similar but involve different preparations. For the cholecystogram, contrast material is taken orally; for a cholangiogram, the contrast material is given intravenously. See Table 11–2.

2. Determine the specific preparatory measures required for the x-ray procedure or scan. For example, before certain x-ray films are taken, a strong laxative needs to be administered to clear the bowel of fecal material, which could prevent proper visualization of a body organ, eg, the kidney or the gallbladder. For other x-ray films, the patient needs to fast for a specific period of time and/or take tablets containing contrast material at prescribed periods of time. Some patients are given a sedative beforehand.

3. Determine where the examination is to be carried out. Most x-ray examinations are performed in a radiology department. However, some scanning procedures that use radioactive materials are carried out in the nuclear medicine department of a hospital.

4. Determine when the examination is scheduled and the approximate time it will take to complete. The anxiety of the patient and support persons can be reduced if they are informed about time schedules.

5. Determine whether medications the patient is receiving are to be given or are canceled prior to the test. For example, a diabetic patient whose diet is altered for a barium enema may have his or her insulin canceled the morning of the test. For a diabetic patient, the roentgenography may be scheduled early in the day to prevent undue disruption of routine insulin administration and diet.

6. Inform the patient about what examination is to be carried out, when and where it will take place, the time involved, and the necessary preparatory measures. Specific instructions that need to be included about common x-ray examinations are outlined in Table 11–2. Patients are generally taken to the hospital radiology department by an escort service.

7. Provide adequate rest periods for the patient following the procedure. Many diagnostic procedures are tiring for the patient, and in some instances several procedures are carried out on consecutive days. For example, a sigmoidoscopy may be done one day, a barium enema the next day, and a barium swallow the third day.

8. Monitor the patient closely for discomfort and potential complications related to the procedure. These are outlined in Table 11–2.

9. Provide the follow-up care that is recommended for each procedure by the agency.

10. Record the procedure in accordance with agency practices, including:

    a. Preparatory measures carried out

TABLE 11-2 ■ Common X-Ray Examinations

Name	Description	Preparation	Follow-up care	Complications
Upper gastrointestinal (GI) series (barium swallow)	The patient swallows barium, and x-ray films are taken of its course through the esophagus, stomach, and duodenum.	The patient fasts 4–6 hours prior to the test. Explain that: ■ No discomfort is involved. ■ The patient will be given a flavored (eg, chocolate) chalky substance to drink in the x-ray department. ■ The procedure usually takes about 30 minutes.	A laxative is given to eliminate the barium. Observe the regularity of bowel elimination and the passage of barium.	Rectal impaction due to retained barium.
Lower gastrointestinal series (barium enema)	A barium enema is given to the patient, and x-ray films are taken of the large intestine.	A clear liquid diet is given 12 or 24 hours before the test to ensure an empty bowel. Enemas are given until returns are clear on the morning of the test, to clean the bowel of all fecal material. Explain that: ■ With the barium enema there will be a feeling of fullness and the urge to defecate. ■ There may be some cramping. ■ Special tubes with balloons are often used to assist the patient to retain the barium. ■ The patient will be asked to assume various positions, eg, lying on the left side, then moving to the right side. ■ The barium is expelled in the x-ray department. ■ The procedure takes about 30 minutes.	Provide a rest period, since this procedure can be tiring. Resume the patient's regular diet. A light snack can be provided as needed. Observe the regularity of bowel elimination and the passage of barium. A cleansing enema may be necessary.	Rectal impaction due to retained barium.
Cholecystogram (oral cholecystography)	X-ray films are taken of the gallbladder after a contrast dye has been given orally.	A fat-free supper is given the evening before. Check for allergy to the contrast dye, which contains iodine. A laxative may be given the evening before, or an enema the morning of the test. Six or more contrast pills (eg, Telepaque) are given at 5-minute intervals the evening before the test, each with 4–6 oz water. The patient fasts from midnight the evening before but may drink water.	Provide a rest period. The patient resumes a regular diet. A snack can be provided if the patient is hungry.	Allergy to the contrast dye.

TABLE 11–2 ■ continued

Name	Description	Preparation	Follow-up care	Complications
Cholecystogram (continued)		Explain that: ■ A fatty drink is given in the x-ray department. ■ No discomfort is usually felt from the x rays. ■ The procedure takes about 30–45 minutes.		
Intravenous cholangiogram	X-ray films are taken of the bile ducts after dye has been administered intravenously.	The patient fasts from midnight the evening before the test but may drink water. The bowel is cleaned with a laxative the evening before or with an enema the morning of the test. Check for allergy to iodine contained in the dye. Explain that: ■ Iodine dye is given intravenously in the x-ray department. ■ The patient may have a test dose in his or her arm first to test for any allergy.	The patient resumes a regular diet. A snack can be provided if the patient is hungry.	Allergy to the contrast dye.
Intravenous pyelography or urography (IVP, IVU)	Visual examination of the urinary system (kidney and ureters) after an intravenous injection of radiopaque material.	A strong laxative (eg, castor oil) is given the afternoon before the test to clear the bowel of fecal material, which can obstruct the view of the urinary structures. The patient fasts from midnight prior to the test. Check for allergy to iodine. Explain that: ■ An intravenous injection will be administered in the x-ray department. ■ The procedure takes about 1 hour.	Encourage fluid intake. The patient resumes a regular diet. Provide for rest, since the effects of the laxative and fasting can cause weakness. Observe for reactions to the radiopaque dye.	Allergic reaction to the radiopaque material, manifested by itching, hives, wheezing, or shock.
Angiography, eg, cerebral angiography (vascular system of the brain), coronary arteriography (coronary arteries of the heart), renal angiography (vascular system of the kidneys), pulmonary angiography (vascular system of the lungs).	Visual examination of portions of the vascular system after a radiopaque material is injected into an artery or vein.	For some of these procedures a catheter may be inserted into an artery or vein prior to the injection of radiopaque material. For some procedures the patient is given a sedative prior to the test. The patient fasts from midnight prior to the test. A strong laxative may be given the evening before certain tests (eg, renal arteriography). Check whether the patient is allergic to iodine. The time needed for these procedures varies. Some may take up to 3 hours.	Bed rest is generally maintained for up to 12 hours. Monitor the patient's radial pulse, respirations, and blood pressure every 15 to 30 minutes until stabilized. Monitor peripheral pulses distal to the injection site. Observe the injection site for bleeding and swelling. Note any discomfort experienced by the patient.	Irritation or bleeding at the injection site. Embolus or thrombus formation.

TABLE 11–2 ■ continued

Name	Description	Preparation	Follow-up care	Complications
Myelogram	A contrast material is injected into the subarachnoid space and x-ray films are taken of the spinal cord, nerve roots, and vertebrae.	Fasting may be required from midnight prior to the test. The patient may be given a sedative prior to the procedure. Explain that: ■ A radiopaque oil dye is injected via a lumbar puncture or a cisternal puncture in the x-ray department. See Technique 11–1 on the lumbar puncture. ■ The patient will assume various positions, eg, on the side for a lumbar puncture, then prone, and then tilted on an x-ray table equipped with shoulder and foot supports. ■ Some pain may be felt when the oil is removed, due to irritation of the nerve roots. ■ The procedure may take about 2 hours.	The patient is generally positioned flat in bed for 24 hours to minimize headache and/or nausea, but may be positioned with the head elevated above the level of the spine if the dye has not been completely removed. This prevents the dye from moving to the head and causing an inflammation of the meninges (meningitis). Monitor vital signs and neurologic status, eg, feeling of numbness, pain, or tingling in the extremities; muscle weakness. Check urinary output.	Postpuncture headache, starting a few hours after the test and lasting for several days up to a week. It characteristically occurs when the patient sits up or moves the head suddenly. Chemical meningitis from the contrast dye, manifested by a stiff neck and fever. Occasional urinary retention.
Organ scan	A scanning examination of a body organ following oral or intravenous administration of a radioactive substance. The specific organ to be examined gives the scan its name, eg, brain scan, liver scan, lung scan.	Restless patients, eg, children, may be given a sedative prior to the procedure. Assure the patient there is no need to fear exposure to radiation; it is less than that acquired from the usual x-ray procedure. A radioactive substance is given orally or intravenously. Depending on the substance used, a blocking agent may also be given to prevent uptake of the radioactive substance by organs other than the one being studied, and to ensure that the substance goes into the organ being studied, eg: ■ Lugol's solution (iodine) is given to block uptake by the thyroid (given orally with juice, since its taste is unpleasant), or a potassium compound may be given to patients allergic to iodine. ■ Mercaptomerin sodium is given (intramuscularly) to block uptake by the kidneys. Check for allergies to the blocking agents used. Explain that:	Additional scans may be performed at subsequent intervals, eg, 2 hours, 24 hours, 48 hours, and 72 hours.	Allergic reaction to the blocking agent. It may range from mild to severe, depending on the agent used.

TABLE 11–2 ■ **continued**

Name	Description	Preparation	Follow-up care	Complications
Organ scan (continued)		■ The scan is performed in the nuclear medicine department. ■ There will be a brief waiting period while the radioactive substance is distributed. ■ There is no discomfort with the procedure. ■ The patient will be asked to assume various positions and must remain still while the scans are taken.		

b. The procedure itself

c. The time the patient is transported to the radiology or nuclear medicine department

d. The time the patient was returned to the unit

e. Follow-up measures provided

f. The response of the patient

Sample Recording

Date	Time	Notes
12/15/86	0700	Clear liquid breakfast given. ————————————Adrian L. Stewart, NS
	0800	3 saline enemas given until returns were clear. Large amount of soft, dark brown stool obtained.——Adrian L. Stewart, NS
	0930	Transported to radiology for barium enema. ——————————Adrian L. Stewart, NS
	1030	Returned to unit. States is tired. No complaints of discomfort.——————————— Adrian L. Stewart, NS

Computerized Axial Tomography (CAT Scan)

Computerized axial tomography is a noninvasive x-ray procedure with the unique capability of distinguishing minor differences in the radiodensity of soft tissues. See Figure 11–20. For example, it can distinguish between liver and tumor or brain and hematoma. In this technique a planar slice of the body is subjected to sequential sweeps or *scans* of a narrow beam of x ray. The unabsorbed beam emerging through the tissues is measured by a radiation detector. Data obtained are stored in a computer, which produces an image on a viewing apparatus or printout machine. The image is referred to as a *tomogram*.

Ultrasound

Ultrasound, another noninvasive technique, uses sound waves well above the upper limit of human hearing. It measures acoustic densities of tissues and has no known harmful effects. In contrast to usual radiography, ultrasound allows the diagnostician to know the depth of a structure below the skin and to determine the anteroposterior dimension of masses. Because sound is very poorly conducted by gases and is reflected very well by bone, however, structures containing air (such as the lung) or surrounded by bone (such as the pelvis) are difficult to examine with ultrasound.

In this technique, a transducer or probe is used as both an emitter and a receiver. Echos or sounds received are translated onto a display unit for observation and photographic recording. Some display units differentiate the ultrasonic reflections by amplitude versus depth; others by brightness versus depth. The latter are referred to as echography or sonography.

Nuclear Medicine

The instruments and radioactive tracers used in nuclear medicine are constantly changing, but the fundamental principles remain the same. One of the most basic principles is that body constituents are dynamic, not static.

In nuclear medicine techniques, radioactive substances that have an affinity for specific body tissues are introduced orally or intravenously. For example, radioac-

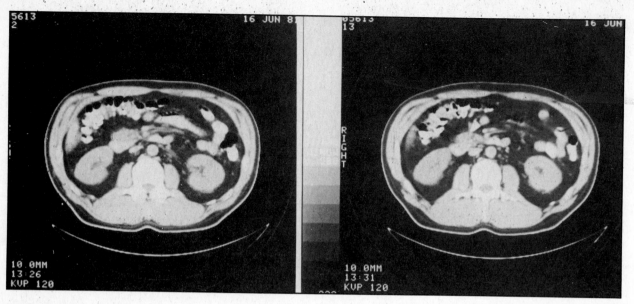

FIGURE 11–20 ■ A CAT scan showing a cross section of the patient at midabdomen. The spine is at the base, with the kidneys to the left and right of it.

tive iodine may be given to measure the function of the thyroid gland. The thyroid gland normally picks up and uses iodine to produce the hormone thyroxine. When radioactive iodine is introduced, the amount of iodine the thyroid actually picks up and how it is distributed can be detected by a scanning device, and any deficiencies in thyroid function can be discovered.

Scanning can be used to measure the concentration of radioactive particles in any body organ to assess the functioning of the organ or detect the existence of a tumor. Organs commonly subjected to diagnostic nuclear medicine include the thyroid, heart, brain, lungs, liver, spleen, bone marrow, bones, and kidneys.

References

Byrne CJ et al: *Laboratory Tests: Implications for Nurses and Allied Health Professionals.* Addison-Wesley, 1981.

French RM: *Guide to Diagnostic Procedures,* 5th ed. McGraw-Hill, 1980.

Harvey AM et al: *The Principles and Practice of Medicine,* 20th ed. Appleton-Century-Crofts, 1980.

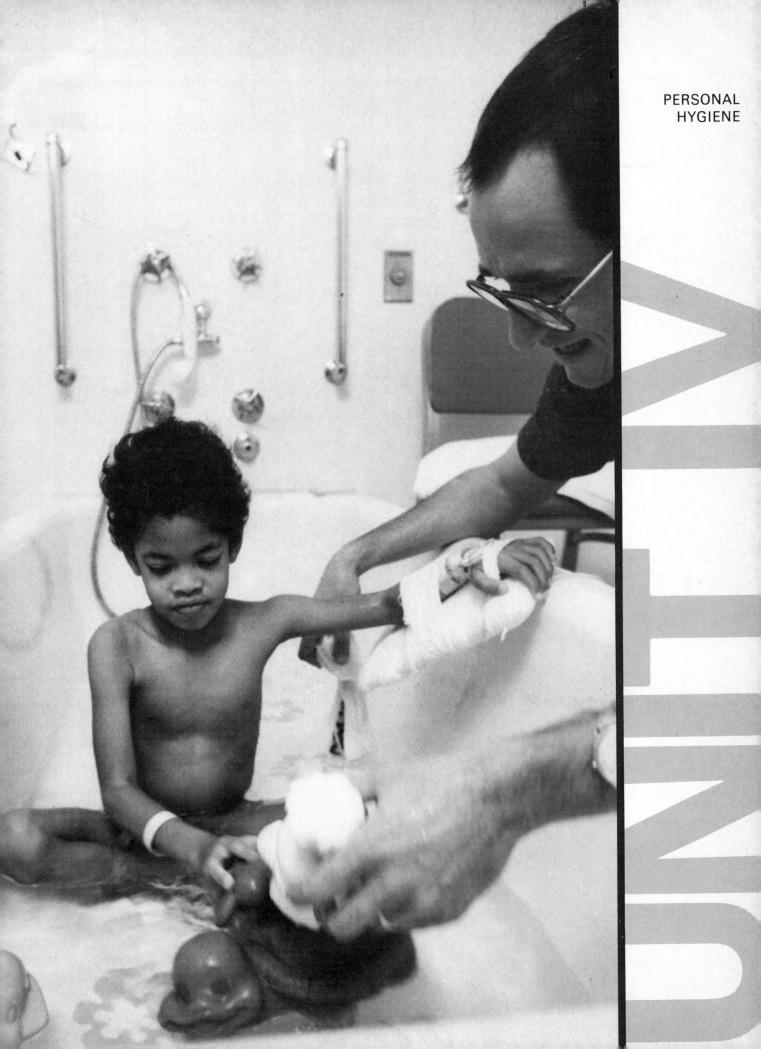

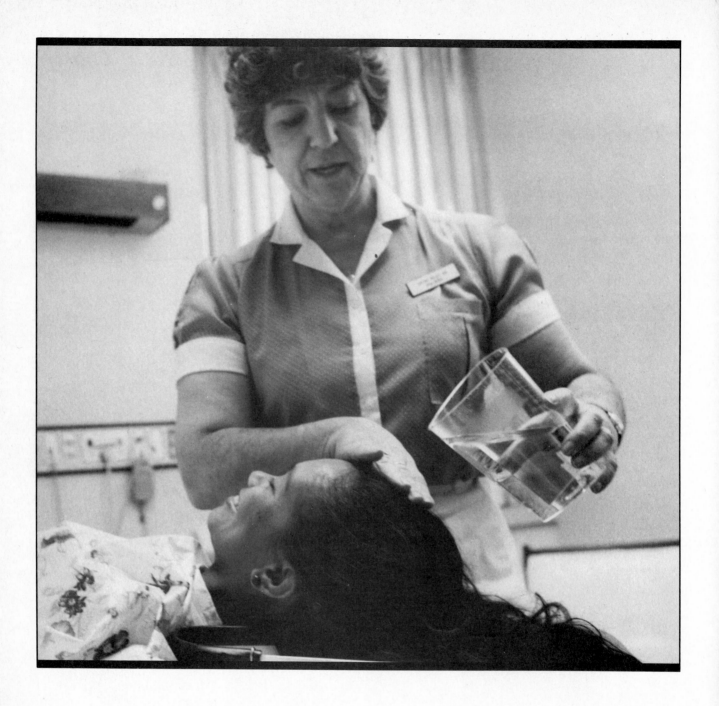

THE HAIR, NAILS, AND FEET

12

Hygiene can be defined as the science of health and its maintenance, including mental, oral, sexual, social, and other aspects of health. *Personal hygiene* is the care that persons take of their own health. Hygiene practices involve care of the skin, hair, nails, teeth, oral and nasal cavities, and, in women, the vagina. The skin, hair, and nails are commonly referred to as the *integumentary system*.

This chapter, the first of four dealing with hygiene practices and techniques, focuses on the hair, nails, and feet. Although hygiene practices are generally done independently and personally, the very young, the elderly, and the physically and mentally ill often require assistance from a nurse. Attending to hygienic needs not only increases the patient's feeling of self-worth but also is effective in maintaining the health of the integument and preventing infection.

Chapter Outline

Hair
- Technique 12–1 Brushing and Combing Hair
- Technique 12–2 Hair Care for Black Patients
- Technique 12–3 Braiding Hair
- Technique 12–4 Shampooing Hair (Bed Patient)

Nails
- Technique 12–5 Cleaning and Trimming Nails

Feet
- Technique 12–6 Foot Care

Objectives

Upon completion of this chapter, the student will:

1. Know essential terms and facts about the hair, nails, and feet
   1.1 Define selected terms
   1.2 Identify selected human structures
   1.3 Identify the function of each structure
   1.4 Identify variations in the hair, nails, and feet from infancy to old age
   1.5 Identify common problems of the hair, nails, and feet
2. Understand facts about techniques used to assist patients with their hair, nails, and feet
   2.1 Identify relevant assessment data
   2.2 Identify nursing diagnoses for which the technique may be implemented
   2.3 Identify nursing goals related to the technique
   2.4 Identify expected and unexpected outcomes from assessment data
   2.5 Identify reasons underlying selected steps of the technique
3. Perform techniques related to hair, nail, and foot care safely

3.1 Assess the patient adequately
3.2 Collect additional data from appropriate sources
3.3 Select pertinent nursing goals for the patient
3.4 Establish relevant outcome criteria for the patient following the technique
3.5 Collect necessary equipment before the technique
3.6 Implement interventions to enhance the effectiveness of the technique and enhance the patient's comfort and safety
3.7 Communicate relevant information about the patient to the appropriate persons
3.8 Determine the evaluative outcomes of the technique
4. Evaluate own performance of specific techniques in a laboratory or clinical setting with the assistance of another
   4.1 Use the performance checklists provided
   4.2 Identify areas of strength and weakness
   4.3 Alter performance in response to own evaluation and that of another

Terms

- alopecia   abnormal loss of hair
- arrector pili muscles   the erector muscle attached to the hair follicle
- athlete's foot   a fungal infection of the foot
- Beau's line   a transverse white line or groove on the nail
- bunion   lateral deviation of the big toe with swelling or callus formation over the metatarsophalangeal joint
- callus   a thickened portion of the skin
- clubbing (of a nail)   elevation of the proximal aspect

of the nail and softening of the nail bed due to a long-term lack of oxygen
- corn   a conical, circular, painful, raised area on the toe or foot
- cradle cap   a yellowish, oily crusting of the scalp of infants
- cuticle   the flat, thin rim of skin surrounding the nail
- dandruff   a dry or greasy scaly material shed from the scalp
- fissure   a cleft or groove

■ hair follicle   a pouchlike depression in the skin enclosing the root of a hair

■ hair shaft   the visible part of the hair

■ hallux valgus (bunion)   lateral deviation of the big toe with swelling or callus formation over the metatarsophalangeal joint

■ hammer toe   a flexed proximal toe joint and hyperextended distal toe joint

■ hangnail   a shred of epidermal tissue at either side of the nail

■ hirsutism   abnormal hairiness

■ ingrown toenail (incurvated nail)   penetration of the edges of the nail plate into the surrounding tissues

■ keratin   the type of protein found in epidermis, hair, and nails

■ lanugo   fine, woolly hair or down on the shoulders, back, sacrum, and earlobes of the unborn child that may remain for a few weeks after birth

■ lice   parasitic insects that infest mammals

■ paronychia   infection of the tissue surrounding the nail

■ pediculosis capitis   infestation with head lice

■ plantar wart   a wart on the sole of the foot

■ seborrheic dermatitis   a chronic disease of the skin, characterized by scaling and crusted patches on various body areas, including the scalp

■ sebum   the oily, lubricating secretion of glands in the skin called *sebaceous glands*

■ spoon nail   a thin nail with a concave profile

■ terminal hair   long, coarse, pigmented body hair

■ thecal whitlow   acute inflammation of the tissue surrounding the nail

■ ticks   parasites that bite into tissue and suck blood

■ tinea pedis (athlete's foot)   a fungal infection of the foot

■ vellus   fine, nonpigmented body hair

HAIR

Hair grows on the whole body surface except the palms of the hands, the soles of the feet, the dorsal surfaces of terminal phalanges, and parts of the genitals (the inner surface of the labia and inner surface of the prepuce of the glans penis).

Surface hair is of two types: *vellus,* which is the fine, nonpigmented hair covering large areas of the body, and *terminal hair,* which is longer, coarser, and pigmented. Hair grows at varying rates and is shed at varying times. The scalp of the average person loses between 20 and 100 hairs per day. Body hair is shed in 3 to 4 months, whereas hair in beards lasts 3 or 4 years (Brown et al, 1973, p 39).

The visible part of a hair is called the *hair shaft.* The root is in a tube known as a *hair follicle.* Muscles known as *arrector pili muscles* are attached to the hair follicles. When these contract, the skin assumes a gooseflesh appearance. Sebaceous glands, which secrete *sebum,* grow from the walls of hair follicles. See Figure 12–1. Sebum is produced in greater quantities on the scalp and the face than elsewhere on the body.

Nutrients carried by the bloodstream to the skin and scalp move into the roots of the hair to nourish it. Protein is very important for healthy hair, and a deficiency can result in dullness, loss of color, and reduced growth.

There are many variations of hair color, texture, and growth. Whether an individual's hair is straight, wavy, curly, kinky, or woolly is usually determined by race or heredity.

Developmental Variables

Newborns may have *lanugo* (the fine hair on the body of the fetus, also referred to as *down* or *woolly hair*) over their shoulders, back, and sacrum. This generally disappears, and the hair distribution becomes noticeable on the eyebrows, head, and eyelashes of young children. Some newborns have hair on their scalps; others are free of hair at birth but grow hair over the scalp during the first year of life.

Pubic hair usually appears in early puberty followed in about 6 months by the growth of axillary hair. Boys develop facial hair in later puberty.

In adolescence the sebaceous glands increase in activity as a result of increased hormone levels. As a result, hair follicle openings enlarge to accommodate the increased amount of sebum, and the adolescent's hair may become more oily.

In elderly people the hair is generally thinner, grows more slowly, and loses its color as a result of aging tissues and diminishing circulation. Men often lose their scalp hair and may become completely bald. This phenomenon may occur even when a man is relatively young. The older person's hair also tends to be drier than normal. With age, axillary and pubic hair becomes finer and scanter, in contrast to the eyebrows, which become bristly and coarse. Most women develop hair on their faces, which may be a problem to them.

Common Problems

Among the common problems of scalp hair are extreme dryness and coarseness, due to the application of hair dyes, rinses, or curling or straightening preparations. Such products can also be allergens that produce scalp itches and rashes. Other problems are dandruff, alopecia, lice, ticks, and hirsutism.

Dandruff is a diffuse scaling of the scalp often accompanied by itching. In severe cases it involves the auditory canals and the eyebrows. Mild cases of dandruff can usually be treated effectively with a commercial shampoo specifically for dandruff. In severe or persistent cases, the patient may need the advice of a physician. Infants during the first month of life may develop this crusting of the scalp, which is referred to as *cradle cap*.

Alopecia is a thinning of the hair or a patchy loss, due, for example, to a disease process, such as hypothyroidism, or to radiation and drug therapy for a malignancy.

Lice are parasitic insects that infest mammals. Hundreds of varieties of lice infest humans. Three that are particularly common are *Pediculus humanus* var *capitis* or the head louse, *P humanus* var *corporis* or the body louse, and *Phthirus pubis* or the crab louse.

P humanus var *capitis* is found on the scalp and tends to stay hidden by the hairs; similarly, *P pubis* stays in pubic hair. *P humanus* var *corporis* tends to cling to clothing, so that, when a patient undresses, the lice may not be in evidence on the body; these lice suck blood from the person and lay their eggs (called *nits*) on the clothing. The nurse can suspect their presence in the clothing from three chief symptoms: (a) the person habitually scratches, (b) there are scratches on the skin, and (c) there are hemorrhagic spots on the skin where the lice have sucked blood.

Head and pubic lice lay their eggs on the hairs; the nits look like oval particles, similar to dandruff, clinging to the hair. Bites and pustular eruptions may also be noticed at the hair lines and behind the ears.

Lice are very small, grayish white, and difficult to see. The crab louse in the pubic area has red legs. Lice may be contracted from infested clothes and direct contact with an infested person.

The treatment now used in most areas is gamma benzene hexachloride (Kwell). It comes in cream, lotion, and shampoo forms. For head lice, the hair is washed with the shampoo, and the bed linens are changed. This treatment is repeated 12 to 24 hours later if needed. For pubic and body lice, the patient takes a bath or shower,

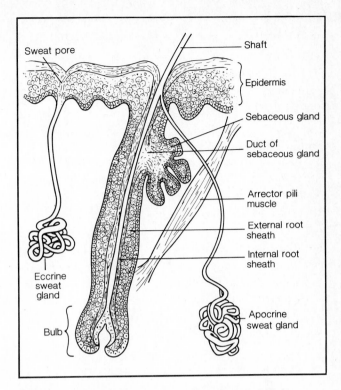

FIGURE 12-1   ■   The anatomic parts of a hair follicle.

dries, and applies the lotion or cream—to the entire body surface for body lice, and to the pubic area and adjacent areas for pubic lice. After 12 to 24 hours, the lotion is washed off, and clean clothing and linens are supplied.

Ticks are small parasites that bite into tissue and suck blood. They take many forms and can adapt to various conditions. The genera *Ornithodoros* and *Dermacentor* are found in North America. They can attach to human beings and are found frequently in the hair. They can be as large as 1.3 cm (0.5 in) and appear gray-brown. They attach to a person with the apparatus by which they suck blood and should not be torn off, because the sucking apparatus will be left in the skin and become infected. If oil is poured on the tick, it loses its hold, because it is deprived of oxygen, and it withdraws its sucker.

Ticks transmit several diseases to people, in particular Rocky Mountain spotted fever and tularemia.

Hirsutism is abnormal hairiness, particularly in women. The cause of excessive body hair is not always known. Elderly women may have some on their faces, and women during menopause may also experience the growth of facial hair. The causes of these conditions may involve the endocrine system. It is also thought that heredity influences both the pattern of hair distribution and the production of androgens by the adrenal glands.

TECHNIQUE 12-1 ■ Brushing and Combing Hair

Hair is normally combed and brushed at least once a day, usually after a bath or morning care. Neat, well-brushed hair usually gives patients a sense of well-being and improves their appearance. Appearance is often particularly important to patients when they have visitors.

For hair care of Black patients, see Technique 12-2.

■ Assessment

See Technique 10-3 on page 169. Assess the patient's personal hygienic practices and learning needs. For example:

1. Young and some older children may need motivation to carry out daily hair care, and the nurse can offer instruction about the importance of it.

2. Adolescents frequently experience oily hair, itchiness, or dandruff and need guidance about methods of control. Skin irritated from oiliness along the scalp line can be cleaned with alcohol. Hair conditioners with oils or petroleum jelly may decrease itchiness and flaking of the scalp but may also produce rashes. Proper fluid and nutrition intake often needs to be encouraged.

3. Elderly persons may need guidance about methods to control dryness of the hair. Often their fluid intake is a factor.

4. Patients who have abnormal alopecia require individual instruction from the nurse, in consultation with their physician, because of the variety of causes of alopecia. A wig is sometimes recomended temporarily until the condition is reversed.

5. Patients with pediculosis and their families need instruction about cleanliness, treatment of infestation, and measures to prevent reinfestation. A public health referral may be necessary, to teach the family how to rid the home of infestation.

6. Parents may need instruction on care of a baby's scalp. See Technique 14-7 on page 346.

■ Nursing Diagnosis

Nursing diagnoses that may indicate the need to brush or comb a patient's hair include:

1. Self-care deficit in grooming related to:
   a. Neuromuscular impairment
   b. Musculoskeletal impairment
   c. Visual disorder
   d. Surgery on upper limb

■ Planning

Nursing goals

1. To stimulate the blood circulation to the scalp through brushing
2. To distribute hair oils and provide a healthy sheen
3. To discover or monitor hair or scalp problems, such as matted hair or dandruff
4. To arrange the hair neatly and attractively

Equipment

1. A clean brush with stiff bristles. These provide the best stimulation to blood circulation in the scalp. The bristles should not be so sharp that they injure the patient's scalp, however. The patient may have a personal brush and comb available.

2. A clean comb with dull, even teeth. A comb with sharp teeth should not be used, because it might injure the scalp. Combs that are too fine can pull and break the hair.

3. Oil, eg, mineral oil, or alcohol to remove mats (optional).

4. A towel to place over the patient's pillow and/or shoulders.

■ Intervention

1. Assist the patient who can sit to move to a chair. Hair is more easily brushed and combed when the patient is in a sitting position. Assist a bed patient to a sitting position by raising the head of the bed, if allowed. Otherwise assist him or her to alternate side-lying positions, and do one side of the head at a time.

2. Place a clean towel over the pillow and the patient's shoulders, if the patient remains in bed. Place it over the sitting patient's shoulders.
   Rationale The towel collects any hair, dirt, and scaly material removed from the head.

3. Remove any pins or ribbons in the hair.

4. For short hair, brush and comb one side at a time. Divide long hair into two sections by parting it down the middle from the front to the back. See Figure 12-2. If the hair is very thick, divide each section into front and back subsections (see Figure 12-3) or into several layers.

5. Holding one section at a time with one hand, brush from the scalp toward the ends. Rotate the wrist in

such a way that the brush massages the scalp. Then comb that section of hair.

Rationale   Massaging stimulates blood circulation in the scalp and thus nourishment of the hair.

6. Brush and comb each section, moving from one side of the head to the other.

7. If the hair is matted or tangled, brush and comb each layer, working from the ends toward the scalp. Mats can usually be pulled apart with fingers or worked out with repeated brushings. If the hair is very tangled, rub alcohol or an oil such as mineral oil on the strands to help loosen the tangles. The hair may then need to be shampooed.

8. Arrange the hair as neatly and attractively as possible, according to the patient's desires. Braiding long hair helps prevent tangles. See Technique 12–3.

9. Record any problems observed, such as excessive dandruff, very dry or very oily hair, or the presence of lice. Daily combing and brushing of hair are not normally recorded.

10. Adjust the nursing care plan as needed to include hygienic learning needs of the patient.

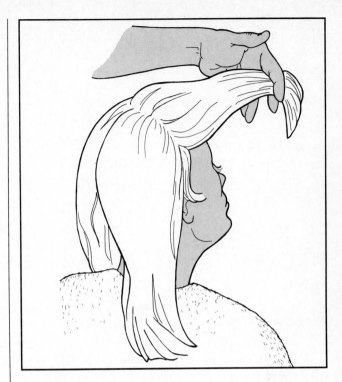

FIGURE 12–3

■ **Evaluation**

Expected outcomes

1. Even hair growth
2. Resilient texture
3. Healthy sheen
4. Absence of mats
5. Absence of dandruff, scalp lesions, or infestations

Unexpected outcomes

1. Hair that is excessively dry or oily
2. Scalp lesions
3. Dandruff
4. Infestation of lice or ticks

Upon observing an unexpected outcome: Report your findings to the responsible nurse and/or physician.

FIGURE 12–2

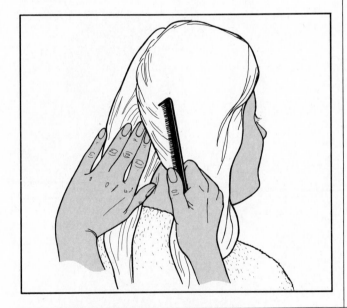

TECHNIQUE 12–2   ■   Hair Care for Black Patients

Black-skinned people often have thicker, drier, curlier hair than white-skinned people. Spiraled or very curly hair usually enters the scalp at a large angle so that the hair stands out from the scalp. Although the shafts of spiraled hair look strong and wiry, they have less strength than straight hair shafts and can be easily broken.

Some Blacks have their spiraled hair straightened. Even if straightened, the hair tends to tangle and mat easily, especially at the back and the sides for bedridden patients. Other Blacks style their hair in cornrows. See Figure 12–4. These cornrows do not have to be unbraided for shampooing and washing. The nurse should obtain the patient's permission before unbraiding such hair.

■ **Assessment**   See Technique 12–1 on page 278.

■ **Nursing Diagnosis**   See Technique 12–1 on page 278.

■ **Planning**

Nursing goals   See Technique 12–1 on page 278.

Equipment

1. A large, open-toothed or long-toothed comb (a pic). The patient may have personal hair care items available.
2. Lubricant (optional) to prevent dryness or loosen tangles. Some Blacks need to oil their hair daily, because it tends to be dry. Oil also prevents the hair strands from breaking and the scalp from becoming too dry.

■ **Intervention**

1. Follow steps 1–3 in Technique 12–1 on page 278.
2. To comb natural (Afro) hairstyles:
   a. Apply a lubricant as the patient indicates or as needed.
   b. Using a large, open-toothed comb, start at the neckline and lift and fluff the hair outward,

moving upward toward the forehead. See Figure 12–5.
   c. Continue fluffing the hair outward and upward until all of the hair is combed on one half of the head. Repeat the procedure for the other half.
3. To remove tangles:
   a. After the hair is lubricated, weave and lift your opened fingers through the hair to ease the tangles free.
      or
   b. Support the hair securely at the base of the scalp, if possible, to prevent pulling and discomfort. Insert a long-toothed comb into the ends of the hair and carefully comb out the ends of the tangles. See Figure 12–6. Repeat this step, each time working the comb farther up the hair shaft toward the scalp, until the hair is untangled.
4. Follow steps 8–10 in Technique 12–1 on page 279.

■ **Evaluation**   See Technique 12–1 on page 279.

FIGURE 12–5

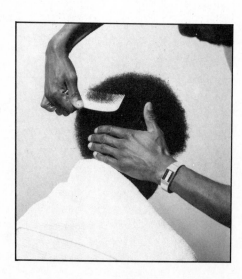

FIGURE 12–4 ■ Black hair styled with cornrow braids.

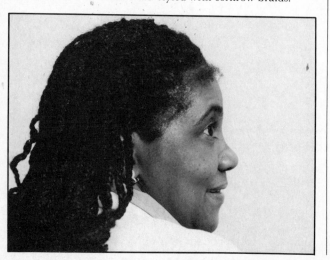

FIGURE 12–6

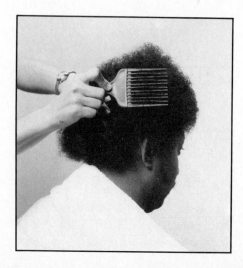

TECHNIQUE 12–3   ■   Braiding Hair

Braiding is a method of entwining hair. For young children who have long hair, two braids can provide a particularly neat and attractive appearance. Before braiding a patient's hair, however, the nurse needs to ascertain that the patient desires a braid or braids. Braids (except cornrows) need to be undone daily, and the hair needs to be brushed and combed.

■ **Assessment**   See Technique 12–1 on page 278.

■ **Nursing Diagnosis**   See Technique 12–1 on page 278.

■ **Planning**

Nursing goals

1. To prevent tangling and matting of hair
2. To maintain a neat appearance

Equipment

1. A brush
2. A comb to divide the hair into sections
3. Ribbon(s) or elastic band(s) to hold the braid(s)
4. A towel to place over the patient's shoulders

■ **Intervention**

1. Assist the patient to a sitting position. If this is not possible, put the patient in alternate side-lying positions, and braid one side of the hair at a time.
2. Place a towel over the patient's pillow and/or shoulders.
   Rationale   The towel collects any hair and debris removed from the hair.
3. Brush and comb the hair to remove any tangles, to stimulate blood circulation to the scalp, to clean the hair, and to assess any problems of the hair or scalp.
4. For one braid, divide the hair into three even sections (strands). For two braids, part the hair down the middle, and then divide one side into three strands.
5. Hold the left strand in the left hand, the center strand by the second finger and thumb of the left hand, and the right strand in the right hand. See Figure 12–7. Hold the strands firmly and tautly, but do not pull.
   Rationale   Pulling can hurt the patient and damage the hair.
6. Lay the right strand (3) over the middle strand (2).

Transfer strand 3 to the left hand and strand 2 to the right hand. See Figure 12–8. Strand 3 is now the middle strand, and strand 2 is the right strand.

FIGURE 12–7

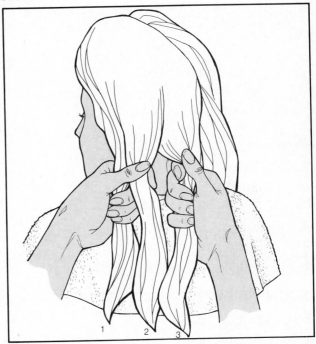

FIGURE 12–8

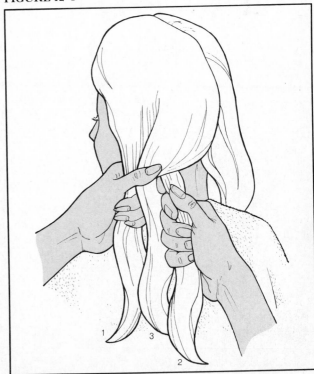

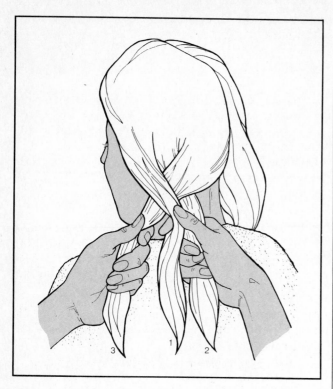

FIGURE 12–9

7. Still holding the strands of hair tautly, cross the left strand (1) over the middle strand (3). See Figure 12–9. Strand 1 is now the middle strand, and strand 3 is the left strand. The left hand holds strand 3, the right fingers hold strand 1, and the right hand holds strand 2.

8. Cross the right strand (2) over the center strand (1). See Figure 12–10. Then cross the left strand (3) over the middle strand (2).

9. Continue crossing the side strands over the center strand, alternating right and left sides until you reach the ends of the strands. See Figure 12–11.

10. When all the hair has been braided, firmly secure the end of the braid with an elastic band or a ribbon so that the strands cannot come undone.

11. Braid the other side of the hair if a second braid is needed.

12. Remove the towel from the patient's shoulders.

13. Record any unusual observations, such as excessive dandruff, very dry or oily hair, or the presence of lice. Braiding hair is not normally recorded.

■ **Evaluation**   See Technique 12–1 on page 279.

FIGURE 12–10

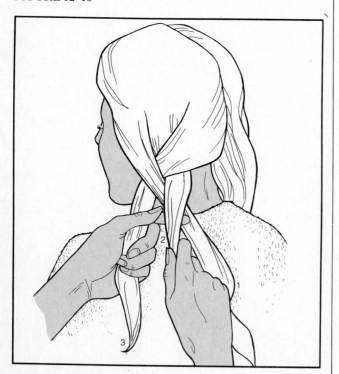

FIGURE 12–11

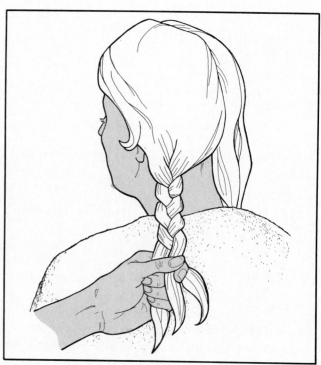

TECHNIQUE 12–4 ■ Shampooing Hair (Bed Patient)

The frequency of shampooing the hair varies considerably among individuals. Many people wash their hair weekly; those who have oily hair may do so more frequently; some shampoo less often than weekly; and a number shampoo daily during a shower.

Patients may shampoo hair in the hospital by several methods, depending on their health, strength, and age. The patient who is well enough to take a shower can conveniently shampoo while in the shower. The patient who is unable to shower may be given a shampoo while sitting on a chair in front of a sink. The back-lying patient who can move to a stretcher can be given a shampoo on a stretcher wheeled to a sink. The patient who must remain in bed can be given a shampoo with water brought to the bedside. This is the least convenient method, but it does provide a shampoo for the patient who is confined to bed.

■ Assessment

See Technique 12–1 on page 278. Other data include:

1. The agency's policies about providing shampoos for bed patients. Some hospitals require a physician's order before a shampoo can be given by nursing personnel.
2. Whether a medicated shampoo is to be used; if so, confirm that it is available.
3. The level of activity appropriate for the patient. This will indicate whether the shampoo must be given in bed or can be given on a stretcher.
4. The best time of day for the shampoo. Discuss this with the patient. A patient who must remain in bed may find the shampoo tiring. Choose a time when the patient is rested and can rest after the procedure.

■ Nursing Diagnosis   See Technique 12–1 on page 278.

■ Planning

Nursing goals

1. To clean the hair
2. To stimulate the blood circulation to the scalp through massage
3. To destroy organisms such as head lice through application of a medicated shampoo

Equipment

1. A comb and a brush.

2. A shampoo basin to catch the water and direct it to the washbasin or other receptacle. Shampoo basins are usually made of plastic or metal. If one is not available, a plastic drawsheet can be rolled up on three sides to make edges about 7 cm (3 in) high. These edges will guide the water to the receptacle, in which the unrolled fourth edge of the sheet is placed.
3. A receptacle for the shampoo water. A pail or a large washbasin can be used. If possible, the receptacle should be large enough to hold all the shampoo water, so that it does not have to be emptied during the shampoo.
4. A pitcher of water. The water should be 40.5 °C (105 °F) for an adult or child to be comfortable and not injure the scalp.
5. A bath thermometer to measure the temperature of the water.
6. Two bath towels.
7. A plastic sheet or pad to protect the bedclothes.
8. A bath blanket to cover the upper part of the patient for warmth.
9. A washcloth or pad to put under the patient's neck.
10. A liquid or cream shampoo. Usually the patient will supply this. If the shampoo is being given to destroy lice, the physician will order the shampoo to be used.
11. A hair dryer.

Arrange the equipment at the bedside for convenient access throughout the procedure.

■ Intervention

1. Assist the patient to the side of the bed from which you will work.
2. Remove pins and ribbons from the patient's hair, and brush and comb the hair to remove any tangles.
3. Remove the pillow from under the patient's head, and place it under the patient's shoulders.
   Rationale   This hyperextends the patient's neck.
4. Put the plastic sheet or pad on the bed under the patient's head.
   Rationale   The plastic keeps the bedding dry.
5. Tuck a bath towel around the patient's shoulders.
   Rationale   The towel keeps the shoulders dry.
6. Place the shampoo basin under the patient's head, putting a folded washcloth or pad where the patient's neck rests on the edge of the basin. If the

patient is on a stretcher, the neck can rest on the edge of the sink with the washcloth as padding.

Rationale Padding supports the muscles of the neck and prevents undue strain and discomfort.

7. Fanfold the top bedding down to the patient's waist, and cover the upper part of the patient with the bath blanket.

Rationale The folded bedding will stay dry, and the bath blanket, which can be discarded after the shampoo, will keep the patient warm.

8. Place the receiving receptacle on a table or chair at the bedside. Put the spout of the shampoo basin over the receptacle.

9. Place a damp washcloth over the patient's eyes. See Figure 12–12.

Rationale The washcloth protects the patient's eyes from soapy water. A damp washcloth will not slip.

10. Place cotton fluffs in the patient's ears if indicated.

Rationale These keep water from collecting in the ear canals.

11. Wet the patient's hair thoroughly with the water.

12. Apply shampoo to the scalp. Make a good lather with the shampoo while massaging the scalp with

the pads of your fingertips. Massage all areas of the scalp systematically, eg, starting at the front and working toward the back of the head.

Rationale Massaging stimulates the blood circulation in the scalp. The pads of the fingers are used so that the fingernails will not scratch the scalp.

13. Rinse the hair briefly, and apply shampoo again.

14. Make a good lather and massage the scalp as before.

15. Rinse the hair thoroughly this time to remove all the shampoo.

Rationale Shampoo remaining in the hair may dry and irritate the hair and scalp.

16. Squeeze as much water as possible out of the hair with your hands.

17. Rub the patient's head with a heavy towel.

18. Remove the shampoo equipment from the bed, and assist the bed patient to a comfortable position.

19. Dry the hair with the dryer.

20. Arrange the hair using a clean brush and comb.

21. If the patient is very tired, arrange for an undisturbed rest period.

22. Record the shampoo and any notable observations on the patient's record. Report problems noted to the responsible nurse.

Sample Recording

Date	Time	Notes
6/2/86	1300	Shampoo given. Abrasion 2.5 cm long on right occipital area. Area appears pink with some bluish discoloration surrounding it. Dr. King notified. White scaly area on left temporal area 4 cm in diameter. ———— Kim L. Krueger, SN

23. Adjust the nursing care plan as needed to include hygienic learning needs of the patient.

■ **Evaluation** See Technique 12–1 on page 279.

FIGURE 12–12

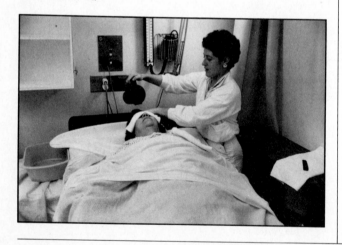

NAILS

The fingernails and toenails are epidermal appendages. Like the hair, they are directly related to the epidermis; they are made of epidermal cells that have been changed to keratin. Today the nails have little functional value except for cosmetic purposes. Nails usually grow regularly, about 1 mm per week, but this growth may stop at times of severe stress or illness. See the discussion of Beau's line on page 286. The nail itself is surrounded by a cuticle,

which tends to grow over the nail and thus regularly requires pushing back. A lost fingernail takes 3½ to 5½ months to regenerate, and a toenail takes 6 to 8 months.

Developmental Variables

Nails are normally present at birth. They continue to grow throughout life, and they change very little until people are old. At that time the nails tend to be tougher, more brittle, and in some cases thicker. The nails of an elderly person will normally grow less quickly than those of a younger person, and they may be ridged and have grooves.

Common Problems

Common problems of nails are hangnails, paronychia, ingrown toenails, and broken nails. Regular nail care can help to prevent these problems. Less common problems are changes in nail plate shape or curvature, changes in texture or thickness, and changes in color.

Hangnails are shreds of epidermal tissue at either side of the nail. A regular schedule of rubbing oil into the tissue around the nails will lubricate the tissue and prevent hangnails. When a hangnail develops and is not infected, it can be either carefully flattened and held in place with collodion or clipped off. Antiseptic should be applied to the area after clipping.

Paronychia is an inflammation of the tissue surrounding the nail. Acute paronychia is called *thecal whitlow;* it is a painful red swelling that develops quickly. It usually follows a hangnail or injury. This condition occurs most frequently in people who have their hands in water a great deal, and it is three times more common in patients who have diabetes. Careful manicuring that does not injure the adjacent soft tissue helps to prevent it.

Incurvated nails (ingrown toenails) are a relatively common condition. The lateral margin of the toenail grows into surrounding soft tissue and produces an inflammatory reaction of the lateral skin fold. The symptoms are pain with walking and when pressure is put on the nail, tenderness, and redness if inflammation has started in the soft tissues. The usual treatment is to remove the part of the nail that has curved into the tissue and to clear any debris and callus tissue in the area. The nail groove is then packed in such a way that the nail will grow forward rather than into the soft tissue. Any secondary infection is generally treated with an antibiotic ointment or powder.

Changes in nail plate shape include clubbing, spoon-shaped nails, and claw nails. *Clubbing* is a reversible proliferation, softening, and loosening of the soft tissues around the nails, which results in an increase in the angle between the nail and the nail bed. The normal angle is slightly less than 180°, giving the nail a nearly straight profile. See Figure 12–13, *A*. In early clubbing, the angle straightens to 180° (see Figure 12–13, *B*); in late clubbing, it increases to more than 180° (see Figure 12–13, *C*). Clubbing usually starts in the thumbs and index fingers and progresses to the remaining fingers and toes. It is generally associated with a long-term lack of oxygen, cardiopulmonary diseases such as emphysema, chronic obstructive lung disease, and congenital heart disease with cyanosis; it may be inherited. When the cause is eliminated, the process is reversible.

Spoon-shaped nails are those in which the lateral edges turn upward, the nail plate is thin, and the nail has a concave profile. See Figure 12–14. This condition is often associated with prolonged iron-deficiency anemia. *Claw nails* are elongated nails that curve over the end of the digit. Because of the difficulty of cutting such nails and the danger of infection, the nurse needs to refer these patients to a podiatrist.

Changes in thickness or texture include hypertrophy, atrophy, and Beau's line. Nail *hypertrophy* (increased

FIGURE 12–13   ■   A, A normal nail showing the convex shape and less than 180° angle; **B,** early clubbing; **C,** late clubbing.

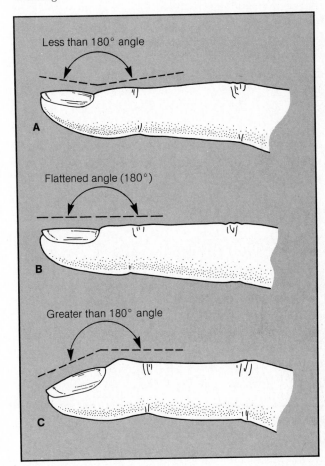

FIGURE 12–14   ■ A spoon-shaped nail.

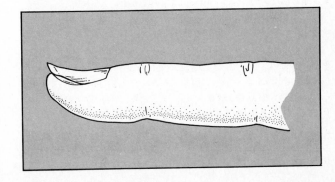

thickness) may be associated with ischemia or chronic fungal infection. Nail *atrophy* (decreased thickness) is often associated with nutritional anemias. *Beau's line* is a transverse white line or groove on the nail that occurs as a result of severe stress or acute illness. Nail growth stops temporarily due to impaired keratin synthesis, and a deep line becomes visible across the nail. See Figure 12–15.

Nail plate color changes may or may not be a problem. See Table 10–6 for normal nail bed colors. Splinter hemorrhages (red or brown longitudinal streaks in the nail) are generally insignificant and may occur with minor trauma or no apparent cause. Striated or streaked white spots, commonly referred to as fortune or love spots, are often of no major concern. Handling certain metals and other substances may cause color changes. Gold produces a brownish black discoloration; silver, a slate-blue one; and tobacco, a yellowish brown one.

Beneath the translucent nail plate, the status of circulation to the extremities can be assessed in the nail bed. Nail bed color acquires a bluish tinge (cyanosis) with a lack of oxygen, instead of its normal pink. The nail beds are one of the first areas of the body where cyanosis is detected. The status of circulation to the extremities can also be determined by checking the rate of capillary refill. See the blanch test discussed in Table 10–6 on page 171.

FIGURE 12–15 ■ A nail with Beau's line.

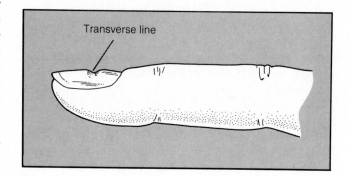

Transverse line

TECHNIQUE 12–5 ■ Cleaning and Trimming Nails

Daily nail care is part of the personal hygiene of most people. Nails are usually cleaned at the time of a bath and filed or cut when they become long. While most patients can attend to their own nail care, the elderly, the very young, the confused, and the blind may require assistance. Often patients enjoy nail care and feel better when it has been done. Some people may require the services of a podiatrist (a specialist in foot care) for nail care.

■ **Assessment**

See Technique 10–4 on page 170. Assess the patient's personal hygienic practices and learning needs. For example:

1. Parents of a newborn may need to learn about infant nail care. The nails are rarely cut during the first few days of life. As the nails become long, and the infant suffers scratches, the parents need to trim the nails. They are cut straight across, using small, blunt scissors. Nails are most readily cut when the infant is sleeping. If cutting is done when the baby is awake, someone else needs to hold the baby. A toothpick protected by absorbent cotton can be used to clean under the baby's nails.

2. School-age children and their parents may need advice on developing nail hygiene habits. Children need to be given a manicure set as soon as they are able to use it. Frequent praise for well-kept hands can motivate youngsters to learn and maintain nail hygiene.

3. Nurses may offer individual counseling about nail biting. This habit is often an indication of nervous tension; it may be learned behavior in a child who imitates a parent with the habit.

4. Patients who have diabetes or circulatory impairments need to be taught safe methods of cutting and filing their nails, particularly their toenails. Prevention of ingrown toenails and injury to the tissues around the nails is of utmost importance to them. See the Intervention and Technique 12–6.

5. Nurses may offer advice on prevention and treatment of hangnails.

6. Nail care can present a challenge to the elderly. Their vision may be impaired, making self-care difficult, or their nails may be too hard or thick to trim easily. The nurse can suggest methods to assist each individual, such as using correct equipment, and may refer some patients to a podiatrist.

Other data include:

1. Whether the patient has diabetes mellitus or impaired circulation to any extremities. These conditions predispose people to infections of the tissues

surrounding the nails, and special precautions are indicated to prevent infection.

2. Whether the patient is scheduled for a general anesthetic or surgical procedure. If so, the patient's nails need to be free of nail polish, so that the nail beds can be observed during the procedure. Impaired oxygen in the body may be reflected by a bluish tinge to the nail beds. A pinkish tinge (or the patient's normal color) indicates adequate oxygen.

■ Nursing Diagnosis

Nursing diagnoses that may indicate the need to clean and trim a patient's nails include:

1. Self-care deficit: grooming, related to:
   a. Impaired vision
   b. Impaired coordination
2. Potential for infection around the nail bed related to vascular disturbance or diabetes

■ Planning

Nursing goals

1. To prevent infections around the nails
2. To improve the patient's appearance and sense of well-being

Equipment

1. A nail cutter or a pair of sharp scissors. Nail cutters are usually used. A file can be used, but it generally takes longer.
2. A nail file or emery board to shape the corners of the nails. Some files have a pointed end, which can be used to clean under the nails.
3. An orange stick to clean under the nails, if a file is not used, and to push back the cuticle.
4. Hand lotion, mineral oil, or petroleum jelly to lubricate the tissues around the nails if they appear to be dry.
5. Polish remover to remove polish, if necessary.
6. A washbasin and water at 40.5 °C (105 °F) to soak the feet or hands, if necessary. The thick, hard nails of the elderly may require softening in warm water before trimming.
7. A plastic sheet to place under the soak basin to catch spilled water, if the toenails need to be soaked while the patient is in bed.
8. A towel to dry the feet or hands if they are to be soaked.
9. A bath blanket to cover the bed patient if the toenails are to be soaked.

■ Intervention

1. Determine agency policy regarding nail care for patients with impaired circulation to the extremities or diabetes mellitus. Some agencies require a physician's order to cut the nails of these patients.
2. Assist the ambulatory patient to a sitting position in a chair or the bed patient to a reclining position with the head of the bed elevated.
3. Remove nail polish, if the patient wishes. If the patient is scheduled for anesthesia, remove colored nail polish. Some agencies permit patients to wear clear nail polish.
   Rationale   Colored nail polish obscures the view of the nail bed so that blood circulation (oxygen) to the extremities cannot be observed.
4. Soak the patient's hands and/or feet in a basin of warm water if the nails are very thick and hard. The toenails of an elderly person are likely to require soaking, and this can be done while you attend to the patient's fingernails.
5. Dry the hand or the foot that has been soaking.
6. Starting with the thumb or large toe, cut or file straight across the nail (see Figure 12–16) beyond the end of the finger or toe. If the patient has diabetes or circulatory problems, file, rather than cut, the nails.
   Rationale   Trimming is done straight across, not down the sides, because of the danger of injuring the tissue around the nail. Filing further reduces the risk of tissue injury for susceptible patients.
7. Shape the fingernail with a file, rounding the corners. Toenails are not shaped because of the danger of damaging the tissues or causing a toenail to grow into the tissues.

FIGURE 12–16

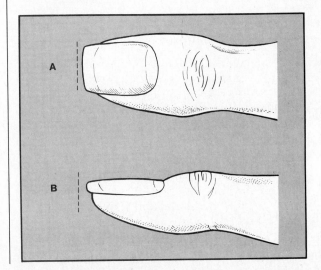

8. Clean under the nail, working from one side to the other, using the pointed end of the file or an orange stick.

9. Proceed to the next finger or toe, and repeat steps 6–8 for all nails.

10. Massage lotion onto the hands and feet, giving particular attention to the cuticles around the nails.
    Rationale Lotion lubricates the cuticles and thus helps to prevent tearing.

11. Gently push the cuticle back around the base of the nail, using the orange stick or a special cuticle tool. Take care not to tear or injure the cuticle, because this could become the site of an infection.

12. Record any abnormalities observed, such as an infected cuticle or inflammation of the tissue around the nail. Daily nail care is not normally recorded.

Sample Recording

Date	Time	Notes
1/14/87	0800	Toenails cut. Reddened swollen area at base of nail on left 2nd toe. States it is tender and feels hot. — Wendy J. Lum, SN

13. Adjust the nursing care plan to include checking the patient's nails daily if indicated. This is usually done during the bath or morning care.

■ Evaluation

Expected outcomes

1. Nails that are smooth to the touch, convex in shape, and have pink nail beds

2. Intact cuticles and surrounding tissues

3. Quick return of nail bed color after the blanch test

Unexpected outcomes

1. Inflammation around the nail

2. Painful ingrown toenails

3. Slow return of nail bed color

4. Clubbing or spoon-shaped nails

Upon observing an unexpected outcome: Report your findings to the responsible nurse.

FEET

The feet are essential for ambulation and merit attention even when patients are confined to bed. Each foot contains 26 bones, 107 ligaments, and 19 muscles. These structures function together for both standing and walking.

During childhood, the bones and small muscles of the feet are easily damaged by tight, binding stockings and ill-fitting shoes. For normal development, it is important that the arches be supported and that the bony structure and the feet grow with no external restrictions.

Developmental Variations

At birth a baby's foot is relatively unformed. The arches are supported by fatty pads and do not take their full shape until 5 or 6 years of age. Feet are not fully grown until about age 20. Healthy feet remain relatively unchanged during life. However, the elderly often require special attention for their feet. Reduced blood supply, accompanying arteriosclerosis, for example, can make a foot prone to infection following trauma.

Common Problems

Foot problems that produce considerable discomfort are commonly observed. Among these are calluses, corns, unpleasant odors, plantar warts, fissures between the toes, fungus infections such as athlete's foot, and deviations in toe contour.

Epidermal problems

A *callus* is a thickened portion of epidermis, a mass of keratotic material. It is flat and usually found on the bottom or side of the foot over a bony prominence. Calluses are usually caused by pressure from shoes. They can be softened by soaking the area in warm water with Epsom salts, and they can be removed by an abrasive substance such as a pumice stone. Creams with lanolin can also be used to keep the skin soft and prevent the formation of calluses.

A *corn* is a keratosis caused by friction and pressure from a shoe. It commonly occurs on a toe, usually the fourth or fifth toe, and usually on a bony prominence such as a joint. Corns are usually conical (circular and raised). The base is the surface of the corn and the apex is in deeper tissues, sometimes even attached to bone. Corns are generally removed surgically. They are prevented from reforming by relieving the pressure on the area and massaging the tissue to promote circulation.

Unpleasant odors occur as a result of perspiration and its interaction with microorganisms. Regular and frequent washing of the feet and wearing clean hosiery help to minimize odor. Foot powders and deodorants also help to prevent this problem.

Plantar warts appear on the sole of the foot. These warts are caused by the virus *papovavirus hominis.* They are moderately contagious. The warts are frequently painful and often make walking difficult. The treatment ordered by a physician may be curettage, freezing with solid carbon dioxide several times, or repeated applications of salicylic acid.

Fissures between the toes occur frequently as a result of dryness and cracking of the skin. The treatment of choice is good foot hygiene and application of an antiseptic to prevent infection. Often a small piece of gauze is inserted between the toes in applying the antiseptic and left in place to assist healing by allowing air to reach the area.

Athlete's foot or *tinea pedis* (ringworm of the foot) is caused by a fungus. The symptoms are scaling and cracking of the skin, particularly between the toes. Sometimes small blisters form, containing a thin fluid. In severe cases the lesions may also appear on other parts of the body, particularly the hands. Treatments vary from potassium permanganate soaks, using a 1:8,000 solution, to commercial antifungal ointments or powders. Prevention is important. Common preventive measures are: keeping the feet well ventilated, wearing clean socks or stockings, and not going barefoot in public showers.

Toe contour deviations

Common deviations in toe contour include hallux valgus and hammer toe. *Hallux valgus* (bunion) is a lateral deviation of the big toe at its metatarsophalangeal joint, with enlargement and development of a bursa or callus over the area, which constitutes the bunion. See Figure 12–17, *A.* If the deviation is severe, the great toe may overlap the second toe. Displacement may cause the second toe to develop hammer toe. A familial tendency toward hallux valgus is apparent, and it is more common in females than in males. Contributing causes include poorly fitted shoes, flat feet, and degenerative arthritic changes. Conservative treatment consists of well-fitted shoes that have a wide forefoot and use of bunion pads to relieve shoe pressure. A severe, painful bursitis may require incising and applying hot, moist compresses or surgical correction. Intraarticular injections of corticosteroids may be given if there is osteoarthritic joint involvement.

Hammer toe is characterized by hyperextension of the metatarsophalangeal joint, flexion of the proximal interphalangeal joint, and hyperextension of the distal interphalangeal joint. See Figure 12–17, *B.* The second toe is most frequently involved, often bilaterally, and it may be associated with hallux valgus. Painful calluses often develop over the proximal interphalangeal joint. Hammer toes may be congenital, linked to a familial

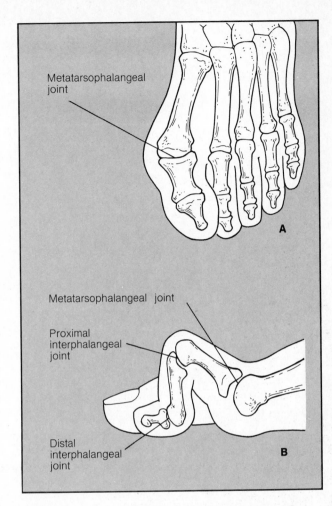

FIGURE 12–17   ■   Toe deviations: **A,** hallux valgus; **B,** hammer toe.

tendency, or acquired. If acquired, they are caused most frequently by poorly fitted shoes that force the involved toe into a flexion deformity. Conservative treatment for hammer toe includes passive stretching exercises and well-fitted shoes, perhaps with padding and inserts to decrease pressure over the proximal interphalangeal joint. Surgical manipulation of the joint into extension and splinting is sometimes necessary.

TECHNIQUE 12–6 ■ Foot Care

Foot care is of particular importance when the patient has an infection or abrasion, diabetes mellitus, or impaired circulation to the extremities. The latter two conditions predispose patients to infections. These patients need to learn proper foot care to prevent problems. Other patients normally care for their own feet. After determining a patient's personal foot care practices, the nurse can identify the patient's learning needs. Foot care is usually provided in conjunction with the patient's bed bath but can be provided at any time, as the patient desires.

■ Assessment

To assess the feet:

1. Inspect each foot for cleanliness, odor, dryness, inflammation, swelling, and abrasions or lesions.
2. Inspect the status of the toenails.
3. Inspect toe contour.
4. Inspect the longitudinal foot arch.
5. Inspect the foot alignment.
6. Assess the patient's ability to perform range-of-motion exercises.
7. Palpate the skin for temperature.
8. Palpate the foot for areas of tenderness and nodules.
9. Palpate the ankle for edema.
10. Palpate the dorsalis pedis pulse.

See Table 12–1. Additional data include:

1. Whether the patient has diabetes mellitus or circulatory disease.
2. Whether the patient has complaints of foot discomfort. If so, determine its onset and location.

■ Nursing Diagnosis

Nursing diagnoses that may indicate the need to provide foot care or instruction include:

1. Altered skin integrity related to:
   a. Corns
   b. Fissures
   c. Plantar wart
   d. Athlete's foot
   e. Ingrown toenail
2. Impaired physical mobility related to:
   a. Painful ingrown toenail
   b. Painful plantar wart
   c. Painful corn
3. Actual or potential altered peripheral tissue perfusion related to:
   a. Diabetes
   b. Inhibited arterial blood flow
   c. Inhibited venous blood flow

■ Planning

Nursing goals

1. To maintain the skin integrity of the feet
2. To prevent foot infections
3. To prevent foot odors
4. To maintain foot function

Equipment

1. A washbasin
2. Soap
3. A washcloth
4. Towels
5. A moisture-resistant disposable pad
6. Lotion
7. Toenail cleaning and trimming equipment (see Technique 12–5 on page 287)

■ Intervention

1. Fill the washbasin with water at 40 °C (105 °F).
   Rationale Warm water promotes circulation, is comforting, and is refreshing.
2. Assist the ambulatory patient to a sitting position in a chair or the bed patient to a supine or semi-Fowler's position.
3. Place a pillow under the bed patient's knees.
   Rationale The pillow provides support and prevents muscle fatigue.
4. Place the washbasin on the moisture-resistant pad at the foot of the bed for a bed patient or on the floor in front of the chair for an ambulatory patient.
5. For a bed patient, pad the rim of the washbasin with a towel.
   Rationale The towel prevents undue pressure on the skin.
6. Place one of the patient's feet in the basin.

TABLE 12–1   ■   Assessing the Feet

Nursing history: Determine presence of diabetes mellitus or peripheral circulatory disease; foot discomfort and its onset and location; and any perceived problems with foot mobility.

Physical assessment	Data	Method	Normal findings	Abnormal findings
Inspection	1. Skin surfaces, for cleanliness, odor, dryness, inflammation, swelling, abrasions or other lesions	Carefully check all skin surfaces, paying particular attention to areas between toes	Intact skin Absence of swelling or inflammation	Excessive dryness Areas of inflammation or swelling, eg, corns, calluses Fissures Scaling and cracking of skin, eg, athlete's foot Plantar warts
	2. Status of toenails	See Technique 10–4 on page 170		
	3. Toe contour	Observe toe profile	Toes are extended (straight and flat)	Bunion (hallux valgus) Hammer toe Claw toe
	4. Longitudinal foot arch	Observe medial foot profile when patient is standing	Presence of medial longitudinal arch, ie, medial concavity, with prominent heel and ball of foot	Flat foot (pes planus) High arch (pes cavus)
	5. Foot alignment	Observe alignment of foot to ankle and tibia, and metatarsal alignment (alignment of forefoot to heel)	Foot in straight alignment	Toeing-in (pes varus) Toeing-out (pes valgus) Abduction of forefoot (metatarsus varus) Adduction of forefoot (metatarsus valgus) Clubfoot
	6. Ability of feet to stand, walk, and perform range-of-motion exercises with each ankle and set of toes	See Technique 19–1 on page 440	Full range of motion	Deformity (eg, foot drop) Impaired range-of-motion in ankle or toes
Palpation	7. Areas of tenderness on body or muscular structures or on plantar surface	Palpate bony and muscular structures of foot and plantar surface to locate points of tenderness	Absence of tenderness and nodules Smooth, firm, fleshy plantar surface	Tenderness in certain areas, related to arthritic changes, muscle strain, or lesions such as plantar warts or bunions
	8. Ankle edema	Palpate anterior and posterior surfaces of ankle	No swelling	Swelling or pitting edema
	9. Circulatory status	Palpate dorsalis pedis pulse on dorsal surface of foot just above longitudinal arch Compare skin temperatures of two feet	Strong, regular pulses in both feet Warm skin temperature	Weak or absent pulses Cool skin temperature in one or both feet

7. Allow the patient's foot to soak for at least 10 minutes. Rewarm the water as needed.
Rationale Soaking softens the skin and nails and loosens debris under the toenails.

8. Wash the foot with soap, and rinse it. Rub callused areas of the foot with the washcloth.
Rationale Friction created by rubbing removes dead skin layers.

9. Remove the foot from the basin and place it on the towel.

10. Blot the foot gently with the towel to dry it thoroughly, particularly between the toes.
   Rationale Harsh rubbing can damage the skin. Thorough drying reduces the risk of infection.

11. Apply lotion to the foot.
   Rationale Lotion moistens dry skin.

12. Assess the foot for any problems.

13. Empty the washbasin, refill it with water, and soak and clean the other foot.

14. While the second foot is soaking, clean and trim the toenails of the first foot (see Technique 12–5), if agency policy permits. In many agencies, toenail trimming is contraindicated for patients with diabetes mellitus, toe infections, and peripheral vascular disease, unless performed by a podiatrist or physician.

15. Record any foot problems observed. Foot care is not generally recorded unless problems are noted.

16. Instruct the patient with diabetes mellitus or peripheral vascular disease about appropriate foot care. Many foot problems can be prevented by having the patient follow simple guidelines:

   a. Wash the feet daily, and dry them well, especially between the toes.

   b. Use creams or lotions to moisten the skin or soak the feet in warm water with Epsom salts to avoid excessive drying of the skin of the feet. Lotion will also soften calluses, which can then be removed with an abrasive such as pumice stone. An effective lotion for reducing dryness is a mixture of lanolin and mineral oil.

   c. To prevent or control an unpleasant odor due to excessive perspiration on the feet, wash them frequently and change socks and shoes at least daily. Special deodorant sprays are also helpful.

   d. File the toenails rather than cutting them to avoid skin injury. File the nails straight across the ends of the toes. If the nails are too thick or misshapen to file, consult a podiatrist.

   e. Check the water temperature before immersing the feet, to prevent burns.

   f. Wear clean stockings or socks daily. Avoid socks with holes or darns that can cause pressure areas.

   g. Wear correctly fitting shoes that neither restrict the foot nor rub on any area; rubbing can cause corns and calluses. For the elderly, an oxford or slip-on style that has a flexible nonskid sole is advised with 2.5 to 5 cm (1 to 2 in) heels. Check worn shoes for rough spots in the lining. Break in new shoes gradually by increasing the wearing time 30 to 60 minutes each day.

   h. Avoid walking barefoot, since injury and infection may result. Wear slippers in public showers and change areas, to avoid contracting common infections such as athlete's foot.

   i. Avoid wearing constricting garments such as knee-high elastic stockings or garters, or sitting with the legs crossed at the knees, which may decrease circulation.

   j. When the feet are cold, use extra blankets and wear warm socks rather than using heating pads or hot water bottles, which may cause burns.

   k. Exercise the feet daily to promote circulation. Point the feet upward, point them downward, and make circles with the feet several times throughout the day.

   l. When washing, check the skin of the feet for breaks or red or swollen areas.

   m. Wash any cut on the foot thoroughly, apply a mild antiseptic, and notify the physician.

   n. Avoid self-treatment for corns or calluses. Pumice stones and some callus and corn applications are injurious to the skin. Consult a podiatrist.

■ Evaluation

Expected outcomes

1. Intact skin
2. Toes are extended
3. Presence of medial longitudinal arch
4. Foot in straight alignment
5. Full range of motion of ankles and toes

Unexpected outcomes

1. Excessive skin dryness
2. Presence of inflammation or swelling
3. Presence of bunion or hammer toe
4. Flat foot
5. Drop foot
6. Tenderness in joints

Upon obtaining an unexpected outcome: Report your findings to the responsible nurse.

References

Bates B: *A Guide to Physical Examination,* 3rd ed. Lippincott, 1983.

Block GJ, Nolan JW, Dempsey MK: *Health Assessment for Professional Nursing: A Developmental Approach.* Appleton-Century-Crofts, 1981.

Bowers AC, Thompson JM: *Clinical Manual of Health Assessment.* Mosby, 1984.

Brown MS et al: Physical examination, part 3: Examining the skin. *Nursing 73* (September) 1973; 3:39–43.

Burns KR, Johnson PJ: *Health Assessment in Clinical Practice.* Prentice-Hall, 1980.

Carpenito LJ: *Nursing Diagnosis: Application to Clinical Practice.* Lippincott, 1983.

Hilt NE, Cogburn SB: *Manual of Orthopaedics.* Mosby, 1980.

Kim MJ, McFarland GK, McLane AM: *Classification of Nursing Diagnoses: Proceedings of the Fifth National Conference.* Mosby, 1984.

Kim MJ, McFarland GK, McLane AM: *Pocket Guide to Nursing Diagnoses.* Mosby, 1984.

Malasanos L et al: *Health Assessment,* 2nd ed. 1981.

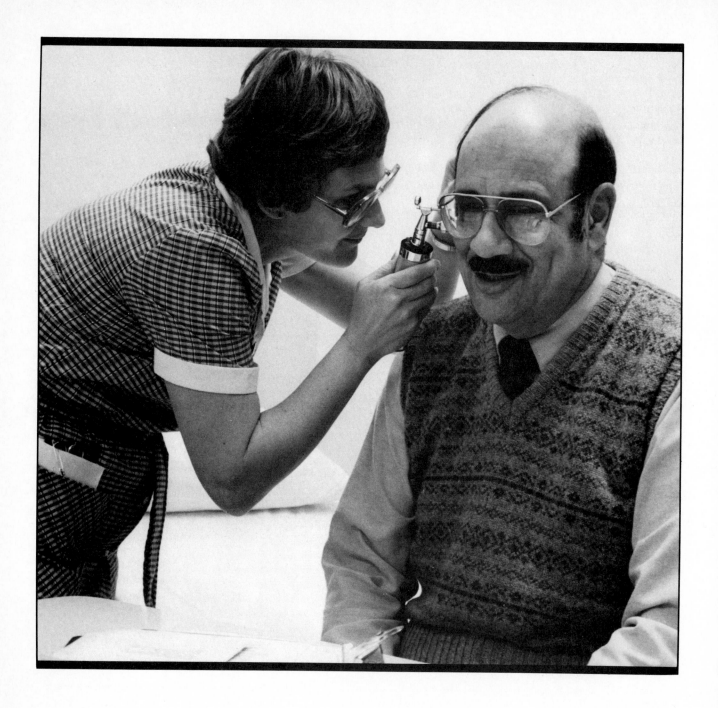

THE MOUTH, EYES, AND EARS

13

This chapter deals with hygiene practices and techniques for the mouth, eyes, and ears. Good oral hygiene is essential for comfort and oral health. Regular brushing and flossing of the teeth need to be stressed for patients who can do their own mouth care. For patients who are unconscious or unable to use their hands, the nurse must provide adequate mouth care.

Eye and ear care is required less than mouth care. However, patients who wear glasses, contact lenses, or hearing aids often require help with and care for these aids.

Chapter Outline

Mouth
- Technique 13–1 Brushing and Flossing Teeth
- Technique 13–2 Cleaning Artificial Dentures
- Technique 13–3 Providing Special Oral Care

Eyes
- Technique 13–4 Removing Contact Lenses (Hard and Soft)
- Technique 13–5 Cleaning Contact Lenses (Hard and Soft)

- Technique 13–6 Inserting Contact Lenses (Hard and Soft)
- Technique 13–7 Removing, Cleaning, and Inserting an Artificial Eye

Ears
- Technique 13–8 Removing, Cleaning, and Inserting a Hearing Aid

Objectives

Upon completion of this chapter, the student will:

1. Know essential terms and facts about the mouth, eyes, and ears
   1.1 Define selected terms
   1.2 Identify selected human structures
   1.3 Identify the function of each structure
   1.4 Identify variations in the mouth, eyes, and ears from infancy to old age
   1.5 Identify common problems of the mouth, eyes, and ears
2. Understand facts about techniques used to assist patients with care of the mouth, eyes, and ears
   2.1 Identify relevant assessment data
   2.2 Identify nursing diagnoses for which the technique may be implemented
   2.3 Identify nursing goals related to the technique
   2.4 Identify expected and unexpected outcomes from assessment data
   2.5 Identify reasons underlying selected steps of the techniques
3. Perform techniques related to mouth, eyes, and ears safely

   3.1 Assess the patient adequately
   3.2 Collect additional data from appropriate sources
   3.3 Select pertinent nursing goals for the patient
   3.4 Establish relevant outcome criteria for the patient following the technique
   3.5 Collect necessary equipment before the technique
   3.6 Implement interventions to enhance the effectiveness of the technique and enhance the patient's comfort and safety
   3.7 Communicate relevant information about the patient to the appropriate persons
   3.8 Determine the evaluative outcomes of the technique
4. Evaluate own performance of specific techniques in a laboratory or clinical setting with the assistance of another
   4.1 Use the performance checklists provided
   4.2 Identify areas of strength and weakness
   4.3 Alter performance in response to own evaluation and that of another

Terms

- anthelix   the anterior curve on the upper aspect of the ear
- astigmatism   a visual refractive error due to differences in curvature of the cornea and the lens
- auricle   the visible part of the ear
- buccal mucosa   the mucous membrane lining the inner surface of the cheeks
- bulbar conjunctiva   the mucous membrane over the eyeball
- canthus   the angular junction of the eyelids at each corner of the eyes
- cataract   an opacity of the lens of the eye

- cementum   calcified tissue covering the root of a tooth
- cerumen   the waxlike substance secreted by glands in the external ear canal
- cochlea   a seashell-shaped structure located in the inner ear; it has numerous apertures for passage of the cochlear division of the auditory nerve
- conjunctiva   the membrane covering the eyelids and eyeball
- conjunctivitis   inflammation of the membrane covering the eyelids and eyeball

■ cornea   a transparent convex avascular structure forming the anterior surface of the eyeball

■ crown (of tooth)   the exposed part of a tooth outside the gum

■ dacryocystitis   inflammation of the lacrimal sac

■ dentifrice   a paste or powder used to clean or polish the teeth

■ dentin   the chief substance of teeth, forming the body, neck, and roots; it is covered by enamel

■ dentures   a natural or artificial set of teeth; usually the term designates artificial teeth

■ emmetropia   normal refraction so that the eyes focus images on the retina

■ enamel (of tooth)   the covering over the crown of the tooth

■ eustachian tube   a channel lined with mucous membrane that connects the middle ear and the nasopharynx; it acts as an air pressure stabilizer

■ external auditory meatus   the entrance to the ear canal

■ frenulum   a midline fold connecting the undersurface of the tongue to the floor of the mouth

■ gingiva   the gum

■ gingivitis   acute or chronic inflammation of the gums

■ glaucoma   an eye disease characterized by increased intraocular pressure, which causes damage to the retina and optic nerve and blindness if left untreated

■ glossitis   inflammation of the tongue

■ halitosis   an unpleasant odor of the breath

■ helix   the posterior curve on the upper aspect of the ear

■ hordeolum (sty)   an inflammation of one or more sebaceous glands of the eyelid

■ hyperopia   farsightedness; abnormal refraction in which light rays focus behind the retina

■ incus   an anvil-shaped ossicle of the middle ear; it communicates sound waves from the malleus to the stapes

■ iris   the colored part of the eye perforated by the pupil

■ iritis   inflammation of the iris

■ lacrimal canal   a passageway from the innermost corner of the eye to the lacrimal sac

■ lacrimal duct   a small passageway from the lacrimal gland draining the tears onto the conjunctiva at the upper outer corner of the eye

■ lacrimal gland   the organ that lies over the upper outer corner of the eye and secretes tears

■ lacrimal sac   a pouchlike structure located in a groove in the lacrimal bone between the inner corner of the eye and the bridge of the nose

■ lobule (of the ear)   earlobe

■ malleus   a hammer-shaped ossicle of the middle ear; it is connected to the tympanic membrane and transmits sound waves to the incus

■ mastication   the act of chewing

■ mastoid   breast shaped; the bony prominence of the temporal bone behind the ear

■ myopia   nearsightedness; abnormal refraction in which light rays focus in front of the retina

■ nasolacrimal duct   the channel between the lacrimal sac and the nose

■ ossicles   the bones of sound transmission in the middle ear

■ otitis externa   inflammation of the external ear canal

■ otitis media   inflammation of the middle ear

■ palate   the roof of the mouth

■ palpebral conjunctiva   the mucous membrane lining the eyelids

■ parotitis   inflammation of the parotid salivary gland

■ periodontal disease   a general term for a number of inflammatory and degenerative diseases that affect the supporting structures of the mouth

■ photophobia   abnormal intolerance to light

■ pinna   see auricle

■ presbyopia   impaired vision, usually farsightedness, as a result of loss of elasticity of the lens due to aging

■ pulp cavity   the cavity in the central part of the crown of a tooth that contains pulp

■ punctum   an extremely small point or spot; the opening into the lacrimal canal

■ pyorrhea   purulent periodontal disease

■ retina   the innermost of three coverings of the eyeball

■ sclera   a tough white covering over about 75% of the eye; it is continuous with the cornea anteriorly and with the external sheath of the optic nerve posteriorly

■ semicircular canals   passages shaped like half circles in the inner ear that control the sense of balance by the effect of fluid moving against hairlike nerves

■ serous otitis   inflammation of the eustachian tube

■ sordes   the accumulation of foul matter (food, microorganisms, and epithelial elements) on the teeth and gums

■ stapes   a stirrup-shaped ossicle of the middle ear; it communicates sound waves from the incus to the internal ear

■ stomatitis   inflammation of the oral mucous membrane

■ strabismus   crossed eyes; squint

■ sulcular technique   a technique of brushing the teeth under the gingival margins; it is also referred to as the Bass method

- **sulcus**   the groove between the surface of the tooth and the gum
- **tragus**   a cartilaginous protrusion at the entrance to the ear canal

- **tympanic membrane**   the eardrum
- **uvula**   a fleshy mass suspended at the midline and back of the palate
- **vestibule (ear)**   a cavity at the entrance to the ear

MOUTH

Mucous membrane, which is continuous with the skin, lines the digestive, urinary, reproductive, and respiratory tracts and the conjunctiva of the eye. It is an epithelial tissue, and it forms mucus, concentrates bile, and secretes or excretes enzymes, for example, in the digestive tract. It serves four general functions:

1. Protection
2. Support for associated structures
3. Absorption of nutrients into the body (in the digestive tract)
4. Secretion of mucus, enzymes, and salts

The mouth (oral cavity) is bordered by the lips anteriorly, the cheeks laterally, and the pharynx posteriorly. The cheeks contain several accessory muscles of *mastication* (chewing), which keep food from escaping the masticating motions of the teeth. The tongue, containing numerous taste buds, extends from the floor of the mouth and is attached to it by a fold of mucous membrane called the *frenulum.* The tongue helps to mix saliva, keeps food pressed between the teeth for chewing, and pushes food into the pharynx for swallowing. The *palate* (roof of the mouth) has two parts: the anterior portion (hard palate) and the posterior portion (soft palate), which ends in a free projection called the *uvula* that marks the opening of the mouth into the pharynx.

The mouth contains two sets of *dentures* (teeth), which are discussed under Developmental Variables. Teeth are necessary to masticate food, so that it can be swallowed and digested in the stomach. Each tooth has a number of parts: the crown, the root, and the pulp cavity. The *crown* is the exposed part of the tooth, which is outside the gum. It is covered with a hard substance called *enamel.* The internal part of the crown below the enamel is ivory colored and is referred to as *dentin.* See Figure 13–1. The *root* of a tooth is embedded in the jaw, and it is covered by a bony tissue called *cementum.* The *pulp cavity* in the center of the tooth contains the blood vessels and nerves.

Assessment of the mouth is covered in chapter 10.

Developmental Variables

Teeth usually appear 5 to 8 months after birth. By the time children are 2 years old, they usually have all 20 of their temporary teeth. See Figure 13–2. At about age 6 or 7, children start losing their deciduous teeth, and these are gradually replaced by the 32 permanent teeth. See Figure 13–3. By age 25, most people have all their permanent teeth.

The incidence of periodontal disease increases during pregnancy, since an increase in female hormones affects gingival tissue and increases its reaction to bacterial plaque. Many pregnant women manifest increased bleeding from the gingival sulcus during brushing and increased redness and swelling of the gums. These gingival changes heighten the pregnant woman's chances of acquiring periodontal disease (Martin, Reeb, 1982, p 391).

Adults of advanced years may have very few permanent teeth left, and many have dentures. Most elderly people have lost all their own teeth by age 70, mainly because of periodontal disease rather than dental caries; however, caries are also common in the middle-aged adult. Preventive dental care is important.

Some receding of the gums and a brownish pigmentation of the gums occur with age. Because saliva production decreases with age, dryness of the oral mucosa is a common finding in older people. A dry mouth can be aggravated by poor fluid intake, heavy smoking, alcohol, high salt intake, anxiety, and many medications. Medica-

FIGURE 13–1 ■ The anatomic parts of a tooth.

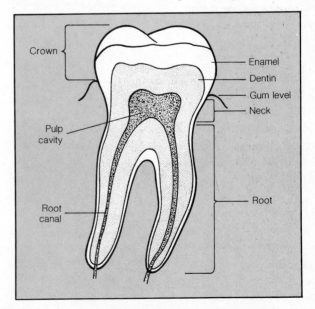

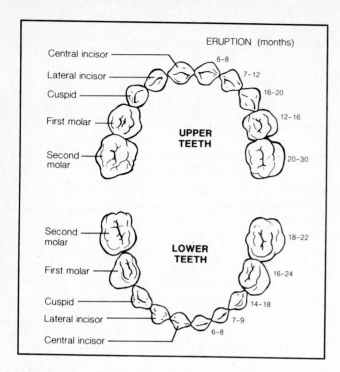

FIGURE 13–2 ■ Temporary teeth and their times of eruption (stated in months).

FIGURE 13–3 ■ Permanent teeth and their times of eruption (stated in years).

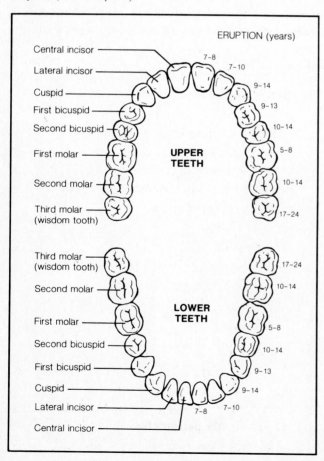

tions that can cause a dry mouth, in addition to the effect for which they are prescribed, include diuretics, laxatives if used excessively, all major tranquilizers (eg, chlorpromazine), some minor tranquilizers (eg, Valium, Librium), some antidepressants (eg, Elavil, Tofranil), some antihypertensives (eg, Arfonad, Inversine), some antispasmodics (eg, Pro-Banthine), and antihistamines used in cold and cough remedies and in analgesics (Todd, 1982, p 122).

Common Problems

Dental caries and periodontal disease are the two problems that most frequently affect the teeth. Periodontal disease (pyorrhea) is characterized by red, swollen gingiva and bleeding. Inflammation of the gums is referred to as *gingivitis*. Another common problem is *halitosis*, which may be caused by poor oral hygiene or a disease process.

Other problems nurses may see in hospitalized patients are *glossitis*, *stomatitis*, and *parotitis*. The accumulation of foul matter (food, microorganisms, and epithelial elements) on the teeth and gums is *sordes*. See also Table 10–9 on page 180.

Oral Hygiene

Good oral hygiene includes daily stimulation of the gums, mechanical scrubbing of the teeth, and flushing of the mouth. Checkups by a dentist every 6 months are also recommended. The nurse is often in a position to help people, young or old, ill or well, to maintain oral hygiene by helping or teaching them to carry out oral practices, by inspecting whether hygiene has been carried out, particularly with children, or by actually providing hygienic measures for patients who are ill or incapacitated. The nurse can also be instrumental in identifying and referring problems that require the services of a dentist.

Teaching situations regarding oral hygienic practices

Oral hygienic practices include brushing teeth or cleaning dentures, flossing teeth, and the use of fluoride. When assessing a patient's practices, the nurse determines the frequency of cleaning and the methods used. Examples of learning needs are:

1. In areas where the water is not fluoridated, nurses may recommend fluoride supplements to parents for their children. Supplements can be started in the first month of a baby's life. If given regularly, they help to prevent but do not necessarily eliminate tooth decay. The supplements need to be taken while the teeth are being formed, that is, from birth to about 14 years of age. Prescriptions are no longer required. It is important to take only the recommended amount and to take it with water, milk, or juice. Recommended dosages are:

- Under 1 year, 2 drops daily
- 1–4 years, 4 drops daily
- 4–8 years, 6 drops daily
- Over 8 years, 8 drops or 1 tablet

2. Parents may need guidance when their baby starts teething at about 6 to 8 months of age. Teething is often accompanied by sore gums, drooling, and fretfulness. Teething babies want to put everything into their mouths, so their safety needs to be monitored. To relieve the baby's sore gums, parents can offer rubber or plastic toys, teething rings, and teething biscuits to chew on. Slightly chilled strained or chopped fruit can also make the mouth feel better. Teething powders or syrups should be avoided unless prescribed by a physician. If the baby becomes too fretful and feverish, the physician should be consulted about a soothing medication that will relieve the gum irritation.

3. The act of brushing teeth needs to be shown to children as soon as their teeth appear. Until the child can manipulate the toothbrush effectively, parents need to help the child brush after each meal and before going to bed.

4. A child's first visit to the dentist should occur at about age 2½ or 3, so that the child becomes used to going to a dentist, preventive measures such as topical fluoride applications can be started, and any defects can be corrected. Primary teeth can decay very rapidly. Dental examinations are needed every 6 months.

5. Patients of all ages may need reinforcement to practice good oral hygiene to prevent dental caries and periodontal disease. The following measures combat tooth decay:

   a. Brush the teeth thoroughly after meals and at bedtime. Assist children or inspect their mouths to be sure the teeth are clean.

   b. Floss the teeth daily.

   c. Ensure an adequate intake of nutrients, particularly calcium, phosphorus, vitamins A, C, and D, and fluoride.

   d. Avoid sweet foods and drinks between meals. Take them in moderation at meals.

   e. Eat coarse, fibrous foods (cleansing foods), such as fresh fruits and raw vegetables.

   f. Take a fluoride supplement daily until age 14 or 16 unless the drinking water is fluoridated.

   g. Have topical fluoride applications as prescribed by the dentist.

   h. Have a checkup by a dentist every 6 months.

TECHNIQUE 13–1   ■   Brushing and Flossing Teeth

Brushing and flossing teeth are integral parts of oral hygiene. Normally people need to brush their teeth at least twice per day and after meals if possible. This removes food particles caught between the teeth and helps prevent tooth decay. While most people carry out these functions independently, the very young, the elderly, and the very ill often require a nurse's assistance.

Patients who must remain in bed need varying degrees of assistance from the nurse, ranging from obtaining water in a cup to brushing the teeth for the patient. Children start to brush their teeth at about 2 years of age when all deciduous teeth have appeared.

Flossing can be done in conjunction with brushing teeth or independently. It is important to employ medical asepsis before and after flossing, to prevent the transmission of microorganisms into and out of the mouth.

■ Assessment   See Technique 10–6 on page 178.

■ Nursing Diagnosis

Examples of nursing diagnoses that may indicate the need to brush and floss a patient's teeth include:

1. Self-care deficit (oral hygiene) related to:
   a. Neuromuscular impairment
   b. Musculoskeletal disorder
   c. Visual disorder
   d. Surgical procedure
2. Alterations in health maintenance related to:
   a. Loss of independence
   b. Lack of knowledge
   c. Inadequate health practices
   d. Lack of supervision (children, elderly)

■ Planning

Nursing goals

1. To remove food particles from around and between the teeth
2. To remove dental plaque
3. To enhance the patient's feelings of well-being
4. To prevent sordes and infection of the oral tissues

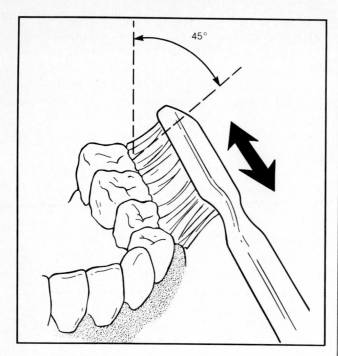

FIGURE 13–4

Equipment

Many patients have these supplies at the bedside; if not, they can be assembled by the nurse.

1. A dentifrice. Most patients have a flavor preference and have their own dentifrice. For the patient who does not have dentifrice and cannot purchase any, a mixture of table salt and baking soda can be used.

2. A curved basin that fits snugly under the patient's chin, such as a kidney basin, to receive the rinse water. A patient who can brush and floss teeth at a sink does not require a basin.

3. A toothbrush. Small toothbrushes are available for children. A soft toothbrush is recommended when using the sulcular technique of cleaning, described in the Intervention, step 5.

4. A cup of tepid water.

5. A towel to protect the patient and the bedclothes.

6. Dental floss, at least two pieces 20 cm (8 in) in length. Waxed floss is less likely to fray than unwaxed floss; particles between the teeth attach more readily to unwaxed floss than to waxed floss. Some believe that waxed floss leaves a residue on the teeth and that plaque then adheres to the wax (Gannon, Kadezabek, 1980, p 16).

7. A floss holder (optional)

8. A mouthwash to rinse the mouth after brushing the teeth. Normally a slightly antiseptic solution is used. Most patients have their own commercial mouthwash. Some hospitals supply a standard mouthwash.

The National Formulary lists the official mouthwash as a preparation of potassium, bicarbonate, sodium borate, thymol, eucalyptol, methyl salicylate, amaranth solution, alcohol, glycerin, and purified water. A mouth rinse of normal saline or diluted hydrogen peroxide can be an effective cleaner and moisturizer.

■ Intervention

1. Assist the patient to a sitting position in bed, if this is permitted. If the patient cannot sit, assist him or her to a side-lying position with the head on a pillow so that the patient can spit out the rinse water.

2. Place the towel under the patient's chin.

3. Moisten the bristles of the toothbrush with tepid water, and apply the dentifrice.
   Rationale Hot water softens the brushes.

4. Place or hold the curved basin under the patient's chin, fitting the small curve around the chin or neck.

5. Hand the toothbrush to the patient, or brush the patient's teeth as follows:

   a. Hold the brush against the teeth with the bristles at a 45° angle. See Figure 13–4. The tips of the outer bristles should rest against and penetrate under the gingival sulcus. See Figure 13–5. The brush will clean under the sulcus of two or three teeth at one time.
   Rationale This sulcular technique removes plaque and cleans under the gingival margins.

   b. Move the bristles back and forth using a vibrating or jiggling motion, from the sulcus to the crowns of the teeth.

   c. Repeat until all outer and inner surfaces of the teeth and sulci of the gums are cleaned.

   d. Clean the biting surfaces by moving the brush back and forth over them in short strokes. See Figure 13–6.

FIGURE 13–5

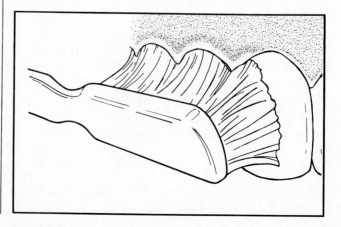

e. If the tongue is coated, brush it gently with the toothbrush.

   Rationale Brushing removes accumulated materials and coatings. A coated tongue may be caused by poor oral hygiene and low fluid intake. Brushing gently and carefully prevents the patient from gagging or vomiting.

6. Hand the patient the water cup or mouthwash to rinse the mouth vigorously. Have the patient spit the water and excess dentifrice into the basin.

   Rationale Vigorous rinsing loosens food particles and washes out already loosened particles.

7. Repeat step 6 until the patient's mouth is free of dentifrice and food particles.

8. Remove the curved basin, and help the patient wipe his or her mouth.

9. Wash your hands before putting them inside the patient's mouth, or assist the patient to wash hands before commencing to floss independently.

10. Wrap one end of floss around the third finger of each hand. See Figure 13–7.

11. To floss the upper teeth, use your thumb and index finger to stretch the floss. See Figure 13–8. Move the floss up and down between the teeth from the tops of the crowns to the gum and along the gum lines as far as possible. Make a "C" with the floss around the tooth edge being flossed. Start at the back on the right side and work around to the back of the left side, or work from the center teeth to the back of the jaw on either side.

12. To floss the lower teeth, use your index fingers to stretch the floss. See Figure 13–9.

13. Give the patient tepid water or mouthwash to rinse the mouth and a curved basin in which to spit the water.

14. Remove the curved basin and assist the patient to wipe his or her mouth.

15. Record any problems of the teeth, tongue, gums, and

FIGURE 13-6

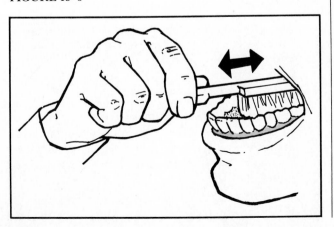

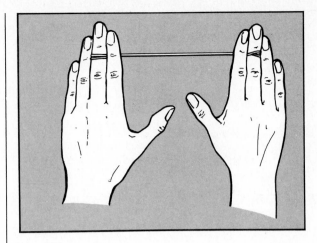

FIGURE 13–7

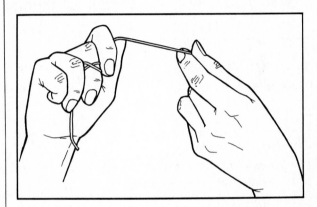

FIGURE 13–8

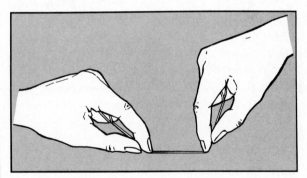

FIGURE 13–9

oral mucosa, such as sordes or inflammation and swelling of the gums. Brushing and flossing teeth are not usually recorded.

■ Evaluation

Expected outcomes

1. Oral mucosa is moist, smooth, and a uniform pink color (or has a brown freckled pigmentation in Blacks).

2. Patient has 32 adult teeth or dentures.

3. Tooth enamel is smooth and white.

4. Gums are moist, firm in texture, and pink (or has bluish or dark patches in Blacks).

5. Tongue is moist, is slightly rough, has thin whitish coating, and is pink (or has some brown pigmentation on tongue borders in Blacks).

Unexpected outcomes

1. Oral mucosa is pale, dry, has white patches, or has ulcerations.

2. Teeth are missing.

3. Teeth have dental caries or discolored enamel.

4. Gums are excessively red, spongy, tender, bleeding, swollen, or receded.

5. Tongue is dry, furry, smooth and red, or ulcerated.

Upon observing an unexpected outcome: Report your findings to the responsible nurse and/or physician.

TECHNIQUE 13-2 ■ Cleaning Artificial Dentures

Some patients have artificial teeth in the form of a plate—a complete set of teeth for one jaw. A person may have a lower plate for the lower jaw and/or an upper plate for the upper jaw. When only a few artificial teeth are needed, the patient is given a bridge, rather than a plate. Artificial teeth are fitted to the individual and cannot be used by another person.

Most patients prefer privacy when they take their artificial teeth out to clean them. Many do not like to be seen without their teeth; one of the first requests of postoperative patients is often, "May I have my teeth in, please?"

Like natural teeth, artificial dentures collect microorganisms and food. They need to be cleaned regularly, at least once a day. They can be removed from the mouth, scrubbed with a toothbrush, rinsed, and reinserted. Some people use a dentifrice, while others use commercial cleaning compounds for plates.

■ Assessment

See Technique 10–6 on page 178. In addition:

1. Note particularly any areas on the mucous membranes irritated by friction from the dentures.

2. Observe the dentures for any rough or sharp areas that could irritate the tongue or mucous membrane.

■ Nursing Diagnosis   See Technique 13–1 on page 299.

■ Planning

Nursing goals

1. To remove food particles and microorganisms from artificial teeth

2. To prevent infection of the oral tissues

3. To enhance the patient's feeling of well-being

Equipment

1. A denture container, such as a small basin or plastic cup, in which to carry the dentures

2. A toothbrush or stiff-bristled brush to scrub the dentures

3. A dentifrice or denture cleaner

4. Tepid water to wash and rinse the dentures

5. A clean washcloth to place in the sink

6. A container of mouthwash for the patient to use while the dentures are removed

7. A curved basin, such as a kidney basin, to receive the mouthwash after use

8. A towel with which the patient can wipe hands and mouth

9. A tissue or piece of gauze to remove the dentures

■ Intervention

1. Assist the patient to a sitting or side-lying position so that the patient can spit out mouthwash readily without swallowing it.

To remove dentures

2. If the patient cannot remove the dentures, use a tissue or a piece of gauze to grasp the upper plate at the front teeth with your thumb and second finger, and move the denture up and down slightly. See Figure 13–10.

   Rationale The slight movement breaks the suction that holds the plate on the roof of the mouth. The tissue prevents the transfer of microorganisms from the dentures to the nurse's hand.

3. Lower the upper plate, move it out of the mouth, and place it in the denture container.

4. Lift the lower plate, turning it so that the left side, for example, is slightly lower than the right, to remove the plate from the mouth without stretching the lips. Place the lower plate in the denture container.

5. Remove a partial denture by exerting equal pressure on the border of each side of the denture, not on the clasps, which can bend or break.

6. Take the denture container to a sink. Take care not to drop the dentures because they may break. Place a washcloth in the bowl of the sink.

   Rationale A washcloth prevents damage to the dentures if the nurse drops them.

To clean dentures

7. Using a toothbrush or special stiff-bristled brush, scrub the dentures with the cleaning agent and tepid water.

   Rationale Hot water is not used because heat will change the shape of some dentures.

8. Brush the outer surfaces using short, back-and-forth strokes.

9. Brush the inner surfaces of the upper and lower front teeth with the brush placed vertically.

10. Brush back and forth over the inner surfaces of the teeth and the roof of the top plate, holding the brush horizontally.

11. Brush back and forth over the biting surface.

12. Rinse the dentures with tepid running water.

    Rationale Rinsing removes the cleaning agent and food particles.

13. If the dentures are stained, soak them in a commercial cleaner. Be sure to follow the manufacturer's directions. To prevent corrosion, dentures with metal parts should not be soaked overnight. Home substitutes for commercial cleaner are the following mixtures:

    a. 5 to 10 ml (1 to 2 tsp) white vinegar and 240 ml (1 cup) warm water.

       or

    b. 5 ml (1 tsp) chlorine bleach, 10 ml (2 tsp) water softener, and 240 ml (1 cup) warm water. It is essential to mix water softener with the bleach to prevent denture corrosion (Gannon, Kadezabek, 1980, p 19).

14. Observe the dentures for any rough, sharp, or worn areas that could irritate the tongue or mucous membranes of the mouth or lips.

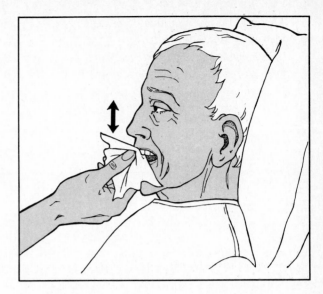

FIGURE 13–10

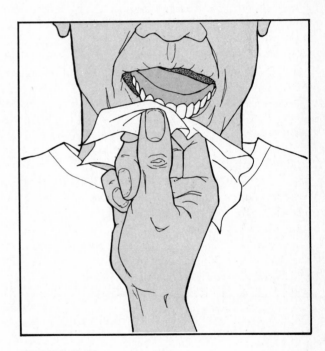

FIGURE 13–11

15. Assess the mouth for any redness, irritated areas, or indications of infection.

16. Return the dentures to the patient. Before inserting them, offer the patient some mouthwash and a curved basin to rinse the mouth. If the patient cannot insert the dentures independently, insert the plates one at a time. Hold each plate at a slight angle while inserting it, to avoid injuring the lips. See Figure 13–11.

17. Assist the patient to wipe hands and mouth with the towel.

18. If the patient does not want to or cannot wear the dentures, store them in a denture container with

water. Label the cup with the patient's name and identification number.

19. Record any problems observed, such as an irritated area on the mucous membranes of the mouth, and report them to the responsible nurse. Cleaning dentures is not normally recorded.

■ **Evaluation**   See Technique 13–1 on page 301.

TECHNIQUE 13–3 ■ Providing Special Oral Care

It may be necessary to clean a patient's oral mucosa and tongue, in addition to cleaning the teeth, if the patient is unconscious or has excessive dryness, sordes, or irritations of the mouth. Agency practices differ in regard to special mouth care and the frequency with which it is provided. Depending on the state of the patient's mouth, special care may be needed every two to eight hours. This technique focuses on oral care for the unconscious patient but may be adapted for conscious patients who are seriously ill or have mouth problems.

Mouth care for unconscious patients is very important, since their mouths tend to become dry and consequently predisposed to infections. Dryness occurs because:

1. The patient cannot take fluids by mouth.
2. The patient often is breathing through the mouth.
3. The patient may be receiving oxygen, which tends to dry the mucous membranes.

The dentures of unconscious patients are normally kept in water in a denture cup labeled with the patient's name and identification number, in the bedside table drawer. In some agencies, dentures are soaked in a commercially prepared solution. The dentures are always cleaned before they are put into the denture cup.

■ **Assessment**   See Technique 10–6 on page 178.

■ **Nursing Diagnosis**   See Technique 13–1 on page 299.

■ **Planning**

Nursing goals

1. To maintain the continuity of the lips, tongue, and mucous membranes of the mouth
2. To prevent oral infections
3. To clean and moisten the membranes of the mouth and lips

Equipment

1. Dentifrice or denture cleaner.
2. A toothbrush.
3. A cup of tepid water.
4. A curved basin, such as a kidney basin.
5. A towel.
6. Mouthwash.
7. A denture container for the patient with dentures.
8. A tissue or piece of gauze to remove dentures.
9. Applicators and cleaning solution for cleaning the mucous membranes. Commercially prepared applicators of lemon juice and oil can be used. If these are not available, a gauze square rolled around the index finger and dipped into lemon juice and oil or into mouthwash solution will usually suffice. Applicator swabs or tongue blades covered with gauze may also be used. Mineral oil is generally contraindicated, because if it is aspirated it can initiate an infection (lipid pneumonia).
10. A rubber-tipped bulb syringe to apply the rinse solution to the mouth.
11. Petroleum jelly (Vaseline) or cold cream to lubricate the lips.
12. A cleaning agent such as hydrogen peroxide for use prior to the lemon juice and oil, if necessary. This agent is effective in removing encrustations that coat the tongue. It should be diluted with water. See Intervention, step 8.
13. A bite-block to hold the mouth open and teeth apart (optional).

Position the equipment on the bedside table within easy reach.

■ **Intervention**

1. Position the unconscious patient on his or her side with the head of the bed lowered, so that the saliva formed in the mouth automatically runs out by

gravity rather than being aspirated into the lungs. This position is the one of choice for the unconscious patient receiving mouth care. If the patient's head cannot be lowered, turn it to one side so that fluid will readily run out of the mouth or pool in the side of the mouth where it can be suctioned.

2. Place the towel under the patient's chin.

   Rationale The towel protects the patient and the bedclothes.

3. Place the curved basin against the patient's chin and lower cheek to receive the fluid from the mouth. See Figure 13–12.

4. If the patient has natural teeth, brush the teeth as in Technique 13–1 on page 300. Brush gently and carefully to avoid injuring the gums. If the patient has artificial teeth, clean them as in Technique 13–2 on page 302.

5. Rinse the patient's mouth by drawing about 10 ml (3 oz) of water or mouthwash into the syringe and injecting it gently into each side of the mouth.

   Rationale If the solution is injected with force, some of it may flow down the patient's throat and be aspirated into the lungs.

6. Watch carefully to make sure that all the rinsing solution has run out of the mouth into the basin. If not, suction the fluid from the mouth. See Technique 37–1 on page 885.

   Rationale Fluid remaining in the mouth may be aspirated into the lungs.

7. Repeat the rinsing until the mouth is free of dentifrice, if used.

8. Inspect the patient's mouth. If the tissues appear dry or unclean, clean them with the applicators or gauze and cleaning solution. If hydrogen peroxide is used, dilute it 1:1 with water, and rinse it thoroughly from the patient's mouth before applying oil and lemon juice.

   Rationale The gums and mucosa can become spongy from prolonged action of hydrogen peroxide.

9. Picking up one oil applicator, wipe the mucous membrane of one cheek. In the absence of commercially prepared applicators, wrap a small gauze square around your index finger, and moisten it with oil and lemon solution. Discard the applicator or gauze in a waste container, and with a fresh one clean the next area. Clean in an orderly manner moving around the mouth, using a fresh applicator or gauze once the previous one becomes soiled or dry.

   Rationale Using separate applicators for each area of the mouth prevents the transfer of microorganisms from one area to another.

10. Clean all the mouth tissues—the cheeks, roof of the mouth, base of the mouth, and tongue. Observe the tissues closely for inflammation and dryness.

11. Rinse the patient's mouth, repeating steps 5–7.

12. Remove the basin, and dry the patient's mouth with the towel. Replace artificial dentures if indicated.

13. Lubricate the patient's lips with petroleum jelly or cold cream.

    Rationale Lubrication prevents cracking and subsequent infection.

14. Record special oral hygiene and pertinent observations. Report problems to the responsible nurse.

Sample Recording

Date	Time	Notes
4/7/87	1500	Special mouth care using oil and lemon q.1h. Outer aspect of lower right gum remains reddened and swollen. ———————————— Sally R. Nolan, SN

15. Establish a plan for the frequency of special mouth care and any specific methods to be used. Record this on the patient's nursing care plan.

■ **Evaluation** See Technique 13–1 on page 301.

FIGURE 13–12

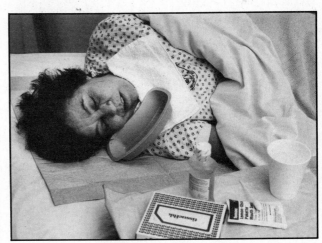

EYES

The eyes are extremely important organs, but they require no special care in daily living. The lacrimal glands, situated in a depression in the frontal bone at the upper outer angle of the eye orbit, produce lacrimal fluid, which continually washes the eyes. See Figure 13-13. This fluid drains through the lacrimal ducts onto the conjunctiva at the upper outer corner of the eye and then through lacrimal canaliculi (canals) to the lacrimal sac, which is situated in the inner canthus. From the lacrimal sac the fluid drains through the nasolacrimal duct to the inferior meatus of the nose. The fluid keeps the eyeball moist and helps wash away foreign particles. Excessive lacrimal fluid forms tears.

The anterior colored portion of the eye (iris) is covered by the cornea, which joins the sclera or white of the eye. See Figure 13-14. The sclera forms the support for the eyeball; it extends posteriorly to cover about 75% of the eyeball. The cornea acts to refract the light rays entering the eye. The iris, which is also located on the anterior eye, regulates the amount of light permitted through the pupil.

Developmental Variables

Visual abilities are present at birth; the newborn can follow large moving objects, is attracted to black–white contrast, can fixate on certain stimuli for 4–10 seconds, and can react to changes in the intensity of light. The pupils of the newborn respond slowly, however, and the eyes cannot focus on close objects. By 3 months of age, vision has developed so that the eyes are coordinated both horizontally and vertically. By 4 months, the infant recognizes familiar objects and follows moving objects. At 6 years of age, visual acuity is comparable to that of an adult. Preschool children are generally farsighted until their eyes grow in length and become *emmetropic* (refracting normally and focusing objects on the retina).

Loss of visual acuity occurs in elderly people as the lens of the eye ages, becomes more opaque, and loses elasticity. Other changes include loss of ability of the iris to accommodate in darkness and dim light, loss of peripheral vision, and difficulty in distinguishing similar colors.

Common Problems

In children, *strabismus* is the most common congenital problem. The muscles of the two eyes are not coordinated, and, when the child has one eye directed straight ahead, the other eye may be directed inward, outward, or upward. The eyes appear crossed. Eyeglasses may be used to correct strabismus; in some cases, surgery is performed on the eye muscles.

Eyeglasses and contact lenses are worn by many children and adults to correct common refractive errors of the lens of the eye. These errors include *myopia* (nearsightedness), *hyperopia* (farsightedness), and *presbyopia* (loss of elasticity of the lens and thus loss of ability to accommodate to close objects). Presbyopia begins at about 45 years of age. People notice that they have

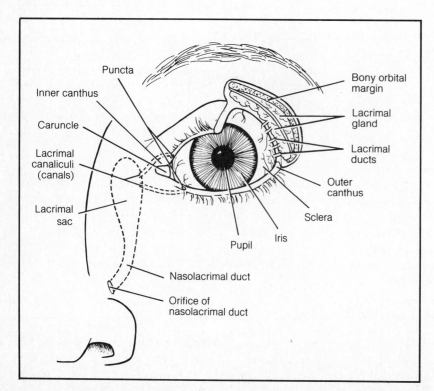

FIGURE 13–13 ■ The left eye showing the external structures and the lacrimal apparatus.

FIGURE 13–14 ■ Anatomic structures of the right eye, lateral view.

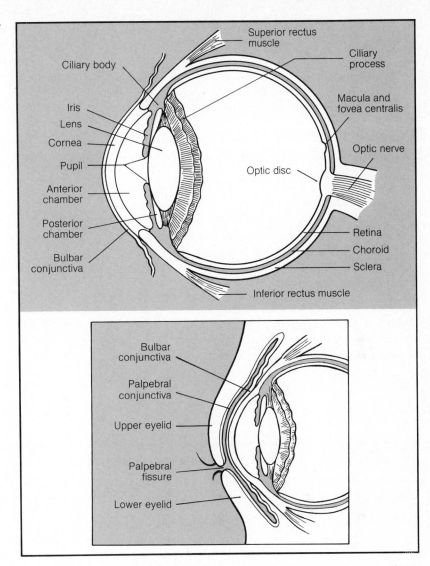

difficulty reading newsprint. Often two corrective lenses (bifocals) are required—one for near vision or reading, and the other for far vision.

Astigmatism, an uneven curvature of the cornea that prevents horizontal and vertical rays from focusing on the retina, is a common problem that may occur in conjunction with myopia and hyperopia.

Common inflammatory problems that nurses may encounter in patients at any age include conjunctivitis, dacryocystitis, hordeolum, iritis, and contusions or hematomas of the eyelids and surrounding structures. *Conjunctivitis* (inflammation of the bulbar and palpebral conjunctiva) may result from foreign bodies, chemicals, allergenic agents, bacteria, or viruses. Redness, itching, tearing, and mucopurulent discharge occur. After sleep, the eyelids may be encrusted and matted together. *Dacryocystitis* (inflammation of the lacrimal sac) is manifested by tearing and a discharge from the nasolacrimal duct. *Hordeolum* (sty) is a redness, swelling, and tenderness of the hair follicles and glands that empty at the edge of the eyelids. *Iritis* (inflammation of the iris) may be caused by local or systemic infections and results in pain,

tearing, and *photophobia* (sensitivity to light). *Contusions* or *hematomas* are "black eyes" resulting from injury.

Cataracts tend to occur in those over 65 years old. This opacity of the lens or its capsule, which blocks light rays, is frequently corrected by surgery. Cataracts may also occur in infants due to a malformation of the lens if the mother contracted rubella in the first trimester of pregnancy.

Glaucoma (a disturbance in the circulation of aqueous fluid, which causes an increase in intraocular pressure) is the greatest cause of blindness in people over 40. It can be controlled if diagnosed early. Danger signs of glaucoma include blurred or foggy vision, loss of peripheral vision, difficulty focusing on close objects, difficulty adjusting to dark rooms, and seeing rainbow-colored rings around lights.

Eye Care

Normally patients do not have hygiene practices for the eyes unless they wear a special appliance such as contact lenses or an artificial eye (discussed later in this chapter).

In newborns the eyes are treated soon after birth to prevent ophthalmia neonatorum (gonorrheal conjunctivitis). Penicillin and silver nitrate are the drugs used. Treatment is mandatory by law in all states in the United States. The method of instilling the drops is the same for babies as for children and adults. See chapter 29.

If dried secretions accumulate on the lashes, they need to be softened and wiped away. In hospitals this is usually done with a sterile cotton ball moistened with sterile water or normal saline. The nurse wipes from the inner canthus of the eye to the outer canthus, to prevent the particles and fluid from draining into the lacrimal sac and nasolacrimal duct. In the home, it is usually not necessary for the fluid to be sterile, and the excess fluid is usually wiped away with a soft tissue.

Teaching situations regarding eye care

1. Parents may need to learn facts about eye care for their children. Children need to have their eyes examined when they are old enough to walk and again when they begin school. Crossed eyes need to be treated, usually with proper eyeglasses and muscle exercises. By school age, children may need glasses for persistent hyperopia or newly developed myopia or astigmatism. Parents may suspect eye problems if a child is unusually clumsy when playing or holds objects close to the eyes to see them.

2. People may need to be encouraged to avoid home remedies for eye problems. Eye irritations or injuries at any age need to be treated medically and immediately. If dirt or dust gets into the eyes, copious cleaning with clean, tepid water can be used as an emergency treatment.

3. Good visual hygiene measures, such as use of adequate lighting when reading and appropriate use of glasses when prescribed, may need to be reinforced by nurses to help prevent eyestrain. Shatterproof lenses are recommended.

4. Middle-aged and older adults may need to be reminded of the importance of regular eye examinations to detect glaucoma or cataracts. Nurses may also remind them of health insurance benefits they may receive for prescribed treatments for visual impairments or problems.

TECHNIQUE 13–4 ■ Removing Contact Lenses (Hard and Soft)

Contact lenses, thin curved discs of hard or soft plastic, fit on the cornea of the eye directly over the pupil, to correct visual defects. They float on the tear layer of the eye. Advantages of contact lenses over eyeglasses for some people are:

1. They cannot be seen and thus have cosmetic value.
2. They are highly effective in correcting some astigmatisms.
3. They are safer than glasses for some physical activities.
4. They do not fog, as eyeglasses do.
5. They provide better vision in many cases.

Contact lenses may be either hard or soft or a compromise between the two—gas permeables. *Hard* contact lenses, introduced in the 1940s, cover part of the cornea and can endure up to 20 years of use. They are made of a rigid, unwettable, airtight plastic that does not absorb water or saline solutions. Hard lenses depend on the tears for lubrication and oxygenation. Disadvantages are that they restrict oxygen supply to the cornea, are not usually worn for more than 12 to 14 hours, and are rarely recommended for first-time wearers.

Soft contact lenses, introduced in the early 1970s, cover the entire cornea. Being more pliable and soft, they mold to the eye for a firmer fit. They are composed of polymers that absorb water, allow through-the-lens oxygen transmission, and are easier on the eyes. There are many varieties: bifocal, toric (for high astigmatism), tinted (to enhance eye color), and extended-wear. The length of extended wear varies by brand from 1 to 30 days or more. Eye specialists and Health and Welfare Canada recommend that long-wear brands be removed and cleaned at least once a week. Extended-wear soft lenses that are ultrathin are comfortable but very flimsy and difficult to keep clean. Disadvantages of soft lenses are that they do not provide vision as crisp as the hard lenses, are more prone to bacterial buildup, are easily ripped, and need to be replaced every year or so. They require scrupulous care and handling.

Gas permeables, introduced in the late 1970s, are rigid enough to provide clear vision but are more flexible than the traditional hard lens. They permit oxygen to reach the cornea, thus providing greater comfort, and will not cause serious damage to the eye if left in place for several days.

Most patients normally care for their own contact lenses. There are a number of ways to place contact lenses on the eyes and to remove them. Patients learn the method that best suits them from their eye specialists. On occasion, illness or emergency treatment may necessitate removal of a person's lenses by the nurse. A hard contact lens wearer who is unconscious and unable to blink can develop corneal abrasions from lack of tears for lubrication. Patients with impaired judgment, for example, from psychiatric illness or substance abuse, are prone to eye damage from prolonged lens wearing. Proper handling of the lenses by the nurse is essential.

■ Assessment

1. Ask the patient the following questions:
   a. What kind of lenses do you wear?
   b. When were the lenses prescribed?
   c. When did you last visit an ophthalmologist?
   d. Have you had any problems with either or both eyes or eyelids, such as excessive tearing, burning, redness, sensitivity to light, swelling, or feelings of dryness? (Have the patient describe them.)
   e. Are you using any eyedrops or ointments? (These medications can combine chemically with *soft* lenses and cause lens damage and eye irritation.)
   f. How often do you wear the lenses? Daily? On special occasions?
   g. What is your lens-wearing time in a given day, including sleep time?
   h. Do you wear lenses alternately with eyeglasses?
   i. Do you remove the lenses for certain activities, eg, contact sports or swimming?
   j. Do you have any problems with the lenses, eg, cleaning, insertion, removal, damage?
   k. Do you carry an emergency identification label to alert others to remove the lenses and ensure appropriate care in an emergency? (If not, advise the patient to acquire one.)
   l. What are your insertion and removal procedures?
   m. What are your cleaning and storage procedures?
2. Inspect the eyes for problems such as redness of the conjunctiva or encrustations of the eyelashes. See Technique 10–8 on page 184.

■ Nursing Diagnosis

Nursing diagnoses that may indicate the need to remove a patient's contact lenses include:

1. Self-care deficit related to:
   a. Nervous system disorder (Parkinson's disease)
   b. Lack of coordination
   c. Paralysis of left arm
   d. Surgery to right shoulder
   e. Central nervous system tumor

■ Planning

Nursing goals

1. To prevent eye irritation and injury
2. To prevent loss of or damage to the lenses

Equipment

1. A lens storage case. Most users have a special container for their lenses. Some contain a solution so that the lenses are stored wet; in others, the lenses are dry. Each lens has a slot with a label indicating whether it is the right or left lens. It is essential that the correct lens be stored in the appropriate slot, since each is ground for a specific eye. The case is placed on the bedside table within easy reach.
   or
2. If a lens storage case is not available, two small medicine cups or specimen containers partially filled with normal saline solution. Mark one cup "L lens," the other "R lens."
3. A flashlight (optional) to help locate the lens.
4. A cotton applicator dipped in saline (optional) to reposition a lens.

■ Intervention

1. Assist the patient to a supine position or a sitting position with the head tilted back.
   Rationale This prevents the lens from falling onto the floor and causing damage or loss.
2. Locate the position of the lens:
   a. Retract the patient's upper eyelid with your index finger and ask him or her to look up, down, and from side to side.
   b. Retract the lower eyelid with your index finger and have the patient look up and down and from side to side.
   c. Use a flashlight if necessary.
   Rationale Some colorless soft lenses are difficult to see. The lens must be positioned directly over the cornea for proper removal.
3. If the lens is displaced:
   a. Ask the patient to look straight ahead.
   b. Using your index fingers, gently exert pressure on the inner margins of the upper and lower lids, and move the lens back onto the cornea.
   or
   c. Using a cotton-tipped applicator dipped in saline, gently move the lens into place.

To remove a hard lens

4. Using both thumbs or index fingers, separate the upper and lower eyelids of one eye until they are

beyond the edges of the lens. See Figure 13–15. Exert pressure toward the bony orbit above and below the eye.

Rationale A two-handed method may be needed for patients unable to cooperate. Retraction of the eyelids against the bony orbit prevents direct pressure, discomfort, and injury to the eyeball.

or

Use the middle finger to retract the upper eyelid and the thumb of the same hand to retract the lower lid.

Rationale Using one hand for retraction keeps the other hand free to receive the lens.

5. Gently move the margins of both the lower eyelid and the upper eyelid toward the lens.

Rationale The margins of the lids trap the edges of the lens.

6. Hold the top eyelid stationary, and lift the bottom edge of the contact lens by pressing the lower lid at its margin firmly under the lens. See Figure 13–16.

Rationale Pressure exerted under the edge of the lens interrupts the suction of the lens on the cornea. The lens then tips forward at the top edge.

7. Slide the lens off and out of the eye by moving both eyelids toward each other.

FIGURE 13–15

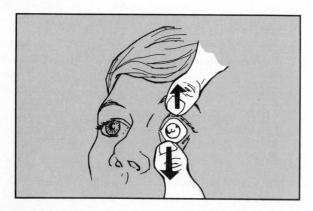

FIGURE 13–16

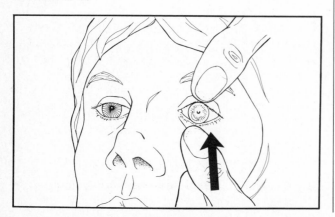

FIGURE 13–17

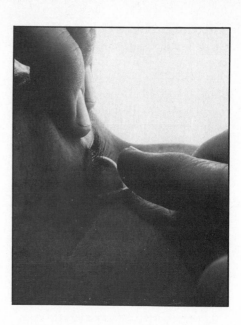

8. Grasp the lens with your index finger and thumb and place it in the palm of your hand.

9. Place the lens in the correct slot in its storage case. The slots are labeled for right and left lenses.

10. Repeat steps 4–9 for the other lens.

11. Be sure each lens is centered well in the storage case. Tighten or close the cover. Proceed to step 21.

Rationale If the lens is not centered, it may crack, chip, or tear.

To remove a soft lens

12. Ask the patient to look upward at the ceiling and keep the eye opened wide.

13. Retract the lower or upper lid with one or two fingers of your nondominant hand.

14. Using the index finger of your dominant hand, move the lens down to the inferior part of the sclera. See Figure 13–17.

Rationale Moving the lens onto the sclera reduces the risk of damage to the cornea.

15. Gently pinch the lens between the pads of the thumb and index finger of your dominant hand, and remove the lens. See Figure 13–18.

Rationale Pinching causes the lens to double up, so that air enters underneath the lens, breaking the suction and allowing removal. The pads of the fingers are used to prevent scratching the eye or the lens with the fingernails.

16. Place the lens in the palm of your hand.

17. For *ultrathin* lenses, slide the lens open with the thumb and index finger *immediately* upon removal.

Rationale It is important to keep the edges from sticking together.

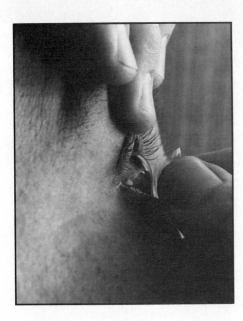

FIGURE 13–18

18. Place the lens in the correct slot in its storage case. The slots are labeled for right and left lenses.

19. Repeat steps 12–18 for the other lens.

20. Be sure each lens is centered well in the storage case. Tighten or close the cover.

    Rationale   If the lens is not centered, it may crack or tear.

21. Place the contact lens container in the drawer of the bedside table.

    Rationale   The lenses and the case should never be exposed to direct sunlight or extreme heat, since these can dry or warp them.

22. Record removal of the lenses prior to surgery or when this is a nursing responsibility. Record any problems observed, such as redness of the conjunctiva, and report problems to the responsible nurse.

Sample Recording

Date	Time	Notes
3/22/87	2100	Contact lenses removed. No redness of the conjunctiva noted.——————— ———— Anita R. Rodriguez, SN

■ Evaluation

Expected outcomes

1.   Eyelids intact without discharge
2.   Conjunctiva clear, sclera white

Unexpected outcomes

1.   Redness of lid margins
2.   Excessive tearing
3.   Redness of conjunctiva
4.   Tenderness of conjunctiva

Upon observing an unexpected outcome:

1.   Report your findings to the responsible nurse and/or physician.
2.   Carry out a more detailed eye assessment, particularly of the external eye structures. See Technique 10–8 on page 184.
3.   Do not insert the lenses until the problem is corrected.

TECHNIQUE 13–5   ■   Cleaning Contact Lenses (Hard and Soft)

Contact lenses need to be cleaned in a sterile, nonirritating wetting solution before they are inserted. The wetting solution helps the lens to glide over the cornea, thus reducing the risk of injury. Some patients use their saliva to wet their lenses. Such practices need to be discouraged since contaminants in saliva can cause bacterial buildup on the lens and infection.

Lenses are cleaned relatively easily with chemical lens cleaning solutions provided with the lenses. Soft lenses can also be cleaned by electric heat disinfecting units. In addition to regular heat disinfection, soft lenses need to be cleaned weekly with an enzymatic solution that dissolves protein deposits. Proper storage of lenses is essential. Soft lenses can become dry, brittle, and permanently damaged if left exposed to the air for an hour or less. Sterile saline is the preferred storage solution, since unsterile solutions facilitate bacterial growth, and the minerals present in tap water can damage a soft lens.

■ Assessment

1.   Assess the lenses for scratches or tears.
2.   Determine the patient's cleaning and storage practices.

■ Planning

Nursing goals

1. To prevent damage to the lens from improper storage
2. To prevent bacterial growth on the lens and the risk of eye infection

Equipment

1. The patient's lens storage case and lenses.

For hard lenses

2. Contact lens cleaner. This is usually a sterile, antiseptic nonirritating solution labeled *lens cleaner*.
3. An absorbent applicator or cotton balls for spreading the cleaning solution (optional).
4. Warm water.
5. Soaking solution (optional).

For soft lenses: Heat disinfection

6. A heat disinfecting case.
7. Saline solution (a salt tablet and distilled water).
8. Cleaning solution (an enzyme tablet and distilled water).

For soft lenses: Chemical disinfection

9. Lens cleaning solution.
10. Rinsing solution.
11. Disinfection and storage solution.

■ Intervention

1. Open the lens container carefully.
   Rationale Soft contact lenses tend to pop out unexpectedly when the case is opened quickly.
2. Pick up one lens from the container.
   Rationale The lenses are cleaned one at a time to make sure they are not put in the wrong slot or wrong eye.

To clean hard lenses

3. Wet the lens by placing a few drops of lens cleaner on both sides of it.
4. Spread the solution on both surfaces with the thumb and index finger or an absorbent applicator or place the lens in the palm of your hand and spread the solution with your index finger.
   Rationale The solution removes dirt and film.
5. Position the lens on the palm side of the index or middle finger.
6. Rinse the lens with warm tap water that feels comfortable to the fingers. If the tap water contains excessive chlorine or minerals, use distilled or puri-

fied water. If rinsing the lens over a sink, be sure the sink drain is closed.
   Rationale Hot water is contraindicated because plastic will warp when exposed to extreme heat. The closer the lens is to body temperature the more comfortable it will feel on insertion. While rinsing removes dirt, it is not necessary to rinse away all of the lens cleaner since this agent has beneficial sterilizing and wetting properties.
7. Place the lens in a soaking solution or store it dry in accordance with the recommendations of the patient's physician.
8. Follow steps 3–7 to clean the second lens.

To clean soft lenses by chemical disinfection

9. Place a few drops of lens cleaner on both sides of the lens and spread it as described in step 4.
10. Position the lens as described in step 5.
11. Rinse the lens thoroughly with rinsing solution.
12. Place the lens in the correct slot of the storage area.
13. Fill the slot with storage and disinfectant solution and tightly close its cap.
14. Follow steps 9–13 for the other lens.
15. Store both lenses for at least four hours.
16. Clean and rinse the lenses before insertion. Follow steps 9–11.
17. Clean the storage slots by emptying the solution and rinsing them with hot water and rinsing solution. Allow them to air dry.

To clean soft lenses by heat disinfection

18. Put a few drops of normal saline solution on each lens and spread it on the lens as described in step 4.
19. Rinse the lenses thoroughly with tap water.
20. Place each lens in the appropriate slot of the heat disinfecting unit, and fill the slots with normal saline solution.
21. Make sure the disinfecting unit is placed on a heat-resistant surface. Plug the unit into an electric outlet, and turn it on. The unit will turn off automatically after disinfection is completed.

To clean soft lenses with an enzymatic solution (weekly)

22. Rinse and fill the plastic or glass wells of the lens storage case with distilled water.
23. Place an enzymatic cleaning tablet in each well.
24. Place one lens in each well and securely close the caps.
25. Shake the wells to dissolve the tablets.
26. Soak the lenses for 6 to 12 hours or overnight.

27. Remove the lenses, and thoroughly rinse them with saline solution.
28. Place the lenses in the heat disinfecting unit and follow steps 20–21.
29. Rinse the storage wells with tap water, and allow them to air dry.
30. Record cleaning of the lenses with removal or insertion of the lenses.

TECHNIQUE 13–6 ■ Inserting Contact Lenses (Hard and Soft)

Seriously ill patients who have had their contact lenses removed will not need them reinserted until they become more active in their care and require their lenses to see properly. When assisting the patient with lens reinsertion, the nurse must ensure that the lenses are adequately cleaned. See Technique 13–5.

■ **Assessment**   See Technique 13–4 on page 309.

■ **Nursing Diagnosis**   See Technique 13–4 on page 309.

■ **Planning**

Nursing goals

1. To prevent injury to the eye
2. To improve the patient's vision

Equipment

1. The patient's lens storage case.
2. A wetting agent to lubricate the lenses. Solutions of methyl cellulose or polyvinyl alcohol are frequently used.

■ **Intervention**

1. Ensure that the lenses are clean.
   Rationale This reduces the chance of introducing an infection to the eye.
2. Ensure that the correct lens is selected for the eye. It is wise always to start with the right eye.
   Rationale Each lens is ground to fit the individual eye and correct its visual defect. Always starting with the right eye establishes a habit so that incorrect placement of each lens is avoided.

To insert hard lenses

3. Put a few drops of wetting solution on the right lens.

Rationale Wetting solution lubricates the lens, facilitates insertion, and lessens the chance of damage to the eye.

4. Spread the wetting solution on both surfaces of the lens using your thumb and index finger, or place the lens in the palm of your hand and spread the solution with your index finger.
5. Place the lens convex side down on the tip of your dominant index finger (right if you are right-handed). See Figure 13–19.
6. Ask the patient to bend her or his head backward.
7. Separate the upper and lower eyelids of the patient's right eye with the thumb and index finger of your nondominant hand. See Figure 13–19. Place your thumb on the skin over the infraorbital bone, your index finger on the skin over the supraorbital bone.
   Rationale Retraction of the eyelids against the bony orbit prevents direct pressure, discomfort, and injury to the eyeball.

FIGURE 13–19

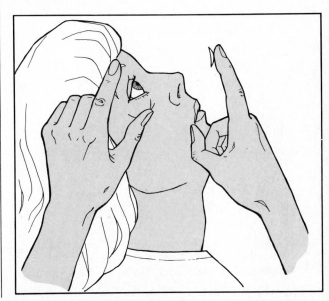

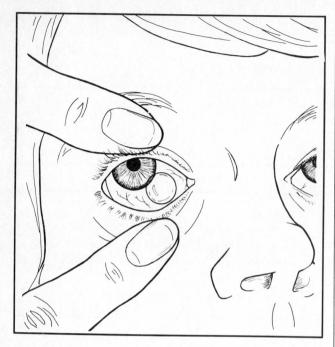

FIGURE 13-20

8. Place the lens as gently as possible on the cornea directly over the iris and pupil.

9. Ask whether the patient's vision is blurred following insertion.

    Rationale If vision is blurred, the lens may be off center.

10. If so, center the lens as follows:

    a. Separate the eyelids using the index or middle finger of the left hand to lift the upper lid and the index or middle finger of the right hand to depress the lower lid. See Figure 13-20.

    b. Locate the lens, and have the patient gaze in the opposite direction. See Figure 13-20.

    c. Gently push the lens in the direction of the cornea, using a finger or the eyelid margins.

    d. Ask the patient to look slowly toward the lens. The lens will slide easily onto the cornea as the patient looks toward it.

11. Repeat steps 3-10 for the other lens. Then proceed to step 22.

To insert soft lenses

12. Remove the lens from its saline-filled storage case with your nondominant hand. If the lens is ultrathin allow it to air dry for a few seconds.

    Rationale The dominant fingers must be kept dry for inserting the lens.

13. Position a regular (not ultrathin) lens correctly for insertion:

    a. Hold the lens at the edge between your thumb and index finger. See Figure 13-21.

    b. Flex the lens slightly. The lens is in the correct position if the edges point inward. It is in the wrong position (ie, inside-out) and must be reversed if the edges point outward. See Figure 13-22.

    Rationale A lens placed on the eye inside-out is less comfortable (an edge sensation may be felt), tends to fold on the eye, can drop to a lower position on the eye, and may move excessively on blinking.

14. Do *not* flex the lens if it is *ultrathin*. Instead put the lens on your placement finger and allow it to dry slightly for a few seconds. Closely inspect the lens to see if the edges turn upward. See Figure 13-23, *A*. If they turn downward, the lens is inside-out and must be reversed. See Figure 13-23, *B*.

    Rationale Flexing an ultrathin lens may cause the lens to fold and stick together.

15. Wet the lens with saline solution as described in step 4, using your nondominant fingers.

16. Ensure that your placement finger is dry. This is particularly important for ultrathin soft lenses.

    Rationale "Water-loving" soft contact lenses have

FIGURE 13-21

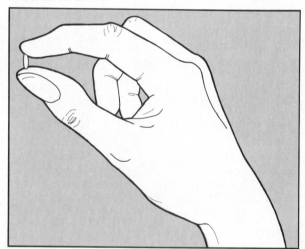

FIGURE 13-22

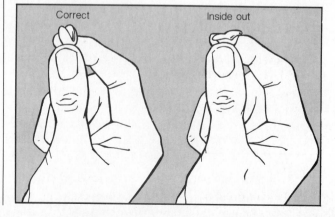

Correct   Inside out

a natural attraction to wet surfaces. Insertion onto the moist eye is facilitated when the finger is dry.

17. Place the lens convex side down on the tip of your dominant index finger.

    Rationale   The concave side of the lens rests against the cornea.

18. Keep the lens parallel with the fingertip, with all edges up and toward the eye. See Figure 13–23, *A*.

    Rationale   Balancing the lens in an upright position facilitates insertion. A lens that rocks forward or sideways allowing one edge to touch the fingertip hinders insertion.

19. If the lens curls and the edges stick together, place the lens in the palm of your hand, wet it thoroughly with saline solution, and gently move the edges apart by rubbing the lens between your thumb and index finger, or soak the lens in saline solution.

20. If the lens flattens or drapes across the finger, move the lens to the palm of your nondominant hand, dry the placement finger, and allow the lens to air dry for a few seconds.

    Rationale   The placement finger on the lens may be too wet.

21. Follow steps 6–8 above for insertion.

22. Replace the patient's lens container, lens cleaner, and wetting solution in the drawer of the bedside table.

23. Record insertion of the contact lenses if a nurse is required to remove them; otherwise this is not

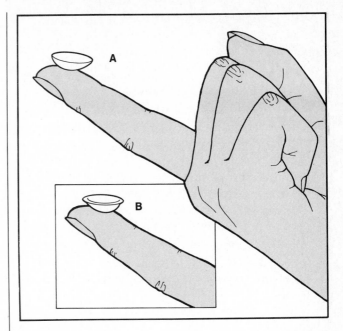

FIGURE 13–23

normally recorded (consult agency policy). Record and report to the responsible nurse any problems observed in the eyes or the lenses.

24. Note on the nursing care plan the time for the lenses to be removed.

■ **Evaluation**   See Technique 13–4 on page 311.

TECHNIQUE 13–7   ■   Removing, Cleaning, and Inserting an Artificial Eye

---

Most patients who have an artificial eye have their own care method. Even for an unconscious patient, daily removal and cleaning is not necessary. If excessive secretions accumulate or the patient is scheduled for surgery, the nurse must remove the eye from the socket, clean the eye, the socket, and the surrounding tissues, and then reinsert the eye. Other patients who may require assistance are those whose mobility is impaired by injury or paralysis.

■ **Assessment**

Assess the socket, surrounding tissues, and eye:

1. Observe the surrounding tissues for signs of redness or irritation and infection.

2. Look for crusting on the eyelashes or drainage from the eye socket.

3. Inspect the artificial eye for rough areas.

In addition, determine the patient's routine eye care practices, so that these can be followed. Some patients may remove and clean the eye and socket daily.

■ **Nursing Diagnosis**   See Technique 13–4 on page 309.

■ **Planning**

Nursing goals

1. To prevent irritation and infection of the socket, surrounding tissues, and artificial eye

2. To assess the socket and the tissues for problems

Equipment

1. A bowl of warm normal saline to clean the eye, the socket, and the surrounding tissues.

2. A soft gauze or cotton wipe to wash and dry the socket and the surrounding tissues. Sterile supplies are normally used in a hospital, but this is not a sterile procedure.

3. A small storage container, such as a denture or specimen container, to hold the eye, if it is not to be reinserted. Line the container with gauze to cushion the eye and prevent scratches.

4. A label for the container.

5. A small rubber bulb to remove the eye (optional). A syringe bulb or medicine dropper bulb can be used.

■ Intervention

To remove the eye

1. Assist the patient to a sitting or supine position.

2. Identify the eye to be removed.

3. If the patient has a specific method for removing the eye, follow that method.

   Rationale Most patients can remove their own eyes under normal circumstances, and they may have a convenient method.

4. Otherwise:

   a. Pull the lower eyelid down over the infraorbital bone with your dominant thumb, and exert slight pressure below the eyelid. See Figure 13–24.

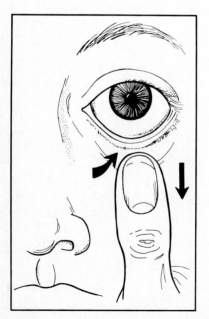

FIGURE 13–24

   Rationale Slight pressure normally breaks the suction, and the eye pops out.

   or

   b. Compress a small rubber bulb, and apply the tip directly on the eye. Gradually decrease the finger pressure on the bulb, and draw the eye out of the socket.

   Rationale Compression squeezes the air out of the bulb, causing a negative pressure inside the bulb. When the finger pressure is released, the suction of the bulb counteracts the suction holding the eye in the socket.

5. Receive the eye with the other hand, and place it carefully in the container. It is important not to scratch or drop the eye.

To clean the eye and the socket

6. Expose the socket by raising the upper lid with the index finger and pulling the lower lid down with the thumb.

7. Clean the socket with soft gauze or cotton wipes and normal saline. Pat dry.

8. Wash the tissue around the eye, stroking from the inner to the outer canthus. Be sure to wash crusts off the upper and lower lids and eyelashes.

   Rationale This direction of stroking avoids washing any debris down the lacrimal canaliculi, if they are still intact.

9. Dry the tissues gently, in the same direction, with dry wipes.

10. Wash the artificial eye gently with the warm normal saline, and dry it with dry wipes.

11. If the eye is not to be inserted, place it in the container filled with water or saline solution, close the lid, label the container with the patient's name and room number, and place it in the drawer of the bedside table.

To insert the eye

12. Ensure that the eye is moistened with water or saline.

    Rationale Moisture facilitates insertion by reducing friction.

13. Using your thumb, gently pull the patient's lower lid down. Rest the thumb on the skin over the infraorbital bone.

14. If the upper lid comes well down over the socket, raise it with your index finger, pressing upward while resting on the skin over the supraorbital bone. See Figure 13–25.

15. With the thumb and index finger of the other hand, hold the eye so that the front of it is toward the palm of your hand. See Figure 13–26. Slip the eye gently

into the socket, and release the lids. The eye should fit securely under the lids.

16. Record the removal, cleaning, and/or insertion of an artificial eye prior to surgery or for a helpless patient. Otherwise these procedures are not usually recorded. Record and report to the responsible nurse any problems observed.

■ **Evaluation**

Expected outcomes

1. Eye socket tissues intact
2. Eyelid skin and mucous membrane intact

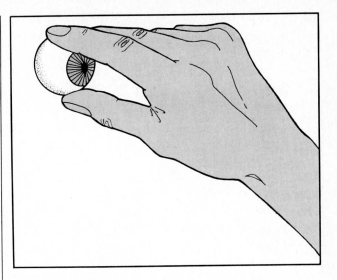

FIGURE 13–26

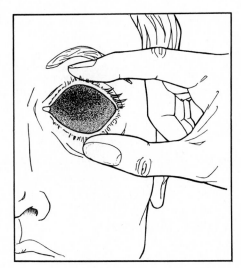

FIGURE 13–25

3. Eye surface smooth and shiny

Unexpected outcomes

1. Redness of socket tissues
2. Redness of eyelids
3. Scratches on surface of artificial eye

Upon observing an unexpected outcome: Report your findings to the responsible nurse and/or physician. Do not reinsert the eye if the socket tissues or eyelids are irritated.

EARS

The ear is divided into three parts: external ear, middle ear, and inner ear. The *external ear* includes the *auricle* or *pinna,* the *external auditory canal,* and the *tympanic membrane* (eardrum). See Figure 13–27. Landmarks of the auricle include the *lobule* (earlobe), *helix, anthelix, tragus, triangular fossa,* and *external auditory meatus.* Although not part of the ear, the *mastoid,* a bony prominence behind the ear, is another important landmark. See Figure 13–28. The external ear canal is curved in shape, is about 2.5 cm (1 in) long in the adult, and ends at the tympanic membrane. It is covered with skin that has many fine hairs, glands, and nerve endings. The glands secrete *cerumen* (earwax), which lubricates and protects the canal.

The *middle ear* is an air-filled cavity that starts at the tympanic membrane and contains three *ossicles* (bones of sound transmission): the *malleus* (the most easily seen), the *incus,* and the *stapes.* See Figure 13–27. The *eustachian*

FIGURE 13–27 ■ Anatomic structures of the external, middle, and inner ear.

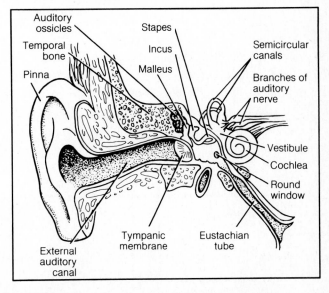

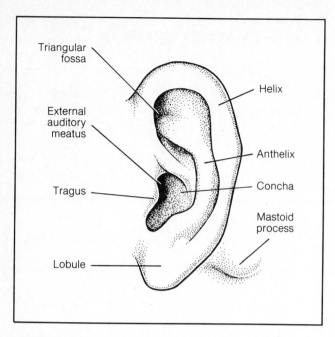

FIGURE 13–28 ■ Landmarks of the external ear.

tube, another part of the middle ear, connects the middle ear to the nasopharynx. This tube stabilizes the air pressure between the external atmosphere and the middle ear, thus preventing rupture of the tympanic membrane and discomfort produced by marked pressure differences.

The *inner ear* contains the *cochlea,* a seashell-shaped structure essential for sound transmission and hearing, and the *vestibule* and *semicircular canals,* which contain the organs of equilibrium. See Figure 13–27.

Sound transmission and hearing are complex processes. In brief, sound can be transmitted by air conduction or bone conduction. *Air-conducted* transmission occurs when:

1. A sound stimulus enters the external canal and reaches the tympanic membrane.

2. The sound waves cross the tympanic membrane and reach the ossicles.

3. The sound waves travel from the ossicles to the opening in the inner ear (oval window).

4. The cochlea receives the sound vibrations.

5. The stimulus travels to the auditory nerve (the eighth cranial nerve) in the cerebral cortex.

Bone-conducted sound transmission occurs when skull bones transport the sound directly to the auditory nerve.

Developmental Variables

The curvature of the external ear canal differs with age. In the infant and toddler, the canal has an upward curvature. By age 3, the ear canal assumes the more downward curvature of adulthood. See Figures 10–41 and 10–42 on page 196.

Audiometric evaluations, which measure hearing at various decibels, are recommended for the elderly. A common hearing deficit with age is loss of ability to hear high-frequency sounds, such as *f, s, sh,* and *ph.* Because this deficit can distort normal conversation, older people may display inappropriate or confused behaviors sometimes. This neurosensory hearing deficit does not respond well to use of a hearing aid.

Common Problems

Localized infections of the external ear canal (*otitis externa*), the middle ear (*otitis media*), and the eustachian tube (*serous otitis*) are most common in children but also occur in adults. In external otitis the patient may experience pain when touching or pressing the tragus or the auricle, and the canal is inflamed. Otitis media is manifested by redness and bulging of the tympanic membrane, and pus or blood in the ear canal. Serous otitis is often associated with otitis media and upper respiratory infections. An amber-colored fluid is usually seen through the eardrum and the patient complains of "ear popping."

Mechanical blockages of the external ear canal most commonly arise from a build-up of cerumen or from foreign bodies lodged in the canal. Children are notorious for inserting small objects in their ears. Signs of blockage are pain and some loss of hearing.

The most common traumatic stress to the eardrum involves exposure to loud noises. Frequent close exposure to loud music or machines is associated with a high potential for hearing loss.

Neurologic disorders that are congenital, inherited, or acquired are responsible for varying degrees of hearing loss. Congenital hearing losses are commonly seen in children who were exposed before birth to rubella, especially in the early months of pregnancy. Most inherited hearing losses do not manifest themselves until adulthood. Acquired hearing losses can occur as a result of mumps, meningitis, or severe reactions to some drugs, eg, streptomycin. Some hearing loss often occurs with the normal aging process.

TECHNIQUE 13–8 ■ Removing, Cleaning, and Inserting a Hearing Aid

A hearing aid is a battery-powered sound amplifying device used by hearing-impaired persons. It consists of

a *microphone* that picks up the sound and converts it to electric energy, an *amplifier* that magnifies the electric

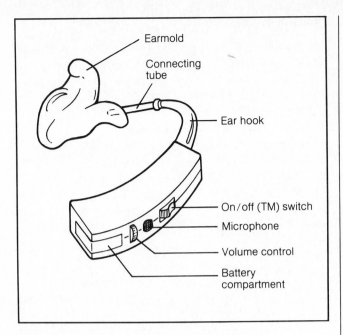

FIGURE 13-29 ■ A behind-the-ear hearing aid.

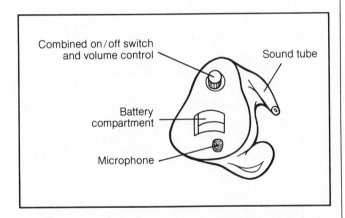

FIGURE 13-30 ■ An in-the-ear hearing aid.

energy electronically, a *receiver* that converts the amplified energy back to sound energy, and an *earmold* that directs the sound into the ear. There are several types of hearing aids:

1. *Behind-the-ear-aid.* This is the most widely used type, since it fits snugly over the ear. The hearing aid case, which holds the microphone, amplifier, and receiver is attached to the earmold by a plastic tube. See Figure 13-29.

2. *In-the-ear-aid.* This one-piece aid is the most compact hearing aid. All its components are housed in the earmold. See Figure 13-30.

3. *Eyeglasses aid.* This is similar to the behind-the-ear aid except that the components are housed in the temple of the eyeglasses. The hearing aid can be in one or both temples of the glasses. See Figure 13-31.

4. *Body hearing aid.* This pocket-sized aid, used for more severe hearing losses, clips onto an undergarment,

shirt pocket, or harness carrier supplied by the manufacturer. See Figure 13-32. The case, containing the microphone and amplifier, is connected by a cord to the receiver, which snaps into the earpiece.

For proper functioning, hearing aids require appropriate handling during insertion and removal, regular cleaning of the earmold, and replacement of dead batteries. Although most patients can look after their hearing aids themselves, some debilitated patients may require assistance. Hearing aids must be removed before surgery.

FIGURE 13-31 ■ An eyeglasses hearing aid.

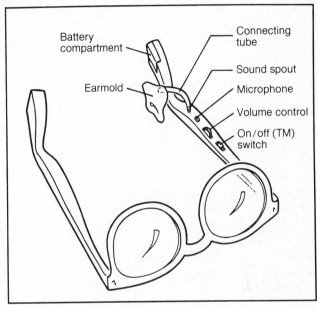

FIGURE 13-32 ■ A body hearing aid.

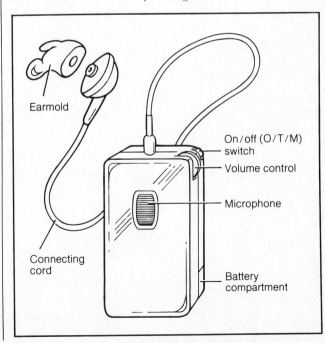

■ Assessment

Determine from the patient:

1. The type of hearing aid worn
2. When and where it was obtained and from whom
3. Maintenance and cleaning methods
4. Any hearing aid problems experienced
5. Any ear problems experienced

■ Nursing Diagnosis

Nursing diagnoses that may indicate the need to assist a patient with hearing aid care include:

1. Self-care deficit related to:
   a. Visual disorder
   b. Neuromuscular impairment of upper extremities
   c. Musculoskeletal impairment of upper extremities
   d. Trauma to or surgery on upper extremities

■ Planning

Nursing goal

To maintain proper hearing aid function.

Equipment

1. The patient's hearing aid
2. A new battery (if needed)
3. A pipe cleaner or toothpick (optional)
4. Soap, water, and towels or a damp cloth

■ Intervention

Removing a hearing aid

1. Turn the hearing aid off and lower the volume. The on/off switch may be designated as "O" (off), "M" microphone, "T" (telephone), or "TM" (telephone/microphone).

   Rationale The batteries continue to be used if the aid is not turned off.

2. Remove the earmold by rotating it slightly forward and pulling it outward.

3. If the aid is not to be used for several days, remove the battery.

   Rationale Removal prevents corrosion of the aid from battery leakage.

4. Store the hearing aid in a safe place. Avoid exposure to heat and moisture.

   Rationale Proper storage prevents loss or damage.

Cleaning the earmold

5. Detach the earmold *if possible*. Disconnect the earmold from the receiver of a body hearing aid or from the hearing aid case of behind-the-ear and eyeglasses aids where the tubing meets the hook of the case. Do not remove the earmold if it is glued or secured by a small metal ring.

   Rationale Removal facilitates cleaning the earmold and prevents inadvertent damage to the other parts.

6. If the earmold is detachable, soak it in a mild soapy solution. Rinse and dry it well.

7. If the earmold is not detachable or is for an in-the-ear aid, wipe the earmold with a damp cloth.

8. Check that the earmold opening is patent. Blow any excess moisture through the opening or remove debris (eg, earwax) with a pipe cleaner or toothpick.

9. Reattach the earmold if it was detached from the rest of the hearing aid.

Inserting the hearing aid

1. Determine from the patient whether the earmold is for the left or the right ear.

2. Check that the battery is inserted in the hearing aid. Turn off the hearing aid, and make sure the volume is turned all the way down.

3. Inspect the earmold to identify the ear canal portion.

   Rationale Some earmolds are fitted for only the ear canal and concha; others are fitted for all the contours of the ear. The canal portion, common to all, can be used as a guide for correct insertion.

4. Line up the parts of the earmold with the corresponding parts of the patient's ear.

5. Rotate the earmold slightly forward and insert the ear canal portion.

6. Gently press the earmold into the ear while rotating it backward.

7. Check that the earmold fits snugly by asking the patient if it feels secure and comfortable.

8. Adjust the other components of a behind-the-ear or body hearing aid.

9. Turn the hearing aid on and adjust the volume according to the patient's needs.

10. If the hearing aid is not functioning properly, ie, the sound is weak or there is no sound:
    a. Ensure that the volume is turned high enough.
    b. Ensure that the earmold opening is not clogged.
    c. Check the battery, by turning the aid on, turning up the volume, cupping your hand over the earmold, and listening. A constant whistling sound indicates the battery is functioning. If necessary, replace the battery. Be sure to match

the negative (–) and positive (+) signs when inserting the new battery.

   d. Ensure that the ear canal is not blocked with wax, which can obstruct sound waves.

11. If the patient reports a whistling sound or squeal after insertion:

   a. Turn the volume down.

   b. Ensure that the earmold is properly attached to the receiver.

   c. Reinsert the earmold.

12. When communicating with the patient, be sure to face the patient, and talk distinctly in natural tones. Do not shout.

   Rationale Facing the patient directly facilitates lip reading by some patients. Natural tones are more easily amplified.

13. Report and record any problems the patient has with the hearing aid. Removal and insertion of a hearing aid are not normally recorded.

■ Evaluation

Expected outcome

Patient hears spoken voice with hearing aid.

Unexpected outcome

Patient is unable to hear spoken voice with hearing aid. Upon obtaining an unexpected outcome: Report your findings to the responsible nurse and/or physician.

References

Block GJ, Nolan JW, Dempsey MK: *Health Assessment for Professional Nursing: A Developmental Approach.* Appleton-Century-Crofts, 1981.

Bowers AC, Thompson JM: *Clinical Manual of Health Assessment,* 2nd ed. Mosby, 1984.

Boyd-Monk H: Examining the external eye: Part 1. *Nursing 80* (May) 1980; 10(5):58–63.

Boyd-Monk H: Examining the external eye: Part 2. *Nursing 80* (June) 1980; 10(6):58–63.

Burns KR, Johnson PJ: *Health Assessment in Clinical Practice.* Prentice-Hall, 1980.

Dyer ED et al: Dental health in adults. *Am J Nurs* (July) 1976; 76:1156–1159.

Eliopoulos C (editor): *Health Assessment of the Older Adult.* Addison-Wesley, 1984.

Gannon ED, Kadezabek E: Giving your patients meticulous mouth care. *Nursing 80* (March) 1980; 10(3):14–19.

Holder L: Hearing aids: Handle with care. *Nursing 82* (April) 1982; 12(4):64–67.

How to examine your patient's ears. *Nursing 84* (January) 1984; 14(1):12–14.

How to test your patient's hearing acuity. *Nursing 80* (July) 1980; 10(7):60–61.

Kamenir S, Fothergill R: Hands-on skills for dealing with hearing aids. *Can Nurse* (December) 1982; 78(11):44–45.

Ludington-Hoe SM: What can newborns really see? *Am J Nurs* (September) 1983; 83(9):1286–1289.

Martin BJ, Reeb RM: Oral health during pregnancy: A neglected nursing area. *Am J Maternal Child Nurs* (November/December) 1982; 7(6):391–392.

Meissner JE: A simple guide for assessing oral health. *Nursing 80* (April) 1980; 10(4):70–75 (Canadian ed. pp 24–25).

Norman S: The pupil check. *Am J Nurs* (April) 1982; 82(4): 588–591.

Osguthorpe NC: If your patient has contact lenses. *Am J Nurs* (October) 1984; 84:1255–1256.

Schweiger JL, Lang JW, Schweiger JW: Oral assessment: How to do it. *Am J Nurs* (April) 1980; 80:654–657.

Slattery J: Dental health in children. *Am J Nurs* (July) 1976; 76:1159–1161.

Todd B: Drugs and the elderly: Dry mouth—causes and cures. *Geriatr Nurs* (March/April) 1982; 3(2):122–123.

Williams PL, Warwick R: *Gray's Anatomy,* 36th ed. Churchill Livingstone, 1980.

Wybar K, Muir MK: *Ophthalmology,* 3rd ed. Bailliere Tindall, Concise Medical Textbooks, 1984.

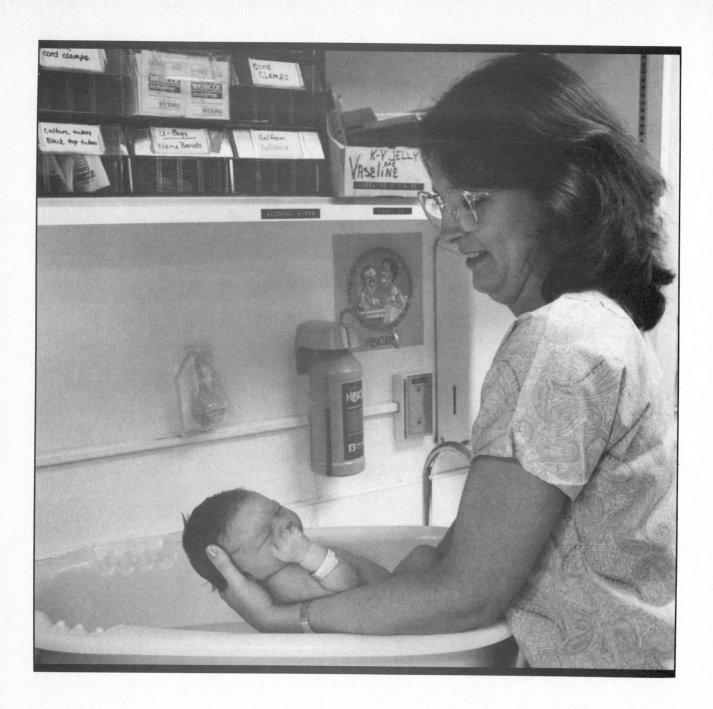

THE SKIN

14

This chapter focuses on measures to maintain the integrity (completeness) and health of the skin, as part of personal hygienic practices and techniques. Nurses frequently give patients baths, provide perineal–genital care, offer back rubs, and shave the facial hair of male patients. Because hygienic practices are learned activities, they can vary considerably among patients. Nurses need to support practices that maintain the patient's health and determine which hygienic practices the patient needs to learn to promote health.

Chapter Outline

Skin

Decubitus Ulcers

Baths

■ Technique 14–1 Bathing an Adult

■ Technique 14–2 Shaving a Male Patient

■ Technique 14–3 Perineal–Genital Care

■ Technique 14–4 Giving a Back Rub

■ Technique 14–5 Changing a Hospital Gown for a Patient with an Intravenous Infusion

■ Technique 14–6 Giving an Infant Sponge Bath

■ Technique 14–7 Giving an Infant Tub Bath

■ Technique 14–8 Changing a Diaper

Objectives

Upon completion of this chapter, the student will:

1. Know essential terms and facts related to the structure, function, and common problems of the skin
   1.1 Define selected terms related to the skin
   1.2 Identify major structures of the skin
   1.3 Identify the major functions of the skin
   1.4 Identify variations that occur in the skin according to age
   1.5 Identify common problems of the skin
   1.6 Identify common causes of skin problems
   1.7 Describe the physiologic basis of decubitus ulcer formation
   1.8 Identify patients at risk for development of decubitus ulcers
2. Know interventions to prevent and relieve skin problems
   2.1 Identify interventions used to prevent the formation of decubitus ulcers
   2.2 Identify interventions used to treat decubitus ulcers
   2.3 Identify general interventions for skin care
   2.4 Identify nursing interventions to prevent excoriated skin
   2.5 Identify nursing interventions for treating diaper rash in infants
3. Understand facts about hygienic techniques
   3.1 Identify relevant assessment data
   3.2 Identify nursing diagnoses for which the technique may be implemented
   3.3 Identify nursing goals related to the technique
   3.4 Identify expected and unexpected outcomes from assessment data
   3.5 Identify reasons underlying selected steps of the technique
4. Perform hygienic techniques safely
   4.1 Assess the patient adequately
   4.2 Collect additional data from appropriate sources
   4.3 Select pertinent nursing goals for the patient
   4.4 Establish relevant outcome criteria for the patient following the technique
   4.5 Collect necessary equipment before the technique
   4.6 Implement interventions to enhance the effectiveness of the technique and enhance the patient's comfort and safety
   4.7 Communicate relevant information about the patient to the appropriate persons
   4.8 Determine the evaluative outcomes of the technique
5. Evaluate own performance of specific techniques in a laboratory or clinical setting with the assistance of another
   5.1 Use the performance checklists provided
   5.2 Identify areas of strength and weakness
   5.3 Alter performance in response to own evaluation and that of another

Terms

■ **acne**   an inflammatory condition of the sebaceous glands

■ **ammonia dermatitis**   diaper rash

■ **axilla**   the armpit

■ **comedo**   a blackhead

■ **cyanosis**   a bluish tinge to the skin and mucous membrane

■ **decubitus ulcer**   a pressure sore or bedsore

■ **dermis (corium)**   true skin, containing blood vessels, nerves, hair follicles, and glands

■ **diaphoresis**   profuse perspiration

■ **ecchymosis**   a bruise

■ **epidermis**   the outermost, nonvascular layer of skin

- **erythema** redness that is associated with a variety of rashes
- **excoriation** loss of superficial layers of the skin
- **foreskin** a covering fold of skin over the glans of the penis
- **genitals** the reproductive organs, usually the external ones
- **hemangioma** a large, persistent, bright red or dark purple vascular area of the skin
- **hypodermis** connective tissue beneath the skin; also referred to as *subcutaneous tissue*
- **jaundice** a yellowish tinge to the skin and mucous membrane
- **keratotic spots** horny growths, such as warts or calluses
- **labia** the fleshy edges of a structure, usually the female genitals
- **melanin** the dark pigment of the skin
- **milia** small, white nodules (whiteheads) usually found over the nose and face of newborns
- **miliaria rubra** a prickly heat rash of the face, neck, trunk, or perineal area of infants
- **mongolian spots** blue or black spots of varying size found largely in the sacral area of Oriental or Black infants

- **orifice** an external opening of a body cavity, eg, the anus is the orifice of the large intestine
- **pallor** the absence of normal skin color
- **penis** the male organ of copulation and urinary excretion
- **perineum** the area between the anus and the posterior (back) aspect of the genitals
- **petechiae** pinpoint red areas in the skin
- **phimosis** a condition in which the opening of the foreskin of the penis is extremely narrow
- **sebaceous gland** a gland of the dermis that secretes sebum
- **smegma** a thick, white, cheeselike secretion that tends to collect between the labia and under the foreskin
- **sudoriferous gland** a gland of the dermis that secretes sweat
- **turgor** the normal fullness and elasticity of the skin
- **vagina** the canal of the female reproductive tract
- **vernix caseosa** the whitish, cheesy, greasy, protective material found on the skin at birth

SKIN

The skin covers the entire surface of the body and thus is the largest organ of the body. At body orifices such as the ears, eyes, nose, rectum, and vagina, the skin is continuous with the mucous membrane that lines these orifices. Skin varies in thickness from about 0.5 mm over the earlobes to 1.5 mm on the palms of the hands and soles of the feet.

Developmental Variables

In early embryonic life, the skin is a single layer of cells. Other layers develop quickly. The skin of an infant is thinner than that of an adult and usually mottled. In Whites it varies from pink to red and becomes ruddy when the baby cries. Babies who are genetically dark-skinned are lightly pigmented at birth. Dark bluish areas are often apparent on the lower back or buttocks of non-Whites, due to the presence of pigmented cells in the deeper skin layers. These are referred to as *mongolian spots* (no relation to mongolism) and usually disappear spontaneously during the first year. Skin pigmentation gradually increases until about 6 or 8 weeks of age. Sweat glands begin to function at about 1 month of age.

In adolescence, the sebaceous glands increase in activity as a result of higher hormone levels. The hair follicle openings enlarge to accommodate the greater amount of sebum. The apocrine glands, which appear at puberty, are thought to enlarge and become more active before and after monthly menses and to secrete less after menopause.

Older people also experience skin changes. The skin tends to become thinner and drier, with fine wrinkling and some inelasticity. This process occurs at various ages, from 40 on. The elderly person's skin typically shows wrinkles, sagging, pigmentations, and keratotic spots (usually on areas exposed to the sun). The skin is also less resilient—that is, when it is pinched, it returns to place more slowly than the skin of a younger person.

Common Problems

Nurses frequently observe skin problems in patients. Some need to be brought to a physician's attention; others require minimal care; and still others eventually disappear spontaneously.

In the newborn, *milia* due to clogged sebaceous glands are commonly present on the nose and sometimes the cheeks for several weeks. *Miliaria rubra* appears most often on the face, neck, and trunk, and in the diaper area of infants. It is due to excessive heat and will disappear if the baby is kept cooler, often with fewer clothes. *Mongolian spots* (discussed earlier under Developmental Variables) generally disappear without treatment as the baby gets older.

Hemangiomas are vascular lesions present at birth. There are several types, and most disappear eventually. However, nurses should refer a child with this problem to a physician for accurate diagnosis of the type and treatment if indicated. The nurse notes and records the size, shape, exact color (such as pink or port wine color), and elevation (whether flat or raised from the skin) of any hemangiomas observed.

Diaper rash, also referred to as *ammonia dermatitis,* is caused by skin bacteria reacting with urea, a product related to ammonia and excreted in the urine. The reaction is irritating to the baby's perineum and buttocks, causing them to become red and sore. Most diaper rashes can be prevented by keeping the buttocks clean and dry. Protective ointments containing zinc oxide may be preventive. Pastes that are difficult to remove are avoided. A treatment for diaper rash is to expose the baby's buttocks to the air and to a 40-watt gooseneck lamp placed 30 cm (12 in) away. This can be done several times a day for about 30 minutes each time. The lamp provides drying as well as warmth. Boiling the diapers to remove the bacteria is helpful; however, most detergents now contain antibacterial agents. Efficient rinsing is essential, since detergent can be irritating to the baby's skin.

Erythema is associated with a variety of rashes and infections. *Petechiae* are caused by intradermal hemorrhages, while *ecchymoses* are collections of blood beneath the skin. Initially ecchymoses are bluish purple, firm, and tender; as the blood is absorbed, they become yellowish and soften.

Acne commonly occurs in adolescence. A number of factors are involved in the development of acne: hormone levels, diet, secondary bacterial infections, exercise, nervous tension, and fatigue. A hair follicle becomes obstructed, causing sebum to accumulate in the follicle, and a comedo forms. The sebaceous gland is eventually destroyed, releasing fatty acids into the surrounding tissues. This causes an inflammation and the acne nodule. Theories about the best treatment for acne vary widely, but cleanliness of the skin is important in all treatments, to prevent secondary infection.

Nursing Interventions for the Skin

1. An intact, healthy skin is the body's first line of defense. It protects the body from invasion by microorganisms and from harmful agents such as chemicals. Nurses need to ensure that all skin care measures provided to patients prevent injury and irritation. Scratching the skin with jewelry or long, sharp fingernails is avoided. Harsh rubbing or use of rough towels and washcloths can cause tissue damage, particularly when the skin is irritated or when circulation or sensation is diminished. Bottom bedsheets are kept taut and free from wrinkles to reduce friction and abrasion to the skin. Top bed linens are arranged to prevent undue pressure on the toes. When necessary bed cradles or footboards are used to keep bedclothes off the feet. See chapter 15.

2. The degree to which the skin protects the underlying tissues from injury depends on the general health of the cells, the amount of subcutaneous tissue, and the dryness of the skin. Skin that is poorly nourished and dry has less ability to protect and is more vulnerable to injury. When the skin is dry, lotions or creams with lanolin are applied, and bathing is limited to once or twice a week. For back rubs, lotion is used, rather than alcohol. The greater the amount of subcutaneous tissue, the more padding there is, particularly over bony prominences. Nurses also assess the patient's nutritional and fluid intake. When either one is deficient, measures are taken to improve it.

3. Moisture in contact with the skin for a period of time can result in increased bacterial growth and irritation. After a bath, the patient's skin is dried carefully, paying particular attention to potential irritation areas, such as the axillae, the groin, beneath the breasts, and between the toes. A nonirritating dusting powder, such as cornstarch, tends to reduce moisture and can be applied to these areas after they are dried. If patients are incontinent of urine or feces or if they perspire excessively, immediate cleaning is provided to prevent skin irritation.

4. Body odors are caused by resident bacteria of the skin acting on body secretions. Cleanliness is the best deodorant. Commercial deodorants and antiperspirants can be applied only after the skin is cleaned. Deodorants diminish odors, whereas antiperspirants reduce the amount of perspiration. Neither is applied immediately after shaving, because of the possibility of skin irritation. They are also withheld from skin that is already irritated.

5. Skin sensitivity to irritation and injury varies among individuals and in accordance with their health. Generally speaking, skin sensitivity is greater in infants, very young children, and the elderly. A person's nutritional status also affects sensitivity. Excessively emaciated or obese persons tend to experience skin irritation and injury. The same tendency occurs among individuals with poor dietary habits and insufficient fluid intake.

Even in healthy persons, skin sensitivity is highly variable. The skin of some may be sensitive to chemicals in skin care agents and cosmetics. Hypoallergenic cosmetic products and special soaps or soap substitutes are now

TABLE 14-1 ■ Agents Commonly Used on the Skin

Type	Description
Soap	Lowers surface tension, and thus helps in cleaning. Some soaps contain antibacterial agents, which can change the natural flora of the skin.
Detergent	Used instead of soap for cleaning. Some people who are allergic to soaps may not be allergic to detergents, and vice versa.
Bath oil	Used in bath water; provides an oily film on the skin that softens and prevents chapping.
Skin cream, lotion	Provides a film on the skin that prevents evaporation and therefore chapping.
Powder	Can be used to absorb water and prevent friction. For example, powder under the breasts can prevent skin irritation. Some powders are antibacterial.
Deodorant	Masks or diminishes body odors.
Antiperspirant	Reduces the amount of perspiration.

available for these people. The nurse needs to ascertain whether the patient has any sensitivities and what agents are appropriate to use.

6. Agents used for skin care have selective actions and purposes. Commonly used agents are described in Table 14-1.

DECUBITUS ULCERS

Decubitus ulcers (also called *pressure sores, bedsores,* or *decubiti*) are ulcerations of the skin. They are chiefly due to deprivation of oxygen and essential nutrients to an area because of prolonged pressure that occludes the blood supply to the tissues. Although they are not a common problem, the potential for them to develop is great, and preventive measures need to be carried out continuously. Decubitus ulcers are frequently seen in people who have difficulty moving in bed or in a chair, and in very emaciated or paralyzed patients.

Decubiti can be categorized as superficial or deep (Ahmed, 1980, p 113). *Superficial* ulcers start with an excoriation caused by a shearing force (such as sliding up and down in a bed or chair), friction from movement on rough surfaces (such as a wrinkled sheet), and maceration produced by urine, feces, or excessive perspiration. Untreated superficial ulcers become infected and painful, but if treated they heal within a few days.

Deep ulcers start as ischemic areas in the muscle or subcutaneous layers and then surface to the skin as black blisters, which change to thick, hard *eschar* (slough). What is apparent to the eye is misleading in terms of the degree of damage, since destruction of the underlying tissues is extensive. The visible eschar is composed of dried plasma, proteins, and dead cells. If this eschar is not removed, the *necrotic* process (dying of the tissues) spreads and becomes a focus of infection.

A number of conditions predispose patients to develop decubitus ulcers. Prolonged pressure is considered the primary cause. Other predisposing factors are moisture, a break in the skin surface, poor nutrition, impaired circulation to the area, lack of subcutaneous and adipose tissue to pad bony prominences, lack of sensation in the area so that the patient cannot feel the tingling (pins and needles) of loss of circulation, and the presence of pathogens.

Assessment of Risk Patients

Assessment of patients at risk for the development of decubiti is essential for prevention. Kerr, Stinson, and Shannon (1981, p 27) have devised a pressure assessment scale with five categories: physical condition, mental condition, activity, mobility, and continence. This scale needs to be used weekly or whenever there is a change in the patient's condition or situation. Patients at risk include:

1. Those with paralysis from either brain or spinal cord injury. Incidence rates for these people are as high as 80%, due to their extensive loss of sensory and motor function.

2. Those with a reduced level of awareness, such as unconscious or heavily sedated patients (those taking analgesics, barbiturates, or tranquilizers). In these patients, the usual perceptions that stimulate changes of position are reduced or absent.

3. Those who are malnourished and whose diet is insfficient in protein and ascorbic acid (vitamin C). Good nutrition is thought essential to promote normal tissue maintenance and healing.

4. Those who are over age 85. These patients have problems with mobility and incontinence and are generally lean. Changes in the circulatory system due to aging also reduce the system's capacity and ability to carry essential nutrients to the skin.

5. Those who are confined to bed or to a wheelchair, particularly if they are dependent on others for movement (ibid, p 24).

Preventive Measures

1. Change the patient's position at least every two hours even when a special support mattress is used, so that another body surface bears the weight. Four body positions can usually be used: prone, supine, and right and left lateral (side-lying) positions. See chapter 17. Prolonged pressure on bony prominences is considered

the primary cause of decubiti. See Figure 14–1 for pressure areas in various positions assumed by bed patients. Prolonged low pressure is potentially more dangerous than high pressure for a short duration, since it is prolonged pressure that alters the tissue's blood supply (Ahmed, 1980, p 113).

FIGURE 14–1 ■ Body pressure areas in: **A,** supine position; **B,** lateral position; **C,** prone position; **D,** Fowler's position.

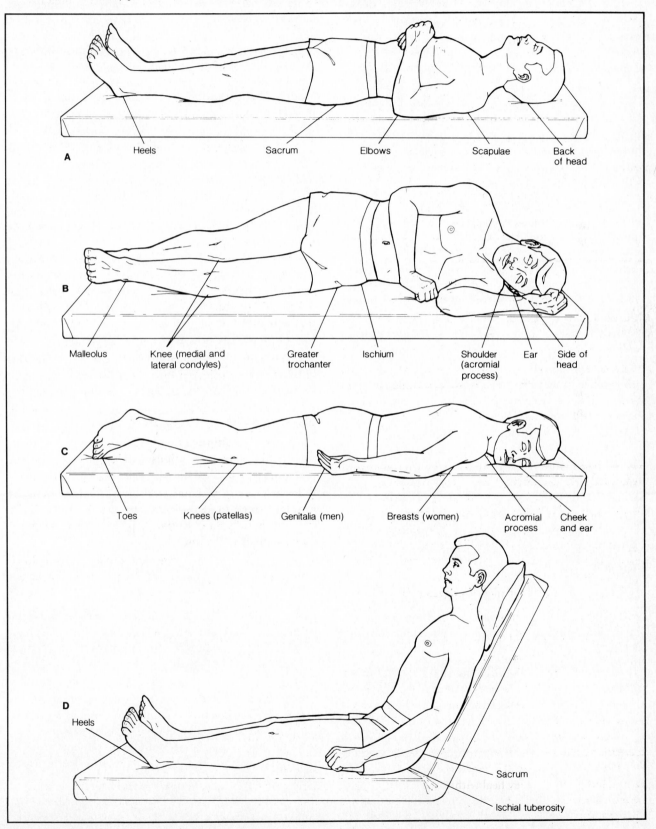

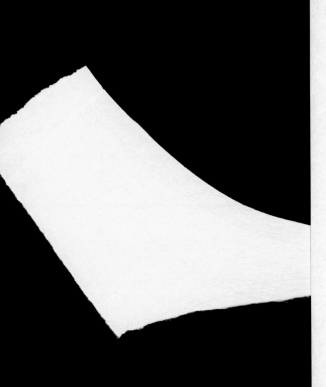

2. Provide good nutrition for the patient, particularly a diet high in protein and vitamin C. Elderly people have increased protein requirements (up to 0.6 g per kg of body weight) to maintain proper nitrogen balance (Kerr, Stinson, Shannon, 1981, p 26).

3. Keep the patient's skin clean and dry, and protect damaged skin from irritation and maceration by urine, feces, sweat, incomplete drying after a bath, soap, or alcohol.

4. Apply powders (rather than astringents, such as alcohol or witch hazel) on tissues with limited blood flow. Astringents constrict the blood vessels and thus inhibit the supply of blood and essential nutrients to the skin. Apply powder carefully to prevent buildup and so that the particles are not inhaled by the patient.

5. Lubricate dry skin areas to prevent cracking. Superfatted soaps and oils may be used.

6. Avoid massaging bony prominences with soap. Research has indicated that the alkalis in soap produce swelling, drying, and loss of natural oils of the skin, thus facilitating skin damage. In addition, prolonged exposure to soap alters the pH of the skin, one of its natural defense barriers (Kerr, Stinson, Shannon, 1981, p 25). Avoid vigorous massage over bony prominences, since it increases tissue damage in deep ulcers that are not apparent to the eye (ibid, p 24).

7. Provide a smooth, firm, wrinkle-free foundation on which the patient can lie.

8. Use foam rubber pads and sheepskins under pressure areas such as the sacrum and heels, and elevate the heels above the bed surface.

9. Avoid the use of rubber rings. Donut-shaped, inflated rubber rings were traditionally placed around actual or potential pressure areas to prevent pressure over bony prominences or actual decubiti. These rings put great pressure on areas of contact, however, and restrict blood flow in both direct contact areas and the enclosed area.

10. Use a special mattress, such as an alternating pressure, eggshell, or flotation mattress, to decrease pressure on body parts.

11. Be alert to early symptoms of pressure sores, particularly over bony prominences: redness or whiteness of an area, tenderness, an unpleasant sensation frequently described as burning, coldness of the area, and localized edema.

12. Teach patients to be aware of discolored areas and of sensations such as tingling, which can indicate pressure.

BATHS

Bathing patterns are highly variable. Some people prefer morning baths, others prefer the evening. Generally, the environment and activity of healthy persons dictate the frequency of bathing. When the weather is hot or strenuous exercise is done, people may take more than one bath daily. Age and the condition of the skin also dictate the frequency of bathing. Elderly people, for example, rarely need a complete bath more than once or twice a week because their skin oil and perspiration are reduced. Any person whose skin is dry usually needs only a partial bath and/or the application of lotion to the skin. Using bath oil in the water and limiting the use of harsh soaps help prevent the skin from drying.

When people are ill, they often need to bathe more frequently. Persons confined to bed are not subjected to the air currents that normally help to evaporate perspiration. This is accentuated for patients who have hyperpyrexia or diaphoresis. Such patients may require complete baths daily and partial sponges more frequently. On the other hand, perspiration may be decreased by some illnesses. Excessive bathing in these instances can interfere with the lubricating effect of sebum, thus aggravating dryness of the skin.

It is not uncommon for patients to require full baths and complete bed linen changes twice a week and partial baths (face, hands, axillae, back, and pubic areas) at least daily. Other baths may be necessitated by illness or recommended in the nurse's judgment. The time for baths in most institutions is morning. For patients who are accustomed to bathing in the evening before retiring, this routine may be a source of frustration.

Kinds of Baths

There are generally two categories of baths given to patients: cleaning and therapeutic. Cleaning baths are given chiefly for hygienic purposes, whereas therapeutic baths are given for a physical effect, such as to soothe irritated skin or to treat an area (eg, the perineum).

Cleaning baths

1. *Complete bed bath.* The nurse washes the entire body of a dependent patient in bed.

2. *Self-help bed bath.* A patient confined to bed is able to bathe himself or herself with help from the nurse for washing the back and perhaps the feet.

3. *Partial bath (abbreviated bath).* Only the parts of the patient's body that might cause discomfort or odor, if neglected, are washed: the face, hands, axillae, perineal area, and back. Omitted are the arms, chest, abdomen, legs, and feet. The nurse provides this care for dependent patients and assists self-sufficient bedridden patients by washing their backs. Some ambulatory patients prefer to take a partial bath at the sink. The nurse can assist by washing the patient's back.

4. *Tub bath.* Tub baths are preferred to bed baths, since washing and rinsing are easier in a tub. Tubs are also

TABLE 14–2 ■ Types of Therapeutic Baths

Bath solution	Directions	Uses
Saline	4 mL (1 tsp) sodium chloride (NaCl) to 500 mL (1 pt) water.	Has a cooling effect. Cleans. Decreases skin irritation.
Oatmeal or Aveeno	720 mL (3 cups) cooked oatmeal in a cheese-cloth bag. Tie the bag securely and twirl it in the tub until the water is opalescent.	Soothes skin irritation. Softens and lubricates dry, scaly skin.
Cornstarch	0.45 kg (1 lb) cornstarch in sufficient cold water to dissolve it; then add boiling water until the mixture is thick. Add to the tub water.	Soothes skin irritation.
Sodium bicarbonate	4 mL (1 tsp) sodium bicarbonate to 500 mL (1 pt) water, or 120–360 mL (4–12 oz) to 120 L (30 gal).	Has a cooling effect. Relieves skin irritation.
Potassium permanganate ($KMnO_4$)	Available in tablets, which are crushed, dissolved in a little water, and added to the bath.	Cleans and disinfects. Treats infected skin areas.

used for therapeutic baths. The amount of assistance offered by the nurse depends on the abilities of the patient. Many agencies have specially designed tubs for dependent patients. These tubs greatly facilitate the work of the nurse in lifting patients in and out of the tub and offer patients greater benefits than a sponge bath in bed.

5. *Shower.* Many ambulatory patients are able to use shower facilities and require only minimal assistance from the nurse.

Therapeutic baths

A therapeutic bath is usually ordered by a physician. Medications may be placed in the water to come in contact with parts of the body, often large skin areas. A therapeutic bath is generally taken in a tub one-third or one-half full, about 114 L (30 gal). The patient remains in the bath for a designated time, often 20 to 30 minutes. If the patient's back, chest, and arms are to be treated, these areas need to be immersed in the solution. The bath temperature is generally ordered by the physician; 37.7 to 40.5 °C (100 to 105 °F) is frequently used for adults and 40.5 °C (105 °F) is usually ordered for infants. See Table 14–2 for types of therapeutic baths.

TECHNIQUE 14–1 ■ Bathing an Adult

The type of bath, the assistance required, and the time of the bath depend largely on the health and preference of the patient. Because adults normally bathe without assistance, nurses must be sensitive to the feelings of the patient who requires assistance with a bath.

■ Assessment

1. Assess the patient's skin. Normal skin exhibits variations in pigment or color; has good tissue turgor and is smooth, soft, and flexible; has a variety of pigmented spots; shows no evidence of cyanosis, jaundice, or pallor; and feels warm to the touch. See Technique 10–2.

a. *Color.* Skin color varies from person to person and from one area of the body to another. Normal skin tones can range from ivory to deep brown (sometimes called *black*). Some people have hues of pink, yellow, or orange. A description of skin color needs to include deviations from the normal, including increased pigmentation. The skin may reflect pallor, flushing, jaundice, or cyanosis. *Pallor* is a whitish-grayish tinge. In a black-skinned person, pallor can appear as ashen gray and in a brown-skinned person as yellowish-brown. In both instances, the skin appears to have lost its underlying red tones. *Flushing* is redness, which may be generalized or restricted to a particular area. In

TABLE 14–3 ■ Skin Lesions

Type of lesion	Description	Examples
Primary		
Macula	A flat, circumscribed area of color with no elevation of its surface; 1 mm to several cm	Freckles, flat nevi
Papule	A circumscribed solid elevation of skin; less than 1 cm	Warts, acne, pimples, flat nevi
Nodule	A solid mass extending deeper into dermis than a papule	Pigmented nevi
Tumor	A solid mass larger than a nodule	Epitheliomas
Cyst	An encapsulated, fluid-filled mass in dermis or subcutaneous tissue	Epidermoid cysts
Wheal	A relatively reddened, flat, localized collection of edema fluid	Mosquito bites, hives
Vesicle	A circumscribed elevation containing serous fluid or blood	Herpes, chickenpox
Bulla	A larger fluid-filled vesicle	Second degree burns
Pustule	A vesicle or bulla filled with pus	Acne vulgaris
Secondary		
Scale	Thickened epidermal cells that flake off	Dandruff
Fissure	A linear crack	Athlete's foot
Erosion	Loss of epidermis that does not extend deeper	Abrasions
Atrophy	A decrease in the volume of epidermis	Striae
Scar	A formation of connective tissue	Keloid
Ulcer	An excavation extending into the dermis or below	Stasis ulcer
Crust	Dried serum on the skin surface	Infected dermatitis

a dark-skinned person, flushing due to a fever may appear at the tips of the ears. *Jaundice* is a yellow tinge to the skin and is often most readily seen in the sclera of the eyes, in both dark- and light-skinned people. However, in darkly pigmented people, jaundice of the sclera needs to be distinguished from deposits of subconjunctival fat; the latter generally appear more concentrated farther from the cornea. The color of the mucous membrane of the hard palate can be checked for

jaundice to confirm it. *Cyanosis* is a bluish color on the lips, around the mouth, in the nails when they are pressed downward, over the cheekbones, and on the earlobes. In black- and brown-skinned people, cyanosis is difficult to detect. Repeated experience observing the patient's palms, soles, nail beds, mouth, and lips often enables the nurse to detect it. The palpebral (eyelid) conjunctiva will also show cyanosis. Increased or decreased pigmentation also needs to be noted. Some increased pigmentation is normal and temporary—for example, brown patches on the forehead and cheeks of some pregnant women (*chloasma gravidarum,* commonly called the *mask of pregnancy*). This particular pigmentation usually disappears spontaneously after childbirth. However, changes in pigmentation may also indicate disease processes.

b. *Texture and turgor.* Although there is some variation in normal skin, it is usually smooth, soft, and flexible. Skin that is dry, flaking, wrinkled, or holding excessive moisture may reflect serious problems. *Turgor* refers to fullness. Skin turgor can be assessed by picking up and pinching the skin. Healthy skin springs back into position, whereas a dehydrated person's skin remains pinched for a short time.

c. *Pigmented spots.* People have a variety of pigmented areas on their bodies. Infants with black and brown skins often have *mongolian spots.* Light-skinned people may have freckles on the face and other parts of the body.

d. *Temperature.* Palpation of the skin reveals whether it is a normal warm temperature or unusually hot or cold. Skin temperature may be similar throughout the body or particular to one area, such as a foot that feels cold due to decreased blood flow.

e. *Lesions.* Many types of lesions occur on the skin. The nurse's main responsibility is to describe them accurately, including (1) distribution and location, (2) size, (3) contour, and (4) consistency. See Table 14–3.

f. *Excoriations and abrasions.* An *excoriation* is the loss of superficial layers of the skin. For example, if a nurse scratches a patient while palpating with long fingernails, the scratch is an excoriation. An *abrasion* is the wearing away of a structure such as the skin or teeth, often by friction (for example, when a patient is dragged instead of rolled across a bed).

2. Assess other pertinent aspects of the patient's health, eg, fatigue, range of motion of joints, and pain.

Additional data include:

1. The type of bath the patient needs, and what assistance the patient requires from the nurse

2. How often the patient requires a bath

3. Other care the patient is receiving, such as roentgenography or physiotherapy, so that the bath can be coordinated with those activities to prevent undue fatigue to the patient

4. The bed linen required by the patient

5. The range of motion of the patient's joints and any other aspects of the patient's health that affect the bathing process

■ Nursing Diagnosis

Nursing diagnoses that may indicate a patient's need for a bath or for assistance with a bath include:

1. Activity intolerance related to congestive heart failure

2. Ineffective breathing pattern related to chest incision and pain

3. Alteration in comfort related to abdominal incision and pain

4. Ineffective individual coping related to loss of limb

5. Impaired physical mobility related to muscle weakness

6. Self-care deficit: inability to bathe self, related to lack of coordination

7. Potential impairment of skin integrity related to immobility of legs

■ Planning

Nursing goals

1. To clean and deodorize the skin by removing accumulated sebum, perspiration, dead skin cells, and some bacteria. When body secretions accumulate they are decomposed by bacterial action, resulting in a pronounced distasteful odor.

2. To stimulate circulation to the skin. Some people take a morning shower for its stimulating effect. A warm or hot bath dilates superficial arterioles, bringing more blood and nourishment to the skin. Vigorous rubbing has the same effect. Rubbing with long smooth strokes from distal to proximal parts of extremities is particularly effective in facilitating venous blood flow.

3. To produce a sense of well-being. Bathing is refreshing and frequently boosts a person's morale, appearance, and self-esteem.

4. To relax tense muscles. Some people take an afternoon or evening bath for its relaxing effect. This relaxation may be greater when a person is ill. It is not uncommon for patients to feel so relaxed and comfortable that they fall asleep after a morning bath.

5. To provide an opportunity to assess the condition of the patient's skin and aspects of the patient's overall physical and mental health, such as mobility, fatigue, strength, hygienic practices, and learning needs.

Equipment

1. Two bath towels, one for the face and one for the remainder of the body.

2. A washcloth.

3. Soap in a soap dish.

4. A basin for the wash water (for a partial or complete bed bath).

5. Hygienic supplies such as lotion, powder, and deodorant.

6. A bath blanket to cover the patient during the bath (for a partial or complete bed bath).

7. Water between 43 and 46 °C (110 and 115 °F) for adults. The water should feel comfortably warm to the patient. People vary in their sensitivity to heat. Most patients will verify a suitable temperature. The water for a bed bath should be changed at least once.

8. A clean gown or pajamas as needed.

9. Additional bed linen and towels, if required.

10. A bedpan or urinal.

■ Intervention

1. Explain what you plan to do. Adjust the explanation to the patient's needs.

   Rationale This reassures the patient by providing knowledge of what will happen, identifies the patient, and allows the nurse to assess whether any special equipment is needed, such as a razor.

2. Close the windows and doors to make sure that the room is free from drafts.

   Rationale Air currents increase loss of heat from the body by convection.

3. Provide privacy by drawing the curtains or closing the door. Some agencies provide signs indicating the need for privacy.

   Rationale Hygiene is a personal matter.

4. Offer the patient a bedpan or urinal or ask whether the patient wishes to use the toilet or commode.

   Rationale The patient will be more comfortable after voiding, and voiding is advisable before cleaning the perineum.

For a bed bath

5. Place the bed in the high position.

   Rationale This avoids undue strain on the nurse's back.

6. Remove the top bed linen, and replace it with the bath blanket. If the bed linen is be reused, place it over the bedside chair. If it is to be changed, place it in the linen hamper.

7. Assist the patient to move near you.

Rationale This facilitates access without undue reaching and straining.

8. Remove the patient's gown.

9. Make a bath mitt with the washcloth (see Figure 14–2):

   a. Triangular method: (1) Lay your hand on the washcloth; (2) fold the top corner over your hand; (3, 4) fold the side corners over the hand; (5) tuck

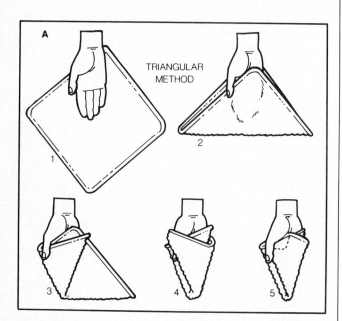

FIGURE 14–2

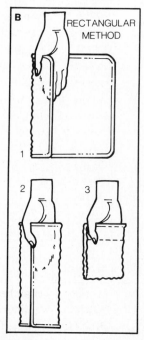

the second corner under the cloth on the palmar side to secure the mitt.

   b. Rectangular method: (1) Lay your hand on the washcloth, and fold one side over your hand; (2) fold the second side over your hand; (3) fold the top of the cloth down, and tuck it under the folded side against your palm to secure the mitt.

   Rationale A bath mitt retains water and heat better than a cloth loosely held.

10. Place one towel across the patient's chest.

11. Wash the patient's eyes with water only, and dry them well. Use a separate corner of the washcloth for each eye, and wipe from the inner to the outer canthus.

   Rationale Using separate corners prevents transmitting microorganisms from one eye to the other. Cleaning from the inner to the outer canthus prevents secretions from entering the nasolacrimal ducts.

12. Ask whether the patient wants soap used on the face. Wash, rinse, and dry the patient's face, neck, and ears.

   Rationale Soap has a drying effect, and the face, which is exposed to the air more than other body parts, tends to be drier.

13. Place the bath towel lengthwise under the patient's arm. Wash, rinse, and dry the arm, using long, firm strokes from distal to proximal areas (from the point farthest from the body to the point closest). Wash the axilla well. Repeat for the other arm. (Omit the arms for a partial bath.) Exercise caution if an IV is present, and check its flow after moving the arm.

   Rationale The bath towel protects the bed from becoming wet. Firm strokes from distal to proximal areas increase venous blood return.

15. Place a towel directly on the bed and put the basin on it. Place the patient's hands in the basin. Assist the patient to wash, rinse, and dry them, paying particular attention to the spaces between the fingers.

   Rationale Many patients enjoy immersing their hands in the basin and washing themselves.

16. Fold the bath blanket down to the patient's pubic area and place the towel alongside the chest and abdomen. Wash, rinse, and dry the patient's chest and abdomen, giving special attention to the skin fold under the breasts. Keep the patient's chest and abdomen covered with the towel between the wash and the rinse. Replace the bath blanket when the areas have been dried. (Omit the chest and abdomen for a partial bath. However, the creases under a woman's breasts may require bathing if they are irritated.) Avoid undue exposure when washing the patient's chest and abdomen. For some patients, it

may be preferable to wash the chest and the abdomen separately. In that case, the bath towel is placed horizontally across the abdomen first and then across the chest.

17. Wrap one of the patient's legs and feet with the bath blanket, ensuring that the pubic area is well covered. See Figure 14–3. Place the bath towel lengthwise under the other leg, and wash that leg. Use long, smooth, firm strokes, washing from the ankle to the knee and from the knee to the thigh. Rinse and dry that leg, reverse the coverings, and repeat for the other leg. (Omit this step for a partial bath.)

    Rationale Washing from distal to proximal areas stimulates venous blood flow.

18. Wash the feet by placing them in the basin of water. Dry each foot. Pay particular attention to the spaces between the toes. If you prefer, wash one foot after that leg, before washing the other leg. (Omit this step for a partial bath.)

19. Obtain fresh, warm bath water now or when necessary.

    Rationale The temperature of the water in the basin cools relatively rapidly, and the water becomes soapy. It needs to be changed often.

20. Assist the patient to turn to a prone position or side-lying position facing away from you. Place the bath towel lengthwise alongside the patient's back and buttocks. Wash and dry the back, buttocks, and upper thighs, paying particular attention to the gluteal folds. Give a back rub. See Technique 14–4. Avoid undue exposure of the patient, as for the abdomen and chest. See step 16.

21. Assist the patient to the supine position, and determine whether the patient can wash the genital–perineal area independently. Say, for example, "I have washed all but your genital area. Would you like to complete your bath?" If the patient cannot do so, drape the patient as shown in Figure 14–5, and wash the area. See Technique 14–3.

    Rationale Many patients prefer to clean their own perineums, if they are able, because it is embarrassing to have this done by another person.

22. Assist the patient to use any hygenic aids desired, such as powder, lotion, or deodorant. Use powder sparingly, because it tends to accumulate.

23. Help the patient to put on a clean gown or pajamas. If intravenous apparatus is attached, see Technique 14–5.

24. Assist the patient with hair, mouth, and nail care. See chapters 12–13. Some patients prefer or need mouth care prior to the bath.

25. Record on the patient's chart significant assessments made during the bath (such as excoriation in the folds beneath the breasts or reddened areas over

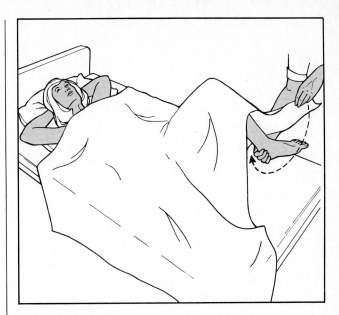

FIGURE 14–3

bony prominences) and progress in relief of previous problems. Bathing is not normally recorded.

For a tub bath or shower

26. Fill the tub about halfway with water at 43 to 46 °C (110 to 115 °F). For a therapeutic bath add the correct medication. See Table 14–2 earlier.

27. Assist the patient to the tub or shower and provide any needed assistance.

    a. Many patients can manage a tub bath or shower independently. Others require assistance only to wash their backs. The patient taking a standing shower may need help initially to adjust the temperature and flow of the water. Explain how the patient can signal for help, and then leave the patient for two to five minutes.

    b. If the patient requires considerable assistance, a second nurse may be needed to help the patient into and out of the tub and/or to hold the patient in a sitting position throughout the bath. When assisting patients into and out of tubs, take safety measures to prevent the patient from falling or slipping. For example, if the patient can step into the tub, he or she should hold the handbar while you support the patient's upper trunk under the axillae. To provide support as the patient sits down in the tub, fold a towel lengthwise and place it around the patient's chest, under both axillae; then hold the ends securely at the back of the patient as the patient sits.

    c. Other patients may need to sit on the edge of the tub or on a chair beside the tub before transferring into the tub. Some tubs have a nonskid surface to prevent the patient's feet from slipping. A rubber mat or a towel placed in the bottom of the tub can provide a secure base for the patient's feet.

28. Wash the patient's back, if necessary, and assist the patient out of the tub.

29. Assist the patient as necessary to dry and to don a clean gown or pajamas.

30. Assist the patient back to the room, and provide a back rub if the patient is spending long periods in bed. See Technique 14–4.

31. Clean the tub or shower in accordance with agency practice, discard used linen in the laundry hamper, and place the "unoccupied" sign on the door.

32. Follow steps 22, 24, and 25.

■ Evaluation

Expected outcomes

1. No evidence of abrasions or reddened skin areas

2. Soft, smooth, flexible skin with good tissue turgor

3. Warm skin temperature

Unexpected outcomes

1. Reddened areas on heels and base of sacrum

2. Broken skin areas

3. Bluish areas

See Table 10–4 on page 169. Upon obtaining an unexpected outcome:

1. Reassess the areas for a detailed description.

2. Refer to the patient's record for pertinent nursing interventions.

3. Report your findings to the responsible nurse and/or physician.

TECHNIQUE 14–2 ■ Shaving a Male Patient

A man who is accustomed to being cleanshaven may feel unkempt and ashamed of his appearance when whiskers grow on his face. Moreover, after two or three days of whisker growth, the skin of the face can become irritated.

■ Assessment

Assess the patient for reddened, bruised, or broken areas on the face. These can be sites of infection and may require cleaning with an antiseptic after shaving. Other data include:

1. The amount of assistance required by the patient.

2. Whether the agency permits nurses to shave male patients. Some hospitals provide barbers for this function, and their labor agreements do not permit nurses to do shaving except in unusual circumstances (eg, when the patient is on precautions for an infection).

3. Whether a physician's order is required before shaving. If so, consult the patient's chart for the order.

■ Nursing Diagnosis

Nursing diagnoses that may indicate the need to shave a male patient include: Self-care deficit: hygiene, related to inability to move upper limbs.

■ Planning

Nursing goal

To remove excess hair growth from the face, to improve the patient's appearance and feeling of well-being.

Equipment

1. A razor and sharp blade or an electric razor. Most patients have their own equipment and have a preference.

2. Shaving cream or shaving soap and a shaving brush. The patient may have a preference.

3. A bath towel, a face towel, and a washcloth. These protect the bed and the patient from moisture and are used for wiping and drying the face.

4. A bath blanket to cover the patient's chest. This maintains warmth and keeps the patient dry.

5. A basin with hot water at 46 °C (115 °F) or the temperature the patient prefers.

6. After-shave lotion or powder, according to the patient's preference.

7. A mirror.

Arrange the equipment for convenient access.

■ Intervention

1. Assist the patient to a sitting position or to as convenient a position as possible for him.

2. Fold the bedclothes to the patient's waist if he is remaining in bed, and place a bath blanket around his shoulders if he feels chilly.

3. If the patient is in bed, place a towel under his head to protect the pillow from moisture.

4. Starting on one side of the face, lather the cheek from below the sideburn to the jaw. Hot water and shaving soap usually provide a good lather. Do not apply soap if you will be using an electric razor.

   Rationale Hot water and shaving soap soften the beard bristles for easier removal and decrease skin irritation from the razor blade.

5. Hold the razor so that the blade is at a 45° angle with the skin. See Figure 14–4.

   Rationale This angle decreases the chances of nicking the skin.

   or

   With an electric razor, start on one side, and work in the direction the hair grows (downward), making short strokes. Empty the razor when it becomes full of hair. Stretch the skin tautly to shave in creases.

6. Shave in the direction of the hair (downward) using short, firm strokes about 2.5 cm (1 in) long.

   Rationale Longer strokes are more likely to pull the hairs.

7. Dip the razor in hot water to remove the lather and hair after each downward set of strokes.

   Rationale These materials can clog the razor and prevent effective cutting.

8. Apply lather and shave the following areas:

   a. The second cheek

   b. The upper lip

   c. The chin

   Pull the skin taut with the other hand before shaving areas with creases, such as the chin.

   Rationale Keeping the skin taut helps prevent cutting the skin.

9. Wipe the patient's face with a wet washcloth to remove any remaining shaving cream and hair.

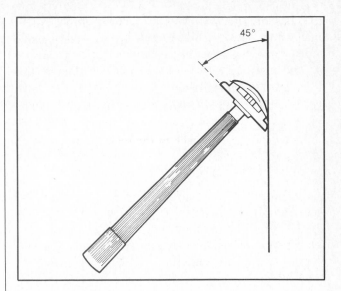

FIGURE 14–4

10. Dry the face well with the face towel.

11. Inspect the face for any unshaven areas and cuts. Assist the patient to inspect the shave in the mirror. If an area was missed, lather and shave it.

12. Apply after-shave lotion or powder (as the patient prefers) to the shaved area of the face, using a patting motion with the fingers.

    Rationale Rubbing can irritate the skin.

13. Record any unexpected response of the patient, such as extreme fatigue, and any facial skin problems. Shaving is not normally recorded.

■ Evaluation

Expected outcome

Smoothly shaven face without abrasions.

Unexpected outcome

Broken areas on the facial skin. See also Table 10–4 on page 169. Upon obtaining an unexpected outcome:

1. Reassess any broken skin area.

2. Report your findings to the responsible nurse and/or physician.

TECHNIQUE 14–3 ■ Perineal–Genital Care

Perineal–genital care is referred to in some agencies as peri-care. For example, the nurse may ask an orderly to "finish the bath" or to provide "peri-care" to a male patient. Other agencies restrict the use of this term to special perineal care provided at prescribed times other than with a bed bath. For example, peri-care is a nursing order commonly prescribed for postdelivery patients, to irrigate or clean the perineal area following each defecation and urination. Because postdelivery patients often have swollen perineal tissues, vaginal discharge of blood, mucus, and tissue from the uterus (lochia), and in some cases an incision of the perineum (episiotomy), frequent cleaning of the perineum is essential to prevent infection.

Perineal care is an embarrassing procedure for most patients. Nurses also may find it embarrassing initially, particularly with patients of the opposite sex. Most patients who require a bed bath from the nurse are able to clean their own genital areas with minimal assistance. The nurse may need to hand a moistened washcloth and soap to the patient, rinse the washcloth, and provide a towel.

Because some patients are unfamiliar with terminology for the genitals and perineum, it may be difficult for nurses to explain what is expected. Most patients, however, understand what is meant if the nurse simply says, "I'll give you a washcloth to finish your bath." Elderly patients may be familiar with the term "private parts." Whatever expression the nurse chooses to use, it needs to be one that the patient understands and one that is comfortable for the nurse to use.

Whenever the nurse provides the perineal care, it needs to be carried out efficiently and matter-of-factly. Some agencies recommend that the nurse wear gloves while providing this care for the comfort of the patient and to protect the nurse from infection.

For information on catheter care, see chapter 27, Technique 27–5.

■ Assessment

Assess the patient for:

1. Complaints of irritation or discomfort in the perineal-genital area
2. Areas of inflammation, excoriation, or swelling, in particular between the labia of females and around the scrotum of males
3. Excessive discharge or secretions from the perineal-genital orifices
4. The presence of odors
5. Areas of irritation or excoriation of the urinary meatus of a patient with an indwelling urinary catheter

Other data include:

1. Recent previous assessments
2. How often the patient needs perineal-genital care, eg, twice a day
3. The amount of assistance the patient requires

4. The physician's or nursing orders for a prescribed solution

■ Nursing Diagnosis

Nursing diagnoses that may indicate the need for perineal-genital care include:

1. Potential impairment of skin integrity related to immobility
2. Self-care deficit: bathing/hygiene, related to fractured legs

■ Planning

Nursing goals

1. To remove normal perineal secretions and odors
2. To prevent infection, eg, when an indwelling catheter is present.
3. To treat an infection

Equipment

When perineal-genital care is provided in conjunction with the bed bath, the following bed bath equipment is used:

1. A bath basin two-thirds filled with water at 43 to 46 °C (110 to 115 °F)
2. Soap in a soap dish
3. A washcloth
4. A bath towel
5. A bath blanket
6. Powder or protective ointment as required

When special perineal-genital care is provided, the equipment listed below may be needed. Some agencies have special peri-care trays for postdelivery patients.

1. A bath towel
2. A bath blanket
3. Disposable gloves
4. Cotton balls or swabs
5. A solution bottle, pitcher, or container filled with warm water or a prescribed solution
6. A bedpan to receive the rinse water
7. A moisture-resistant bag or receptacle for used cotton swabs
8. A perineal pad

■ Intervention

1. Offer an appropriate explanation, being particularly sensitive to any embarrassment felt by the patient.

2. Fold the top bed linen to the foot of the bed, and fold the patient's gown up to expose the genital area.

3. Place a bath towel under the patient's hips so that the lower end can be used to dry the anterior perineum, while the upper end can dry the rectal area.

   Rationale The bath towel prevents the bed from becoming soiled.

For females

4. Position the patient in a back-lying position with the knees flexed and spread well apart (abducted).

5. Cover the patient's body and legs with the bath blanket. Drape the patient's legs by tucking the bottom corners of the bath blanket under the inner sides of the legs. See Figure 14–3 earlier. The middle portion of the base of the blanket is then brought up over the pubic area. See Figure 14–5.

   Rationale Minimum exposure lessens the patient's embarrassment and provides warmth.

6. Wash and dry the upper inner thighs.

7. Clean the labia majora. Then spread the labia to wash the folds between the labia majora and the labia minora. See Figure 14–6. Use separate corners of the washcloth for each fold, and wipe from the pubis to the rectum. For menstruating women and patients with indwelling catheters, use cotton balls or gauze. Take a clean ball for each stroke.

   Rationale Smegma, which tends to collect around the labia minora, facilitates bacterial growth. Using separate corners of the washcloth or new cotton balls or gauzes prevents the transmission of microorganisms from one area to the other. Wiping is done from the area of least contamination (the pubis) to the area of greatest contamination (the rectum).

8. Rinse the area well. You may place the patient on a bedpan and pour a pitcher of warm water over the area.

9. Dry the perineum thoroughly, paying particular attention to the folds between the labia.

   Rationale Moisture supports the growth of many microorganisms.

10. Inspect the labia and perineal orifices for intactness. Inspect particularly around the urethra for patients who have indwelling catheters. Apply a protective ointment if necessary.

    Rationale A catheter may tend to cause excoration around the urethra.

11. To clean between the buttocks, assist the patient to turn on her side facing away from you. Pay particular attention to the anal area. Clean the anus with toilet tissue before washing it, if necessary. Dry the area well.

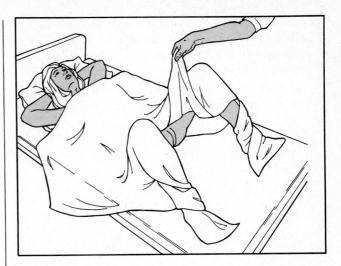

FIGURE 14-5

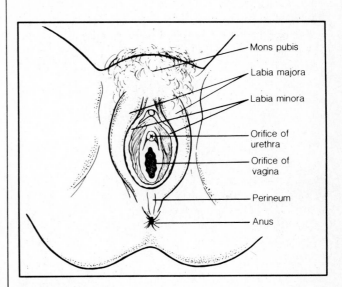

Mons pubis
Labia majora
Labia minora
Orifice of urethra
Orifice of vagina
Perineum
Anus

FIGURE 14-6

12. Apply powder or protective ointments, such as petroleum jelly, if necessary.

    Rationale Powder tends to absorb moisture. Petroleum jelly can protect excoriated areas.

13. For postdelivery patients, apply a perineal pad from front to back.

    Rationale This prevents contamination of the vagina and urethra from the anal area.

14. Record on the patient's chart any significant observations, such as redness, swelling, or discharge.

For males

15. Position the patient in a supine position with knees slightly flexed and hips slightly externally rotated.

16. Wash and dry the upper inner thighs.

17. Put on gloves (optional). Wash and dry the penis using firm strokes. If the patient is uncircumcised,

retract the prepuce (foreskin) to expose the glans penis (the tip of the penis) for cleaning. Replace the foreskin after cleaning the glans penis. See Figure 14–7.

Rationale By handling the penis firmly, the nurse may prevent an erection. Having the nurse wear gloves may also be more comfortable for the patient. Retracting the foreskin is necessary to remove the smegma that collects under the foreskin and facilitates bacterial growth.

18. Wash and dry the scrotum. The posterior folds of the scrotum may need to be cleaned with the buttocks.

Rationale The scrotum tends to be more soiled than the penis because of its proximity to the rectum; thus it is usually cleaned after the penis.

FIGURE 14–7

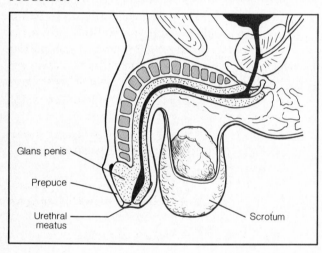

19. Clean the buttocks in the manner described for female patients (steps 11–12 above).

20. Record on the patient's chart any significant observations, such as redness, swelling, or discharge.

Sample Recording

Date	Time	Notes
7/10/86	0900	Perineal care given. Circular reddened area about 2.5 cm diameter to left of urethral orifice. No discharge apparent.———— ———————— Patricia L. Snow, SN

■ Evaluation

Expected outcomes

1. No evidence of reddened areas
2. No abnormal discharge
3. No foul odor

Unexpected outcomes

1. Any reddened, excoriated, or swollen areas
2. Any discharge from perineal–genital orifices
3. Complaints of discomfort in perineal–genital area

Upon obtaining an unexpected outcome:

1. Reassess the area for a detailed description.
2. Refer to the patient's record for pertinent nursing interventions.
3. Report your findings to the responsible nurse and/or physician.

TECHNIQUE 14–4 ■ Giving a Back Rub

The back rub is a massage of the back, with two chief objectives: to relax and relieve tension (sedative effect), and to stimulate blood circulation to the tissues and the muscles. Friction from the rubbing produces heat at the skin surface. This causes the peripheral blood vessels in the area to dilate, thus increasing the blood supply to the area. Because tissues are under pressure when a patient is in bed and muscles are usually relaxed, stimulation of the circulation is essential so that the tissues obtain nutrients and oxygen.

Five types of massage can be used to rub the back and the bony prominences of the body:

1. In the *tapotement,* the little-finger side of each hand is used in a sharp, hacking movement on the back. Care must be taken not to bruise the patient. This method is not advised for the elderly, debilitated patients, or patients who have pathologic back conditions.
2. The *petrissage* is a kneading or large, quick pinch of the skin, subcutaneous tissue, and muscle. Pinches are taken first up the vertebral column and then over the entire back. The tapotement and the petrissage are primarily stimulating, especially if done quickly, with firm pressure.

3. The *friction* stroke is a circular stroke using both thumbs. The back is massaged from the buttocks to the shoulders using smooth, tiny circles.
4. The *effleurage* is a smooth, long stroke, moving the hands up and down the back. The hands move lightly down the sides of the back, maintaining contact with the skin, but move firmly up the back. This rub has a relaxing, sedative effect if slow movement and light pressure are used.
5. The *three-handed effleurage* is a smooth, stroking motion that gives the patient an impression of three hands. The nurse starts with one hand at the base of the patient's neck and moves it to the lateral aspect of the shoulder. The other hand then makes the same movement to the other shoulder before the first hand is removed from shoulder to return to the base of the neck. This rub is particularly effective in relieving tension of the neck muscles.

Effleurage with circular motions is the method usually used by nurses for patients in hospitals.

■ Assessment

Assess the patient for:

1. Whitish or reddened skin areas, caused by pressure, that do not disappear after a few minutes of rubbing.
2. Broken or raw skin areas caused by friction (rubbing). These frequently occur on the elbows or heels which rub against the base of the bed.

See also Table 10–4. Other data include:

1. Previous assessments of the skin
2. How often the patient needs skin care
3. Any special lotions used by the patient

■ Nursing Diagnosis

Nursing diagnoses that may indicate the need for rubbing the back and bony prominences include:

1. Alteration in comfort related to chronic arthritic pain
2. Impaired physical mobility related to fractured legs

■ Planning

Nursing goals

1. To relax and relieve muscle tension
2. To stimulate blood circulation to the tissues in the area, thereby preventing decubitus ulcers
3. To relieve pain

Equipment

1. Lotion, alcohol, or powder depending on the patient's preference. Often patients have a container of back rub solution at the bedside. Unless another agent is specifically ordered by the physician, lotion is preferred because of its lubricating action on the skin. Alcohol has a cooling, refreshing effect, but it tends to be drying and is therefore not indicated for people with dry skin, particularly the elderly.
2. A towel to remove excess moisture.

■ Intervention

1. Assist the patient to move to the near side of the bed within your reach.
2. Establish which position the patient prefers. The prone position is recommended for a back rub. If this position cannot be assumed, a side-lying position is used, although that makes it difficult to massage the lateral aspect of the hip on which the patient is lying. The patient will need to turn to the other side for you to complete that part of the back rub.
3. Expose the patient's back from the shoulders to the inferior sacral area.
4. Pour a small amount of lotion onto the palms of your hands and hold it for a minute, or place the container in a bath basin filled with warm water.
   Rationale   Back rub preparations tend to feel uncomfortably cold to patients. Holding warms the solution slightly, so that it will be more comfortable.
5. Rub in a circular motion over the sacral area.
6. Move your hands up the center of the back and then over both scapulae.
7. Massage in a circular motion over the scapulae.
8. Move your hands down the sides of the back.
9. Massage the areas over the right and left iliac crests. See Figure 14–8.
10. Repeat steps 5–9 for three to five minutes. Repeat step 4 as necessary.
11. While massaging the patient's skin, watch for:
    a. Whitish or reddened skin areas that do not disappear after rubbing.
    b. Broken or raw skin areas, especially on the elbows or heels.
12. Provide extra rubbing on any reddened areas on the body.
    Rationale   It is important to stimulate blood circulation to these areas.
13. Pat dry any excess solution with a towel.
14. Record on the patient's chart any redness, broken skin areas, and bruises.

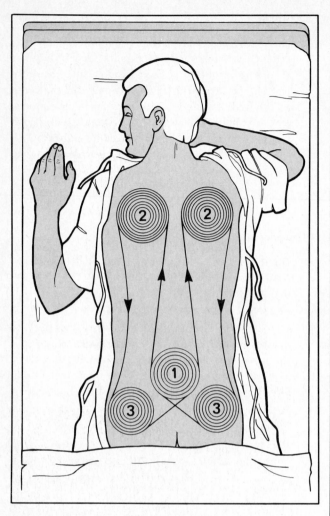

FIGURE 14–8

■ Evaluation

Expected outcomes

1. Skin surface is unbroken and unbruised.
2. Reddened areas disappear with rubbing.

Unexpected outcomes

1. Broken and/or bruised areas on the skin surface
2. Reddened areas that remain red after rubbing

Upon obtaining an unexpected outcome:

1. Reassess the appearance and location of any broken, bruised, or reddened areas.
2. Report your findings to the responsible nurse and/or physician.
3. Adjust the nursing care plan for regular skin care and position changes.

TECHNIQUE 14–5 ■ Changing a Hospital Gown for a Patient with an Intravenous Infusion

A patient may require a gown change while an intravenous (IV) infusion is running into a vein in the patient's arm. Some hospitals provide special gowns for patients receiving IVs. These gowns open from the neck over the shoulders and down the sleeves. The openings are closed with ties or Velcro fasteners that can be undone on the side with the IV, so that the sleeve slips readily off the patient when the gown needs to be removed. Another practice is to remove the gown sleeve from the patient's arm before an IV is started. Again, this makes it simple to change the gown.

However, many patients wear standard hospital gowns. The arm receiving the IV is placed through the sleeve, and nurses need to follow a special sequence of steps to change the gown.

■ Assessment

Assess the following:

1. The intravenous site and the arm for:
   a. Discoloration
   b. Swelling
   c. Fluid leakage
   d. Coldness of the skin

2. The amount of IV solution remaining in the container and the amount that should be in the container. If another bottle needs to be attached, report this to the responsible nurse before changing the gown.

3. The rate of the intravenous infusion before removing the gown and after putting on the clean gown. The counts should be the same. On regulating intravenous flow rates, see chapter 25.

4. Whether the patient's bedding requires changing.

Other data include:

1. The correct infusion rate and the type of infusion ordered.

2. Whether another container has been ordered to follow the one currently running.

■ Nursing Diagnosis

Nursing diagnoses that may indicate the need to change the patient's gown without interrupting the infusion include: Self-care deficit: inability to dress self, related to restricitve intravenous infusion.

■ Planning

Nursing goal

To change a patient's gown without interrupting the flow of the intravenous solution.

Equipment

1. A clean hospital gown
2. Clean bed linen if required
3. A basin of water, soap, a washcloth, and a towel, if needed for washing the patient

■ Intervention

1. Count the rate of flow of the infusion.
   Rationale   It should be running at the designated rate.

Removing a soiled gown

2. Remove the gown from the arm without the infusion.
   Rationale   It is easier to remove the sleeve from the arm with the infusion next.

3. Slip the gown down the arm with the IV and onto the tubing. See Figure 14–9.

4. Take the intravenous container off the hook and slide the sleeve over it. See Figure 14–10. Maintain the position the container was in when hanging, and

hold it above the patient's arm. Do not pull on the tubing.
Rationale   Maintaining the container's position prevents the backflow of blood from the vein into the tubing. Pulling on the tubing can dislodge the needle in the vein.

5. Remove the soiled gown. Rehang the intravenous container. Wash and dry the patient as necessary.

Putting a clean gown on the patient

6. Put the gown in front of the patient as it would be worn.

7. Take the intravenous container off the hook, and pass it through the sleeve from the inside to the cuff. See Figure 14–11. Maintain the position the container was in on the stand, and keep it above the level of the arm.

8. Rehang the intravenous container.

9. Carefully guide the patient's arm and the tubing into the sleeve. Be careful not to pull on the tubing.

FIGURE 14–9

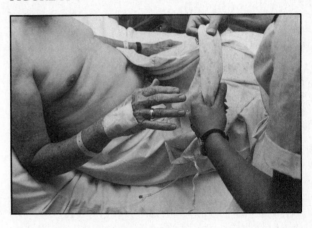

FIGURE 14–10

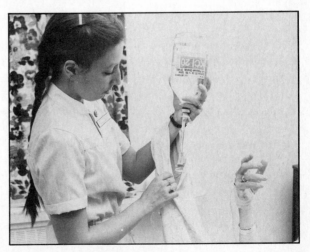

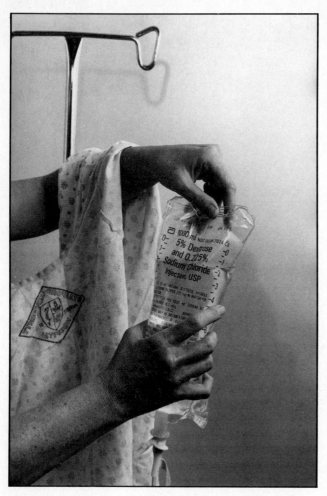

FIGURE 14–11

10. Arrange the tubing so that it is gently coiled. Avoid any kinks.

    Rationale Kinks can stop the flow of the solution into the patient's vein.

11. Assist the patient to put the other arm into the second sleeve of the gown.

12. Secure the ties on the gown at the back of the neck.

13. Count the rate of flow of the infusion to make sure it is correct.

■ Evaluation

Expected outcome

The infusion rate remains unchanged.

Unexpected outcomes

1. The infusion rate is changed or the infusion has stopped.

2. The infusion is leaking.

Upon obtaining an unexpected outcome:

1. Reassess the rate of flow of the infusion.

2. Reassess that there is nothing obstructing the tubing.

3. Correct the rate of flow.

4. Report your findings to the responsible nurse.

TECHNIQUE 14–6 ■ Giving an Infant Sponge Bath

Practices in the hygienic care of infants vary considerably. For example, some agencies provide a bath when the newborn is first admitted to the nursery, while others simply remove any birth debris from the infant's face, for aesthetic reasons, and then diaper and wrap the baby warmly in a blanket. Some remove the vernix caseosa, while others do not. When the newborn's status is stabilized, daily hygienic care often includes a sponge bath until the umbilical cord stump falls off. Cord care and, for some male infants, circumcision care are also required. The cord stump usually falls off spontaneously in five to eight days, but it may last up to 2 weeks. After it disappears and the umbilicus appears well healed, the infant is usually given tub baths.

■ Assessment

During a bath, you have an opportunity to assess many aspects of the infant's health, such as reflexes, responses, and the color and consistency of stools. This section, however, focuses on assessment of the infant's skin. Assess the infant for:

1. Skin areas that are dry, cracked, or peeling. Peeling generally occurs 2 to 4 weeks following birth.

2. Cradle cap on the scalp.

3. Signs of redness at the cord stump or a foul-smelling discharge around the umbilicus, which may indicate infection.

4. Diaper rash (reddened and chafed areas) on the buttocks and perineum.

5. Healing of the circumcision incision or signs of bleeding and infection.

6. Overall color of the skin. Physiologic jaundice normally occurs about three or four days following birth, since the large numbers of red blood cells necessary for fetal life are no longer needed and undergo destruction. When jaundice occurs within the first 24 hours after birth, it may indicate a blood incompatibility between mother and baby. This is called *pathologic jaundice*. The physician needs to be notified of this, and medical therapy can then be initiated.

See also Table 10–4. Other data include:

1. Whether the infant's eyes, face, and scalp are to be washed before or after the infant is undressed. Practices vary from agency to agency.

2. Whether the infant requires a complete or partial bath. Some agencies recommend daily washing of the scalp, washing of the genital area as necessary, and a complete sponge bath less frequently.

3. Whether the baby's weight is to be taken in conjunction with the bath.

4. Whether the infant's temperature is to be taken after the bath.

■ Nursing Diagnosis

Nursing diagnoses that may indicate the need to give an infant a sponge bath include:

1. Self-care deficit: bathing/hygiene, related to maturation

2. Potential impairment of skin integrity related to diaper rash

■ Planning

Nursing goals

1. To remove the vernix caseosa that covers the skin of the fetus, particularly from creases and folds, such as under the foreskin of the glans penis in male babies and between the labia in female babies, if required

2. To clean the skin, including the scalp, genitals, and buttocks

3. To provide care for the umbilical cord stump

4. To assess the skin, healing of the cord stump and circumcision incision, and general physical growth and functioning

Equipment

1. A washbasin or other container with bath water. Some agencies provide disposable cups for bath water, to maintain strict aseptic technique. The water should be 38 to 40 °C (100 to 105 °F) if measured with a bath thermometer, or it should feel slightly warm when tested against the inside of the nurse's wrist or elbow.

2. A soft washcloth or absorbent pad for sponging and drying.

3. Mild, nonperfumed soap in a container.

4. Cotton balls.

5. A moisture-resistant bag in which to dispose of used cotton balls.

6. A towel to place under the baby during the bath.

7. A bath blanket or towel to cover the infant during the bath.

8. A soft-bristled brush or baby comb for cleaning the infant's scalp.

9. A diaper.

10. A shirt and/or nightgown.

11. Mild lotion or baby oil if needed for dry skin.

■ Intervention

When caring for newborns, you should be free of pathogenic microorganisms, including any in the respiratory tract. Employ strict medical aseptic practices, including washing hands, before handling a newborn, because infants have few defenses against unfamiliar microorganisms.

1. Ensure that the room is warm and free of drafts. This is particularly important when caring for newborns, because their temperature-regulating mechanisms are not completely developed.

2. Remove the infant's diaper, and wipe away any feces on the baby's perineum with tissues.

3. Reassure the infant before and during the bath by talking in soothing tones, and hold the infant firmly but gently.

4. Undress the infant, and bundle him or her in a supine position in a towel.

5. Place small articles such as safety pins out of the infant's reach.

6. Ascertain the infant's weight and vital signs. They are often measured in conjunction with a bath.

7. Clean the baby's eyes with water only, using a washcloth or cotton balls. Use a separate corner of the washcloth or a separate ball for each eye. Wipe from the inner to the outer canthus. In some agencies

the infant's eyes, face, and scalp are cleaned *before* the infant is undressed.

Rationale Using a separate corner or ball prevents the transmission of microorganisms from one eye to the other. Wiping away from the inner canthus avoids wiping debris into the nasolacrimal duct.

8. Wash and dry the baby's face using water only. Soap may be used to clean the ears.

Rationale Soap can be very irritating to the eyes.

9. Pick the baby up using the football hold (that is, hold the baby against your side, supporting the body with your forearm and the head with the palm of your hand). See Figure 24–7 on page 528. Position the baby's head over the washbasin, and lather the scalp with a mild soap. Massage the lather over the scalp using the soft-bristled brush, the baby comb, or your fingertips.

Rationale This loosens any dry scales from the scalp and helps to prevent cradle cap. If cradle cap is present, it may be treated with baby oil, a dandruff shampoo, or ointment prescribed by the physician.

10. Rinse and dry the scalp well. Place the baby supine again.

11. Wash, rinse, and dry each arm and hand, paying particular attention to the axilla. Avoid excessive rubbing. Dry thoroughly.

Rationale Rubbing can cause skin irritation, and moisture can cause excoriation of the skin.

12. Wash, rinse, and dry the baby's chest and abdomen. Keep the baby covered with the bath blanket or towel between washing and rinsing.

Rationale Covering the infant prevents chilling.

13. Clean the base of the umbilical cord with a cotton ball dipped in 70% ethyl alcohol. Some agencies use other antiseptics, such as povidone-iodine (Betadine).

Rationale Alcohol promotes drying and prevents infection.

14. Wash, rinse, and dry the baby's legs and feet. Expose only one leg and foot at a time. Give special attention to the areas between the toes.

Rationale Keeping exposure to a minimum maintains the baby's warmth.

15. Turn the baby on her or his stomach or side. Wash, rinse, and dry the back.

16. Place the baby on his or her back. Clean and dry the genitals and anterior perineal area from front to back.

Rationale The rectal area is cleaned last, since it is the most contaminated.

a. Clean the folds of the groin.

b. For females, separate the labia, and clean between them. Clean the genital area from front to back, using moistened cotton balls. Use a clean swab for each stroke.

Rationale The smegma that collects between the folds of the labia (and under the foreskin in males) facilitates bacterial growth and must be removed. Lotions, powders, etc, can also accumulate between the labia and need to be removed. Clean swabs are used to avoid spreading microorganisms from the rectal area to the urethra.

c. If a male infant is uncircumcised, retract the foreskin if possible, and clean the glans penis, using a moistened cotton ball. If the foreskin is tight, do not forcibly retract it. Gentle pressure on a tight foreskin over a period of days or weeks may accomplish eventual retraction. Phimosis may require correction by circumcision. After swabbing, replace the foreskin to prevent edema (swelling) of the glans penis. Clean the shaft of the penis and the scrotum. In some agencies, the foreskin is not retracted.

d. If a male infant has been recently circumcised, clean the glans penis by gently squeezing a cotton ball moistened with clear water over the site. Note any signs of bleeding or infection. In some agencies, petroleum jelly or a bacteriocidal ointment is applied to the circumcision site. Avoid applying excessive quantities of ointment.

Rationale Excess ointment may obstruct the urinary meatus.

e. Apply A and D Ointment (lanolin and petrolatum) to the perineum according to agency practice.

Rationale This helps prevent diaper rash.

17. To clean the posterior perineum and buttocks, grasp both of the baby's ankles, raise the feet, and elevate the buttocks. Wash and rinse the area with the washcloth. Dry the area, and apply ointment, according to agency policy. Do not apply powder.

Rationale The baby may inhale particles of powder, which would irritate the respiratory tract.

18. Check for dry, cracked, or peeling skin, and apply a mild baby oil or lotion according to agency policy.

19. Clothe the baby in a shirt (if the temperature of the environment warrants it) and/or nightgown and a diaper. Place the diaper below the cord site.

Rationale Exposing the cord site to the air will promote healing.

20. Until the umbilicus and circumcision are healed, position the baby on his or her side in the crib with a rolled towel or diaper behind the back for support.

Rationale This position allows more air to circulate around the cord site, facilitates drainage of mucus from the mouth, and is more comfortable for circumcised babies.

When the umbilicus and circumcision are healed, place the baby in the prone position.

21. Cover and bundle the baby with a blanket, if the environmental temperature permits.

    Rationale   This gives the baby a sense of security as well as keeping him or her warm.

22. Record any significant observations, such as reddened areas or skin rashes, the color and consistency of the stool, the state of the cord stump, and the state of the circumcision incision.

■ Evaluation

Expected outcome

Normal healthy skin, with good tissue turgor, normal color, and soft, smooth, flexible texture.

Unexpected outcome

Abrasions, poor tissue turgor, and/or abnormal color. Upon obtaining an unexpected outcome:

1. Reassess the skin for a detailed description.
2. Report your findings to the responsible nurse and/or physician.
3. Plan specific nursing interventions for problems assessed, and record these on the infant's care plan.

TECHNIQUE 14-7   ■   Giving an Infant Tub Bath

After the cord stump has separated and the umbilicus is healed, the infant's body can be immersed in a tub of water. New parents need information from the nurse about this basic hygienic care. Many agencies provide bath demonstration and opportunities for new parents to ask questions before they leave the hospital.

■ Assessment

See Technique 14–6 on page 342 and Table 10–4 on page 169. In addition:

1. Detemine how often the infant requires a tub bath.
2. Determine whether the baby's weight and temperature are to be measured in conjunction with giving the bath.
3. From the infant's record, obtain information about skin problems and what progress assessments are to be made.

■ Nursing Diagnosis

Nursing diagnoses that may indicate the need to give an infant tub bath include:

1. Self-care deficit: bathing/hygiene, related to maturation
2. Potential impairment of skin integrity related to presence of urine and diaper rash

■ Planning

Nursing goals

1. To clean and deodorize the skin
2. To stimulate circulation to the skin
3. To provide a sense of well-being
4. To assess the skin, reflexes, etc

Equipment

Assemble all supplies needed within easy reach. A baby left unattended or out of sight for even a few seconds can move and fall from the bath area. Keep supplies out of reach of the infant, however. Small articles, such as safety pins, can be hazardous to an active and curious infant.

The equipment required for an infant tub bath is similar to that for a sponge bath. It includes:

1. A tub with bath water at 38 to 40 °C (100 to 105 °F). Measure the temperature with a bath thermometer, or test it against the inside of your wrist or elbow. Some parents add a few drops of baby oil to the bath water. Because this makes the tub slippery, they should place a small towel in the bottom of the tub.
2. A soft washcloth or absorbent pad for sponging and drying.
3. Mild, nonperfumed soap in a container.

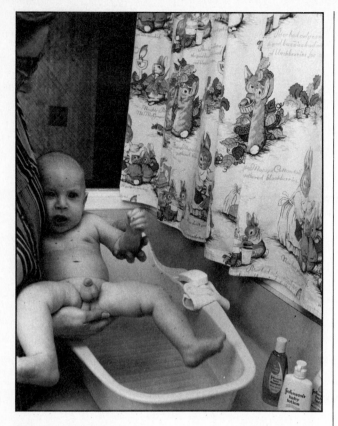

FIGURE 14–12

4. Cotton balls.

5. A bag in which to dispose of used cotton balls.

6. A towel to place under the baby before and after the bath and to dry the infant.

7. A bath blanket or towel to cover the infant before and after the bath.

8. A soft-bristled brush for cleaning the scalp.

9. A diaper.

10. A shirt and/or nightgown.

11. Mild lotion or baby oil, if necessary, for dry skin.

■ **Intervention**

1. Prepare a flat, padded surface in the bath area, on which to dress and undress the infant. It should be high enough so that you or the parent can avoid stooping, which can produce back strain. Usually parents use a counter or table top in the bathroom or kitchen, unless a bathinette is available. Cover the surface with a towel.

2. Place the tub near the dressing surface to prevent exposure and chilling when transferring the baby in and out of the tub. Be sure the room is warm and free from drafts.

3. Follow Technique 14–6, Intervention steps 7–8.

4. Pick up and hold the baby securely, with the head

and shoulders supported on one forearm and the hips and buttocks supported on the other hand. See Figure 14–12.

Rationale Young infants have not developed sufficiently to hold their heads up alone.

5. Gradually immerse the baby into the tub, giving the infant time to adjust to the water.

6. Keeping the baby's head and back supported on your forearm (see Figure 14–13), lather the scalp with a mild soap. Massage the lather over the scalp, using the soft-bristled brush or your fingertips. Rinse the scalp well.

Rationale This loosens any dry scales from the scalp and helps prevent cradle cap. If cradle cap is present, it may be treated with mineral oil, a dandruff shampoo, or ointment prescribed by the physician.

7. Soap and rinse the baby's trunk, extremities, genitals, and perineal area with your free hand. Hold the baby as shown in Figure 14–13 throughout. If the baby enjoys the bath, this technique can be done in a leisurely manner.

8. Remove the baby from the tub by the hold shown in Figure 14–12, and quickly bundle the baby in a towel.

Rationale It is important to avoid chilling the infant.

9. Gently pat the baby dry, giving special attention to the body creases and folds.

Rationale Rubbing can cause skin irritation.

10. Apply baby oil or lotion to dry, cracked, or peeling areas.

11. Clothe the baby in a shirt (if the temperature of the environment warrants it) and/or a nightgown and a diaper.

12. Place the baby in a prone or side-lying position in the crib.

FIGURE 14–13

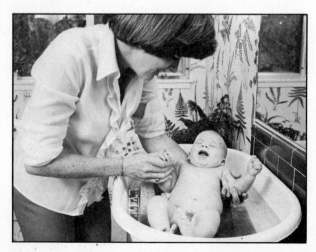

Rationale   These positions facilitate the drainage of mucus from the mouth.

13. Cover and bundle the baby with a blanket, if the environmental temperature permits.

    Rationale   This gives the baby a sense of security as well as keeping him or her warm.

14. Record any significant observations, such as reddened areas or skin rashes, and the color and consistency of the stool.

■ **Evaluation**   See Technique 14–6 on page 345.

TECHNIQUE 14–8   ■   Changing a Diaper

When a diaper becomes soiled with either urine or feces, it should be changed promptly, so that the baby's skin does not become irritated by the waste products. The infant's perineal–genital area is washed and thoroughly dried before a clean diaper is applied.

■ **Assessment**

Assess the infant for:

1. The condition of the skin. See Table 10–4 on page 169. Inspect for excoriation, irritations, etc, especially around the perineum and buttocks.
2. The amount, color, and odor of the urine and feces.
3. The state and progress of any health problem, such as a swollen abdomen or healing of a circumcision.
4. Any behavior that could reflect pain. Assess this before, during, and after changing the diaper.
5. Emotional reactions, eg, fear, friendliness, suspicion.

Other data include:

1. The type of diaper required by the infant
2. Any special precautions to take while changing the diaper, such as not elevating the infant's buttocks by lifting the legs, or the need to obtain a stool specimen

■ **Planning**

Nursing goals

1. To maintain the infant's comfort and cleanliness
2. To maintain the integrity of the skin by preventing irritation from urine and/or feces

Equipment

1. A clean diaper. Commercial disposable diapers are used in many agencies and homes. However, soft absorbent cloth can also be folded as a diaper. Three methods can be used to fold diapers: triangular (see Figure 14–14), rectangular (see Figure 14–15), or kite (see Figure 14–16). When the rectangular method is used, an extra thickness of material is provided either at the front (for boys) or the back (for girls) for additional absorbency. It may also be placed at the front for girls who are positioned on their stomachs for sleep (so that the urine runs to the front).
2. Commercially prepared wipes or a basin with warm water, 38 to 40 °C (100 to 105 °F).
3. Soap.
4. A washcloth.
5. A towel.
6. Mild lotion or protective ointment, eg, zinc oxide, to protect the infant's buttocks and perineal area.
7. A receptacle for the soiled diaper.

■ **Intervention**

1. Place the infant in a supine position on a clean, flat surface near the assembled supplies. Handle the infant slowly and securely, and speak in soothing tones.

    Rationale   Slow movements and soothing voice tones will help calm any of the infant's fears.

Removing a soiled diaper

2. Placing your fingers between the baby's skin and the diaper, unpin the diaper on each side. Close the pins and place them out of reach of the infant.

    Rationale   The fingers protect the baby from being pricked as the pins are removed. Babies may grab the pins and place them in their mouths if the pins are within reach.

3. Pull the front of the diaper down between the infant's legs.

4. Grasp the infant's ankles with one hand and lift the baby's buttocks. See Figure 14–17.

5. Use the clean portion of the diaper to wipe any excess urine or feces from the buttocks. Wipe from anterior to posterior.

   Rationale Wiping toward the posterior of the infant wipes away from the urethral orifice and decreases the possibility of transferring microorganisms to the urinary tract.

6. Remove the diaper. Lower the baby's buttocks. Dispose of the diaper. Do not let the infant out of your sight or reach.

   Rationale The infant could roll over and off the changing surface.

FIGURE 14–14 ■ The triangular method of folding a diaper: **A,** fold a square cloth to a rectangular shape; **B,** fold the cloth again to the correct size square; **C,** bring opposite corners together to form a triangle; **D,** apply the triangle with the fold at the waist.

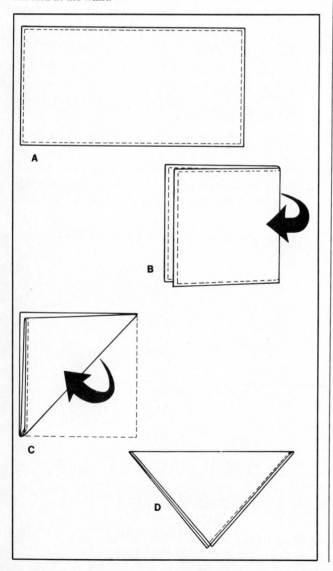

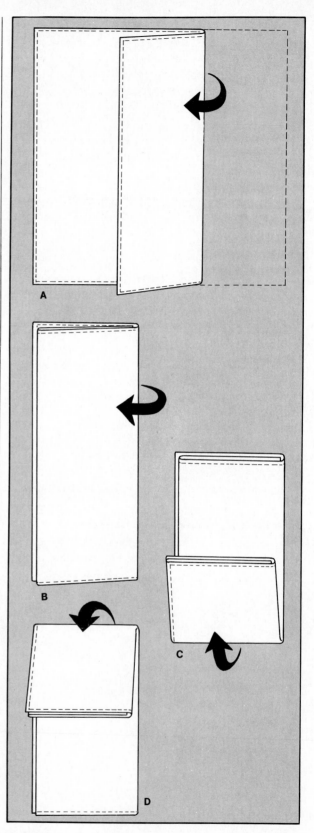

FIGURE 14–15 ■ The rectangular method of folding a diaper: **A, B,** fold the diaper into a rectangle by bringing the sides over; **C,** fold the bottom edge up to provide the thickness in front; or **D,** fold the top edge down to provide the thickness at the back.

7. Clean the buttocks and the anal–genital area with warm water and soap or commercial cleansing tissues. Clean toward the posterior as in step 5. Rinse and dry the area well with the towel.

   Rationale Cleaning removes remaining urine and feces, which can irritate the skin. Drying well prevents irritation of the skin by moisture.

8. Apply a protective ointment or lotion to the perineum and buttocks, especially to the skin creases.

Applying a clean diaper

9. Lay the diaper flat on a clean surface with the folded edges up, and place the baby on the center of the diaper width so that the back edge of the diaper is at waist level.

   or

   Grasp the baby's ankles with one hand and raise the baby's legs and buttocks. Place the diaper under the baby so that the back edge is at waist level.

FIGURE 14–16 ■ The kite method of folding a diaper: **A,** make a triangle by folding the side corners to the center; **B,** bring the bottom corner up to the center; **C,** fold down the top corner.

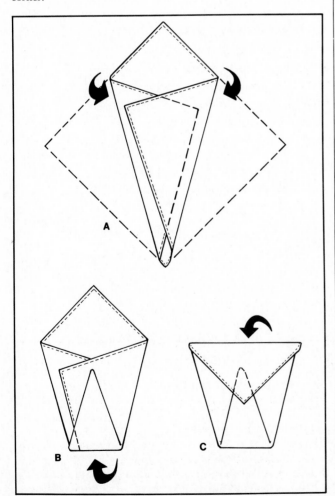

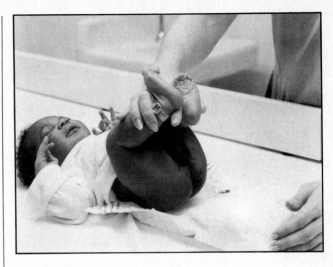

FIGURE 14–17

10. Draw the diaper up between the baby's legs to the waist in front.

11. Fasten the diaper at the waist so that it fits snugly. If safety pins are used, hold your fingers between the baby and the diaper while pinning.

    Rationale The nurse's fingers protect the baby from being pricked with the pins.

    The pins may be positioned vertically or horizontally. See Figure 14–18.

    Rationale The horizontal position is suggested when the child is old enough to sit. The pins are then less likely to poke the body. The vertical position is suggested for diapers pinned at the sides rather than at the front, if the infant does not yet sit up.

    Insert the diaper pins so that they face upward or outward.

    Rationale If a pin then opens inadvertently, it will not puncture the baby's thigh or abdomen.

12. Dress the infant with additional clothes as required.

13. Return the infant to the crib.

14. Record stool and/or urine observations on the record sheet and/or the infant's chart. Record other pertinent observations, such as skin redness, on the patient's record.

■ Evaluation

Expected outcomes

1. Skin is clean and soft with no excoriation.

2. Urine and feces are normal.

3. The infant appears comfortable.

4. The infant exhibits no signs of fear.

FIGURE 14-18

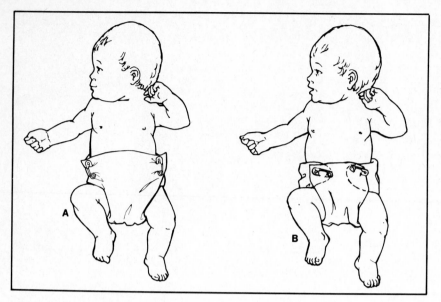

Unexpected outcomes

1. Excoriated skin.
2. Abnormal amount or appearance of urine and/or feces. See chapters 26–27, for characteristics of normal urine and feces.

Upon obtaining an unexpected outcome:

1. Adjust the nursing care plan for regular skin care.
2. Report your findings to the responsible nurse and/or physician.

Teaching Situations Regarding Skin Care

Examples of situations in which patients or families may have learning needs are:

1. New parents usually need the following instruction about hygienic care of the newborn:

a. How to give a sponge bath and a tub bath

b. The frequency of bathing

c. Cord care

d. Preventive measures for diaper rash

e. Preventive measures for cradle cap and how to treat it if it occurs

f. Care of the infant's nails (see chapter 12, Technique 12–5)

g. Circumcision care

h. Preventive measures for heat rash

2. For a patient confined to bed at home, family members may need guidance about:

a. How to prevent decubitus ulcers. The nurse needs to emphasize the importance of frequent turning in bed, keeping the patient clean and dry, and providing regular back rubs. Early recognition of tissue breakdown and the most common sites of breakdown are also stressed.

b. How to provide a sponge bath in bed, or what safety aids, such as handbars or rails, to install for a tub bath.

References

Cahn MM: The skin from infancy to old age. *Am J Nurs* (July) 1960; 60:993–996.

Chrisp M: New treatment for pressure sores. *Nurs Times* (August 4) 1977; 73:1202–1205.

Feustel DE: Pressure sore prevention: Aye there's the rub. *Nursing 82* (April) 1982; 12:78–83 (Canadian ed. pp 18–23).

Judd CO: The prevention and treatment of pressure sores. *Can Nurse* (July/August) 1981; 77:32–33.

Kerr JC, Stinson SM, Shannon ML: Pressure sores: Distinguishing fact from fiction. *Can Nurse* (July/August) 1981; 77:23–28.

Lang C, McGrath A: Gelfoam for decubitus ulcers. *Am J Nurs* (March) 1974; 74:460–461.

Morley MH: Decubitus ulcer management—a team approach. *Can Nurse* (October) 1973; 69:41–43.

Morley MH: 16 steps to better decubitus ulcer care. *Can Nurse* (July/August) 1981; 77:29–31.

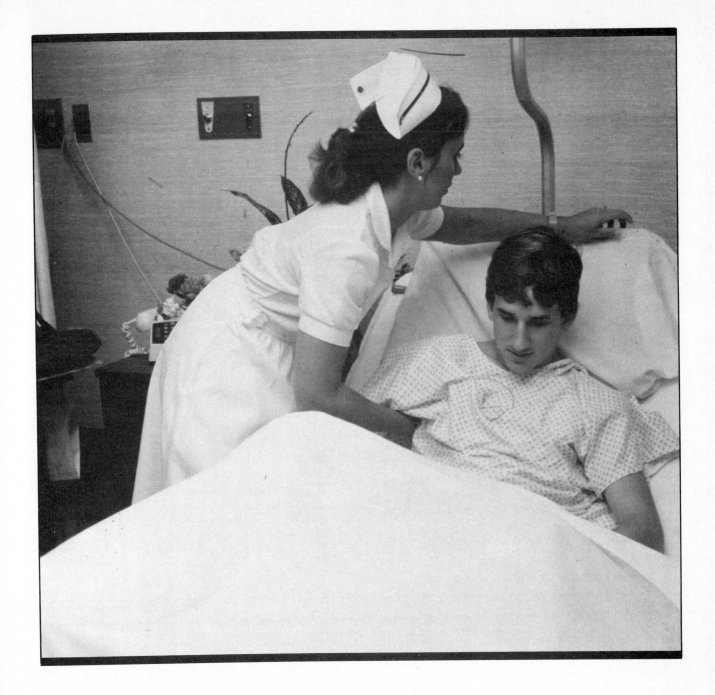

THE BED UNIT AND MAKING BEDS

15

Bed units usually have: a bed, a bedside table, an overbed table, a closet or locker, a set of drawers, one or two chairs, lights, and a signal light or intercom. Long-term care units often have more storage space for clothes and personal effects than acute care units.

The special equipment in a bed unit varies from one hospital to another. The modern acute care hospital unit often has built-in wall outlets for oxygen, suction, and a blood pressure manometer. Long-term care facilities often do not have special built-in equipment.

Chapter Outline

Objectives

Upon completion of this chapter, the student will:

1. Know essential terms and facts related to bed units and hospital beds
   1.1 Identify essential furniture and equipment for a hospital bed unit
   1.2 Identify various positions to which a hospital bed can be adjusted
   1.3 Identify types of beds (closed, open, occupied, and surgical)
   1.4 Identify accessory devices for hospital beds that are required by some patients (eg, footboards)
2. Understand facts about techniques for making beds
   2.1 Identify relevant assessment data
   2.2 Identify nursing diagnoses for which the technique may be implemented
   2.3 Identify nursing goals related to the technique
   2.4 Identify expected and unexpected outcomes from assessment data
   2.5 Identify reasons underlying selected steps of the technique
3. Perform techniques for preparing beds effectively for patients

   3.1 Assess the patient adequately
   3.2 Collect additional data from appropriate sources
   3.3 Select pertinent nursing goals for the patient
   3.4 Establish relevant outcome criteria for the patient following the technique
   3.5 Collect necessary equipment before the technique
   3.6 Implement interventions to enhance the effectiveness of the technique and enhance the patient's comfort and safety
   3.7 Communicate relevant information about the patient to the appropriate persons
   3.8 Determine the evaluative outcomes of the technique
4. Evaluate own performance of bed-making techniques in a laboratory or clinical setting with the assistance of another
   4.1 Use the performance checklists provided
   4.2 Identify areas of strength and weakness
   4.3 Alter performance in response to own evaluation and that of another

Terms

■ **bed foundation** the mattress and the frame supporting the mattress

■ **caster** a small wheel, often made of rubber or plastic, that permits furniture, such as a bed, to be moved easily

■ **closed bed** an unoccupied bed with the top covers drawn up to the top of the bed under the pillows

■ **contour position** a position with the head and foot sections of the bed elevated, creating a break of about 15°

■ **drawsheet (half sheet)** a special sheet, made of cotton, plastic, or rubber, that is placed across the center of the foundation of a bed

■ **Fowler's position** a bed sitting position with the head of the bed raised to 45°

■ **Gatch bed** a bed fitted with movable joints beneath the hips and knees of the patient

■ **hyperextension position** a position with the head and foot sections of the bed lowered to form a 15° angle in the bed foundation

■ **miter** a method of folding the bedclothes at the corners to maintain them securely

■ **occupied bed** a bed currently being used by a patient

■ **open bed** a bed not presently being used by its occupant, with the top covers folded back

■ **reverse Trendelenburg's position** a position with the head of the bed raised and the foot lowered, while the bed foundation remains unbroken

■ **surgical bed (anesthetic, recovery, or postoperative bed)** a bed with the top covers fanfolded to one side or to the end of the bed

■ **toe pleat (tuck)** a fold made in the top bedclothes to provide additional space for the patient's toes

■ **Trendelenburg's position** a position with the head of the bed lowered and the foot raised, while the bed foundation remains unbroken; in some agencies this position involves elevation of the knees, with the feet lowered and the head lowered

■ unoccupied bed   a bed not currently being used by a patient

FURNITURE AND EQUIPMENT

Hospital Beds

When people are ill they are often confined to bed for days, weeks, or even months. The bed, then, becomes a very important piece of furniture; it becomes the patient's territory. A bed at home is usually satisfactory if illness does not confine the patient to bed for long periods of

FIGURE 15–1 ■ Cranks commonly used to change the position of a hospital bed.

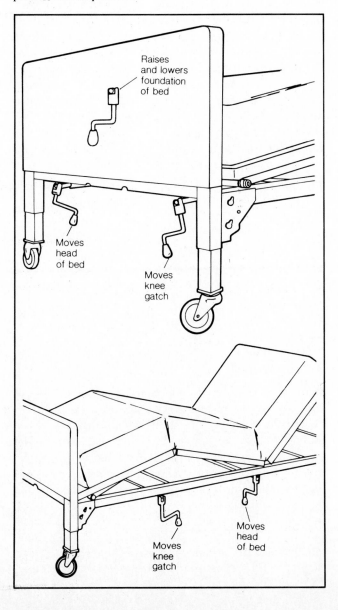

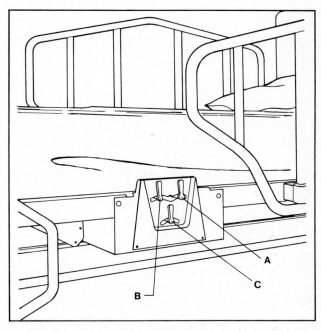

FIGURE 15–2 ■ Controls for a motor-operated hospital bed: **A,** raises and lowers the backrest; **B,** raises and lowers the knee gatch; **C,** raises and lowers the foundation of the bed.

time. Hospital beds are often preferred by people who are ill for more than several weeks and are more convenient for care giving by nursing personnel because of the following characteristics:

1. Hospital beds can be adjusted to a variety of positions (see Bed Positions later in this chapter). Most hospitals use Gatch beds. When the gatches, or joints, are flexed, the patient is raised to a sitting position with the knees elevated. The cranks that operate the gatches are usually at the bottom or side of the bed. See Figure 15–1. Manual cranks are left in the retracted position under the bed when they are not being used. Otherwise, people walking by the bed might easily hit their legs against the cranks. Some hospital beds have electric motors to operate the gatches. The motor is activated by pressing a button or moving a small lever, located either at the side of the bed or on a small panel separate from the bed but attached to it by a cable. See Figure 15–2.

2. Hospital beds are usually 66 cm (26 in) high. (Long-term care facilities for ambulatory patients usually have low beds to facilitate movement in and out of bed.) Some hospital beds have "high" and "low" positions that can be adjusted either mechanically by a crank at the center of the foot of the bed or electrically by a button or lever on the same panel as the gatch controls. The high position

permits the nurse to reach the patient without undue stretching or stooping. The low position allows the patient to step easily to the floor.

3. A hospital bed is normally 0.9 m (3 ft) wide, which is narrower than the usual bed. This permits the nurse to reach the patient from either side of the bed without undue stretching. The length is usually 1.9 m (6.5 ft). Some beds can be extended in length, if required.

4. Most hospital beds have casters that permit people to move the bed easily and quietly.

Mattresses

Most mattresses used in hospitals have innersprings, which give even support to the body. When changing a bed, nurses need to note any unevenness of the mattress surface, which might indicate a broken spring. Mattresses are usually covered with a water-repellent material that resists soiling and can be cleaned easily, to maintain a medical aseptic environment. Most mattresses have handles on the sides called *lugs* by which the mattress can be moved.

Foam rubber "egg crate" surface mattresses are also used for hospital mattresses. They provide support and have the advantage of relieving pressure on the body's bony prominences, such as the heels. Foam mattresses are particularly helpful for patients who are in bed for a long time.

Another option is the air mattress, a mattress attached to a motor that fluctuates the air pressure within the mattress. It is also called the *alternating pressure mattress*.

A fourth type of mattress, which has become popular recently, is the water mattress, which consists of a plastic bag filled with water. The principle behind use of this mattress is displacement. The body loses an amount of weight equal to the fluid it displaces. If the body displaces 9 kg (20 lb) of water it is 9 kg (20 lb) lighter, and there is less pressure on the weight-bearing areas.

When air and water mattresses are used, their surfaces must not be broken, or the air or water will escape. It is therefore inadvisable to use pins on the sheets covering these mattresses.

Special mattresses are placed on a standard bed mattress, although the water mattress may be placed on the base springs.

Bed Boards

A bed board, or *fracture board* as it is sometimes called, is a board placed directly under a mattress to give added support to a patient's body. Physicians often order bed boards for patients with back injuries.

The bed board is usually the size of the mattress. Some are plain flat boards while others are hinged so that the head of the bed, and sometimes the knees, can be elevated.

Side Rails

Side rails, or safety sides, are used on both hospital beds and stretchers. They are of various shapes and sizes and are usually made of metal. Devices to raise and lower them differ. Often one or two knobs are pulled to release the side and permit it to be moved.

Side rails have a number of functions:

1. To prevent patients from rolling or falling out of bed. This is a danger particularly for the elderly, young children, restless patients, and unconscious patients.

2. To give some patients, especially the elderly, the blind, and the sedated, a sense of security.

3. To provide a hand hold with which a patient can move up in bed or turn over.

4. If they are half rails, to provide support for a patient who is getting out of bed.

When side rails are being used, it is important that the nurse never leave the bedside while the rail is lowered. Some side rails have two positions: up and down. Others have three: high, intermediate, and low. The down and low positions are employed when a side rail is not needed. For some models, the bed foundation has to be raised to put the side rail in the low position; otherwise the side rail might hit the floor and be damaged. The intermediate position is used when the bed is in the low position and the nurse is present. The up or high side rail position is used when a patient is in bed and requires protection from falling. See Figure 15–3.

Footboards

A footboard is a flat panel, often made of wood or plastic, that is placed at the foot end of a bed. It serves three purposes:

1. To provide support for the patient's feet, maintaining a natural foot position while the patient is in bed. See Figure 15–4.

2. To keep the top bed covers off the patient's feet, relieving pressure from the weight of the covers.

3. To facilitate foot comfort (for example, when a patient has a painful foot).

Without the support of a footboard, a patient's feet will "drop" from the normal right angle with the legs to a *plantar flexion position* with the toes pointing toward the foot of the bed. See Figure 15–5. Prolonged assumption of this position results in permanent shortening of the muscles and tendons at the back of the legs. When that happens, the patient is unable to stand flat-footed on the floor, and walking is seriously impaired.

Footboards are often made in an L shape, so that the base of the L fits under the foot of the mattress. Some footboards are adjustable—the board can be moved along the mattress to adjust to the patient's height. If a board cannot be adjusted, sandbags and rolled pillows or blankets can be used to fill the space between the patient's feet and the board.

Bed Cradles

A bed cradle, sometimes called an *Anderson frame,* is a device designed to keep the top bedclothes off the feet, legs, and even abdomen of a patient. The bedclothes are arranged over the device and may be pinned in place. There are several types of bed cradles. One of the most common is a metal rod in an arch shape that extends from one side of the bed to the other. Part of the cradle fits under the mattress, and small metal brackets press down on each side of the mattress to keep the cradle in place. The frame on some cradles runs above only one leg, extending over half of the bed.

Intravenous Rods

Intravenous rods (poles, stands, standards), usually made of metal, are used to support intravenous infusion

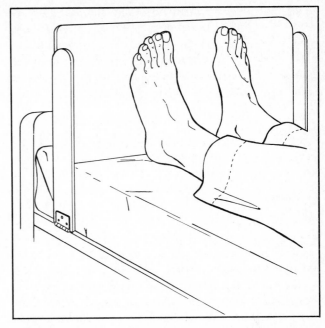

FIGURE 15–4 ■ A footboard that can be adjusted to the patient's height.

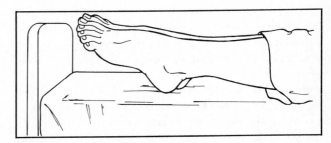

FIGURE 15–5 ■ Feet in plantar flexion.

containers while fluid is being administered to a patient. These rods were traditionally freestanding on the floor beside the patient's bed. Now hospital beds often have intravenous rods attached to the bed. Some hospital units have overhead hanging rods on a track for IVs.

Bedside Tables

The bedside table is a small table placed beside the bed. It frequently has a drawer, in which a patient can keep personal articles, and a cupboard beneath the drawer, containing a washbasin, soap dish and soap, mouthwash container, and emesis or kidney basin. Some bedside tables also have a place for a bedpan or urinal and a rod at the back for washcloths and towels.

Overbed Tables

The overbed table stands on the floor but fits over the patient's bed. It is usually on casters, so it can be easily moved. It can be raised or lowered to suit the patient, usually by turning a handle at the side. Some overbed

FIGURE 15–3 ■ Positions of the side rails: **A,** high position; **B,** intermediate position; **C,** low position.

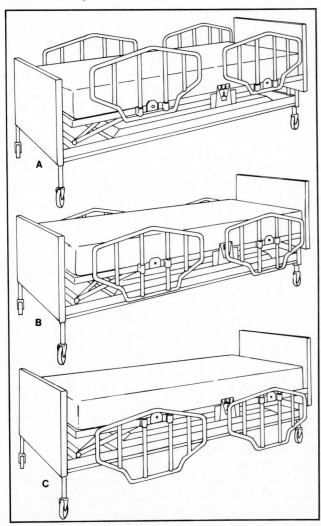

tables have a mirror and a small compartment for personal articles beneath the table top. Overbed tables are often used for the patient's meal tray. A patient who can assume a sitting position in bed can eat from that table in relative comfort. Nurses also use these tables for sterile supplies.

Chairs

Most bed units have chairs for patient and visitor use. Often one chair is without arms and is kept near the bed. There may also be an easy chair that is more comfortable to sit in for long periods.

Clothing Storage Spaces

Hospital bed units generally contain a locker or closet for the storage of clothes. These facilities are usually larger in a long-term care unit than in an acute care setting. Some units also have a chest of drawers or other drawer space for clothing.

Lights

Each bed unit has one or more lights. Often a light at the head of the bed has an extendable neck that allows it to be moved. Some rooms have overhead lights as well. Most bed units also have a signal light. When a patient pulls a switch or presses a button, a light goes on at a specific place in the hospital unit, such as the nurses' station or a service area. Patients generally turn on their signal lights when they require assistance. It is important for nurses to be aware of the signal light areas, so that they can note when a light goes on and answer quickly. Some acute hospitals are equipped with intercoms that permit the nurse at the nursing station to talk with the patient before going to the bedside. Intercom signal lights can also be turned off from the nurse's station. Nursing units generally have night lights, which provide subdued lighting during the night. Some also have emergency signal lights.

FIGURE 16–6 ■ A bed in the flat position.

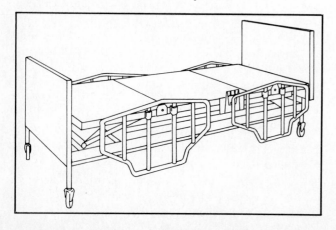

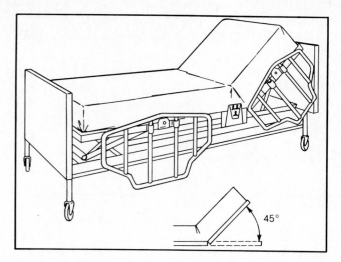

FIGURE 15–7 ■ A bed in Fowler's position.

Other Equipment

Hospitals vary in the equipment provided as part of the bed unit. Long-term care facilities may have very little additional equipment, whereas an acute facility may have several commonly used devices built into each unit. Three types of equipment are often installed on the wall at the head of the bed: a suction outlet for several kinds of suction, an oxygen outlet for most oxygen equipment, and a sphygmomanometer to measure the patient's blood pressure.

Some long-term care agencies also permit patients to have personal equipment, such as a television, a chair, and lamps, at the bedside.

BED POSITIONS

The Flat Position

In the flat bed position, the mattress is completely horizontal with no breaks in it. See Figure 15–6. In some agencies, no pillows are used, while in others, one or even two pillows are permitted in the flat bed position. It is important to check agency practice when a flat position is required.

Fowler's Position

Fowler's position is a semisitting bed position that is frequently used in hospitals. It gives patients relief from the lying positions and is convenient for eating, reading, etc. In Fowler's position the head of the bed is raised to at least 45°. In some hospitals, the term *Fowler's position* refers to elevation of the head of the bed alone (see Figure 15–7), while in other agencies it includes elevation of the knee gatch (see Figure 15–8). In some agencies, the

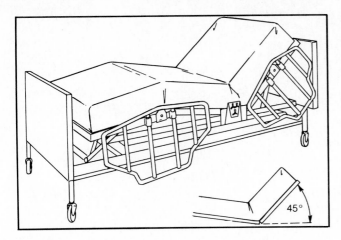

FIGURE 15–8 ■ A bed in Fowler's position with the knee gatch elevated.

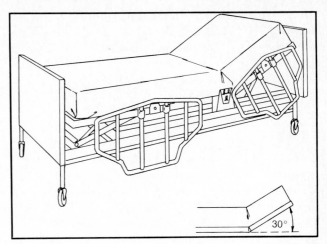

FIGURE 15–10 ■ A bed in semi-Fowler's position.

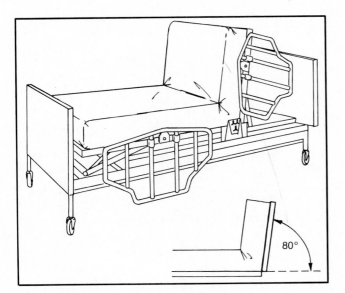

FIGURE 15–9 ■ A bed in high Fowler's position.

term *semi-Fowler's* is used for the position with the knees elevated. It is important for nurses to determine what is meant by these terms in the particular agency.

Two adaptations of the Fowler's position are the high Fowler's and semi-Fowler's positions. In the *high Fowler's position* the head of the bed is elevated to approximately 80°, that is, at nearly a right angle to the foundation of the bed. See Figure 15–9. This position is the one most closely analogous to sitting in a chair, when the back of the chair is at a right angle to the seat. *Semi-Fowler's position* usually means elevation of the head of the bed to about 30°. See Figure 15–10.

Trendelenburg's Position

In Trendelenburg's position, the head of the bed is lowered and the foot of the bed is elevated, while the foundation of the bed remains unbroken. See Figure 15–11. If the foundation cannot be raised mechanically, this position may be obtained by placing blocks under

the legs at the foot of the bed or pins in extendable legs. The blocks are often referred to as *shock blocks,* because this position was used some years ago for patients in shock. It is now contraindicated for patients suffering from head injuries, respiratory distress, chest injuries, or shock. Currently it is used for some postural drainage.

Reverse Trendelenburg's Position

Reverse Trendelenburg's position is a tilt in the opposite direction—the head of the bed is elevated and the foot of the bed is lowered, while the foundation of the bed remains unbroken. See Figure 15–12. Sometimes the legs at the head of the bed are raised by blocks or by pins if the foundation cannot be raised mechanically. This position may be used for patients experiencing problems with arterial circulation to the legs.

The Contour Position

In the contour bed position, the head and foot sections of the bed are elevated, permitting a break of about 15° between them. See Figure 15–13. On some hospital beds, it is necessary to raise both the knee and the foot sections of the bed to obtain this position.

FIGURE 15–11 ■ A bed in Trendelenburg's position.

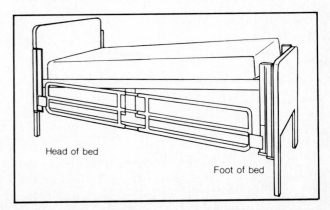

Head of bed

Foot of bed

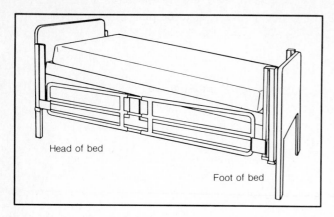

FIGURE 15-12 ■ A bed in reverse Trendelenburg's position.

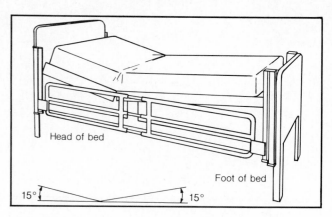

FIGURE 15-13 ■ A bed in contour position.

The Hyperextension Position

For the hyperextension bed position, both the head and the foot sections are lowered to create a 15° angle in the bed foundation. See Figure 15–14. This position is sometimes used for patients who have spinal fractures. It should be used only with specific orders from the physician, and continuous nursing assessment of the patient is important. Not all hospital beds assume this position.

MAKING BEDS

Nurses need to be able to prepare hospital beds in different ways for specific purposes. In most instances, beds are made after hygienic care of the patient and when they are unoccupied. At times, however, nurses need to make an occupied bed or a bed for a patient who is having surgery (an anesthetic, postoperative, or surgical bed).

Concepts Basic to Bed Making

1. Linens and equipment that have been soiled with a patient's secretions and excretions harbor microorganisms that can be transmitted to others directly or by the nurse's hands or uniform. Therefore, nurses wash hands thoroughly after handling a patient's bed linen. They also hold soiled linen away from their uniforms.

2. Neither clean nor soiled linen for one patient is ever placed on another patient's bed. Clean linen can inadver-

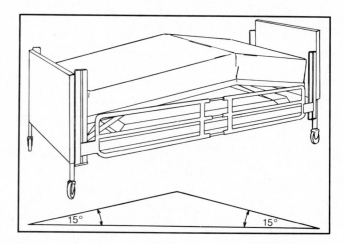

FIGURE 15-14 ■ A bed in hyperextension position.

tently become soiled, and soiled linen can contaminate the other patient's bed linen. In addition, soiled linen is not shaken in the air, because infectious materials could inadvertently be spread to others.

3. The floor is considered more contaminated with microorganisms. Therefore no linen is placed on the floor. Soiled linen is placed directly in a portable linen hamper or tucked in at the end of the bed before it is gathered up for disposal in the linen hamper or linen chute.

4. When stripping and making a bed, nurses complete as much as possible on one side of the bed before going to the other side, to conserve time and energy.

5. Nurses gather all needed linen before starting to strip a bed, to save the time and energy required by extra trips to the linen supply area.

TECHNIQUE 15-1 ■ Changing an Unoccupied Bed

There are two types of unoccupied beds: closed and open. Generally the top covers of an open bed are folded back for the patient to get in. See Figure 15–15. For a closed bed, the top sheet, blanket, and bedspread are drawn up to the top of the bed under the pillows. Otherwise, open and closed beds are made the same way.

■ Assessment

Assess the patient for:

1. Pulse rate, volume, and regularity if the patient's condition indicates this precaution. In some instances —when the patient is getting up for the first time after surgery or after 24 hours or more of bed rest—it is necessary to assess the pulse before the patient leaves the bed and after she or he sits in a chair.

2. Present health status to ensure that it is safe for the patient to get out of bed. Note respirations, color, and any other significant data indicated on the nursing care plan. If your assessment differs substantially from the baseline data or the nursing care plan, report this to the responsible nurse before assisting the patient out of bed.

3. The need for specific nursing interventions prior to having the patient get out of bed, eg, rest, analgesic.

Other data include:

1. Baseline data regarding the above assessments

2. Nursing or physician's orders indicating whether the patient can get out of bed, the length of time the patient can stay up, the activity permitted and any position the patient must maintain, eg, elevation of a leg

3. Other assessments needed, eg, the presence of cyanosis or dyspnea

4. Whether special bed or linen adaptations are required, such as a footboard, a special mattress, an anesthetic bed, unbleached bed linen (for a patient who is allergic to substances in bleached linen), incontinence pads, or orthopedic sheets

5. The need for clean linen

■ Planning

Nursing goals

1. To provide a clean bed for the patient

2. To make a bed that will be comfortable and maintain a neat appearance while it is occupied

Equipment

1. A mattress pad, if used. Some agencies do not use pads, so check agency practice. Some mattress pads are attached to the bed by elastic or ties at the corners. Some lie freely on the mattress.

2. Two large sheets. Fitted sheets, which do not require mitering, are being used increasingly in hospitals.

3. A plastic or rubber drawsheet, if required, to place across the center of the bed to protect the bottom sheet from drainage, urine, or feces. In some agencies drawsheets are used only when the nurse decides it is necessary.

4. A cloth drawsheet to be placed over the plastic or rubber drawsheet, if required.

5. One blanket.

6. One bedspread.

7. Two pillowcases for the two head pillows. Additional pillowcases may be needed if additional pillows are used.

8. Portable linen hamper for the soiled linen, if available.

■ Intervention

1. Place the fresh linen on the patient's chair or overbed table; do not use another patient's bed.
   Rationale   It is important to prevent cross-contamination (the movement of microorganisms from one patient to another) via soiled linen.

2. Make sure that this is an appropriate and convenient time for the patient to be out of bed.

3. Assist the patient to a comfortable chair.

Stripping the bed

4. Starting at the head of the bed, on the side nearer the clean linen, loosen the bedding, including the foundation, moving down the bed, working around the foot, and moving up to the other side of the head. Remove the call signal, if it is attached to the linen.

**FIGURE 15–15   ■   An open bed with the top covers: A, fanfolded; B, pie-folded.

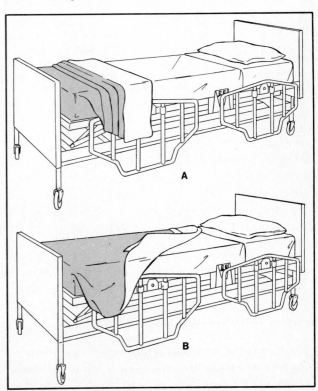

5. Return to the first side.

6. Remove the pillowcases, if soiled, and place the pillows on the bedside chair near the foot of the bed.

   Rationale The bedside chair can be used to hold bedding that can be reused.

7. Using both hands, grasp the top edge of the spread, one hand at the center, the other at the mattress edge. See Figure 15–16. Fold it in half by bringing the top edge even with the bottom edge.

   Rationale Linens folded this way are readily reapplied to the bed later.

   If the spread is soiled, place it in the linen hamper, if the agency has portable linen hampers that can

FIGURE 15–16

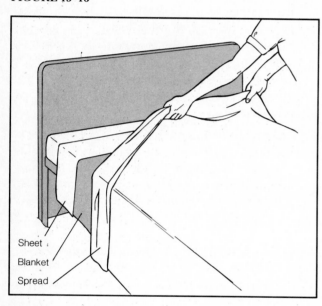

Sheet

Blanket

Spread

FIGURE 15–17

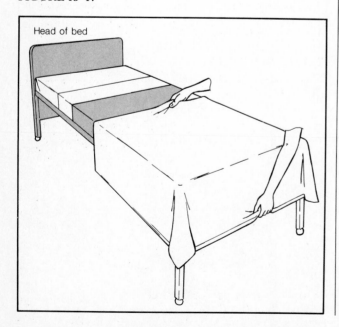

Head of bed

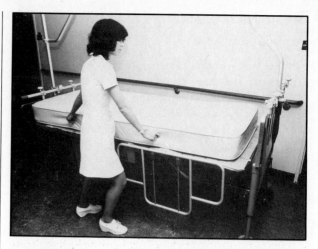

FIGURE 15–18

be taken to the bed unit. If the agency has a central disposal chute for linen, tuck in the soiled spread at the foot of the bed, and collect all the soiled linen here to take to the chute. Take care to prevent soiled bed linen from touching your uniform.

Rationale The uniform can become soiled and transmit microorganisms to other patients.

8. If the spread is not soiled, pick it up carefully by grasping it at the center of the middle fold and the bottom edges. See Figure 15–17.

   Rationale It is useful to fold the spread in such a way that it can be readily reapplied.

9. Lay the spread over the back of the bedside chair if it is to be reused.

10. Repeat steps 7–9, first for the blanket and then for the top sheet.

11. Pick up the cotton drawsheet at the center of the top and bottom edges, and lay it over the back of the bedside chair or, if soiled, discard it in the hamper.

12. Repeat step 11 for the plastic or rubber drawsheet.

13. Repeat steps 7–9 for the bottom sheet if it is to be changed.

14. Grasp the mattress lugs and, using good body mechanics, move the mattress up to the head of the bed. If there are no lugs, grasp the lower edge of the mattress. See Figure 15–18.

Making the bed

15. Standing at the same side of the bed as the linen supply, place the mattress pad on the bed.

16. Smooth the mattress pad so that it is free of wrinkles.

    Rationale Wrinkles can irritate the patient's skin and feel uncomfortable.

17. Working from the foot of the bed, place the bottom sheet, folded into four layers, on the bed so that the vertical center fold of the sheet is at the center line

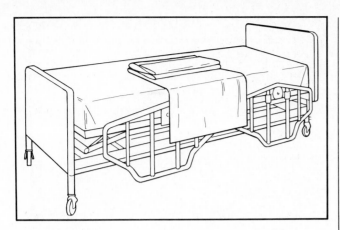

FIGURE 15–19

of the mattress and the bottom edge of the sheet extends about 2.5 cm (1 in) over the end of the mattress.

Rationale Unless a contour sheet is used, the sheet is not tucked in at the foot of the bed so that it can be changed without removing the top bedcovers.

Make sure that the hem of the sheet is facing down.

Rationale The hem edge can be irritating to the patient's skin.

Open the sheet across the bottom of the bed, and then pull the top layer up to the top of the bed, so that the sheet is fully spread. (Agency practice may vary on methods of folding and spreading sheets on beds. This is one common method. In some agencies the sheet is spread over only one side of the bed at a time.)

18. Move to the head of the bed on the same side. Tuck the excess sheet under the mattress at the near side of the head of the bed. If a contour sheet is used, fit it under the corner of the mattress.

19. Miter the sheet at the top corner on that side, and tuck the sheet under the mattress side, working from the head of the bed to the foot. See Technique 15–3.

20. Lay the plastic or rubber drawsheet on the bed, folded in half, with the center fold at the center line of the bed. Fanfold the uppermost half of the drawsheet at the center of the bed. Place the top edge of the drawsheet 30 to 37 cm (12 to 15 in) from the head of the bed. See Figure 15–19.

21. Tuck in the drawsheet on the near side.

22. Repeat steps 20–21 for the cloth drawsheet, making sure that it completely covers the rubber or plastic sheet at both top and bottom edges.

Rationale Any exposed plastic or rubber can be irritating to the patient's skin.

23. Move to the opposite side of the bed.

24. Starting at the head of the bed, tuck the excess bottom sheet under the head of the mattress.

25. Pulling the sheet firmly, miter the side corner at the head of the bed or fit a contour sheet under the mattress corner.

26. Tuck in the bottom sheet, working toward the foot of the bed. Pull the sheet firmly so that there are no wrinkles in it.

27. Pull the plastic or rubber drawsheet over firmly, and tuck it in at the side. See Figure 15–20.

28. Repeat step 27 for the cotton drawsheet.

29. Return to the first side of the bed. The foundation of the bed is now complete.

30. Place the top sheet on the bed so that the vertical center fold is at the center line of the bed, the top edge is even with the top edge of the mattress, and the hems of the sheet will be facing up when unfolded.

Rationale With the hems facing up, the edges of the sheet will not rub against the patient's skin.

31. Spread the sheet over the bed as described in step 17 or according to agency practice.

32. Tuck in the sheet at the bottom of the bed on the near half (optional).

33. Make either a vertical or a horizontal toe pleat in the sheet:

   a. Vertical toe pleat: Standing at the foot of the bed, make a fold in the sheet 5 to 10 cm (2 to 4 in), perpendicular to the foot of the bed. See Figure 15–21. Tuck in the end of the sheet at the foot of the bed. See Figure 15–22.

   b. Horizontal toe pleat: Make a fold in the sheet 5 to 10 cm (2 to 4 in), across the bed, 15 to 20 cm (6 to 8 in) from the foot. Tuck in the sheet at the foot. See Figure 15–23.

   Rationale A toe pleat provides additional room for a patient's feet. It is an optional comfort measure. Additional toe space can also be provided by

FIGURE 15–20

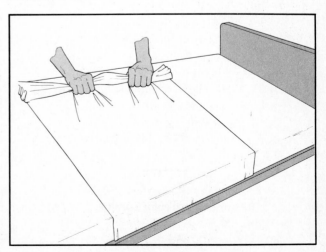

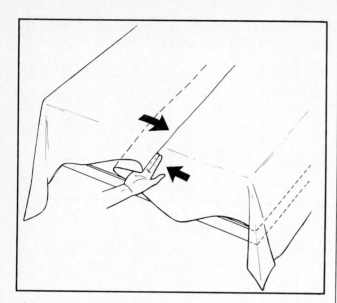

FIGURE 15–21

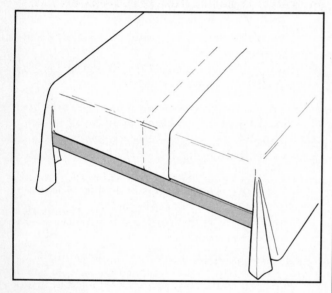

FIGURE 15–22

loosening the top covers around the feet after the patient is in bed.

34. Place the blanket on the bed so that the top edge is about 15 cm (6 in) from the head of the bed and the center fold is at the center of the bed.

Rationale This allows a cuff of sheet to be folded over the blanket and spread.

35. Tuck in the blanket at the foot of the bed on the near side. Make a toe pleat if needed. See step 33.

36. Put the bedspread on the bed so that the center fold is at the center of the bed and the top edge extends about 2.5 cm (1 in) beyond the blanket. Tuck the top edge of the spread under the top edge of the blanket. See Figure 15–24.

37. Fold the top of the top sheet down over the spread,

providing a cuff of about 15 cm (6 in). Smooth the spread, working from the top to the foot of the bed.

Rationale The cuff of sheet protects the patient's face from rubbing against the blanket or bedspread, thus preventing skin irritation.

38. Tuck in the spread at the foot of the bed on the near side.

39. Miter the bottom corner of the bed using all three layers of linen (top sheet, blanket, and spread). Leave

FIGURE 15–23

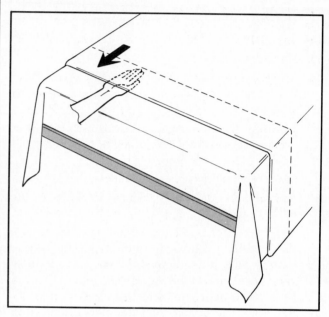

FIGURE 15–24

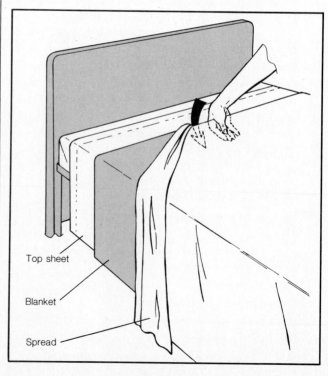

Top sheet

Blanket

Spread

the sides of the top sheet, blanket, and spread hanging freely.

Rationale Mitering makes the corner of the bed-clothes secure even though they are left hanging freely to permit easy access by the patient.

40. Walk around the foot of the bed to the far side, pulling the blanket and spread over the bed. Work toward the head of the bed on the second side.

41. Fold the remainder of the spread under the top of the blanket. Fold the remainder of the top sheet over the spread to make a cuff.

42. Going to the foot of the bed tuck in the top sheet, blanket, and spread at the bottom of the bed on the second side. Maintain the toe pleat if one was made.

43. Miter this corner as in step 39.

44. Moving to the first side of the bed put clean pillowcases on the pillows:

   a. Grasp the closed end of the pillowcase at the center with one hand.

   b. Gather up the sides of the pillowcase, and place them over the hand grasping the case. Then grasp the center of one short side of the pillow through the pillowcase. See figure 15–25.

   c. With the free hand, pull the pillowcase over the pillow.

   d. Adjust the pillowcase so that the pillow fits into the corners of the case and the seams are straight.

   Rationale A smoothly fitting pillowcase is more comfortable than a wrinkled one.

45. Place the pillows at the head of the bed in the center, with the open ends of the pillowcases facing away from the door of the room.

   Rationale This provides a neat appearance.

46. Attach the signal cord so that the patient can conveniently use it. Some cords have clamps that attach to the sheet or pillowcase. Others are attached by a safety pin.

47. If the bed is currently being used by a patient, either fold back the top covers at one side or fanfold them down to the center of the bed.

   Rationale This makes it easier for the patient to get into the bed.

48. Put the bedside table and the overbed table in order so that they are available to the patient.

49. Put the bed in the low position. (Place the bed in the high position if the patient is returning by stretcher.)

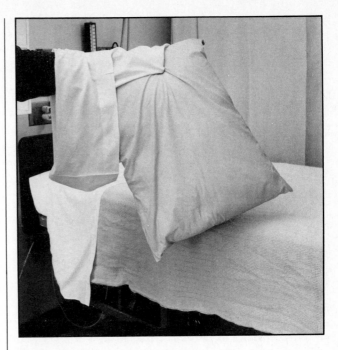

FIGURE 15–25

50. Record assessment data on the patient's record. Bed making is not normally recorded.

■ Evaluation

Expected outcomes

1. Pulse rate, volume, and rhythm within the patient's normal range

2. No significant change in the patient's current health status

Unexpected outcomes

1. Pulse rate, volume, and rhythm outside the patient's normal range

2. Excessive fatigue, dyspnea, or cyanosis, for example, depending on the patient's health

Upon obtaining an unexpected outcome:

1. Reassess the patient's response ten minutes after returning to bed.

2. Report your findings to the responsible nurse and/or physician.

TECHNIQUE 15–2 ■ Changing an Occupied Bed

Not all patients are able to leave their beds. Those who cannot must remain in bed when the linen is changed. In most acute care hospitals, the beds are made once a day. The linen is changed at that time and whenever it becomes soiled. Long-term and nonacute agencies change bed linens less often. Use the following guidelines when making an occupied bed:

1. Maintain the patient in good body alignment.
2. Move the patient gently, smoothly, and appropriately for the condition. Rough handling can cause the patient discomfort and abrade the skin.
3. Throughout the procedure, explain what you plan to do before you do it. Use terms that the patient can understand.
4. Never move or position a patient in a manner that is contraindicated for his or her health or comfort. For example, the patient who is dyspneic should be maintained in Fowler's position and not placed in a supine position.
5. Use the bed-making time, like the bed bath time, to assess and meet the patient's needs (for example, the need for information about a forthcoming operation).

■ Assessment

Assess the patient for:

1. Readiness to have the bed changed (eg, is the patient free of pain, rested after a meal?)
2. Significant data according to the patient's health, eg, pulse, respirations, color

Other data include:

1. Baseline data regarding the above assessments
2. Information regarding the positions the patient can safely assume
3. Whether special linen or bed adaptations are required
4. Whether clean linen is needed

■ Planning

Nursing goals

1. To provide a clean bed for the patient
2. To make a bed that is comfortable and neat
3. To change the bed with minimum disturbance to the patient

Equipment

Hospital beds are often changed after bed baths. The linen can be collected before the bath. Some hospitals do not change all the linen unless it is soiled. For example, you may use the top sheet as a bottom sheet and provide a clean top sheet, drawsheet, and pillowcases.

The following equipment is usually required for a complete bed change:

1. A mattress pad, if necessary
2. Two large sheets
3. A bedspread
4. A plastic or rubber drawsheet, if necessary
5. A cloth drawsheet
6. Two pillowcases
7. Bath blanket (optional)

■ Intervention

1. Place the fresh linen on the bedside chair or overbed table within easy reach and in order of use.
2. Remove any equipment attached to the bed linen, such as a call light.

Removing the top bedding

3. Loosen all the top linen at the foot of the bed.
4. Using both hands, grasp the top edge of the spread, one hand at the center, the other at the mattress edge. Fold it in half by bringing the top edge even with the bottom edge.
   Rationale Linens folded this way are readily reapplied to the bed later.
5. Pick up the spread carefully by grasping it at the center of the middle fold and the bottom edges.
6. If the spread is soiled, place it in the linen hamper or tuck it in at the bottom of the bed. Some agencies have portable linen hampers that can be taken to the bed unit. If the agency has a central disposal chute for linen, collect all the soiled linen at the foot of the bed to take to the chute. Take care to prevent the soiled linen from touching your uniform.
   Rationale The uniform can become soiled and transmit microorganisms to other patients.
7. If the spread is not soiled and is to be reused, lay it over the back of the bedside chair.
8. Repeat steps 4–7 for the blanket.
9. Leave the top sheet over the patient (the top sheet can remain over the patient if it is being discarded

and if it will provide sufficient warmth) *or* replace it with a bath blanket as follows:

a. Spread the bath blanket over the top sheet.

b. Ask the patient to hold the top edge of the blanket.

c. Reaching under the blanket from the side, grasp the top edge of the sheet and draw it down to the foot of the bed, leaving the blanket in place.

d. Remove the sheet from the bed and place it with the soiled linen.

Moving the mattress up on the bed

10. Place the bed in the flat position if the patient can tolerate this.

11. Loosen the foundation on the near side to expose the mattress.

12. Grasp the mattress lugs and, using good body mechanics, move the mattress up to the head of the bed. Have the patient assist, if able, by grasping the head of the bed and pulling as you push. If the patient is heavy, you may need help from another nurse.

    Rationale   When the head of the bed is raised, the mattress tends to slide toward the foot of the bed, thus moving the patient toward the foot of the bed.

Changing the foundation of the bed

13. Assist the patient to turn on her or his side facing away from the linen supply and on the far side of the bed. Raise the side rail on the far side.

    Rationale   This leaves the near half of the foundation free to be changed. The raised side rail protects the patient from falling. If there is no side rail, have another nurse support the patient at the edge of the bed.

14. Returning to the first side of the bed, loosen the foundation linen at the side. Fanfold the two drawsheets and the bottom sheet at the center of the bed, as close to the patient as possible.

    Rationale   Close fanfolding makes room for the new linen.

15. Smooth the matress pad, if it is to be retained. If not, fanfold it, and place a new pad on the bed, with the center fold at the center of the bed and the uppermost half fanfolded at the center.

    Rationale   Smoothing removes wrinkles that could irritate the patient's skin.

16. Place the new bottom sheet on the bed so that the lower edge extends slightly, eg, 2.5 cm (1 in), over the end of the mattress. Make sure that the hem of the sheet is facing down.

    Rationale   The hem edge can irritate the patient's skin.

17. Moving from the foot to the head, open the sheet lengthwise.

18. Fanfold the uppermost half of the clean bottom sheet vertically at the center of the bed.

19. Tuck the sheet under the near half of the head of the bed. Miter the sheet at the top corner of the side of the bed or fit the corner of a contour sheet under the mattress. See Technique 15–3.

    Rationale   A mitered corner holds the sheet firmly in place.

20. Moving toward the foot of the bed, tuck the bottom sheet under the side of the mattress, smoothing the sheet at the same time.

    Rationale   Wrinkles could irritate the patient's skin.

21. Pull the plastic or rubber drawsheet from the center of the bed where it was fanfolded. Tuck it under the side of the mattress. If a clean plastic drawsheet is to be used:

    a. Lay it on the bed with the center fold at the center of the bed. The drawsheet should extend from midway down the patient's back to midway down the thighs.

    b. Fanfold the uppermost half vertically at the center of the bed.

    c. Tuck the near side edge under the side of the mattress.

22. Repeat step 21 for the cloth drawsheet, making sure that it covers the plastic or rubber drawsheet at the top and bottom edges.

    Rationale   Exposed plastic or rubber can irritate the patient's skin.

23. Assist the patient to roll over toward you onto the clean side of the bed. The patient rolls over the fanfolded linen at the center of the bed.

24. Move the pillows to the clean side for the patient.

    Rationale   Pillows provide comfort.

25. Raise the side rail, if necessary, before leaving the side of the bed.

    Rationale   The side rail provides safety and a sense of security for the patient.

26. Move to the other side of the bed and lower the side rail if it was raised.

27. Loosen the foundation linen on that side. Fanfold the drawsheets if they are being reused, and remove the soiled bottom sheet. Remove the drawsheets with the bottom sheet if they are being changed. Roll the linens so that the patient does not see the soiled parts.

    Rationale   Sight of the soil might be embarrassing to the patient.

28. Place the soiled linen at the foot of the bed or in the portable linen hamper.

    Rationale   This helps to prevent the spread of

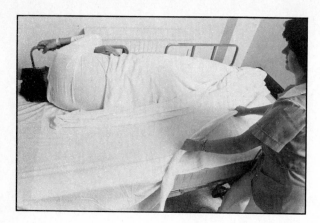

FIGURE 15–26

microorganisms contained in linens soiled with the patient's excretions or other body discharges.

29. Smooth out the mattress cover to remove any wrinkles.

30. Unfold the fanfolded bottom sheet from the center of the bed.

31. Tuck the top of the sheet under the near half of the head of the bed. Miter the sheet at the top corner of the side of the bed.

32. Facing the side of the bed, use both hands to pull the bottom sheet so that it is smooth, and tuck the excess under the side of the mattress. See Figure 15–26.
    Rationale Pulling at an angle removes wrinkles.

33. Unfold the plastic or rubber drawsheet fanfolded at the center of the bed, and pull it tightly with both hands. Pull the sheet in three sections: Face the side of the bed to pull the middle section, face the far top corner to pull the bottom section, and face the far bottom corner to pull the top section. See Figure 15–27. Tuck the excess sheet under the side of the mattress.

34. Repeat step 33 for the cloth drawsheet.

35. Reposition the pillows at the center of the bed. If a pillowcase is soiled, remove it and place it with the soiled linen. Put on a clean pillowcase as follows:
    a. Grasp the closed end of the pillowcase at the center with one hand.
    b. Gather up the sides of the pillowcase, and place them over the hand grasping the case. Then grasp the center of one short side of the pillow through the pillowcase.
    c. With the free hand, pull the pillowcase over the pillow.
    d. Adjust the pillowcase so that the pillow fits into the corners of the case and the seams are straight.
    Rationale A smoothly fitting pillowcase is more comfortable than a wrinkled one.

36. Assist the patient to the center of the bed. Determine what position the patient requires or prefers, and assist him or her to that position.

37. Raise the side rail on the second side of the bed, if required, and return to the first side. Lower the side rail on the first side.

FIGURE 15–27

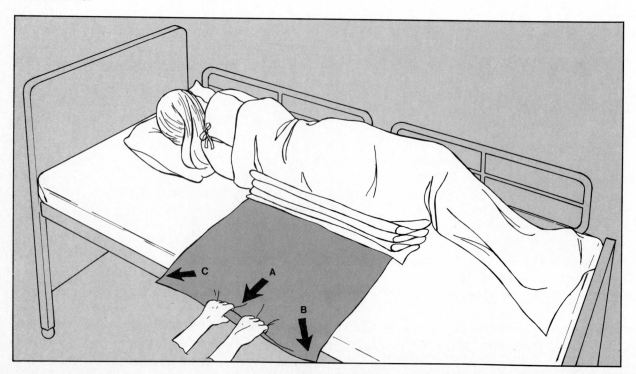

Making the top of the bed

38. Spread the top sheet over the patient so that the center crease is in the center of the bed and the top edge is at the patient's shoulders. There should be enough sheet at the top so that a cuff can be folded over the blanket and spread.

39. Ask the patient to hold the top edge of the sheet or tuck it under her or his shoulders. The sheet should remain over the patient when the bath blanket or used sheet is removed.

40. Reaching under the fresh sheet, grasp the bottom edge of the bath blanket or used sheet and remove it by pulling it to the foot of the bed.

41. Fold the bath blanket and put it in the bedside table if it is to be reused, or place the used sheet with the soiled linen.

42. Complete the top of the bed as described in Technique 15–1, page 361.

43. Attach the signal cord to the bed linen within the patient's reach. Some cords have clamps that attach to the sheet or pillowcase; others are attached by a safety pin.

44. Put the bedside table and the overbed table in order. Put items used by the patient within easy reach.

45. Adjust the side rails and the height of the bed for the patient's needs and according to agency policy. Some hospitals require that the side rails be raised for all patients 70 years old and older.

46. Record pertinent assessment data about the patient on the patient's record. Changing bed linen is not normally recorded.

■ **Evaluation**   See Technique 15–1.

TECHNIQUE 15–3 ■ Mitering the Corner of a Bed

Mitering is used to secure the corners of sheets, blankets, and bedspreads on a bed. Fitted sheets do not require mitering.

■ **Planning**

Nursing goal

To secure bedclothes in place.

FIGURE 15–28

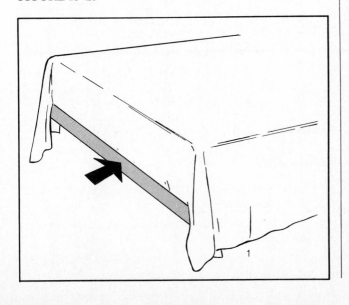

Equipment

Bedding as required, eg, sheets, blankets.

■ **Intervention**

1. Tuck in the bedcover firmly under the mattress at the bottom or top of the bed. See Figure 15–28.

2. Lift the bedcover at point 1 to form a triangle, so that the edge of the bedcover is parallel with the end of the bed. See Figure 15–29.

FIGURE 15–29

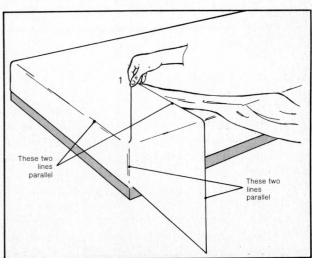

These two lines parallel

These two lines parallel

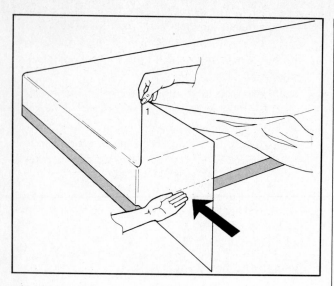

FIGURE 15–30

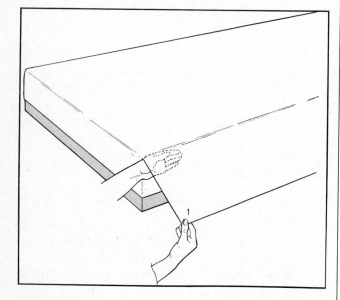

FIGURE 15–31

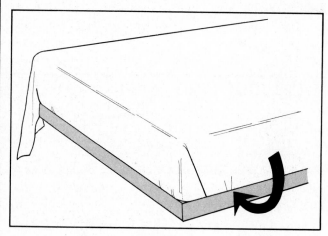

FIGURE 15–32

3. Tuck the hanging edge under the mattress while continuing to hold point 1. See Figure 15–30.

4. Bring the top of the triangle down while holding the fold with the other hand parallel to the bed surface. See Figure 15–31.

5. Optional: Tuck the remainder of the bedcover under the mattress while removing your hand. See Figure 15–32. Top bedcovers are often not tucked in but left hanging freely.

TECHNIQUE 15–4 ■ Making a Surgical Bed

The surgical bed is also referred to as the *recovery bed, anesthetic bed,* or *postoperative bed.* It may be used not only for patients who have undergone surgical procedures but also for patients who have been given anesthetics for certain examinations.

Determine from the patient's record or from the responsible nurse whether special equipment, such as suction or oxygen apparatus, is required for the surgical unit. Connect any equipment that will be required, so that it is ready for use.

■ Planning

Nursing goals

1. To arrange the top bed linen so that the patient can be readily transferred to the bed

2. To provide as clean an environment as possible for the patient

3. To provide a bed foundation that can be changed quickly and easily if it becomes soiled

4. In some instances, to provide extra warmth through the use of flannelette sheets

Equipment

While supplies vary from one agency to another, the following are generally needed:

1. Two clean sheets
2. A clean cotton drawsheet
3. A clean flannelette sheet for the foundation of the bed if this is agency practice
4. A clean bedspread
5. A disposable incontinence or drainage pad (optional)

At some agencies these supplies are arranged in a surgical bundle.

■ Intervention

1. Place the supplies within easy reach in the order in which they will be used.
2. Place and leave the pillows on the bedside chair.
    Rationale Pillows are not put onto the bed to facilitate transferring the patient into the bed.
3. Arrange the furniture and equipment so that there is room near the bed for a stretcher or room to move the bed out of the room if the bed is to be transported to the operating room.
4. Strip the bed according to Technique 15–1, steps 4–14.
5. Make the foundation of the bed as shown in Technique 15–1, steps 15–29.
6. Place the flannelette sheet on the foundation of the bed, if this is agency practice.
    Rationale A flannelette sheet provides additional warmth.
7. Place a disposable pad for the patient's head (optional).
8. Spread the top covers on the bed. Do not tuck them in, miter the corners, or make a toe pleat.
9. Fold the hanging edges of the top covers up over the top of the bed so that the folds are at the mattress edge (fold the sides first, then the top and bottom). See Figure 15–33. Then fanfold the covers in either of the following ways:
    a. Fanfold them lengthwise at one side of the bed. See Figure 15–34.
    b. Fanfold them crosswise at the bottom of the bed. See Figure 15–35.
    Rationale The covers are fanfolded for ease in transferring the patient into bed.
10. Lock the wheels of the bed if the bed is not to be

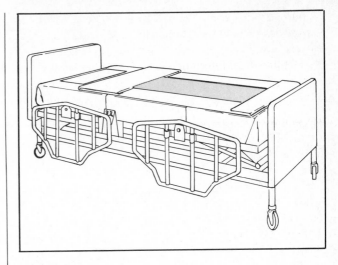

FIGURE 15–33

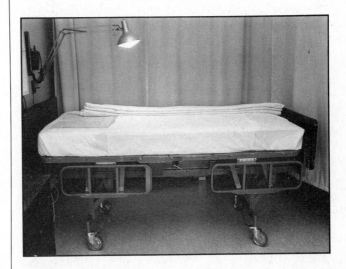

FIGURE 15–34

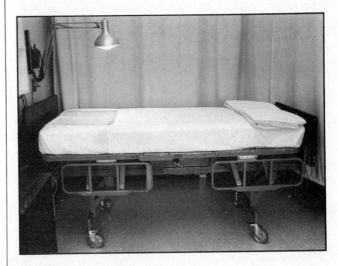

FIGURE 15–35

moved, and leave the bed in the high position to meet the level of the stretcher.

Rationale Locking the wheels keeps the bed from rolling. The high position facilitates the transfer of the patient.

11. Notify appropriate people that the surgical bed is ready. In some hospitals, a porter service or the like takes the bed to the recovery room.

12. Place any additional equipment, eg, suction, in readiness for use when the patient returns from surgery.

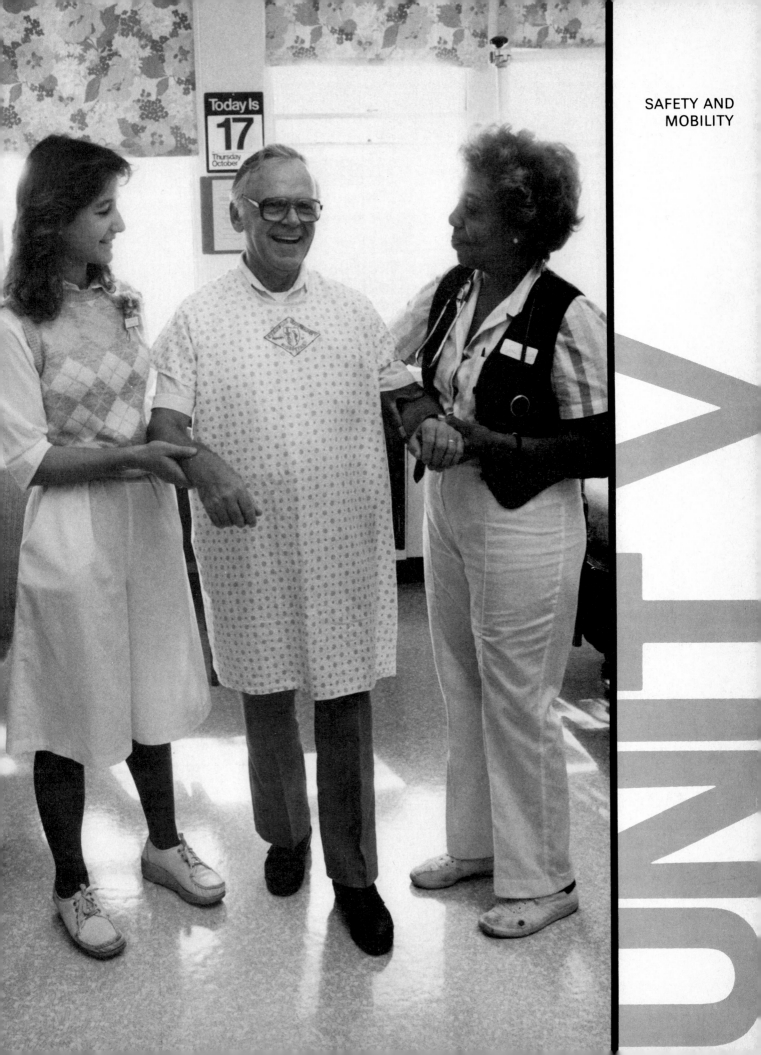

Today Is
17
Thursday
October

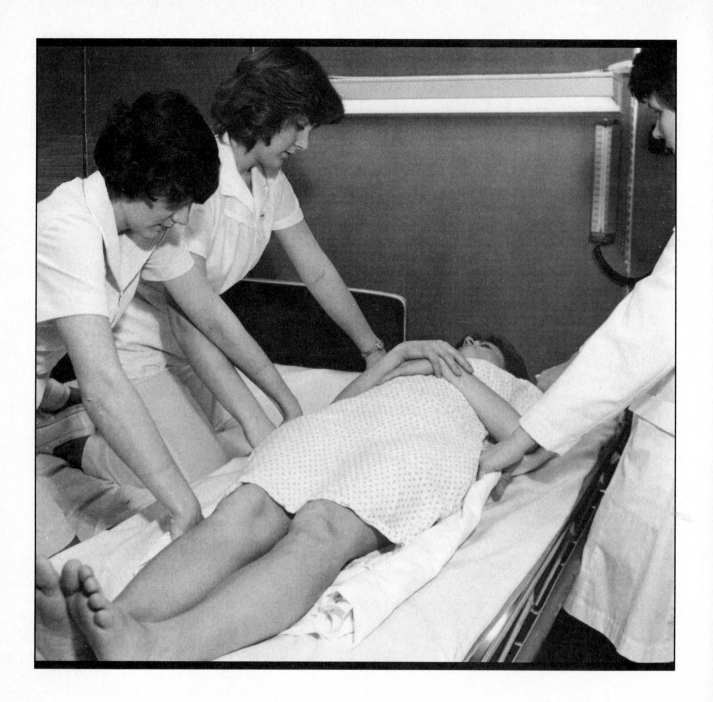

MOVING PATIENTS

16

A healthy person usually takes for granted that he or she can change body position and go from one place to another with little effort. However, ill people may have difficulty moving even in bed. The ability to move easily is associated with feelings of independence; inability to move is often associated with feelings of dependence and frustration.

In a number of situations a nurse can anticipate that a patient will require assistance to move. Some of the common ones are:

1. When the patient is unconscious, paralyzed, or debilitated from illness or surgery

2. When the patient has had a prolonged illness or been inactive for a long period of time

3. When the patient is elderly or very young

4. When certain disease conditions are present, such as multiple sclerosis or Parkinson's disease

5. When rest is essential or exertion is contraindicated, such as for a patient with acute congestive heart failure

How much assistance patients require depends on their own ability to move and the extent to which they can safely exert themselves. In general, nurses should be sensitive to both the need of patients to function independently and their need for assistance to move. Frequently a patient will accept help if the nurse explains the reason for it and, if possible, offers reassurance about future independent functioning.

When a nurse assists a patient to move, good body mechanics need to be employed so that the nurse is not injured. Proper body alignment for the patient is also maintained, so that undue stress is not placed on the patient's musculoskeletal system. Body mechanics, the efficient and coordinated uses of the body in resting positions and motions, involve three basic elements:

1. Proper alignment (posture)

2. Balance (stability)

3. Coordinated body movement

Good body mechanics are essential to nurses, to prevent strain and injury. They also prevent fatigue, because a minimum amount of energy is required.

Chapter Outline

Objectives

Upon completion of this chapter, the student will:

1. Know essential terms and facts about body mechanics and moving patients
   1.1 Define specific terms about body mechanics
   1.2 Identify the large muscle groups used in body mechanics
   1.3 Identify the normal standing and sitting positions
   1.4 Describe two methods to improve the balance of the body
   1.5 Identify three physical forces that influence body movement
   1.6 Identify essential guidelines for safe and efficient body movements
2. Understand facts about techniques used to move patients
   2.1 Identify relevant assessment data
   2.2 Identify nursing diagnoses for which the technique may be implemented
   2.3 Identify nursing goals related to the technique
   2.4 Identify expected and unexpected outcomes from assessment data
   2.5 Identify reasons underlying selected steps of the techniques
3. Perform techniques for moving and transferring patients safely
   3.1 Assess the patient adequately
   3.2 Collect additional data from appropriate sources
   3.3 Select pertinent nursing goals for the patient
   3.4 Establish relevant outcome criteria for the patient following the technique
   3.5 Collect necessary equipment before the technique
   3.6 Implement interventions to enhance the effectiveness of the technique and enhance the patient's comfort and safety
   3.7 Communicate relevant information about the patient to the appropriate persons

3.8 Determine the evaluative outcomes of the technique

4. Evaluate own performance of specific techniques in a laboratory or clinical setting with the assistance of another

4.1 Use the performance checklists provided

4.2 Identify areas of strength and weakness

4.3 Alter performance in response to own evaluation and that of another

Terms

■ alignment (posture)   the proper relationship of body segments to one another

■ balance   stability; steadiness

■ base of support   the area on which an object rests

■ body mechanics   the movement and coordination of the body in response to stimuli and the body's coordinated efforts to maintain its balance while responding to these stimuli

■ cartilage   a firm connective tissue found throughout the body

■ center of gravity   the point at which the mass (weight) of the body is centered

■ dorsal   of, toward, or at the back

■ Fowler's position   a bed sitting position with the head of the bed raised to 45°

■ friction   rubbing; the force that opposes motion

■ gravity   the force that pulls objects toward the earth

■ internal girdle   tensed (or tightened) gluteal and abdominal muscles

■ joint   the place where two or more bones join

■ kyphosis   an exaggerated convexity in the thoracic region of the vertebral column

■ lateral position   a side-lying position

■ lever   a rigid bar that moves on a fixed axis called a *fulcrum*

■ leverage   force applied with the use of a lever

■ ligament   a broad, fibrous band that holds two or more bones together

■ line of gravity   an imaginary vertical line running through the center of gravity

■ lordosis   an exaggerated concavity in the lumbar region of the vertebral column

■ pronation   turning the palm of the hand downward

■ prone position   lying on the abdomen

■ scoliosis   a lateral curvature of a part of the vertebral column

■ supination   turning the palm of the hand upward

■ supine position   a back-lying position

■ torsion   twisting

■ trapeze bar   a triangular handgrip suspended from an overbed frame, used by the patient

BODY ALIGNMENT

A person's body alignment or posture and body movement are dependent upon skeletal development, muscular coordination, a sense of balance, and learning. In addition posture can be affected to some extent by a person's emotions. The depressed person may slouch, bend the head forward, hunch the shoulders, and adopt a slow gait, for example.

Normal body alignment or good posture is essential to the effective functioning of the body. When the body is well aligned, no undue strain is placed on any aspect, and the person can maintain balance. Assessment of body alignment is discussed in Technique 16–1 on page 379.

Proper body alignment is essential to body balance. When there is poor alignment, the body can become unbalanced, the pull of gravity can overcome it, and the person may tip and fall. It is difficult to separate body balance from body alignment, although balance is the result of proper alignment. Both depend on the same three factors:

1. A base of suport that stabilizes the body

2. A center of gravity that lies within the base of support

3. A line of gravity that runs from the center of gravity through the base of support

The body's center of gravity is located on the midline, halfway between the umbilicus and the pubic symphysis. See Figure 16–1. A vertical line drawn from the body's center of gravity falls between the feet (the body's base of support). See Figure 16–2. Whenever the line of gravity and the center of gravity lie outside the base of support, the body becomes unbalanced and strained. See Figure 16–3.

Body balance can be greatly enhanced by altering two of the three factors governing it: the base of support and

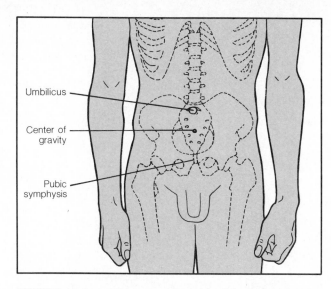

FIGURE 16–1 ■ The center of gravity of the body.

the center of gravity. The base of support can be *widened,* and the center of gravity can be *lowered,* bringing it closer to the base of support. The base of support is easily widened by spreading the feet farther apart. See Figure

FIGURE 16–2 ■ The line of gravity in a well-aligned adult standing.

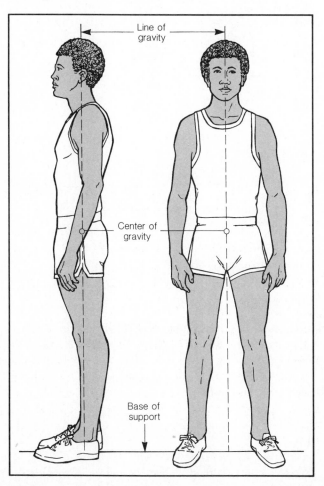

16–4. The center of gravity is readily lowered by flexing the hips and knees until a squatting position is achieved. See Figure 16–5. The importance of these alterations cannot be overemphasized for nurses. Practice of good body mechanics is basic to all techniques that assist patients to move and that require lifting and transporting objects.

Common Problems

Common problems of the musculoskeletal system often relate to misalignments and abnormal curvatures of the vertebral column. One abnormal curvature is *lumbar lordosis,* an exaggerated concavity in the lumbar region (see the discussion of the posture of pregnant women, earlier). *Kyphosis* is an exaggerated convexity in the thoracic region. Slight kyphosis is quite common in elderly people. *Scoliosis* is a lateral curvature in a part of the vertebral column. It is usually a developmental problem.

FIGURE 16–3 ■ **A,** a balanced body, with the line of gravity within the base of support; **B,** an unbalanced body, with the line of gravity outside the base of support.

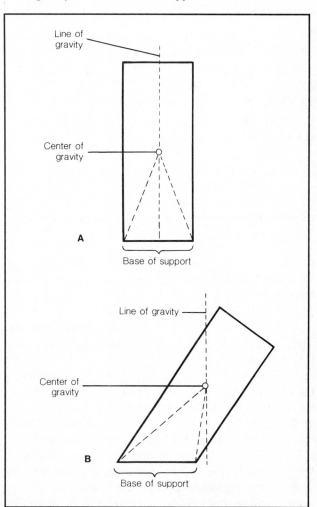

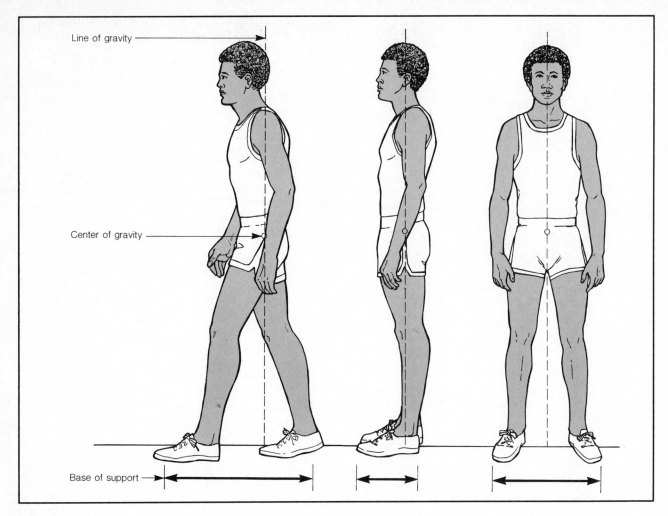

FIGURE 16–4 ■ Widening the base of support.

Poor posture is even more common. This places pressure on the vertebral column, frequently straining the muscles of the back and leading to the common complaint, "My back aches."

BODY MOVEMENT

Every nursing activity uses the musculoskeletal system, either to stand, walk, sit, or squat, or to carry, lift, push, or pull objects. When the body is used effectively, muscle strain, fatigue, and injury are avoided. To move effectively, the body works with the physical forces of friction, leverage, and gravity.

Friction increases the amount of effort required to move an object. It can be reduced by using a smooth, dry, clean surface in contrast to a rough, wet, or soiled surface. To reduce friction when moving (sliding) a patient up in bed, for example, the nurse provides a smooth, dry, firm bed foundation.

Leverage is a force that can be used by nurses to increase their lifting power and to make lifting easier. There are three basic types of levers. See Figure 16–6. The simplest, shown in Figure 16–6, *A,* is a seesaw (teeter-totter), on which a child can lift a heavier person. Nurses frequently use leverage to lift objects. The resisting force or weight is held in the hands or on the forearms, the fulcrum is the elbow, and the force is applied by contraction of the biceps (flexor) muscles of the arm. See Figure 16–7. The lifting power is increased when the elbow (fulcrum) is supported on a bed surface or a countertop.

The force of *gravity* frequently has to be overcome when the nurse lifts and moves objects or patients. To work effectively against gravity, the nurse needs to use the major muscle groups rather than weaker ones. These major groups include:

1. Flexors, extensors, and abductors of the thighs
2. Flexors and extensors of the knees
3. Flexors and extensors of the upper and lower arms
4. Flexors of the abdominal cavity and the pelvic floor

For the specific muscles used and their functions, see Table 16–1. For information about body movements, eg, flexion, extension, see Table 19–2 on page 428.

Guidelines for Body Movement

1. Start any body movement with proper alignment and balance. Increase the body's stability as necessary, by enlarging the base of support and/or lowering the center of gravity toward the base of support.

2. Adjust the working area to waist level and keep your body close to the area. Elevate adjustable beds and

FIGURE 16–5 ■ **A,** The center of gravity remains high during stooping; **B,** the center of gravity is lowered by squatting.

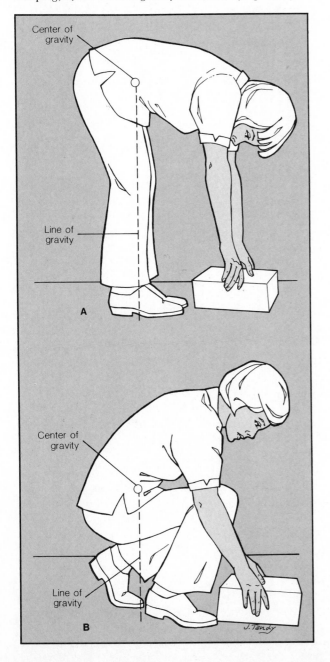

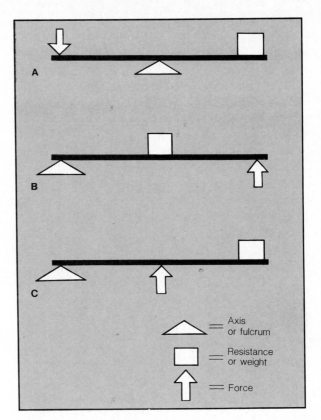

FIGURE 16–6 ■ Types of levers.

overbed tables, and lower the side rails to prevent stretching and reaching. Stretching creates unnecessary muscle fatigue and strain and places the line of gravity outside the base of support, resulting in instability.

FIGURE 16–7 ■ Using the arm as a lever.

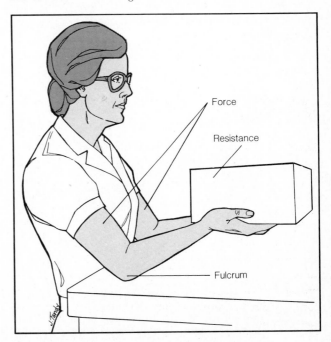

3. Face in the direction of the task. If a change of direction is required, turn the body and extremities as a single unit by pivoting. Avoid twisting the spinal column, which can produce back strain or injury. To pivot, place one foot ahead of the other, raise the heels very slightly, and put the body weight on the balls of the feet. When the weight is off the heels, the frictional surface is decreased and the knees are not twisted when turning. Keeping the body aligned, turn (pivot) about 90° in the desired direction. The foot that was forward will now be behind.

4. When moving a heavy object, face in the direction of the force. For example, when assisting a patient to move up in bed, face toward the head of the bed. This avoids torsion of the spine.

5. Tighten the gluteal and abdominal muscles before lifting or moving any object. This is often referred to as "putting on the internal girdle." The abdominal muscles pull upward, and the gluteal muscles (buttocks) pull downward. The "internal girdle" helps to support the abdomen and stabilizes the pelvis. These muscles also assist other large muscle groups to lift and push. The abdominal muscles are less likely to be injured if they are tightened ahead of time.

6. Avoid working against gravity whenever possible. It takes less effort to slide, push, or pull objects than it does to lift or carry them. Less effort is required to move a patient up in bed if the head of the bed is lowered first. In many instances, patients can be encouraged to push against the bed surface with their heels, or to grasp the bed rungs at the top of the bed and pull themselves up.

7. Carry objects close to the body and to the base of support. Holding objects close to the body prevents strain of the arm muscles, because the larger muscles of the thighs and legs carry some of the weight. Body stability is enhanced if the object is close to the base of support. See Figure 16–8.

8. Use the palmar grip when grasping and lifting objects. Extend the fingers and the hand around an object when you lift it. Fingers alone have little power; the strength of the entire hand should be used.

9. When lifting heavy objects, squat rather than stoop. Bending from the waist (stooping) to lift a heavy load is a major cause of back strain, since it forces the sacrospinal muscles to pull the body upright and to lift the weight. These are relatively small muscles. The squatting position uses the larger and stronger gluteal and femoral muscles of the buttocks and thighs. See Figure 16–5 earlier. In the squatting position, the abdominal muscles are also tensed, supporting the internal organs and preventing inguinal herniation. Better balance is maintained in the squatting position, since the center of gravity is lower than in the stooping position and the line of gravity falls within the base of support.

When squatting, place one foot ahead of the other, to distribute the body weight on the front foot and the ball of the back foot. Lower the body by flexing the knees, and keep the back straight. When returning to the standing position, lift the body using the muscles of the thighs and hips.

10. Use the body's own weight to push or pull objects. Body weight adds power to muscle action. When pushing an object (eg, a stretcher), lean toward it; when pulling an object, lean away from it. Take a broad stance and use the thigh muscles to enhance stability and power. Use your body's weight when assisting patients to move. For example, when helping a patient to stand, rock your own body backward to counterbalance the patient's weight.

TABLE 16–1 ■ Major Muscles Used in Moving Patients

Body part	Muscles	Function
Forearm	Biceps brachii	Flexes the forearm
	Triceps brachii	Extends the forearm
Upper arm	Deltoid	Abducts the upper arm; assists in flexion and extension of the upper arm
	Pectoralis major	Flexes the upper arm upward
	Latissimus dorsi	Extends the upper arm downward
Thigh	Gluteal group	
	Gluteus maximus	Extends and rotates the thigh outward
	Gluteus medius	Abducts the thigh and rotates it outward
	Gluteus minimus	Abducts the thigh and rotates it inward
	Iliopsoas	Flexes the thigh
	Rectus femoris	Flexes the thigh and extends the lower leg
Lower leg	**Quadriceps** Femoris group	
	Rectus femoris	Flexes the thigh and extends the leg
	Vastus lateralis	Extends the leg
	Vastus medialis	Extends the leg
	Vastus intermedius	Extends the leg
	Hamstring group	
	Biceps femoris	Flexes the leg and extends the thigh
Abdomen	External oblique	Compresses the abdomen
	Internal oblique	Compresses the abdomen
	Transversus abdominis	Compresses the abdomen
	Rectus abdominis	Flexes the trunk
Pelvic floor	Levator ani	Supports the floor of the pelvic cavity
	Coccygeus	Supports the floor of the pelvic cavity

11. Before moving a patient, lock the wheels of the bed or stretcher to keep it stable during the move. Unexpected movement can upset your balance.

12. Whenever possible, encourage the patient to assist with the move so that he or she maintains some sense of independence or control and obtains some exercise. The patient's force often helps to overcome friction impeding the move.

13. Make your body movements smooth and rhythmic. Sudden, jerky movements expend more energy than controlled smooth motions and put more strain on the muscles.

14. Use other mechanical aids or other persons to move heavy loads. Many mechanical aids are available to assist nurses when moving patients. The mechanical lifter is discussed in Technique 16–12.

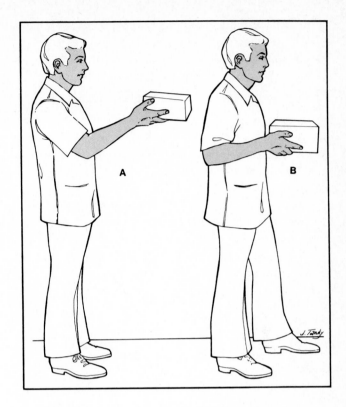

FIGURE 16-8 ■ Carrying an object: **A,** away from the base of support, which can strain arm muscles; **B,** close to the base of support, which uses leg and thigh muscles as well, and improves stability.

TECHNIQUE 16–1 ■ Assessing Body Alignment and Body Movement

Body alignment is usually assessed during an initial physical examination. Periodic reassessments may need to be conducted for patients with a long-term illness or physical disability.

Body alignment can be assessed when the person is standing, sitting, or lying. Alignment in standing and sitting positions is discussed here; alignment in lying positions is noted here and discussed more thoroughly in chapter 17.

■ Planning

Nursing goals

1. To identify postural deviations
2. To identify normal developmental postural deviations
3. To identify the body's functional balance
4. To identify factors contributing to poor body alignment
5. To identify impaired body movement
6. To identify learning needs of the patient

■ Intervention ✗

Normal standing position

1. Attempt to put the patient at ease.
   Rationale A tense person may assume an unnatural position.

2. Facing the patient to view him or her anteriorly, assess whether:
   a. The arms are at the sides with the elbows slightly flexed.
   b. The hands are positioned midway between pronation and supination with the fingers slightly flexed, and the wrists are neither flexed nor extended.
   c. The toes point forward.
   d. The feet are slightly apart to maintain a base of support.
   e. The line of gravity is at the body's midline, running from a midpoint on the forehead to a midpoint between the feet.
   f. The head is erect, neither flexed forward nor extended backward nor flexed laterally.

g. The main body weight is borne well forward on the outer sides of the feet.

3. From a lateral view, assess whether:

   a. The chin is held in, not protracted.

   b. The vertebral curves are not exaggerated.

   c. The hips are straight.

   d. The lower abdomen is pulled up and in.

   e. The knees are slightly flexed, and a line drawn through the middle of the patella (kneecap) and the ankle ends at the second or third toe.

   f. The body appears to be fully stretched but relaxed and poised, with minimal muscle strain.

4. From a posterior view, assess whether:

   a. The shoulders are at the same level.

   b. The hips are straight.

5. If the person is elderly, the usual posture is one of flexion. The head and neck are slightly flexed, and the eyes are turned downward. The spinal column is flexed in the thoracic and lumbar areas, producing a mild dorsal kyphosis and loss of the normal lumbar lordosis. See Figure 16–9. The hips and knees are slightly flexed. The ability to balance is reduced because of decreased strength of the hip and knee extensor muscles.

Normal sitting position

6. From an anterior view, assess whether:

   a. The forearms are supported on the lap, the armrests, or a table in front.

FIGURE 16–9 ■ Dorsal kyphosis in an elderly person.

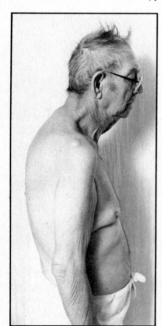 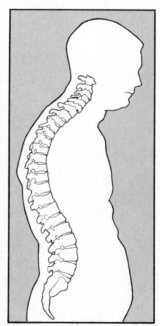

   b. The thighs are in a horizontal position.

   c. The weight of the body from the head to the buttocks is centered on the buttocks and thighs.

   d. Both feet are on the floor with the same ankle flexion as in a standing position. One foot may be slightly ahead of the other for comfort.

   e. The buttocks are against the back of the chair.

7. From a lateral view, assess whether:

   a. The head is erect, neither flexed forward nor extended backward.

   b. The vertebral curves are not exaggerated (see Common Problems earlier in this chapter).

   c. The popliteal spaces (backs of the knees) are at least 2.5 cm (1 in) from the edge of the chair, to avoid pressure on the nerves and blood vessels there.

Normal lying position

8. From a posterior view, with the patient lying in a lateral position with a small pillow under the head, assess whether:

   a. The vertebral column is in straight alignment without lateral curves.

Movement

9. Assess the patient's gait, range of motion of joints, and exercise capacity. See chapter 19.

10. Assess the patient rising from a lying position to a sitting position on the edge of the bed. The patient can normally rise without support from the arms; however, a patient with muscle weakness may roll to the side and push with the arms or pull with the arms on side rails or nearby furniture to rise.

11. Assess the patient rising from a chair to a standing position. Normally this can be done without pushing with the arms; however, a person with weak muscles may use the arms to push upward and may thrust the upper body forward before rising.

12. Assess the patient moving in the bed, and observe the amount of assistance required for turning:

    a. From a supine position to a lateral position.

    b. From a lateral position on one side to a lateral position on the other.

    c. From a supine position to a prone position.

    d. From a supine position to a sitting position in bed.

See chapter 17 for discussion of positions.

TECHNIQUE 16–2 ■ Moving a Patient Up in Bed

Moving a patient up toward the head of the bed is facilitated if the patient can safely tolerate having the head of the bed lowered to a flat position and the head pillow removed for a few minutes. If this is not possible, it is wise to obtain a second person to help from the other side of the bed. With this assistance, the patient will experience less exertion and less discomfort. The steps presented here are followed by either one or two nurses.

■ Assessment

Prior to moving a patient, assess:

1. How the patient's illness influences her or his ability to move. Unconscious patients and those with generalized muscular weakness, loss of or injury to one or both lower extremities, acute spinal cord injury, paralysis of one or both lower extremities, or paralysis of one or both upper extremities will need assistance by one, two, or more nurses.

2. Whether the patient's illness contraindicates exertion. Patients with severe cardiac or respiratory impairments often cannot tolerate what would be minor exertion to most people.

3. The patient's mental status, ie, ability to comprehend instructions and to participate in the move. Obviously, unconscious patients are unable to participate and to assist the nurse. Patients, for example, who are medicated for pain postoperatively or who have suffered brain changes with age or disease may be too lethargic or mentally impaired to understand instructions.

4. The patient's degree of comfort. Patients who have severe discomfort when moving, such as those with painful burns, acute inflammatory disease of the joints (eg, arthritis), or recent surgery, require more help to move them with the least possible discomfort. These patients may require an analgesic at least 30 minutes before they are moved, to help them relax and move with minimal discomfort.

5. The patient's weight. Lifting and moving an obese patient may result in injury to the nurses and the patient if extra assistance or mechanical devices are not used.

6. Your own strength and ability. It is wise to request assistance from another person whenever your ability is doubtful.

■ Nursing Diagnosis

Nursing diagnoses that may indicate the need to assist a patient to move include:

1. Impaired physical mobility related to:
   a. Neuromuscular impairment (eg, multiple sclerosis)
   b. Musculoskeletal impairment (eg, muscle weakness)
   c. Surgical procedure
   d. Nonfunctioning limb (eg, leg fracture)
   e. Missing limb (eg, amputation)
   f. Decreased motor agility (eg, elderly)
2. Activity intolerance related to:
   a. Alterations in the oxygen transport system (eg, myocardial infarction, chronic obstructive pulmonary disease, malnutrition, anemia, chronic hepatic or renal disease)
   b. Prolonged bed rest
   c. Pain

■ Planning

Nursing goal

To move the patient up toward the head of the bed safely and comfortably.

■ Intervention

1. Adjust the head of the bed to a flat position or make it as low as the patient can tolerate.
   Rationale The patient then does not have to move against gravity.

2. Remove all pillows; then place one at the head of the bed.
   Rationale The pillow will protect the patient's head from inadvertent injury against the top of the bed.

3. Facing the head of the bed, assume a broad stance with the foot nearest the bed behind the other foot.
   Rationale A broad stance increases balance. Proper foot placement prevents unnecessary twisting of the body when the patient is moved.

4. Ask the patient to flex both knees, bringing both heels up to the buttocks, and to flex the neck so that the chin is tilted toward the chest.
   Rationale Flexed knees ensure that the patient uses the femoral muscles when subsequently asked to

push. The chin pulled toward the chest prevents hyperextension of the neck as the head resists moving against the bed surface.

5. If the patient is able to assist, have him or her:

   a. Grasp the bed head with both hands.

   or

   b. Grasp the trapeze bar.

   or

   c. Push the hands on the bed surface by flexing the elbows and hyperextending the shoulder joints.

   Rationale Patient assistance provides additional power to overcome friction when the move is made.

6. If the patient cannot assist, place his or her arms across the chest.

   Rationale This prevents them from dragging on the bed surface and thus decreases friction.

7. Flex your knees and hips to bring your forearms to the level of the bed surface.

   Rationale Flexed knees and hips allow the nurse to use the major muscle groups of the thighs and legs to move the patient and also brings the nurse's center of gravity closer to the patient's.

8. Place one arm under the patient's shoulders and the other arm under the patient's thighs. See Figure 16–10.

   Rationale This placement of the arms distributes the patient's weight and supports the heaviest part of the body (the buttocks).

9. Tighten your gluteal and abdominal muscles.

FIGURE 16–10

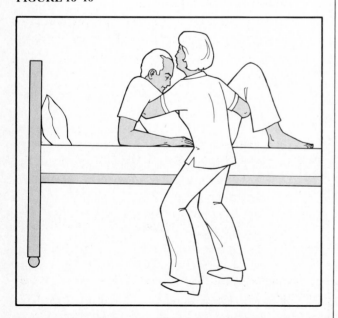

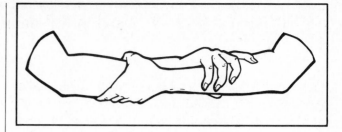

FIGURE 16–11

Rationale These muscles assist other large muscle groups to lift and push; they are less likely to be injured if tightened.

10. Rock from the back leg to the front leg and back again; then shift weight to the front leg as the patient pushes with the heels and pulls with the arms, moving the patient toward the head of the bed.

    Rationale Rocking helps to attain a balanced, smooth motion and to overcome inertia. The nurse's weight shift helps to counteract the patient's weight.

11. Elevate the head of the bed. Provide appropriate support devices for the patient's new position. See the discussion of the supine position or Fowler's position in chapter 17.

Variation: Two nurses using a hand–forearm interlock

Two people are required to move a patient who is unable to assist because of his or her condition or weight. Using the technique described above, with the second nurse on the opposite side of the bed, the two nurses interlock their forearms under the patient's thighs and shoulders. See Figure 16–11.

Variation: Two nurses using a turn sheet

Two nurses can use a turn sheet to move a patient up in the bed. A turn sheet distributes the patient's weight more evenly, decreases friction, and exerts a more even force on the patient during the move. In addition, it prevents injury of the patient's skin, since the friction created between two sheets when one is moved is less than that created by the patient's body moving over the sheet.

A drawsheet or a full sheet folded in half is placed under the patient, extending from the shoulders to the thighs.

Each nurse rolls up or fanfolds the turn sheet close to the patient's body on either side. The nurses then grasp the sheet close to the shoulders and buttocks of the patient. This draws the weight closer to the nurses' base of support, and increases the nurses' balance and stability, permitting a smoother movement. The method described in steps 7, 9, and 10 is then used to move the patient up in the bed.

Chapter 16 Moving Patients ■ 383

TECHNIQUE 16–3 ■ Moving a Patient to the Side of the Bed in Segments

Occasionally a patient who must remain on his or her back needs to be moved to the side of the bed. This may be necessary when changing a bed or carrying out some treatment for the patient within easy reach. In this movement, the nurse's weight is used to counteract the patient's weight; the nurse's arms serve as connecting bars between the patient and the nurse.

■ **Assessment** See Techniques 16–1 and 16–2 on pages 379 and 381.

■ **Nursing Diagnosis** See Technique 16–2 on page 381.

■ **Planning**

Nursing goal

To move the patient closer to the nurse safely and comfortably.

■ **Intervention**

1. Adjust the head of the bed to a flat position or make it as low as the patient can tolerate.
   Rationale The patient will move more easily with the head of the bed lowered.
2. Position yourself at the side of the bed toward which the patient will be moved and opposite the patient's chest.
   Rationale This position reassures the patient that he or she cannot fall and avoids the need for the nurse to reach.
3. Place the patient's near arm across his or her chest.

Rationale This reduces resistance to the patient's movement and prevents injury to the arm.

4. Assume a broad stance, with one foot in front of the other, and flex your knees.
   Rationale The broad stance provides balance. Flexing the knees lowers the center of gravity (increasing stability) and ensures use of the large muscle groups in the legs during movement.
5. Place one of your arms under the patient's far shoulder so that the patient's head rests on your forearm and elbow crease. Place your other arm under the patient's lumbar curvature.
   Rationale The arm under the patient's shoulder securely supports the head and shoulders. The other arm supports the trunk.
6. Tighten your gluteal and abdominal muscles.
   Rationale Tensing these muscles prepares them for use and protects the internal organs against injury.
7. Pull the patient's head, shoulders, and thorax to the near side of the bed by rocking backward and shifting your weight to the rear foot.
   Rationale Pulling avoids lifting against gravity. Rocking backward uses the nurse's body weight in the direction of the pull.
8. To move the patient's buttocks, place one arm under the patient's lumbar region, the other under the patient's thighs. Repeat steps 6 and 7, pulling the buttocks.
   Rationale This placement of the arms centers the weight of the buttocks.
9. To move the patient's legs and feet, place one arm under the patient's thighs, the other under the calves. Repeat steps 6 and 7, pulling the legs.

TECHNIQUE 16–4 ■ Moving a Patient to a Lateral Position in Bed

Movement to a lateral (side-lying) position is most easily accomplished if the patient is lying on a flat bed; however, it can be accomplished if the head or the foot of the bed is raised. It is easiest if the patient is in a supine position. Before moving a patient to a lateral position, the nurse moves the patient closer to the side of the bed opposite the side the patient will face when turned. See Technique

16–3. This ensures that the patient will be positioned safely in the center of the bed after turning.

■ **Assessment** See Techniques 16–1 and 16–2 on pages 379 and 381.

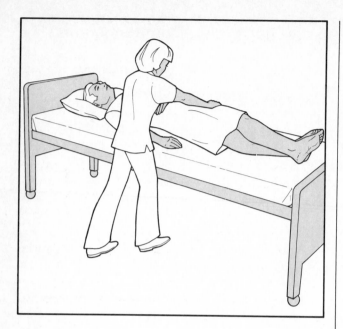

FIGURE 16–12

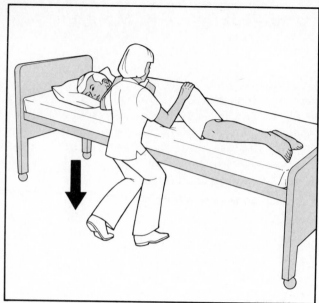

FIGURE 16–13

■ **Nursing Diagnosis**   See Technique 16–2 on page 381.

■ **Planning**

Nursing goal

To move the patient to a lateral position safely and comfortably.

■ **Intervention**

1. Adjust the head of the bed to a flat position, or make it as low as the patient can tolerate.

   Rationale   The patient will turn more easily with the head of the bed lowered.

2. Elevate the side rail on the side nearest the patient if there is any danger that the patient might roll off the bed.

3. Position yourself opposite the patient's abdomen on the side of the bed toward which the patient will turn.

   Rationale   This position prevents spinal torsion by the nurse when moving the patient and centers the nurse's weight opposite the patient's central weight.

4. Assume a broad stance with one foot ahead of the other.

   Rationale   A broad stance enhances balance.

5. Place the patient's arm nearest you away from his or her body.

Rationale   This prevents the patient from rolling onto that arm.

6. Flex the patient's far arm over the chest; place the far leg over the near leg. See Figure 16–12.

   Rationale   These positions facilitate turning by the patient.

7. Tighten your gluteal and abdominal muscles, and flex your knees.

   Rationale   Tensing the muscles prepares them for use and prevents injury. Flexing the knees lowers the center of gravity (increasing stability) and ensures use of the large muscle groups in the legs during movement.

8. Place one hand on the patient's far hip and the other hand on the far shoulder.

   Rationale   This placement of the hands distributes the patient's weight and supports the heaviest part of the body.

9. Roll the patient toward you:

   a. Rock backward and shift your weight to the rear foot.

   b. Increase your knee flexion and lower your pelvis. See Figure 16–13.

   Rationale   Rocking backward makes use of the nurse's body weight in the direction of the movement. Increased knee flexion lowers the nurse's center of gravity, enhancing stability.

10. Align the patient appropriately. See the discussion of the lateral position in chapter 17 on page 408.

TECHNIQUE 16–5   ■   Moving a Patient to a Prone Position

The prone position is seldom used for bed patients except for special therapeutic reasons, such as changing a dressing on the sacrum, avoiding body pressure on a decubitus ulcer in the sacral area, or administering an intramuscular injection into the gluteus maximus muscle (buttock).

■ **Assessment**   See Techniques 16–1 and 16–2 on pages 379 and 381.

■ **Nursing Diagnosis**   See Technique 16–2 on page 381.

■ **Planning**

Nursing goal

To turn the patient safely and comfortably to a prone position.

■ **Intervention**

1. Follow Technique 16–4, steps 1–4.
2. Keep the patient's near arm alongside the body for the patient to roll over. Place the patient's far leg over the near leg.

    Rationale   Keeping the arm alongside the body prevents it from being pinned under the patient in the prone position.
3. Follow Technique 16–4, steps 7–9. Roll the patient completely onto his or her abdomen.
4. Center the patient in the bed. See Technique 16–3.

    Rationale   The patient is centered for comfort and safety.
5. Align the patient appropriately. See Technique 17–5 on page 406.

TECHNIQUE 16–6   Logrolling a Patient

Logrolling is a technique used to turn a patient whose body must at all times be kept in straight alignment (like a log). An example is the patient who has a spinal injury. This technique requires two nurses or, if the patient is large, three nurses.

■ **Assessment**   See Techniques 16–1 and 16–2 on pages 379 and 381.

■ **Nursing Diagnosis**   See Technique 16–2 on page 381.

■ **Planning**

Nursing goal

To turn the patient while maintaining the alignment of the back.

■ **Intervention**

1. The nurses stand on the same side of the bed. Assume a broad stance with one foot ahead of the other.

    Rationale   A broad stance enhances balance.
2. Place the patient's arms across his or her chest.

    Rationale   The patient's arm then will not be injured or become trapped under him or her.
3. Flex your knees.

    Rationale   Flexing the knees ensures use of the large muscle groups in the legs when moving and lowers the center of gravity (enhances stability).
4. Place your arms under the patient as shown in Figure 16–14 or Figure 16–15 depending upon the patient's size.

    Rationale   Each nurse then has a major weight area of the patient centered between the arms.
5. Tighten your abdominal and pelvic muscles.

    Rationale   Tensing these muscles prepares them for action and avoids injury.
6. One nurse counts "one, two, three, go." Then, at the same time, all nurses pull the patient as a unit to the side of the bed by shifting weight to the back foot and flexing the knees.

    Rationale   Moving the patient as a unit maintains the patient's body alignment.

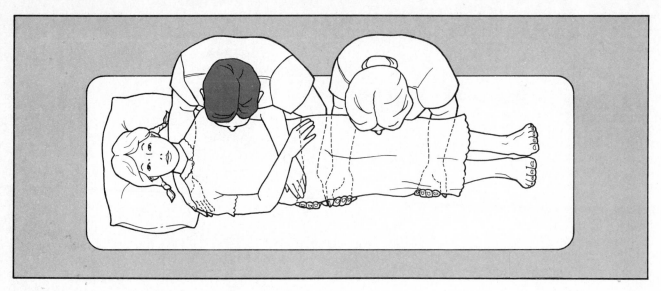

FIGURE 16–14

7. Elevate the side rail on this side of the bed.

   Rationale Elevating the side rail prevents the patient from falling while lying so close to the edge of the bed.

8. All nurses move to the other side of the bed.

9. Place a pillow where it will support the patient's head after he or she is turned.

   Rationale The pillow will prevent lateral flexion of the neck and ensure alignment of the cervical spine.

10. Place one or two pillows between the patient's legs to support the upper leg when the patient is turned.

    Rationale A pillow between the patient's legs prevents adduction of the upper leg and keeps the legs parallel and aligned.

11. All nurses flex the knees and assume a broad stance with one foot forward.

12. All nurses reach over the patient and place hands as shown in Figure 16–16 or Figure 16–17.

    Rationale This centers a major weight area of the patient between each nurse's arms.

13. One nurse counts "one, two, three, go." Then, at the same time, all nurses roll the patient as a unit to a lateral position.

14. Place pillows in front of and behind the patient's trunk to support the patient's alignment in the lateral position. See Technique 17–6 on page 408.

Variation: Using a turn sheet

Logrolling can be facilitated with the use of a turn sheet, described in Technique 16–2. The patient is first moved to the side of the bed by two nurses who stand on the

FIGURE 16–15

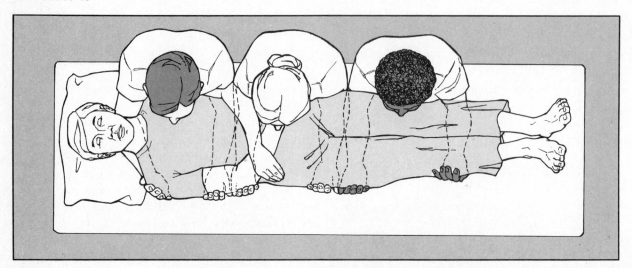

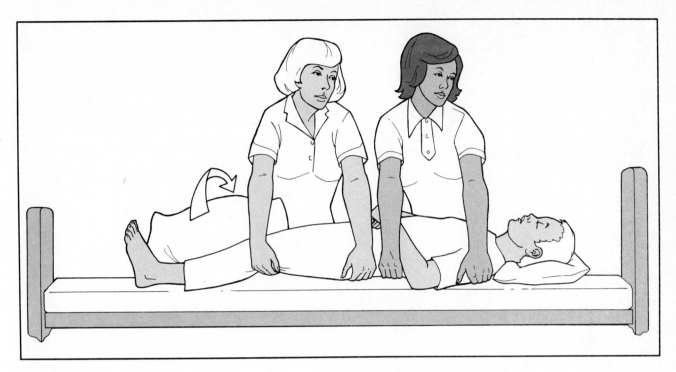

FIGURE 16-16

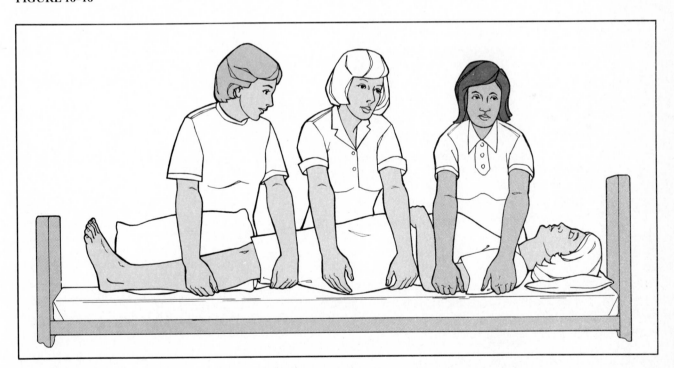

FIGURE 16-17

same side of the bed. Each nurse assumes a broad stance with one foot forward and grasps half of the fanfolded or rolled edge of the turnsheet. On a signal, the nurses pull the patient toward them. See Figure 16-18. Pulling is easier when the nurses flex their knees and brace their forward thighs against the bed frame.

Before the patient is turned, pillow supports are placed for the head and the legs, as described in steps 9-10, to maintain the patient's alignment when turning. One nurse then goes to the other side of the bed (farthest from the patient) and assumes a stable stance. Reaching over the patient, this nurse grasps the far edges of the turn sheet and rolls the patient toward her or him. See Figure 16-19. The second nurse (behind the patient) helps to turn the patient as needed and provides pillow supports to ensure good alignment in the lateral position.

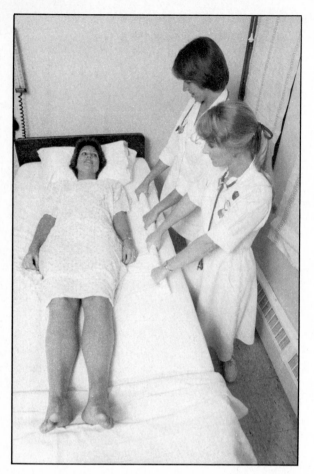

FIGURE 16–18

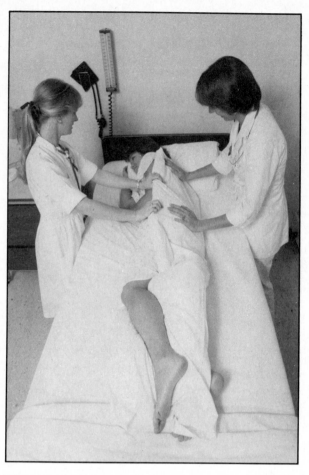

FIGURE 16–19

TECHNIQUE 16–7 ■ Moving a Patient to a Sitting Position in Bed

Patients may need assistance to sit in bed while pillows are rearranged or, in some instances, for back care. The degree of assistance required depends on the patient's condition. When assisting patients to a sitting position, the nurse uses her or his own weight to counteract the patient's weight. In one method, the nurse's arm serves as a lever, with the elbow as the fulcrum.

■ **Assessment** See Techniques 16–1 and 16–2 on pages 379 and 381.

■ **Nursing Diagnosis** See Technique 16–2 on page 381.

■ **Planning**

Nursing goal

To move the patient to a sitting position safely and comfortably.

■ **Intervention**

1. Assist the patient to a supine position.
2. Adjust the bed to a low Fowler's position as tolerated by the patient. See chapter 17.
3. Ask the patient to place his or her arms at the sides with the palms of the hands against the surface of the bed.

   Rationale The patient can push against the bed surface to assist the nurse.

4. Facing the head of the bed, stand at the side of the bed and opposite the patient's buttocks. Assume a broad stance with the foot nearest the bed behind the other foot.

   Rationale Facing the head of the bed prevents twisting of the nurse's body in the motion that follows. A broad stance enhances balance.

5. If the patient is helpless, place your hand farthest

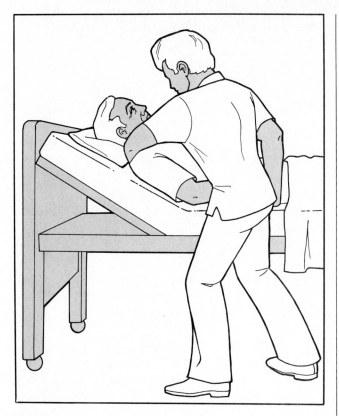

FIGURE 16–20

FIGURE 16–21

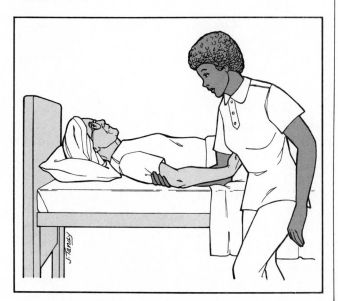

from the patient over his or her near shoulder at a point between the shoulder blades. Place the hand of your free arm on the bed surface. See Figure 16–20.

Rationale   This hand placement is designed to lift the patient's upper trunk evenly. The hand on the bed provides balance and leverage.

   or

If the patient can assist, ask the patient to flex the knees. Then the patient and you grasp the backs of each other's arms. Rest your elbow on the bed surface when lifting the patient. See Figure 16–21.

Rationale   Having the patient flex the knees facilitates upward movement of the trunk against gravity. The nurse's elbow is the fulcrum for the lever action of the arm.

6.   Raise the patient to a sitting position by shifting your weight to the back leg and flexing your knees to bring your hips downward. At the same time have the patient who can assist push with the arm that is not grasping your arm. See Figure 16–22.

Rationale   The nurse uses her or his own weight to counteract the patient's weight.

7.   Support the patient appropriately.

FIGURE 16–22

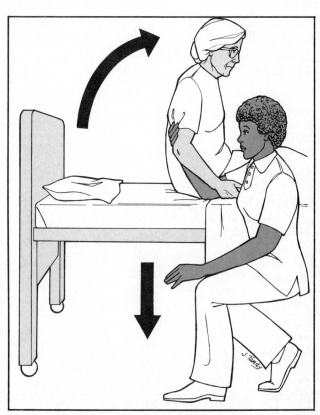

TECHNIQUE 16–8 ■ Moving a Patient to a Sitting Position on the Edge of the Bed 🏠

The nurse's weight is used to counterbalance the patient's weight in moving to a sitting position on the edge of the bed. It is crucial that the nurse's balance be maintained while shifting weight from the front leg to the rear one.

■ **Assessment**   See Techniques 16–1 and 16–2 on pages 379 and 381.

■ **Nursing Diagnosis**   See Technique 16–2 on page 381.

■ **Planning**

Nursing goal

To move the patient safely and comfortably to a sitting position on the edge of the bed.

■ **Intervention**

1. Assist the patient to a lateral position facing the nurse. See Technique 16–4.
2. Raise the head of the bed to about 60°.
    Rationale   Raising the head of the bed decreases the distance that the patient needs to move to sit up.

3. Facing the patient and the far bottom corner of the bed, stand opposite the patient's hips. Assume a broad stance, placing the foot nearest the bottom of the bed to the rear.
    Rationale   This position enhances balance and prevents twisting of the nurse's body.
4. Place the patient's feet and lower legs just over the edge of the bed.
    Rationale   This position prevents the feet from resisting the sitting movement.
5. Place one arm under the patient's shoulders and the other arm over the patient's far thigh, with your hand resting on the posterior aspect of the thigh. See Figure 16–23.
    Rationale   This hand placement prevents the patient from falling backward when sitting up.
6. Pivot toward your rear leg so that the patient's legs swing downward and your weight shifts to the rear leg. See Figure 16–24.
    Rationale   The nurse's weight counteracts the patient's weight.
7. Maintain support of the patient until he or she is balanced and comfortable.
    Rationale   This movement may cause some patients to feel faint.

FIGURE 16–23

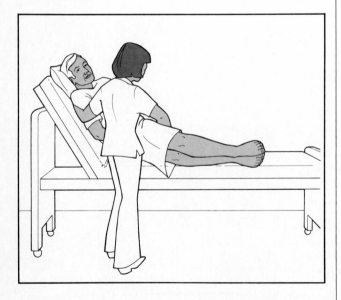

FIGURE 16–24

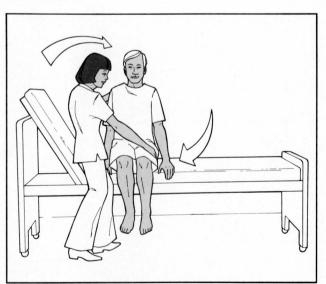

TECHNIQUE 16–9 ■ Raising the Buttocks of a Patient in Bed

Frequently the buttocks are raised to assist the patient onto a bedpan. In this movement, the nurse's arm acts as a lever, with the elbow on the bed surface as the fulcrum. The nurse's body weight is the force applied to the lever and hence to the patient.

■ **Assessment**   See Techniques 16–1 and 16–2 on pages 379 and 381.

■ **Nursing Diagnosis**   See Technique 16–2 on page 381.

■ **Planning**

Nursing goal

To raise the patient's buttocks safely and comfortably.

Equipment

A bedpan or other supplies depending on the purpose of lifting the patient's buttocks.

■ **Intervention**

1. Place the bedpan or other required supplies within easy reach.
2. Lower the head of the bed as far as the patient can tolerate.
   Rationale   Less of the patient's weight will then be centered at the buttocks.
3. Assume a broad stance at the patient's side opposite the buttocks.
   Rationale   A broad stance provides stability.
4. Have the patient flex the knees to bring the feet toward the buttocks.
   Rationale   This allows the patient to use his or her femoral and gluteal muscles to raise the buttocks.
5. Have the patient place her or his arms at the sides, with elbows slightly bent, and palms facing down against the bed, ready to push. See Figure 16–25. For patients who are on restricted bed rest, a trapeze may be helpful and require less effort.
   Rationale   Patient assistance lessens the energy required by the nurse.
6. Place your forearm and hand (palm upward) that are nearer the head of the bed under the patient's sacrum. Rest your elbow on the mattress.
   Rationale   The elbow serves as a fulcrum and the forearm as a lever.
7. Flex your knees and lower your hips at the same time as the patient pushes to elevate his or her buttocks. See Figure 16–26.
   Rationale   The arm acts as a lever and your weight counteracts the patient's weight.
8. With your free hand, provide the necessary nursing intervention, eg, put the bedpan in place.
9. Lower the patient and assist him or her to a comfortable position, eg, adjust the head of the bed.

FIGURE 16–25

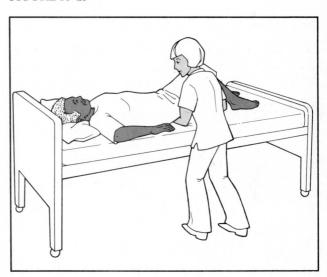

FIGURE 16–26

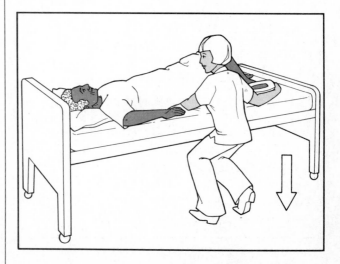

TECHNIQUE 16–10 ■ Transferring a Patient between a Bed and a Chair

For transferring a patient to a chair, the bed should be in the low position so that the patient can step easily to the floor. If the bed is not adjustable in this way, a broad-based and stable footstool can be used; the patient needs to step initially onto the stool and then step down to the floor.

■ **Assessment**   See Techniques 16–1 and 16–2 on pages 379 and 381.

■ **Nursing Diagnosis**   See Technique 16–2 on page 381.

■ **Planning**

Nursing goal

To transfer a patient between a bed and a chair safely and comfortably.

■ **Intervention**

1. Obtain a dressing gown and slippers or shoes for the patient. The slippers or shoes should have nonskid soles.

2. Assist the patient to a sitting position on the edge of the bed. See Technique 16–8.

3. Assist the patient to put on the dressing gown and slippers or shoes.

4. Lower the bed to the low level or obtain a broad-based, stable footstool.

5. Assume a broad stance facing the patient, and place your foot that is nearer the direction of the movement ahead of the other foot.
   Rationale   The broad stance provides stability and a smooth, balanced movement when turning; it also prevents twisting of the body.

6. Flex your knees and hips.
   Rationale   This ensures use of major muscle groups of the thighs and legs if the patient requires lifting or holding up.

7. Have the patient place his or her hands on your shoulders and put your hands on either side of the patient's waist.
   Rationale   This hand placement provides balance and support for the patient.

8. When the patient steps to the floor or the footstool, brace your front knee against the patient's knee. See Figure 16–27.

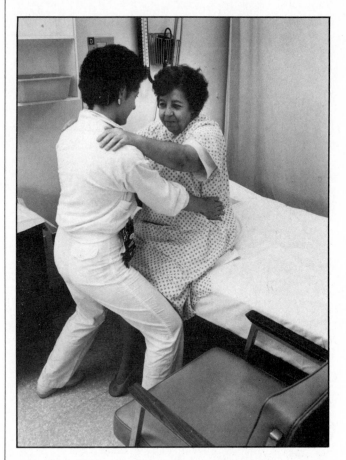

FIGURE 16–27

Rationale   This prevents the patient's knee from buckling and keeps the patient from falling.

9. After the patient feels steady, step back with your forward leg and guide the patient forward until the back of his or her legs are against the chair. Keep your knee against the patient's knee.

10. Assist the patient to lower into the chair by flexing your knees and hips as the patient flexes his or her knees and hips. See Figure 16–28.
    Rationale   Flexing the knees and hips prevents strain to the arm and back muscles.

11. Align the patient properly in the chair.

Variation: Using two nurses

Another method of assisting a patient from a bed to a chair uses two nurses. In this method, the bed is left in the raised position.

The patient is assisted to a sitting position on the edge of the bed and suitably attired for sitting in a chair. The chair is placed at the side of the bed with its back toward the foot of the bed, about 30 to 60 cm (1 to 2 ft) from the bed.

The nurses assume a broad stance with knees flexed, on opposite sides of the patient. Each nurse places an arm under the patient's near axilla, reaching from front to back, with the nurse's arm extending behind the back of the patient to the far axilla. The nurses can either hold the patient†s back just below the far axilla or grasp each other's forearms. Each nurse's other arm is placed under the patient's thighs, and the nurses grasp each other's forearms.

The patient places his or her arms around the nurses' shoulders if possible. The nurses together extend their knees to lift the patient and then move the patient to the chair with coordinated movements. The nurse nearer the chair sidesteps in front of the chair to the side farther from the bed, while the other nurse moves forward to the side of the chair near the bed. The patient is now over the chair. Each nurse flexes the knees to lower the patient into the chair.

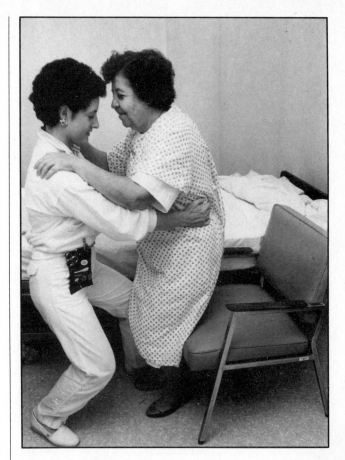

FIGURE 16–28

TECHNIQUE 16–11 ■ Transferring a Patient between a Bed and a Stretcher

Lifting and carrying the average adult from a bed to a stretcher or to another bed and at the same time maintaining the patient's horizontal position generally requires three people. A child may be moved by just two persons, and a baby by one person safely.

■ **Assessment**   See Techniques 16–1 and 16–2 on pages 379 and 381.

■ **Nursing Diagnosis**   See Technique 16–2 on page 381.

■ **Planning**

Nursing goal

To transfer a patient safely and comfortably while maintaining a supine position.

Equipment

A stretcher or a second bed.

■ **Intervention**

1. Place the stretcher to receive the patient at a right angle to the patient's bed, with the head near the foot of the patient's bed. Lock the wheels of the stretcher, and confirm that the wheels of the bed are locked.
   Rationale The right-angle, head-to-foot position decreases the distance the nurses must move during the transfer. The wheels are locked so that the bed and stretcher will not slip out from under the patient.

2. All nurses stand on the same side of the bed. The tallest person stands beside the patient's shoulders and the strongest person stands opposite the patient's hips.

Rationale The tallest person has the longest arms and can best support the head and shoulders. The strongest person can best support the heaviest part of the patient's body. The third person supports the legs and feet.

3. Assume a broad stance, with one foot ahead of the other. If the stretcher is to the right of the nurses, the right foot of each nurse is placed in front of the left foot.

Rationale A broad stance enhances balance. Placing the feet as described allows the nurses to step backward in unison, in a smooth, coordinated fashion, to the stretcher.

4. Place the patient's arms across his or her chest.

Rationale Putting the arms across the chest prevents injury to them during the transfer.

5. Flex your knees.

Rationale Flexing the knees lowers the center of gravity (enhancing stability) and ensures use of the large muscle groups of the legs when moving.

6. Place your arms under the patient as shown in Figure 16–14 or Figure 16–15, earlier. The first and third nurses place their arms close to the middle nurse's arms.

Rationale Placing the arms close together assists the middle nurse in lifting the heaviest weight (the buttocks).

7. If the patient is lying uncomfortably far from you, pull him or her closer to you before lifting for the transfer.

Rationale If the patient is too far, it will be difficult to lift him or her for the transfer.

8. On a signal from one nurse, all three nurses roll (do not pull) the patient toward their chests, resting their elbows against the bed.

Rationale The patient is rolled close to the base of support. The elbows act as a fulcrum for leverage.

9. On a signal, lift the patient as a unit while shifting your weight to the rear foot, then step backward in unison and walk to the stretcher. See Figure 16–29.

10. On a signal, flex your knees and lower the patient to the stretcher, until your elbows rest on the stretcher or bed.

FIGURE 16–29

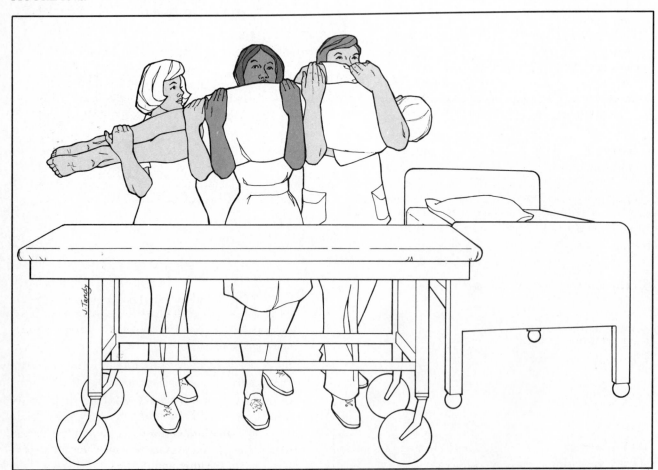

11. In unison, extend your elbows until the patient is lying flat.

Variation: Using a turn sheet

The bed or stretcher is aligned with the bed on which the patient is lying. Reaching across the bed to which the patient is to be moved, two or three nurses grasp the turn sheet close to the patient's body and pull the sheet (and the patient on it) onto the bed or stretcher, using their own weight to counteract the patient's weight. See the variation using a turn sheet in Technique 16–2 earlier.

TECHNIQUE 16–12 ■ Transferring a Patient to a Chair Using a Mechanical Lifter

Various types of mechanical lifters are used to lift and move patients. It is important that nurses be familiar with the model used and the practices that accompany use. Before using the lifter, the nurse ensures that it is in working order and that the hooks, chains, straps, and canvas seat are in good repair. Most agencies recommend that two nurses operate a lifter. Agency policy should be checked in this regard.

Before lifting the patient, the nurse explains the procedure and demonstrates the lifter. Some patients are afraid of being lifted and will be reassured by a demonstration.

The lifter may have a one- or two-piece canvas seat. See Figure 16–30. The one-piece seat stretches from the patient's head to the knees. The two-piece seat has one canvas strap to support the patient's buttocks and thighs and a second strap to support the back, extending up to the patient's axillae.

■ **Assessment**   See Techniques 16–1 and 16–2 on pages 379 and 381.

■ **Nursing Diagnosis**   See Technique 16–2 on page 381.

■ **Planning**

Nursing goal

To transfer the patient safely and comfortably using a mechanical lifter.

Equipment

1. A mechanical lifter
2. A chair

■ **Intervention**

1. Place the chair that is to receive the patient beside

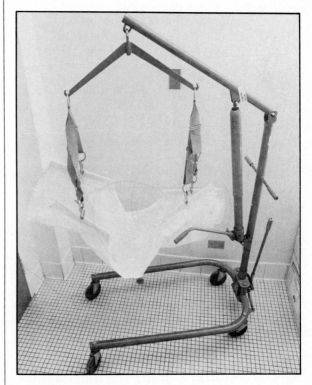

FIGURE 16–30 ■ A mechanical lifter with a one-piece seat.

the bed. Allow room for the lifter and the patient to clear the bed and the chair.

2. Lock the wheels, if a chair with wheels is used.
   Rationale This prevents the chair from moving under the patient.

3. Put the canvas seat or straps exactly in place under the patient.
   Rationale Correct placement permits the patient to be lifted evenly with minimal shifting.

4. Wheel the lifter into position at a right angle to the side of the bed, with the footbars under the bed. Lock the wheels of the lifter and the bed.

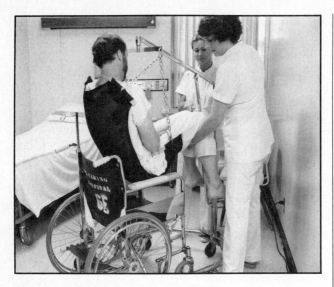

FIGURE 16-31

5. Ask the patient to remove his or her glasses, and put them in a safe place.

   Rationale The patient should not wear glasses because the swivel bar may come close to his or her face.

6. Attach the lifter straps or hooks to the corresponding openings in the canvas seat. Check that the hooks are correctly placed and that matching straps or chains are of equal length.

7. a. Nurse 1: Close the pressure valve, and gradually pump up the lift until the patient is above the bed surface.

   Rationale Gradual elevation of the lift is less frightening to the patient than a rapid rise.

   b. Nurse 2: Assume a broad stance and tighten your abdominal and pelvic muscles. Guide the patient with your hands as he or she is lifted.

   Rationale The nurse prepares to hold the patient and provide control during the movement.

8. a. Nurse 1: With the pressure valve securely closed, slowly roll the lifter until the patient is over the chair.

   b. Nurse 2: Guide the patient by hand until he or she is directly over the chair. See Figure 16-31.

   Rationale Slow movement decreases swaying and is less frightening. Guidance also decreases swaying and gives a sense of security.

9. a. Nurse 1: Release the pressure valve very gradually.

   b. Nurse 2: Guide the patient into the chair.

   Rationale Gradual release lowers the patient slowly and is less frightening than being lowered quickly.

10. Remove the hooks from the canvas seat. Leave the seat in place.

    Rationale The seat is left in place in preparation for the lift back to bed.

11. Align the patient properly in a sitting position. See the section on the adult sitting position in Technique 16-1. Give the patient his or her glasses if appropriate.

References

Drapeau J: Getting back into good posture: How to erase your lumbar aches. *Nursing 75* (September) 1975; 5:63–65.

Ford JR, Duckworth B: Moving a dependent patient safely, comfortably, part I: Positioning. *Nursing 76* (January) 1976; 6:27–36.

Ford JR, Duckworth B: Moving a dependent patient safely, comfortably, part 2: Transferring. *Nursing 76* (February) 1976; 6:58–65.

Foss G: Use your head and your back . . . body mechanics. *Nursing 73* (May) 1973; 3:25–32.

Klabak L: Getting the grip on the transfer belt technique. *Nursing 78* (February) 1978; 8:10.

Leinweber E: Belts to make moves smoother. *Am J Nurs* (December) 1978; 78:2080–2081.

Long BC, Buergin PS: The pivot transfer. *Am J Nurs* (June) 1977; 77:980–982.

Owen BD: How to avoid that aching back. *Am J Nurs* (May) 1980; 80:894–897.

Works RF: Hints on lifting and pulling. *Am J Nurs* (February) 1972; 72:260–261.

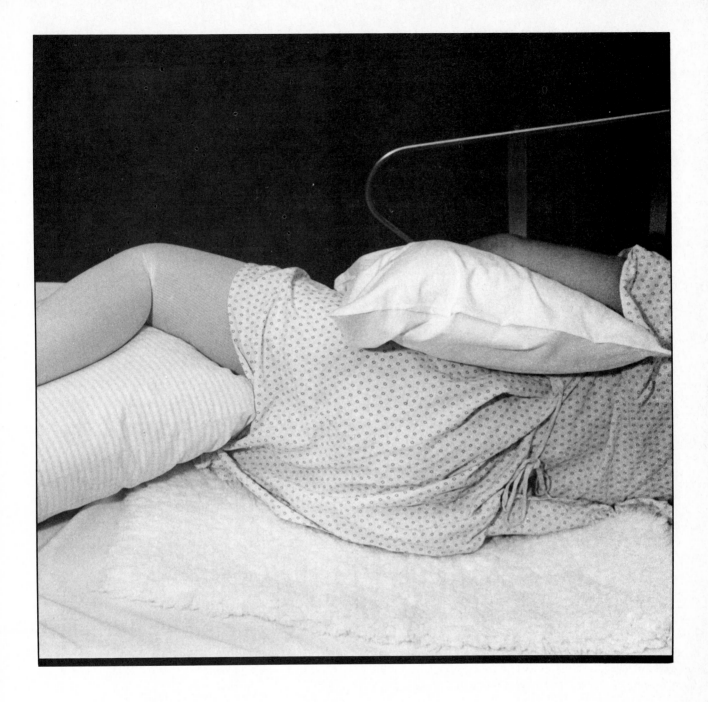

PATIENT POSITIONS

17

Positioning a bed-confined patient in body alignment and changing his or her position regularly and systematically are essential nursing functions. Patients who can move easily in bed automatically reposition themselves for comfort. Such patients generally require minimal positioning assistance from nurses other than guidance about ways to maintain body alignment and to exercise their joints. See chapter 19. However, patients who are weak, frail, in pain, paralyzed, or unconscious rely on nurses to provide or assist with position changes.

Frequent position changes are essential to prevent decubiti (pressure sores) and contractures.

Bed patients can assume a variety of positions for both comfort and therapeutic reasons. Each position has advantages and disadvantages in terms of body alignment and pressure areas. Supportive aids such as pillows, towels, foam rubber, and footboards are used to maintain the patient in the best alignment possible and to cushion pressure points. Some patients are required to assume special positions for physical assessments. These are discussed in chapter 10.

Chapter Outline

Objectives

Upon completion of this chapter, the student will:

1. Know essential terms and facts related to positioning patients in bed
   1.1 Define selected terms
   1.2 Identify positions that patients assume in bed
   1.3 Identify alignment problems to be prevented in various positions
   1.4 Identify appropriate supportive devices to support the patient in good body alignment
   1.5 Identify essential criteria for selecting supportive devices to position a patient
   1.6 Identify the pressure points created by various positions

2. Understand facts about techniques used to support patients in selected positions
   2.1 Identify relevant assessment data
   2.2 Identify nursing diagnoses for which the technique may be implemented
   2.3 Identify nursing goals related to the technique
   2.4 Identify expected and unexpected outcomes from assessment data
   2.5 Identify reasons underlying steps of the technique

3. Perform techniques related to supporting patients in various positions
   3.1 Assess the patient adequately
   3.2 Collect additional data from appropriate sources
   3.3 Select pertinent nursing goals for the patient
   3.4 Establish relevant outcome criteria for the patient following the technique
   3.5 Collect necessary equipment before the technique
   3.6 Implement interventions to enhance the effectiveness of the technique and enhance the patient's comfort and safety
   3.7 Communicate relevant information about the patient to the appropriate persons
   3.8 Determine the evaluative outcomes of the technique

4. Evaluate own performance of specific techniques in a laboratory or clinical setting with the assistance of another
   4.1 Use the performance checklists provided
   4.2 Identify areas of strength and weakness
   4.3 Alter performance in response to own evaluation and that of another

Terms

■ anterior   in the front

■ contracture   a permanent shortening of a muscle

■ decubitus ulcer   an ulcer of the skin and underlying tissues produced by prolonged pressure

■ dehydration   insufficient fluid in the body

■ diaphragm   a musculomembranous partition that separates the abdominal and thoracic cavities

■ dorsal   referring to the back

■ dorsal flexion   movement of the ankle so that the toes are pointing up

■ dorsal recumbent position   a back-lying position with the head and shoulders slightly elevated

■ flaccid paralysis   impaired muscle function with loss of muscle tone

■ foot drop   plantar flexion of the foot with permanent contracture of the gastrocnemius (calf) muscle and tendon

■ Fowler's position   a bed sitting position in which the head of the bed is elevated to at least 45°

■ hydration   the act of combining or being combined with water

■ lateral   to the side, away from the midline

■ lateral position   a side-lying position

■ malleolus   a rounded prominence on the distal end of the tibia or fibula

■ medial   toward the midline

■ orthopneic position   a position that enables breathing

■ plantar flexion   movement of the ankle so that the toes point downward

■ posterior   in the back

■ process (of bone)   a prominence or projection

■ prone   lying on the abdomen with the face turned to one side

■ sacrum   a triangular bone located at the base of the vertebral column

■ semi-Fowler's position   a bed sitting position in which the head of the bed is elevated to at least 30°, with or without knee flexion

■ Sims's position   semiprone position

■ supine position   a position lying on the back with the face upward, without support for the head and shoulders; also called *dorsal position*

■ thorax   the chest cavity

■ trochanter   either of two processes below the neck of the femur

■ tubercle   a rounded eminence of bone

GUIDELINES FOR POSITIONING PATIENTS IN BED

1. Ensure the best possible body alignment to prevent strain on the patient's muscles and joints. This is achieved by placing supportive devices (pillows, towel rolls, foam rubber supports, etc) in specified areas according to the patient's position. Common alignment problems are:

   a. Flexion or hyperextension of the neck

   b. Internal rotation of the shoulder

   c. Adduction of the arm

   d. Flexion of the wrist

   e. Anterior or posterior convexity of the lumbar spine

   f. External or internal rotation and adduction of the legs

   g. Hyperextension of the knees

   h. Plantar flexion of the foot

See Table 19–2 on page 428 for definitions of these types of joint movements.

2. Not all patients require identical supports. Adapt supportive devices to the individual's body and physical ability. A patient who is muscular and has adequate adipose tissue in the lumbar region may not require support in this area, while an emaciated person with a marked lumbar curvature will. A person who has a paralyzed leg will require a support against the thigh and hip to prevent external rotation. A patient with a paralyzed arm may require a wrist and hand splint.

3. Plan a systematic 24-hour schedule for position changes. See Table 17–1. Frequent changes are essential for helpless patients to prevent decubiti. See chapter 14.

Usually such patients are repositioned every two hours throughout the day and night, and more frequently when there is concern about skin breakdown. This schedule is usually outlined on the patient's nursing care plan. The example in Table 17–1 specifies longer intervals at night to allow for the patient's sleep.

4. Provide skin care to pressure areas created by the previous position whenever a patient is repositioned. The bony prominences that absorbed the body weight need to be massaged with lotion.

5. Ensure that the foundation of the bed is firm, clean, and dry. Wrinkled or damp sheets increase the risk of decubitus ulcer formation.

6. Encourage or provide range-of-motion (ROM) exercises for the patient's major joints, unless contraindicated, each time the position is changed. ROM exercises prevent the formation of *contractures* (permanent shortening of a

TABLE 17–1   ■   Example of a Turning Schedule

Time	Position
0300	Supine
0600	Left lateral
0800	Left Sims's
1000	Right lateral
1200	Right Sims's
1400	Supine
1600	Left lateral
1800	Left Sims's
2000	Right lateral
2400	Right Sims's

muscle). These exercises may be contraindicated if the patient cannot tolerate the movement, for example, if the patient has an acute illness or an extensive malignancy. See chapter 19 for information about ROM exercises.

CRITERIA FOR SELECTING SUPPORTIVE DEVICES

1. *The patient's adipose tissue.* A patient who has ample adipose tissue generally requires less support and cushioning than the emaciated patient while in a back-lying position, but greater support to maintain a lateral position.

2. *The patient's skeletal structure.* Both the amount and the type of support needed vary according to the individual's skeletal structure. A patient with a marked lumbar lordosis requires more lumbar support than one with a slight lumbar curvature.

3. *The patient's state of health.* A patient with a paralyzed arm or leg requires more supportive devices to maintain body alignment than the patient who can move his or her limbs.

4. *The patient's discomfort.* A patient who experiences pain when he or she moves requires more support to prevent movement than one who can move without pain.

5. *The condition of the patient's skin.* Patients with nutritional problems and/or impaired circulation require more cushioning of the pressure points to prevent skin breakdown than do healthy persons.

6. *The patient's ability to move.* A patient who can move in bed can change position frequently. The patient who is unable to move requires considerable support so that muscles do not become strained because of immobility.

7. *The patient's hydration.* Dehydrated patients are more at risk for decubitus ulcer formation than well-hydrated patients and therefore need more support under pressure areas. For further information on decubitus ulcer formation, see chapter 14.

TECHNIQUE 17-1 ■ Assessing Pressure Areas of the Body

It is important to assess pressure areas for a number of factors before, while, and after a patient is moved.

■ Nursing Diagnosis

Nursing diagnoses that may indicate the need to assess a patient before or after a move include:

1. Actual impairment of skin integrity related to pressure ulcer
2. Potential impairment of skin integrity related to immobility

■ Planning

Nursing goals

1. To obtain data on the condition of a patient's skin pressure areas
2. To obtain data about the patient's mobility
3. To develop a plan for moving the patient if a turning schedule has not been developed for the patient

Equipment

1. A good light, preferably natural or fluorescent, since incandescent lights can give a transilluminating effect.

2. A room that is not too hot or too cold. Heat can cause the skin to flush; cold can cause the skin to blanch or become cyanotic.

■ Intervention

1. Inspect the pressure areas (see Figure 14–1 on page 327) for any whitish or reddened spots.
   Rationale This discoloration can be caused by impaired blood circulation to the area. It should disappear in a few minutes when rubbing restores circulation.

2. Inspect the pressure areas for abrasions and excoriations.
   Rationale An abrasion (wearing away of the skin) can occur when skin rubs against a sheet, eg, when the patient is pulled. Excoriations (loss of superficial layers of the skin) can occur when the skin has prolonged contact with body secretions or excretions or with dampness in skin folds.

3. Identify the stage of any cell damage:
   Stage I. Redness for a prolonged period with intact skin
   Stage II. Redness for a prolonged period with excoriation
   Stage III. Diminished thickness of the skin and serosanguineous drainage

Stage IV. Damage to the subcutaneous tissue and/or muscle, visible necrotic tissue and bone in some cases, and purulent drainage in some cases

4. With warm hands, palpate the surface temperature of the skin over the pressure areas. Normally the temperature is the same as that of the surrounding skin. Increased temperature is abnormal.
   Rationale   Warm hands are more pleasant for the patient than cold hands. An increased temperature may be due to inflammation or blood trapped in the area.

5. With warm hands, palpate over bony prominences and dependent body areas for the presence of edema.
   Rationale   Edema will feel spongy upon palpation.

6. For further assessment data about the skin, see Technique 10–2 on page 168 and Table 10–4 on page 169.

7. Record the assessment data on the patient's record.

■ Evaluation

Expected outcome

Skin appears normal. See Table 10–4 on page 169.

Unexpected outcomes

1. Abnormal pressure area
2. Patient discomfort in pressure area

Upon obtaining an unexpected outcome:

1. Reassess the patient's pressure areas.
2. Report your findings to the responsible nurse and/or physician.
3. Adjust the nursing care plan appropriately.

TECHNIQUE 17–2   ■   Supporting a Patient in Fowler's Position

Fowler's position is a bed sitting position with the head of the bed raised to at least 45°. The knees may or may not be flexed. In some agencies, the term *Fowler's position* refers to elevation of the upper part of the body without knee flexion. See Figure 17–1. The term *semi-Fowler's* is then used to refer to a sitting position with slight knee flexion. The knees can be flexed by placing a pillow under the thighs or by elevating the knee gatch on the bed. Some agencies do not permit elevation of the knee gatches because pressure on the popliteal spaces could impair

FIGURE 17–1 ■ Fowler's position without knee flexion.

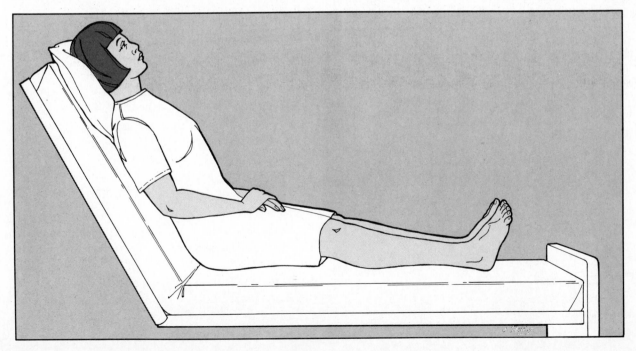

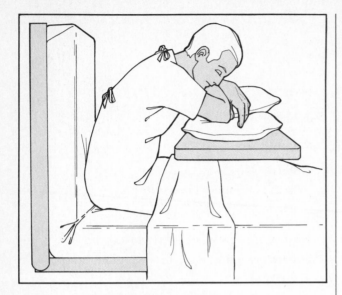

FIGURE 17–2 ■ An orthopneic position.

blood circulation to and from the feet. If the knee gatch is raised, it should be done for only a short time (15 to 30 minutes).

There are two adaptations of Fowler's position: high Fowler's and semi-Fowler's. For *high Fowler's position,* the head of the bed is elevated to almost 90°, ie, at a right angle to the foundation. This position is most analogous to sitting in a chair. An adaptation of high Fowler's position is the *orthopneic position.* The patient sits either in bed or on the side of the bed with an overbed table placed across his or her lap. The table is elevated to a comfortable height and padded with a pillow. See Figure 17–2. The high Fowler's and orthopneic positions are often helpful to patients who have problems exhaling, because they can press the lower part of the chest against the overbed table.

FIGURE 17–3 ■ The diaphragm and adjacent organs.

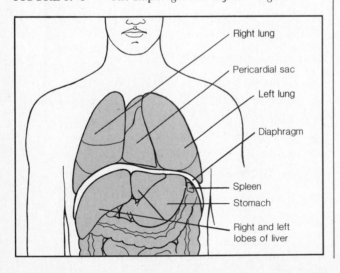

For *semi-Fowler's position,* the head of the bed is usually raised to about 30°. This position allows some chest expansion and is often indicated for patients who have cardiac and respiratory problems.

■ Assessment

See Technique 17–1 on page 400. Assess the patient for:

1. Pressure areas of particular concern in Fowler's position (see Figure 14–1 on page 327):
   a. The calcaneus (the heel)
   b. The olecranon (the protrusion of bone at the elbow)
   c. The sacrum (the bone at the base of the vertebral column)
   d. The scapulae (the shoulder blades)
   e. The toes and knees (which may sustain pressure from the top bedclothes)
2. Significant clinical signs, eg, pulse, color, dyspnea

Other data from the nursing care plan include:

1. Whether there is a turning schedule for the patient
2. Which supportive devices the patient requires to maintain body alignment
3. The skin care required
4. The joint exercises required

■ Nursing Diagnosis See Technique 17–1 on page 400.

■ Planning

Nursing goals

1. To enhance the functioning of the cardiopulmonary system (the heart and lungs). In any variant of Fowler's position the lungs expand more easily because the abdominal organs are not pressing upward against the diaphragm. See Figure 17–3.
2. To provide comfort and convenience. Patients confined to bed usually find it easier to eat, watch television, and talk with others in this position.

Equipment

1. Pillows:
   a. One or two pillows for the back. One pillow should be the correct size to fit under the lumbar curvature.
   b. One small pillow to go under the thighs.
   c. One small pillow or rolled towel for the ankles.
   d. Two pillows to support the arms (optional).

2. Two trochanter rolls, one for each hip (optional). See Technique 17–3.

3. A footboard to support the feet.

4. A roll or pillow to place between the footboard and the patient's feet if the footboard is not adjustable.

■ **Intervention**

See Figure 17–4.

1. Provide skin care for all pressure areas.

2. Provide ROM exercises as needed.

3. Assist the patient to a supine position and make sure his or her head is near the head of the bed.
   Rationale   Patients in Fowler's position tend to slide toward the foot of the bed.

4. Raise the head of the bed to 30°, 45°, or the angle required or ordered for the patient.

5. Place a small pillow or roll under the lumbar region of the back.
   Rationale   This pillow prevents posterior convexity of the lumbar curvature.

6. Place one or two pillows to support the upper back, shoulders, and head.
   Rationale   These pillows prevent hyperextension of the neck and support the cervical curvature of the vertebral column.

7. Place a small pillow under the thighs.
   Rationale   This pillow prevents hyperextension of the knees.

8. Put a trochanter roll lateral to each femur (optional). See Technique 17–3.
   Rationale   Trochanter rolls prevent external rotation of the hips.

9. Place a small pillow under the ankles to raise the heels off the bed.
   Rationale   This reduces pressure on the heels.

10. Put a footboard on the bed to support the feet. See chapter 15.
    Rationale   The footboard prevents plantar flexion.

11. Place pillows to support both arms and hands if the patient does not have normal use of them.
    Rationale   These pillows prevent shoulder and muscle strain, dislocation of the shoulder, edema (an excess amount of interstitial fluid) of the hands and arms, and flexion contracture of the hand at the wrist.

12. Normally each change in a patient's position is not recorded. At the end of the shift, however, record a summary statement, including the patient's response to the position.

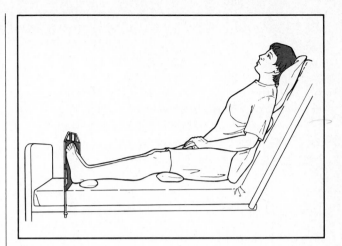

FIGURE 17–4

Sample Recording

Date	Time	Notes
3/19/87	1300	Fowler's position maintained and skin care given q.2h. ——————— Stacy M. Stiles, NS

■ **Evaluation**

Expected outcomes

1. Verbalized feeling of comfort

2. Relief of dyspnea and improvement of cyanosis of the lips and mucous membranes

3. Intact skin over bony prominences and pressure areas

Unexpected outcomes

1. Increased discomfort described or indicated by restlessness

2. No relief of dyspnea or cyanosis

3. Reddened, abraded, or excoriated areas over bony prominences and weight-bearing areas

Upon obtaining an unexpected outcome:

1. Reassess the significant clinical signs.

2. Reassess the patient's alignment, and adjust the supportive devices if indicated.

3. Position the patient in another position.

4. Report your findings to the responsible nurse.

5. Adjust the nursing care plan appropriately.

TECHNIQUE 17–3 ■ Making and Applying a Trochanter Roll 🏠

A trochanter roll is a roll of cloth, frequently a towel, that is placed against the greater trochanter of the femur to prevent external rotation of the hip. Trochanter rolls are made commercially or can be constructed as described here. A commercial roll only needs to be covered before it is used.

■ **Assessment**

Assess the alignment of the patient's legs.

■ **Planning**

Nursing goals

To maintain the femur in anatomic position

Equipment

1. A bath towel for each hip
2. Three safety pins or tape for each towel

■ **Intervention**

1. Fold the bath towel in half lengthwise. See Figure 17–5, *A.*

FIGURE 17-5

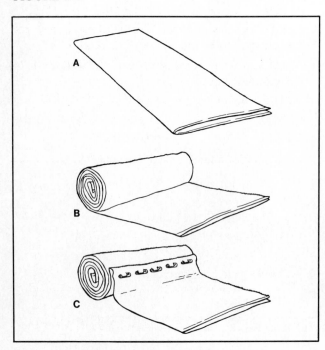

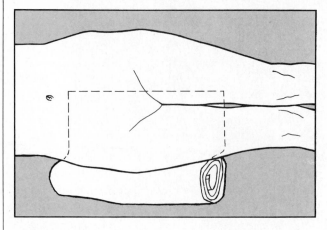

FIGURE 17-6

2. Roll the towel tightly, starting at one narrow edge and rolling to within about 30 cm (1 ft) of the other edge. See Figure 17–5, *B.*
3. Secure the roll with safety pins or tape. See Figure 17–5, *C.*
4. Align the patient's hip so that the toes are pointing upward, ie, the hip is neither externally nor internally rotated.
5. Invert the roll, and place the flat part of the towel under the patient's hip. See Figure 17–6. The safety pins or tapes are now on the underside, away from the patient's skin.
6. Turn the roll to tighten it against the leg, so that the thigh remains well aligned.
7. Repeat for the other leg.

■ **Evaluation**

Expected outcome

The patient's leg remains aligned, not externally rotated.

Unexpected outcome

The patient's leg rotates externally. Upon obtaining an unexpected outcome, remove the trochanter roll and reapply it firmly to the leg.

TECHNIQUE 17–4   ■   Supporting a Patient in Dorsal Recumbent Position

The *dorsal recumbent* position is one in which the patient's head and shoulders are slightly elevated on a small pillow. Although in some agencies the terms *dorsal recumbent* and *supine* are used interchangeably, strictly speaking, in the *supine* or *dorsal* position the head and shoulders are not elevated. In both, the patient's forearms may be elevated on pillows or placed at the patient's sides with the hands pronated. Supports are similar in both positions, except for the head pillow.

■ Assessment

See Technique 17–1 on page 400. Assess the patient for:

1. Pressure areas of particular concern in this position:
   a. The heels
   b. The sacrum
   c. The elbows
   d. The scapulae
   e. The posterior aspect of the skull
   f. The toes (pressure from the top bedclothes)

For other data, see Technique 17–2 on page 402.

■ Nursing Diagnosis   See Technique 17–1 on page 400.

■ Planning

Nursing goals

1. To provide comfort for rest or sleep.
2. To maintain alignment of the vertebral column, eg, following spinal injury or surgery.
3. To prevent backache or headache following a lumbar puncture (spinal tap). Spinal fluid is removed in this procedure, and time is required to replace it.
4. To support blood circulation to vital structures (eg, the heart and brain) in cases of severe hemorrhage or hypotension (low blood pressure).
5. To maintain certain skin tractions, eg, Buck's extension or a pelvic girdle. See chapter 21.

Equipment

1. Pillows:
   a. A moderate-sized pillow to place under the patient's head and shoulders
   b. A small pillow to place under the thighs
   c. One pillow to support the ankles if sheepskin is not used under the heels
2. One or two trochanter rolls for the legs
3. One towel rolled or folded or a small pillow to place under the lumbar curvature
4. A footboard to support the feet

■ Intervention

See Figure 17–7.

1. Provide skin care for all pressure areas.
2. Provide ROM exercises as needed.
3. Assist the patient to a supine position.
4. Place a pillow of suitable thickness under the patient's head and shoulders as needed.
   Rationale The pillow prevents hyperextension or flexion of the neck.
5. Place a small pillow under the patient's thighs.

FIGURE 17–7

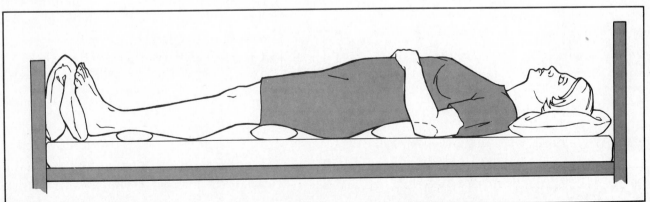

Rationale The pillow flexes the knees slightly and prevents hyperextension of the knees.

6. Place trochanter rolls laterally against the femurs (optional).

   Rationale The trochanter rolls prevent external rotation of the legs.

7. Place a rolled towel or small pillow under the lumbar curvature (optional).

   Rationale This prevents flexion of the lumbar spine.

8. Place a small pillow under the patient's ankles to raise the heels off the bed.

   Rationale This prevents pressure sores on the heels.

9. Put a footboard or rolled pillow on the bed to support the feet.

   Rationale This support prevents plantar flexion of the feet.

10. A position change is usually not recorded. At the end of the shift, however, record a summary statement to indicate the frequency of position changes, the response of the patient to the position, skin care, and ROM exercises.

■ Evaluation

Expected outcomes

1. Verbalized feeling of comfort
2. Intact skin over bony prominences and pressure areas

Unexpected outcomes

1. Complaints of increased discomfort
2. Reddened, abraded, or excoriated skin over bony prominences and weight-bearing areas

Upon obtaining an unexpected outcome:

1. Reassess the patient's alignment, and adjust the supportive devices if indicated.
2. Position the patient in another position.
3. Report your findings to the responsible nurse.
4. Adjust the nursing care plan appropriately.

TECHNIQUE 17–5 ■ Supporting a Patient in Prone Position

In the prone position, the patient lies on his or her abdomen, with the legs extended and the face turned to the side. The hips are not flexed. Both children and adults frequently sleep in this position, sometimes with one or both arms flexed over their heads.

■ Assessment

See Technique 17–1 on page 400. Assess the patient for:

1. Pressure areas of particular concern in this position:
   a. The toes
   b. The knees
   c. The anterior aspects of the pelvis
   d. The acromial process and the head of the humerus at the shoulders
   e. The medial epicondyle of the humerus at the elbows
   f. The temporal and parietal bones of the skull
   g. The ears
   h. The heels (pressure from the top bedclothes)

   i. The scapulae (pressure from the top bedclothes)

For other data, see Technique 17–2 on page 402.

■ Nursing Diagnosis
See Technique 17–1 on page 400.

■ Planning

Nursing goals

1. To provide a position for comfort and for sleeping
2. To maintain the normal alignment of the hips
3. For the unconscious patient, to facilitate the drainage of mucus from the mouth

Equipment

1. Pillows:
   a. A small pillow for the head. So that mucus can drain freely from the mouth of an unconscious

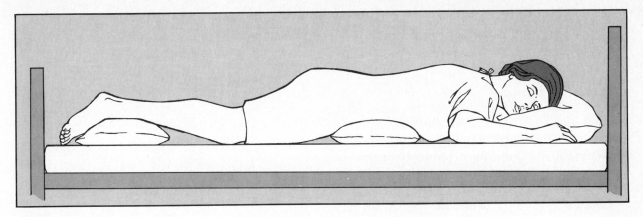

FIGURE 17–8

patient, a small rather than a large pillow, or no pillow, may be indicated.

b. A small pillow or roll to put under the abdomen. A roll can be made by tightly rolling up a towel.

c. A small pillow to put under the lower legs.

■ Intervention

See Figure 17–8.

1. Provide skin care for all pressure areas.

2. Provide ROM exercises as needed.

3. Assist the patient to a prone position. See Technique 16–5 on page 385.

4. Place a small pillow under the patient's head, unless contraindicated (eg, for the drainage of mucus), so that the face is turned to the side and the neck is slightly flexed.
   Rationale The pillow prevents acute flexion or hyperextension of the neck.

5. Place a small pillow or roll under the abdomen just below the diaphragm.
   Rationale This pillow prevents hyperextension of the lumbar curvature, difficulty breathing, and pressure on a woman's breasts.

6. Place a small pillow under the lower legs, or position the patient on the bed so that the feet extend in a normal anatomic position over the foot of the mattress.
   Rationale The pillow raises the toes off the bed surface and flexes the knees slightly. It also reduces plantar flexion.

7. A patient's position is not normally recorded. At the end of the shift, however, record a summary statement, including the frequency of position changes, the response of the patient to the position, skin care, and ROM exercises.

Sample Recording

Date	Time	Notes
7/13/86	1400	Prone and lateral positions alternated q.2h. Skin care given q.2h. Skin areas appear intact. Large amount of thick white drainage from mouth. Unresponsive to voice. ——————————————— Leslie L. Beck, NS

■ Evaluation

Expected outcomes

1. Verbalized feeling of comfort

2. Intact skin over bony prominences and pressure areas

Unexpected outcomes

1. Complaints of increased discomfort by the patient

2. Reddened, abraded, or excoriated skin over bony prominences and/or weight-bearing areas

Upon obtaining an unexpected outcome:

1. Reassess the patient's alignment and adjust the supportive devices if indicated.

2. Place the patient in another position.

3. Report your findings to the responsible nurse.

4. Adjust the nursing care plan appropriately.

TECHNIQUE 17–6 ■ Supporting a Patient in Lateral Position 🏠

In the lateral (side-lying) position, the body weight is borne by the greater tubercle of the humerus, the acromial process of the clavicle, the ischium, and the greater trochanter of the femur. Both arms lie in front of the patient. If appropriate supportive devices are used, this is a comfortable position and a welcome change for the patient who has been lying in the prone or supine position for a period of time. The major disadvantage is the tendency for the shoulders and uppermost thigh to rotate inward.

■ Assessment

See Technique 17–1 on page 400. Assess the patient for:

1. Pressure areas of particular concern in this position:
   a. The ear.
   b. The shoulder (greater tubercle of the humerus). See Figure 17–9.
   c. The lateral aspect of the ilium. See Figure 17–10.
   d. The medial aspect of the uppermost ankle (medial malleolus).

FIGURE 17–9 ■ Anterior view of the bony prominences of the right shoulder.

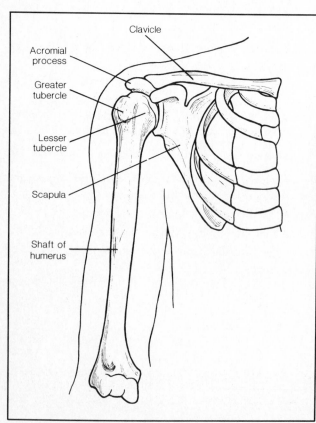

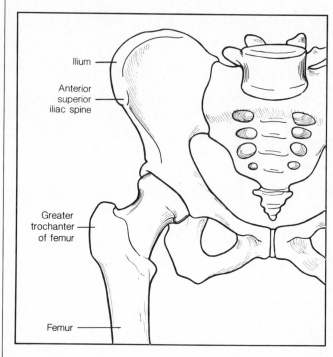

FIGURE 17–10 ■ Anterior view of the bony prominences of the right ilium and femur.

   e. The lateral aspect of the lower ankle (lateral malleolus). See Figure 17–11.
   f. The medial aspect of the uppermost knee.
   g. The lateral aspect of the lower knee.

For other data, see Technique 17–2 on page 402.

■ Nursing Diagnosis
See Technique 17–1 on page 400.

■ Planning

Nursing goals

1. To provide a position for comfort and sleep
2. To relieve pressure from the back of the head, scapulae, sacrum, and heels
3. To promote drainage of salivary secretions in the unconscious patient, to prevent aspiration of these secretions

Equipment

1. Four pillows:
   a. One to put under the patient's head
   b. One to put under the upper leg and thigh

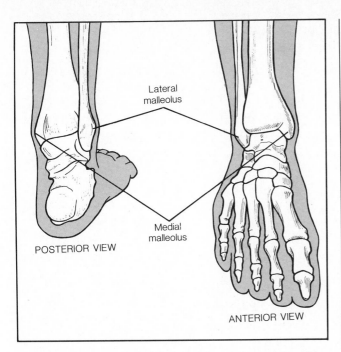

FIGURE 17-11 ■ The bony prominences of the right ankle.

c. One to put under the upper arm
d. One to put at the patient's back

■ **Intervention**

See Figure 17-12.

1. Provide skin care for all pressure areas.
2. Provide ROM exercises as needed.
3. Assist the patient to a lateral position. See Technique 16-4 on page 383.
4. Place a pillow under the patient's head.
   Rationale This pillow prevents lateral flexion and fatigue of the sternocleidomastoid muscles.

5. Place a pillow under the upper leg and thigh.
   Rationale This pillow prevents internal rotation of the thigh and adduction of the leg.
6. Place a pillow under the upper arm.
   Rationale This pillow prevents internal rotation of the shoulder and adduction of the arm.
7. Place a rolled pillow at the patient's back (optional).
   Rationale When necessary, eg, for an emaciated patient, a pillow supports the back and helps to maintain the position.
8. A position change is normally not recorded. At the end of the shift, however, record a summary statement, indicating the frequency of position changes, skin care, ROM exercises, and the response of the patient.

■ **Evaluation**

Expected outcomes

1. Verbalized feeling of comfort
2. Intact skin over bony prominences and pressure areas

Unexpected outcomes

1. Complaints of increased discomfort by the patient
2. Reddened, abraded, or excoriated skin over bony prominences and/or weight-bearing areas

Upon obtaining an unexpected outcome:

1. Reassess the patient's alignment and adjust the supportive devices, if indicated.
2. Position the patient in another position.
3. Report your findings to the responsible nurse.
4. Adjust the nursing care plan appropriately.

FIGURE 17-12

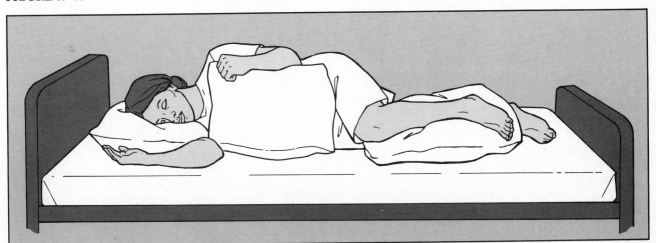

TECHNIQUE 17–7 ■ Supporting a Patient in Sims's Position

Sims's position or semiprone position is a variation of the lateral position. It differs chiefly in that the weight is borne by the anterior aspects of the ilium and the humerus and clavicle rather than by the lateral aspects of the ilium. In Sims's position the patient's lower arm is behind him or her, and the upper arm is flexed at the shoulder and the elbow. Both legs are flexed in front of the patient. The upper leg is more acutely flexed at both the hip and the knee than the lower one.

■ Assessment

See Technique 17–1 on page 400. Assess the patient for:

1. Pressure areas of particular concern in this position:

   Undermost side

   a. The side of the skull (the temporal and parietal bones and the ear).

   b. The anterior aspects of the humerus (the lesser tubercle) and the acromial process of the clavicle. See Figure 17–9 earlier.

   c. The anterior superior iliac spine and the greater trochanter of the femur. See Figure 17–10.

   d. The lateral aspect of the knee.

   e. The lateral malleolus of the ankle. See Figure 17–11.

   Uppermost side

   f. The medial epicondyle on the medial aspect of the elbow.

   g. The medial aspect of the knee.

   h. The medial malleolus of the ankle. See Figure 17–11.

For other data, see Technique 17–2 on page 402.

■ Planning

Nursing goals

1. To facilitate drainage from the mouth for the unconscious patient
2. To provide comfort for sleeping
3. To provide comfort for the pregnant patient in the last trimester of pregnancy or for the patient who has a large abdominal tumor

Equipment

1. Pillows:

   a. One small pillow for the head

   b. One pillow for under the upper arm

   c. One pillow for under the upper leg

   d. One pillow to place in front of the abdomen (optional)

2. A support device for the feet

■ Intervention

See Figure 17–13.

1. Provide skin care for all pressure areas.

2. Provide ROM exercises as needed.

3. Assist the patient to turn as for a prone position. See Technique 16–5 on page 385.

4. Place a small pillow under the patient's head, unless drainage from the mouth is being encouraged.

   Rationale This pillow prevents lateral flexion of the neck and cushions the cranial and facial bones and the ear. It is contraindicated if mucus drainage is required.

5. Place a pillow under the upper arm.

   Rationale This pillow prevents internal rotation of the upper arm and pressure on the chest that could restrict chest expansion and breathing.

6. Place a pillow under the upper leg.

   Rationale This pillow prevents internal rotation and adduction of the hip and leg.

7. Place a rolled pillow against the abdomen if needed by an emaciated patient.

   Rationale This pillow supports the trunk.

8. Place a support device, eg, a rolled towel, against the lower foot.

   Rationale This roll prevents foot drop.

9. A position change is not usually recorded. At the end of the shift, however, record a summary statement including the patient's response to the position.

Sample Recording

Date	Time	Notes
6/9/86	2300	Sims's position maintained. Sides alternated and skin care given q.2h. Skin on right anterior superior iliac spine appears reddened. No apparent breaks in skin.————— Ann-Marie Miles, SN

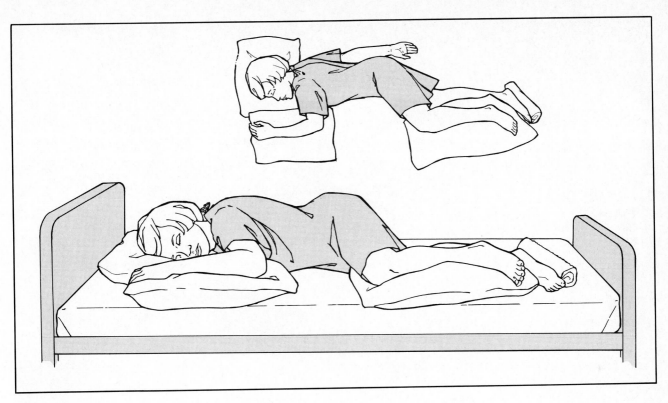

FIGURE 17–13

■ **Evaluation**

Expected outcomes

1. Verbalized feeling of comfort
2. Intact skin over bony prominences and pressure areas

Unexpected outcomes

1. Complaints of increased discomfort by the patient

2. Reddened, abraded, or excoriated skin over bony prominences and/or weight-bearing areas

Upon obtaining an unexpected outcome:

1. Reassess the patient's alignment and adjust the supportive devices if indicated.
2. Place the patient in another position.
3. Report your findings to the responsible nurse.
4. Adjust the nursing care plan appropriately.

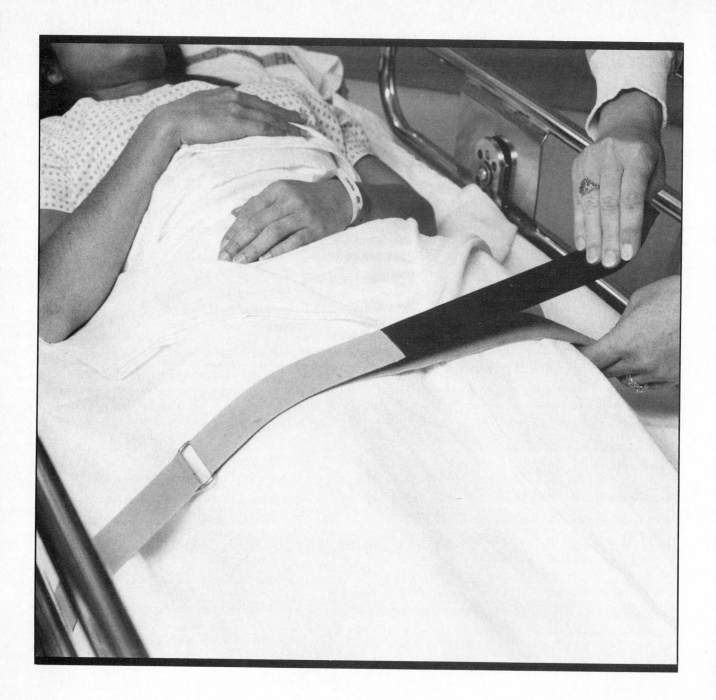

RESTRAINTS

18

Restraints are protective devices used to limit the physical activity of the patient or a part of the body. They are applied to safeguard the patient against injury, eg, from falling, or movements that would disrupt therapy to a limb that is connected to tubes or appliances. Because people tend to resist restraint of any kind and consider it a violation of their right to move about freely, nurses need to ensure that patients understand the reason for using a restraint, that it is a protective device, and that the body part has to be kept relatively still.

Recently, there has been a shift toward means other than restraints to protect patients. Restrained patients often become restless and anxious as a result of the loss of self-control. Sometimes nurses can remain with the restrained patient and speak quietly to give reassurance and allay distress.

Chapter Outline

Legal Implications of Restraints

When to Use a Restraint

Selecting a Restraint

Nursing Interventions Accompanying Restraints

Kinds of Restraints

Knots Used with Restraints

■ Technique 18–1   Applying Restraints

Objectives

Upon completion of this chapter, the student will:

1. Know essential terms and facts about restraints
   1.1   Define selected terms
   1.2   Identify criteria for selecting a restraint
   1.3   Identify when to use a restraint
   1.4   Identify nursing interventions accompanying restraints
   1.5   Identify various kinds of restraints
   1.6   Identify knots used with restraints
2. Understand facts about techniques used to apply restraints
   2.1   Identify relevant assessment data
   2.2   Identify nursing diagnoses for which the technique may be implemented
   2.3   Identify nursing goals related to the technique
   2.4   Identify expected and unexpected outcomes from assessment data
   2.5   Identify reasons underlying steps of the technique
3. Perform techniques for applying restraints
   3.1   Assess the patient adequately

   3.2   Collect additional data from appropriate sources
   3.3   Select pertinent nursing goals for the patient
   3.4   Establish relevant outcome criteria for the patient following the technique
   3.5   Collect necessary equipment before the technique
   3.6   Implement interventions to enhance the effectiveness of the technique and enhance the patient's comfort and safety
   3.7   Communicate relevant information about the patient to the appropriate persons
   3.8   Determine the evaluative outcomes of the technique
4. Evaluate own performance of specific techniques in a laboratory or clinical setting with the assistance of another
   4.1   Use the performance checklists provided
   4.2   Identify areas of strength and weakness
   4.3   Alter performance in response to own evaluation and that of another

LEGAL IMPLICATIONS OF RESTRAINTS

Because restraints restrict an individual's ability to move freely, their use has legal implications. In some settings, the decision to use a restraint is made by the nurse; in others, it must be made by a physician. Often a nurse can apply a restraint in an emergency; however, the physician must order subsequent use of the restraint. It is important for nurses to know their agency's practices and the state or provincial laws about restraining patients.

Before restraining a patient, a nurse needs to try (and document) other nursing interventions, eg, reorienting the patient to reality. The nurse has to describe in the record what patient behavior led to the decision to use a restraint. This information documents that restraints were applied for the patient's safety, not for the nurse's convenience.

The nurse must document the type of restraint used, the exact times the restraint was applied and removed, the patient's behavior before and with the restraint, care given while the restraint was applied, and notification of the physician. It is important to explain the need for the restraint both to the patient and to support persons; the nurse also should document the substance of these explanations.

WHEN TO USE A RESTRAINT

Restraints are used in a number of situations to limit a patient's movement. Some of these are:

1. To prevent patients from falling out of bed or out of a chair (eg, an elderly confused person)

2. To remind patients to restrict movement (eg, restraining an arm while an intravenous infusion is running or limiting the movement of patients who are likely to fall if they get out of bed alone)

3. To prevent confused patients or children from harming themselves (eg, by pulling out urinary catheters or pulling off surgical dressings)

4. To prevent patients from harming others through aggressive actions (eg, placing mitts on patients who hit out at others)

SELECTING A RESTRAINT

Before selecting a restraint, nurses need to understand its purpose clearly. Then they can choose a restraint that best meets the needs of the patient. Restraints should be measured against the following criteria in the process of selection:

FIGURE 18–1 ■ Posterior view of the bony prominences of the wrist.

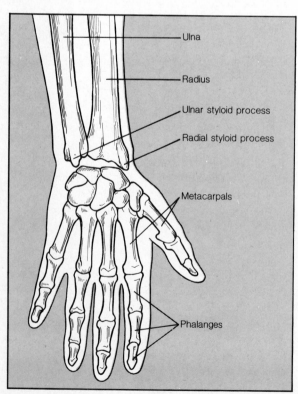

1. It restricts the patient's movement as little as possible. If a patient needs to have one arm restrained, do not restrain his or her entire body.

2. It is the least obvious to others. Both patients and visitors are often embarrassed by a restraint, even though they understand why it is being used. The less obvious the restraint, the more comfortable people feel. A crossover jacket restraint may be less conspicuous than arm and leg restraints.

3. It does not adversely affect the patient's treatment or health problem. If a patient has poor blood circulation to the hands, apply a restraint that will not aggravate that circulatory problem.

4. It is readily changeable. Restraints need to be changed frequently (see the next section), and more often if they become soiled. Keeping other guidelines in mind, choose a restraint that can be changed with minimal disturbance to the patient.

5. It is safe for the particular patient. Choose a restraint with which the patient cannot self-inflict injury. For example, a physically active child could incur injury trying to climb out of a crib if one wrist is tied to the side of the crib. A jacket restraint would restrain the child more safely.

NURSING INTERVENTIONS ACCOMPANYING RESTRAINTS

1. Explain the restraint and the reasons for its use to the patient and the patient's support persons. Often people are very disturbed when they visit a hospital and find "grandfather tied down." A simple explanation and assurance that the restraint is temporary, that it is a protection for the patient rather than a punishment, are usually sufficient. A restraint must never be applied as punishment for any behavior or merely for the nurse's convenience.

2. Apply the restraint in such a way that the patient can move as freely as possible without defeating the purpose of the restraint. For example, a jacket restraint need not pin the patient against the bed. It may permit some movement, such as bending forward or turning slightly to one side, while still preventing the patient from falling out of bed.

3. Ensure that limb restraints are applied securely but not so tightly that they impede blood circulation to any body area or extremity.

4. Pad bony prominences (eg, wrists and ankles) before applying a restraint over them. The movement of a restraint without padding over such prominences can quickly abrade the skin (damage it by friction). See Figure 18–1 here and Figure 17–11 on page 409.

5. Always tie a limb restraint with a knot that will not tighten when pulled. For example, a clove hitch applied to a wrist will stay secure, while a slip knot will tighten with pulling. The clove hitch is discussed later in this chapter.

6. Tie the ends of a body restraint to the part of the bed that moves when the head is elevated. Never tie the ends to a side rail or to the fixed frame of the bed if the bed position is to be changed. The patient could be injured if the restraint is pulled tight when the side rail or bed part is moved.

7. Remove most limb restraints at least every four hours, and provide range-of-motion (ROM) exercises (see chapter 19) and skin care (see chapter 14). For elderly patients, restraints may need to be removed more often, eg, every two hours, to maintain blood circulation and mobility of the joints.

8. When a restraint is temporarily removed, do not leave the patient unattended.

9. Immediately report to the responsible nurse and record on the patient's chart any persistent reddened or broken skin areas under the restraint.

10. At the first indication of cyanosis or pallor, coldness of a skin area, or a patient's complaint of a tingling sensation, pain, or numbness, loosen the restraint, and exercise the limb. Impaired blood circulation can cause these symptoms.

11. Apply a restraint in such a way that it can be released quickly in case of an emergency. For example, secure a body restraint to a place on the bed that is easily reached.

12. Apply a restraint so that the body part can assume a normal anatomic position, eg, the elbow is slightly flexed.

13. Provide emotional support verbally and through touch for the patient. Being restrained causes a great deal of anxiety in some people, and they can exhaust themselves fighting the restraint. Stay with the patient as required.

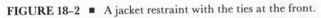

FIGURE 18–2 ■ A jacket restraint with the ties at the front.

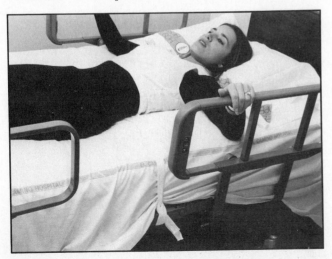

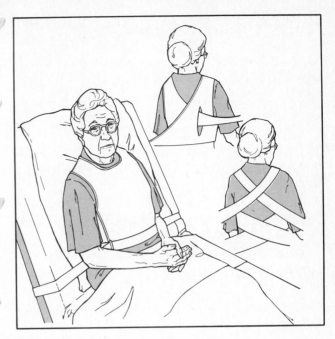

FIGURE 18–3 ■ A jacket restraint with the ties at the back.

KINDS OF RESTRAINTS

Jacket Restraint

While jacket restraints vary, they are all essentially sleeveless jackets (vests) with straps (tails) that can be tied to the bed frame under the mattress or to the legs of a chair. The jacket may be put on with the ties at the front or at the back, depending on the type. See Figures 18–2 and 18–3. These body restraints are used for confused or sedated patients to prevent them from falling out of a bed or chair.

Belt Restraint

Belt or safety strap body restraints are used to ensure the safety of all patients who are being moved on stretchers or in wheelchairs. They may also be used for certain patients lying in bed or sitting in a chair. See Figure 18–4. Some are equipped with buckles and a lock. The key to the lock is usually kept at the nurse's station.

Mitt or Hand Restraint

A mitt or hand restraint is used to prevent confused patients from using their hands or fingers to scratch and injure themselves. For example, a confused patient may need to be prevented from pulling at intravenous tubing or a head bandage following brain surgery. Hand or mitt restraints allow the patient to be ambulatory and/or to move the arm freely rather than be confined to a bed or a chair. Mitt restraints are commercially available. See

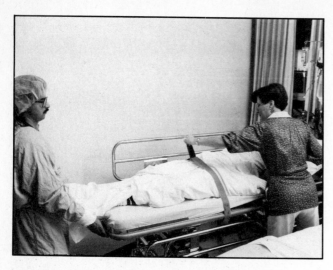

FIGURE 18-4 ■ A belt restraint.

Figure 18-5. Hand restraints can also be made using large dressings and stockinette. See Technique 18-1.

Wrist or Ankle Restraint

Wrist and ankle restraints, generally made of cloth, are also referred to as *limb-holder* restraints, since they are used to immobilize a limb, primarily for therapeutic reasons (eg, to maintain an intravenous infusion). Some commercially prepared restraints are available. See Figure 18-6. A restraint can also be improvised using padded dressings and gauze. See Technique 18-1.

Crib Net

A crib net is simply a net placed over the top of a crib, to prevent active young children from climbing out of the crib. At the same time, it allows them freedom to move about in the crib. See Figure 18-7.

Elbow Restraint

Elbow restraints are used to prevent infants or small children from flexing their elbows to touch or scratch a surgical incision or skin lesion, eg, eczema. See Figure 18-8. This restraint consists of a piece of material with pockets into which plastic or wooden tongue depressors are inserted to provide rigidity. After the restraint is applied it is sometimes pinned to the child's shirt to prevent it from sliding down the arm.

Mummy Restraint

The mummy restraint is a blanket restraint used to protect an infant from moving and possibly causing injury during special treatments or examinations, such as a scalp vein infusion. The head is exposed and has to be held still but the remainder of the body is restricted. See Technique 18-1.

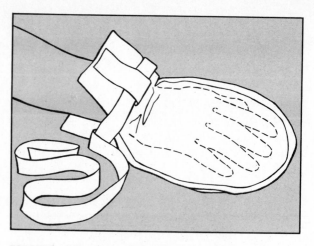

FIGURE 18-5 ■ A commercial mitt restraint.

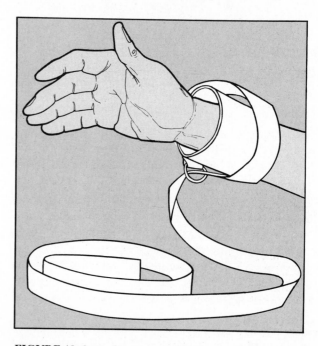

FIGURE 18-6 ■ A commercial wrist restraint.

FIGURE 18-7 ■ A crib net.

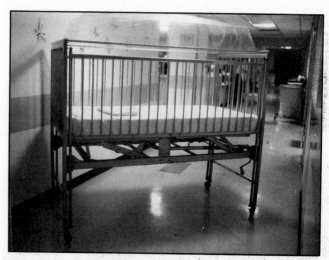

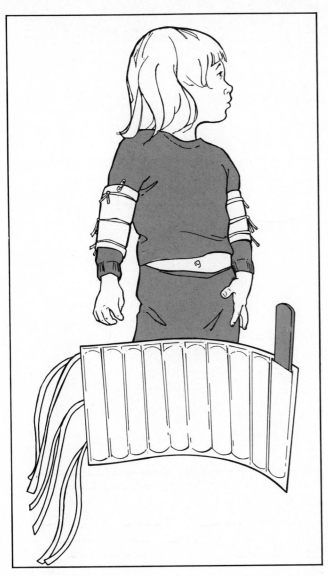

FIGURE 18–8 ■ An elbow restraint.

KNOTS USED WITH RESTRAINTS

Three types of knots are commonly used with restraints: the clove hitch, the square knot, and the half-bow knot.

Clove Hitch

The clove hitch is used for waist and ankle restraints. Its advantages are:

1. It does not tighten with pulling.
2. It is readily released.
3. It permits the patient some mobility.

To make this knot, form a figure eight. See Figure 18–9, *A*. Pick up the two loops. See Figure 18–9, *B*. Put the limb through the loops and secure it by pulling the ends. See Figure 18–9, *C*.

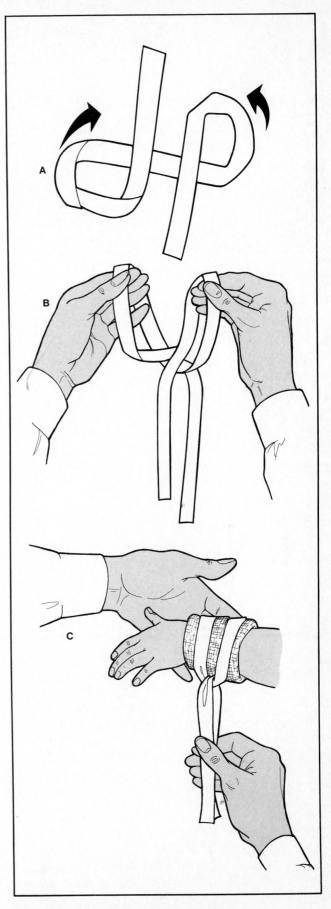

FIGURE 18–9 ■ Making a clove hitch restraint.

Square (Reef) Knot

The square knot is useful when tying two restraint tails together around a bed frame or chair leg. Its advantages are:

1. It does not tighten with pulling.
2. It does not slip when pressure is released.

To make this knot, form a "U" loop. See Figure 18–10, *A*. Pass one end (*1*) over and under the other (*2*). See Figure 18–10, *B*. Take the same end (*1*), and pass it over, under, and over the other. See Figure 18–10, *C*. Pull the knot tight. See Figure 18–10, *D*. When the knot is tied correctly, the ties on each side are both either above or below the loop. See Figure 18–10, *E*.

FIGURE 18–10 ■ Tying a square (reef) knot.

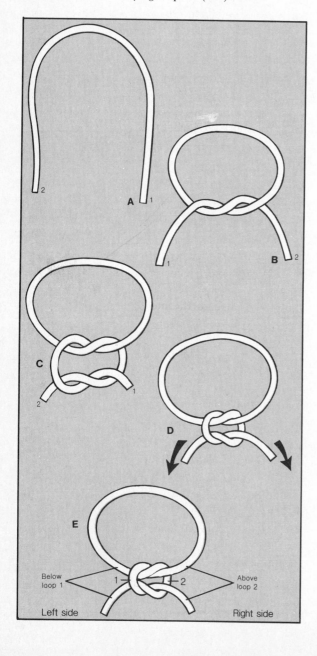

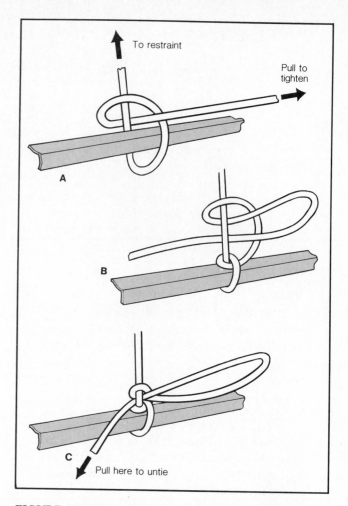

FIGURE 18–11 ■ Tying a half-bow knot.

Half-Bow Knot

This knot resembles a shoelace bow except that only one half of the bow is made. It is useful for attaching one restraint tie to a bed or chair frame. Its advantages are:

1. It will not slip with pulling.
2. It is easy to untie.

To make a half-bow knot, place the restraint tie under the bed side frame (or around a chair leg), bring it up around, over, and under the tie, and pull it tight. See Figure 18–11, *A*. Again take it over and under the tie, but this time make a half-bow loop. See Figure 18–11, *B*. Tighten the free end of the tie and the bow, until the knot is secure. To untie the knot, pull the end of the tie, and then loosen the first cross over the tie. See Figure 18–11, *C*.

TECHNIQUE 18–1 ■ Applying Restraints

■ Assessment

Assess the patient for:

1. The behavior that might indicate the need for a restraint, eg, mental confusion.
2. Status of the skin in the area to which a restraint would be applied, eg, an ankle or wrist. An excoriated area may necessitate the choice of another type of restraint. The skin should be clean and free from redness and abrasions.

Other data include:

1. The physician's order for the restraint, on the patient's chart. Most agencies require a physician's order to apply a restraint, although nurses are expected to take appropriate action if a patient's safety is threatened.
2. Whether other measures have been taken to assist the patient instead of using a restraint. Restraining a person is a serious matter, because it denies the individual the freedom to move about. Many agencies require that nurses document on the patient's chart the patient behavior that necessitates a restraint and the other protective measures that were tried and found ineffective.

■ Nursing Diagnosis

Nursing diagnoses that may indicate the need to use a restraint include:

1. Ineffective individual coping related to brain tumor
2. Potential for injury related to altered blood chemistry due to inadequate urine output

■ Planning

Nursing goals

1. To prevent a patient in a bed, stretcher, or chair from falling
2. To prevent the interruption of selected therapy, eg, an intravenous infusion
3. To prevent the patient from injuring self, for example, by pulling out a urinary catheter
4. To prevent the patient from injuring others

Equipment

Select the kind and size of restraint required by the patient. See Selecting a Restraint, earlier in this chapter.

If a commercial hand, wrist or ankle restraint is not available, the following supplies are needed:

Mitt restraint

1. Four large padded dressings, eg, ABD pads
2. Pieces of thick gauze to put between the patient's fingers
3. A stockinette dressing or elastic bandage
4. Adhesive tape

Wrist or ankle restraint

1. A padded or thick gauze dressing, eg, an ABD pad
2. A strip of gauze bandage or cloth tie 5 to 8 cm (2 to 3 in) wide and 90 to 120 cm (3 to 4 ft) long

■ Intervention

1. Explain to the patient and support persons how the restraint is used and its purpose. Give the explanation even to disoriented and unconscious patients; they may understand what you are saying.

Jacket restraint

2. Put the jacket on over the patient's gown and bring the ties to the sides.
3. Ensure that the patient's gown and the jacket are not wrinkled.

   Rationale Wrinkles could irritate the patient's skin.

4. Secure each tie to the movable portion of the bed, using a half-bow knot. See Figure 18–11.

   Rationale If tied to the movable part of the bed, the jacket will not tighten when the bed is elevated. The half-bow knot does not tighten or slip when the attached end is pulled but unties easily when the loose end is pulled.

Belt restraint (safety belt)

5. Determine that the safety belt is in good order. If a Velcro safety belt is to be used, make sure that both pieces of Velcro are intact.
6. Place the long portion of the belt behind (under) the patient and secure it to the movable part of the bed frame.

   Rationale The long attached portion will then move up when the head of the bed is elevated and will not tighten around the patient.

7. Place the shorter portion of the belt around the patient's waist, over the gown. There should be a finger's width between the belt and the patient.

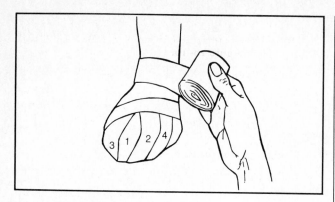

FIGURE 18-12

8. If a locked safety belt is used, secure the buckle or lock, and put the key in the appropriate place.

Mitt or hand restraint

9. Apply the mitt to the hand to be restrained. Make sure the fingers can be slightly flexed and are not caught under the hand. Some patients may require only one restraint if, for example, the other hand is paralyzed or already secured by a wrist restraint for an IV.

10. If there is no commercial mitt, make a mitt as follows:

    a. Place a large folded dressing, such as an abdominal (ABD) pad, in the patient's palm for him or her to grasp. Ensure that the hand is in a natural position with the fingers slightly flexed.

    b. Separate the fingers with pieces of large dressing or thick gauze, to prevent skin abrasion.

    c. Put a padded dressing around the patient's wrist to prevent pressure and skin abrasion.

    d. Place two large dressings (ABD pads) over the hand. Place the first one from the back of the hand over the fingers to the palm; then wrap the other from side to side around the hand.

    e. Cover these dressings by placing a stockinette dressing over the hand or wrapping them with an elastic bandage, using a recurrent pattern. See Figure 18-12. See also chapter 33 for basic turns used in bandaging.

    f. Secure the stockinette or elastic bandage with adhesive tape.

11. If a mitt is to be worn for several days, remove it at least every 12 hours. Wash and exercise the patient's hand, then reapply the mitt. Check agency practices about recommended intervals for removal. Assess the patient's circulation to the hands shortly after the mitt is applied and at regular intervals. Feelings of numbness, discomfort, or inability to move the fingers could indicate impaired circulation to the hand.

Wrist or ankle restraint

12. Apply the padded portion of a commercially prepared restraint around the ankle or wrist.
    or
    Improvise a restraint as follows:

    a. Cushion the wrist or ankle with a padded or thick gauze dressing, eg, an ABD pad.

    b. Wrap a long, narrow strip of gauze bandage or a cloth tie around the padding.

13. Pull the tie of the commercially made restraint through the slit in the wrist portion or through the buckle.
    or
    Use a clove hitch to secure the gauze strip or cloth tie of the improvised restraint. See Figure 18-10, earlier.

14. Using a half-bow knot or a square knot, as appropriate, attach the other end of the commercial restraint (or the two ends of the improvised restraint) to the movable portion of the bed frame. See Figures 18-11 and 18-12 for how to tie these knots.

    Rationale If the ties are attached to the movable portion, the wrist or ankle will not be pulled when the bed position is changed.

Crib net

15. Place the net over the sides and ends of the crib.

16. Secure the ties to the springs or frame of the crib.

    Rationale The crib sides can then be freely lowered without removing the net.

17. Test with your hand that the net will stretch if the child stands in the crib against it.

Elbow restraint

18. Examine the restraint to make sure that the tongue depressors are intact, ie, all in place and not broken.

19. Place the infant's elbow in the center of the restraint. Make sure that the ends of the tongue depressors are covered by the padded material so they will not irritate the skin.

20. Wrap the restraint smoothly around the arm.

21. Secure the restraint, using safety pins, ties, or tape. Ensure that it is not so tight that it obstructs blood circulation.

Mummy restraint

22. Obtain a blanket or sheet large enough so that the distance between opposite corners is about twice the length of the infant's body. Lay the blanket or sheet on a flat dry surface.

23. Fold down one corner, and place the baby on it in the supine position. See Figure 18-13.

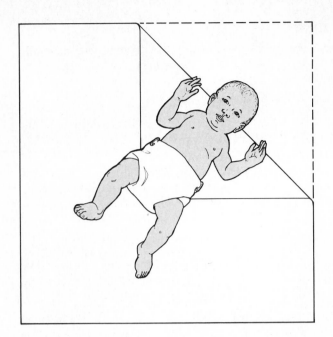

FIGURE 18–13

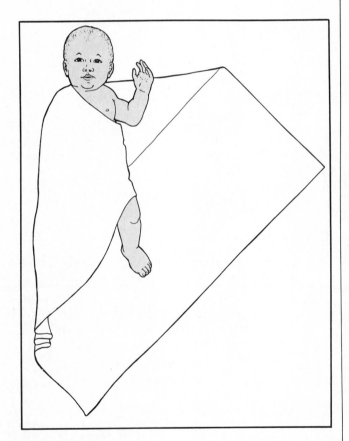

FIGURE 18–14

24. Fold the right side of the blanket over the infant's body and tuck it under the back, leaving the left arm free. See Figure 18–14. The right arm is in a natural position at the side.

25. With the left arm in a natural position at the baby's side, fold the left side of the blanket over the infant, including the arm, and tuck the blanket under the body. See Figure 18–15.

26. Fold the excess blanket at the bottom up under the infant. See Figure 18–16.

27. Remain with the infant who is in a mummy restraint until the specific procedure is completed.

For all kinds of restraints

28. Record on the patient's chart the type of restraint, the time it was applied, where on the body it was applied, and any problems noted when assessing the response.

29. If there is no order for a restraint, notify the physician so that he or she can assess the situation and supply the appropriate order. You may put a note on the patient's chart to draw the physician's attention to the matter. Some hospitals have on-call physicians, who should be notified when the restraint is applied.

FIGURE 18–15   **FIGURE 18–16**

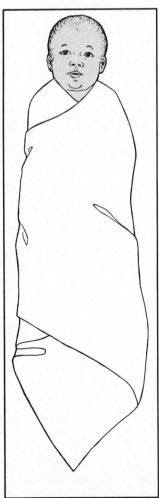

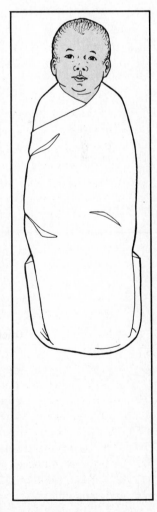

30. Adjust the nursing care plan as required, eg, to include releasing the restraint q.4h., providing skin care, and providing ROM exercises.

31. Note on the chart to discuss the restraint with the patient's support persons when they visit, if it has not already been discussed.

Sample Recording

Date	Time	Notes
9/29/86	0320	Found climbing over side rails. Explained possibility of falling and injury. Sat with patient for 10 minutes. She continued to try to climb over side rails. Jacket restraint applied. Stated "Don't know where I am." Resting comfortably. Dr. Singh notified. — ———————— Edward R. King, NS

■ Evaluation

Expected outcomes

1. Verbal acceptance of the restraint by the patient and reduced restlessness

2. Body position in normal alignment

3. No verbalized discomfort or irritated skin surfaces

4. Body extremities warm and normal color

Unexpected outcomes

1. Increased restlessness and verbal objection to the restraint; stated "Take this off"

2. Nonalignment of body position

3. Discomfort verbalized

4. Reddened or excoriated skin surfaces

5. Body extremities cold and pale or cyanotic

Upon obtaining an unexpected outcome:

1. Explain the reasons for the restraint to the patient.

2. Remove the restraint, provide ROM exercises and skin care, then reapply the restraint.

3. Report your findings to the responsible nurse and/or physician.

4. Adjust the nursing care plan as necessary for ROM exercises and skin care.

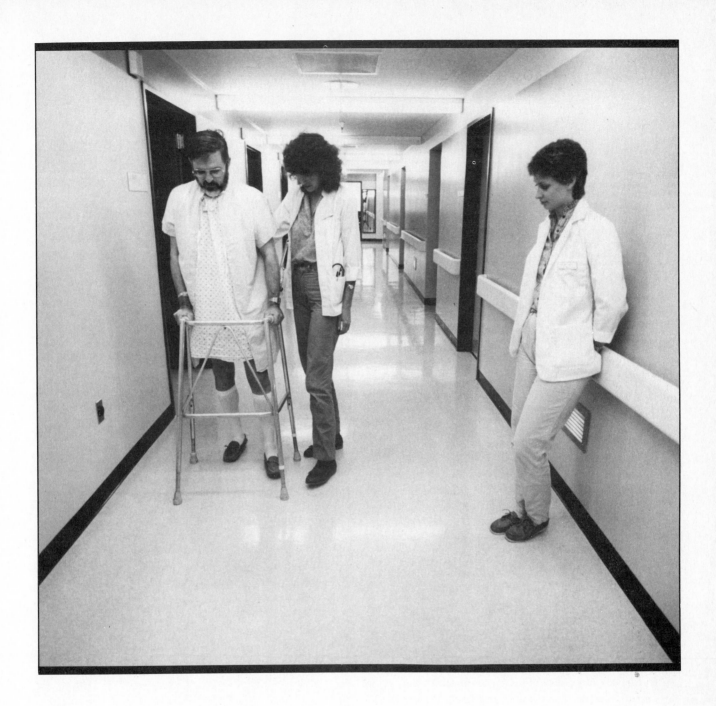

EXERCISE AND AMBULATION

19

The importance of exercise and ambulation to a person's health cannot be overemphasized. The overall benefits of exercise and the ability to carry out the activities of everyday life by walking and moving are often taken for granted by a healthy person. Being ill and confined to bed soon weakens the body and can result in serious impairments not only to movement but also to the functioning of other body systems. This chapter focuses on ways the nurse can maintain the patient's optimal muscle tone and joint mobility for daily functioning.

Chapter Outline

Objectives

Upon completion of this chapter, the student will:

1. Know essential terms and facts about exercise and ambulation
   1.1 Define selected terms
   1.2 Identify the effects of exercise on various body systems
   1.3 Identify physical and psychologic problems associated with immobility
   1.4 Identify five major kinds of exercise
   1.5 Identify the normal range of motion for each body joint
   1.6 Identify guidelines for providing passive exercises
   1.7 Identify exercises requisite to ambulation and using crutches
2. Understand facts about techniques for assisting patients to exercise and ambulate
   2.1 Identify relevant assessment data
   2.2 Identify nursing diagnoses for which the technique may be implemented
   2.3 Identify nursing goals related to the technique
   2.4 Identify expected and unexpected outcomes from assessment data
   2.5 Explain reasons underlying steps of the technique
   2.6 Identify interventions taken to maintain the patient's physical comfort and safety during the technique

   2.7 Identify interventions implemented to enhance the patient's psychologic comfort
3. Perform techniques related to assisting patients with exercise and ambulation
   3.1 Assess the patient adequately
   3.2 Collect additional data from appropriate sources
   3.3 Select pertinent nursing goals for the patient
   3.4 Establish relevant outcome criteria for the patient following the technique
   3.5 Collect necessary equipment before the technique
   3.6 Implement interventions to enhance the effectiveness of the technique and enhance the patient's comfort and safety
   3.7 Communicate relevant information about the patient to the appropriate persons
   3.8 Determine the evaluative outcomes of the technique
4. Evaluate own performance of specific techniques in a laboratory or clinical setting with the assistance of another
   4.1 Use the performance checklists provided
   4.2 Identify areas of strength and weakness
   4.3 Alter performance in response to own evaluation and that of another

Terms

- active exercise exercise carried out by the patient that moves the body parts
- ambulation the act of walking
- ankylosis permanent fixation of a joint
- atrophy a decrease in muscle size
- brace a leather, fabric, plastic, or metal appliance used to support a specific body part
- contraction normal, active shortening or tensing of a muscle

- contracture permanent shortening of a muscle and subsequent shortening of tendons and ligaments
- crutch a device with hand and arm supports used to facilitate walking
- crutch palsy weakness of the hand, wrist, and forearm induced by prolonged pressure of a crutch on the axillary nerves
- gait the way a person walks
- goniometer an instrument used to assess joint angles

■ **hemiplegia**   paralysis of one side of the body as a result of a stroke

■ **hypertrophy**   physical enlargement of a muscle

■ **isometric muscle contraction**   tensing of the muscle against an immovable outer resistance, a contraction that does not change muscle length or produce joint motion

■ **isotonic muscle contraction**   shortening of the muscle in the process of doing work (eg, ROM exercises, weight lifting), which produces joint motion

■ **osteoblast**   a bone-building cell

■ **osteoclast**   a cell associated with bone resorption and breakdown

■ **osteoporosis**   demineralization of the bones

■ **pace**   the distance covered in a step when walking, or the number of steps taken per minute

■ **passive exercise**   exercise in which the nurse supplies the energy to move the patient's body part

■ **range of motion**   the degree of movement possible for each joint

■ **resistive exercise**   exercise in which the patient contracts a muscle against an opposing force, eg, a weight

■ **rigidity**   stiffness or inflexibility of a muscle

■ **spasticity**   a sudden, prolonged, involuntary muscle contraction that occurs in patients with damage to the central nervous system

■ **station**   the way a person stands

■ **walker**   a metal, rectangular frame used to assist a person to walk

MOBILITY

Being mobile—that is, being able to move about freely—is a basic human need. To carry out most of life's activities, a person needs to be able to move. However, movement is not limited to moving the body from place to place; a person's gestures, facial expressions, and mannerisms also depend on the ability to move.

A number of aspects of mobility are of particular relevance in health care: joint mobility, station and gait, exercise, and activity tolerance.

Joint Mobility

A joint is the functional unit of the musculoskeletal system. It is where the bones of the skeleton articulate. Most of the skeletal muscles attach to the two bones at the joint. These muscles are categorized according to the type of joint movement they produce upon contraction. Muscles are therefore called *flexors, extensors, internal rotators,* etc. The flexor muscles are stronger than the extensor muscles. Thus, when a person is inactive, the joints are pulled into a flexed (bent) position. If this is not counteracted with exercise and position changes, permanent shortening (contracture) of the muscles develops, and the joint becomes fixed in a flexed position.

Range of motion

The range of motion of a joint is the maximum movement that is possible for that joint. Not all people possess a similar range of motion. Each person's range is determined by genetic inheritance, developmental patterns, the presence or absence of disease, and the amount of physical activity the person normally does. See Technique 19–1.

Types of synovial joints

A *synovial joint* is freely movable and characteristically has a cavity enclosed by a capsule. Within this capsule is a lining of synovial membrane, which secretes synovial fluid to lubricate the joint. Cartilage of a joint provides a smooth surface upon which a bone can glide during movement. Thick bands of collagenous fibers extending from one bone to another are called *ligaments;* they provide strength for the joint, and they are usually stretched tautly when the joint is in the position of greatest stability. The muscles surrounding the joint provide the most stability for the joint. Synovial joints of the body serve primarily to bear weight and to provide for movement. The body has six types of synovial joints, and certain movements are normally possible for each type. See Table 19–1.

Synovial joint movements

Each type of synovial joint is capable of specific movements. These movements are described in relation to the anatomic body position and the three body planes: sagittal, transverse, coronal. See Figure 19–1. The sagittal plant is a vertical line or plane dividing the body or its parts into right and left portions. The transverse plane is a horizontal line or plane dividing the body or its parts into superior and inferior portions. The frontal or coronal plane is any plane dividing the body into anterior (ventral) and posterior (dorsal) portions at right angles to the sagittal plane. For descriptions of the movements of synovial joints, see Table 19–2.

TABLE 19–1 ■ Types of Synovial Joints

Type	Description	Examples	Movement
Ball-and-socket	The ball-shaped head of one bone fits into the concave socket of another bone.	The hip and shoulder joints.	Movement in three planes. Greatest range of all joints: flexion and extension; abduction and adduction; rotation.
Hinge	The convex, spool-shaped end of one bone fits into the concave surface of another bone.	The elbow, knee, ankle, finger, and toe joints.	Movement in one plane. Flexion and extension.
Pivot	An arch-shaped surface rotates in a rounded or longitudinal axis.	The axis and atlas joints of the vertebral column, the joints between the radius and the ulna.	Movement in one plane. Rotation only.
Condyloid (ovoid)	The oval-shaped part of one bone fits into an elliptical cavity.	The wrist joints.	Movement in two planes at right angles to each other. Flexion and extension; abduction and adduction.
Saddle	Two bones have opposite concave-convex surfaces that fit together.	The base of the thumb only.	Same movements as for condyloid joints but freer.
Gliding	Two flat bone surfaces glide over each other.	The carpal bones, the tarsal bones, the medial end of the clavicle with the sternum, the ribs with the bodies of the vertebrae, the sacrum and the ilia, the fibula with the tibia.	Gliding only.

Station and Gait

Station, or stance, is the way a person stands; gait is the way a person walks or ambulates. A desirable station for a person provides good body alignment. However, a poor stance can develop because of postural habits or disease processes. Poor body alignment places undue strain on some of the muscles and bones of the body. For information on body alignment, see chapter 17. Further information on gait is provided later, in Technique 19–3 and Table 19–5.

Exercise

Exercise has a number of purposes: (a) to restore, maintain, or increase the tone and strength of the muscles; (b) to maintain or increase the flexibility of the joints; (c) to maintain or promote the growth of bones through the application of physical stressors; and (d) to improve the functioning of other body systems, such as the cardiovascular and gastrointestinal systems.

Effects of exercise

Exercise and adequate movement of the joints have many positive effects on the body as a whole. Immobility creates many physical and psychologic problems. Promoting exercise to maintain a patient's muscle tone and joint mobility is one of the essential functions of nursing personnel.

Musculoskeletal system

1. The size, shape, tone, and strength of muscles (including the heart muscle) are maintained with mild exercise and increased with strenuous exercise. With strenuous exercise, muscles hypertrophy, and the efficiency of muscular contraction increases. Hypertrophy is commonly seen in the arm muscles of a tennis player, the leg muscles of a skater, the arm and hand muscles of a carpenter, and the body muscles of weight lifters.

2. Joint mobility is maintained.

3. Bone density is maintained through weight bearing. The stress of weight bearing maintains a balance between *osteoblasts* (bone-building cells) and *osteoclasts* (bone-resorption and breakdown cells).

Cardiovascular system

1. The heart rate increases.

2. Arterial (systolic) blood pressure increases.

3. Blood is shunted from the nonexercising tissues to the heart and the muscles.

4. Cardiac output (the amount of blood pumped by the heart) increases due to the redirection of the blood flow. Exercise can increase cardiac output to 22 L/min in the average person (Guyton, 1981, p 286). Normal cardiac output is 5 to 7 L/min.

Respiratory system

1. Ventilation (the amount of air circulating into and out of the lungs) increases. In strenuous exercise, the intake

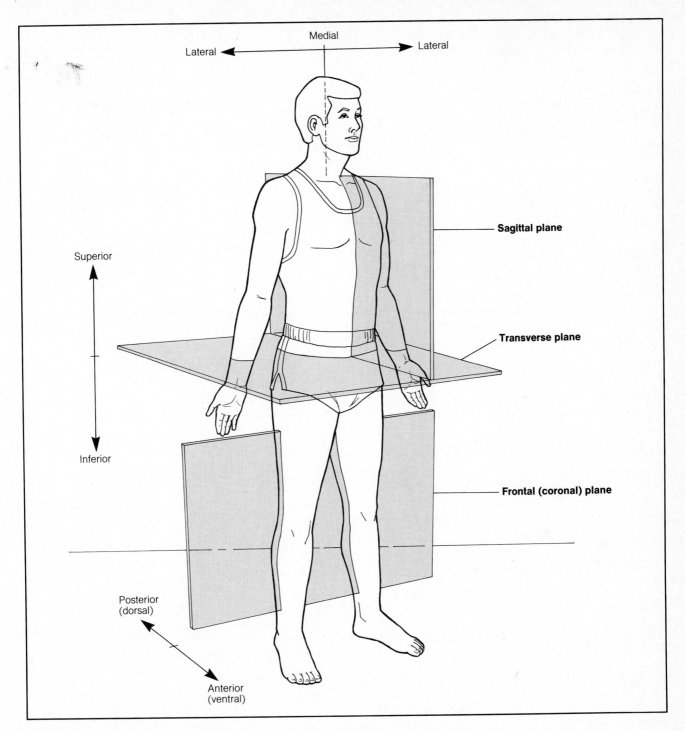

FIGURE 19–1 ■ Planes of the body.

of oxygen increases to as much as 20 times normal intake (Guyton, 1981, p 505). Normal ventilation is about 5 or 6 L/min.

2. Adequate exercise prevents pooling of secretions in the bronchi and bronchioles.

Gastrointestinal system

1. Appetite improves.

2. Gastrointestinal tract tone increases, improving digestion and elimination.

Urinary system

1. Body wastes are excreted more effectively with efficient blood flow.

2. Stasis of urine in the bladder is prevented.

Metabolism   Metabolism refers to all physical and chemical processes of the body. Basal metabolism is the minimal energy expended for the maintenance of these processes. The metabolic rate is the rate of basal metabolism expressed in calories per hour per square meter of

TABLE 19-2 ■ Types of Synovial Joint Movements

Movement	Action
Flexion	Decreasing the angle of the joint (eg, bending the elbow)
Extension	Increasing the angle of the joint (eg, straightening the arm at the elbow)
Hyperextension	Further extension or straightening of a joint (eg, bending the head backward)
Abduction	Movement of the bone away from the midline of the body
Adduction	Movement of the bone toward the midline of the body
Rotation	Movement of the bone around its central axis
Circumduction	Movement of the distal part of the bone in a circle while the proximal end remains fixed
Eversion	Turning the sole of the foot outward by moving the ankle joint
Inversion	Turning the sole of the foot inward by moving the ankle joint
Pronation	Moving the bones of the forearm so that the palm of the hand faces downward when held in front of the body
Supination	Moving the bones of the forearm so that the palm of the hand faces upward when held in front of the body
Protraction	Moving a part of the body forward in the same plane parallel to the ground
Retraction	Moving a part of the body backward in the same plane parallel to the ground

body surface. During very strenuous exercise the metabolic rate can increase to as much as 20 times the normal rate. Lying in bed and eating an average diet utilizes 1,850 calories per day (Guyton, 1981, p 882).

Psychoneurologic system Exercise produces a sense of relaxation and restores well-being.

Effects of immobility

Although the term *immobility* denotes complete lack of movement, it is frequently used in nursing to refer to a decrease in activity from a person's normal level. Several psychologic and physical problems ensue with immobility (Olson, 1967). They are presented here to help nurses appreciate the importance of regular exercise for patients.

Psychologic and social problems

1. Self-esteem is lowered when a person is unable to carry out the usual activities related to his or her role (eg, as breadwinner, husband, mother, or athlete).

2. Exaggerated emotional reactions occur due to frustration and decreased self-esteem. Emotional reactions vary considerably. Some individuals become apathetic and

withdrawn, some regress, and some become angry and aggressive.

3. Hunger and sex drives are diminished.

4. Perception of time intervals deteriorates, since participation in life is much narrower and the variety of stimuli is decreased.

5. Motivation to learn and retain information is decreased.

6. Motivation to solve problems is decreased.

7. Anxiety occurs due to loss of control over events.

Musculoskeletal problems

1. *Osteoporosis.* Without the stress of weight-bearing activity, the bones demineralize. They are depleted chiefly of calcium, which gives the bones strength and density. Regardless of the amount of calcium in a person's diet, the demineralization process continues with immobility. The bones become spongy and may gradually deform and fracture easily.

2. *Disuse atrophy.* Unused muscles atrophy, losing most of their strength and normal function.

3. *Contractures.* When the muscle fibers are no longer able to shorten and lengthen, contractures limit joint mobility. This process eventually involves the tendons, ligaments, and joint capsules; it is irreversible except by surgical intervention. Joint deformities occur when a stronger muscle dominates the opposite muscle.

4. *Stiffness and pain in the joints.* Without movement, the collagen (connective) tissues at the joint become ankylosed. In addition, as the bones demineralize, excess calcium may be deposited in the joints, contributing to stiffness and pain.

5. *Skin breakdown.* Normal blood circulation relies on muscle activity. Immobility impedes circulation and diminishes the supply of nutrients to specific areas. As a result, skin breakdown and formation of decubitus ulcers can occur. See chapter 14.

Cardiovascular problems

1. *Venous stasis and orthostatic hypotension.* After a patient has remained in a supine position for a period of time there is often reduced peripheral vasoconstriction, thus permitting pooling of the venous blood in the lower extremities. In addition the ability of the autonomic nervous system to equalize the blood supply is diminished. This, together with reduced muscle tone, decreases venous blood return to the heart. Therefore, upon assuming a sitting or standing position, the patient may experience a drop in blood pressure (orthostatic, or postural, hypotension) resulting in feelings of dizziness and faintness. Orthostatic hypotension is a drop of 15 mm Hg or more in the blood pressure, when the patient rises from a sitting to a standing position.

2. *Increased cardiac work load.* The heart also loses muscle tone with decreased activity. In the supine position, grav-

ity assists in returning to the heart the venous blood that is normally pooled in the lower extremities, thus increasing the amount of blood the heart has to pump. Both the heart rate and the stroke volume (amount of blood ejected with each contraction) increase to accommodate the increased volume of blood.

3. *Dependent edema.* Inactivity and loss of muscle tone cause fluid to accumulate in the interstitial spaces that are lower than the heart (dependent edema). This is the result of poor venous return and venous stasis. Stasis creates a higher than normal hydrostatic pressure in the veins and allows fluid to flow from the veins into the tissues rather than from the tissues back into the veins. Edema can be seen in the back and sacral area in bedridden patients and in the legs and feet when the person is standing or sitting.

4. *Thrombus formation.* A thrombus (blood clot) can develop in the veins as a result of venous stasis arising from inactivity. Thrombi are also thought to occur as a result of increased blood viscosity (thickness) as pooled venous fluid is lost into the tissues. Prolonged pressure on the veins, from, for example, raising the knee gatch on the bed, can also damage the veins.

5. *Increased use of the Valsalva maneuver.* The Valsalva maneuver refers to holding the breath while moving. For example, patients tend to hold their breath when attempting to move up in bed or sit on a bedpan. This builds up sufficient pressure on the large veins in the thorax to interfere with the return blood flow to the heart and coronary arteries. When the patient exhales, pressure is suddenly released and a surge of blood flows to the heart. Tachycardia (increased heart rate) and cardiac arrest can result, if the patient has cardiac pathology.

Respiratory problems

1. *Decreased respiratory movement.* With inactivity, the patient's respirations are shallow, and lung expansion is limited. Lung expansion is further limited by the positions the patient assumes in bed. For example, in the supine position, the diaphragm is pressed upward by the abdominal organs; in the lateral position, expansion of the lower lung and rib cage is restricted.

2. *Pooling of respiratory secretions.* Secretions of the respiratory tract are normally expelled by changing position or posture and by coughing. Inactivity allows secretions to pool by gravity, interfering with the normal diffusion of oxygen and carbon dioxide in the alveoli. The ability to cough up secretions may also be hindered by loss of respiratory muscle tone, dehydration (which thickens secretions), or sedatives that depress the cough reflex.

3. *Hypostatic pneumonia.* Pooled (hypostatic) secretions provide excellent media for bacterial growth, and pneumonia can result. Symptoms are fatigue; rapid, shallow respirations; diminished chest expansion; and fever.

Gastrointestinal problems

1. *Anorexia.* Loss of appetite (anorexia) occurs as a result

of the decreased metabolic rate and increased protein breakdown (catabolism) that accompany immobility.

2. *Constipation.* Inactivity decreases the peristaltic movement of the intestines, and constipation is a common result. Constipation can be aggravated when patients ignore the defecation reflex because they dislike using a bedpan. Constipation is accompanied by abdominal distention and malaise, increasing the problem of anorexia.

Urinary problems

1. *Stasis of urine in the kidney pelvis.* When a person is erect, gravity helps most of the urine flow out of the kidney pelvis. In the supine position pooling of urine occurs. See Figure 19-2.

2. *Urinary calculi and infections.* The inactive patient is

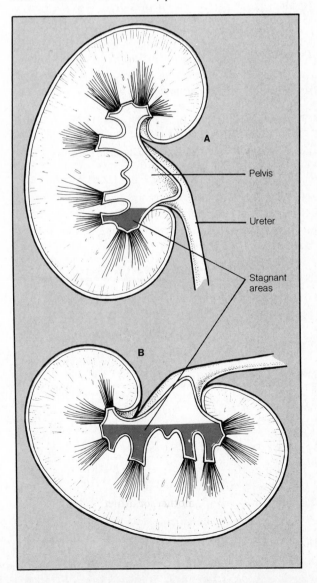

FIGURE 19-2   ■   The position of the kidney in the body: **A**, standing position; **B**, supine position, showing the increased stasis of the urine in the kidney pelvis.

Pelvis

Ureter

Stagnant areas

susceptible to urinary infection and calculus (stone) formation in the kidney as a result of urine stagnation and increased levels of minerals (eg, calcium) in the urine. An excess of calcium elevates the pH of the urine (makes it more alkaline). This also predisposes the patient to urinary infection.

3. *Urinary retention and incontinence.* With lack of activity, urinary control is diminished. Normal urination is reflexively dependent on effective contraction of the bladder (the detrusor muscle of the bladder wall), which increases the pressure within the bladder and in turn relaxes the bladder sphincters so that urination occurs. However, in immobilized patients, this sequence of events is suppressed by reduced muscle tone of the bladder and inability to relax the perineal muscles for the bladder to empty. Urine is retained in the bladder, which then becomes distended. Increasing distention leads to urinary incontinence.

Types of exercise

There are five major kinds of exercise that may be chosen according to the patient's health and strength. These are: active (isotonic); passive; active-assistive; static (isometric, muscle setting); and resistive. The first three types of exercise (active, passive, and active-assistive) are used primarily for the range-of-motion (ROM) exercises, discussed in Techniques 19–1 and 19–2. The latter two are used primarily for muscle conditioning.

1. Active exercise causes the muscles to contract, thus maintaining the size, shape, and strength of the muscles, and joint mobility. Whenever possible, active exercise is encouraged for patients to prevent disuse atrophy and contractures.

2. Passive exercise maintains and prevents contractures and joint stiffness. This type of exercise is necessary for patients with paralyzed limbs. However, it does not prevent muscle atrophy and weakness because the muscles do not contract.

3. Active-assistive exercise encourages normal muscle function in that the patient moves the body part as far as he or she is able, and then the nurse moves it up to its normal range. Active-assistive exercises are useful for patients whose muscle strength is diminished (eg, from disuse or a bone fracture).

4. Static (isometric) exercise maintains muscle tone and strength and prevents atrophy. It does not maintain joint mobility. The patient consciously tenses the muscles, holds the contraction for a specified time (5 to 10 seconds), and then relaxes the muscles. This type of exercise is useful for the patient who has a cast.

5. Resistive exercise increases muscle size, shape, and strength, and provides the stress and strain necessary to maintain bone strength, ie, prevent osteoporosis. Examples are pushing against a footboard, lifting weights, or doing pushups.

Activity Tolerance

Activity tolerance or endurance is the ability to withstand activity in terms of duration. It generally increases with repeated activity over a period of time. Tolerance is affected by a number of factors: pain, physical strength, cardiopulmonary status, age, life-style, and emotional state.

A person who experiences pain with activity will normally tolerate the activity for a shorter time than one who experiences no pain. Physical strength is directly proportional to activity tolerance; the weaker the person, the greater the energy required to carry out the activity, and the sooner the person experiences muscle fatigue. Impaired functioning of the cardiopulmonary system can limit the flow of oxygen and nutrients to the exercising muscles, decreasing activity tolerance. The elderly often tolerate exercise less well than younger persons. With increasing age the body's muscle mass, and thus the person's strength, is reduced. People with a less active life-style tire sooner with exercise than those who have good muscle tone. A positive attitude and the desire to carry out an activity also increase an individual's tolerance. The depressed person often tires sooner than an emotionally healthy person.

TECHNIQUE 19–1 ■ Assessing Joint Mobility (Range of Motion)

The range of motion of a joint is the maximum amount of movement of which it is capable. Joint mobility is determined by the patient's bones, muscles, and ligaments as well as by disease processes. Certain movements are specific to each plane in which a joint can move. See Table 19–3.

■ Planning

Nursing goals

1. To assess the degree of mobility of the joints
2. To maintain joint mobility

TABLE 19-3   ■   The Three Body Planes and Joint Movements

Plane	Joint movement	Example
Transverse	Pronation	Elbow
	Supination	Elbow
	Internal rotation	Hip, shoulder
	External rotation	Hip, shoulder
	Flexion (dorsiflexion)	Ankle
	Extension (plantar flexion)	Ankle
Saggital	Flexion	Hip, knee
	Extension	Hand, elbow
	Hyperextension	Hip, neck
Frontal (coronal)	Abduction	Wrist, shoulder
	Adduction	Wrist, shoulder
	Inversion	Foot
	Eversion	Foot

3. To maintain muscle size, tone, and strength
4. To prevent muscle atrophy and contractures
5. To enable the patient to carry out the activities of everyday living as independently as possible

Equipment

The amount of movement of a joint can be measured by a goniometer, a device that measures the angle of the joint in degrees. See Figure 19–3.

■ Intervention

1. While the patient performs the range-of-motion exercises described for each joint, assess:
    a. The degree of movement of the joint.
    b. Any discomfort experienced by the patient.
    c. Any joint swelling or redness, which could indicate the presence of an injury or an inflammation.
    d. The muscle development associated with each joint and the relative size of the muscles on each side of the body.
    e. The patient's tolerance of the exercise.
    Range-of-motion exercises should not be unduly fatiguing to the patient. An elderly patient, for example, may require several sessions to do the exercises without becoming overtired.
2. Assist the patient to either a standing or a supine position, with the heels parallel and the arms placed along the sides.
    Rationale Active joint range-of-motion exercises can be carried out in either position. When the patient is lying down, the prone or lateral position

is required for hyperextension of the neck, hips, and shoulders.
3. Make sure that the patient is wearing unrestrictive clothing.
    Rationale The clothing then will not limit the joint movement, and the joint motion can be clearly observed.
4. Ask the patient to perform the motions you request smoothly, slowly, and rhythmically and not to force any joint.
    Rationale Uneven, jerky movement and forcing can injure the joint and the muscles and ligaments surrounding it.

Neck—pivot joint

5. Flexion: Move the head from the upright midline position forward, so that the chin rests on the chest. See Figure 19–4. Normal range: 45° from midline. Major muscle: sternocleidomastoideus.
6. Extension: Move the head from the flexed position to the upright position. See Figure 19–5. Normal range: 45° from the midline. Major muscle: trapezius.

FIGURE 19–3   ■   A goniometer used to measure joint angles.

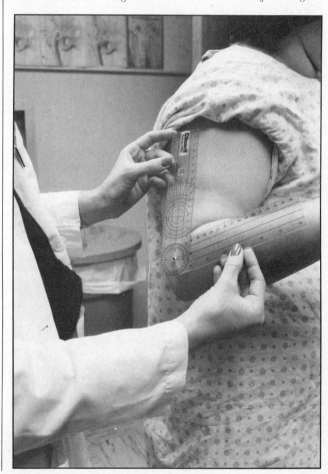

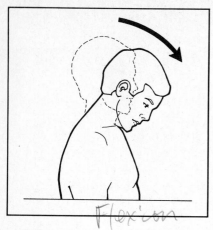

FIGURE 19-4

Flexion

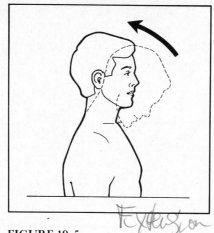

FIGURE 19-5

Extension

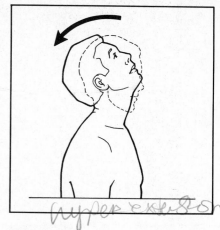

FIGURE 19-6

hyper extension

7. Hyperextension: Move the head from the upright position back as far as possible. See Figure 19-6. Normal range: 10°. Major muscle: trapezius.

8. Lateral flexion: Move the head laterally to the right and left shoulders, while facing front. See Figure 19-7. Normal range: 40° from the midline. Major muscle: sternocleidomastoideus.

9. Rotation: Turn the face as far as possible to the right and left. See Figure 19-8. Normal range: 70° from the midline. Major muscles: sternocleidomastoideus and trapezius.

Shoulder—ball-and-socket joint

10. Flexion: Raise each arm from a position by the side forward and upward to a position beside the head. See Figure 19-9. Normal range: 180° from the side. Major muscles: pectoralis major, coracobrachialis, and deltoideus.

11. Extension: Move each arm from a vertical position beside the head forward and down to a resting position at the side of the body. See Figure 19-10. Normal range: 180° from a vertical position beside the head. Major muscles: latissimus dorsi, deltoideus, and teres major.

12. Hyperextension: Move each arm from a resting side position to behind the body. See Figure 19-11. Normal range: 50° from side position. Major muscles: latissimus dorsi, deltoideus, and teres major.

13. Abduction: Move each arm laterally from a resting position at the sides to a side position above the head, palm of the hand away from head. See Figure 19-12. Normal range: 180°. Major muscles: deltoideus and supraspinatus.

14. Anterior adduction: Move each arm from a position beside the head downward laterally and across the front of the body as far as possible. See Figure 19-13. Normal range: 230°. Major muscles: pectoralis major and teres major.

15. Posterior adduction: Move each arm from a position beside the head downward laterally and across

FIGURE 19-7

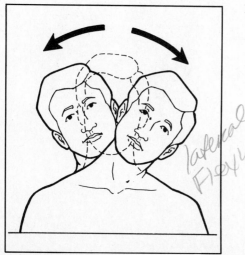

lateral Flexion

FIGURE 19-8

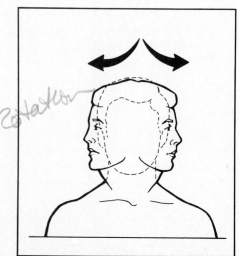

Rotation

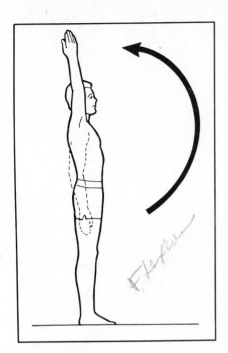

FIGURE 19-9

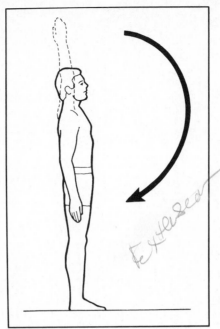

FIGURE 19-10

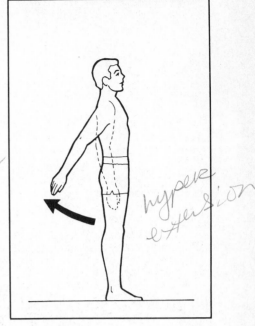

FIGURE 19-11

behind the body as far as possible. See Figure 19–14. Normal range: 230°. Major muscles: latissimus dorsi and teres major.

16. Horizontal flexion (horizontal adduction): Extend each arm laterally at shoulder height and move it through a horizontal plane across the front of the body as far as possible. See Figure 19–15. Normal

range: 130°–135°. Major muscles: pectoralis major and coracobrachialis.

17. Horizontal extension (horizontal abduction): Extend each arm laterally at shoulder height and move it through a horizontal plane as far behind the body as possible. See Figure 19–16. Normal range:

FIGURE 19-12

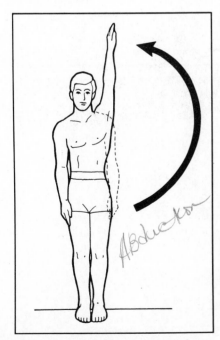

FIGURE 19-13

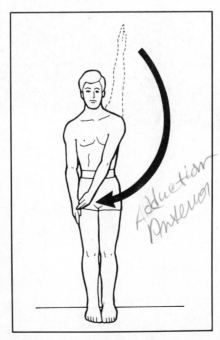

FIGURE 19-14

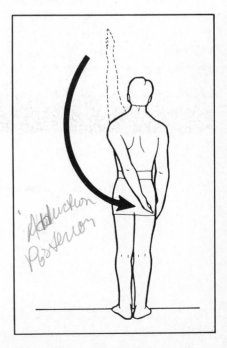

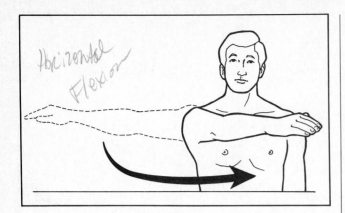

FIGURE 19–15

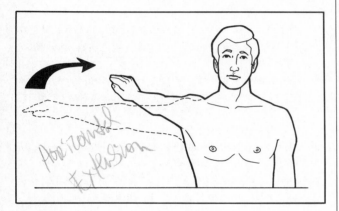

FIGURE 19–16

45°. Major muscles: latissimus dorsi, teres major, and deltoideus.

18. Circumduction: Move each arm forward, up, back, and down in a full circle. See Figure 19–17. Normal range: 360°. Major muscles: deltoideus, coracobrachialis, latissimus dorsi, and teres major.

19. External rotation: With each arm held out to the

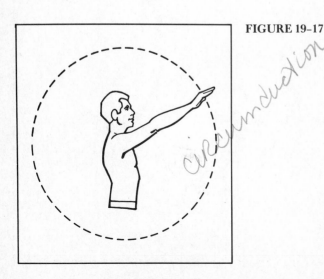

FIGURE 19–17

side at the shoulder level and the elbow bent to a right angle, fingers pointing down, move the arm upward so that the fingers point up. See Figure 19–18. Normal range: 90°. Major muscles: infraspinatus and teres minor.

20. Internal rotation: With each arm held out to the side at shoulder level and the elbow bent to a right angle, fingers pointing up, bring the arm forward and down so that the fingers point down. See Figure 19–19. Major muscles: subscapularis, pectoralis major, latissimus dorsi, and teres major.

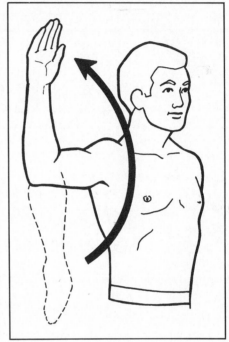

FIGURE 19–18

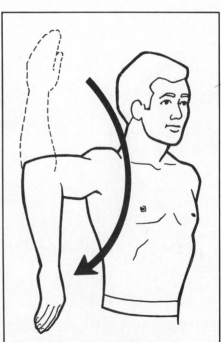

FIGURE 19–19

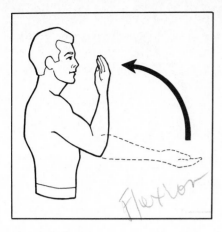

FIGURE 19–20

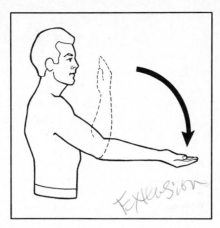

FIGURE 19–21

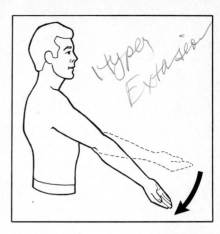

FIGURE 19–22

Elbow—hinge joint

21. Flexion: Bring each lower arm forward and upward so that the hand is at the shoulder. See Figure 19–20. Normal range: 150°. Major muscles: biceps brachii, brachialis, and brachioradialis.

22. Extension: Bring each lower arm forward and downward, straightening the arm. See Figure 19–21. Range of motion: 150°. Major muscle: triceps brachii.

23. Hyperextension: Move each lower arm farther backward from the straightened position. See Figure 19–22. Normal range: 0°–15°. Major muscle: triceps brachii.

24. Rotation for supination: Turn each hand and forearm so that the palm is facing upward. See Figure 19–23. Normal range: 70°–90°. Major muscles: biceps brachii and supinator.

25. Rotation for pronation: Turn each hand and forearm so that the palm is facing downward. See Figure 19–24. Normal range: 70°–90°. Major muscles: pronator teres and pronator quadratus.

FIGURE 19–23

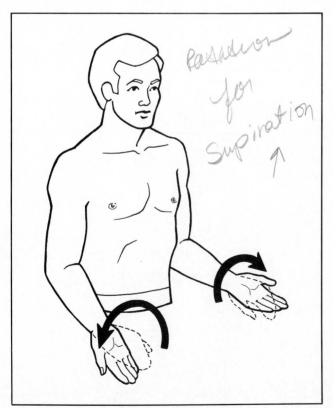

FIGURE 19–24

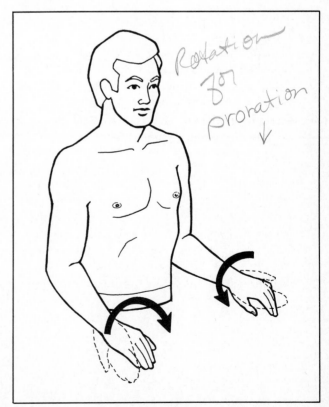

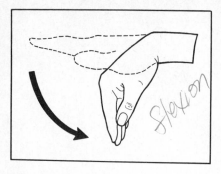

FIGURE 19-25

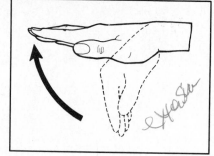

FIGURE 19-26

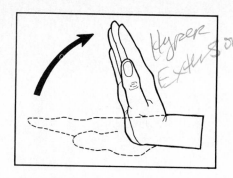

FIGURE 19-27

Wrist—condyloid joint

26. Flexion: Bring the fingers of each hand toward the inner aspect of the forearm. See Figure 19–25. Normal range: 80°–90°. Major muscles: flexor carpi radialis and flexor carpi ulnaris.

27. Extension: Straighten each hand to the same plane as the arm. See Figure 19–26. Normal range: 80°–90°. Major muscles: extensor carpi radialis longus, extensor carpi radialis brevis, and extensor carpi ulnaris.

28. Hyperextension: Bend the fingers of each hand back as far as possible. See Figure 19–27. Normal range: 70°–90°. Major muscles: extensor carpi radialis longus, extensor carpi radialis brevis, and extensor carpi ulnaris.

29. Abduction (radial flexion): Bend each wrist laterally toward the thumb side with the hand supinated. See Figure 19–28. Normal range: 0°–20°. Major muscle: extensor carpi radialis longus.

30. Adduction (ulnar flexion): Bend each wrist laterally toward the fifth finger with the hand supinated. See Figure 19–29. Normal range: 30°–50°. Major muscle: extensor carpi ulnaris.

Hand and fingers: metacarpophalangeal joints—condyloid; interphalangeal joints—hinge

See Figure 19–30.

31. Flexion: Make a fist with each hand. See Figure 19–31. Normal range: 90°. Major muscles: interossei dorsales manus and flexor digitorum superficialis.

32. Extension: Straighten the fingers of each hand. See Figure 19–32. Normal range: 90°. Major muscles: extensor indicis and extensor digiti minimi.

33. Hyperextension: Bend the fingers of each hand back as far as possible. See Figure 19–33. Normal range: 30°. Major muscles: extensor indicis and extensor digiti minimi.

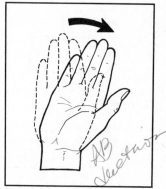

FIGURE 19-28

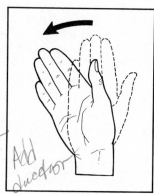

FIGURE 19-29

FIGURE 19-30

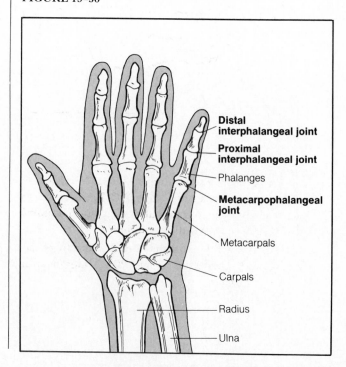

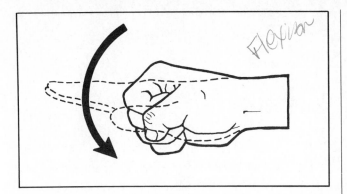

FIGURE 19–31

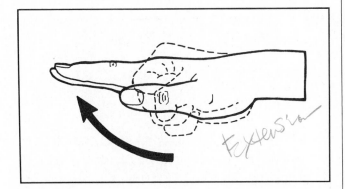

FIGURE 19–32

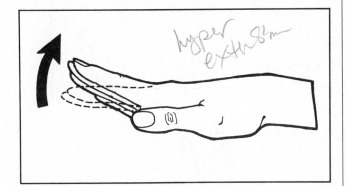

FIGURE 19–33

34. Abduction: Spread the fingers of each hand apart. See Figure 19–34. Normal range: 20°. Major muscles: interossei dorsales manus, abductor digiti minimi manus, and opponens digiti minimi.

35. Adduction: Bring the fingers of each hand together. See Figure 19–35. Normal range: 20°. Major muscle: interossei palmares.

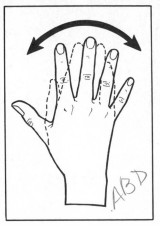   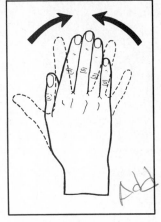

FIGURE 19–34   **FIGURE 19–35**

Thumb—saddle joint

36. Flexion: Move each thumb across the palmar surface of the hand toward the fifth finger. See Figure 19–36. Normal range: 90°. Major muscles: flexor pollicis brevis and opponens pollicis.

37. Extension: Move each thumb away from the hand. See Figure 19–37. Normal range: 90°. Major muscles: extensor pollicis brevis and extensor pollicis longus.

38. Abduction: Extend each thumb laterally. See Figure 19–38. Normal range: 30°. Major muscles: abductor pollicis brevis and abductor pollicis longus.

39. Adduction: Move each thumb back to the hand. See Figure 19–39. Normal range: 30°. Major muscle: adductor pollicis.

FIGURE 19–36   **FIGURE 19–37**

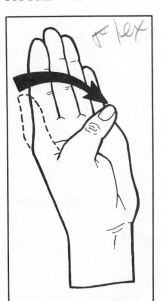   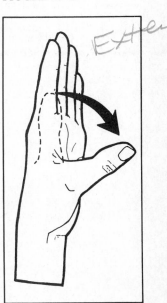

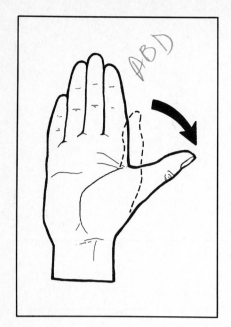

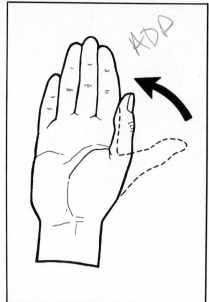

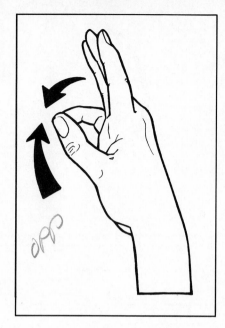

FIGURE 19–38　　　　　**FIGURE 19–39**　　　　　**FIGURE 19–40**

40. Opposition: Touch each thumb to the tip of each finger of the same hand. The thumb joint movements involved are: abduction, rotation, and flexion. See Figure 19–40. Major muscles: opponens pollicis and flexor pollicis brevis.

Hip—ball-and-socket joint

41. Flexion: Move each leg forward and upward. The knee may be extended or flexed. See Figure 19–41.

Normal range: knee extended, 90°; knee flexed, 120°. Major muscles: psoas major and iliacus.

42. Extension: Move each leg back beside the other leg. See Figure 19–42. Normal range: 90°–120°. Major muscles: gluteus maximus, adductor magnus, semitendinosus, and semimembranosus.

43. Hyperextension: Move each leg back behind the body. See Figure 19–43. Normal range: 30°–50°. Major muscles: gluteus maximus, semitendinosus, and semimembranosus.

FIGURE 19–41

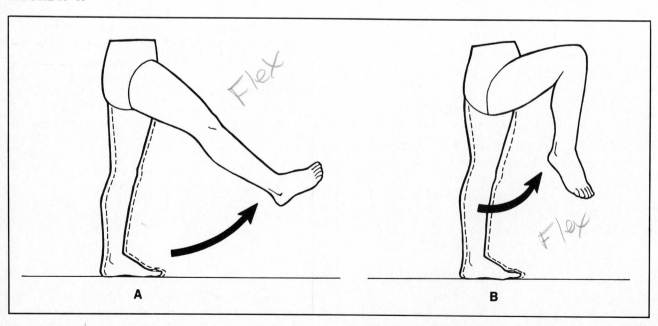

A　　　　　　　　　　　　　　　B

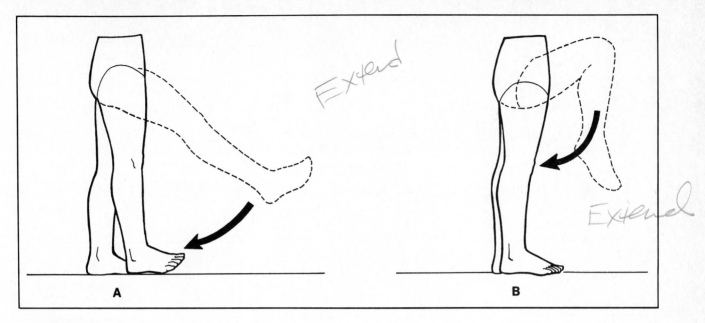

FIGURE 19–42

44. Abduction: Move each leg out to the side. See Figure 19–44. Normal range: 45°–50°. Major muscles: gluteus medius and gluteus minimus.

45. Adduction: Move each leg back to the other leg and beyond in front of it. See Figure 19–45. Normal range: 20°–30° beyond the other leg. Major muscles: adductor magnus, adductor brevis, and adductor longus.

46. Circumduction: Move each leg backward, up, to the side, and down in a circle. See Figure 19–46. Normal range: 360°. Major muscles: psoas major, gluteus maximus, gluteus medius, and adductor magnus.

47. Internal rotation: Turn each foot and leg inward so that the toes point as far as possible toward the other leg. See Figure 19–47. Normal range: 90°. Major muscles: gluteus minimus and tensor fasciae latae.

48. External rotation: Turn each foot and leg outward so that the toes point as far as possible away from the other leg. See Figure 19–48. Normal range: 90°. Major muscles: obturator externus, obturator internus, and quadratus femoris.

FIGURE 19–45   **FIGURE 19–46**

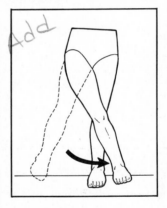   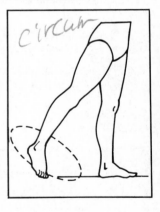

FIGURE 19–43   **FIGURE 19–44**

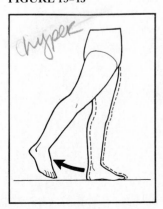   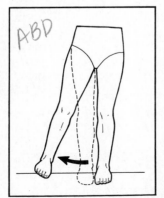

FIGURE 19–47   **FIGURE 19–48**

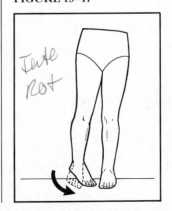   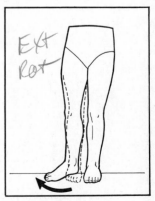

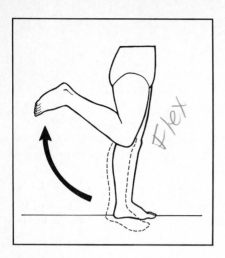

FIGURE 19-49

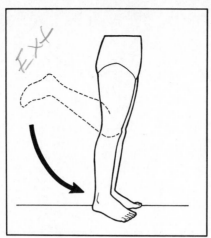

FIGURE 19-50

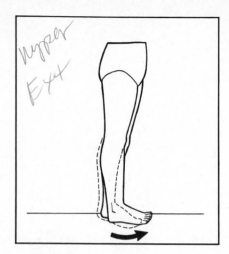

FIGURE 19-51

Knee—hinge joint

49. Flexion: Bend each leg, bringing the heel toward the back of the thigh. See Figure 19-49. Normal range: 120°–130°. Major muscles: biceps femoris, semitendinosus, semimembranosus, and popliteus.

50. Extension: Straighten each leg, returning the foot to its position beside the other foot. See Figure 19-50. Normal range: 120°–130°. Major muscles: rectus femoris, vastus lateralis, vastus medialis, and vastus intermedius.

51. Hyperextension: Some people can also hyperextend the knee 10°. See Figure 19-51. Major muscles: rectus femoris, vastus lateralis, vastus medialis, and vastus intermedius.

Ankle—hinge joint

52. Extension (plantar flexion): Point the toes of each foot downward. See Figure 19-52. Normal range: 45°–50°. Major muscles: gastrocnemius and soleus.

53. Flexion (dorsiflexion): Point the toes of each foot upward. See Figure 19-53. Normal range: 20°. Major muscles: peroneus tertius, tibialis anterior.

Foot and toes: interphalangeal joint—hinge; metatarsophalangeal joint—hinge; intertarsal joint—gliding

See Figure 19-54.

54. Eversion: Turn the sole of each foot laterally. See Figure 19-55. Normal range: 5°. Major muscles: peroneus longus and peroneus brevis.

55. Inversion: Turn the sole of each foot medially. See Figure 19-56. Normal range: 5°. Major muscles: tibialis posterior and tibialis anterior.

56. Flexion: Curve the toe joints of each foot downward. See Figure 19-57. Normal range: 35°–60°. Major

FIGURE 19-54

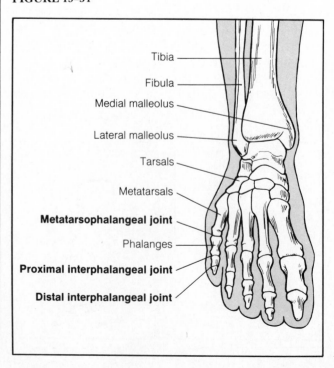

FIGURE 19-52

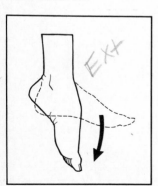

FIGURE 19-53

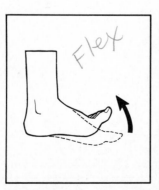

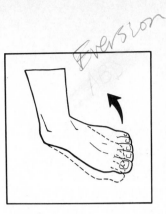

FIGURE 19-55

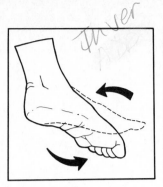

FIGURE 19-56

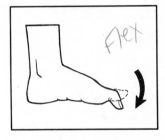

FIGURE 19-57

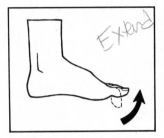

FIGURE 19-58

Trunk—gliding joint

60. Flexion: Bend the trunk toward the toes. See Figure 19–61. Normal range: 70°–90°. Major muscles: rectus abdominis, psoas major, and psoas minor.

61. Extension: Straighten the trunk from a flexed position. See Figure 19–62. Normal range: 70°–90°. Major muscles: longissimus thoracis, iliocostalis thoracis, iliocostalis lumborum, erector spinae, and longissimus cervicis.

62. Hyperextension: Bend the trunk backward. See Figure 19–63. Normal range: 20°–30°. Major muscles: longissimus thoracis, iliocostalis thoracis, iliocostalis lumborum, erector spinae, and longissimus cervicis.

muscles: flexor hallucis brevis, lumbricales pedis, and flexor digitorum brevis.

57. Extension: Straighten the toes of each foot. See Figure 19–58. Normal range: 35°–60°. Major muscles: extensor digitorum longus, extensor digitorum brevis, and extensor hallucis longus.

58. Abduction: Spread the toes of each foot apart. See Figure 19–59. Normal range: 0°–15°. Major muscles: interossei dorsales pedis and abductor hallucis.

59. Adduction: Bring the toes of each foot together. See Figure 19–60. Normal range: 0°–15°. Major muscles: adductor hallucis, interossei plantares.

FIGURE 19-59

FIGURE 19-60

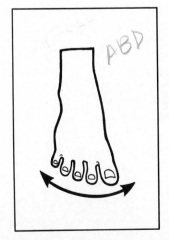

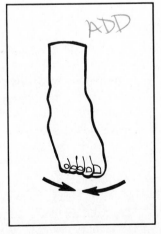

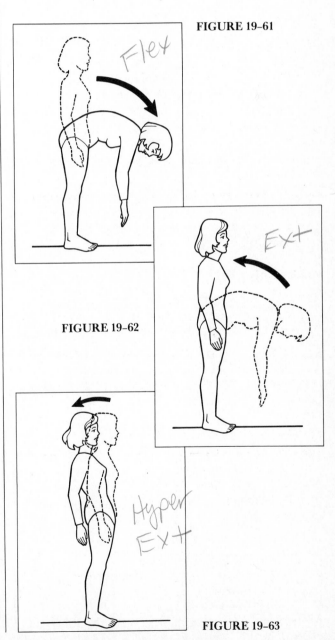

FIGURE 19-61

FIGURE 19-62

FIGURE 19-63

63. Lateral flexion: Bend the trunk to the right and to the left. See Figure 19–64. Normal range: 35° on each side. Major muscle: quadratus lumborum.

64. Rotation: Turn the upper part of the body from side to side. See Figure 19–65. Normal range: 30°–45° to each side. Major muscle: erector spinae.

For all joint movements

65. Record your findings on the appropriate record.

■ **Evaluation**

Expected outcomes

1. Joint movements are similar on the two sides of the body.

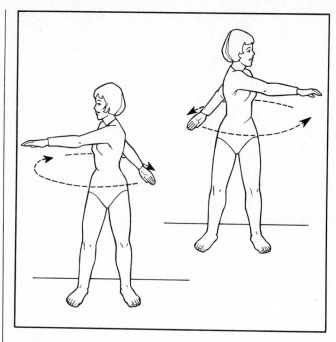

FIGURE 19–65

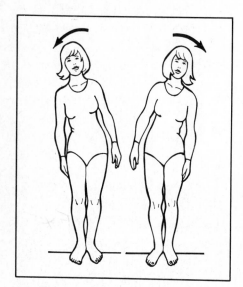

FIGURE 19–64

2. All joint movements are within the normal range.

Unexpected outcomes

1. Joint movements on left side of body are less than on right side of body.

2. Left shoulder flexion is 90°.

Upon obtaining an unexpected outcome: Report your findings to the responsible nurse and/or physician.

 TECHNIQUE 19–2 ■ Providing Passive Range-of-Motion Exercises

Passive or active-assistive exercises are often provided by nurses for patients who have paralysis or muscle weakness of a body part. Specific exercises selected depend on the patient's limitations. Guidelines for providing passive exercises include:

1. Ensure that the patient understands the reason for doing range-of-motion exercises.

2. Use good body mechanics when providing ROM exercises, to avoid muscle strain or injury to both yourself and the patient.

3. Expose only the limb being exercised, to avoid embarrassing the patient.

4. Support the patient's joints and limbs as needed to prevent muscle strain or injury. This is done by cupping joints in the palm of the hand or cradling limbs along the forearm. If a patient's joint is painful (eg, arthritic), support the limb in the muscular areas above and below the joint.

5. Use a firm, comfortable grip when handling the limb.

6. Move the body parts smoothly, slowly, and rhythmically. Jerky movements cause discomfort and possibly injury. Fast movements can cause spasticity or rigidity in some patients.

7. Avoid moving or forcing a body part beyond the patient's existing range of motion. Muscle strain, pain, and injury can result. This is particularly important for patients with flaccid (limp) paralysis, whose muscles can be stretched and joints dislocated without the patient's awareness.

8. If muscle spasticity occurs during movement, stop the movement temporarily but continue to apply slow, gentle pressure on the part until the muscle relaxes; then proceed with the motion.

9. If a contracture is present, apply slow firm pressure without causing pain, to stretch the muscle fibers.

10. If rigidity occurs, apply pressure against the rigidity, and continue the exercise slowly.

■ Assessment

Assess the patient for:

1. Ability to tolerate exercise. A planned program of passive ROM exercises should not create excessive fatigue for the patient.

2. A baseline pulse rate before beginning the passive exercises.

3. The activities he or she is not able to do, so that appropriate movements can be stressed in the exercise program. For some patients (eg, the elderly) it is not essential to achieve full range of motion in all joints. Instead, emphasize achieving a sufficient range of motion to carry out the activities of daily living, such as walking, dressing, combing hair, showering, and preparing a meal.

Additional data include:

1. The restrictions placed on passive ROM exercises. Obtain the physician's approval before beginning any exercise program.

2. The agency's policies and practices about providing passive ROM exercises. In some agencies a physiotherapist is responsible for some aspects of this care.

■ Nursing Diagnosis

Nursing diagnoses that may indicate the need to provide passive exercises include:

1. Impaired physical mobility related to:
   a. Neuromuscular impairment
   b. Musculoskeletal impairment
   c. Skeletal surgery
   d. Aging

■ Planning

Nursing goals

1. To maintain joint mobility and prevent contractures

2. To promote ultimate independence in everyday activities

■ Intervention

1. Assist the patient to a supine position on your side of the bed, and expose the body parts requiring exercise. Place the patient's feet together, place the arms at the sides, and leave space around the head and the feet.

   Rationale Positioning the patient close to the nurse prevents excessive reaching.

2. Return to the starting position after each motion. Repeat each motion three times.

Shoulder and elbow movement

Begin each exercise with the patient's arm at his or her side. Grasp the patient's arm beneath the elbow with one hand and beneath the wrist with the other hand unless otherwise indicated. See Figure 19–66.

3. Flex, externally rotate, and extend the shoulder: Move the arm up to the ceiling and toward the head of the bed. See Figure 19–67. The elbow may need to be flexed if the headboard is in the way.

FIGURE 19–66

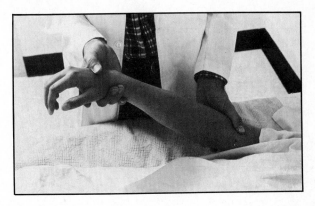

FIGURE 19–67

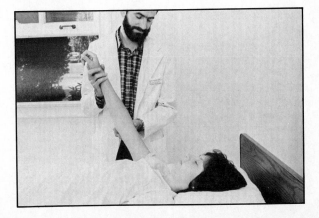

4. Abduct and externally rotate the shoulder: Move the arm away from the body (see Figure 19–68) and toward the patient's head until the hand is under the head (see Figure 19–69).

5. Adduct the shoulder: Move the arm over the body until the hand touches the patient's other hand. See Figure 19–70.

FIGURE 19–68

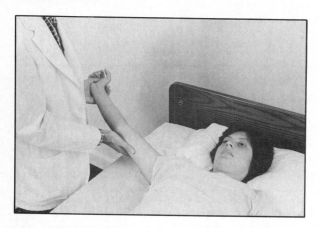

FIGURE 19–69

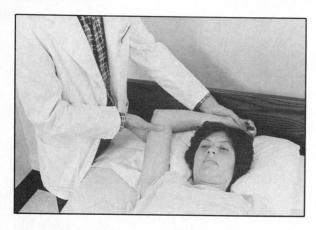

FIGURE 19–70

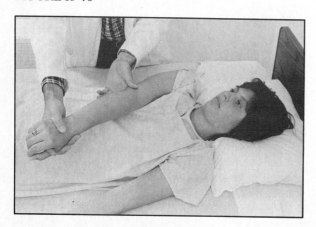

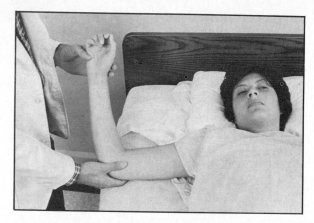

FIGURE 19–71

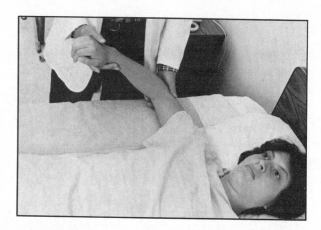

FIGURE 19–72

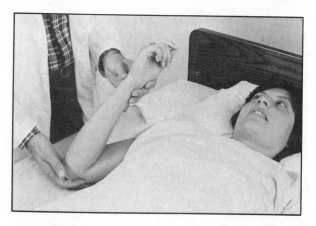

FIGURE 19–73

6. Rotate the shoulder internally and externally: Place the arm out to the side at shoulder level (90° abduction), and bend the elbow so that the forearm is at a right angle to the mattress. See Figure 19–71. Move the forearm down until the palm touches the mattress and then up until the back of the hand touches the bed. See Figure 19–72.

7. Flex and extend the elbow: Bend the elbow until the fingers touch the chin, then straighten the arm. See Figure 19–73.

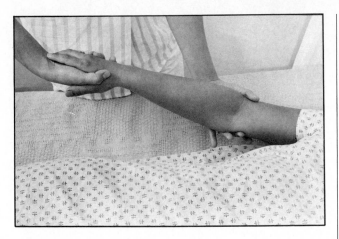

FIGURE 19–74

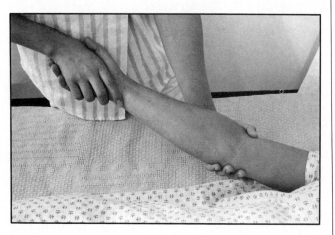

FIGURE 19–75

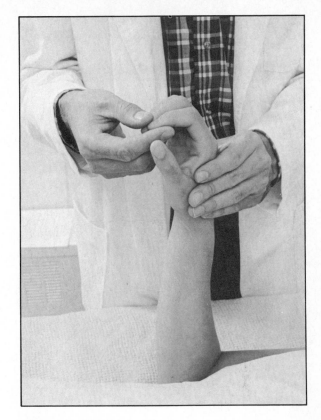

FIGURE 19–76

FIGURE 19–77

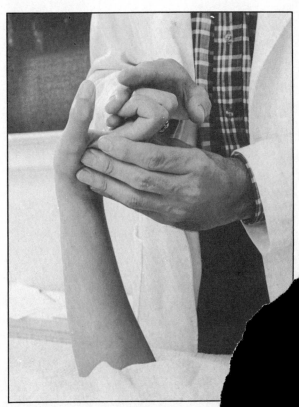

8. Pronate and supinate the forearm: Grasp the patient's hand as for a handshake and turn the palm upward (see Figure 19–74) and downward (see Figure 19–75), ensuring that only the forearm moves (not the shoulder).

Wrist and hand movement

For wrist and hand exercises, flex the patient's arm at the elbow until the forearm is at a right angle to the mattress. Support the wrist joint with one hand while your other hand manipulates the joint and the fingers. See Figure 19–76.

9. Hyperextend the wrist, and flex the fingers: Bend the wrist backward and at the same time flex the fingers, moving the tips of the fingers to the palm of the hand. See Figure 19–77. Align the wrist in a straight line with the arm and place your fingers over the patient's fingers to make a fist.

10. Flex the wrist and extend the fingers: Bend the wrist forward and at the same time extend the fingers. See Figure 19–78.
11. Abduct and oppose the thumb: Move the thumb away from the fingers and then across the hand toward the base of the little finger. See Figure 19–79.

FIGURE 19–78

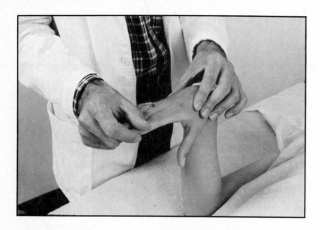

FIGURE 19–79

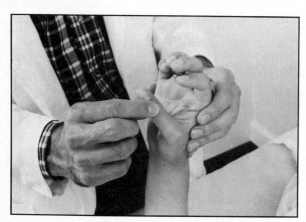

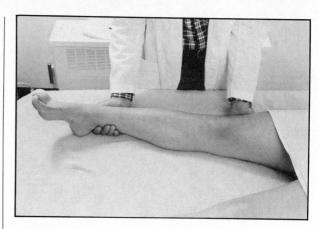

FIGURE 19–80

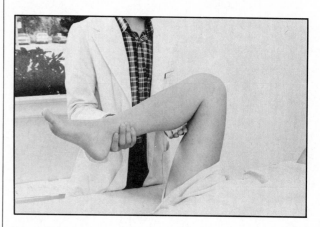

FIGURE 19–81

FIGURE 19–82

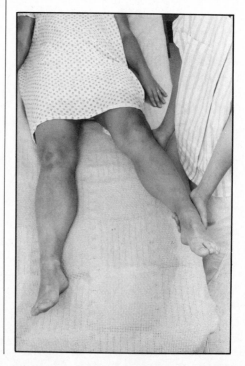

Leg and hip movement

To carry out leg and hip exercises, place one hand under the patient's knee and the other under the ankle. See Figure 19–80.

Flex and extend the hip and knee: Lift the leg and the knee, moving the knee up toward the chest as possible. Bring the leg down, straighten the and lower the leg to the bed. See Figure 19–81.

and adduct the leg: Move the leg to the side, the patient (see Figure 19–82) and back ont of the other leg (see Figure 19–83).

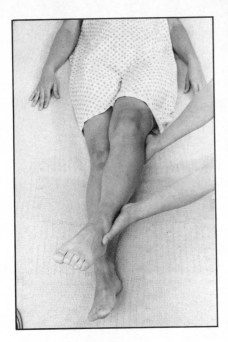
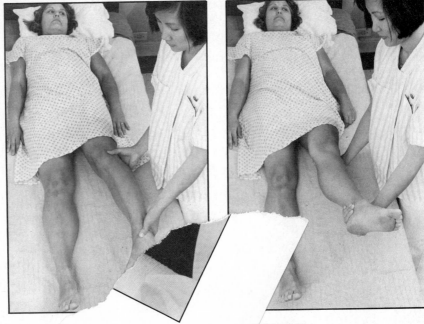

FIGURE 19–83   **FIGURE** ...   ...**RE 19–85**

14. Rotate the hip internally and externally: Roll the leg inward (see Figure 19–84), then outward (see Figure 19–85).

Ankle and foot movement

For ankle and foot exercises, place your hands in the positions described, depending on the motion to be achieved.

15. Dorsiflex the foot and stretch the Achilles tendon (heel cord): Place one hand under the patient's heel, resting your inner forearm against the bottom of the patient's foot. Place the other hand under the knee to support it. Press your forearm against the foot to move it upward toward the leg. See Figure 19–86.

16. Invert and evert the foot: Place one hand under the patient's ankle and the other over the arch of the foot. Turn the whole foot inward (see Figure 19–87), then turn it outward (see Figure 19–88).

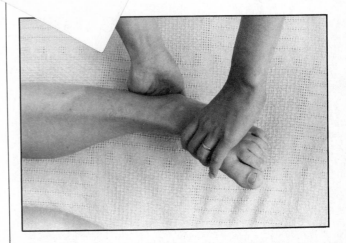

FIGURE 19–88

FIGURE 19–86

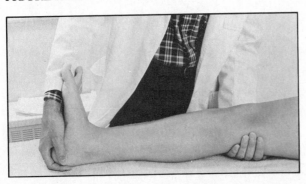
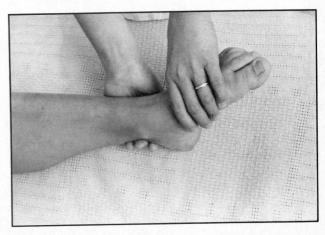

FIGURE 19-89

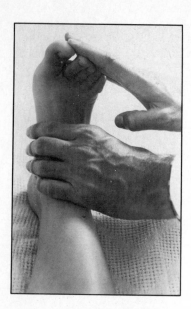

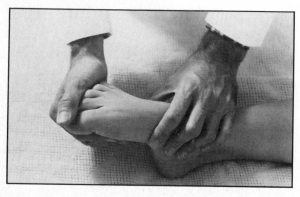

FIGURE 19-90

17. Plantar flex the foot and extend and flex the toes: Place one hand over the arch of the foot to push the foot away from the leg. Place the fingers of the other hand under the toes, to bend the toes upward (see Figure 19-89), and then over the toes, to push the toes downward (see Figure 19-90).

Neck movement

Remove the patient's pillow.

18. Flex and extend the neck: Place the palm of one hand under the patient's head and the palm of the other hand on the patient's chin. Move the head forward until the chin rests on the chest, then back to the resting supine position without the head pillow. See Figure 19-91.

19. Laterally flex the neck: Place the heels of the hands on each side of the patient's cheeks. Move the top of the head to the right and to the left. See Figure 19-92.

Hyperextension movements

20. Assist the patient to a prone or lateral position on your side of the bed.

21. Hyperextend the shoulder: Place one hand on the shoulder to keep it from lifting off the bed and the other under the patient's elbow. Pull the upper arm up and backward. See Figure 19-93.

22. Hyperextend the hip: Place one hand on the hip to stabilize it and keep it from lifting off the bed. With the other arm and hand, cradle the lower leg over the forearm, and cup the knee joint with the hand. Move the leg backward from the hip joint. See Figure 19-94.

23. Hyperextend the neck: Remove the pillow. With the patient's face down, place one hand on the forehead and the other on the back of the skull. Move the head backward. See Figure 19-95.

Following the exercises

24. Take the patient's pulse rate to assess her or his endurance of the exercise.

FIGURE 19-91

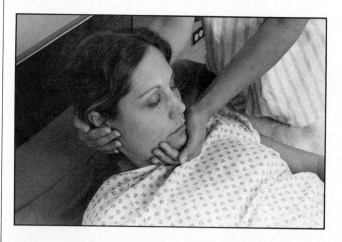

FIGURE 19-92

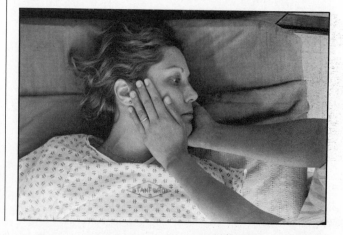

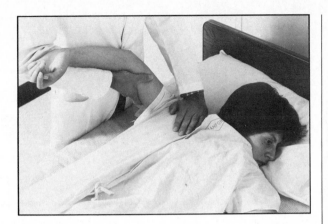

FIGURE 19–93

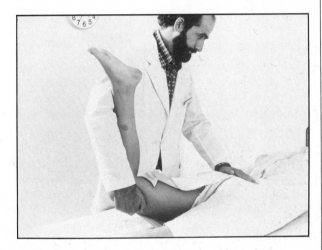

FIGURE 19–94

25. Report to the responsible nurse unusual problems or notable changes in the patient's movements, eg, rigidity or contractures.
26. Record appreciable changes or difficulties in the patient's movements.

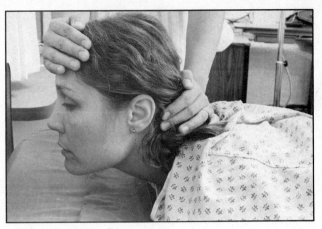

FIGURE 19–95

Sample Recording

Date	Time	Notes
6/14/87	1100	Passive exercises provided to R leg and foot. Full ROM in hip, knee, and ankle. ——— Sally S. Ames, SN

■ Evaluation

Expected outcome

Full ROM in joints selected for exercise

Unexpected outcomes

1. Limited ROM in one joint
2. Contracture
3. Spasticity
4. Rigidity

Upon obtaining an unexpected outcome: Report your findings to the responsible nurse.

AMBULATION

Ambulation is a function that most people take for granted. However, when people are ill they are often confined to bed and are thus nonambulatory. The longer a person is in bed the more difficulty he or she may have walking.

Mechanics of Ambulation

Body alignment is very important for walking. Poor body alignment causes the individual to place undue strain on some muscles and bones. Balance and coordination are also affected. As a result, the person's walk is frequently jerky and uneven and expends extra energy.

The mechanics of walking take place in two phases: the swing phase and the weight-bearing phase. From a standing (double-stance) position (both feet bearing weight), the individual starts the swing phase by shifting the body weight to one foot while lifting the other foot and bringing it forward. The foot that is brought forward is dorsiflexed. See Figure 19–96. The heel of that foot is placed on the ground, completing the swing phase. The ball of the foot then touches the floor, and the person's weight shifts to the front foot. During the swing phase the body turns slightly, but balance is maintained by moving the arm on the opposite side.

The weight-bearing phase includes shifting the body weight to the forward heel, moving the weight along the outer edge of the foot to the ball of the foot and then to the toes, from which the individual starts the next step.

The chief muscles used in walking are the muscles of the thighs and legs. Table 19–4 lists some of these muscles and their specific actions.

Common Problems

Common problems that affect walking include pathology of the muscles, disease or injury of the bones of the

TABLE 19–4 ■ Muscles Used in Walking

Muscle	Action
Psoas major	Flexes the thigh
Biceps femoris	Flexes the knee
Gluteus maximus	Extends the thigh
Quadriceps femoris	Extends the knee, flexes the thigh
Tibialis anterior	Dorsiflexes the foot
Gastrocnemius	Plantar flexes the foot
Soleus	Plantar flexes the foot

FIGURE 19–96 ■ Swing phase of walking: the foot is dorsiflexed as it is brought forward; then the heel is placed on the ground first.

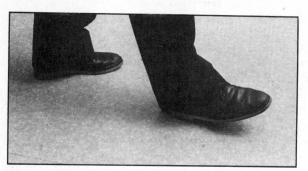

lower extremities, and impaired balance—for example, as a result of an inner ear infection or a cerebrovascular accident (CVA), which produces *hemiplegia* (loss of movement on one side of the body). Other diseases, such as multiple sclerosis and Parkinson's disease, affect walking through impairment of muscle function. A less serious and more common problem is muscle weakness. When muscles are not used for as short a period as 24 hours, they can weaken, and the joints can stiffen. Patients with a prolonged acute illness can become considerably weakened.

Nurses frequently need to assist patients in walking, and a variety of devices can be used for this purpose.

TECHNIQUE 19–3 ■ Assisting a Patient to Walk

Even patients who have been in bed for only a few days may feel weak and need assistance to walk. The amount of assistance will depend on the patient's condition, eg, age, health status, and length of inactivity.

■ Assessment

Assess the patient for:

1. Gait. The normal person is well aligned and balanced when walking. See Table 19–5 for normal and abnormal findings and some associated conditions.
2. Pace. The normal walking pace for an adult is 70 to 100 steps per minute. A fast pace is 120 steps per minute. An elderly person often has a slow pace, perhaps 40 steps per minute.
3. Vital signs for baseline data before walking, especially if this is the patient's first time walking. Note the pulse rate, respiratory rate, and blood pressure.

4. Activity tolerance when walking. In addition to the vital signs, note facial color, shortness of breath, feelings of dizziness, and weakness when ambulating.

Other data include:

1. If the patient has been confined to bed ("on bed rest"), whether there is a nursing or physician's order on the patient's chart for him or her to get up or to walk.
2. Whether the assistance of a second nurse will be required.
3. Whether the walk is to be progressively longer each time. If so, this needs to be planned with and understood by the patient.
4. The patient's medication intake. Many medications (eg, narcotics, sedatives, tranquilizers, and antihistamines) cause drowsiness, dizziness, weakness, and orthostatic hypotension, which can seriously hinder a patient's ability to walk safely.

TABLE 19–5 ■ Assessing Gait

Normal findings	Abnormal findings	Some associated conditions
Head is erect, and vertebral column straight.	Body is rigid and bent forward.	Parkinsonism
Gaze is straight ahead.	Gaze is toward ground.	Fear of falling
Toes point forward.	Toes are everted.	Flat-footedness
Kneecaps point forward.	Legs are knock-kneed with feet apart (normal until age 3 or 4).	Rickets; congenital bone disorders
	Legs are bowlegged with feet together (normal until age 2 or 2½).	Rickets; congenital bone disorders
Elbows are slightly flexed.	One elbow is flexed and held close to body.	Hemiplegia
Foot is dorsiflexed in swing phase.	One foot is plantar flexed and drags.	Hemiplegia
Arm opposite swing-through foot moves forward at same time.	Arms swing forward and do not swing with steps.	Parkinsonism
Steps are smooth, coordinated, and rhythmic.	Steps are weaving, uncoordinated, and uneven.	Alcohol or barbiturate intoxication; cerebellum disorder
	Steps are short, shuffling, and often on tiptoes.	Parkinsonism
	Gait starts slowly, gradually increases, and may be difficult to stop.	Parkinsonism
	Steps are stiff, jerking, and uncoordinated, with legs held stiffly together.	Spastic paraplegia; multiple sclerosis; spinal cord tumor
	Exaggerated lateral leaning accompanies steps.	Hip disorder

5. Whether the patient uses walking aids such as a walker, a cane, or crutches.

■ Nursing Diagnosis

Nursing diagnoses that may indicate the need to assist a patient to walk include:

1. Impaired physical mobility related to:
   a. Neuromuscular impairment
   b. Musculoskeletal impairment
   c. Surgical procedure
   d. Pain
   e. External device (eg, cast, IV tubing)
   f. Decreased motor agility
2. Sensory–perceptual alteration related to:
   a. Visual disorder
   b. Neurologic alteration
   c. Impaired oxygen transport

■ Planning

Nursing goals

1. To exercise the muscles and joints and thereby regain strength

2. To increase the patient's sense of independence
3. To increase mobility

Preambulatory exercises

Patients who have been in bed for long periods of time often need a plan of muscle tone exercises to strengthen the muscles used for walking (see Table 19–4), before attempting to walk. One of the most important muscle groups is the quadriceps femoris, which extends the knee and flexes the thigh. This group is also important for elevating the legs, eg, when walking upstairs. To strengthen these muscles the patient consciously tenses them, which draws the kneecap upward and inward. The popliteal space of the knee is pushed against the bed surface, and this raises the heels off the bed surface. See Figure 19–97. On the count of 1, the muscles are tensed; they are held during the counts of 2, 3, 4; and they are relaxed at the count of 5. The exercise should be done within the patient's tolerance—that is, without fatiguing the muscles. Carried out several times an hour during the waking day, this simple exercise significantly strengthens the muscles used for walking.

■ Intervention

1. Ensure that the patient is appropriately dressed to walk and wears shoes or slippers with nonskid soles.

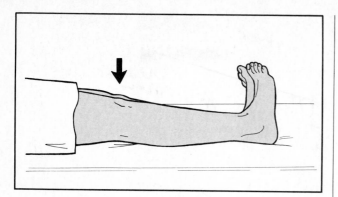

FIGURE 19-97

Rationale Proper attire and footwear prevent chilling and falling.

2. Assist the patient to sit on the edge of the bed and then to stand by the side of the bed until he or she feels secure. See chapter 16.

3. Plan the length of the walk with the patient, in light of the nursing or physician's orders. Be prepared to shorten the walk according to the patient's tolerance.

One nurse

4. Position yourself behind the patient and support him or her by the waist.

   Rationale Standing behind the patient assists the patient to stand erect, maintaining his or her center of gravity within the base of support (between the feet), instead of leaning to one side for support from the nurse.

5. If the patient has a pronounced weakness on one side, provide more support by assuming a position on the patient's affected side.

   a. Place your near arm around the patient's waist and the patient's near arm over your far shoulder. Grasp the patient's hand. This position is advisable only if the patient's height is similar to the nurse's and the patient can bear weight on both legs.

   b. Step forward with the patient, using the opposite leg to that used by the patient.

   Rationale This provides as wide a base of support as possible for the weak leg.

6. Optional: Wrap a towel (folded lengthwise) or a walking belt around the patient's waist. See Figure 19-98.

   Rationale These aids provide a firmer hold for the nurse and more support for the patient.

7. Take a couple of steps with the patient, then check that the patient has his or her balance and feels well enough to continue.

8. Ambulate the patient for the time and/or distance planned. Walk with an even gait, at the same speed as the patient, and with the same size steps.

   Rationale An even gait gives the patient a greater sense of security.

9. If the patient starts to fall and cannot regain his or her strength or balance, assume a broad stance with one foot in front of the other, and bring the patient backward so that he or she is supported by your body. Lower the patient gently to the floor, making sure that the patient's head does not hit any objects. See Figure 19-99.

   Rationale The nurse's broad stance widens the base of support for stability. One foot behind the other allows the nurse to rock backward and use the femoral muscles when supporting the patient's weight and lowering his or her center of gravity, thus preventing back strain. Bringing the patient's weight backward against the nurse's body allows gradual movement to the floor without injury to the patient.

10. Verbally recognize the patient's achievement, eg, "You walked the entire distance very well."

   Rationale Recognition enhances the patient's sense of achievement.

FIGURE 19-98

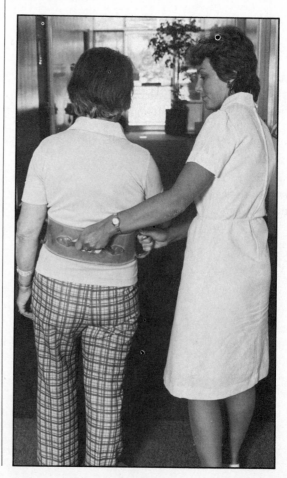

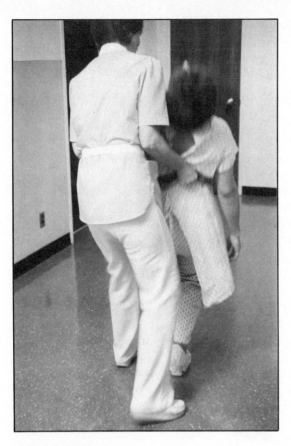

FIGURE 19-99

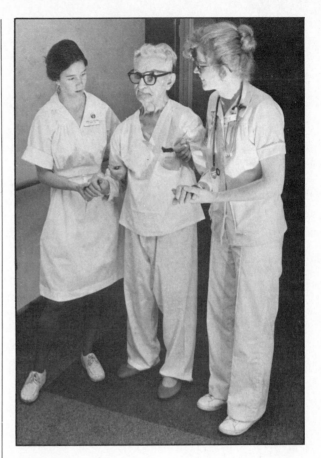

FIGURE 19-100

FIGURE 19-101

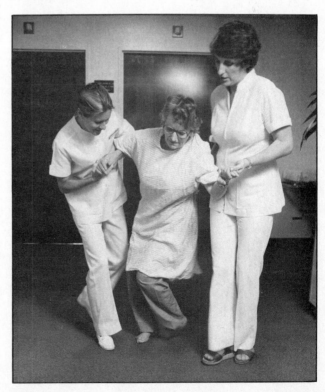

Two nurses

11. After the patient is standing, assume a position with one nurse at either side of the patient. Grasp the inferior aspect of the patient's upper arm with your nearest hand and the patient's lower arm or hand with your other hand. See Figure 19-100.

    Rationale   This provides a secure grip for each nurse.

12. Optional: Place a walking belt around the patient's waist. Each nurse grasps the side handle with the near hand and the lower aspect of the patient's upper arm with the other hand.

13. Walk in unison with the patient, using a smooth, even gait, at the same speed and with steps the same size as the patient's.

    Rationale   This gives the patient a greater feeling of security.

14. If the patient starts to fall and cannot regain his or her strength or balance, slip your arms under the patient's axillae, grasping the patient's hands, and lower the patient gently to the floor or to a nearby chair. See Figure 19-101.

    Rationale   Placing the nurses' arms under the patient's axillae evenly balances the patient's weight between the two nurses, preventing injury to both the nurses and the patient.

15. Verbally recognize the patient's achievement, eg, "You walked farther than yesterday."

    Rationale Recognition enhances the patient's sense of achievement and well-being.

16. After the walk, align the patient comfortably in the bed or a chair, whichever is appropriate.

17. Assess the patient's pulse and blood pressure to compare with baseline data before the walk.

18. Record the time of the walk, the distance walked or time taken, and the patient's response.

19. Adjust the nursing care plan, if necessary, to indicate the need for walking aids, assistance required by the nurse, etc.

■ Evaluation

Expected outcomes

1. Walked the specified distance with or without support

2. Pulse rate and blood pressure stable

3. Respirations normal

4. Gait well aligned and balanced

5. Pace 70 steps/minute

Unexpected outcomes

1. Unable to stand unsupported

2. Unable to walk the specified distance with or without support

3. Shortness of breath with slight exertion

4. Pulse rate 20 beats/minute higher after walk

5. Systolic blood pressure dropped 20 mm Hg from lying to standing position

6. Excessive fatigue with walking

7. Gait disturbance (see Table 19–5 on page 451)

Upon obtaining an unexpected outcome:

1. Readjust the patient's goals.

2. Report your findings to the responsible nurse or physician.

TECHNIQUE 19–4 ■ Assisting a Patient to Use a Cane

Three main types of canes are used today: the simple straight-legged cane, the tripod or crab cane, which has three prongs, and the quad cane, which has four legs and provides the most support. See Figure 19–102. Canes should have rubber caps on the tips of the legs to improve traction and prevent slipping. The four-legged cane may be equipped with two tips and two wheels, permitting the patient to keep it in contact with the ground all the time. The patient tilts the cane toward the body, which lifts the tips while the wheels remain on the ground, and then pushes the cane forward. The standard cane is 91 cm (36 in) long; aluminum canes are available that can be adjusted from 56 to 97 cm (22 to 38 inches). Patients use either one or two canes depending on the amount of support they require.

■ Assessment

Assess the patient for:

1. Ability to walk with a cane. Note whether the patient requires instruction about using a cane.

2. Body alignment standing and walking with a cane.

FIGURE 19–102 ■ A quad cane.

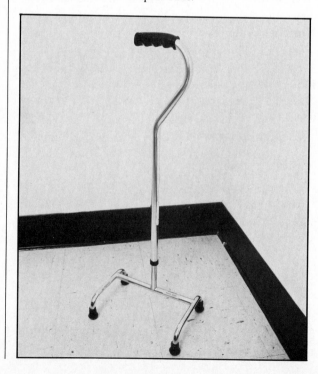

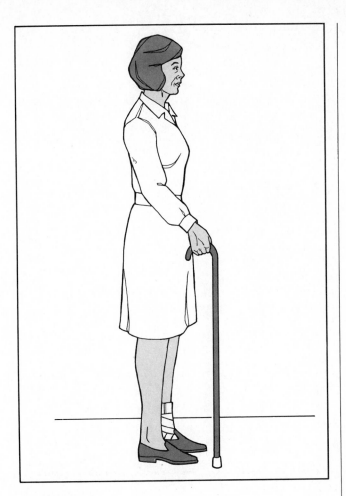

FIGURE 19-103

3. Gait when walking with the cane. See Table 19-5 on page 451.

■ **Nursing Diagnosis** See Technique 19-3 on page 451.

■ **Planning**

Nursing goals

1. To enhance the patient's balance and gait alignment
2. To provide additional support, for example, when the patient has weakness on one side of the body even though weight bearing is possible

Equipment

An appropriate cane with rubber tips

■ **Intervention**

1. Have the patient hold the cane on the stronger side of the body.
   Rationale This provides more balance and support. The arm opposite the advancing foot normally

swings forward when walking, so the hand holding the cane will come forward and the can will support the weaker leg.

2. Have the patient stand so that the cane is 15 cm (6 in) to the side and 15 cm (6 in) in front of the near foot, and so that the elbow is slightly flexed. See Figure 19-103.
   Rationale This provides the best balance and prevents the patient from leaning on the cane. In this position the patient stands erect, with her or his center of gravity within the base of support.

3. Ensure that the patient has his or her balance and feels well enough to walk.

4. For maximum support:
   a. The patient moves the cane forward about 30 cm (1 ft), or the distance that is comfortable to the patient. See Figure 19-104, *A*. The weight is borne by both legs.
   b. The patient moves the affected leg forward to the cane. See Figure 19-104, *B*. The weight is now borne by the unaffected leg and the cane.
   c. The patient moves the unaffected leg forward ahead of the cane and the affected leg. See Figure

FIGURE 19-104

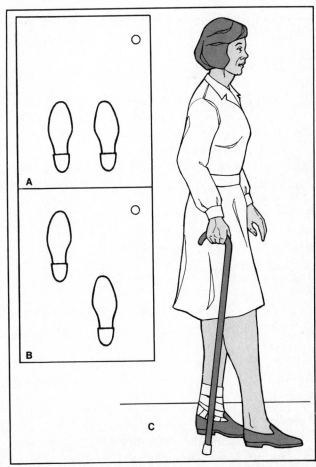

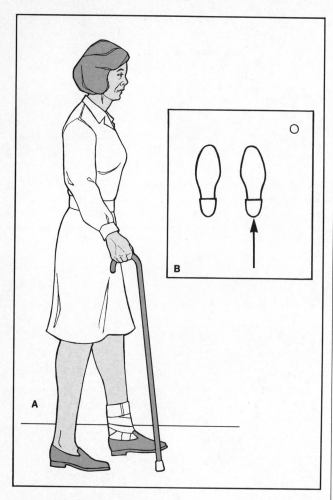

FIGURE 19-105

19–104, *C.* The weight is now borne by the affected leg and the cane.

5. For less support:

   a. The patient moves the cane and the affected leg forward at the same time. See Figure 19–105, *A.* The weight is borne by the unaffected leg.

   b. The patient moves the unaffected leg forward. See Figure 19–105, *B.* The weight is now borne by the cane and the affected leg.

6. Walk beside the patient on the affected side.

   Rationale The patient is most likely to fall toward the affected side.

7. Walk the patient for the time or distance indicated on the nursing care plan.

8. If the patient loses his or her balance or strength and is unable to regain it, slide your hand up to the patient's axilla, and take a broad stance to provide a base of support. Have the patient rest against your hip until assistance arrives, or gently lower yourself and the patient to the floor.

9. Verbally recognize the patient's achievement.

   Rationale Recognition enhances the patient's sense of achievement and well-being.

10. After returning from the walk, align the patient suitably and comfortably in the bed or a chair.

11. Record relevant assessment data on the patient's record.

■ **Evaluation** See Technique 19–3 on page 454.

TECHNIQUE 19-5 ■ Assisting a Patient to Use a Walker

Walkers are mechanical devices for ambulatory patients who need more support than a cane provides. There are many types of walkers of different shapes and sizes, with devices suited to individual needs. The standard type is made of polished aluminum. It has four legs with rubber tips and plastic hand grips. See Figure 19–106. Many walkers have adjustable legs.

The standard walker needs to be picked up to be used. The patient therefore requires partial strength in both hands and wrists, strong elbow extensors, such as the triceps brachii, and strong shoulder depressors, such as the pectoralis minor. The patient also needs the ability to bear at least partial weight in both legs. Four-wheeled models of walkers do not need to be picked up to be moved, but they are less stable than the standard walker.

■ **Assessment**

Assess the patient for:

1. Ability to walk with a walker. Note the strength in the hands, arms, and shoulders as well as the ability to walk.

2. Body alignment, standing and walking with a walker.

3. Understanding about use of the walker. Provide an explanation and demonstration if needed.

■ **Planning**

Nursing goals

1. To provide stability and support for the patient when walking
2. To enhance the patient's balance
3. To provide a sense of security to the patient

■ **Nursing Diagnosis**   See Technique 19–3 on page 451.

■ **Intervention**

1. Help the patient to stand in front of the walker and grasp the hand grips.
2. Adjust the height of the walker so that the hand bar is just below the patient's waist and the patient's elbows are slightly flexed.
   Rationale   This position helps the patient assume a more normal stance. A walker that is too low causes the patient to stoop; one that is too high makes the patient stretch and reach.
3. For a patient with two weak legs:
   a. The patient moves the walker ahead about 15 cm (6 in). The weight is borne by both legs.
   b. The patient moves the right foot up to the walker. The weight is borne by the left leg and both arms.
   c. The patient moves the left foot up to the right foot. The weight is borne by the right leg and both arms.
4. For a patient with one affected leg:
   a. The patient moves the walker and the weak leg ahead together about 15 cm (6 in). The weight is borne by the stronger leg.
   b. The patient moves the stronger leg ahead. The weight is borne by the affected leg and both arms.
5. Walk closely behind and slightly to the side of the patient.
   Rationale   In this position the nurse can provide support if the patient loses balance and falls.

6. Ambulate the patient for the time or distance recommended on the nursing care plan. Carefully observe the patient's tolerance to activity.
7. If the patient starts to fall, hold him or her under the axillae, and take a broad stance. Have the patient rest against your body until assistance comes, or lower yourself and the patient gently to the floor.
8. Verbally recognize the patient's achievement.
   Rationale   Recognition enhances the patient's sense of achievement and well-being.
9. After the walk, align the patient suitably and comfortably in the bed or a chair.

■ **Evaluation**   See Technique 19–3 on page 454.

FIGURE 19–106   ■   A standard walker.

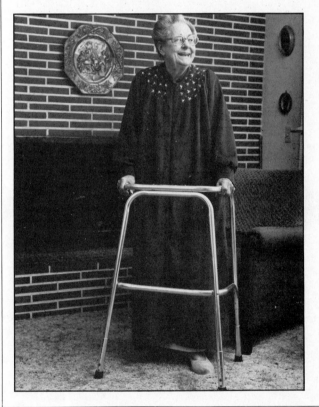

Crutches

Walking with crutches may be a temporary situation for some people and a permanent one for others. Crutches should enable a person to ambulate independently; therefore, it is important to learn to use them properly.

There are a number of kinds of crutches. The most frequently used are the *underarm* or *axillary crutch* with hand bars and the *Lofstrand crutch,* which extends only to the forearm. The underarm crutch can be extended. It has double uprights, an underarm bar, and a hand bar. See Figure 19–107, *A.* The Lofstrand crutch is a single adjustable tube of aluminum to which are attached a curved piece of steel, a rubber-covered hand bar, and a metal forearm cuff. See Figure 19–107, *B.* This type of

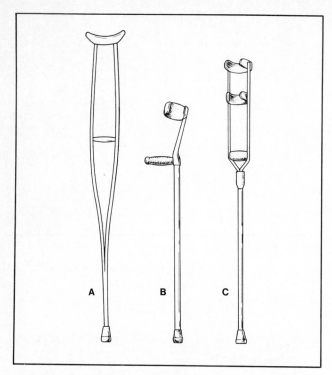

FIGURE 19–107 ■ Three types of crutches: **A**, axillary crutch; **B**, Lofstrand crutch; **C**, Canadian (elbow extensor) crutch.

crutch is most useful as a substitute for a cane. The metal cuff around the forearm and the metal bar stabilize the wrists and thus make walking safer and easier. The person can release the hand bar to use his or her hand, and the metal cuff will hold the crutch in place, while a cane would fall.

The *Canadian* or *elbow extensor crutch* is like the Lofstrand in that it is made of a single tube of aluminum with lateral attachments, a hand bar, and a cuff for the forearm, but it also has a cuff for the upper arm. See Figure 19–107, *C*. This crutch is usually used by patients who require support for weak extensor muscles of the forearm and trunk, (eg, weak triceps brachii).

All crutches require suction tips, which are usually made of rubber. The tips help prevent the crutches from slipping on a floor surface.

Measuring patients for crutches

When measuring patients for axillary crutches it is most important to obtain the correct length for the crutches and the correct placement of the hand piece. If the crutches are too long, the shoulders are forced upward, and the patient cannot push his or her body off the ground. If the crutches are too short, the patient hunches over uncomfortably and has poor body alignment. There are two methods of measuring crutch length:

1. Have the patient lie in a supine position, and measure from the anterior fold of the axilla to a point 10 cm (4 in) lateral from the heel of the foot. See Figure 19–108.
2. Have the patient stand erect, and position the crutch tips 5 cm (2 in) in front of and 15 cm (6 in) to the side of the feet. See Figure 19–109. Make sure the shoulder rest of the crutch is at least 3 finger widths, ie, 2.5 to 5 cm (1 to 2 in), below the axilla. See Figure 19–110.

To determine the correct placement of the hand bar:

1. Have the patient stand upright and support his or her weight by the hand grips of the crutches.
2. Measure the angle of elbow flexion. It should be about 30°. A goniometer (see Figure 19–3 earlier) may be used to verify the correct angle.

Guidelines about crutches

1. The weight of the body should be borne by the arms rather than the axillae. Pressure on the axillae can injure the radial nerve and eventually cause crutch palsy, a paresis (weakness of the muscles) of the forearm, wrist, and hand.
2. The patient should maintain erect posture, to prevent strain on muscles and joints and to maintain balance.

FIGURE 19–108 ■ Measuring for crutch length while the patient is in the supine position.

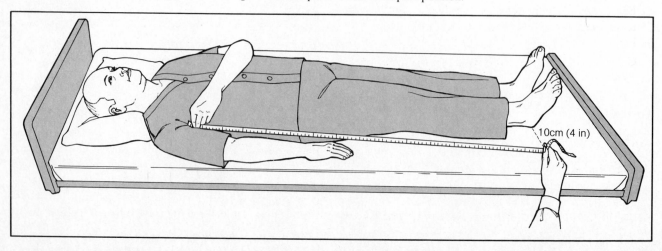

10cm (4 in)

Five major muscle groups are used:

1. The flexor muscles of the arms (eg, the pectoralis major and brachialis) move the crutches forward.

2. The extensor muscles of the forearms (eg, the triceps brachii) hold the elbows up at an angle while the body weight is raised off the ground.

3. The finger and thumb flexors (eg, the flexor pollicis brevis) allow the hands to grasp the hand bars.

4. The muscles that dorsiflex the wrists (eg, the flexor carpi radialis) maintain the hands in the correct position on the hand bars.

5. The shoulder girdle depressors and the downward rotators (eg, the pectoralis minor) support the body weight off the floor.

Exercises are suggested for patients before crutch walking to develop and strengthen these muscle groups. A plan of exercises should be developed for each patient. The following exercises are recommended:

1. The patient flexes and extends the arms in several directions.

2. The patient comes from a supine position to a sitting position by flexing the elbows and pushing the hands against the bed surface. See Figure 19–111. This exercise strengthens the flexor and extensor muscles of the arms and the muscles that dorsiflex the wrist.

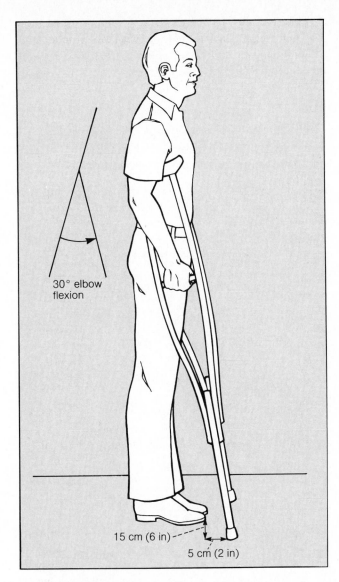

FIGURE 19–109 ■ The standing position to measure the correct length of crutches.

30° elbow flexion

15 cm (6 in)

5 cm (2 in)

FIGURE 19–110 ■ The three-finger space between crutch top and axilla.

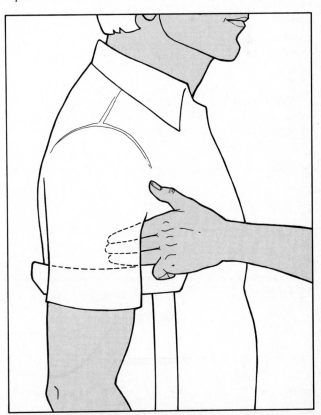

3. The shoulder rests of axillary crutches can be slightly padded for comfort, but the padding must not press against the axillae.

4. Each step taken with crutches should be a comfortable distance for the patient. It is wise to start with a small rather than a large step.

5. Crutches should have rubber (suction) tips to prevent slipping.

6. Crutch tips should be inspected regularly and replaced if worn.

7. Crutch tips should be kept dry to maintain their surface friction. If they become wet, the patient should dry them well before use.

Exercises for crutch walking

In crutch walking, the patient's weight is borne by the muscles of the shoulder girdle and the upper extremities.

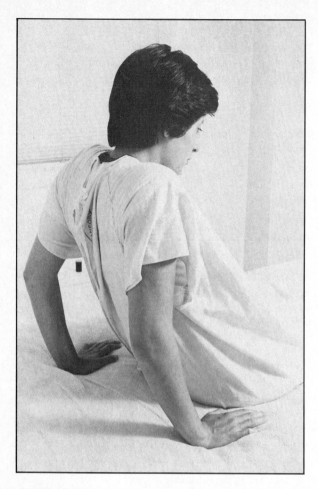

FIGURE 19-111 ■ Strengthening the flexor and extensor muscles of the arms and the muscles that dorsiflex the wrist.

3. The patient pushes his or her body off the bed surface by pushing down with the hands and extending the elbows. See Figure 19-112. This exercise is particularly useful in strengthening the extensor muscles of the arms.

4. The patient squeezes a rubber ball or a gripper with the hands. This exercise strengthens the flexor muscles of the fingers.

Crutch gaits

The crutch gait is the gait a person assumes on crutches by alternating his or her weight on one or both legs and the crutches. The gaits discussed in Technique 19-6 are the four-point gait, three-point gait, two-point gait, swing-to, and swing-through gaits. The gait used depends on the following individual factors:

1. Ability to take steps
2. Ability to bear weight and keep balance in a standing position on both legs or only one
3. Ability to bear weight and keep balance with the upper body, eg, to push off from a chair or bed by using the crutches
4. Ability to hold the body erect

FIGURE 19-112 ■ Strengthening the extensor muscles of the arms in preparation for crutch-walking.

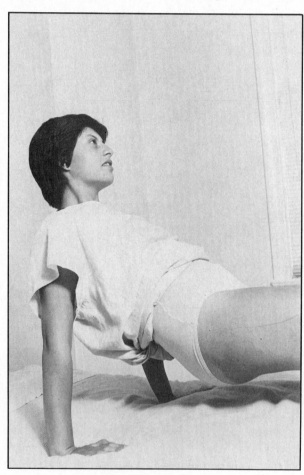

TECHNIQUE 19-6 ■ Assisting a Patient to Use Crutches

The choice of a crutch gait for a specific patient to learn is usually made by a physiotherapist or a physician. Nurses are increasingly involved in these decisions, however. Often a physiotherapist teaches the crutch gait initially, but nurses give follow-through lessons. In some instances, nurses alone teach the patient the technique.

Patients also need instruction about how to get into and out of chairs and go up and down stairs safely. All of these crutch skills are best taught before the patient is discharged and preferably before the patient has surgery.

■ Assessment

Assess the patient for:

1. Leg or foot disability. Can the patient bear weight on one leg only or partially on the affected leg or foot?
2. Ability to maintain balance in an erect standing position.
3. Muscle strength, particularly in the arms and unaffected leg. See Technique 10–17 on page 233.
4. Previous experience with crutches, and learning needs.

■ Nursing Diagnosis   See Technique 19–3 on page 451.

■ Planning

Nursing goals

1. To help the patient walk with crutches safely and with minimum expenditure of energy
2. To help the patient on crutches move safely into and out of a chair or bed
3. To help the patient on crutches go safely up and down stairs

Equipment

1. Crutches with suction tips, hand grips, and axillary pads
2. A walking belt (optional)

■ Intervention

1. Ensure that the patient is wearing supportive, nonskid shoes with laces or buckles.

Tripod position

This is the basic crutch stance used before crutch walking.

2. Have the patient stand erect, facing straight ahead, and place the tips of the crutches 15 cm (6 in) in front of the feet and 15 cm (6 in) to the side of each foot. See Figure 19–113.

    Rationale   The tripod position provides a wide base of support and enhances stability and balance.

3. Stand slightly behind the patient and on his or her

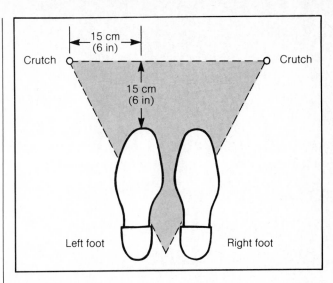

FIGURE 19–113

affected side. If the patient is unsteady, place a walking belt around his or her waist; grasp it from above, not from below.

Rationale   The patient is more likely to fall toward the affected side. In this position the nurse can support the patient if he or she loses balance and falls. A walking belt provides more psychologic support to the patient. It is held from above to counteract a fall more effectively.

Four-point alternate gait

This is the most elementary and safest gait, providing at least three points of support at each time, but it requires coordination. It can be used when walking in crowds because it does not require much space. For this gait the patient needs to be able to bear weight on both legs. See Figure 19–114 (reading from bottom to top).

4. Have the patient:
    a. Move the right crutch ahead a suitable distance, eg, 10 to 15 cm (4 to 6 in).
    b. Move the left foot forward, preferably to the level of the left crutch.
    c. Move the left crutch forward.
    d. Move the right foot forward.

Three-point gait

For this gait the patient must be able to bear her or his entire weight on the unaffected leg. The two crutches and the unaffected leg bear weight alternately. See Figure 19–115 (reading from bottom to top).

5. Have the patient:
    a. Move both crutches and the weaker leg forward.
    b. Move the stronger leg forward.

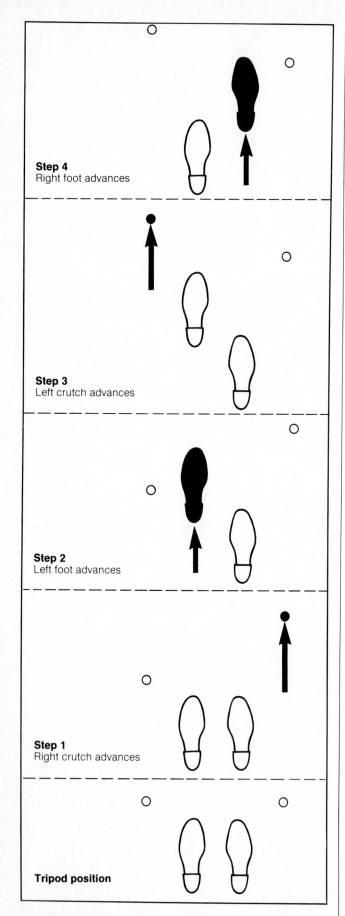

FIGURE 19–114

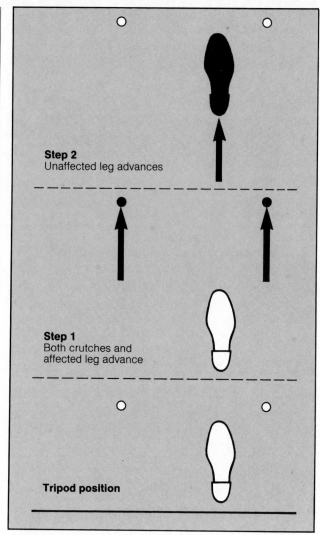

FIGURE 19–115

Two-point alternate gait

This gait is faster than the four-point gait. It requires more balance, because only two points support the body at one time; it also requires at least partial weight bearing on each foot. In this gait, arm movements with the crutches are similar to the arm movements during normal walking. See Figure 19–116 (reading from bottom to top).

6. Have the patient:

    a. Move the left crutch and the right foot forward together.

    b. Move the right crutch and the left foot ahead together.

Swinging-to gait

The swing gaits are used by patients with paralysis of the legs and hips. The swing-to gait is the easier of these two gaits. See Figure 19–117.

7. Have the patient:

    a. Move both crutches ahead together.

b. Lift his or her weight by the arms and swing to the crutches.

Swinging-through gait

This gait requires considerable skill, strength, and coordination. See Figure 19–118.

8. Have the patient:
   a. Move both crutches forward together.
   b. Lift his or her weight by the arms and swing through and beyond the crutches.

Getting into a chair

9. Ensure that the chair has armrests and is secure or braced against a wall. Have the patient:
   a. Stand with the back of the unaffected leg centered against the chair. See Figure 19–119.

   Rationale The chair helps support the patient during the next steps.

FIGURE 19–116

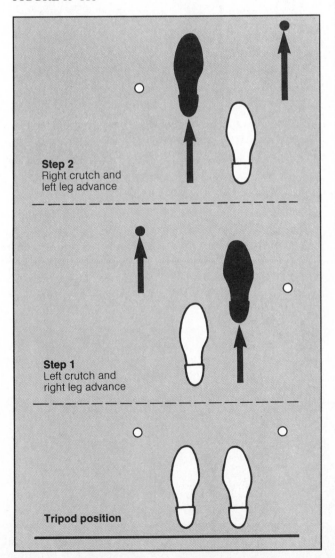

FIGURE 19–117

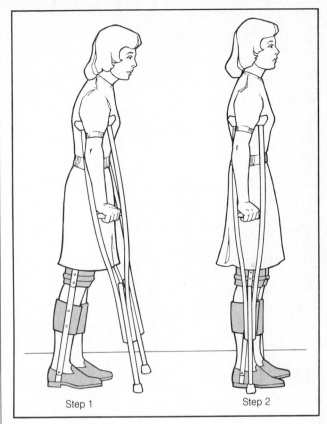

FIGURE 19–118

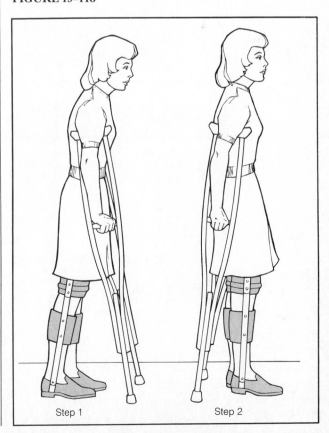

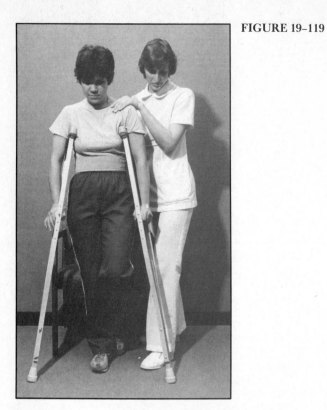

FIGURE 19–119

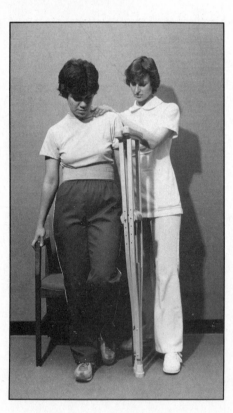

FIGURE 19–120

b. Transfer the crutches to the hand on the affected side. Hold the crutches by the hand bars. Grasp the arm of the chair with the hand on the unaffected side. See Figure 19–120.

Rationale This allows the patient to support the body weight on the arms and the unaffected leg.

c. Lean forward, flex the knees and hips, and lower into the chair.

Getting out of a chair

10. Have the patient:
    a. Move forward to the edge of the chair, and place the unaffected leg slightly under or at the edge of the chair.

    Rationale This position facilitates standing up from the chair and achieving balance, since the unaffected leg is supported against the edge of the chair.

    b. Grasp the crutches by the hand bars in the hand on the affected side, and grasp the arm of the chair by the hand on the unaffected side.

    Rationale The body weight is placed on the crutches and the hand on the armrest, to provide additional support to the unaffected leg when rising to stand.

    c. Push down on the crutches and the chair armrest while elevating his or her body out of the chair.

    d. Assume the tripod position before moving.

Going up stairs

11. Stand behind the patient and slightly to the affected side.
12. Have the patient:
    a. Assume the tripod position at the bottom of the stairs.
    b. Transfer the body weight to the crutches and move the unaffected leg onto the step. See Figure 19–121.
    c. Transfer the body weight to the unaffected leg on the step and move the crutches and affected leg up to the step.

    Rationale The affected leg is always supported by the crutches.

    d. Repeat steps b and c until the top of the stairs is reached.

Going down stairs

13. Stand one step below the patient on the affected side.
14. Have the patient:
    a. Assume the tripod position at the top of the stairs.
    b. Take the body weight on the unaffected leg, and move the crutches and affected leg down onto the next step. See Figure 19–122.
    c. Transfer the body weight to the crutches, and move unaffected leg to that step.

    Rationale The affected leg is always supported by the crutches.

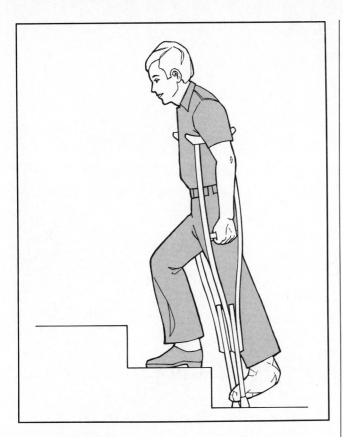

FIGURE 19-121

    d. Repeat steps b and c until the bottom of the stairs is reached.

For all crutch skills

15. Record on the patient's chart your teaching and any problems the patient had.
16. Adjust the nursing care plan as needed to indicate learning achievements and needs.

■ Evaluation

Expected outcomes

1. Walked to end of hall and back, using three-point crutch gait

2. Moved from chair to standing position without assistance, using crutches
3. Went up and down three stairs using crutches

Unexpected outcomes

1. Unable to move from a chair to a standing position using crutches without assistance
2. Unable to balance on crutches without assistance

Upon obtaining an unexpected outcome: Report your findings to the responsible nurse and/or physician.

FIGURE 19-122

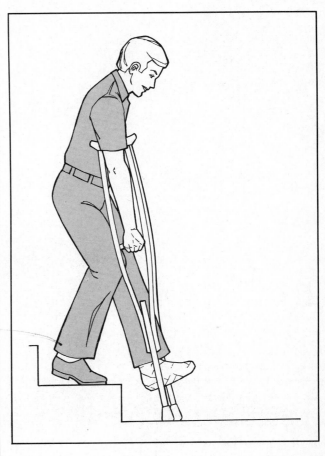

TECHNIQUE 19-7 ■ Applying and Removing Braces

A brace is a supportive appliance used for one of the following reasons:

1. To support the body weight
2. To prevent deformities
3. To correct deformities
4. To prevent abnormal movement

There are many types of braces. They are usually made of a combination of leather, plastic, metal, and/or cloth.

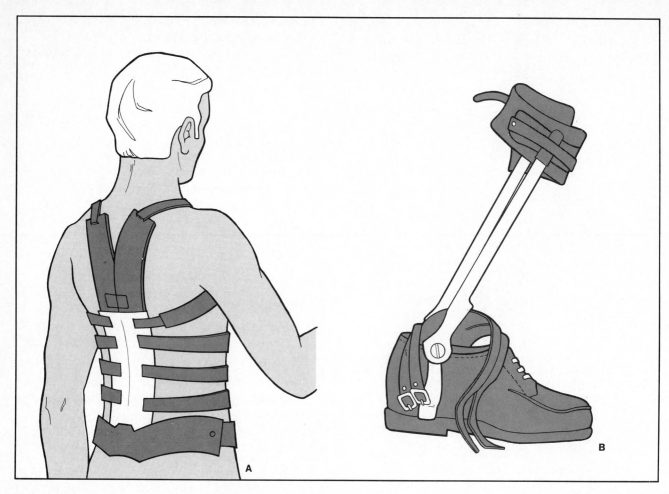

FIGURE 19-123 ■ **A,** one type of back brace; **B,** a short leg brace.

Some braces worn over a joint, such as an ankle or a knee, are hinged to permit movement of the joint. These hinges require weekly lubrication with grease. Because braces are usually made to fit a specific person, they are not interchangeable among people. It is very important that a brace be worn correctly if the purpose of the brace is to be accomplished. Commonly used braces are those worn on the lumbar region of the back (eg, the Knight spinal brace) and on a leg (eg, the Klenzak short leg brace). See Figure 19-123.

■ **Assessment**

Assess:

1. The bony prominences under the brace and the skin areas on the upper and lower edges of the brace. These can become irritated from the brace and may require special skin care. See chapter 14. A thin piece of sponge rubber can be used to pad these areas.

2. How the brace fits the patient.

3. The brace for any missing parts, eg, screws, lining, or hooks.

■ **Planning**

Nursing goals

1. To restrict motion of a joint

2. To support weakened muscles

3. To support paralyzed muscles, for example, the abdominal musculature

4. To prevent a contracture (eg, a brace for the lower extremities may be applied to prevent hip flexion contractures)

Equipment

The patient's brace

■ **Intervention**

Applying a back brace

1. Assist the patient to put on a shirt.
   Rationale The shirt provides comfort and prevents the brace from becoming soiled with perspiration.

2. Assist the patient to a supine position on the bed.
3. Roll the patient to his or her side facing toward you. Maintain the alignment of the patient's neck and back.
4. Fit the brace on the side and back. Make sure that the upper edge of the brace is in place and that it fits the curves of the patient's back.
5. Roll the patient again to his or her back, maintaining the head and back alignment.
6. Bring the straps from under the patient to the front.
7. Secure the straps so that the brace fits firmly.
8. Check for pressure areas created by the brace or straps, particularly over bony prominences, such as the hips (the iliac spines), the scapulae, and the sternum (breastbone).

Removing a back brace

9. Assist the patient to a supine position on the bed.
10. Unfasten the straps at the front.
11. Tuck the straps closest to the near side under the patient.
12. Turn the patient toward you on her or his side, maintaining the alignment of the head and back.
13. Remove the brace.
14. Assist the patient to a comfortable position, and align him or her correctly.

Applying a short leg brace

15. Assist the patient to a sitting position on the edge of the bed. Assist the patient to dress.
16. If the brace has a hinge, check that it is functioning, and grease it if necessary.

FIGURE 19–124

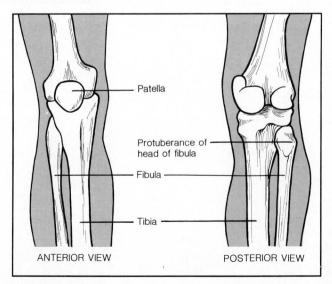

ANTERIOR VIEW   POSTERIOR VIEW

- Patella
- Protuberance of head of fibula
- Fibula
- Tibia

17. Put the patient's foot into the shoe attached to the brace. Ensure that the foot is correctly and comfortably in place and that the toes are not caught on the side or curled under the foot.
18. Fasten the shoe firmly but not so tightly that it interferes with the blood circulation.
19. Put the upper cuff of the brace around the calf of the patient's leg.
20. Secure the brace so that it is snug but not tight. There should be about 1 cm (0.5 in) space between the cuff and the skin.
21. Check for any pressure areas created by the brace, particularly over bony prominences, eg, the medial and lateral malleoli of the ankle. For a long leg brace, check the protuberance of the head of the fibula on the lateral aspect of the knee. See Figure 19–124.

Removing a short leg brace

22. Assist the patient to a sitting position on the edge of the bed.
23. Unfasten the cuff and the shoe.
24. Remove the brace and the shoe.
25. Assist the patient to a comfortable position, and align him or her appropriately.

For all braces

26. Assess the response of the patient to use of the brace, including ability to move with the brace, discomfort, relief of pain, perceptions of support, irritated skin areas, and fatigue.
27. Record on the patient's chart the use of the brace, including any assessment data.
28. Adjust the nursing care plan as needed.

Sample Recording

Date	Time	Notes
2/24/87	1200	Wore back brace for 30 min. Stated felt support and no discomfort. No reddened skin areas noted. ————————— ——————Muriel B. Rawlings, NS

■ Evaluation

Expected outcomes

1. Moved effectively with brace on
2. Skin over bony prominences intact
3. No complaints of discomfort with brace on

Unexpected outcomes

1. Irritated skin over bony prominences

2. Discomfort or pain when wearing brace

3. Difficulty moving with brace on

Upon obtaining an unexpected outcome:

1. Report your findings to the responsible nurse.

2. Do not apply the brace again until the problem is corrected.

References

Carnevali D, Brueckner S: Immobilization: Reassessment of a concept. *Am J Nurs* (July) 1970; 70:1502–1507.

Ciuca R, Bradish J: Passive range-of-motion exercises encore: A handbook. *Nursing 78* (July) 1978; 8:59–65.

Deaver GG: *Abnormal Gait Patterns Etiology, Pathology, Diagnosis and Methods of Treatment: Crutches, Braces, Canes and Walkers.* Rehabilitation Monograph No. 30. Institute of Rehabilitation Medicine, New York University Medical Center, nd.

Gordon M: Assessing activity tolerance. *Am J Nurs* (January) 1976; 76:72–75.

Guyton AC: *Textbook of Medical Physiology,* 6th ed. Saunders, 1981.

Olson EV: The hazards of immobility. *Am J Nurs* (April) 1967; 67:780–797.

Ranalls J: Crutches and walkers. *Nursing 72* (December) 1972; 2:21–24.

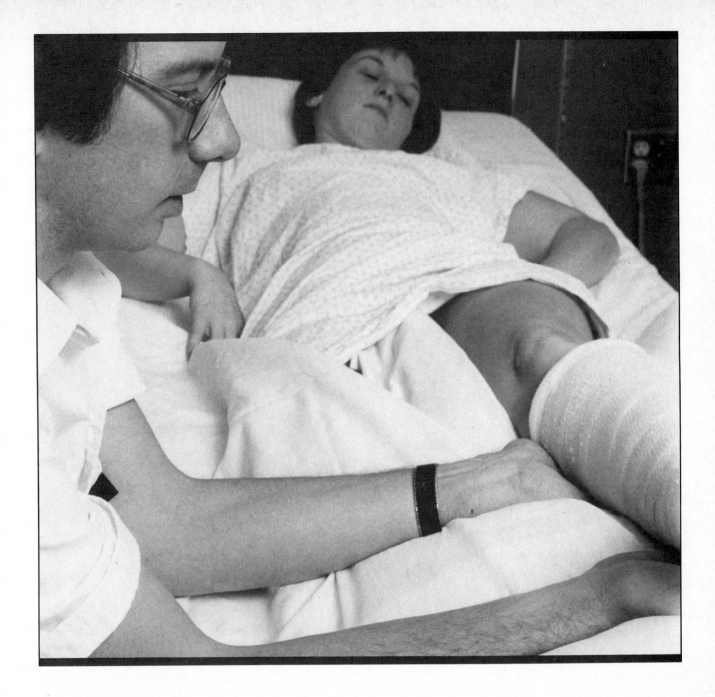

CAST CARE

20

Casts are generally applied to immobilize a body part so that healing can take place without further injury. The degree of immobilization of the person varies with the type of cast. Some people are confined to bed for weeks or even months, while others are able to resume most daily activities with only slight inconvenience from the cast. Although casts are applied for reasons other than fractures, this chapter focuses on patients with fractures.

Essential nursing care for patients who have casts includes interventions to prevent pressure on underlying blood vessels, nerves, and the skin; to maintain the integrity of the cast itself; and to prevent problems associated with immobility.

Chapter Outline

Fractures

Casts

■ Technique 20–1 Assisting with a Cast Application

Objectives

Upon completion of this chapter, the student will:

1. Know essential terms and facts about fractures and casts, and the nurse's responsibilities in regard to them
   1.1 Identify differences between closed and open fractures
   1.2 Describe fracture repair
   1.3 Describe three ways fractures are reduced
   1.4 Identify various cast materials
   1.5 Identify selected types of casts
   1.6 Identify essential aspects of assisting with cast application
   1.7 Identify ways a cast is supported, elevated, and handled before it is dry
   1.8 Identify interventions used to enhance the drying of a cast
   1.9 Identify observations required to detect neurovascular impairments and skin irritation following cast application
   1.10 Identify interventions required to prevent skin irritation following cast application
   1.11 Identify interventions required to keep a cast dry
   1.12 Identify essential considerations for positioning patients with casts
2. Understand facts about techniques used to assist patients with casts
   2.1 Identify relevant assessment data
   2.2 Identify nursing goals related to the technique
   2.3 Identify expected and unexpected outcomes from assessment data
   2.4 Identify reasons underlying steps of the technique
3. Perform techniques related to cast application and care
   3.1 Assess the patient adequately
   3.2 Collect additional data from appropriate sources
   3.3 Select pertinent nursing goals for the patient
   3.4 Establish relevant outcome criteria for the patient following the technique
   3.5 Collect necessary equipment before the technique
   3.6 Implement interventions to enhance the effectiveness of the technique and enhance the patient's comfort and safety
   3.7 Communicate relevant information about the patient to the appropriate persons
   3.8 Determine the evaluative outcomes of the technique
4. Evaluate own performance of specific techniques in a laboratory or clinical setting with the assistance of another
   4.1 Use the performance checklists provided
   4.2 Identify areas of strength and weakness
   4.3 Alter performance in response to own evaluation and that of another

Terms

■ callus   early bone, formed following fracture of a bone, that is normally ultimately replaced by hard bone

■ cast   a stiff cylindrical dressing or casing made of bandages impregnated with hardening material; used to immobilize various parts of the body

■ ecchymosis   a blotchy area or discoloration of the skin; a bruise

■ endosteum   the lining membrane of a hollow bone

■ fracture   a break in the continuity of bone

■ lacerate   to tear, rather than cut, a body tissue

■ periosteum   the connective tissue covering all bones and possessing bone-forming potential

■ reduction   realignment of fractured bone fragments to their normal position

■ traction   exertion of a pulling force

FRACTURES

Fractures are breaks in the continuity of bones. They are described in terms of type, location, and special features.

Types of Fractures

All fractures are designated either simple (closed) or compound (open).

1. *Simple* or *closed* fractures are the most common. The bone is broken in one place only, and there is no skin wound. Hence the bone is protected from contamination.

2. In a *compound* or *open* fracture, there is a skin wound, and the bone is therefore vulnerable to infection through the opening in the skin. The skin wound may be caused from the outside (eg, a gunshot, which breaks the skin before it fractures the bone) or from the inside (the fracture occurs first, and it lacerates the tissues and skin).

Fracture Repair

Bleeding at the fracture site produces a hematoma (blood clot), which is the basis for repair. This clot becomes an interlacing mesh composed of fibrin from the clotted blood, lymph, and inflammatory exudate. It forms a bridge across the fracture site, and eventually granulation tissue is formed. Calcium is deposited into this tissue, and when this occurs the tissue is called *callus* (early bone). The callus is usually more abundant than appears necessary. Callus will not stand much muscle stress, strain, or weight bearing. The process of calcium depositing goes on until the callus becomes hard bone. The larger the bone, the longer the healing process. A radius or ulna heals in about 2 months, a humerus in about 3 months, and a femur in about 6 months. Age and blood circulation are also significant. Children heal much more rapidly than adults, and healing is delayed without a good blood supply. With normal use, the bone eventually assumes a shape that resembles the original bone. This takes place over a period of months, and frequently a year is needed to complete the process.

Reduction and Immobilization of Fractures

Reduction can be accomplished by three methods:

1. *Closed reduction* is manual traction and manipulation of the bone fragments. The patient may be given a general anesthetic. After reduction, a cast is applied to immobilize the part. See Technique 20-1.

2. *Open reduction* includes surgical exposure of the fracture. The bone may be immobilized by pins, nails, screws, plates, or rods.

3. *Traction* for a period of days or weeks may be necessary to reduce some fractures, eg, of the femur or humerus where the large muscles make manual traction and manipulation impossible. See chapter 21 for further discussion.

CASTS

Cast Materials

In addition to the traditional plaster of paris (POP) cast material, several synthetic materials are now available: polyester and cotton, fiberglass, and thermoplastics. See Table 20-1. Advantages of the synthetic casts compared to POP casts include:

1. They dry and set quickly, so they can bear weight within a short period of time.

2. They are lightweight, so they restrict mobility less.

3. They are less bulky, so regular clothing can be worn over them.

4. They are less likely to become indented while drying.

5. They do not crumble at the edges, and any rough cast edges can be smoothed with a nail file or emery board.

6. They can be immersed in water if the physician permits and if a nonabsorbent synthetic lining such as polypropylene stockinette and polyester padding is used. (POP is weakened by moisture and must be kept dry at all times.) Synthetic casts must be thoroughly dried, however (see disadvantage 4, later).

7. They are easily kept clean with water and small amounts of a mild, nonirritating soap.

8. Foreign particles that gain entrance to the cast can be flushed out with water.

Disadvantages of the synthetic casts include:

1. They are more expensive (3 to 8 times more than POP material).

2. They cannot be molded as readily as POP to fit limb contours, so they are not as effective for immobilizing severely displaced fractures or fractures that produce excessive edema.

3. Their surfaces are rougher than POP, so that they can snag clothes, scratch furniture, and abrade the skin on the opposite extremity.

4. There is an increased chance of skin maceration if proper drying procedures are not followed. When the cast becomes wet, excess water must be blotted with a towel, and a blow dryer must be used, on the cool or warm setting, over the entire cast until it is completely dry.

5. Vigorous activity can misalign the fracture or break the cast.

TABLE 20–1 ■ **Characteristics of Cast Materials**

Characteristics	Plaster of paris (POP)	Synthetics		
		Polyester and cotton (eg, Cutter Cast)	Fiberglass; water-activated (eg, Scotch-cast, Delta-lite) or light-cured (eg, Lightcast II)	Thermoplastic (eg, Hexcelite)
Description	Open-weave cotton rolls or strips saturated with powdered calcium sulfate crystals (gypsum)	Open-weave polyester and cotton tape permeated with water-activated polyurethane resin	Open-weave fiberglass tape impregnated with water-activated polyurethane resin (Scotchcast) or photosensitive polyurethane resin (Lightcast II)	Knitted thermoplastic polyester fabric in rigid rolls
Application	Applied after being soaked in tepid water for a few seconds until bubbling stops	Applied after being soaked in cool water, 26 °C (80 °F)	Applied after being soaked in tepid water (Scotchcast); applied with silicone type hand cream to keep it from sticking (Lightcast II)	Applied after being heated in water at 76 to 82 °C (170 to 180 °F) for 3 to 4 minutes to make the rolls soft and pliable
Setting time and weight-bearing restrictions	Dries in 48 hours, no weight bearing allowed until dry	Sets in 7 minutes, weight bearing allowed in 15 minutes	Sets in 15 minutes, weight bearing allowed in 30 minutes (Scotchcast); sets after being exposed for 3 minutes to a special ultraviolet lamp, weight bearing allowed immediately (Lightcast II)	Sets in 5 minutes, weight bearing allowed in 20 minutes

Source: PL Lane, MM Lee: New synthetic casts: What nurses need to know. *Orthop Nurs* (November/December) 1982; 1(6):13–20.

Types of Casts

The following are types of casts for the arm, leg, and trunk of the body:

1. The hanging arm cast extends from the axilla to the fingers of the hand, usually allowing for elbow flexion. See Figure 20–1, *A*. It immobilizes the wrist, the humerus, the radius, and the ulna.

2. The short arm cast extends from below the elbow to the fingers. See Figure 20–1, *B*. It immobilizes the wrist, the radius, and the ulna.

3. The shoulder spica cast extends around the chest and the entire arm to the fingers. The arm is usually abducted to immobilize the shoulder bones, eg, the clavicle. See Figure 20–1, *C*.

4. The long or full leg cast extends from above the knee to the toes. See Figure 20–1, *D*.

5. The short leg cast begins just below the knee and extends to the toes. See Figure 20–1, *E*.

6. The hip spica cast begins at waist level or above. It immobilizes the hip joint and the femur, extends down one entire leg, and may cover all or part of the second leg. A single spica covers one leg only. See Figure 20–1, *F*. A one-and-one-half hip spica covers the second leg to the knee. See Figure 20–1, *G*. A double hip spica covers both legs to the toes.

7. The body cast extends from the axillae to encompass the entire trunk. It is often used to immobilize the spine.

TECHNIQUE 20–1 ■ Assisting with a Cast Application

Casts are usually applied, adjusted, split, and removed only by physicians. The major role of the nurse during cast application is to hold and support the fractured extremity. Additional assistance may be required depending on the size and location of the cast and the age and condition of the patient. Manually holding an extremity is not an easy task because of the weight of the extremity and the time involved in cast application.

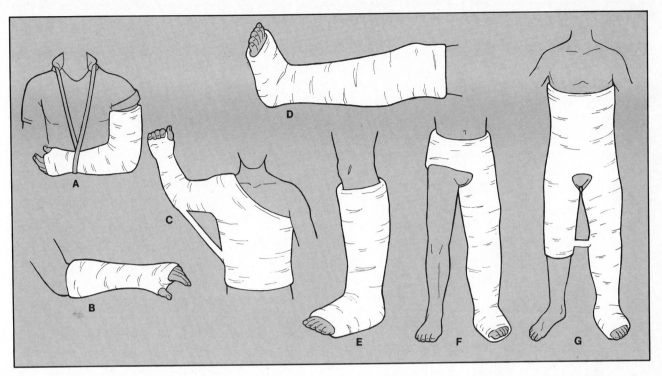

FIGURE 20–1 ■ Types of cylindrical casts: **A,** hanging arm cast; **B,** short arm cast; **C,** shoulder spica; **D,** long leg cast; **E,** short leg cast; **F,** single hip spica; **G,** one and one half hip spica.

■ **Assessment**

Assess the patient for:

1. Discomfort and blood circulation to the area. Note any clinical signs of restricted circulation, eg, skin pallor, cyanosis, coldness to the touch, and numbness.
2. General response to the fracture in terms of color of the skin and mucous membranes, blood pressure, pulse, respirations, and perspiration.

Additional data include:

1. The body area to be put in a cast, and the purpose of the cast
2. The type of cast material to be used

■ **Planning**

Nursing goals

1. To provide physical and emotional support to the patient during the cast application
2. To expedite application of the cast by the physician
3. To assess the patient's response during the cast application

Equipment

1. Rolls of cast material. See Table 20–1 on page 472.
2. A plastic-lined bucket of water at the prescribed temperature:

a. Tepid water for POP and water-activated fiber-glass
b. Cool water at 26 °C (80 °F) for a polyester and cotton cast

or

A thermostatically controlled hydrocollator or a boiler or cooking pot with a temperature-regulating thermometer for a thermoplastic cast. The water is heated to 76 to 82 °C (170 to 180 °F). Follow the cast manufacturer's directions.

3. Stockinette, a soft, flexible, tubular, cloth material to place over the body part before the cast material is applied. The most common sizes are 5 to 25 cm (2 to 12 in) in flattened width. Usually one thickness of stockinette is used for extremity casts and two thicknesses for casts covering the trunk of the body. Two thicknesses may also be used beneath thermo-plastic casts to protect the skin from this hot application. If the patient's fracture is severe and the limb very painful, stockinette may not be used since its application is difficult and may enhance pain.

4. Cotton sheet wadding or padding to apply directly over the skin or stockinette or to pad bony promi-nences or between skin surfaces. Sheet wadding clings and molds to the contours of the limb. It is available in 2-, 3-, and 4-inch rolls.

5. Felt padding (optional) to apply over bony promi-nences or joints that are vulnerable to skin break-down. Padding is available in ½- or ¼-inch thick-nesses, is cut to fit the desired area, and is incor-

porated within the folds of cotton sheet wadding.

6. Plaster splints (optional) to add strength over areas susceptible to breakage, eg, over a knee joint or the heel. Splints are flat strips of cast material 3 × 15, 4 × 15, or 4 × 30 inches in length. They are prepared like the POP cast rolls and may be applied in four to eight layers.

7. Moisture-resistant drapes to protect the patient's clothing and bedding.

8. Rubber gloves to protect the hands from the casting material.

9. Plastic aprons to protect the clothing.

10. Water-soluble lubricant to lessen the tack on the physician's gloves when molding the cast.

11. Plaster knife to trim the edges of the cast after application.

12. Large plaster scissors to cut felt padding or to trim the cast after application.

13. Pillows to support the cast after application.

14. A damp cloth to remove excess plaster, or swabs and alcohol, acetone, or nail polish remover for synthetic cast materials.

FIGURE 20–2

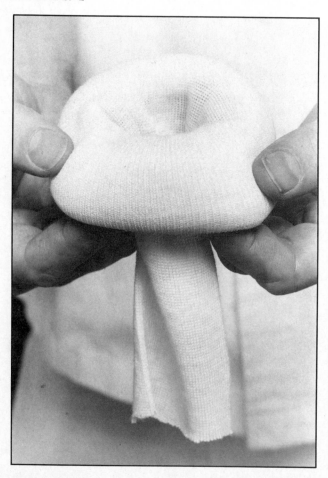

■ Intervention

1. Explain the technique to the patient, including the length of time the cast material requires for drying. Explain that the patient may feel warmth during and after application.

   Rationale Different cast materials require different drying times. Weight bearing or pressure will cause a wet cast to change shape. Only when a cast is dry does it become hard and inflexible. POP, Cutter Cast, and light-cured fiberglass give off heat as they set, and thermoplastics are hot when applied.

2. Provide an analgesic as ordered by the physician, if the bones need to be set before the cast is applied. Otherwise, applying a cast is not usually uncomfortable. If pain can be anticipated, make sure that the patient knows this.

3. Assist the patient to a comfortable sitting or lying position.

4. Remove clothing from the body area before the cast is applied.

   Rationale Often clothes cannot be removed over a cast.

5. Support the part to receive the cast, eg, support an arm with a plastic-covered pillow.

6. Wash the skin area, and dry it thoroughly. If there is no open wound, powder may be applied.

7. Provide stockinette of the correct size, if used, and cut it several inches longer than the length of the extremity so that it will extend beyond the plaster edges. Then roll the stockinette to facilitate its application. See Figure 20–2. The physician will fit the stockinette smoothly to avoid folds or creases that could irritate the skin. Stockinette for body and hip spica casts is usually applied at the patient's bedside.

8. Provide sheet wadding and felt pads as needed. Usually two or three layers are applied. Additional padding may be applied over bony prominences.

9. Provide gloves for the physician prior to application of the cast material.

   Rationale Gloves protect the hands from irritation or tacky resin. POP is irritating to the hands. The residue from polyester and cotton material is difficult to remove. Fiberglass resin becomes tacky when wet and adheres to the skin. Thermoplastic material is difficult to handle without gloves because of its high temperature.

10. Hand the physician the cast material or place the material within his or her reach. Preparation of cast material varies:

    a. Rolls of plaster of paris bandage with the corner of the roll turned back are immersed in tepid water and removed when the bubbles stop. One or two rolls are usually prepared at a time and they are first pressed to remove excess water. Splints are usually submerged in layers of four to eight and are fanfolded to remove excess water.

b. Polyester and cotton knit rolls are opened one at a time and must be used within 2 to 3 minutes since exposure to the humidity in the air hardens the tape. They are immersed in cold water and squeezed with one hand four successive times while immersed to ensure uniform wetting of the innermost layers of tape. They are left dripping wet when removed from the water to provide a cooling effect and facilitate handling. Cutter Cast gives off heat as it sets, like POP.

c. Water-activated fiberglass rolls are immersed in tepid water for only 10 to 15 seconds. This initiates the chemical reaction between the polyurethane and water, which produces heat and hardening of the tape. Open only one roll at a time and do not squeeze excess water from the roll before application.

d. Light-cured fiberglass remains soft and pliable during application. No setting (hardening) occurs until it is exposed to ultraviolet light.

e. Thermoplastic rolls must be heated before application. Remove excess water from the rolls by squeezing them between two layers of towel.

11. Squeeze a generous amount of water-soluble lubricant on the physician's gloves as requested or special silicone cream for a light-cured fiberglass cast.

12. Support the limb while the physician applies the stockinette, padding, and cast material. With one hand grasp the patient's toes for a leg cast or fingers for an arm cast, and with the other hand support beneath the limb in areas on which the physician is not working. See Figure 20–3. Maintain the limb in the same position throughout the procedure.

Rationale Failure to support the limb in the one position could produce wrinkles on the inside of the cast, which could subsequently cause pressure areas.

13. After the cast is applied, pull the stockinette out over the proximal and distal cast opening edges, while the physician secures it in place with one or two layers of cast material.

Rationale The stockinette covers rough cast edges.

14. Remove any excess cast material deposited accidentally on the patient's skin. A cloth dampened with water will remove plaster of paris effectively. The resin of synthetic casting materials is best removed with a swab moistened with alcohol, acetone, or nail polish remover. Check the manufacturer's directions.

Rationale Cast material is most easily removed while it is still wet.

15. Assess the patient's response to the cast in terms of

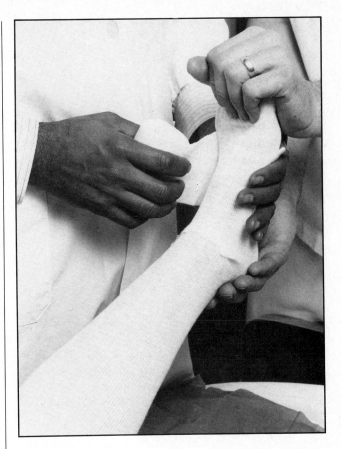

FIGURE 20–3

discomfort, chilling, and restrictions of blood circulation.

16. Provide firm support for the cast. See Technique 20–2.

17. Gather and dispose of the used materials appropriately. Plaster of paris and some plastics can obstruct plumbing and should be disposed of in a waste container. Pour the water through a strainer to prevent plaster from entering the drains.

18. Record the technique on the patient's chart, including the physician's name, the site, the type of cast, and the patient's response.

Sample Recording

Date	Time	Notes
12/5/86	1400	Plaster of paris hanging arm cast applied to L arm by Dr. G. Rodriguez. Aching sensation with occasional sharp pains throughout arm. Arm moderately elevated. Fingers warm, good mobility, color normal. ——— ——————— Paula O. Sayewich, NS

19. See Technique 20–3 for cast and skin care.

TECHNIQUE 20–2 ■ Patient Care Immediately after Cast Application

Nursing interventions immediately after cast application include:

1. Neurovascular assessment of affected limbs
2. Supporting and handling the cast appropriately until it sets
3. Actions to reduce swelling
4. Actions to promote drying of the cast
5. Monitoring any drainage or bleeding
6. Assessing pain and signs of pressure beneath the cast

■ Assessment

Rapid swelling under a cast can cause neurovascular problems necessitating frequent neurovascular assessments by the nurse to prevent these problems. Assess the toes and fingers for nerve or circulatory impairments every 30 minutes for several hours following application and then every 3 hours for the first 24 to 48 hours or until all signs and symptoms of impairment are negative. Check the following:

1. Color of the skin. Compare it to the color of the unaffected extremity. Pallor or cyanosis can indicate circulatory impairment.
2. Temperature of the skin. Feel both extremities (affected and unaffected), and compare the temperatures. Excessive coldness can indicate circulatory impairment.
3. Degree of swelling. Some swelling can be expected, and swelling does not always indicate circulatory impairment.
4. Blanching sign (capillary refill). Compress the nail of the thumb or large toe for a few seconds until it blanches, and note the return flow of blood. Blood should return instantly on release of pressure. If it returns too slowly there may be venous congestion or arterial insufficiency.
5. When obtainable, palpate the distal pulse of the extremity in the cast for presence and strength and compare it with the pulse in the opposite extremity. A weak or absent pulse may indicate decreased circulation to the area.
6. Motor ability or movement. Have the patient move the fingers and wrist or toes and ankle as indicated in Table 20–2. Inability to do so suggests compression of a nerve and potential paralysis. Commonly affected nerves are the peroneal, tibial, radial, median, and ulnar nerves. See Figure 20–4. If the peroneal nerve is compressed, the patient is unable to dorsiflex the foot. With compression of the tibial nerve, the patient is unable to plantar flex the foot. With compression of the radial nerve, the patient is unable to hyperextend the thumb or wrist. With compression of the ulnar nerve, the patient is unable to abduct all the fingers in unison. With compression of the median nerve the patient is unable to flex the wrist and oppose the thumb and little finger.

7. Sensation. Ask the patient about the presence or absence of sensation, eg, numbness, tingling, or inability to feel pain. These symptoms can indicate increasing pressure within the cast. Pinch all toes or fingers and ask the patient to identify which one you are pinching. All toes and fingers must be checked since they are innervated by different nerves. If the patient does not feel sensation in one or more digits, conduct the sensory function tests outlined in Table 20–2. Have the patient close his or her eyes, use the pointed end of a safety pin to prick the specific areas, and ask the patient if he or she feels the stimulus. Lack of sensation in any of the areas noted can indicate impaired function of the associated nerves.

TABLE 20–2 ■ Nerve Function Assessments

Nerve	Motor function tests	Sensory function tests
Radial	Instruct patient to hyperextend thumb or wrist and straighten all four fingers.	Prick web space between thumb and index finger.
Median	Instruct patient to oppose thumb and little finger and flex wrist.	Prick distal fat pad of index finger.
Ulnar	Instruct patient to abduct all fingers.	Prick fat pad at distal end of small finger.
Peroneal	Instruct patient to dorsiflex ankle and extend toes.	Prick web between great toe and second toe or lateral surface of great toe and medial surface of second toe.
Tibial	Instruct patient to plantar flex ankle and flex toes.	Prick medial and lateral surfaces of sole of foot.

Sources: J Farrell: *Illustrated Guide to Orthopedic Nursing*, 2nd ed. (Lippincott, 1982), p 66; PL Swearingen: *The Addison-Wesley Photo-Atlas of Nursing Procedures* (Addison-Wesley, 1984), pp 519–521.

■ Planning

Nursing goals

1. To support a cast in the correct alignment until it dries and hardens
2. To avoid or reduce excessive swelling
3. To promote drying of the cast
4. To monitor neurovascular function of the affected extremity or drainage or pressure areas beneath the cast

Equipment

1. Soft, pliable pillows

■ Intervention

Supporting and handling the cast

1. Immediately after the cast is applied, place it on pillows. Avoid using plastic or rubber pillows.

   Rationale The pillows provide even pressure and support the curves of the cast. Plastic or rubber pillows do not allow the heat of a drying cast to dissipate and cause discomfort for the patient.

2. Until a cast has set or hardened (10 to 20 minutes), support the cast in the palms of your hands rather than with the fingertips. Some authorities advocate that you extend your fingers so that your fingertips do not touch the plaster (Farrell, 1982, p 60). See Figure 20–5. When the cast is set continue to handle the cast in your palms, but you may then wrap your fingers around the contour of the cast.

   Rationale Fingertip pressure can cause dents in unset plaster and subsequent skin pressure areas.

Reducing swelling

3. Control swelling by elevating arms or legs on pillows or, for a leg fracture, by elevating the foot of the bed. Immediately after injury and surgery, elevate the limb well above the level of the patient's heart. Generally three pillows are needed to achieve high elevation of a leg. As circulation improves and healing progresses, the elevation can be gradually reduced to two pillows (moderate elevation) and then to one pillow (low elevation).

   Rationale Elevation of an extremity aids venous blood flow, prevents or reduces swelling, and prevents potential neurovascular impairment.

4. Report excessive swelling and indications of neurovascular impairment to the physician or responsible nurse. The physician may bivalve a cast if it appears to be too tight. Bivalving a cast is cutting the cast and the underlying padding on each side, thus making two separate shells. See Figure 20–6, *A*. This

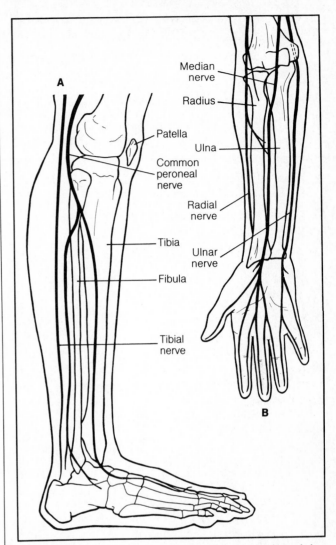

FIGURE 20–4   ■   The peroneal and tibial nerves (**A**) and the radial, median, and ulnar nerves (**B**) can be injured by prolonged compression in a cylindrical cast.

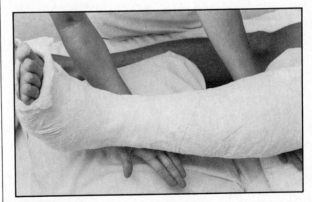

FIGURE 20–5

relieves the pressure of the cast but still provides support. Bivalved casts are usually fastened in place with Velcro straps or buckled webbing straps. See Figure 20–6, *B*.

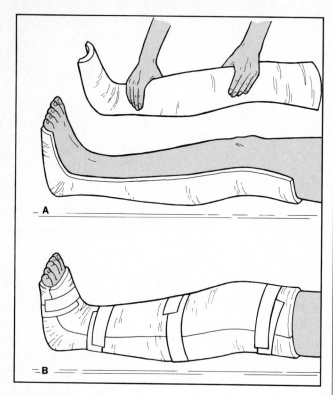

FIGURE 20–6

5. Apply ice packs to control perineal edema associated with a hip spica cast. Although ice packs are a less effective method of control, elevation of the area is obviously not as possible.

Drying the cast

Extremity plaster of paris casts usually take 24 to 48 hours to dry completely; spica or body casts require 48 to 72 hours. Drying time depends on the temperature, humidity, size of the cast, and method used for drying. The cast is dry when it no longer feels damp. A dry cast feels dry and looks white and shiny and is odorless, hard, and resonant when tapped.

6. Expose the cast to the circulating air. Place sheets and blankets only over areas that do not have the cast.

7. Check agency policy about the recommended turning frequency for patients with different kinds of casts.

   Rationale Frequent turning promotes even drying of the cast.

8. Turn the patient with an extremity cast or body spica every two to four hours. See Technique 20–3, step 13 on page 482.

9. Use regular pillows.

   Rationale Plastic or rubber pillows hinder drying and do not allow the heat of a drying cast to dissipate.

10. Avoid the use of artificial methods to facilitate drying such as a fan, hair dryer, infrared lamp, or electric heaters.

    Rationale Artificial methods dry the outer surface of the cast while the inner portion remains soft and spongy. Such a cast cracks readily at points of strain. Natural methods dry the cast evenly.

Monitoring drainage

11. If an open reduction has been done or if the injury was a compound fracture, bleeding may occur, and the cast may become stained with blood.

    a. Monitor such drainage for 24 to 72 hours after surgery or injury or longer if necessary.

    b. Outline the stained area with a ball point pen every 8 hours or at the change of shift, and note the time and date, so that any further bleeding can be determined. See Figure 20–7.

Assessing pain and pressure areas

12. Never ignore any complaints of pain, burning, or pressure by the patient. If a patient is unable to communicate, be alert to changes in temperament, restlessness, or fussiness.

13. Note particularly whether the pain is persistent and if it occurs over a bony prominence or joint. See Table 20–3 for common pressure points associated with various casts.

14. Give pain medications selectively.

    Rationale Pain medication can mask symptoms.

15. Do not disregard the cessation of persistent pain or discomfort complaints.

    Rationale Cessation of complaints can indicate a skin slough. When a skin slough occurs superficial skin sensation is lost and the patient no longer feels pain.

16. When a pressure area under the cast is suspected the physician may either bivalve the cast so that all of the skin beneath the cast can be inspected or cut a "window" in the cast over only the area of concern. When a cast is "windowed":

    a. Retain the piece (cast and padding) that was cut out and tape it securely back in place.

       Rationale Putting back the piece prevents "window" edema, which occurs when skin pressure at the window is not equal to that from the remainder of the cast.

    b. Inspect the skin under the window at scheduled intervals.

17. Record each assessment whether or not there are problems. Examples include: "Toes warm to touch, color pink," or "Toes cold, pale, and edematous"; "Blanching sign satisfactory," or "Slow return of blood from blanching sign"; "Moves toes readily; states no numbness or tingling; states leg painful,"

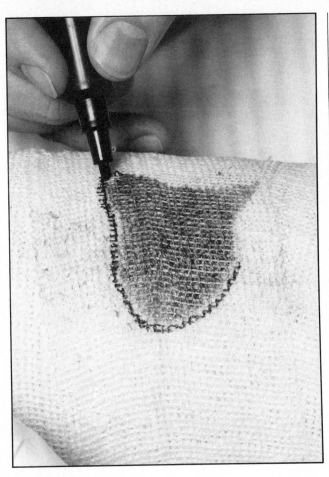

FIGURE 20-7

or "C/o numbness and tingling in toes; movement decreased." Record specific nerve function asssessments such as "Able to hyperextend R thumb"; "Sensation felt at web space between R thumb and index finger."

18. Record care provided.

■ Evaluation

Expected outcomes

1. Skin color of toes or fingers of affected extremity same as opposite extremity

2. Skin temperature of toes or fingers of affected extremity same as opposite extremity

3. Satisfactory blanching sign

4. Able to move fingers or toes of affected extremity appropriately

Unexpected outcomes

1. Pallor or cyanosis of toes or fingers

2. Coldness of skin on fingers or toes

3. Excessive swelling

4. Inability to move fingers or toes

5. Loss of sensation, numbness, or tingling in toes or fingers

6. Bleeding through cast

Upon obtaining an unexpected outcome:

1. Report your findings to the responsible nurse and/or physician.

2. Adjust the nursing care plan as required.

TABLE 20-3   ■   Common Cast Pressure Areas

Type of cast	Common pressure areas
Short arm cast	Radial styloid
	Ulnar styloid
	Joint at base of thumb
Hanging arm cast	Radial styloid
	Ulnar styloid
	Olecranon
	Lateral epicondyle
Short leg cast	Heel
	Achilles tendon
	Malleolus
Long leg cast	Heel
	Achilles tendon
	Malleolus
	Popliteal artery behind knee
	Peroneal nerve at side of knee
Hip spica	As above for long leg cast
	Sacrum
	Iliac crests

TECHNIQUE 20-3   ■   Continuing Care for Patients with Casts

Continuing care for patients with casts involves (a) providing meticulous skin care, (b) keeping the cast clean and dry, (c) turning and positioning the patient appro-

priately, (d) encouraging active exercise, and (e) teaching cast care.

■ **Assessment**

Assess the patient for:

1. Skin irritation at the edge of the cast
2. Complaints of a burning sensation or pain beneath the cast
3. A foul odor emanating through the cast

See also Technique 20–2 on page 476.

■ **Planning**

Nursing goals

1. To prevent skin irritation at the edges of a cast
2. To keep the cast dry
3. To prevent the formation of pressure areas
4. To prevent respiratory problems resulting from immobility
5. To prevent joint stiffness and muscle atrophy

Equipment

For skin care

1. Rubbing alcohol
2. Mineral, olive, or baby oil to apply to the skin after cast removal

For covering rough cast edges

3. Adhesive tape 2.5 cm (1 in) wide or 5 to 7 cm (2 to 3 in) wide
4. Scissors

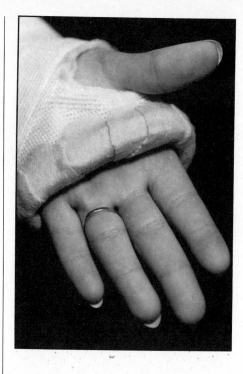

FIGURE 20–9

For keeping the cast clean and dry

5. A damp washcloth for plaster of paris casts
6. Warm water and a mild soap for synthetic casts

For comfort

7. Pillows
8. A slipper pan

■ **Intervention**

Skin care

The skin near and under the cast edges is inspected whenever neurovascular assessments are made and/or whenever the patient is turned. To prevent skin irritation at the edges of a cast, implement the following measures.

1. Wash crumbs of plaster from the skin with a damp cloth and feel along the cast edges to check for rough edges or areas that press into the patient's skin. It may be necessary to use a duckbilled cast bender to bend cast edges that may irritate the skin. See Figure 20–8. Excessive bending or trimming of the cast should not be done without a physician's order.

   Rationale As a plaster of paris cast dries, small bits of plaster frequently break off from its rough edges. If they fall inside the cast they can cause discomfort and irritation.

2. Cover any rough edges of the cast when it is dry. If stockinette has not been used to line the cast, "petal" the edges with small strips of adhesive tape as follows (see Figure 20–9):

   a. Cut several strips of 2.5 cm (1 in) *non*waterproof

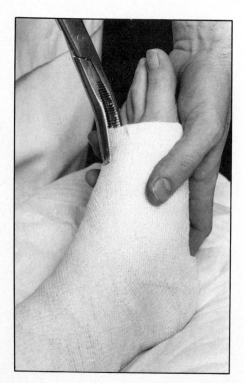

FIGURE 20–8

adhesive, 5 to 7.5 cm (2 to 3 in) long. Then curve all corners of each strip. See Figure 20–10.

Rationale   Square or pointed ends tend to curl. Nonwaterproof adhesive is more adherent.

b. Insert one end of each strip as far as possible inside the cast, and bring the other end out over the cast edge. See Figure 20–11.

c. Press the petals firmly against the plaster. See Figure 20–12.

d. Overlap successive petals slightly.

3.   Check the cast daily for a foul odor.

Rationale   This kind of odor may indicate skin excoriation from pressure or an infected area beneath the cast.

4.   Provide skin care, using alcohol, to all areas vulnerable to pressure and breakdown at least every four hours. For patients with sensitive skin or potential skin problems provide care every two hours during the day and every three hours at night.

Rationale   Alcohol cleans and toughens the skin and evaporates without making the cast soggy.

a. Reach under the cast edges as far as possible and massage the area.

b. Also provide skin care over all bony prominences not under the cast, eg, the sacrum, heels, ankles, wrists, elbows, and feet.

Rationale   These are potential pressure areas while the patient is confined to bed.

5.   Itching is a common problem.

a. Discourage the patient from using long sharp objects to scratch under the cast.

Rationale   These objects can break the skin and cause an infection, since bacteria flourish in the warm, dark, moist environment under the cast.

b. Suggest that the patient tap the cast, or at home to use a hair dryer on cool, or a vacuum cleaner on reverse.

Rationale   These are safer ways to resolve itching and less irritating to the skin.

6.   When healing is complete and the cast is removed, the underlying skin is usually dry, flaky, and encrusted, since layers of dead skin have accumulated. Remove this debris gently and gradually.

a. Apply oil (eg, mineral, olive, or baby oil).

b. Soak the skin in warm water and dry it.

c. Caution the patient not to rub the area too vigorously.

Rationale   Vigorous rubbing can cause bleeding or excoriation.

d. Repeat steps a and b for several days.

Rationale   Gradual removal of skin exudate avoids skin irritation.

Keeping the cast clean and dry

7.   Plaster of paris casts. Because this cast is porous and will absorb water or urine, every effort is made to keep the cast dry. Casts that become wet soften, and their function is impaired; thus tub baths and showers are contraindicated. Casts that become soiled with feces develop an unremovable odor. Elimination presents a particular problem for patients with long leg, body, and hip spica casts.

FIGURE 20–10

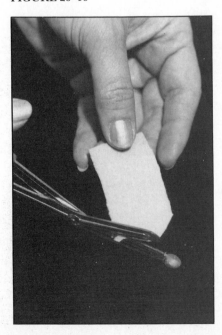

FIGURE 20–11

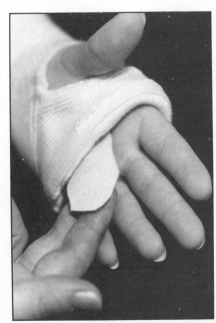

FIGURE 20–12

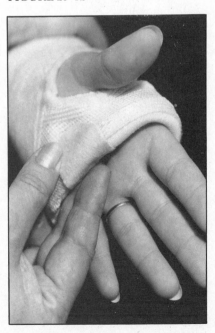

There is no effective way to keep a POP cast clean other than wiping it with a damp cloth. Before a patient is discharged, a cast may be cleaned by applying more wet plaster over the soiled area. The best approach is to prevent soils and stains, especially those from food spills, urine, and feces.

a. Place a bib or towel over a body cast to catch spills. If a spill does wet the cast, allow the area to air dry.

b. Use a slipper (fracture) bedpan for patients with long leg, hip spica, or body casts.

   Rationale The flat end placed correctly under the patient's buttocks lessens the chance of spillage and minimizes the amount of lifting required by the patient and/or nurse.

c. Before placing the patient on the bedpan, tuck plastic or other waterproof material around the top of a long leg cast or in around the perineal cutout. For a perineal cutout funnel one end of the plastic into the bedpan.

d. Remove the plastic when elimination is completed.

   Rationale If left in place, waterproof material makes the cast edge airtight and prevents evaporation of perspiration, which is irritating to the skin.

e. For patients with long leg casts, keep the cast supported on pillows while the patient is on the bedpan.

   Rationale If the cast dangles urine may run down the cast.

f. For patients with hip spica casts, support both extremities and the patient's back on pillows so that they are as high as the buttocks.

   Rationale This prevents urine from running back into the cast.

g. When removing the bedpan, hold it securely while the patient is turning or lifting his or her buttocks.

   Rationale This prevents dripping and spilling.

h. After removing the bedpan, thoroughly clean and dry the perineal area.

8. Synthetic casts. Synthetic casts can be cleaned readily and may, with the doctor's permission, be immersed in water if polypropylene stockinette and padding were applied.

   a. Wash the soiled area with warm water and a mild soap.

   b. Thoroughly rinse the soap from the cast.

   c. Dry thoroughly to prevent skin maceration and ulceration under the cast.

   d. If the cast is immersed in water, the cast and underlying padding and stockinette must be dried thoroughly. First blot excess water from the cast with a towel. Then use a hand-held blow dryer on the cool or warm setting, directing the air stream in a sweeping motion over the exterior of the cast for about one hour or until the patient no longer feels a cold clammy sensation like that produced by a wet bathing suit.

   Rationale This drying procedure is essential to prevent skin maceration and ulceration.

Turning and positioning patients

Proper body alignment, turning, and positioning are absolutely necessary to prevent the formation of pressure areas.

9. Place pillows in such a way that:

   a. Body parts press against the cast edges as little as possible.

   b. Toes, heels, elbows, etc, are protected from pressure against the bed surface.

   c. Body alignment is maintained.

10. Plan and implement a turning schedule incorporating all possible positions. Generally patients can be placed in lateral, prone, and supine positions unless surgical procedures or other factors contraindicate them.

    Rationale Repositioning prevents pressure areas.

11. Turn patients with large casts or those unable to turn themselves at least once every four hours. If the patient is at risk for skin breakdown turn him or her every one to three hours as needed.

12. When turning the patient in a long leg cast to the unaffected side, place a pillow between the legs to support the cast.

13. At least three persons are needed to turn a patient in a damp hip spica cast. When the cast is dry the patient can usually turn with the assistance of one nurse. To turn a patient from the supine to prone position follow these steps:

    a. Remove the support pillows only when an assistant is supporting the cast.

    b. Move the patient to one side of the bed.

    c. Have the patient place his or her arms above the head or along the sides.

    d. Have two assistants go to the other side of the bed while you remain to provide security for the patient who is at the edge of the bed.

    e. Place pillows along the bed surface to receive the cast when the patient turns.

    f. Roll the patient toward the two assistants onto the pillows.

    g. Adjust the pillows as needed so that they provide proper support and comfort, and prevent pressure areas.

Exercise

14. Unless contraindicated, encourage active range of motion exercises for all joints on the unaffected extremities, as well as on the joints proximal and distal to the cast. If active exercises are contraindicated, implement active-assisted or passive exercises depending on the patient's abilities and disabilities.

    Rationale Exercise prevents joint stiffness and muscle atrophy.

15. Encourage the patient to move toes and/or fingers of the casted extremity as frequently as possible.

    Rationale Moving these extremities enhances peripheral circulation and decreases swelling and pain.

16. With the physician's approval, teach the patient isometric (muscle setting) exercises. See chapter 19, page 430.

    Rationale Isometric exercise will minimize muscle atrophy in the affected limb.

    a. Teach the isometric exercises on the patient's unaffected limb before the patient applies it to the affected limb.

    b. Demonstrate muscle palpation while the patient is carrying out the exercise. See Figure 20–13.

       Rationale Palpation enables the patient to feel the changes that occur with muscle contraction and relaxation.

Meeting the patient's learning needs

Common learning needs include cast care, ways to move effectively with casts, and instructions before discharge.

17. Teach parents of young children ways to prevent the child from placing small items under the cast. One approach is to avoid giving the child small play items such as marbles, pencils, or crayons. Parents also need to ensure that the top of a body cast is well covered during meals, so that food does not fall inside the cast.

18. Teach patients immobilized in bed with large body casts ways to turn and to move safely by using a trapeze, the side rails, etc.

19. Instruct patients with leg casts about ways to walk effectively with crutches. See Technique 19–6 on page 460.

20. Instruct patients with arm casts how to apply slings. See Technique 33–1 on page 795.

21. Instruct all patients about isometric exercises for extremities in a cast, to prevent muscle atrophy. See the discussion earlier in this chapter.

22. Before the patient's discharge from the hospital, instruct the patient to:

    a. Observe for indications of nerve or circulatory impairment such as extreme coldness or blueness

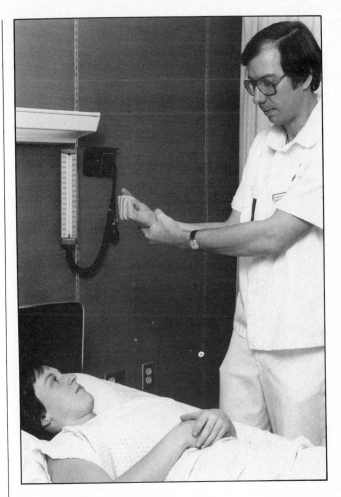

FIGURE 20–13

of toes or fingers; extreme continuous swelling of casted toes or fingers; numbness or tingling ("pins and needles" sensation) in casted toes or fingers; continuous complaints of pain; or inability to move the toes or fingers.

    b. Keep the cast dry.

    c. Avoid strenuous activity and follow the physician's advice about exercises.

    d. Elevate the arm or leg frequently to prevent dependent edema.

    e. Move the toes or fingers frequently.

    f. Observe the skin around the cast edges frequently, and keep it clean and dry.

    g. Report to the physician any increase in pain, unexplained fever, foul odor from within the cast, decreased circulation, numbness, inability to move the fingers or toes, or a weakened, cracked, loose, or tight cast.

23. Record nursing care given and relevant assessments made on the appropriate records.

■ **Evaluation**

Expected outcomes

See Technique 20–2 on page 479.

1. Intact skin around cast edges
2. No complaints of discomfort

Unexpected outcomes

1. Skin irritation at edge of cast

2. Complaints of burning sensation beneath cast
3. Complaints of pain
4. Foul or musty odor emanating through cast
5. Excessive swelling

See also Technique 20–2 on page 479. Upon obtaining an unexpected outcome:

1. Report your findings to the responsible nurse and/or physician.
2. Adjust the nursing care plan appropriately.

References

Farrell J: *Illustrated Guide to Orthopedic Nursing,* 2nd ed. Lippincott, 1982.

Hilt NE, Cogburn SB: *Manual of Orthopedics.* Mosby, 1980.

Lane PL, Lee MM: New synthetic casts: What nurses need to know. *Orthop Nurs* (November/December) 1982; 1(6):13–20.

Lane PL, Lee MM: Special care for special casts. *Nursing 83* (July) 1983; 13(7):50–51.

Swearingen PL: *Photo-Atlas of Nursing Procedures.* Addison-Wesley, 1984.

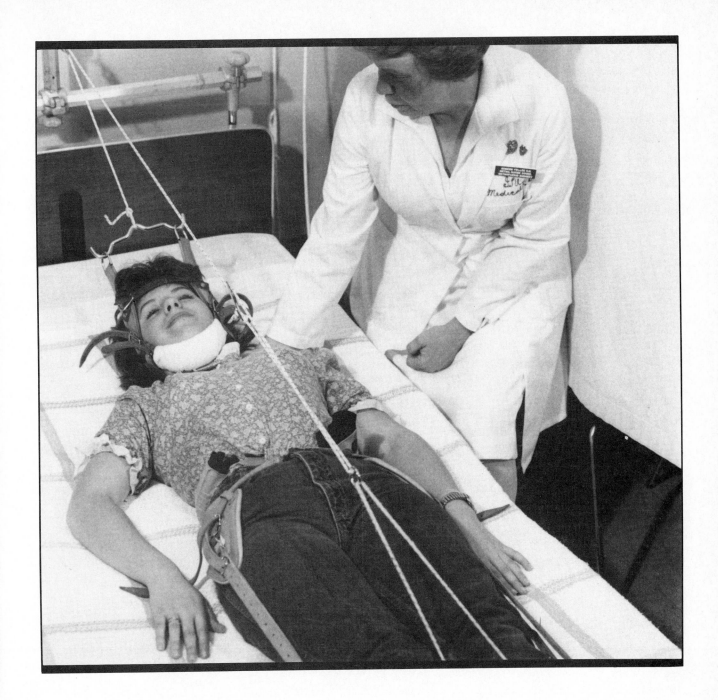

TRACTION CARE

21

Traction, like a cast, is a device by which a part of the body is immobilized. But unlike a cast, traction involves a pulling force that is applied to a part of the body, while a second force, called *countertraction*, pulls in the opposite direction. The pulling force of traction is provided through a system of pulleys, ropes, and weights attached to the patient; the countertraction is often supplied by the patient's body. In balanced traction, the amount of force in the traction is equal to the amount of force in the countertraction. A *suspension* is a mechanism that suspends a body part by using traction equipment, but it does not involve a pulling force. However, traction may be added to a suspension.

In *straight* or *running traction,* the traction force is pulled against the long axis of the body, and the countertraction is supplied by the patient's body. In a *suspension* or in a *balanced traction,* the affected part is supported by a sling, hammock, or ring splint, and countertraction is supplied partly by the body and partly by a system of weights attached to an overhead frame with pulleys and ropes.

Patients who have traction are often confined to bed for weeks or even months. Nursing therefore involves activities of daily living, maintenance of the traction, and the prevention of problems such as pressure sores.

Chapter Outline

Purposes of Traction

Types of Traction

Traction Equipment

Guidelines for Traction

Specific Tractions

■ Technique 21–1 Applying Nonadhesive Skin Traction

■ Technique 21–2 Assisting a Patient in Traction

Objectives

Upon completion of this chapter, the student will:

1. Know essential terms and facts about traction
   1.1 Differentiate between skin and skeletal traction
   1.2 Identify six common types of skin traction
   1.3 State the purposes of selected tractions
   1.4 Identify potential problems associated with specific tractions
2. Understand facts about techniques related to traction care
   2.1 Identify relevant assessment data
   2.2 Identify nursing diagnoses for which the technique may be implemented
   2.3 Identify nursing goals related to the technique
   2.4 Identify expected and unexpected outcomes from assessment data
   2.5 Identify reasons underlying selected steps of the technique
3. Perform traction care techniques safely
   3.1 Assess the patient adequately

   3.2 Collect additional data from appropriate sources
   3.3 Select pertinent nursing goals for the patient
   3.4 Establish relevant outcome criteria for the patient following the technique
   3.5 Collect necessary equipment before the technique
   3.6 Implement interventions to enhance the effectiveness of the technique and enhance the patient's comfort and safety
   3.7 Communicate relevant information about the patient to the appropriate persons
   3.8 Determine the evaluative outcomes of the technique
4. Evaluate own performance of specific techniques in a laboratory or clinical setting with the assistance of another
   4.1 Use the performance checklists provided
   4.2 Identify areas of strength and weakness
   4.3 Alter performance in response to own evaluation and that of another

Terms

■ **carrier**   a mechanism used in traction attached to the rope and upon which weights are placed

■ **countertraction**   a force that counteracts the direct pull of traction

■ **footplate**   a device that provides both support for a foot and a place to attach the rope of a traction apparatus

■ **spreader bar**   a bar designed to spread traction tape away from the bony prominences of the involved body part, eg, the lateral and medial malleoli of the leg; the bar must be wider than the involved part

■ **traction**   an apparatus designed to immobilize and to apply a pulling force to an area or areas of the body

■ **traction tape (strap)**   adhesive or nonadhesive tape, made of various materials (some are elastic and porous), which is applied lengthwise along a limb and attached to a spreader bar

PURPOSES OF TRACTION

1. To reduce and/or immobilize a fracture for healing. To *reduce* a fracture is to realign the bones.
2. To correct, reduce, or prevent deformities.
3. Prior to surgery, eg, hip replacement, to provide more space within the hip joint.
4. To decrease muscle spasm before a fracture is reduced.
5. To treat inflammatory conditions by immobilizing a joint, eg, for arthritis or tuberculosis of a joint.

TYPES OF TRACTION

There are four types of traction: manual, skin, skeletal, and encircling.

1. *Manual traction* is applied by the hands, ie, the nurse holds the limb while exerting pulling force. It is a temporary measure used while skin traction is being prepared, eg, when a cast is being applied, or in an emergency, eg, when a traction rope breaks.
2. *Skin traction* is a pulling force applied to the skin and soft tissues through the use of tape or traction straps and a system of ropes, pulleys, and weights. The traction strap is often made of vented foam rubber or cloth, and it may have either an adhesive or nonadhesive backing. Adhesive skin traction is used only for continous traction. Nonadhesive skin traction is used intermittently; it can easily be removed and applied.
3. *Skeletal traction* is applied by inserting metal pins or wires directly into or through a bone. The metal device is then attached to a system of ropes, pulleys, and weights by means of a metal frame attached to the bed.
4. *Encircling traction* is often considered a type of skin traction. A halter or sling is placed around a body part and attached by means of a rope and pulley to a weight that pulls in a straight line. Examples of encircling traction are cervical head halter traction and pelvic traction.

Traction can be either continous or intermittent. Continuous traction (skeletal or skin) should be applied and released by a physician, and a physician should be responsible for handling the affected part when it is not in traction (Hilt, Cogburn, 1980, p 518). Intermittent traction (nonadhesive skin traction), on the other hand, can be applied and released by nursing personnel with the appropriate order.

TRACTION EQUIPMENT

The following equipment is required for all traction:

1. An overhead frame. This frame is attached to the hospital bed and provides a means for attachment of the traction apparatus (see Figure 21–1). There are a number of kinds of overhead frames, which attach to the bed in different ways; each frame, however, has at least two upright bars and one overhead bar.
2. A trapeze. Attached to the overhead frame, the trapeze can be used by the patient for moving in bed, unless contraindicated by the patient's condition.
3. A firm mattress. To maintain body alignment and the efficiency of the traction, a firm mattress is essential. Some beds are manufactured with a solid bottom instead of springs, to provide firm support. If a firm bed is not available, a bed board can be used to provide the needed support.

GUIDELINES FOR TRACTION

1. All traction should have countertraction to prevent the patient from being pulled by the force of traction against the pulleys or the bed, thus negating the traction.
2. To apply and maintain the correct amount of traction, all traction weights should be hanging freely and the ropes should not touch any part of the bed.
3. The traction force should follow an established line of pull. The line of pull determines the position and alignment of the body as prescribed by the physician. All ropes should be on the center track of a pulley, and the line of pull should always be from (a) the point of attachment to the patient, to (b) the first pulley. See Figure 21–1.
4. Traction should always be applied while the patient is in good body alignment in a supine position.

SPECIFIC TRACTIONS

Specific tractions that nurses may see in a hospital include the following. See Table 21–1 for the uses of these tractions, the nursing interventions involved, and other key considerations.

1. *Buck's extension.* This is a simple traction that can be applied to one leg (unilateral) or both legs (bilateral). See Figure 21–1. It is a skin traction and may use either

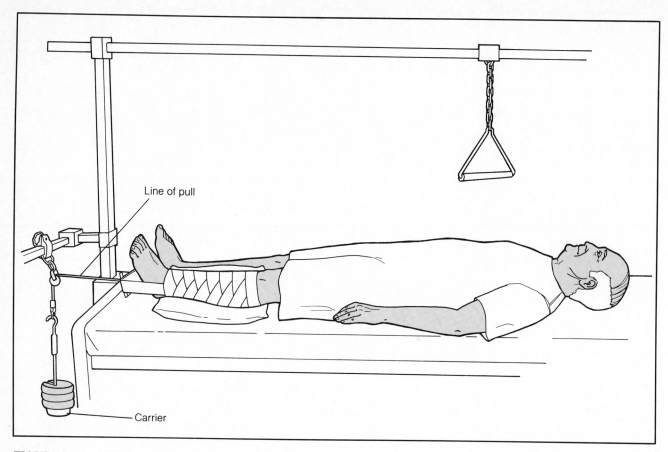

Line of pull

Carrier

FIGURE 21-1 ■ Unilateral Buck's extension traction.

adhesive or nonadhesive tape. Sometimes commercially made foam rubber boot-type splints with self-adhering straps are used (see Figure 21–2).

2. *Russell traction.* This is a skin traction (adhesive or nonadhesive) applied to one or both legs. A sling is used under the knee to suspend the limb. See Figure 21–3.

The pull on the limb is both vertical through the sling and horizontal through the footplate. The degree of flexion of the knee depends on the angle needed as

FIGURE 21-2 ■ A commercially made Buck's boot.

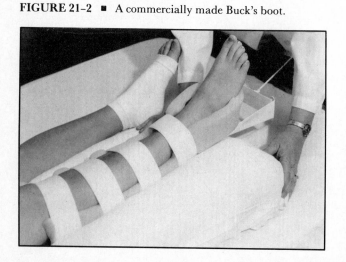

FIGURE 21-3 ■ Russell traction.

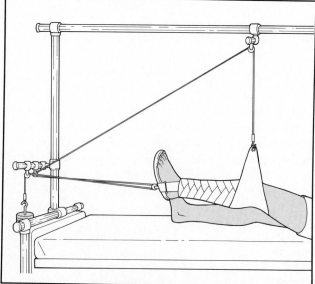

TABLE 21–1   ■   Specific Tractions: Uses and Nursing Interventions

Traction	Uses	Key considerations	Nursing interventions
Buck's extension	Prior to surgery for fractured femur Knee and hip contractures Disease processes of knee and hip	Bandages applied too tightly can cause: ■ Constriction of circulation in the extremity. Symptoms: numbness and coldness. ■ Pressure on and possible damage to peroneal nerve. Symptoms: tingling or pain of anterior aspect of lower leg and dorsal surface of foot; foot inversion and inability to extend toes. Pressure areas: skin over the tibia, if bandage slips; popliteal space; hamstring tendon; heels.	Provide regular back care, especially for the buttocks, because patient is confined to a back-lying position. Two nurses may be required to place and remove a bedpan if patient has pain or is obese. Because traction is often temporary, exercises are generally restricted to turning (eg, for back care), deep breathing, coughing, and foot movement.
Russell traction	Fractured femur Knee and hip contractures	See Buck's extension, first consideration. Pressure areas: popliteal space, due to sling; sole of foot, due to footplate.	Provide regular back care. Place and remove bedpan from the unaffected side. Teach exercises in preparation for crutch walking; see chapter 19.
Thomas leg splint and Pearson attachment	Fractured femur Pre- or postoperative immobilization	Pressure areas: the groin (adductor muscle and ischial area), from ring; popliteal space; Achilles tendon; heel; peroneal nerve, if splint and Pearson attachment slip to one side.	Provide regular skin care of the leg, foot, and back. Teach exercises in preparation for crutch walking; see chapter 19.
Pelvic belt (girdle) traction	Lower back pain	Belt will slip if too loose or incorrectly applied, causing uneven pull. Pressure areas: iliac crests, back.	Teach exercises to move extremities through full range of motion. Teach exercises to strengthen back muscles. Evaluate back pain: type, relief, etc.
Cervical head halter traction	Cervical injuries "Whiplash"	Pressure areas: chin, occiput of the head, ears, mandible.	Provide regular skin care, eg, every two hours. Keep the chin dry, using alcohol or cornstarch. Closely monitor food and fluid intake to ensure adequate diet, since eating and chewing are often difficult. A soft diet may be easier for patient to take. Assess for neck discomfort and for numbness and tingling in arms and hands.
Halo-thoracic vest traction	Thoracic and cervical spine injuries	Head pin migration (anchoring pin shifts in position), resulting in misalignment and loosening of halo. Discomfort from metal objects striking the metal traction rods. Conduction of sound through skull bones is discomforting, so care should be taken to avoid hitting rods with metallic objects. Pressure areas: where jacket edges touch the skin.	Meticulous pin site care with hydrogen peroxide and water in equal amounts needs to be given at least twice a day. Povidone-iodine is not used (may corrode pins). Some agencies advocate use of antibiotic ointment after cleaning with hydrogen peroxide. Infection at pin site is evidenced by increased drainage, inflammation, elevated body temperature, and headache.

TABLE 21–1 ■ continued

Traction	Uses	Key considerations	Nursing interventions
Halo-thoracic vest traction (continued)			Encourage deep breathing and coughing exercises q.4h., and auscultate chest sounds periodically. Incentive spirometry can be used also. (Respiratory complications from the vest and from decreased mobility can occur.)
			Open or remove vest daily to inspect the skin and provide skin care. At other times, inspect and massage skin around vest edges at least q.4h. Change or clean the sheepskin lining at least weekly.
			Assess for neurologic impairment of upper extremities due to the thoracic disorder. Check patient's hand grasps and sensation in fingers and hands q.4h. for first few days, then daily.
			Assess for cranial nerve impingement by the pins and traction forces. See Table 10–25 on page 235.
Side-arm traction	Fracture of the humerus Contractures or fracture of the elbow	Muscle stiffness due to maintenance of one position. Pressure areas: soft tissues near shoulder; anterior surface of elbow joint, due to bandages.	Do a neurovascular assessment of the arm and hand. Provide regular skin care of the back, arm, and hand. Encourage regular range-of-motion exercises for the unaffected extremities to prevent thrombophlebitis.

determined by the physician. The placement of the overhead pulley and the pulley on the foot of the bed will vary. The latter may be raised so that it is in line with the pulley on the footplate. The foot of the bed may or may not be elevated for countertraction. A pillow may or may not be ordered to support the lower leg. A variation of Russell traction is called *Split Russell.* In this traction, the weights are applied to the knee and the foot using separate cords; the cord from the sling usually runs to the overhead frame and then to the head of the bed.

3. *Thomas leg splint and Pearson attachment.* The Thomas leg splint consists of a full ring or a half ring around the thigh with two rods on either side of the leg. A sling is attached to the rods of the splint. A foam rubber pad or sheepskinlike material is used in some agencies for the sling. The Pearson attachment is a sling construction that supports the lower leg off the bed and permits the knee to be flexed. Countertraction is supplied mostly by the body's weight. This is a suspension that can be used with skin and/or skeletal traction. See Figure 21–4 for a balanced suspension using a Thomas splint and Pearson attachment in conjunction with both skin and skeletal traction.

4. *Pelvic belt traction.* Pelvic belts (girdles) provide traction to the patient's lower back. See Figure 21–5. The belts in common use today are disposable and adjustable, with self-adhering straps. The belt is fitted directly on the skin over the iliac crests (ie, the top margin is at the level of the umbilicus) and fastened over the abdomen. The straps, which attach to the pulley and weight system, may be attached either at the patient's sides, so that the pull of the traction is toward the foot of the bed, or at the back (under the patient), so that the traction pull is downward and toward the foot of the bed. Countertraction is provided by elevating the foot of the bed. This type of traction requires a supine position, unless otherwise ordered, and is frequently intermittent.

5. *Cervical head halter traction.* The cervical head halter provides skin (encircling) traction on the cervical spine. See Figure 21–6. The head halter is attached to a spreader bar wide enough to prevent the halter from pressing on the patient's ears, jaws, or sides of the head. Countertraction from the patient's body weight is provided by elevating the head of the bed. Head halter traction may be applied intermittently or continously. If traction is required for long periods of time, however, skeletal traction is applied.

6. *Halo-thoracic vest traction.* The halo-thoracic traction consists of a circular metal band (tiara or halo) that is fixed to the head by four pins (two anterior and two

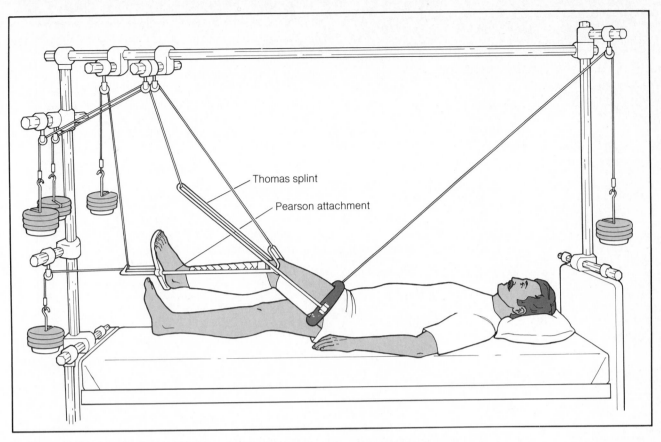

FIGURE 21–4 ■ Balanced suspension with Thomas ring splint and Pearson attachment.

FIGURE 21–5 ■ Pelvic belt.

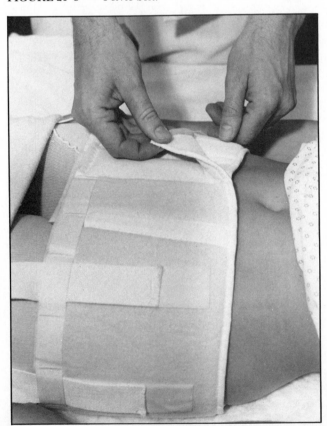

posterior). See Figure 21–7. These pins penetrate the skull only a fraction of an inch. The halo clears the head by about 1½ cm (½ in). Attached to the halo are metal rods that are in turn attached to either a plaster cast or plastic vest worn on the patient's trunk. Some vests extend to the patient's pelvic girdle. The vest, which is well padded with sheepskin, supports and suspends the weight of the entire apparatus around the patient's chest.

Halo traction is applied under local anesthetic. It provides firm stabilization of the thoracic spine. Trac-

FIGURE 21–6 ■ Cervical head halter traction.

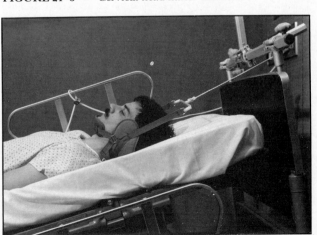

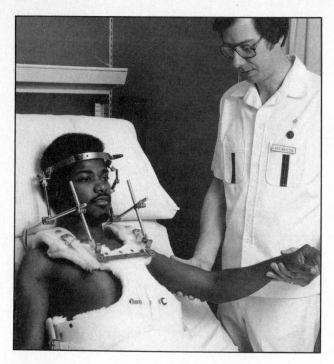

FIGURE 21-7 ■ Halo-thoracic vest traction.

tion to the thoracic spine is achieved by adjusting the nuts and bolts that attach the metal bars to the halo apparatus. By increasing or decreasing the distance between the halo and the vest, traction is increased or decreased. The advantage of this traction over other types of head and neck traction is that it allows the patient to sit, stand, and walk, thus decreasing the respiratory, circulatory, and muscular problems associated with prolonged immobility.

7. *Side-arm traction.* Side-arm traction may be skeletal or skin traction, depending on the site of the fracture, the presence of other injuries, and the physician's choice. The traction pull is outward from the upper arm and upward from the forearm. Countertraction is provided by the positioning of the body, eg, a folded blanket placed under the mattress on the side of the traction frame will augment countertraction (Farrell, 1982, p 137).

TECHNIQUE 21-1 ■ Applying Nonadhesive Skin Traction 🏠

Nonadhesive skin traction does not cause the skin irritations that are associated with adhesive tape. Furthermore, with the appropriate order, it can be released and applied by nurses. This type of traction is applied to an extremity.

■ Assessment

Assess for:

1. Bruises and abrasions in the area where the traction is to be applied. Report any open areas to the responsible nurse and/or physician before proceeding to apply the traction.

2. The neurovascular status of the extremity, ie, color, amount of movement, temperature, capillary filling, edema, numbness, sensation. See Technique 20-2 and Table 20-2 on page 476.

3. The presence of pain in the area: exact location, degree, duration, and description of the pain (eg, sharp, needlelike, etc) and identification or any movement or activity that would initiate the pain.

Other data include:

1. Any history of circulatory problems and skin allergies

2. The order to apply and/or remove the nonadhesive skin traction, including times and amount of weight

■ Planning

Nursing goals

1. To promote and maintain alignment of a lower extremity

2. To prevent neurovascular impairment

Equipment

1. Folded stockinette to place over the malleoli of the ankle.

2. 2-in or 3-in elastic bandage, depending on the circumference of the extremity.

3. Nonadhesive traction straps.

4. Adhesive tape to secure the elastic bandage.

5. Footplate (see Figure 21-8) or spreader bar (see Figure 21-9) wide enough to prevent the traction straps from irritating the skin over the sides of the foot and ankle. A footplate will also help keep the foot in a normal position, ie, neither acutely flexed nor extended.

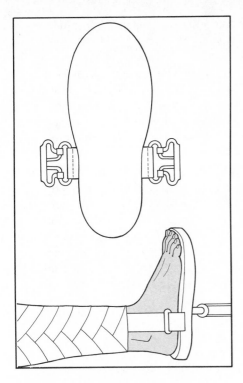

FIGURE 21–8 ■ A footplate.

FIGURE 21–9 ■ A spreader bar.

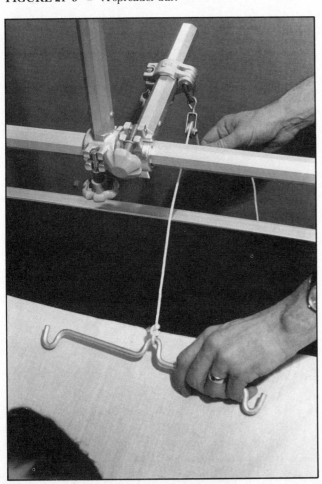

■ Intervention

1. Wash and dry the extremity, ie, the foot and leg.
2. Apply a piece of folded stockinette over the malleoli of the ankle.
    Rationale   This protects the skin from abrasion and pressure.
3. Place the nonadhesive traction strap down the inner aspect of the leg, around the foot, and up the lateral aspect of the leg, leaving the tape slack around the foot.
    Rationale   The slack of the tape will be taken up by the spreader bar or footplate.
4. Secure an elastic bandage over the strap, starting just above the ankle, using spiral-reverse or modified figure-eight turns. See Figure 21–10.
    Rationale   Starting just above the ankle avoids placing pressure on the Achilles tendon, and a spiral-reverse or modified figure-eight secures the bandage better than a simple spiral.
5. Secure the elastic bandage with adhesive tape.
6. Attach the spreader bar or footplate to the traction straps.
7. Check the amount of weight to be used.
8. Attach the rope to the spreader bar or footplate.
9. Slowly place the weight on the carrier (see Figure 21-1).
    Rationale   Sudden weight can jar the extremity and cause pain.

■ Evaluation

Expected outcomes

1. Skin intact and normal color
2. Neurovascular signs normal (see Table 20–2 and Assessment in Technique 20–2)

FIGURE 21–10

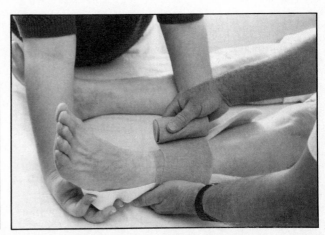

Unexpected outcomes

1. Skin reddened or abraded
2. Unable to dorsiflex ankle and extend toes
3. Unable to feel sensation on the web between the greater and second toes
4. Toes cold to touch

5. Capillary refill sluggish

Upon obtaining an unexpected outcome:

1. Report your findings to the responsible nurse and/or physician.
2. Revise the nursing care plan as necessary.

TECHNIQUE 21–2 ■ Assisting a Patient in Traction

After the application of traction, it is important for the nurse to assess the patient's physical condition as well as provide support. If the patient has had skeletal traction applied in the operating room, postoperative care is usually needed as well. See chapter 32.

■ Assessment

Assess the patient for:

1. Clinical signs of constipation, hypostatic pneumonia, and muscle atrophy.
2. Clinical signs of emboli. Fat emboli may occur as a result of fractures of long bones such as the femur. Regularly assess the patient's pulse, blood pressure, and respirations for evidence of emboli. A pulmonary embolus can occur secondary to thrombophlebitis or by itself. See Table 32–1 on page 777 for potential postoperative complications.
3. Need for diversional activities.
4. Signs of skin irritation or pressure on the skin areas. Note in particular:
    a. Bony prominences, such as the heels, ankles, sacrum, elbows, chin, and shoulders
    b. Areas susceptible to pressure from the traction, eg, the iliac crests for a pelvic girdle or the legs for Buck's extension
5. The correct position of the traction and the body alignment.
6. Neurovascular condition. For patients who have adhesive skin traction or skeletal traction, provide a neurovascular assessment every hour for the first 24 hours. If the patient's status is "normal," then assess every four hours during the traction. If the patient's status is not normal, continue hourly assessments. For patients who have nonadhesive skin traction, provide a neurovascular assessment 30 minutes following reapplication of the bandage, then every two hours for the first 24 hours, then every four hours if the patient's status is normal. For details

about a neurovascular assessment, see chapter 20 on page 476.
7. Inflammation and drainage at the pin sites for skeletal traction.

Other data include:

1. The type of traction and the degree of movement permitted
2. Any special precautions, eg, bed positions permitted

■ Nursing Diagnosis

Nursing diagnoses that may indicate the need to assist a patient with traction include:

1. Impaired physical mobility related to traction devices
2. Impairment of skin integrity related to immobility

■ Planning

Nursing goals

1. To support the patient psychologically
2. To maintain the traction
3. To assist the patient with activities of daily living, as required
4. To prevent the occurrence of complications, such as pressure sores, pneumonia, and muscle contractures

Equipment

1. Protective skin devices, eg, heel protectors.
2. Trapeze if needed.
3. Rubbing alcohol.
4. Supplies for pin care in skeletal traction, eg, alcohol to clean the pin site or antiseptic recommended at the agency. Sterile technique is required. See chapter 35 for sterile dressing supplies.

■ Intervention

1. Inspect the traction to ensure that appropriate countertraction is provided and that the correct weights are applied. The physician determines the amount of weight required for the traction.

2. Inspect the traction apparatus regularly, ie, whenever you are at the patient's bedside, or at prescribed intervals, such as every two hours. Ensure that:

   a. There is free play of the ropes on the pulleys, ie, the groove of the pulley supports the rope.

   b. All weights hang freely and do not rest against or on the bed or floor.

   c. Ropes are not frayed, knotted, or kinked between their points of attachment.

   d. The line of the traction is straight and in the same plane as the long axis of the bone.

   e. Bedclothes and other objects do not impinge on the traction.

   f. The footplate is positioned above, not resting against, the end of the bed.

   Rationale   Any articles that impinge on the traction can negate its effectiveness.

3. Provide protective devices and measures to safeguard the skin. For example, place heel protectors or sheepskins under the heels, sacrum, shoulders, and other pressure areas. Massage the skin with rubbing alcohol every four hours and, if redness and signs of pressure appear, every two hours.

   Rationale   Alcohol tends to toughen the skin and leave it less vulnerable to breakdown (Hilt, Cogburn, l980, p 532).

4. Ensure that the ropes are securely attached with slip knots, which can be untied easily and rapidly. Figure 21–11 shows how to tie a slip knot. Check that the short ends of the ropes are also attached with tape to prevent them from slipping. When taping the ends of the ropes, make a folded tab at the end of the tape to facilitate its removal. See Figure 21–12.

5. Provide a trapeze to assist the patient to move and lift the body for back care if he or she is unable to turn, eg, if the patient has balanced suspension traction.

6. Maintain the patient in the supine position unless there are other orders.

   Rationale   Changing position can change the body alignment and the amount of force supplied by the traction.

7. Maintain body alignment when turning the patient. In some cases, the patient can turn to a lateral position if body alignment is maintained by a pillow placed between the legs. Refer to the patient's chart for information about permitted movement.

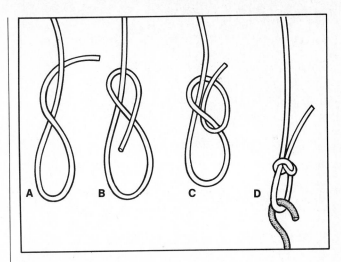

FIGURE 21–11   ■   Tying a slip knot: **A**, make a figure eight; **B**, bring the free end of the rope through the lower loop; **C**, bring the free end of the rope under and through the upper loop; **D**, tighten the knot by pulling on the free end.

8. Do not remove skeletal and adhesive skin traction.

   Rationale   A reduced fracture, for example, can become malpositioned if traction is removed; therefore, removal is a physician's responsibility (Hilt, Cogburn, 1980, p 518).

9. Nonadhesive skin traction is intermittent and can be removed; check agency policy about any orders required. Remove the weights first; then unwrap the bandage and provide skin care. Rewrap the limb and slowly reattach the weights.

FIGURE 21–12

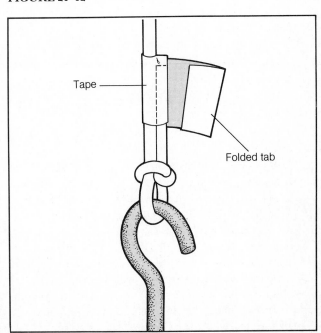

Tape

Folded tab

10. Make sure the spreader bar is wide enough to prevent the traction tape from rubbing on the patient's bony prominences.

11. Provide pin site care. This varies with different authorities. Five principles recommended for such care are:

    a. Carefully inspect the site.

    b. Use sterile technique.

    c. Remove crusts with a rolling technique.

    d. Cover sites with a sterile barrier.

    e. Determine frequency of care by amount of drainage (Celeste, Folcik, Dumas, l984, p 20).

Regular inspection of the site ensures early detection of minor infections, eg, serosanguinous drainage, crusting, swelling, and erythema. Sterile technique for cleaning helps protect the patient from infection. Infection at the site can spread to the bone. Removing all crusted secretions permits the pin site to drain freely. Initial crusts around Steinmann's pins do not create a problem and can be left, but accumulated crusts around external fixator pins can cause secondary infection (Sproles, l985, p 18). These crusts can be removed by using hydrogen peroxide twice daily. Using a gentle rolling technique reduces irritation to the tissue.The site is then covered with a sterile barrier, ie, sterile gauze or sterile ointment. One method is to soak 2 × 2 sterile gauze with povidone-iodine solution after the gauze has been applied around the pin (Celeste, Folcik, Dumas, l984, p 20). Procedures vary, so check agency practices regarding pin site care.

12. Teach the patient deep breathing and coughing to prevent hypostatic pneumonia. See chapter 31.

13. Teach the patient appropriate exercises to maintain and develop muscle tone, prevent muscle atrophy, and promote blood circulation. Isometric exercises are discussed in chapter 19, page 430. Specific exercises are designed to strengthen the biceps and triceps muscles in preparation for using crutches. For example, raising the buttocks off the bed by pushing down with the arms develops the triceps, and pulling the body up with a trapeze develops the biceps. Isometric exercises to strengthen the quadriceps muscles include tightening the knees; by pushing the knees down without moving them the hamstring muscles are also strengthened. Tensing the buttocks and the inner thighs promotes stabilization of the hips; tensing the inner thighs also helps stabilize the knees. Circulation to the extremities is promoted by flexing and extending the feet as well as by the isometric exercises.

■ Evaluation

Expected outcomes

1. Pin site clean, small amount of serous drainage
2. Absence of redness on pressure areas
3. Patient performs isometric exercises q.4h. as taught
4. Patient uses trapeze to move

Unexpected outcomes

1. Pin site erythematous, moderate serosanguinous drainage
2. Skin irritated, eg, right heel reddened, skin broken

Upon obtaining an unexpected outcome:

1. Report your findings to the responsible nurse and/or physician.
2. Revise the nursing care plan, eg, increase the frequency of skin care.

References

Celeste SM, Folcik MA, Dumas KM: Identifying a standard for pin site care using the quality assurance approach. *Orthop Nurs* (July/August) 1984; 3:17–24.

Farrell J: *Illustrated Guide to Orthopedic Nursing*, 2nd ed. Lippincott, 1982.

Hilt NE, Cogburn SB: *Manual of Orthopedics.* Mosby, 1980.

Jobes, RD: Cranial nerve assessment with halo traction. *Orthop Nurs* (July/August) 1982; 1:11–15.

Milazzo V: An exercise class for patients in traction. *Am J Nurs* (October) 1981; 81:1842–1844.

Preventing problems at pin sites. *Am J Nurs* (February) 1980; 80:259.

Rutecki B et al: Caring for the patient in a halo apparatus. *Nursing 80* (October) 1980; 10:73–77 (Canadian ed. pp 19–23).

Sproles KJ: Nursing care of skeletal pins: A closer look. *Orthop Nurs* (January/February) 1985; 4:11–12, 15–19.

York N et al: Halo traction. *Can Nurse* (January) 1980; 76:28–31.

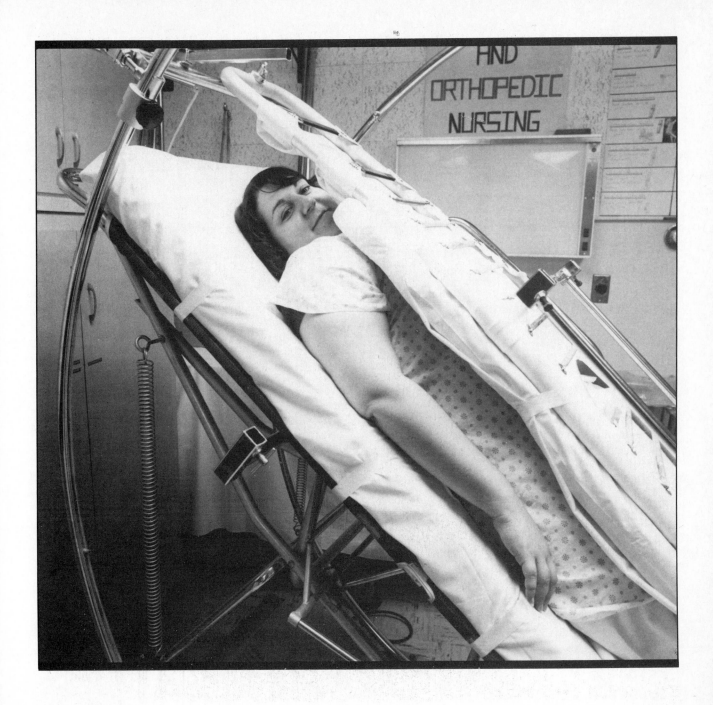

TURNING FRAMES

22

Specially designed turning frames, such as the Stryker frame and the CircOlectric bed, are used for patients in hospitals who cannot be positioned in a conventional hospital bed because of their injury or illness. To operate these devices, the nurse requires an understanding not only of their mechanics but also of precautions essential to the patient's safety. Patients are often apprehensive when initially placed on a different bed frame, especially when turned. Fear of falling and concern about immobility and dependence on others are not uncommon. To allay such fears, the patient needs reassurance from the nurse and confidence in the nurse's competence in operating the bed. The nurse's explanations of what will happen can alleviate patient apprehension.

Chapter Outline

Objectives

Upon completion of this chapter, the student will:

1. Know essential facts about turning frames and some of the techniques related to them
   1.1 Identify two types of turning frames
   1.2 Identify essential parts of turning frames
   1.3 Identify safety precautions essential to turning patients
   1.4 Identify measures necessary to enhance the patient's sense of security
2. Understand facts about techniques used to assist patients on turning frames
   2.1 Identify relevant assessment data
   2.2 Identify nursing diagnoses for which the technique may be implemented
   2.3 Identify nursing goals related to the technique
   2.4 Identify expected and unexpected outcomes from assessment data
   2.5 Identify reasons underlying the steps of the technique
3. Perform nursing interventions for patients on turning frames

   3.1 Assess the patient adequately
   3.2 Collect additional data from appropriate sources
   3.3 Select pertinent nursing goals for the patient
   3.4 Establish relevant outcome criteria for the patient following the technique
   3.5 Collect necessary equipment before the technique
   3.6 Implement interventions to enhance the effectiveness of the technique and enhance the patient's comfort and safety
   3.7 Communicate relevant information about the patient to the appropriate persons
   3.8 Determine the evaluative outcomes of the technique
4. Evaluate own performance of specific techniques in a laboratory or clinical setting with the assistance of another
   4.1 Use the performance checklists provided
   4.2 Identify areas of strength and weakness
   4.3 Alter performance in response to own evaluation and that of another

TURNING FRAMES

Whenever a patient's body alignment must be strictly maintained, a specially designed bed that rotates on an axis is used to turn the patient from the supine to the prone position and vice versa. Two such beds are the Stryker wedge frame and the CircOlectric bed. The Stryker wedge frame turns the patient laterally through the side-lying position and is manually operated by the nurse. The CircOlectric bed rotates the patient vertically through the standing position and is operated electrically by the nurse using a push button. These turning frames are used for patients with certain types of spinal injuries, extensive burns, arthritis, pressure sores, etc., who require position changes that cannot be effectively managed in the standard bed.

THE STRYKER FRAME AND STRYKER WEDGE FRAME

The *Stryker frame* consists of two removable rectangular metal frames (anterior and posterior) with canvas stretched across them. Thin, sponge-rubber mattresses, covered with special sheets with ties, are placed over the canvas. The frames are fastened by a knurled nut to a metal attachment at the head and the foot. See Figure 22–1.

To allow use of the bedpan, the canvas and mattress on the posterior frame (used for the supine position) have a section that can be removed or a split under the buttocks. An opening in the canvas and mattress of the anterior frame (used for the prone position) may be used to allow a male patient to void. In the prone position, the canvas and mattress should extend from below the shoulders to the ankles. Narrow forehead and chin straps are provided to support the head. The bed is also equipped with armboard and footboard attachments. Three restraining straps (often fastened with Velcro) are placed around both frames when turning the patient. Since the bed is so narrow, these restraints may also be fastened around the patient as a safety precaution either continuously or at night.

An adaptation of the Stryker frame is the *Stryker wedge frame*, which by design requires only one nurse to turn

FIGURE 22–1 ■ A standard Stryker turning frame.

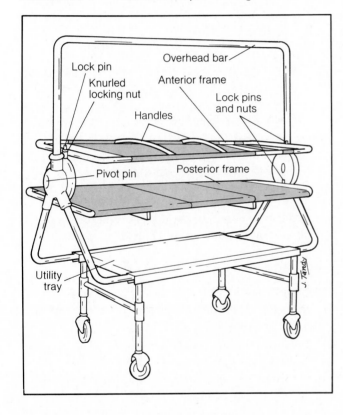

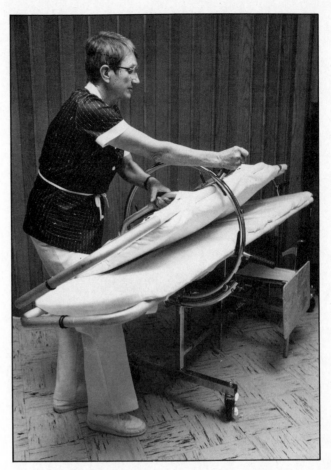

FIGURE 22–2 ■ A Stryker wedge frame. Note the wedge shape formed by the anterior and posterior frames.

the patient (two nurses are required for the standard Stryker frame). See Figure 22–2. This frame has a wedge shape because the upper frame is angled toward the lower frame at the side on which the frame will turn. This wedge prevents the patient from sliding out between the frames during the turn. The frames are attached to a turning ring that can be adjusted to tighten the frame snugly over the patient. The turning ring opens to form anterior and posterior rings, ie, two half rings.

TECHNIQUE 22–1 ■ Turning a Patient on a Stryker Wedge Frame

Patients on turning frames are generally turned every two hours, but the frequency of turning depends on the patient's diagnosis, care requirements, and tolerance. The schedule for turning the patient needs to be established with the patient and recorded on the nursing care plan. The usual plan schedules turns so that the patient can sleep on the posterior frame and have meals on the anterior one.

The technique for turning a patient on a standard Stryker frame is similar to that for the Stryker wedge frame discussed here, except that only *one* nurse is required for the Stryker wedge frame. *Two* nurses are essential to turn the patient on standard frames; one nurse stands at the foot, the other at the head, and on a signal they turn the patient in unison.

■ Assessment

Assessment depends on the patient's diagnosis and condition. Check the patient's nursing care plan. Assessments commonly include the following:

1. Note the patient's body alignment.
2. Assess the condition of the patient's skin for irritation and pressure areas.
3. Note specific complaints of discomfort.
4. Assess the patient's neurologic status, eg, feelings of numbness or tingling in the extremities, ability to move extremities, and motor strength of extremities. Most agencies have a checklist for such assessments. See also Table 20–2 on page 476.
5. Note the patient's tolerance for specific positions. For example, some patients tolerate the supine position for longer periods than the prone position.

Additional data include:

1. Skin care or other special needs required by the patient, eg, range-of-motion (ROM) exercise.
2. Position of pillows. Some patients may be allowed a small pillow under their heads and others not.
3. Scheduled times for the turn.
4. Whether restraining straps are applied continuously or only at night.

■ Nursing Diagnosis

Nursing diagnoses that may indicate the need for the use of a special turn bed include:

1. Impaired physical mobility related to:
   a. neuromuscular impairment
   b. musculoskeletal impairment
   c. surgical procedure to the spine
   d. multiple trauma
   e. severe burns
2. Actual or potential impairment of skin integrity related to immobility

■ Planning

Nursing goals

1. To maintain the patient's body alignment while changing her or his position

2. To prevent skin, respiratory, and circulatory problems related to immobility

Equipment

1. The anterior or posterior frame, depending on the turn. These are usually kept at the bedside.
2. Clean linen for the frame, as required. Special sheets with ties are available.
3. Positioning devices, eg, pillow supports, footboards.
4. Protective devices for the skin, eg, sheepskin.
5. Incontinence pads, if required.
6. Restraining straps.

■ Intervention

1. Even though the Stryker wedge frame can be operated by one nurse, it is a policy in many agencies that there should always be two nurses present when turning any bed frame. Check the agency policies.
2. Before turning the patient, ensure that all nursing care requirements are completed. For example, if the patient is on the posterior frame, the nurse can bathe all but the patient's back and place a clean gown on the patient.
3. Explain to the patient the direction in which the turn will take place, eg, to the patient's right or left.
4. If the patient has suction or drainage tubes, place them carefully at the head of the bed before the turn. Be sure that the tubing is long enough to accommodate the turn. Place urinary drainage bags on the mattress beside the patient; they must not be elevated above the level of the patient's bladder.

Turning from supine to prone position

5. Ensure that the wheels of the frame are locked.
   Rationale The wheels are locked to prevent the frame from moving during the turn.
6. Remove the armboards and bed linen or bath blanket.
7. Place a pillow lengthwise over the lower legs.
   Rationale The pillow provides security during the turn and maintains the alignment of the feet and legs.
8. Ensure that the anterior frame has clean linen on it.
9. Place the anterior frame over the patient, and tighten the knurled nut at the head of the frame. See Figure 22–3. The anterior frame will be angled with the posterior frame to form a wedge. If a standard Stryker frame is used, rather than the wedge frame, knurled nuts are fastened at *both* the head and the foot of the frame, and the frames are not angled.

Rationale   Tightening the knurled nut(s) will keep the frame securely in place during the turn.

10. Ensure that the forehead and chin bands are placed appropriately. See Figure 22–4.

    Rationale   Avoid obstructing the nose, mouth, and eyes.

11. Close the turning ring over the anterior frame, making sure that it is locked securely and that the frame fits snugly over the patient. The nuts on the anterior turning ring can be adjusted to tighten the frame against the patient. Directions for doing this are written on the frame.

12. Place the two restraining straps around both the frame and the patient's legs and chest. If the standard Stryker frame is used, a third restraining strap is placed over the hips (on the wedge frame, the turning ring is positioned over the hips).

    Rationale   The straps prevent the patient from slipping, especially his or her arms, if the patient is unable to use them.

13. Turn the patient:

    a. Have the patient wrap her or his arms around the anterior frame, if able. Otherwise make sure that the patient's arms are restrained.

       Rationale   This provides greater security for the patient when turning.

    b. Pull out the positive lock pin at the head of the frame. See Figure 22–5.

       Rationale   The frame can pivot when this pin is out.

    c. Pull out the red turning lock knob on the turning ring. See Figure 22–6.

       Rationale   This allows the frame to turn.

    d. Grasp the handle on the turning ring, and inform the patient that you will turn on the count of three.

    e. Count to three, and turn the frame toward you and toward the narrower side of the wedge, using a smooth, gradual motion.

FIGURE 22–3

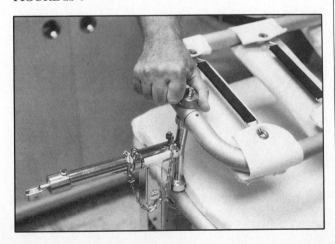

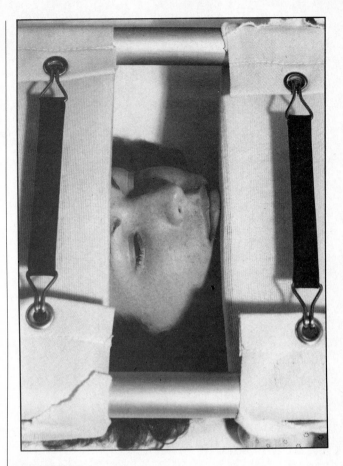

FIGURE 22–4

Rationale   Patients feel more secure when turned toward the nurse.

14. Replace the positive lock pin.

    Rationale   The pin stabilizes the frame and prevents it from pivoting.

FIGURE 22–5

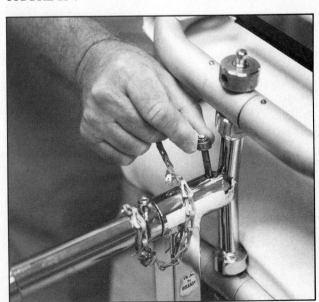

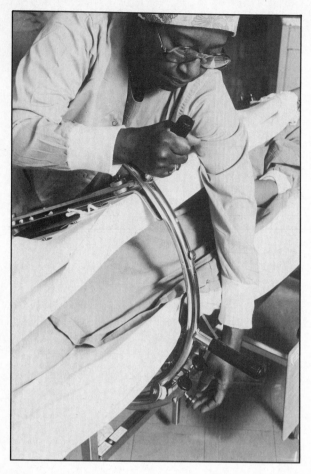

FIGURE 22-6

15. Push in the circular silver lock knob. See Figure 22-7. This opens the turning ring.
16. Release the knurled nut and remove the posterior frame.
17. Provide necessary care, and position the patient.

FIGURE 22-7

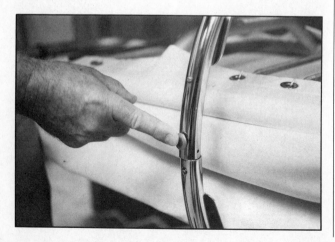

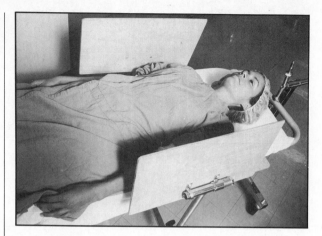

FIGURE 22-8

Turning from prone to supine position

18. Follow steps 1–6.
19. Place incontinence pads or sheepskins over the patient's sacrum, if necessary, and put a small pillow under the lumbar curvature, if required.
20. Place the posterior frame over the patient, and fasten it securely by the knurled nut at the head of the frame.
21. Follow steps 11–16, adjusted for the patient moving from the prone to the supine position.

For either position

22. Provide skin care to pressure areas as required.
23. Position the patient in good body alignment. See chapter 17. Check the physician's and nursing orders about the positioning supports that are recommended and permitted. Footboards are generally attached, to prevent foot drop when the patient is in the supine position. When the patient is prone, the feet should hang over the end of the canvas in a flexed position. To prevent external rotation of the hips, a sandbag or trochanter roll may be placed against the hips. See chapter 17.
24. Attach the armboards, and position the patient's arms appropriately to prevent adduction contractures of the shoulders and flexion contractures of the elbows. The armboards should be slightly below the level of the frame when the patient is in the prone position and level with the frame when the patient is in the supine position. In the supine position, the armboards may also be used as protective side rails. See Figure 22-8.
25. Cover the patient appropriately for warmth.
26. Place restraining straps around the patient as a protective measure if required. Generally, one restraining strap is placed around the hips for

patients receiving narcotics or sedatives and for all patients at bedtime.

27. Instruct the patient about foot or leg exercises, eg, dorsiflexion and plantar flexion, inversion and eversion of the foot, if not contraindicated.

28. Put clean linen and a pillow on the frame that was removed, in readiness for the next turn.

29. Record relevant assessments and interventions on the appropriate records.

■ Evaluation

Expected outcomes

Although these depend on the patient's pathology, outcomes generally include:

1. Skin intact over bony prominences
2. Adequate range of motion in all joints
3. Neurologic status intact

4. Ability to tolerate specific position for specified periods of time

Unexpected outcomes

1. Skin irritation or redness over bony prominences
2. Pain unrelieved by position change
3. Limited range of motion in joints
4. Impaired neurologic status, eg, numbness or tingling in extremities, decreased motor strength, inability to move extremities
5. Inability to tolerate specific position for specified time period

Upon obtaining an unexpected outcome:

1. Report your findings to the responsible nurse and/or physician.
2. Adjust the nursing care plan as required, eg, to incorporate skin care or to change the frequency of turning.

THE CIRCOLECTRIC BED

The CircOlectric bed (see Figure 22–9) is similar in purpose to the Stryker frame but offers a greater variety of positions. For example, patients can be placed in standing position, Trendelenburg's position, and even sitting positions. Positions that tilt the patient vertically toward the standing position are particularly useful for preventing postural hypotension and preparing the patient for ambulation. From the standing position, the patient can walk directly off the bed without changing the spinal alignment. Another advantge of the CircOlectric bed is that it can be operated independently by the patient. Even a very helpless patient may be able to adjust his or her position slightly and assume a greater degree of independence.

A CircOlectric bed consists of the following equipment (see Figure 22–10):

1. An electrically operated circular framework and motor, which can be operated manually in case of a power failure.

2. A posterior (basic) frame, for lying in the supine position, with a foam mattress, a mattress cover, and a headboard. A circular section of the mattress and a metal plate under the perineal area can be removed to insert a bedpan. The bedpan is held in place by special fasteners.

3. An anterior frame, for lying in the prone position, with a foam mattress and cover.

FIGURE 22–9 ■ A CircOlectric bed.

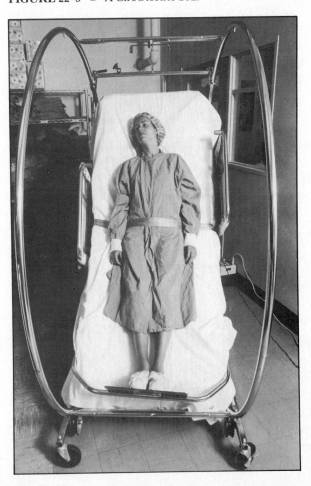

4. Special sheets that fasten to the mattresses with elastic bands.

5. A footboard that attaches to the frame.

6. A control switch to adjust the bed and a hand crank if it needs to be operated manually. The control switch has two labels, "Face" and "Back." The face switch turns the bed slowly to the prone position while the back switch turns it to supine position.

7. Adjustable side rails.

8. Forehead and chin supports for the anterior frame.

Accessory equipment includes traction bars, an IV pole, exercise apparatus, and canvas arm slings to support the arms.

Placing a patient on the bed

Prepare the bed before the patient is placed on it. Cover the mattress sections with the special sheets, and lock the wheels to prevent the bed from rolling. Test the bed to make sure it is in good working order before the patient is placed on it. It is important to explain to the patient and support persons how the bed works. If possible, give a demonstration of the bed before the patient is moved. Then lift the patient onto the posterior frame, using a three-person or four-person lift. See Technique 16–11 on page 393. A fourth person may be required, for example, to hold the head of a patient who has had a neck injury and cannot control his or her head movements. Center the patient on the frame so that the buttocks are over the bedpan opening. Adjust the footboard to the patient's height, and place pillows and rolls as needed to support the patient's body in proper alignment.

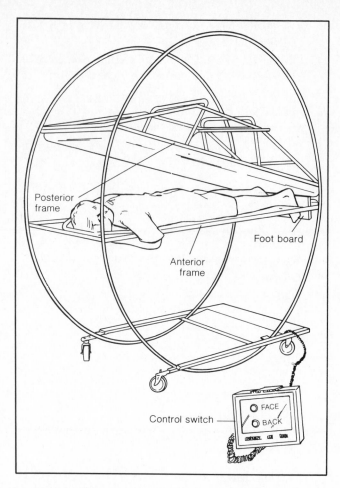

FIGURE 22–10 ■ Some of the functional parts of a CircOlectric bed.

TECHNIQUE 22–2 ■ Turning a Patient on a CircOlectric Bed

A CircOlectric bed can turn 210°, thus permitting a patient to assume a variety of positions.

■ **Assessment** See Technique 22–1 on page 500.

■ **Nursing Diagnosis** See Technique 22–1 on page 500.

■ **Planning**

Nursing goals See Technique 22–1 on page 500.

Equipment

1. Restraining straps for the patient in a prone position (side rails cannot be used).

2. Canvas slings and/or safety belt to protect the patient's arms if they cannot be held around the frame.

3. Skin care materials, including padding for bony prominences, if needed. See chapter 14.

4. Positioning devices, eg, pillows, folded bath blankets, towels. See chapter 17.

■ **Intervention**

1. Lock the wheels of the bed.
   Rationale Locking the wheels will prevent the bed from moving during turning.

2. Describe the technique and the sensations the patient may experience. Patients often need considerable reassurance the first few times they are turned,

because they experience vertigo (dizziness) from the turning. They also feel helpless and sometimes imagine that they will fall. It is important to discuss these sensations and reassure the patient that the turning is carefully controlled and can be stopped at any time.

3. Free any tubing, and arrange tubing and containers appropriately prior to the turn.

    Rationale Tubing can become tangled during the turn if it is not arranged beforehand.

4. Maintain eye contact with the patient during any turn.

    Rationale Maintaining eye contact is reassuring to the patient and allows the nurse to become immediately aware of any problem.

5. Do not stop a turn until the patient reaches the intended position unless absolutely necessary.

    Rationale Stopping and starting a turn can increase a patient's nausea and vertigo.

6. Maintain traction (eg, skull tongs) while turning the patient.

    Rationale Lack of traction can result in nonalignment of the vertebral column.

Turning from supine to upright or prone position

7. Measure the distance from the patient's shoulders to ankles, and adjust the canvas of the anterior frame to fit the patient.

    Rationale The anterior frame should support the patient from the shoulders to the ankles.

8. Remove the restraining strap and top covers from the patient.

9. Place a pillow or folded bath blanket lengthwise over the lower legs.

    Rationale This padding maintains their alignment and prevents movement during the turn.

10. Remove the pillow under the patient's head.

11. Place the anterior frame over the patient and fasten the bolts at both ends. See Figure 22–11.

12. Adjust the head support, and pad it if necessary.

13. Determine that the patient's feet are placed where they will not be injured by the footboard.

14. Assist the patient to place her or his arms around the anterior frame. If the patient cannot grasp the frame, place the arms alongside the body and secure them with a restraining strap, or place the arms in the canvas slings. See Figure 22–12.

15. Inform the patient, then turn on the control marked "Face." The bed will move slowly, turning the patient toward a prone position. (For an upright position, stop the bed when the patient is vertical. The upright position for a patient is first established with the anterior frame in place. When the patient

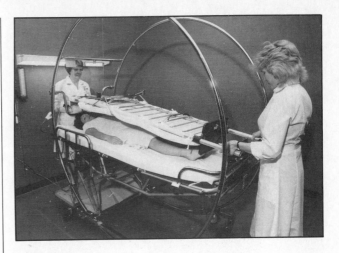

FIGURE 22–11

tolerates standing between the frames for five to ten minutes, the patient then progresses to standing with only restraining straps at the waist and the knee.)

16. Release the switch when the patient is horizontal. See Figure 22–13.

17. Release the locks on the posterior frame, and push the frame upward until it locks in its gatched (raised) position.

18. Adjust the patient's body to ensure correct alignment.

19. Place a restraining strap on the patient to prevent a fall.

    Rationale The side rails cannot be used in the prone position, but a restraining strap offers a sense of security and will prevent the patient from falling off the bed.

FIGURE 22–12

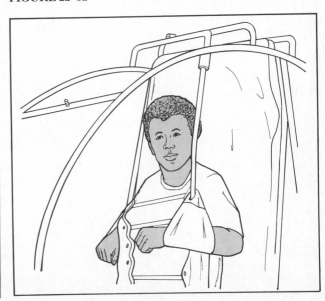

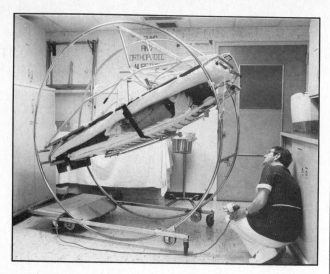

FIGURE 22–13

Turning from prone to supine position

20. Remove the restraining strap and the bedclothes from the patient.
21. Make sure that the footboard is placed against the patient's feet.

    Rationale The footboard helps to stabilize the patient during the turn.
22. Disengage the posterior frame from its raised position by releasing the lock and pushing the frame upward.
23. Lower the frame so that it fits over the patient, then fasten the bolts at both ends.
24. Secure the patient's arms as in step 14.
25. Inform the patient, then turn on the control marked "Back." The bed will move slowly to turn the patient toward a supine position.
26. Release the switch when the bed is horizontal or in the desired position.

27. Release the locks on the anterior frame, and remove the frame.
28. Remove the pillow or bath blanket over the patient's legs.
29. Adjust the patient's body for correct alignment. Provide supports, eg, a head pillow, if permitted.
30. Adjust the side rails, if necessary.

For all turns

31. Provide skin care to bony prominences before and after the turn.

    Rationale Skin care before a turn will treat the pressure areas onto which the patient will be moved; after a turn it will treat pressure areas she or he has been lying on.
32. Adjust the bedclothes.
33. Assess the patient's response to the turn in terms of discomfort, vertigo, syncope, nausea, and pallor.
34. Record relevant assessments and interventions on the patient's chart. In many agencies, turns are recorded in a summary statement at the end of a shift.

Sample Recording

Date	Time	Notes
11/6/86	1600	Alternated prone and supine positions q.2h. Sacrum remains reddened, no breaks in the skin. No discomfort with turns, but states still fearful.—Metsa C. Iwasaki, RN

35. Adjust the nursing care plan as needed.

■ **Evaluation**   See Technique 22–1 on page 503.

References

Allan D: Care of the patient in a wedge turning frame . . . Stryker frame. *Nurs Times* (August 15–21) 1984; 80(33): 40–41.

Hilt NE, Cogburn SB: *Manual of Orthopedics.* Mosby, 1980.

Hrobsky A: The patient on a CircOlectric bed. *Am J Nurs* (December) 1971; 71:2352–2353.

Nursing 82 Photobook: *Coping with Neurologic Disorders.* Intermed Communications, 1981.

Zejdlik CP: *Management of Spinal Cord Injury.* Wadsworth, 1983.

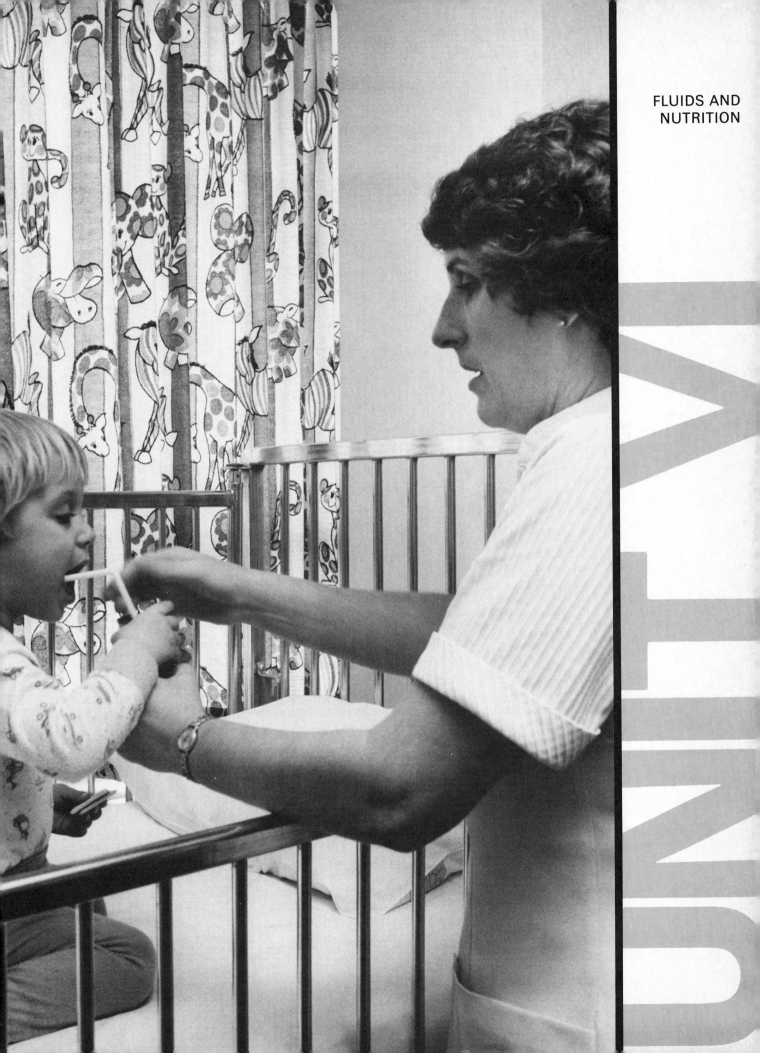

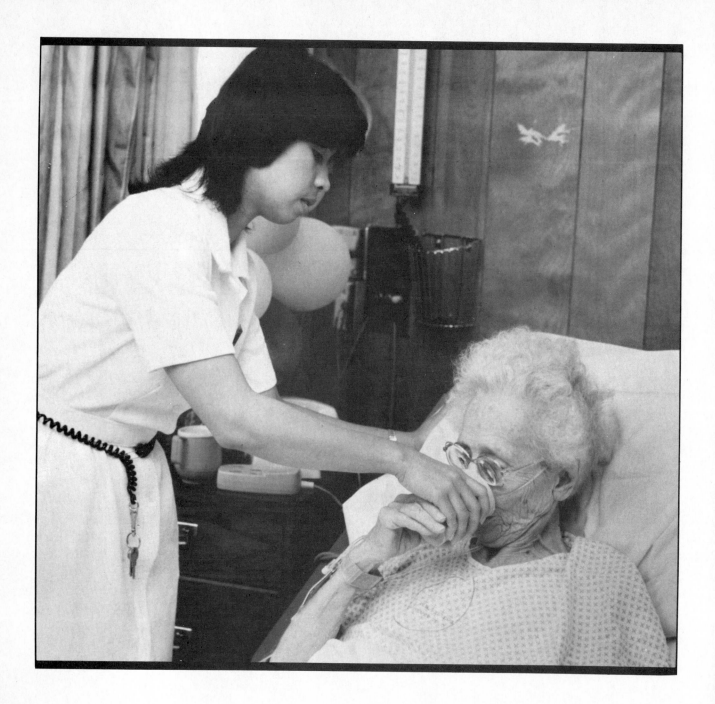

FLUID INTAKE AND OUTPUT

23

It is necessary to measure fluid intake and output for many hospital patients. Usually both intake and output are measured over a 24-hour period and the totals are compared for information about fluid balance. Measured fluid intake includes fluids taken by mouth, intravenous feedings, nasogastric feedings, and gastrostomy feedings. Measured fluid output usually includes urine and any drainages, such as drainage from gastric suction. Outputs of sweat, feces, and respirations are described in general terms rather than specific measurements. Sweat may be profuse, moderate, or slight. Feces are described as liquid, semisolid, or solid, in large, moderate, or small amounts. Respirations are described

according to rate, depth, rhythm, and character. Rate is particularly significant for fluid loss in the breath.

Chapter Outline

Body Fluid

Normal Fluid Intake

Normal Fluid Output

■ Technique 23–1 Monitoring Fluid Intake and Output

Objectives

Upon completion of this chapter, the student will:

1. Know essential terms and facts about body fluid and fluid balance
   1.1 Define selected terms
   1.2 Identify factors affecting the proportion of body weight that is fluid
   1.3 Identify the body's fluid compartments
   1.4 Identify three major sources of body fluids
   1.5 Identify unusual sources of fluid intake during illness
   1.6 Identify four sources of fluid output
   1.7 Identify unusual sources of fluid output during illness
   1.8 Identify normal daily fluid intakes and outputs
2. Understand facts about techniques used to monitor a patient's fluid intake and output
   2.1 Identify relevant assessment data
   2.2 Identify nursing diagnoses for which the technique may be implemented
   2.3 Identify nursing goals related to the technique
   2.4 Identify expected and unexpected outcomes from assessment data
   2.5 Identify reasons underlying steps of the technique

3. Perform techniques related to monitoring a patient's fluid intake and output effectively
   3.1 Assess the patient adequately
   3.2 Collect additional data from appropriate sources
   3.3 Select pertinent nursing goals for the patient
   3.4 Establish relevant outcome criteria for the patient following the technique
   3.5 Collect necessary equipment before the technique
   3.6 Implement interventions to enhance the effectiveness of the technique and enhance the patient's comfort and safety
   3.7 Communicate relevant information about the patient to the appropriate persons
   3.8 Determine the evaluative outcomes of the technique
4. Evaluate own performance of specific techniques in a laboratory or clinical setting with the assistance of another
   4.1 Use the performance checklists provided
   4.2 Identify areas of strength and weakness
   4.3 Alter performance in response to own evaluation and that of another

Terms

■ dehydration insufficient fluid in the body

■ dependent edema edema of the lowest or most dependent parts of the body

■ diaphoresis profuse perspiration

■ diuretic an agent that increases the production of urine

■ edema excess interstitial fluid

■ electrolyte (ion) a chemical substance that develops an electric charge and conducts an electric current when placed in water

■ excretion waste produced by the body cells

■ extracellular fluid (ECF) fluid found outside the body cells

■ hematocrit the percentage of red blood cell mass in proportion to whole blood

■ hemorrhage the escape of blood from the blood vessels

■ interstitial fluid fluid found between the body cells

■ intracellular fluid (ICF) fluid found within the body cells (cellular fluid)

■ intravascular within a blood vessel

■ lymph transparent, slightly yellow fluid found within the lymphatic vessels

■ pitting edema edema that leaves a small depression or pit after finger pressure is applied to the swollen area

■ plasma   the fluid portion of blood

■ secretion   the product of a gland, eg, saliva is the secretion of the salivary glands

■ shock   acute peripheral circulatory failure

■ solute   a substance dissolved in a liquid

■ solvent   the liquid in which a solute is dissolved

BODY FLUID

Proportions

The proportion of fluid in the human body varies with age, body fat, and sex. As age increases, the proportion of body water decreases. For example, while 77% of a newborn's body weight is fluid, only 55% of an adult female's body weight is fluid. See Table 23–1. Because body fat is essentially free of fluid, the amount of fat substantially alters the total volume of fluid in proportion to a person's weight. For example, an obese person's body may have only 50% fluid in relation to weight while a thin person's may have 60% fluid. This variable of body fat also accounts for the difference in total body fluid between the sexes. Adult females have a higher proportion of body fat than adult males, and thus less fluid.

Distribution

The body's fluid is divided into two major reservoirs, intracellular and extracellular. The *intracellular fluid* (ICF), also called the *cellular fluid,* is fluid found within the cells of the body. It comprises two thirds to three quarters of the total body fluid. The *extracellular fluid* (ECF) is fluid found outside the cells; it is subdivided into two compartments, *intravascular* (plasma) and *interstitial.* Plasma is fluid found within the vascular system; interstitial fluid is fluid that surrounds the cells, and it includes lymph. Extracellular fluid comprises one third to one fourth of the total body fluid. Interstitial fluid comprises three quarters of extracellular fluid. Normal body functioning requires that the volume of each fluid compartment remain relatively constant.

Secretions and excretions are also part of the body's total fluid volume and provide essential functions. They

TABLE 23–1 ■ Fluid Percentage of Body Weight by Age

Age (developmental stage)	Approximate percentage of fluid
Early human embryo	97
Newborn	75
Adult male	57
Adult female	55
Elderly adult	45

TABLE 23–2 ■ Secretions of the Adult Alimentary Tract

Secretion	Volume (mL/day)
Saliva	1,200
Gastric secretions	2,000
Pancreatic secretions	1,200
Bile	700
Succus entericus	2,000
Brunner's gland secretion	50
Large intestine secretions	60
Total	7,210

Source: Adapted from AC Guyton: *Textbook of Medical Physiology,* 6th ed, Saunders, 1981, p 803.

are part of the extracellular fluid. A *secretion* is the product of a gland, for example, the salivary glands. Some specific secretions are cerebrospinal fluid, synovial fluid, pericardial fluid, and alimentary secretions. An *excretion* is waste produced by the cells of the body. Just as balances exist between cellular and extracellular compartments, balances occur among plasma and secretions and excretions. Alimentary secretions for an adult, for example, are estimated to be about 7,200 mL per day. See Table 23–2.

Nurses need to be aware of abnormal amounts of secretions and excretions. Excessive losses can seriously deplete first the extracellular fluid volume and then the intracellular fluid volume. Excessive or inadequate secretions interfere with a number of body processes, such as digestion and elimination.

Composition

All body fluids contain important substances, such as salts, oxygen from the lungs, dissolved nutrients (glucose, fatty acids, and amino acids) from the digestive tract, and waste products of metabolism (eg, carbon dioxide).

The salts in solution break into one or more electrically charged particles called *ions* or *electrolytes.* For example, sodium chloride breaks into one ion of sodium (Na) and one ion of chloride (Cl). Ions that carry a positive charge are called *cations,* and those carrying a negative charge are called *anions.* Examples are:

Cations	*Anions*
Sodium (Na^+)	Chloride (Cl^-)
Potassium (K^+)	Bicarbonate (HCO_3^-)
Calcium (Ca^{++})	Phosphate (HPO_4^{--})
Magnesium (Mg^{++})	Sulfate (SO_4^{--})

TABLE 23-3 ■ Electrolyte Composition of Secretions and Excretions Compared to Plasma

| Substance | Electrolyte (mEq/L) | | | |
	Sodium (Na$^+$)	Potassium (K$^+$)	Chloride (Cl$^-$)	Bicarbonate (HCO$_3^-$)
Plasma	135–145	3.6–5.0	95–108	21–28
Gastric secretions	70	5+	140	5
Pancreatic juice	140+	5	35	115+
Hepatic duct bile	140+	5	100+	40
Jejunal secretions	140	5	135	30
Perspiration	80	5	85	—
Diarrhea in children	15	18	10	No method of determining; thought to be as high as K$^+$

In solution, positive and negative ions are attracted to one another until a balance is attained.

The electrolyte composition of the fluid compartments varies from one to another. For example, the principal ions of the extracellular compartment are sodium and chloride, while the principal ions of the intracellular compartment are potassium and phosphate. Just as the fluid volumes within the compartments must be maintained, so must the electrolyte compositions of the various compartments. Although the specific numbers of cations and anions may differ in the fluid compartments, in a state of homeostasis the total number of cations equals the total of anions within each compartment.

Body secretions and excretions also contain electrolytes. This is of particular concern when excretions are abnormally increased or decreased or when a secretion is lost from the body (for example, when gastric suction removes the gastric secretions). Fluid and electrolyte imbalance can result from prolonged loss through these routes. See Table 23–3 for the electrolyte composition of some body secretions and excretions.

Sources of Fluids and Electrolytes

The healthy person obtains fluids and electrolytes from three major sources:

1. Solid foods account for about half the fluid requirement of the average adult (750 mL). The water content of fresh vegetables is approximately 90% and of fresh fruits about 85%. Electrolytes are also found in foods. Table 23–4 shows the chief sources of some of the major electrolytes needed by the body.

2. Ingested fluids, such as water and juices, account for most of the other half of fluid requirements. The needed intake varies with the age and health of the individual.

3. Oxidation of food within the body also produces water. Oxidation is a chemical process by which a substance combines with oxygen; energy is released, and other substances are formed.

Table 23–5 shows the sources of a healthy adult's average daily fluid intake (2,500–2,600 mL). Note the 4:2:1 ratio, which assists recall.

The ill person, who cannot ingest food or fluids, may receive fluids through unusual routes:

1. Intravenous fluids (see chapter 25)
2. Nasogastric tube feedings (see Technique 24–6)
3. Gastrostomy or jejunostomy feedings (see Technique 24–6)

TABLE 23-4 ■ Major Food Sources of Selected Electrolytes

Electrolyte	Sources
Sodium (Na)	Table salt, cheese, ham, processed meats, canned foods, fish
Potassium (K)	Dark leafy greens, bananas, oranges, nuts, meat, fish, liver
Calcium (Ca)	Milk, cheese, yogurt
Magnesium (Mg)	Nuts, peanut butter, whole grains
Phosphorus (P)	Milk, poultry, fish, cereals

TABLE 23-5 ■ Sources of Adult Average Daily Fluid Intake

Source	Amount (mL)	Ratio
Water consumed as fluids	1,500	4
Water present in food	750	2
Water produced by oxidation	350	1
Total	2,600	

NORMAL FLUID INTAKE

Age is an important factor in establishing the individual's needed fluid intake. Infants and growing children have a much larger turnover of fluid than adults—that is, greater water needs and greater water losses. For this reason, an infant can become seriously dehydrated much more quickly than an adult. Some of the causes of the greater losses of fluids in infants are:

1. Less efficient kidneys
2. Rapid respirations
3. An increased metabolic rate due to activity and growth

Needed fluid intake can be calculated by determining the body surface area, which is derived from height and weight measurements, or according to body weight and age. Table 23–6 provides approximate fluid requirements at different ages according to body weight.

The health and activity of an individual also affect fluid needs. Because fluid intake is counterbalanced by fluid output, anything that affects output also affects the need for intake. For example, a patient who has a fever will have an abnormally high metabolic rate, which increases the activity of the kidneys and fluid loss. Because of the fever, increased amounts of fluid are also lost through breathing and diaphoresis. As a result of all these factors, the individual with a fever requires additional fluid intake to maintain the body's fluid balance. Activity also increases the metabolic rate, breathing, and diaphoresis, which increase fluid intake needs.

NORMAL FLUID OUTPUT

The fluid output of an individual counterbalances the fluid intake. The sources of normal fluid output are:

1. Urine excreted through the kidneys
2. Feces excreted from the intestine
3. Perspiration from the skin
4. Insensible loss in the water vapor of exhaled air and through the skin by diffusion

Table 23–7 shows the average daily fluid output for an adult. The major source of fluid output is urine. In an adult it accounts for about 1,500 mL per day. Fluid loss occurring through the skin and lungs is called *insensible* because it is usually not noticeable.

In illness, there are other sources of fluid loss and excessive losses from normal routes:

1. Drainage from catheters or suction tubes
2. Vomitus
3. Diarrhea
4. Diaphoresis
5. Hemorrhage
6. Ileostomy, cecostomy, or colostomy drainage
7. Excessive urine output

TABLE 23–6 ■ Average Daily Water Requirements by Age and Weight

Age	Water requirement	
	mL	mL/kg body weight
3 days	250– 300	80–100
1 year	1,150–1,300	120–135
2 years	1,350–1,500	115–125
4 years	1,600–1,800	100–110
10 years	2,000–2,500	70– 85
14 years	2,200–2,700	50– 60
18 years	2,200–2,700	40– 50
Adult	2,400–2,600	20– 30

Sources: RE Behrman, VC Vaughan: *Nelson Textbook of Pediatrics,* 12th ed, Saunders, 1979, p 138; RB Howard, NH Herbold, *Nutrition in Clinical Care,* 2nd ed, McGraw-Hill, 1982, p 153.

TABLE 23–7 ■ Average Daily Fluid Output for an Adult

Route	Amount (mL)
Urine	1,400–1,500
Insensible losses	
Lungs	350– 400
Skin	350– 400
Sweat	100
Feces	100– 200
Total	2,300–2,600

TECHNIQUE 23–1 ■ Monitoring Fluid Intake and Output

The physician or responsible nurse may order the monitoring (measurement) of a patient's fluid intake and output (I & O) for a variety of reasons. It is commonly measured for patients who:

1. Are postoperative
2. Are permitted nothing by mouth (NPO) and have intravenous infusions

3. Have retention catheters and urinary drainage systems
4. Have special drainages or suctions, such as a nasogastric suction
5. Are receiving diuretics
6. Have excessive fluid losses and require increased fluids
7. Have fluid retention and may require restricted fluids
8. May not be taking in the fluids they need, eg, the elderly

Units of measurement

The unit used to measure intake and output is the milliliter (mL) or cubic centimeter (cc); these are equivalent metric units of measurement. In household measures, 30 mL is roughly equivalent to 1 fluid ounce, 500 mL is about 1 pint, and 1,000 mL is about 1 quart. To measure fluid intake, household measures such as a glass, cup, or soup bowl need to be converted to metric units. Most agencies provide conversion tables, since the sizes of dishes vary from agency to agency. A table is often provided on or with the bedside I & O record. Examples of equivalents are:

Water glass	200 mL
Juice glass	120 mL
Cup	180 mL
Soup bowl	
Adult	180 mL
Child	100 mL
Teapot	240 mL
Creamer	
Large	90 mL
Small	30 mL
Water pitcher	1,000 mL
Jello, custard dish	100 mL
Ice cream dish	120 mL
Paper cup	
Large	200 mL
Small	120 mL

Intake and output forms

Most agencies have two forms for recording I & O: (a) a bedside worksheet record for a list of all items measured and their quantities per shift (see Figure 23–1), and (b) a 24-hour permanent record on the patient's chart, noting the totals for an 8-hour or 24-hour period (see Figure 4–5 on page 45). Some agencies have another form to record the specifics of intravenous fluids, such as the type of solution, additives, time started, amounts absorbed, and amounts remaining per shift. However, the total amounts for a specific period (eg, per shift) are then recorded on the permanent I & O record.

■ Assessment

Assess the patient for:

1. Clinical signs of fluid imbalances.
2. Body weight. Weigh the patient daily at the same time and with the same clothing, to assess weight gain or loss accurately (eg, before breakfast, dressed in a hospital gown, dressing gown, and slippers).
3. Observe the patient's urine for color, odor, clarity, and the presence of unusual constituents. See Table 27–1 on page 622.
4. Presence and degree of edema. To assess ankle edema daily, measure the ankle circumference with a measuring tape.
5. Fluid likes and dislikes, particularly if the patient is on forced fluids.
6. Any problems with voiding or ingesting fluids.

■ Nursing Diagnosis

Nursing diagnoses that may indicate the need to monitor fluid intake and output include:

1. Fluid volume deficit related to:
   a. Diarrhea
   b. Vomiting
   c. Restricted fluid intake
   d. Blood loss
2. Fluid volume excess related to:
   a. Kidney disorder
   b. Hormonal disturbances
   c. Low protein intake

■ Planning

Nursing goals

1. To assess the body's fluid balance
2. To determine whether a patient is taking adequate fluids to meet normal requirements
3. To verify an increased fluid intake
4. To verify a restricted fluid intake
5. To determine voiding patterns and urinary function
6. To assess the effectiveness of a medication, such as a diuretic, that increases urinary output

Equipment

1. A bedside I & O form and a pencil
2. A bedside bedpan, commode, or urinal for the patient
3. A calibrated container in which to measure the urine

BEDSIDE INTAKE-OUTPUT RECORD

Mary Brown
Name

747-2
Room No.

7/11
Date

Time		INTAKE		OUTPUT		
	Liquids		Intravenous	Urine	Emesis	Drainage etc.
8-4	0900	Juice 120		0700 - 250		
		Coffee 180		1100 - 400		
		Cream 90		1500 - 350		
	0930	Water 90				
	1200	Tea 180				
		Cream 90				
		Jello 50				
	1400	Juice 180				
Total		980		1000		
4-12						
Total						
12-8						
Total						

FIGURE 23-1 ■ A sample bedside fluid intake and output record.

■ Intervention

1. Explain to the patient that an accurate measurement of his or her fluid intake and output is required, the reason for it, and the need to use a bedpan or urinal (unless a urinary drainage system is in place). Many patients wish to be involved in recording these measurements and need to be given further information about how to compute the values and what foods are considered fluids.

2. Establish with the patient a plan for ingesting the required amount of fluid. Generally one half the total volume is ingested on the day shift, and the other half is divided between the evening and night shifts, with the majority on the evening shift.

To measure fluid intake

3. Following meals, record on the I & O form the amount of each fluid item taken, if the patient has not already done so. Specify the kind of fluid and the time. Measure all obvious fluids, such as water, milk, juice, soft drinks, coffee, tea, cream, soup, sherry, and wine. Also include such foods as ice cream, sherbet, custard, and gelatin (Jello). Do not measure foods that are pureed.

   Rationale Pureed foods are simply solid foods prepared in a different form.

4. Confirm with the patient any other fluids ingested between meals, and add the amounts to the form. Include water that is taken with medications. To assess the amount of water used from a water pitcher, measure what remains, and subtract this amount from the full amount of the pitcher. Then refill the pitcher.

5. Total the measurements at the end of the shift (every 8 or 12 hours), and transfer these totals to the correct column on the permanent record. Include the total volumes of intravenous fluids, including blood

transfusions. In some critical care settings you may need to record intake hourly.

To measure fluid output

6. Following each voiding, pour the urine into the measuring container, observe the amount, and record it and the time of voiding on the bedside I & O form. Clean the bedpan and measuring container, and return the bedpan to the patient.

7. For patients with retention catheters, note and record the amount of urine at the end of the shift, and then empty the drainage bag. The drainage bag usually has markings that indicate the amount of urine. If there is any doubt about the amount in the drainage bag, empty it first into an accurate measuring container.

8. Record any other output, such as emesis, liquid feces, and other drainage. Specify the type of fluid and the time.

9. If the patient is incontinent of urine or is extremely diaphoretic, estimate and record these "outputs." For example, of an incontinent patient you might record "Incontinent × 3," or "Drawsheet soaked in 12-in diameter." Of a diaphoretic patient you might record: "Perspiring profusely [or + + +]. Gown and drawsheet changed × 2." Follow agency practices in this regard.

10. At the end of the shift (every 8 or 12 hours), total the measurements, and transfer the totals to the correct column on the permanent record. In some critical care units you may need to total the fluid measurements hourly.

11. Compare the total fluid output measurement with the total fluid intake measurement and compare both measurements to previous measurements.
    Rationale Determine whether the fluid output reflects the fluid intake and any changes in fluid balance.

12. Observe the patient for signs of dehydration or overhydration. Weigh the patient daily, if indicated.

13. Report to the responsible nurse inadequate intakes and outputs. An adult urine output of less than 500 mL in 24 hours is considered inadequate.

14. Record pertinent assessment data on the patient's record.

15. Adjust the nursing care plan as needed to ensure appropriate fluid intake for the patient and appropriate measurement of I & O.

■ Evaluation

Expected outcomes

1. Fluid intake of 1,500 mL in 24 hours if solid foods are ingested and tolerated
2. Fluid intake of 3,000 mL in 24 hours if diet is restricted to fluids
3. Fluid output of 1,500 mL in 24 hours
4. Stable body weight
5. Clear, amber-colored urine

Unexpected outcomes

1. Fluid intake less than 1,000 mL in 24 hours
2. Fluid output less than 500 mL in 24 hours
3. Specific signs associated with fluid loss or excess
4. Diarrhea
5. Vomiting
6. Diaphoresis
7. Sudden weight gain

Upon obtaining an unexpected outcome:

1. Report your findings to the responsible nurse and/or physician.
2. Adjust the nursing care plan appropriately, eg, if a patient has inadequate intake, establish the reasons for it, and encourage increased fluid intake.

References

Behrman RE, and Vaughan VC: *Nelson Textbook of Pediatrics,* 12th ed. Saunders, 1983.

Burke SR: *The Composition and Function of Body Fluids,* 3rd ed. Mosby, 1980.

Grant MM, Kubo WM: Assessing a patient's hydration status. *Am J Nurs* (August) 1975; 75:1306–1311.

Guyton AC: *Textbook of Medical Physiology,* 6th ed. Saunders, 1981.

Harvey AM et al: *The Principles and Practice of Medicine,* 20th ed. Appleton-Century-Crofts, 1980.

Howard RB, Herbold NH: *Nutrition in Clinical Care,* 2nd ed. McGraw-Hill, 1982.

Twombly M: The shift into third space. *Nursing 78* (June) 1978; 8:38–41.

Whitney EN, Cataldo CB: *Understanding Normal and Clinical Nutrition.* West, 1983.

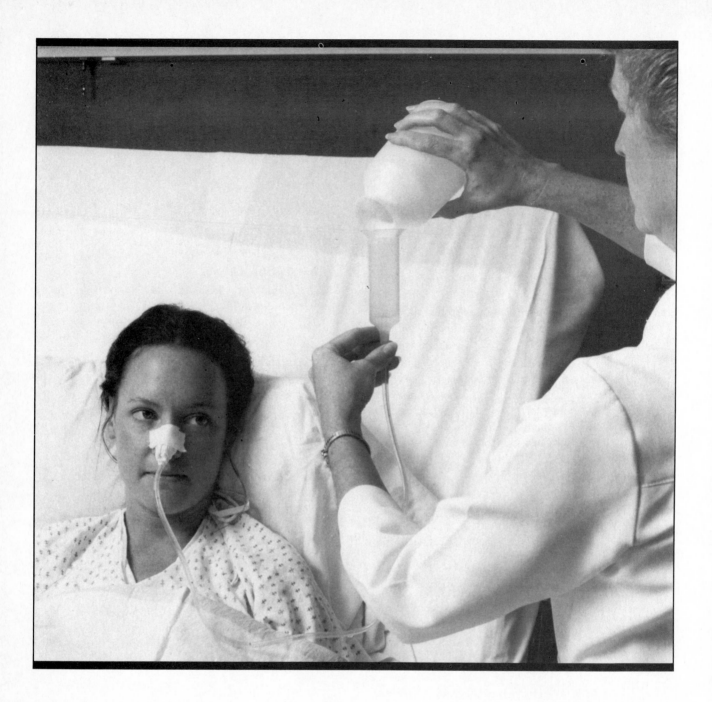

ASSISTING WITH NUTRITION

24

During illness or injury, the body requires more nutrients than usual. Yet, because of illness or age, many patients are unable to feed themselves part or all of a meal. Thus, nurses need to become skillful in assisting patients to eat. Because patterns of eating vary considerably among people, the nurse needs to determine each person's food habits when planning nursing care. The nurse also needs to be able to assess the nutritional status of patients. To meet learning needs, nurses may teach new parents how to breast- or bottle-feed their infants.

Chapter Outline

Objectives

Upon completion of this chapter, the student will:

1. Know essential terms and facts about nutrition
    1.1 Define selected terms
    1.2 Identify information required to assess the nutritional status of a person
    1.3 Identify advantages of breast-feeding
    1.4 Identify three types of breast milk
    1.5 Identify essential aspects of assisting patients with meals
2. Understand facts about techniques used to assist patients with nutrition
    2.1 Identify relevant assessment data
    2.2 Identify nursing diagnoses for which the technique may be implemented
    2.3 Identify nursing goals related to the technique
    2.4 Identify expected and unexpected outcomes from assessment data
    2.5 Identify reasons underlying steps of the technique
3. Perform techniques related to nutrition
    3.1 Assess the patient adequately
    3.2 Collect additional data from appropriate sources
    3.3 Select pertinent nursing goals for the patient
    3.4 Establish relevant outcome criteria for the patient following the technique
    3.5 Collect necessary equipment before the technique
    3.6 Implement interventions to enhance the effectiveness of the technique and enhance the patient's comfort and safety
    3.7 Communicate relevant information about the patient to the appropriate persons
    3.8 Determine the evaluative outcomes of the technique
4. Evaluate own performance of specific techniques in a laboratory or clinical setting with the assistance of another
    4.1 Use the performance checklists provided
    4.2 Identify areas of strength and weakness
    4.3 Alter performance in response to own evaluation and that of another

Terms

■ anorexia   lack of appetite

■ anthropometry   a system of measurement of the size and makeup of the body and specific body parts

■ appetite   a pleasant sensation in which the person desires and anticipates food

■ areola   the darkened area surrounding the nipple of the breast

■ cachexia   a state of emaciation, weakness, and malnutrition

■ calipers   an instrument used to measure the thickness of folds of skin

■ colic   paroxysmal cramplike intestinal pain

■ colostrum   a yellow, milky fluid secreted by the mother's mammary glands a few days before or after childbirth

■ esophagus   the muscular tube that extends from the pharynx to the stomach

■ fistula   an abnormal passage between two organs or between an organ and the body surface

■ gastric   pertaining to the stomach

■ gavage   administration of nourishment to the stomach through a nasogastric or orogastric tube; tube feeding

■ jejunum   the portion of the small intestine that extends from the duodenum to the ileum

■ letdown reflex (milk ejection reflex)   a pattern of

stimulation, hormone release, and resulting muscle contraction that forces milk into the lactiferous ducts of the breasts, making it available to the infant

■ **malnutrition** any disorder connected with nutrition

■ **mastitis** inflammation of the breast

■ **nausea** the urge to vomit

■ **nutrient** an organic or inorganic substance in food that is digested and absorbed in the gastrointestinal tract and then used in the body's metabolic processes

■ **-ostomy** a suffix meaning to form an opening or outlet

■ **oxytocin** a hormone normally produced by the posterior pituitary that is responsible for stimulating

uterine contractions and the release of milk into the lactiferous ducts

■ **pharynx** the musculomembranous sac behind the nose and mouth that connects with the esophagus and bronchi

■ **protein** any of the large, complex compounds of carbon, hydrogen, oxygen, and nitrogen essential to body maintenance

■ **rooting reflex** an infant's tendency to turn the head and open the lips to suck when one side of the mouth or cheek is touched

■ **satiety** a feeling of fullness as a result of satisfying the desire for food

ASSESSING NUTRITIONAL STATUS

To assess the nutritional status of a person, the nurse follows the "ABCD" approach: she or he takes *anthropometric measurements* (A) (see Technique 24–1), looks at *biochemical data* (B), assesses the *clinical signs* of nutritional status (C), and obtains a *dietary history* (D).

Anthropometric Measurements

Anthropometric measurements provide a quick and easy way to assess a person's protein and calorie reserves. Protein–calorie malnutrition (PCM) is a common problem among hospitalized patients; it is estimated to occur in as many as 50% (Bistrian et al, 1974, p 858; Weinsier et al, 1979, p 418). Common anthropometric measurements taken are discussed in Technique 24–1 on page 519.

Biochemical Data

Biochemical data also contribute to a nutritional assessment of an individual. Malnutrition may be suspected in certain patients either upon admission to a hospital or during hospitalization. Many laboratory studies can reveal information about nutrition. Some of the most common are:

1. Hematocrit, hemoglobin, and red blood cell indices provide evidence of iron deficiency anemia.

2. The presence of multilobular granulocytes among the white blood cells suggest vitamin B_{12} and folate deficiencies. A lymphocyte count of less than 1,500 suggests protein–calorie malnutrition.

3. Serum albumen concentration of less than 1,500 suggests protein malnutrition.

4. A low blood urea nitrogen suggests inadequate protein intake.

5. Serum cholesterol and serum triglyceride concentrations are indices of fat nutrition.

6. Urine creatinine levels can suggest malnutrition.

Clinical Signs

Since nutrition affects most body systems, an assessment of these systems can reveal nutritional problems. Table 24–1 lists some of the data that can be collected to assist nursing personnel in determining a patient's nutritional status. This list is not exhaustive; for more detailed information, consult nutrition and assessment texts. A thorough assessment is usually done with the initial physical examination when the patient is admitted to the agency. The data obtained serve as baseline data for comparison with later findings during the patient's stay.

Dietary History

A dietary history generally includes data about the patient's usual eating patterns and habits, food preferences and restrictions, daily fluid intake, use of vitamin or mineral supplements, any dietary problems (such as difficulty chewing or swallowing), physical activity, health history, and concerns related to food buying and preparation. See Figure 24–1 for a sample nutritional history tool for an adult. To obtain data about eating patterns and habits, the nurse elicits a typical 24-hour diet history. More detailed records of the patient's food intake can be kept over a three-day period, including one weekend day. Such a record enables the nurse and the patient to compare the data listed with recommended daily allowances to determine whether the patient is receiving a nutritionally balanced diet. The nurse also acquires the patient's perspective of his or her nutritional

TABLE 24–1   ■   Clinical Signs Indicating Nutritional Status

Body part or system	Normal signs	Abnormal signs
Hair	Shiny, neither dry nor oily	Oily, dry, dull, patchy in growth
Skin	Smooth, slightly moist, good turgor	Dry, oily, broken out in rash, scaly, rough, bruised
Eyes	Bright, clear	Dry, reddened
Tongue	Pink, moist	Reddened in patches, swollen
Mu_us membranes	Reddish pink, moist	Reddened, dry, cracked
Cardiovascular	Heart rate and blood pressure within normal ranges, heart rhythm regular	Rapid heart rate, elevated blood pressure, irregular heart rhythm
Muscles	Firm, well developed	Poor in tone, soft, underdeveloped
Gastrointestinal	Appetite good, elimination regular and normal	Manifesting anorexia, indigestion, diarrhea, constipation
Neurologic	Reflexes normal, alert, good attention span, emotionally stable	Reflexes decreased, irritable, inattentive, confused, emotionally labile
Vitality	Vigorous, energetic, able to sleep well	Lacking energy, tired, apathetic, sleeping poorly
Weight	Normal for age, build, and height	Overweight, underweight

status. It is important not to judge differences from the nurse's own practices. A question about what foods the patient considers harmful or helpful to health is beneficial in eliciting cultural data. For example, people of Asian and Hispanic origins may classify foods as *hot* or *cold* on the basis of inherent characteristics of the food, and not on their actual temperature. According to these cultures, the hot and cold foods need to be balanced for

optimum health. If a person has a "cold" illness or condition, such as colic or earache, he or she should eat "hot" foods to balance the condition. Data about the patient's medication intake are also important, especially in relation to mealtimes. Many medications are to be taken only before or after meals, so variations from the usual breakfast–lunch–dinner mealtimes need to be documented.

TECHNIQUE 24–1   ■   Taking Anthropometric Measurements

Anthropometric measurements are measurements of the size and composition of the body. They include measurements of height, weight, skin folds (fat folds), and arm circumference. The triceps, subscapular, biceps, and suprailiac skin folds can be measured with special calipers. The site most commonly used is the triceps fold. This technique includes only mid-upper-arm circumference and triceps and subscapular skin fold measurements. The arm muscle circumference is calculated from the triceps skin fold and upper-arm circumference. See chapter 9 for height and weight measurements.

■ Planning

Nursing Goal

To assess nutritional status by specific body measurements.

Equipment

1. A flexible steel tape measure calibrated in millimeters.
2. Proper calipers to measure the thickness of skin folds. Plastic calipers are more subject to measurement error.

■ Intervention

1. Assist the patient to a comfortable sitting position.
2. Remove the patient's upper clothing so that the upper nondominant arm and the subscapular area are exposed.

Mid-upper-arm circumference (MUAC)

The mid-upper-arm circumference provides information about the individual's muscle mass.

NUTRITIONAL HISTORY

Name _____

Age _____ Height _____

WEIGHT

Current weight _____

Weight history (obesity, onset, fluctuations) _____

Percentage of

  Overweight _____

  Underweight _____

OTHER ANTHROPOMETRIC DATA

Triceps skin fold measurement _____

Arm muscle circumference _____

EATING PATTERNS AND HABITS

1. Typical day's food intake

Time	Item	Portion
_____	_____	_____
_____	_____	_____
_____	_____	_____
_____	_____	_____
_____	_____	_____
_____	_____	_____
_____	_____	_____
_____	_____	_____
_____	_____	_____
_____	_____	_____
_____	_____	_____
_____	_____	_____

2. Food likes _____

3. Food dislikes _____

4. Food allergies _____

5. Foods considered harmful or beneficial to health

  Harmful _____

  Beneficial _____

6. Food restrictions

  Special diet _____

  Religious _____

  Cultural _____

7. Fluid intake

  Number of glasses of water per day _____

  Number of cups of tea or coffee per day _____

  Number of soft drinks per day _____

  Amount of alcohol or wine per day _____

8. Use of vitamins

  Kind _____

  Frequency _____

9. Use of minerals (eg, calcium, iron)

  Kind _____

  Frequency _____

10. Perception of diet

  Nutritionally balanced _____

  Not nutritionally balanced _____

DIETARY PROBLEMS

1. Describe appetite (usual, increased, decreased) _____

2. Foods causing indigestion, diarrhea, or gas _____

3. Difficulty following special diet

  Yes _____ No _____

  If yes, how _____

4. Chewing difficulties

  Number of teeth

  Upper _____ Lower _____

  Dentures

  Partial _____

  Complete _____

  Fit of dentures _____

5. Swallowing difficulties _____

6. Usual bowel movements _____

HEALTH HISTORY

1. Physical activity

  Type _____

  Frequency _____

2. Medication intake

  Name _____

  Time _____

3. History of diseases, surgical procedures, or weight problems

	Yes	No
Diabetes	___	___
Heart problems	___	___
Surgery (specify) _____	___	___
Cancer	___	___
Kidney stones	___	___
Gallstones	___	___
Ulcers	___	___
Intestinal disorder	___	___
Allergies other than food (specify) _	___	___
Weight problems	___	___

4. Perception of general health

  Good _____

  Satisfactory _____

  Poor _____

FOOD BUYING AND PREPARATION

1. Ingredients used

  Salt _____

  Soy _____

  MSG _____

  Other _____

2. Methods most used

  Boil _____

  Bake _____

  Fry _____

  Broil _____

  Steam _____

  Other _____

3. Shopping/cooking capabilities

  Is able to shop _____

  Relies on others _____

  Is able to cook _____

  Relies on others _____

4. Living situation

  Number of family members _____

  Lives alone _____

5. Do food costs affect diet?

  Yes _____ No _____

  How? _____

FIGURE 24-1 ■ A sample adult nutritional history tool.

3. Make sure the upper arm hangs freely in a dependent position and the forearm is positioned horizontally.

4. Locate the midpoint of the upper arm, that is, halfway between the acromial process and the olecranon process. See Figure 24–2.

5. Use the tape measure to measure the circumference of the arm at the midpoint to the nearest millimeter. Maintain the tape in a horizontal plane and avoid distortion of the skin surface.

Triceps skin fold

A skin fold measurement indicates the amount of body fat, the main storage form of energy. This measurement can be considered an index of the body's energy stores.

6. Locate the midpoint of the upper arm.

7. Grasp the skin on the back of the upper arm along the long axis of the humerus. See Figure 24–3.

8. Placing the calipers 1 cm (0.4 in) below your fingers, measure the thickness of the fold to the nearest millimeter. The fold of skin includes the subcutaneous tissue but not the underlying muscle.

Subscapular skin fold

9. Pick up the skin below the scapula. Three fingers should be on top of the fold just below the scapula, the thumb below the fold and the forefinger at the lower tip of the scapula. The skin fold should be angled about 45° from the horizontal, upward medially and downward laterally. See Figure 24–4.

10. Placing the calipers about 1 cm (0.4 in) above or below your fingers, measure the skin fold.

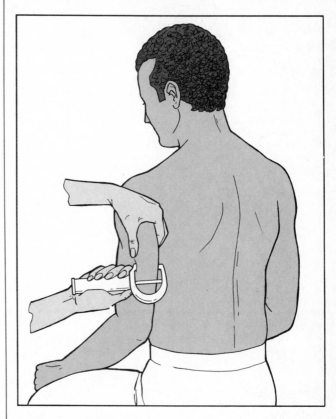

FIGURE 24–3

FIGURE 24–4

FIGURE 24–2

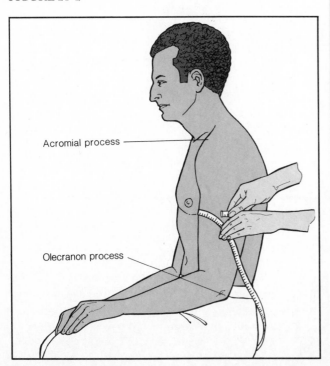

Acromial process

Olecranon process

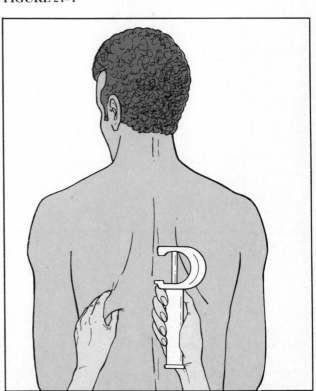

TABLE 24–2 ■ American Standards for Anthropometric Measures*

Measurement	Age	Male Mean	Male 5th percentile	Male 95th percentile	Female Mean	Female 5th percentile	Female 95th percentile
Mid-upper-arm circumference in centimeters	18–24	30.9	25.7	37.4	27.0	22.1	34.3
	25–34	32.3	27.0	37.6	28.6	23.3	37.2
	35–44	32.7	27.8	37.1	30.0	24.1	38.5
	45–54	32.1	26.7	37.6	30.7	24.3	39.3
	55–64	31.5	25.6	36.6	30.7	23.9	38.2
	65–74	30.5	25.3	36.5	30.1	23.8	37.2
Triceps skin fold thickness in millimeters	18–24	11.2	4.0	23.0	19.4	9.4	34.0
	25–34	12.6	4.5	24.0	21.9	10.5	37.0
	35–44	12.4	5.0	23.0	24.0	12.0	39.0
	45–54	12.4	5.0	25.5	25.4	13.0	40.0
	55–64	11.6	5.0	21.5	24.9	11.0	39.0
	65–74	11.8	4.5	22.0	23.3	11.5	36.0
Mid-upper-arm muscle circumference in centimeters	18–24	27.4	23.5	32.3	20.9	17.7	24.9
	25–34	28.3	24.2	32.9	21.7	18.3	26.6
	35–44	28.8	25.0	33.0	22.5	18.5	27.4
	45–54	28.2	24.0	32.6	22.7	18.8	27.8
	55–64	27.8	22.8	31.8	22.8	18.6	28.1
	65–74	26.8	22.5	30.7	22.8	18.6	28.1

Source: National Center for Health Statistics, *Health and Nutrition Examination Survey of 1971 to 1974,* DHEW Pub No. (PHS) 79–1310, nd.

*These values are representative of the adult noninstitutionalized civilian population of the United States as of November 1, 1972, and were developed from measurements obtained from the right arm.

Arm muscle circumference (AMC)

Since muscle serves as the major protein reserve of the body, this measurement can be considered an index of the body's protein reserves.

11. a. Use the following formula to calculate the AMC in millimeters:

    AMC = MUAC (mm) – [3.14 × triceps skin fold (mm)]

    or

    b. Use available tables.

12. Record all measurements on the appropriate records. See Table 24–2 for standards for these measurements.

■ Evaluation

Expected outcomes   See Table 24–2.

Unexpected outcomes

1. Arm circumference too small or large
2. Skin folds too small or large
3. Muscle circumference too small

Upon obtaining an unexpected outcome:

1. Report your findings to the responsible nurse.
2. Adjust the patient's care plan appropriately to correct protein–calorie malnutrition or obesity.

TECHNIQUE 24–2 ■ Assisting a Mother to Breast-Feed

Three types of breast milk are produced: (a) colostrum, (b) transitional milk, and (c) mature milk. *Colostrum* is a yellowish or creamy-appearing fluid that is thicker than later milk and contains more protein, fat-soluble vitamins, and minerals. It also contains high levels of immunoglobulins, which may be a source of immunity for the newborn. *Transitional milk* is produced from two to four days after delivery (during which colostrum is produced) until approximately two weeks postpartum. This milk contains higher levels of fat, lactose, water-soluble vitamins, and calories than colostrum. *Mature milk* has a high percentage of water and although it appears similar to skim milk it has more calories: 20 calories per ounce, whereas skim milk provides only 10 calories per ounce.

Breast-feeding is advantageous to both the mother and the baby because:

1. Sucking stimulates the release of oxytocin in the mother so that uterine involution (retrogression) occurs more quickly after delivery.
2. It is convenient and economical, negating the need to purchase and prepare formula.
3. It facilitates psychologic closeness between the mother and the baby.
4. It offers some antibody protection to the infant.

■ Assessment

Assess the infant for:

1. General nutritional status
2. Weight gain or loss
3. Eagerness to nurse or fatigue
4. Urinary output

Assess the mother for:

1. Soreness or cracking of the nipples
2. Breast engorgement
3. Signs of mastitis: red, tender, or warm breasts and fever
4. Pleasure or problems from the feeding relationship
5. Influence of the father's attitudes about breast-feeding

■ Planning

Nursing goals

1. To provide the nutrients the infant requires for growth and life
2. To establish an adequate milk supply in the mother
3. To prevent trauma to the nipples
4. To help the mother provide feelings of love and warmth to the infant

Equipment

1. A nursing or support bra for breast support
2. Pillows
3. A towel or other protective cover for the pillows (optional)
4. Breast pads (optional)
5. A water-based cream or hydrous lanolin (optional)

■ Intervention

1. Check whether the infant needs a diaper change. If so, change the diaper, and wash your hands.
   Rationale A clean diaper is conducive to a pleasurable feeding period.
2. Make sure that the mother voids immediately before the feeding.
   Rationale This will prevent discomfort during or disruption of the feeding.
3. Help the mother to assume a comfortable feeding position.
   Rationale A comfortable position aids the letdown reflex.
   a. The *madonna* or *cradle position* is usually preferred. See Figure 24–5.
      ■ The mother sits comfortably in a chair or in bed with the infant.
      ■ She supports the infant on her lap and her forearm on the side of the exposed breast.
      ■ The infant's neck rests on the antecubital space of her arm.

FIGURE 24–5

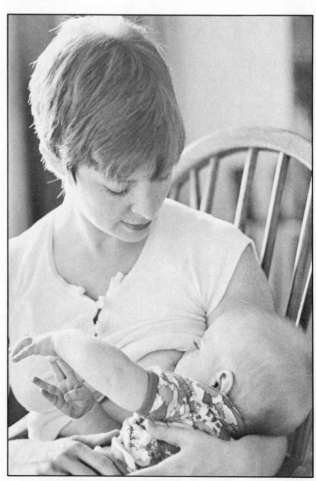

■ She supports her forearm with a pillow (optional).

Rationale This allows the mother a free hand to manipulate her breast and thus facilitate breastfeeding.

b. The *side-lying position* is particularly useful for a mother who has had a cesarean section and cannot tolerate having the infant rest against her abdomen for long periods or for a mother who has had an episiotomy and cannot sit comfortably for long periods. See Figure 24–6.

FIGURE 24–6

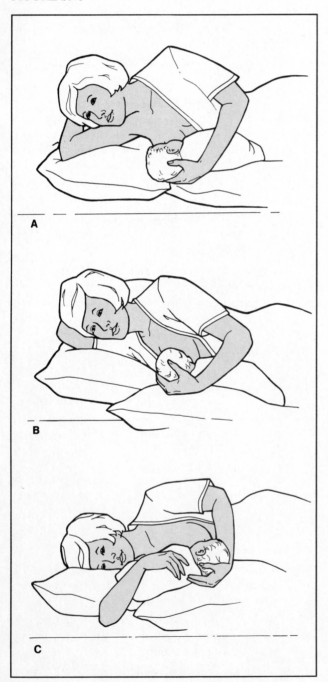

■ The mother lies on her side.
■ She raises her lower arm and flexes it beneath her head on a pillow.
■ The infant is positioned with the feet either away from the mother's head (see Figure 24–6, *A–B*) or toward her head (see Figure 24–6, *C*).
■ The mother feeds the infant on either breast.

4. Help the mother expose her breast and insert the nipple into the infant's mouth.

a. Help her position the infant so that the child's entire body is turned toward the mother and the mouth is adjacent to the nipple.

Rationale This prevents the mother from having to lift her shoulder or breast when directing the nipple into the mouth and ensures the comfort of both mother and infant during the feeding.

b. Have her place her thumb above the nipple on the areolar tissue and two fingers below the nipple, or place her index finger above and middle finger below the nipple to guide the nipple into the infant's mouth.

c. Have her stroke the infant's cheek closest to the breast with the nipple. She should avoid touching the other cheek or both cheeks together.

Rationale Touching the cheek nearest the breast stimulates the *rooting reflex*. Touching the other cheek may make the infant turn away from the breast. Touching both cheeks confuses the infant.

d. She should avoid pushing the back of the infant's head against the breast.

Rationale This also confuses the infant and may make him or her resist the breast.

e. As the infant is rooting for the nipple, have her insert the nipple, including as much areolar tissue as possible, into the baby's mouth. Direct the nipple straight into the mouth, not toward the tongue or palate.

Rationale As much areolar tissue as possible is inserted so that, as the baby sucks, sufficient pressure is exerted by the lips, gums, and cheek muscles to compress the milk sinuses directly beneath the areola.

5. Have the mother check for occulsion of the infant's nostrils while nursing. If they are occluded, have her press her finger on the breast below the infant's nostrils.

Rationale This pushes the breast away to make breathing room for the infant.

6. Instruct the mother to nurse from both breasts at each feeding. She should begin with five minutes on each side and progress to seven minutes and then ten minutes on each side within three days.

Rationale A ten-minute period usually empties the breast.

7. Advise the mother to alternate breasts at each feeding, ie, start with the breast used last at the previous feeding. Have her fasten a small safety pin to the bra cup on the side used last for nursing.

   Rationale   The safety pin reminds her to start nursing on that side at the next feeding. Alternating ensures stimulation of both breasts to produce milk.

8. To remove the infant from the breast, instruct the mother to insert a finger into the side of the infant's mouth.

   Rationale   Inserting the finger breaks the suction seal and allows the nipple to be removed without trauma.

9. Have the mother burp the infant before feeding on the other breast and at the end of the feeding. If the infant has been crying, burp the infant before the feeding. See Technique 24–3, step 10, on page 528, for burping techniques.

   Rationale   Burping helps the infant expel swallowed air and therefore consume maximum amounts of milk.

10. If the infant remains awake and the mother wishes, allow the mother to nurse the infant longer than ten minutes.

    Rationale   This satisfies the infant's need to suck and promotes bonding.

11. If the infant is either too sleepy or too active to suck and feed, have the mother rub the infant's feet, change the diaper, loosen the clothing, and/or change her position or the infant's.

    Rationale   Stimulation and activity will arouse the sleepy infant. These activities may also assist an active newborn to calm down.

12. If the infant is initially reluctant to nurse or uninterested in breast-feeding, instruct the mother:

    a. That it may take several days for the infant to adjust.

    b. To express a small amount of milk and then encourage the infant to suck.

       Rationale   Already flowing milk encourages some infants to suck eagerly.

13. When the mother has finished nursing, encourage her to hold the infant if desired, to enhance bonding. Then place the infant in the lateral position, with a roll at the back for support, or in the prone position.

    Rationale   These positions prevent aspiration of vomitus should regurgitation occur.

14. Have the mother air-dry her nipples for at least 15 minutes and apply lanolin or cream, if desired.

    Rationale   These measures prevent nipple irritation and cracking or relieve existing irritation.

15. Although there is no need to remove the lanolin or cream before the next feeding, the infant may object to the taste of the substance. If so, have the mother wash her nipples with water. Avoid use of soap and a washcloth.

    Rationale   Soap and washcloths may remove the natural oils and keratin layer buildup on the areolar tissue.

16. If the mother has a problem with leakage of milk between feedings, instruct her:

    a. To insert absorbent breast pads in her bra. Avoid the use of plastic-lined breast pads.

       Rationale   Plastic liners interfere with air circulation and may cause nipple irritation. Breast pads without plastic liners absorb secretions.

    b. To change the breast pads frequently.

       Rationale   Moist pads can contribute to nipple irritation or infection.

    c. To apply direct pressure to the breast with her fingers, hand, or forearm.

       Rationale   Pressure stops the leaking.

    d. That milk leakage will cease when the supply of milk meets the demands of the infant. Initially more milk is being produced than the infant requires.

17. Recognize and support the mother's breast-feeding efforts.

18. Provide patient teaching material about breast-feeding. Many pamphlets are available. Some general instructions include:

    a. Newborns are generally put to the breast as soon as possible after birth. Although some infants are not interested this soon, the experience can be soothing to those who are and provides the mother with psychologic and physiologic benefits.

    b. Colostrum has sufficient nutrients to satisfy the infant until milk is established. (However, some cultures, eg, Mexican-American, Navajo, Filipino, and Vietnamese, do not offer colostrum to the newborn. In these cultures, breast-feeding begins when the milk flow is established, several days after delivery.)

    c. Establishment of lactation depends on the frequency of nursing and the strength of the infant's sucking.

    d. Breast milk is more easily digested than formula, so breast-fed infants become hungry sooner, and the frequency of feeding is greater.

    e. Fatigue or excitement may decrease the milk supply temporarily, but increasing the frequency of feeding will alleviate this problem.

    f. The infant will probably demand more frequent feedings during growth spurts: at 10 to 14 days, 5 to 6 weeks, and 3 months.

    g. Infants routinely lose several ounces during their

first few days of life. This weight loss is no cause for alarm.

h. The mother can expect some cramping of the uterus during breast-feeding until it returns to its original size. The release of oxytocin, which contracts the muscles of the uterus and initiates the letdown reflex, causes this cramping.

i. Relaxation promotes the letdown reflex, which may take three minutes to activate. When this reflex occurs, the mother may feel a tingling sensation, and milk may spray or drip from her nipples.

j. Developing a breast-feeding routine takes time. There is no standard schedule.

k. Adequacy of intake is difficult to determine with breast-fed babies, since there is no visual assurance of the amounts consumed. Intake is adequate if the baby gains weight and has six or more wet diapers a day. The mother can also listen for and hear the sounds of the baby swallowing during nursing.

l. Supplementary feedings, such as glucose and water, are unnecessary for breast-fed infants. Frequent supplemental bottle feedings often confuse the infant and weaken the sucking reflex; the infant may also become used to the artificial nipple and reject the mother's breast. If an infant fails to nurse sufficiently, it is preferable to express milk manually and offer it through a small syringe or medicine dropper.

m. Manual expression of milk may be necessary if the mother will be absent for a scheduled feeding or if she is advised to forgo a feeding because of breast discomfort. The milk is manually expressed by squeezing the nipple between the thumb and index finger. Because milk supply decreases if the breasts are not emptied regularly, manual expression of milk maintains the milk supply. Manually expressed milk can be frozen in a plastic bottle for a future feeding. Use of glass bottles is discouraged because the antibodies in milk adhere to the sides of glass bottles, thus depleting the milk of some of its benefits.

n. Some nipple soreness is to be expected initially with breast-feeding. It is most pronounced during the first few minutes until the letdown reflex is established. Nipple soreness can be relieved by having the infant change feeding positions, from the cradle hold to side-lying positions. In the side-lying position, the infant can be positioned with either the feet toward or away from the mother's head. See Figure 24–6 earlier. Nipple trauma and soreness can also be decreased if the mother nurses more frequently and for less lengthy periods.

o. Breast engorgement (breasts that are hard, painful, warm to the touch, and taut and shiny in appearance) may occur when the milk initially comes in. Engorgement is initially caused by venous congestion due to the increased vascularity in the breasts. The problem is compounded by the pressure of accumulating milk. Comfort and corrective measures include application of hot compresses to the breasts, massage of the breasts, wearing a supportive nursing bra, frequent nursing if possible, manual expression of milk, use of a nontraumatic breast pump to initiate milk flow, and judicious use of analgesics. Engorgement is generally relieved in 12 to 24 hours.

p. The mother should be encouraged to take a nap every day, especially for the first few weeks after delivery.

q. The mother needs to eat a balanced diet and drink plenty of fluids (8 glasses per day) while breast-feeding.

r. The mother should avoid taking medications that can be secreted in milk, eg, aspirin, antibiotics, alcohol, addicting drugs, and cathartics. If the mother requires medical treatment, her physician should be informed that she is nursing.

19. Record the teaching provided and any problems experienced by mother or baby.

20. Adjust the patient's nursing care plan to include areas in which she needs further assistance.

■ Evaluation

Expected outcomes

1. Infant:
   a. Appropriate weight gain
   b. Six or more wet diapers daily
   c. Interest in and effective nursing
2. Mother:
   a. Nipples intact
   b. Some breast engorgement
   c. Some milk leakage
   d. Relaxed feeling when nursing

Unexpected outcomes

1. Infant:
   a. Insufficient weight gain
   b. Insufficient urine output
   c. Signs of dehydration
   d. Disinterest in nursing
2. Mother:
   a. Cracked, sore nipples

b. Severe breast engorgement

c. Tension when nursing

Upon obtaining an unexpected outcome: Report your findings to the responsible nurse and/or physician.

TECHNIQUE 24–3 ■ Bottle-Feeding an Infant

A variety of formula preparations are used to feed infants. Some are powdered or concentrated formulas that are mixed with water; others are prepared by mixing prescribed amounts of evaporated milk, dextrose (sugar) or corn syrup, and water; still others are ready-to-use formulas in bottles or cans. The physician prescribes the type of formula.

■ Assessment

Assess the infant for:

1. General nutritional status
2. Weight gain or loss
3. Eagerness to take fluids
4. Fatigue

Other data (from the mother or the infant's chart) include:

1. The type of formula used (powder, concentrate, ready-to-use), or whether evaporated milk is used
2. The amount per feeding, eg, 4 to 5 oz
3. The type of bottle and nipple used
4. The frequency of feeding, eg, every four hours, and the specific times of day
5. How the formula is prepared, ie, at what dilution
6. What other fluids, eg, water, apple juice, are given at scheduled times per day and the amounts
7. The type of vitamins or other supplements given and the time of day
8. Who feeds the baby or who helps with feeding
9. Any problems experienced with feeding

■ Planning

Nursing goals

1. To provide the nutrients required for normal growth and life.
2. To provide feelings of love and security to the infant for sound psychologic development. Holding the infant securely and lovingly during feeding gives the infant a sense of security and trust.

Equipment

1. A bottle containing the correct formula. If the formula is refrigerated, warm it to room temperature. The formula should feel lukewarm to the inner wrist when a few drops are shaken onto it. Babies digest formula at room temperature more quickly than cold formula and are less likely to develop abdominal cramps.

2. A nipple with holes of appropriate size. The nipple holes need to be large enough to allow the baby to get formula with normal sucking but not large enough to allow milk to flow freely, which can cause choking and regurgitation. Nipple holes that are too small require too much energy to suck and too much air is sucked with them. The size of the nipple holes can be tested by turning the bottle upside down. If a drop of milk appears at the tip of the nipple, the holes are the correct size. If no milk appears or if milk flows out freely, the nipple needs to be changed.

3. A bib or clean cloth to place under the infant's chin.

■ Intervention

1. Check whether the infant needs a diaper change. If so, change the diaper. Handle the infant calmly, gently, and unhurriedly.

    Rationale A clean dry diaper is conducive to pleasurable feeding. Calm, gentle handling soothes the infant.

2. Wash hands, if the diaper was changed.

3. Arrange a quiet, comfortable environment in which to feed the infant.

    Rationale A calm environment is conducive to successful feeding.

4. Carry the infant, using the football hold, to the feeding chair. See Figure 24–7.

    Rationale The football hold supports the infant's head and back, yet it frees one of the nurse's hands to carry the bib and formula.

5. Sit comfortably in the chair and relax.

    Rationale Discomfort and tension can be transmitted to the infant and can interfere with feeding and digestion.

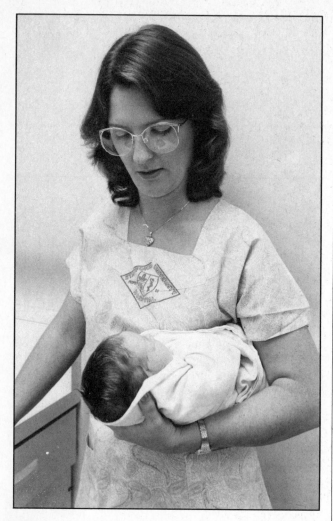

FIGURE 24-7

FIGURE 24-8

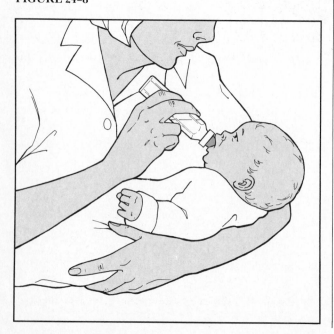

6. Tuck the bib or clean cloth under the infant's chin.

7. Cradle the baby in your arms, with the head slightly elevated. Support the head and neck in the bend of your elbow while the buttocks rest on your lap. If the baby cannot be removed from an isolette or crib because of therapy (eg, an oxygenated croupette or traction), provide as much hand contact as possible, and stay with the infant during the feeding.

Rationale Elevating the head facilitates swallowing. Infants need to be held while being fed to feel warm and loved.

8. Never leave an infant with a propped bottle.

Rationale The infant can suck in excessive air or ingest the formula too quickly. Both circumstances induce regurgitation and possible aspiration of fluid into the lungs, which can cause pneumonia.

9. Insert the nipple gently along the infant's tongue and hold the bottle at about a 45° angle so that the nipple is filled with formula and not air. See Figure 24-8.

Rationale Excessive swallowed air causes gas, abdominal distention, discomfort, and possible regurgitation.

10. Remove the bottle periodically, place it on a clean surface, and burp (bubble) the baby.

Rationale Periodic burping helps the infant expel swallowed air and therefore consume the maximum amount of formula. Small infants may need to be burped after every ounce or at least at the middle and end of the feeding. With some collapsible feeding bottles, infants suck in very little air and may need to be burped only at the end of the feeding. The infant who was crying before the feeding may have swallowed air and may need to be burped before the feeding begins or after taking just enough formula to calm down.

a. Place the baby either:
   ■ Over your shoulder. See Figure 24-9.
   ■ In a supported sitting position on your lap. See Figure 24-10.

   Rationale This position is often preferred because the infant's responses can be observed continuously.

   ■ In a prone position over your lap. See Figure 24-11.

b. Place the bib where it will protect your clothing.

   Rationale Newborns frequently regurgitate small amounts of feedings. This normal occurrence may be due initially to excessive mucus and gastric irritation from foreign substances in the stomach from birth. Later, regurgitation may occur when the infant feeds too rapidly and swallows air or when the infant is overfed and the cardiac sphincter allows the excess to be regurgitated.

c. Rub or pat the infant's back gently.

Rationale Patting encourages relaxation of the cardiac sphincter of the stomach and the expulsion of air.

11. Continue with the feeding until the formula is finished and/or the baby is satisfied. An infant feeding generally takes about 30 minutes. Prolonged feeding times tend to foster lazy eating habits.

12. For newborns who need encouragement to continue sucking during initial feedings, provide gentle tactile stimulation to the feet and hands.

Rationale Stimulation helps maintain sucking for a sufficient time to complete a feeding.

13. Once feedings are established, encourage the infant to set his or her own pace.

14. Avoid overfeeding or feeding the infant every time he or she cries.

Rationale Overfeeding results in infant obesity. A fat baby is not necessarily healthy.

15. Return the infant to the crib or isolette.

16. Check whether the diaper needs changing, and change it if necessary. Smaller infants commonly move their bowels while feeding because of the gastrocolic reflex.

17. Position the infant on his or her side or on the abdomen with the head to one side.

Rationale In these positions, the infant is less likely to aspirate any fluid that may be regurgitated. For infants in whom regurgitation is a problem, a right side-lying position tends to facilitate the expulsion of air without regurgitation, since the cardiac sphincter is located on the left side of the stomach.

18. Ensure that the crib sides are elevated before leaving the infant.

19. Observe whether the infant seems satisfied after each feeding and rests quietly.

20. Record the type and the amount of the feeding taken, your assessments, the responses of the infant (eg, amount and frequency of regurgitation), and the color and characteristics of the feces or urine. Some agencies require these data to be recorded on flow sheets.

Sample Recording

Date	Time	Notes
6/6/87	0700	5 oz Similac taken well. Regurgitated small amount formula × 1. Resting quietly on right side.————— Sally R. Duprez, SN

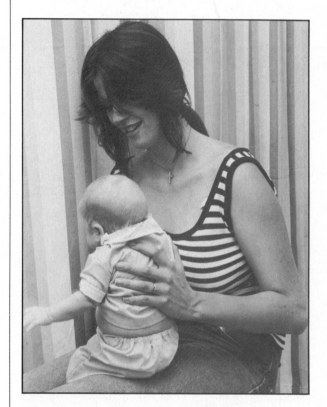

FIGURE 24–10

FIGURE 24–11

FIGURE 24–9

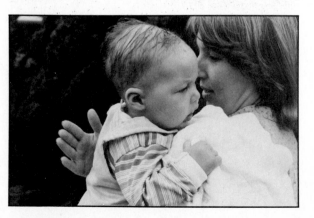

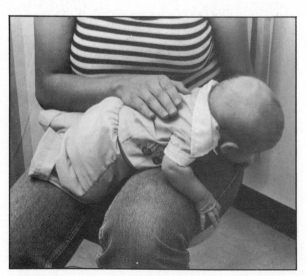

■ Evaluation

Expected outcomes

1. Rested quietly after feeding
2. Manifested an appropriate daily weight gain

Unexpected outcomes

1. Cried, fussed, and was irritable after feeding

2. Showed a weight loss

Upon obtaining an unexpected outcome:

1. Report your findings to the responsible nurse and/or physician.
2. Alter the infant's nursing care plan as required.

TECHNIQUE 24–4 ■ Feeding Solid Foods to an Infant

Infants may be fed solids while being held in the arms, as for bottle-feeding, or while seated and restrained in an infant seat. When old enough to sit unsupported, the infant can sit on the nurse's or another person's lap rather than in an infant seat. Young children progress to a high chair.

■ Assessment

Assess:

1. The infant's developmental abilities in relation to feeding:
    a. The extrusion reflex is normally present for the first 4 months. At 4 months, because infants can reach their mouths with their hands, the hands may get in the way during feeding.
    b. By 5 to 6 months, infants can sit with support, can grasp objects in a mittenlike fashion, can bring their lips to the rim of a cup and begin drinking, and can begin to chew.
    c. At 7 months, infants can feed themselves a biscuit, like to play with food and smear it, bang cups and objects on the table, and enjoy finger foods (eg, pieces of banana).
    d. At 9 months, infants can hold their bottles, sit erect unsupported in a high chair, and develop finger-to-thumb (pincer) movements to pick up food.
    e. At 10 months, infants poke at food with their index fingers, reach for food and utensils, and like to hold a spoon and push objects with it.
    f. Beyond 10 months, infants show an increased desire to feed themselves. They begin to use a spoon and to hold a cup with both hands, but frequently spill food. Between 2 and 3 years of age,

self-feeding is completed with only occasional spilling.
2. The infant's appetite.
3. The infant's likes and dislikes for specific foods.
4. Whether the infant has any specific food allergies and specially ordered foods.

■ Planning

Nursing goals

1. To provide the necessary calories and nutrients to meet the growing infant's needs
2. To promote muscular development of the mouth and tongue

Equipment

1. A small feeding spoon and unbreakable dishes
2. The proper food (eg, pureed or diced), at room temperature
3. A bib
4. An infant seat or high chair, if required

■ Intervention

1. Determine whether the infant's diaper needs changing, and change it if required.
2. Wash your hands if the diaper was changed.
3. Approach the infant with a pleasant, relaxed attitude and provide a calm environment. An infant old enough to eat solids will be well aware of this, because his or her interest in the surroundings is increasing.
4. Put the bib on the infant and place him or her on your lap or in the infant seat or high chair.

5. Seat yourself comfortably, and relax.

    Rationale   Feeding times need to be unhurried and relaxed to promote good eating habits and proper digestion.

6. Control the infant's hands with your free hand by giving her or him something to hold or by gently holding the arms. See Figures 24–12 and 24–13.

    Rationale   Holding the arms prevents young infants from smearing their food.

7. Offer plain foods before sweet ones, eg, cereal and vegetables before fruits.

    Rationale   Infants may reject plain foods after eating the sweeter tasting ones.

8. Place small spoonfuls of food well back on the infant's tongue.

    Rationale   Putting food well back in the mouth overcomes the extrusion reflex, if it is present.

9. Scrape up any food that is pushed back out of the mouth, and refeed it.

10. Continue to feed at a pace appropriate for the infant until she or he is satisfied. Hungry infants tend to eat quickly and show frustration if the food is given too slowly.

11. Talk with the infant throughout the meal.

    Rationale   Friendly talk at mealtimes is conducive to digestion and socialization.

12. Wash and dry the infant's face and hands.

13. Feed a young infant his or her formula.

14. Change the diaper, if required.

15. Place the infant in a safe position in the crib. See Technique 24–3, step 17. Encourage the child to nap or rest. Ensure that the crib sides are elevated before leaving the infant.

16. Record your assessments, the type and amount of feeding taken, and the infant's responses.

■ Evaluation

Expected outcomes

1. Ingested all foods provided without difficulty
2. Showed appropriate weight gain

Unexpected outcomes

1. Refused all or some foods
2. Vomited food taken in
3. Showed weight loss

Upon obtaining an unexpected outcome:

1. Report your findings to the responsible nurse.
2. Adjust the nursing care plan appropriately.

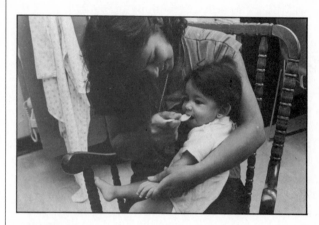

FIGURE 24–12

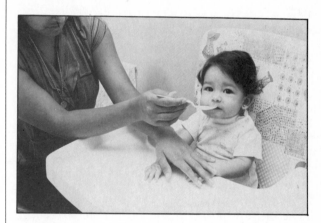

FIGURE 24–13

NURSING INTERVENTIONS ASSOCIATED WITH PATIENTS' MEALS

Arrangements for the provision of food to patients vary considerably. Some hospitals serve meals to ambulatory patients in a special dining area, and the patients are expected to go there to eat. Other agencies, eg, day-care centers, have a coffee shop for food or machines from which patients can obtain sandwiches and beverages. However, because patients are frequently confined to their beds, particularly in acute care settings, most hospitals must have meals brought to the patient. Often the patient receives a tray that has been assembled in a central hospital kitchen or a kitchen adjacent to the nursing unit. Nursing personnel may be responsible for giving out and collecting the trays; in some settings this is done by special personnel. In either case, nurses have the following responsibilities associated with the provision of meals for patients:

1. Check on the patient's chart or Kardex whether the patient is fasting for laboratory tests or surgery or whether the physician has ordered "nothing by mouth" (NPO). For patients who are fasting or on NPO, ensure that the appropriate signs are placed on either the room door or the patient's bed, according to agency practice.

2. For patients who are experiencing considerable pain, check the nursing care plan, and arrange for analgesics to be provided about 30 minutes before the meal. Pain usually takes away a patient's appetite.

3. Some patients require medications before or with their meals. Check the patient's chart, and provide the prescribed medication, or check that this has been done.

4. If there is a change in the type of food the patient is to receive, notify the dietary staff. Some hospitals have a form with the patient's name that indicates any change in diet. This form is placed in a special location for the dietary staff.

5. Prior to mealtime, determine if the patient needs to urinate or defecate. Assist him or her to the bathroom or onto a bedpan or commode, as appropriate.

6. Ensure that the patient washes his or her hands prior to a meal. If the patient has problems with oral hygiene, brushing the teeth or using a mouthwash can improve the taste in his or her mouth and hence the appetite.

7. Provide good ventilation and good light, and remove any unpleasant room odors. A spray deodorizer can help.

8. Remove any unpleasant sights, such as a full bedpan or a soiled dressing, which could disturb the patient's appetite.

9. Assist the patient to a comfortable position for eating. Sitting is used by most people during a meal; if it is permitted, assist the patient to sit in bed or in a chair, whichever is appropriate. Make sure that a patient who must remain in a supine or lateral position is comfortable.

10. Overbed tables are often used for patients sitting in bed or on bedside chairs. Clear the table so that there is space for the tray. If the patient must remain in a lying position in bed, arrange the overbed table close to the bedside, so that the patient can see the food.

11. Trays are usually delivered to the nursing unit on a movable trolley or a special lift. If nursing personnel are expected to deliver the trays, the unit will have a method of notifying the nurses that the trays have arrived, eg, a bell.

12. Check each tray for the patient's name, the type of diet, and whether the tray contains everything needed. In some agencies, the patient's name and bed number are written on a colored card. Different colors are used to represent different diets, eg, white for the general diet and blue for the soft diet. If the diet does not seem to be correct, check it against the patient's chart. Confirm the patient's name by checking the wristband before leaving the tray. Do not leave an incorrect diet for a patient to eat.

13. Assist the patient as required, eg, to remove the food covers, butter the bread, pour the tea, and cut the meat.

14. Patients who need to be fed may receive their trays before or after other patients. It is important that the patients be fed as soon as the trays are out and while the food is hot. Some agencies arrange for these trays to come out 30 minutes earlier, and nursing personnel are designated to feed specific patients.

15. After the patient has completed the meal, replace the food covers, and note how much and what the patient has eaten and the amount of fluid taken. If the patient's intake and output of fluid is being recorded, record the fluid ingested. See chapter 23. If a calorie count has been ordered, record the exact amount of each food eaten. A special form is usually provided by the dietitian.

16. Assist the patient to a comfortable position. For some patients eating is a tiring process, and they will need to rest after a meal.

17. Return the tray to the trolley.

18. If the patient is on a special diet or is having problems eating, record on the chart the pertinent data, such as amount of food eaten and any pain, fatigue, or nausea experienced.

Sample Recording

Date	Time	Notes
5/13/87	0800	Refused all solid food. Ingested 120 mL milk. Nauseated. Dull crampy pain persists in epigastric region.—Wendy B. Low, SN

19. If the patient is not eating, notify the responsible nurse so that the diet can be changed or other nursing measures can be taken, eg, providing an analgesic before meals.

TECHNIQUE 24–5   ■   Assisting an Adult to Eat   🏠

Some patients in a hospital setting require assistance in eating. How much and what kind of assistance is needed depend on the physical and mental limitations of the patients. Two groups of people frequently require help: the elderly, who are weakened and quickly fatigued when they are ill; and the handicapped, eg, blind patients, those who must remain in a back-lying position, or those who do not have use of their hands. The patient's nursing care plan will indicate that assistance is required with meals.

Because adults are normally able to eat independently, the patient may find assistance of any kind embarrassing and difficult to accept. Often patients become depressed because they require help and because they believe they are burdensome to busy nursing personnel. It is very important not to convey either verbally or nonverbally impatience or annoyance with patients who require assistance eating. Rather, appear unhurried and convey that you have ample time.

■ Assessment

Assess the patient for:

1. Eating skills retained and assistance required.
2. Appetite for and tolerance of food and fluid.
3. Amounts of food and fluid ingested.
4. Nutritional status for baseline data. See Technique 24–1 on page 519.

Other data include: whether a special diet is required by the patient.

■ Nursing Diagnosis

Examples of nursing diagnoses that may indicate the need to assist a patient to eat include:

1. Self-care deficit (feeding) related to:
   a. Neuromuscular impairment
   b. Musculoskeletal disorder
   c. Visual disorder

■ Planning

Nursing goals

1. To assist the patient to obtain nourishment and fluid
2. To teach the patient needed eating skills

Equipment

1. A meal tray with the correct food and fluids.
2. An extra napkin or small towel to protect the patient's clothes and the bedclothes.
3. A straw, special drinking cup, or weighted glass, if the patient has difficulty taking fluids. See Figure 24–14.

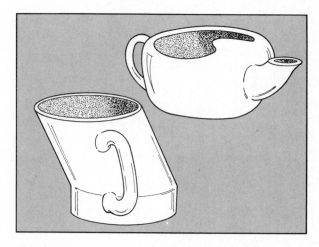

FIGURE 24–14   ■   Two types of special drinking cups.

■ Intervention

1. Assist the patient to a sitting position if possible, or to a lateral position if he or she is unable to sit.
   Rationale The patient will swallow more easily in these positions than in a back-lying position. A sitting position in bed is a near-normal position for eating.
2. If possible, assume a sitting position beside the patient.
   Rationale The nurse's sitting conveys a more relaxed presence to the patient, which is more conducive to eating.
3. Assist the patient to identify the food on the tray, if needed. For a blind person, identify the placement of the food as you would describe the time on a clock. See Figure 24–15.
4. Ask the patient in which order he or she desires to eat the food.
5. Use normal utensils whenever possible.
   Rationale Using ordinary utensils enhances the patient's self-esteem.

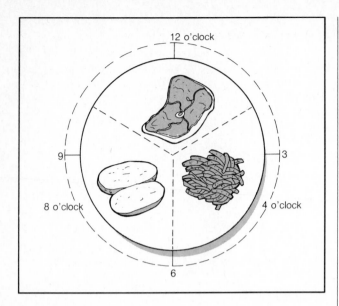

12 o'clock

9 | 3

8 o'clock | 4 o'clock

6

FIGURE 24-15

6. Encourage the patient to eat independently, assisting where needed. Do not take over feeding from the patient.
   Rationale Participation by the patient enhances feelings of independence.

7. Warn the patient if the food is hot or cold.

8. If the patient cannot see, tell him or her which food you are giving.

9. Allow ample time for the patient to chew and swallow the food before offering more.

10. Provide the patient with fluids as requested, or, if he or she is unable to tell you, offer fluids after every three or four mouthfuls of solid food.

11. Use a straw or special drinking cup for fluids if they would spill from normal containers.

12. Make the time a pleasant one, choosing topics of conversation that are of interest to the patient, if he or she wants to talk.

13. Demonstrate any new skills the patient needs to learn, and encourage the patient to practice. For example, the patient may need to learn to cut food with one hand or to feed himself or herself with the nondominant hand.

14. After the meal, assist the patient to clean his or her mouth and hands.

15. Record the amount of fluids taken, if measurement of the patient's fluid intake and output is required.

16. Record any significant assessments, such as the exact amounts of food consumed by a patient if a calorie count is needed, anorexia, or nausea.

■ Evaluation

Expected outcomes

1. Triceps skin fold measurement within predetermined range or at baseline level

2. Arm muscle circumference (AMC) within predetermined range or at baseline level

3. Stable daily weight or, if on reducing diet, prescribed weekly weight loss

4. Fluid intake at prescribed level or 1,500 mL/day

5. Urinary output in balance with fluid intake

6. Tolerated food and fluids provided

Unexpected outcomes

1. Triceps skin fold measurement below predetermined or baseline level

2. AMC below predetermined or baseline level

3. Weight gain or loss

4. Fluid intake below 1,000 mL/day
   Urinary output below 500 mL/day

5. Complaints of anorexia, nausea, or abdominal discomfort after eating

Upon obtaining an unexpected outcome:

1. Report your findings to the responsible nurse.

2. Adjust the nursing care plan appropriately.

TECHNIQUE 24-6   Administering a Nasogastric Tube Feeding (Gastric Gavage) 🏠

A *nasogastric feeding,* or *gastric gavage,* is the instillation of specially prepared nutrients into the stomach through a nasogastric tube. It usually requires a physician's order. A tube is inserted through one of the nostrils, down the nasopharynx and esophagus, into the stomach. See Figure 24-16. Nasogastric feedings are indicated for patients who cannot eat by mouth or swallow a sufficient diet without aspirating food or fluid into the lungs. Feedings may be given continously over a 24-hour period or at prescribed intervals, eg, four times per day.

■ Assessment

Assess the patient for:

1. Any feeling of abdominal distention, belching, loose stools, flatus, or pain. The lack of bulk in liquid feedings may cause constipation. The presence of concentrated ingredients may cause diarrhea and flatulence. A distended abdomen could indicate the patient's intolerance to a previous feeding.
2. Bowel sounds, by auscultating the patient's abdomen. Bowel sounds reflect intestinal movement.
3. Hydration status. Dehydration may cause constipation.
4. Allergies to any foods, such as eggs. Check the contents of the feeding for these foods. Report any significant problems to the responsible nurse.
5. Glucose tolerance and response to the feedings, as ordered. Assess glucose tolerance by monitoring the patient's blood and urine glucose levels. Assess response to therapy by monitoring serum electrolytes, doing other ordered blood tests, and taking anthropometric measurements.

Other data include:

1. The physician's order for the feeding on the patient's record. This should include the type of feeding, the amount to be fed, and the frequency of feedings.
2. Any information on the nursing care plan related to the feeding, eg, the position in which the patient best tolerates the feeding.

■ Planning

Nursing goal

To maintain the patient's hydration and nutritional status.

Equipment

1. The correct amount of feeding solution ordered by the physician (300 to 500 mL per meal is usual for an adult). Check the expiration date on a commercially prepared formula or the preparation date and time if the solution was prepared in the agency. Discard an agency solution that is more than 24 hours old or a commercial formula that has passed the expiration date. The standard gastric feeding contains 1 cal/mL of solution, with protein, fat, carbohydrate, minerals, and vitamins in specified proportions. Commonly included foods are milk, sugar, water, eggs, and vegetable oil. Feedings are usually administered at room temperature unless the order specifies otherwise. Warm the specified amount of solution in a basin of warm water or let it stand for a while until it reaches room temperature. Continuous feeding should be kept cold (see item 7 below). Excessive heat coagulates feedings of milk and egg, and hot liquids can irritate the mucous membranes. On the other hand, excessively cold feedings can reduce the flow of digestive juices by causing vasoconstriction and may cause cramps. Commercially prepared feedings are available in cans and bottles ready for administration. Some containers are designed so that ice chips can be placed in an outer section to keep the formula cooled.

2. A 20- to 50-mL syringe with an adapter. The syringe is used to check that the tube is in the stomach.
3. An emesis basin to collect the aspirated stomach contents.
4. If an intermittent feeding is being given, a bulb syringe. The bulb is removed from the syringe, and the barrel is attached to the tube.

    or

    A burette (calibrated plastic bag) and a drip chamber, which can be attached to the tubing.

    or

    A prefilled bottle with a drip chamber, tubing, and a flow regulator clamp.

FIGURE 24–16 ■ A nasogastric tube in place.

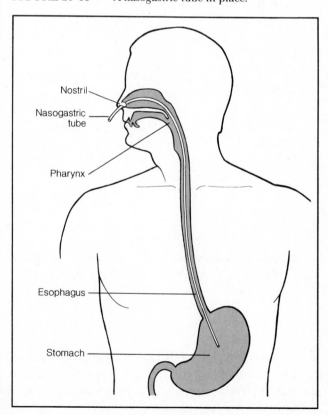

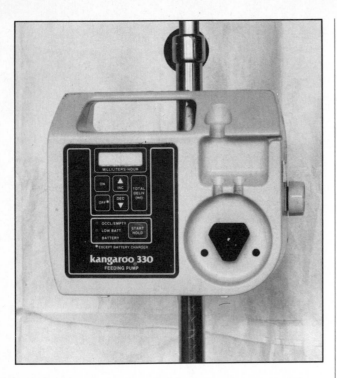

FIGURE 24–17

5. A measuring container from which to pour the feeding if the syringe or burette method is used.

6. Water at room temperature (60 mL unless otherwise specified) to clean the inside of the tube after the feeding.

7. Optional: a feeding pump, which can be used with a prefilled tube-feeding set to regulate the exact amount of feeding for the patient. See Figure 24–17. The pump can also be used to administer the feeding in instances when smaller-bore gastric tubes are used or when gravity flow is insufficient to instill the feeding. Because the feeding is administered over a long time period, a formula that is warmed can grow microorganisms. It should not hang longer than the manufacturer recommends, eg, 3 to 4 hours. If it will hang longer, it should be kept cool with ice chips.

■ **Intervention**

1. Explain the technique to the patient. A feeding should not cause any discomfort, but it may cause a feeling of fullness. For an adult, the usual intermittent feeding takes about 10 minutes; the exact length of time depends largely on the volume of the feeding.

2. Provide privacy for this procedure if the patient desires it. Nasogastric feedings are embarrassing to some people.

3. Assist the patient to a Fowler's position in bed or a sitting position in a chair, the normal position for eating. If a sitting position is contraindicated, a slightly elevated right side-lying position is acceptable.

Rationale These positions enhance the gravitational flow of the solution and prevent aspiration of fluid into the lungs.

4. If the patient does not have a nasogastric tube in place, insert one. See Technique 31–3 on page 766.

5. Confirm that the nasogastric tube is in the stomach. Attach the syringe to the open end of the nasogastric tube, and aspirate stomach contents. See Table 31–3 on page 769 for other methods to determine placement of a nasogastric tube.

6. If the nasogastric tube is maintained in the patient:

    a. Aspirate all the stomach contents and measure the amount prior to administering the feeding.

    Rationale This is done to evaulate absorption of the last feeding, ie, whether undigested formula of a previous feeding remains.

    b. If 50 mL or more of undigested formula is withdrawn, check with the responsible nurse before proceeding.

    Rationale At some agencies a feeding is withheld if 50 mL or more of formula remains in the stomach.

    c. Reinstill the gastric contents into the stomach if this is the agency or physician's practice. Remove the syringe bulb or plunger, and pour the gastric contents via the syringe into the nasogastric tube.

    Rationale Removal of the contents could disturb the patient's electrolyte balance.

7. If a bulb syringe is being used:

    a. Remove the bulb from the syringe, and connect the syringe to a pinched or clamped nasogastric tube.

    Rationale Pinching or clamping the tube prevents excess air from entering the stomach, causing distention.

    b. Add the feeding to the syringe barrel. See Figure 24–18.

    c. Permit the feeding to flow in slowly. Raise or lower the syringe to adjust the flow as needed. Pinch or clamp the tubing to stop the flow for a minute if the patient experiences discomfort.

    Rationale Quickly administered feedings can cause flatus, crampy pain, and/or reflex vomiting.

    d. After the feeding has been administered, instill 60 mL of water through the tube. Be sure to add the water before the feeding solution has drained from the neck of the syringe.

    Rationale Water cleans the lumen of the tube and prevents future blockage. Adding water before the syringe is empty prevents instillation of air into the stomach.

    e. Clamp the tube before removing the syringe.

    Rationale Clamping prevents any reflux of the feeding.

8. If a burette is being used:

   a. Hang the burette from an infusion pole about 30 cm (12 in) above the tube's point of insertion into the patient.

   b. Clamp the tubing, and pour the formula into the burette.

   c. Open the clamp, run the formula through the burette tubing, and reclamp the tube.

   Rationale   The formula will displace the air in the burette and its tubing, thus preventing the instillation of excess air into the patient's stomach.

   d. Confirm placement of the nasogastric tube by withdrawing stomach contents (see step 6) or injecting air through the nasogastric tube while listening for a whooshing sound with a stethoscope placed over the patient's stomach.

   e. After completing step 6, attach the burette tubing to the nasogastric tube (see Figure 24–19), and regulate the drip by adjusting the clamp.

   f. Just before all the formula has run through and the burette is empty, add 60 mL of water to the burette and run it through the nasogastric tube.

   Rationale   The water rinses the nasogastric tube and maintains its patency by removing sticky formula that can occlude the tube.

   g. Clamp the burette tube before all the water has gone through the tube.

   Rationale   Clamping the tube prevents air from entering the stomach.

9. If a prefilled tube-feeding set is being used:

   a. Remove the sealed cap from the container, and replace it with the screw-on cap to which the drip chamber and tubing are attached. See Figure 24–20.

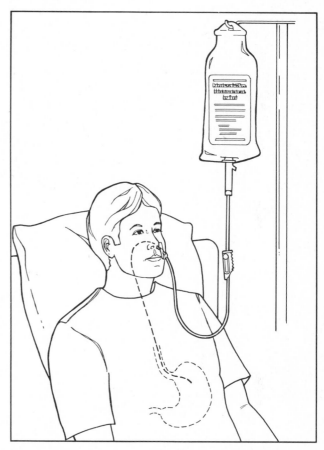

FIGURE 24–19

FIGURE 24–18

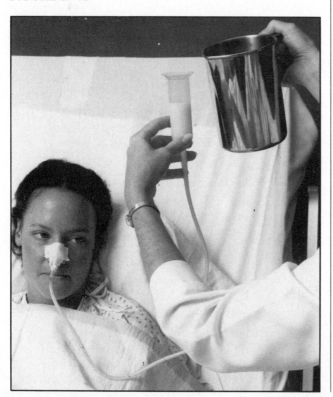

FIGURE 24–20

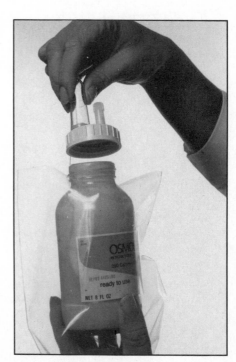

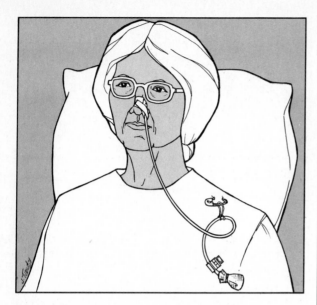

FIGURE 24–21

b. Close the clamp on the tubing.

c. Hang the container on an intravenous pole about 30 cm (12 in) above the tube's insertion point into the patient.

Rationale   At this height the formula should run at a safe rate into the stomach.

d. Squeeze the drip chamber to fill it to one-third to one-half its capacity.

e. Open the tubing clamp, run the formula through the tubing, and reclamp the tube.

Rationale   The formula will displace the air in the tubing, thus preventing the instillation of excess air into the patient's stomach.

f. Follow step 6 above. Then attach the feeding set tubing to the nasogastric tube, and regulate the drip rate to deliver the feeding over the desired length of time. Some prefilled tube-feeding sets can be attached to a feeding pump.

g. Just before all the formula has run through the tubing, clamp the feeding tube and the nasogastric tube and disconnect the two.

h. Using a 50-mL syringe, instill 30 to 50 mL of water through the nasogastric tube to rinse it.

10. If the feeding is a continuous-drip tube feeding, discontinue the feeding at least every 6 hours, or as indicated by agency policy, and aspirate and measure the gastric contents. Then flush the tubing with 30 to 50 mL of water.

Rationale   This ensures adequate absorption and verifies correct placement of the tube.

11. After the feeding and tube rinsing, clamp the patient's tube, if this is agency practice; some tubes are left unclamped.

Rationale   Clamping prevents leakage from the tube.

12. Cover the end of the tube with gauze held by an elastic band, and pin the tubing to the patient's gown. See Figure 24–21.

Rationale   Covering the tube end prevents contamination.

13. Have the patient remain sitting upright, in Fowler's position, or in a slightly elevated right lateral position for at least 30 minutes.

Rationale   These positions facilitate digestion. A right lateral position facilitates movement of the feeding from the stomach into the small intestine.

14. If the equipment is to be reused, wash it thoroughly with soap and water so that it is ready for reuse. Change equipment every 24 hours or according to agency policy.

15. Check the agency's policy on the frequency of changing the nasogastric tube and the use of smaller-lumen tubes.

Rationale   These measures prevent irritation and abrasion of the pharyngeal and esophageal mucous membrane.

16. Record the feeding, including the amount and kind of solution taken and the response of the patient.

Sample Recording

Date	Time	Notes
6/9/86	1210	350 mL Meritene feeding administered. Eructated small amount of flatus. Tolerated feeding well. No discomfort. —————————————— ——————————Juan S. Ramirez, SN

■ Evaluation

Expected outcomes

1. Stated felt comfortable after feeding
2. Bowel sounds normal following feeding
3. Absence of abdominal distention and constipation
4. Anthropometric measurements within predetermined range or at baseline level
5. Normal blood and urine glucose
6. Normal serum electrolytes

Unexpected outcomes

1. Complained of abdominal cramps following feeding
2. Bowel sounds minimal
3. Diarrhea
4. Abdominal distention

5. Anthropometric measurements below predetermined or baseline level
6. Elevated blood and urine glucose
7. Abnormal serum electrolytes

Upon obtaining an unexpected outcome:

1. Report your findings to the responsible nurse.
2. Adjust the nursing care plan appropriately.

TECHNIQUE 24–7 ■ Administering a Gastrostomy or Jejunostomy Feeding

A *gastrostomy feeding* is the instillation of liquid nourishment through a tube that enters a surgical opening through the abdominal wall into the stomach (called a *gastrostomy*). A *jejunostomy feeding* is the instillation of liquid nourishment through a tube that enters a surgical opening through the abdominal wall into the jejunum (a *jejunostomy*). These feedings are usually temporary measures. When there is an obstruction in the esophagus, they may become permanent measures, for example, after removal of the esophagus.

For gastrostomies and jejunostomies, a surgeon inserts a plastic or rubber tube or catheter into either the stomach or the jejunum. The surgical opening is sutured tightly around the tube or catheter to prevent leakage. Care of this opening before it heals requires surgical aseptic technique. When the incision heals (10 to 14 days), the tube or catheter can be removed and reinserted for each feeding. Between feedings, a prosthesis may be used to close the "ostomy" opening. It consists of a shaft 4 to 6 cm (1½ to 2 in) long, with internal and external flanges and a screw cap.

Gastrostomy and jejunostomy feedings are used as alternatives to intravenous infusions and nasogastric feedings. They allow the patient greater mobility and enable self-feeding.

■ Assessment

Assess the patient for:

1. Allergies to any food in the feeding. Commonly included foods are milk, sugar, water, eggs, and vegetable oil.
2. Bowel sounds before each feeding.
3. Abdominal distention at least daily. Measure the patient's abdominal girth at the umbilicus.
4. Regurgitation and feelings of fullness after a feeding.
5. Hydration status. Measure the patient's fluid intake and output, and note complaints of thirst.
6. Changes in anthropometric measurements, ie, weight, triceps skin fold, and arm muscle circumference. See Technique 24–1.

7. Status of peristomal skin. Gastric or jejunal drainage contains digestive enzymes that can irritate the skin. Any redness and broken skin areas need to be reported and recorded.
8. Dumping syndrome. Jejunostomy patients may experience nausea, vomiting, diarrhea, cramps, pallor, sweating, heart palpitations, increased pulse rate, and fainting after a feeding. These are signs of dumping syndrome, which results when hypertonic foods and liquids suddenly distend the jejunum. To make the intestinal contents isotonic, body fluids shift rapidly from the patient's vascular system. Smaller, more frequent feedings and a longer adjustment period may relieve dumping.

Other data include:

1. The physician's order for the feeding. This should include the type of feeding, the amount to be instilled, and the frequency of feedings.
2. Any information on the patient's chart related to the feeding, eg, the position in which the patient best tolerates the feeding.

■ Planning

Nursing goal

To maintain the patient's hydration and nutritional status.

Equipment

1. The correct amount of feeding solution. Amounts are gradually increased from about 200 to 800 mL. Check the expiration date on a commercially prepared formula or the preparation date and time if the solution has been prepared in the agency. Discard a solution that has passed the expiration date or an agency formula that is more than 24 hours old. Gastric and jejunal feedings differ. Jejunal feedings contain nutrients that can be absorbed in the small intestine without gastric and duodenal

digestive processes. All feedings generally contain 1 cal/mL of solution with protein, fat, carbohydrate, minerals, and vitamins in specified proportions. Warm the solution in a basin of warm water or let it stand for a while until it reaches room temperature. Feedings are generally administered at room temperature unless the order specifies otherwise.

2. A large bulb syringe.

3. A graduated container to hold the feeding.

4. A graduated container with 60 mL of water to flush the tubing.

5. For a tube sutured in place:

   a. Some 4 × 4 gauze squares to cover the end of the tube.

   b. An elastic band.

6. For tube insertion:

   a. Water-soluble lubricant to lubricate the tube.

   b. Clean disposable gloves.

   c. A #18 Fr. whistle-tip catheter or other feeding tube.

   d. A tubing clamp.

   e. A moisture-proof bag.

7. For a prosthesis:

   a. Water-soluble lubricant.

   b. A #18 Fr. whistle-tip catheter or other feeding tube.

8. For cleaning the peristomal skin and dressing the stoma:

   a. Mild soap and water.

   b. Petrolatum, zinc oxide ointment, or other skin protectant.

   c. Precut 4 × 4 gauze squares.

   d. Uncut 4 × 4 gauze squares.

   e. Abdominal pads.

   f. An abdominal binder or Montgomery straps.

■ Intervention

1. Provide privacy for this technique. Gastrostomy and jejunal feedings involve exposing the abdomen, which is embarrassing to many people, and this method of feeding may in itself be embarrassing.

2. Assist the patient to a Fowler's position in bed, a sitting position on a chair, or, if sitting is contraindicated, a slightly elevated right lateral position.

   Rationale These positions promote digestion and prevent esophageal reflux of a gastric feeding.

3. If a tube is already in place:

   a. Remove the gauze from the end of the tube.

   b. Remove the clamp from the tube unless agency policy indicates otherwise. Some agencies leave the tube clamped until the syringe is attached.

Rationale A clamped tube prevents excess air from distending the stomach or duodenum and causing discomfort.

   c. Attach the bulb syringe to the tube.

   d. Pour 15 to 30 mL of water into the syringe, remove the tube clamp, and allow the water to flow into the tube.

   Rationale This determines the patency of the tube. If water flows freely, the tube is patent; if it does not, notify the responsible nurse and/or physician.

4. If a tube is not in place, and one needs to be inserted:

   a. Lubricate the insertion end of the tube.

   b. Wearing gloves, remove the ostomy dressing, being careful not to pull or dislodge the tube. Discard the dressing and gloves in the moisture-proof bag.

   c. Insert the tube into the ostomy opening about 10 to 15 cm (4 to 6 in).

   d. Attach the bulb syringe to the tube.

5. If a prosthesis is in place:

   a. Remove the screw cap on the prosthesis.

   b. Lubricate and insert the feeding tube into the ostomy opening about 10 to 15 cm (4 to 6 in).

   c. Attach the syringe to the end of the feeding tube.

6. Aspirate and measure the stomach or jejunal contents as follows:

   a. Compress the bulb on the syringe, and withdraw the stomach or jejunal contents.

   b. Measure the amount of aspirated contents in a graduated pitcher.

   Rationale To evaluate absorption of the previous feeding, the aspirated amount is compared with the amount instilled. If the amount is significant (eg, more than half of the last feeding) the amount or frequency of the feeding may be changed.

   c. If 50 mL or more of undigested formula is withdrawn, check with the responsible nurse before proceeding.

   Rationale At some agencies a feeding is withheld if 50 mL or more of formula remains in the stomach.

   d. Reinstill the gastric or jejunal contents if this is the agency or physician's practice. Remove the bulb and pour the contents via the syringe into the tube.

   Rationale The removed formula is reinstilled to prevent electrolyte imbalance.

7. To administer the feeding solution:

   a. Hold the syringe about 7 to 15 cm (3 to 6 in) above the ostomy opening.

   b. Slowly pour the solution into the syringe, and allow it to flow through the tube by gravity.

c. Just before all the formula has run through and the syringe is empty, add 30 mL of water.

Rationale   Water rinses the tube and preserves its patency.

d. If the tube is sutured in place, hold it upright, remove the syringe, and then clamp the tube to prevent leakage. Cover the end of the tube with a 4 × 4 gauze, and secure the gauze with a rubber band.

e. If the tube was inserted for the feeding, remove it, and either apply the screw cap to a prosthesis or apply a dressing over the ostomy.

8. After the feeding, have the patient remain in the sitting position, or a slightly elevated right lateral position, for at least 30 minutes.

Rationale   This prevents leakage and enhances the normal digestive process.

9. Check agency policy about cleaning the peristomal skin, applying a skin protectant, and applying appropriate dressings. Generally the peristomal skin is washed with mild soap and water at least once daily. Petrolatum, zinc oxide ointment, or other skin protectant may be applied around the stoma, and precut 4 × 4 gauze squares may be placed around the tube. The precut squares are then covered with regular 4 × 4 gauze squares, and the tube is coiled over them. The coiled tube is covered with abdominal pads and secured with either an abdominal binder or Montgomery straps.

10. Record the date, the time, the type and amount of each feeding, the amount of water instilled, and any relevant assessment data.

11. When appropriate, instruct the patient about self-care of the stoma and tube, and how to administer a feeding.

■ **Evaluation**   See Technique 24–6 on page 538.

References

Bishop CW, Bowen PE, Ritchey SJ: Norms for nutritional assessments of American adults by upper arm anthropometry. *Am J Clin Nutr* (November) 1981; 34(11):2530–2539.

Bistrian BR et al: Protein status of general surgical patients. *JAMA* 1974; 230:858.

Brody JE: *Jane Brody's Nutrition Book.* Norton, 1981.

Caly JC: Helping people eat for health: Assessing adults' nutrition. *Am J Nurs* (October) 1977; 77:1605–1610.

Frisancho AR: New norms of upper limb fat and muscle areas for assessment of nutritional status. *Am J Clin Nutr* (November) 1981; 34(11):2540–2545.

Glaser S: How to improve the first stage of digestion. *Geriatr Nurs* (September/October) 1981; 2:350–353.

Gray EG, Gray LK: Anthropometric measurements and their interpretation: Principles, practices, and problems. *J Am Diet Assoc* (November) 1980; 77(5):534–539.

Griggs BA, Hoppe MC: Update—nasogastric tube feeding. *Am J Nurs* (March) 1979; 79:481–485.

Halpern SL: *Quick Reference to Clinical Nutrition.* Lippincott, 1979.

Keithley JC: Proper nutritional assessment can prevent hospital malnutriton. *Nursing 79* (February) 1979; 9:68–72.

Konstantinides NN, Shronts E: Tube feeding: Managing the basics. *Am J Nurs* (September) 1983; 83:1312–1318.

Metheny MM: 20 ways to prevent tube-feeding complications. *Nursing 85* (January) 1985; 15:47–50.

National Center for Health Statistics: *Plan and operation of the Health and Nutrition Examination Survey (HANES), United States, 1971–1973.* Vital and Health Statistics, Series 1: Programs and Collection Procedure, No. 10a, DHEW Pub No. (PHS) 79–1310, 1979.

US Department of Agriculture, Science and Education Administration, Human Nutrition: *Ideas for Better Eating: Menus and Recipes to Make Use of Dietary Guidelines.* US Government Printing Office, January 1981.

Weinsier RL et al: Hospital malnutrition: A prospective evaluation of general medical patients during the course of hospitalization. *Am J Clin Nutr* 1979; 32:418.

White JH, Schroeder MA: When your client has a weight problem: Nursing assessment. *Am J Nurs* (March) 1981; 81:550–552.

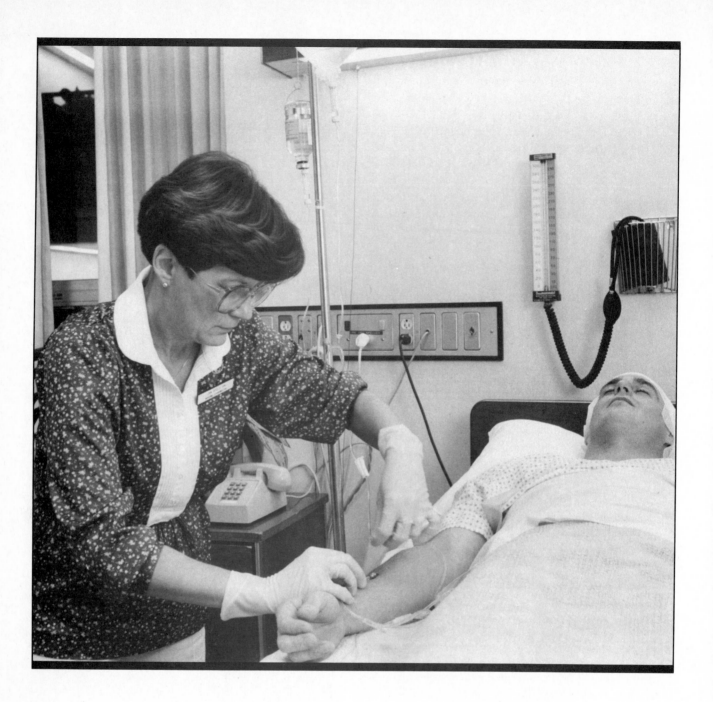

INTRAVENOUS THERAPY

25

Intravenous infusion is one of the more common methods of providing fluids, nutrients, and medications to patients. Intravenous solutions are the sole source of nourishment and fluid for many patients who are acutely ill. In acute care settings, nurses are responsible for many aspects of intravenous therapy, including setting up the equipment, monitoring the patient, maintaining the infusion and changing solution containers and tubing as necessary, and discontinuing infusions when the ordered amount of fluid has been administered.

Chapter Outline

Objectives

Upon completion of this chapter, the student will:

1. Know essential terms and facts about intravenous infusions
   1.1 Identify selected terms associated with intravenous therapy
   1.2 Identify common types of intravenous infusions
   1.3 Identify purposes of intravenous therapy
   1.4 Identify various venipuncture sites
   1.5 Identify methods for calculating infusion rates
   1.6 Identify potential problems associated with intravenous therapy
   1.7 Identify factors influencing infusion rates
   1.8 Identify differences between IV pumps and controllers
   1.9 Identify four main human blood groups
   1.10 Explain why various blood groups are incompatible
   1.11 Identify risks associated with blood transfusions
   1.12 Identify three types of transfusion reactions
   1.13 Identify the differences in purpose and technique between TPN and IV therapy
   1.14 Identify various solutions used in TPN
   1.15 Identify catheters used in central venous lines
   1.16 Identify sites used for central venous lines
   1.17 Identify reasons for use of central venous lines
   1.18 Identify reasons for taking a central venous pressure measurement
2. Understand facts about intravenous infusion techniques
   2.1 Identify relevant assessment data
   2.2 Identify nursing diagnosis for which the technique may be implemented
   2.3 Identify nursing goals related to the technique
   2.4 Identify expected and unexpected outcomes from assessment data
   2.5 Identify reasons underlying selected steps of the technique
3. Perform intravenous infusion techniques safely
   3.1 Assess the patient adequately
   3.2 Collect additional data from appropriate sources
   3.3 Select pertinent nursing goals for the patient
   3.4 Establish relevant outcome criteria for the patient following the technique
   3.5 Collect necessary equipment before the technique
   3.6 Implement interventions to enhance the effectiveness of the technique and enhance the patient's comfort and safety

3.7 Communicate relevant information about the patient to the appropriate persons through records or reports

3.8 Determine the evaluative outcomes of the technique

4. Evaluate own performance of specific techniques

in a laboratory or clinical setting with the assistance of another

4.1 Use the performance checklists provided

4.2 Identify areas of strength and weakness

4.3 Alter performance in response to own evaluation and that of another

Terms

■ antecubital fossa or space   the point on the arm located in front of the elbow

■ central venous line   a catheter inserted into a large vein located centrally in the body, eg, the superior vena cava

■ central venous pressure (CVP)   a measurement of the pressure of the blood, in centimeters of water, within the vena cava or right atrium of the heart

■ embolus   (1) a clot (in a blood vessel) that has moved from its place of origin; (2) a clot or substance such as air (air embolus) that is obstructing a blood vessel

■ hematoma   a collection of blood in a tissue, organ, or body space due to a break in the wall of a blood vessel

■ heparin   a substance that prevents the coagulation of blood

■ heparin flush   irrigation of a central venous line using a saline solution containing heparin

■ heparin lock   the airtight cap covering the end of a patient's intravenous or central venous tubing

■ hydration   the act of combining with water

■ hyperalimentation   *see* total parenteral nutrition

■ infusion   the introduction of fluid into a vein or other part of the body

■ infusion controller   a device used with intravenous infusions to obtain the desired infusion rate; it regulates gravitational flow by counting drops per minute and compressing the IV tubing

■ infusion pump   a device used with intravenous infusions to obtain the desired infusion rate; it delivers a measured amount of solution at a constant high pressure

■ intravenous   within a vein

■ intravenous hyperalimentation (IVH)   *see* total parenteral nutrition

■ knotted (referring to veins)   knoblike

■ manometer   an instrument used to measure the pressure of fluids or gases

■ metacarpal   referring to the part of the hand between the wrist and the fingers

■ plasma   the fluid portion of the blood in which the blood cells are suspended

■ pneumothorax   accumulation of air or gas in the pleural cavity

■ port   an opening or entrance

■ serum (in blood)   the clear liquid portion of the blood that does not contain fibrinogen

■ stopcock   a valve that controls the flow of fluid or air through a tube

■ thrombophlebitis   inflammation of a vein followed by formation of a blood clot

■ thrombus   a solid mass of blood constituents in the circulatory system

■ tortuous   twisted

■ total parenteral nutrition (TPN) (intravenous hyperalimentation)   administration of a hypertonic solution of carbohydrates, amino acids, and lipids by an indwelling intravenous catheter placed into the superior vena cava via the jugular or subclavian vein

■ tourniquet   a device, eg, a rubber strip, that is wrapped around a body extremity to compress the blood vessels

■ transfusion   the introduction of whole blood or its components, eg, serum, erythrocytes, or platelets, into the venous circulation

■ venipuncture   puncture of a vein for collection of a blood specimen or for therapeutic purposes

INTRAVENOUS INFUSIONS

An *intravenous (IV) infusion* is the instillation into a vein of fluid and/or electrolytes or nutrient substances. It is given to patients who require extra fluid or who cannot take fluids and/or nutrients orally. A physician is responsible for ordering the type of solution to be administered, the amount to be given, and the rate at which it is to be infused.

Purposes of Intravenous Therapy

1. To supply fluid when patients are unable to take adequate fluids by mouth

2. To provide salts needed to maintain electrolyte balance

3. To provide glucose (dextrose), the main fuel for metabolism

4. To provide water-soluble vitamins and medications

5. To provide a lifeline for rapidly needed medications

Common Types of IV Solutions

Common IV solutions include nutrient solutions, electrolyte solutions, alkalizing and acidifying solutions, and blood volume expanders.

Nutrient solutions

Nutrient solutions contain some form of carbohydrate (eg, dextrose, glucose, or levulose) and water. Water is supplied for fluid requirements and carbohydrate for calories and energy. For example, 1 L of 5% dextrose provides 170 calories. Common nutrient solutions are:

1. 5% dextrose in water (D5W)

2. 3.3% glucose in 0.3% sodium chloride (NaCl) (glucose in saline)

3. 5% dextrose in 0.45% sodium chloride (dextrose in half-strength saline)

Nutrient solutions are useful in preventing dehydration and ketosis but do not provide sufficient calories to promote wound healing, weight gain, or normal growth in children.

Electrolyte solutions

Electrolyte solutions are either saline (NaCl) or multiple electrolyte solutions containing varying amounts of specific cations and anions. Commonly used solutions are:

1. Normal saline (0.9% sodium chloride solution).

2. Ringer's solution, which contains sodium (Na^+), chloride (CL^-), potassium (K^+), and calcium (Ca^{++}).

3. Lactated Ringer's solution, which contains sodium, chloride, potassium, calcium, and lactate. Lactate is a salt of lactic acid that is metabolized in the liver to form bicarbonate (HCO_3^-).

Normal saline solutions are frequently used as initial hydrating solutions. Multiple electrolyte solutions approximate the ionic profile of plasma and are used to prevent dehydration or to restore or correct fluid and electrolyte imbalances.

Alkalizing and acidifying solutions

Alkalizing solutions are administered to counteract metabolic acidosis. One commonly used solution is lactated Ringer's solution. Acidifying solutions, in contrast, are administered to counteract metabolic alkalosis. Examples of acidifying solutions are 5% dextrose in 0.45% sodium chloride; and 0.9% sodium chloride solution.

The body fluids are normally maintained within a precise pH range of 7.35 to 7.45. This is a slightly alkaline state. However, in conditions such as prolonged diarrhea, starvation, or renal impairment, metabolic acidosis can occur. Metabolic alkalosis can occur with prolonged vomiting and in other conditions that result in an excessive amount of bicarbonate ions in the bloodstream.

Blood volume expanders

Blood volume expanders are used to increase the volume of blood following severe loss of blood (eg, from hemorrhage) or plasma (eg, from severe burns, which draw large amounts of plasma from the bloodstream to the burn site). Common blood volume expanders are:

1. Dextran

2. Plasma

3. Human serum albumin

VENIPUNCTURE SITES

The site chosen for venipuncture varies with the patient's age, the infusion time, the type of solution used, and the condition of the veins. For adults, veins in the arm are commonly used; for infants, veins in the scalp are used. The larger veins of the forearm are preferred to the metacarpal veins of the hand, for infusions that need to be given rapidly and for solutions that are hypertonic, are highly acidic or alkaline, or contain irritating medications.

Adults

The most convenient veins for venipuncture in the adult are the basilic and median cubital veins in the crease of the elbow (antecubital space). See Figure 25–1. These large superficial veins are frequently used by laboratory technicians to withdraw blood for examination. Unfortunately, use of these veins for prolonged infusions limits arm mobility, because a splint is needed to stabilize the elbow joint. For prolonged therapy, veins on the back of the hand and on the forearm are preferred. The metacarpal, basilic, and cephalic veins are commonly used. Forearm sites are equipped with the natural splints of the ulna and radius and allow the patient more arm movement for activities such as eating.

Ideally, for long-term therapy, sites at the distal end of the arm should be used first. If these veins have been used for prolonged periods or have developed thrombi,

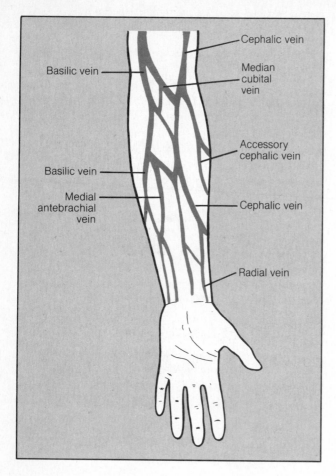

FIGURE 25-1 ■ Venipuncture sites of the arm.

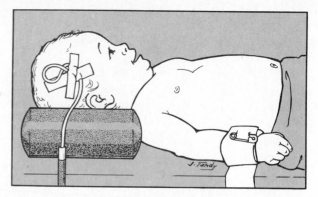

FIGURE 25-2 ■ For an infant, the temporal vein of the scalp is often used to administer intravenous fluids for a prolonged period.

other more proximal sites may be required. If arm veins are inaccessible, veins in the feet and legs may be used, although they are more prone to thrombus formation and subsequent emboli.

Infants

Because infants do not have large veins in the antecubital fossa, blood specimens for examination are usually taken from the external jugular vein and femoral veins. If an infusion is to be maintained for a long period , veins in the temporal region of the scalp (see Figure 25-2), or sometimes the back of the hand or the dorsum of the foot, are used.

TECHNIQUE 25-1 ■ Setting Up an Intravenous Infusion

A nurse usually sets up an intravenous infusion, even though it may actually be started by a physician or the responsible nurse. The preparation centers primarily on readying the patient and assembling the equipment.

◗ Assessment

Assess the patient for:

1. Vital signs (pulse, respirations, and blood pressure) for baseline data if not already available. Because fluid is instilled directly into the circulatory system, problems such as too much fluid can be reflected in the vital signs.
2. Oral fluid intake.
3. Skin turgor. Lifting the skin over the anterior chest with two fingers. An inverted V, called *tenting,* that remains after the skin is released indicates decreased turgor and possible fluid deficit.

4. Amount of urine output and its specific gravity.
5. Other objective and subjective data pertinent to the patient's hydration and electrolyte status.
6. Allergy to tape or povidone-iodine.

■ Planning

Nursing goals

1. To prepare the patient for an intravenous infusion
2. To assemble the equipment and supplies required for the intravenous infusion

Equipment

1. The container(s) of sterile intravenous solution. IV solutions are supplied in bottles and plastic bags. See Figure 25-3.

a. Select the size ordered. Do not select containers with greater volumes than ordered. For example, if 750 mL 5% D/NS (750 mL of 5% dextrose in normal saline) has been ordered, obtain one 500-mL container and one 250-mL container, which total 750 mL. Do not obtain a 1,000-mL container with the intention of stopping the solution after 750 mL has been administered. Too often the incorrect amount can be instilled. If a 1,000-mL solution container *must* be used, remove 250 mL before starting the IV.

b. Some solution bottles have a tube inside the bottle that serves as an air vent so that, as the solution runs out of the bottle, it is replaced with air. See Figure 25–4. Containers without air vents require a vent on the administration set. See Figure 25–5. Air vents usually have filters to remove any contamination from the air that enters the container.

2. An administration set, consisting of an insertion spike, a drip chamber, a roller valve or screw clamp, tubing, and a protective cap over the needle adapter. See Figure 25–6. The insertion spike is kept sterile and inserted into the solution container when the IV is set up and ready to start. The drip chamber

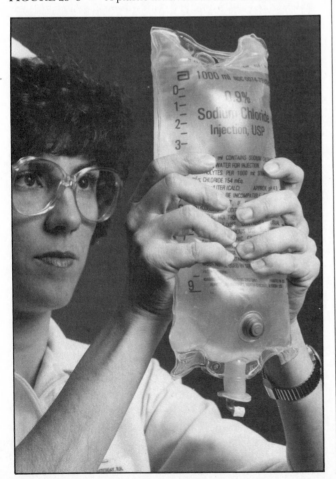

FIGURE 25–3 ■ A plastic intravenous fluid container.

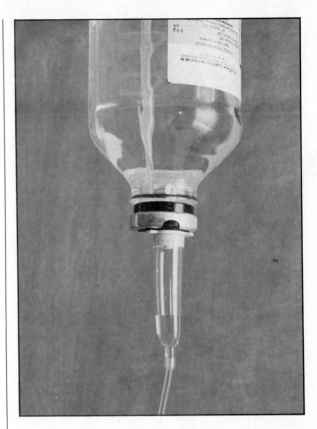

FIGURE 25–4 ■ An intravenous container with an indwelling vent. Note that the tubing does not have a vent.

FIGURE 25–5 ■ An intravenous container without an indwelling vent. Note the vent on the tubing just below the container.

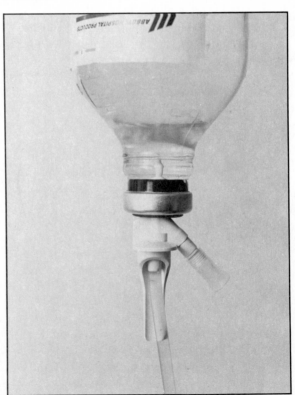

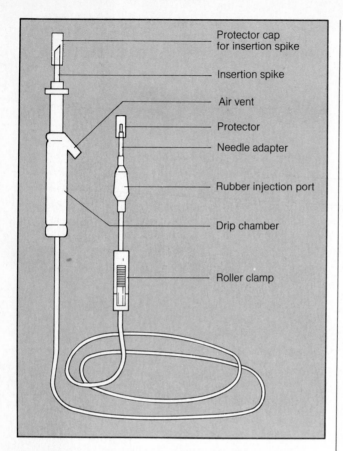

FIGURE 25–6 ■ An intravenous administration set, consisting of an insertion spike with a protector cap, an air vent (optional), a drip (drop) chamber, plastic tubing with a roller control clamp, rubber injection port, and a needle adapter covered by a protective cap.

Labels:
- Protector cap for insertion spike
- Insertion spike
- Air vent
- Protector
- Needle adapter
- Rubber injection port
- Drip chamber
- Roller clamp

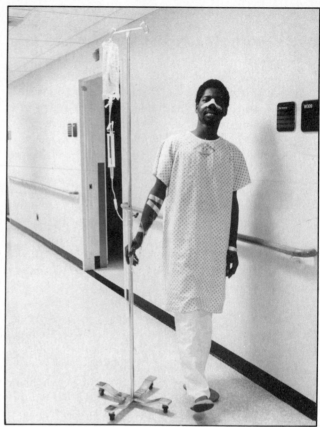

FIGURE 25–7 ■ An IV pole with wheels facilitates a patient's ambulation.

permits a predictable amount of fluid to be delivered to the patient. A commonly used drip chamber is the macrodrip, which provides 10 to 20 drops per mL of solution. This information will be on the package. There are also microdrip sets, which provide 60 drops per mL of solution. The roller valve or screw clamp is used to control the rate of flow of the solution by compressing the lumen of the tubing. The protective cap over the needle adapter maintains the sterility of the end of the tubing so that it can be attached to a sterile needle inserted in the patient's vein.

3. IV poles (rods) for hanging the solution container. Some poles are attached to hospital beds. Others stand on the floor or hang from the ceiling. There are floor models with casters that can be pushed along when a patient is up and walking. See Figure 25–7. The height of most poles is adjustable. The higher the solution container is suspended, the greater the force of the solution as it enters the patient and the faster the rate of flow.

4. An intravenous needle or catheter. These are usu-

ally packaged separately. Butterfly or wing-tipped needles, with wings attached to the shaft, are commonly used. See Figure 25–8. They vary in length from 1.5 to 3 cm (½ to 1¼ in), and from #25 to #17 gauge in diameter. The larger the gauge number, the smaller the diameter of the shaft. Needles of #20 to #22 gauge and short lengths are commonly used for adults. Some practitioners prefer to use a needle bevel that is short, to minimize injury to the tissues and discomfort on insertion. A catheter or angiocatheter is a plastic tube that is inserted into the patient's vein. Some catheters fit over a needle during insertion, while others fit inside a needle. See Figure 25–9. An angiocatheter has a metal stylet (needle), which is used to pierce the skin and vein and is then withdrawn, leaving the catheter in place.

5. An arm board if needed to help immobilize the patient's arm. Arm boards are made of plastic, metal, or wood. They are usually padded with a towel, for comfort. Tape or wrapping is required to secure the board to the patient's arm.

6. An intravenous tray containing all the supplies

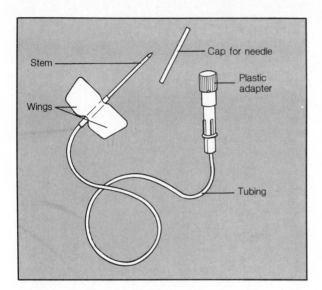

FIGURE 25–8   ■   An intravenous butterfly (wing-tipped) needle.

required to start an IV. It should include sterile swabs, antiseptic solution, plastic or paper tape, and a tourniquet.

7.   Sterile 2 × 2 gauze squares and/or transparent tape to place over the insertion site.

8.   A local anesthetic, eg, 1% lidocaine without epinephrine, and a small syringe with a #27 gauge needle, if this is to be used before the venipuncture.

Additional equipment is required for variations from the standard infusion. Secondary sets are required when more than one solution is running at the same time.

9.   In a tandem setup, a second container is attached to the line of the first container at the lower, secondary port. See Figure 25–10, A. It permits medications to be administered intermittently or simultaneously with the first solution.

10.   In the piggyback alignment, a second set connects the second container to the tubing of the first at the upper port. This setup is used solely for intermittent drug administration. See Figure 25–10, B. Various manufacturers describe these sets differently, so check the manufacturer's labeling and directions carefully.

11.   Another variation is a volume-control set, which is used if the volume of fluid administered is to be carefully controlled. The set is attached below the solution container, and the drip chamber is placed below it. See Figure 25–11. Volume control sets are frequently used in pediatric settings where the volume administered is critical.

Agencies have different policies about when to take the equipment to the bedside prior to starting an intravenous

infusion. Normally it is not taken to the bedside in advance if it will produce anxiety in the patient.

■ Intervention

1.   Check the patient's record for the physician's order indicating the type of solution, the amount to be administered, and the rate of flow of the infusion.

2.   Determine the types of solutions used by the agency and the container sizes that are available. Intravenous solutions are supplied in 150-mL, 250-mL, 500-mL, and 1,000-mL sizes. Some agencies use abbreviations to describe commonly used solutions, eg, DW (distilled water), NS (normal saline), D5W (5% dextrose in water), D5NS (5% dextrose in normal saline). Check the abbreviations used by the agency.

3.   Check the order for any special equipment required, eg, a microdrip set is usually required if the fluid is to be administered at a rate of 50 to 75 mL/hr or less, for accurate regulation.

4.   Determine the agency practice or the physician's order about the type of needle or catheter to be used for intravenous infusions.

5.   Determine what equipment is contained in an intravenous set. Some agencies have special trays for use by personnel who start infusions. These are normally kept in a central place and taken to the bedside when the infusion is to be started.

6.   Explain the procedure to the patient. A venipuncture can cause discomfort for a few seconds, but there should be no discomfort while the solution is flowing.

FIGURE 25–9   ■   A, An over-the-needle catheter—after insertion in the vein, the needle is removed, and the plastic catheter remains; B, an inside-the-needle catheter (intracatheter)—the plastic catheter is threaded through the needle after the venipuncture.

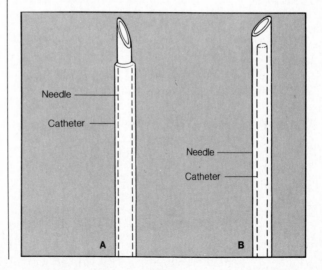

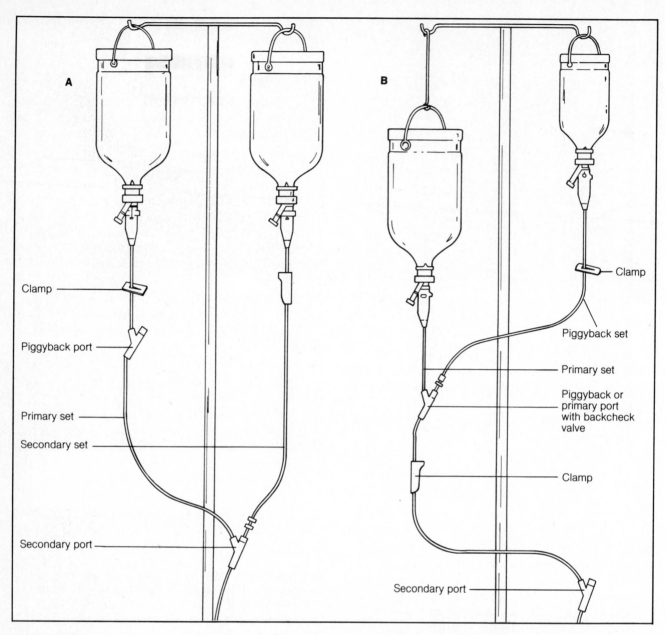

FIGURE 25-10 ■ **A,** A tandem intravenous alignment—the secondary set connects to the secondary (lower) port of the primary set; **B,** a piggyback intravenous alignment—the secondary set connects to the primary (upper) port of the primary set.

Patients often want to know how long the process will last. The physician's order may specify the length of time of the infusion, eg, 3,000 mL over 24 hours.

7. Provide any scheduled care before establishing the IV, to minimize movement of the affected limb during the procedure, since moving the limb after the IV is established could dislodge the needle.

8. Make sure that the patient's gown can be removed over the IV apparatus if necessary. Some agencies provide special gowns that open over the shoulder and down the sleeve for easy removal.

9. Determine that the solution is sterile and in good condition, ie, clear. Check the expiration date on the label. Examine the other packages to confirm their sterility. Inspect and squeeze a plastic solution bag for any leaks or hairline cracks. Return any unsatisfactory container to the central supply or distributing department, indicating the reason for the return.
Rationale Cloudiness, evidence that the container has been opened previously, or leaks indicate possible contamination.

10. Open the administration set, maintaining the sterility of the ends of the tubing. The ends of the tubing may be covered with plastic caps, which are left in place until the IV is started.

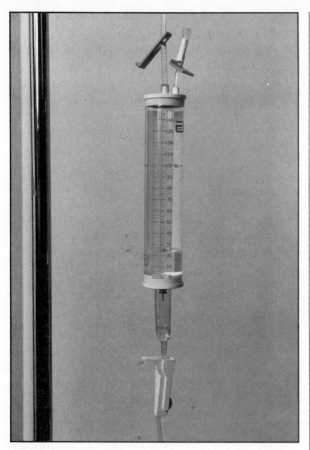

FIGURE 25–11 ■ A volume-control set above the drip chamber of an intravenous infusion.

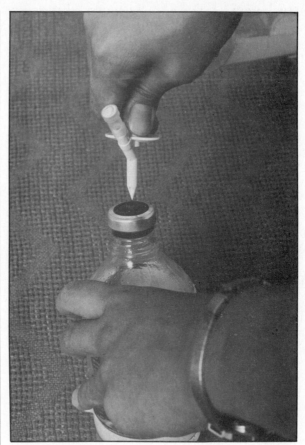

FIGURE 25–12

FIGURE 25–13

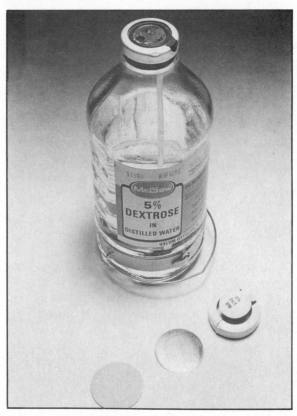

11. Slide the tubing clamp along the tubing until it is just below the drip chamber.

12. Close the clamp.

13. If using an intravenous bottle with a rubber stopper, remove the metal disc while maintaining the sterility of the stopper. If the stopper becomes contaminated while you are removing the metal disc, swab it with disinfectant. Remove the cap from the tubing, and insert the spike firmly through the rubber stopper into the port, maintaining sterile technique. See Figure 25–12.

    or

    If using a bottle with an indwelling vent, remove the metal disc and the rubber diaphragm, keeping the stopper sterile, and listen for a hissing sound as the air rushes into the bottle. If there is no hissing sound, discard the container because it was probably not sealed. Insert the spike into the larger hole (the one without the vent.) See Figure 25–13.

    or

    For spiking a plastic bag, read the manufacturer's directions. Some bags are hung on the pole before spiking.

14. Hang the solution container on the pole, usually about 1 m (3 ft) above the patient's head.

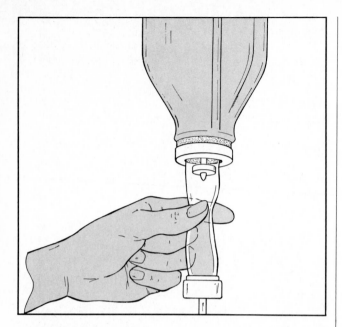

FIGURE 25–14

Rationale This height is needed to enable gravity to overcome venous pressure and facilitate flow of the solution into the vein.

15. If using a flexible drip chamber, squeeze it gently until it is half full of solution. See Figure 25–14.

    or

    If the drip chamber is firm, it will usually fill automatically.

    Rationale The drip chamber is partly filled with solution to prevent air from moving down the tubing.

16. To prime the tubing, remove the protective cap, and hold the tubing over a cup or basin. Maintain the sterility of the end of the tubing and the cap. Release the clamp and let the fluid run through the tubing until all bubbles are removed. Tap the tubing with your fingers to help the bubbles move.

    Rationale The tubing is primed to prevent the introduction of air into the patient, because air bubbles can act as emboli in the bloodstream.

17. Reclamp the tubing.

18. Replace the tubing cap, maintaining sterile technique.

19. Label the solution container, applying the label upside down on the container. Include the following information: the patient's name, identification number, room, and/or bed number; any medication and dosage; the drip rate; the date, the time the container is being started; the container number; and the name of the person starting it. See Figure 25–15. Labeling may be done when the IV is started.

Rationale The label is applied upside down so it can be read easily when the container is hanging up. The IV bottles are numbered consecutively.

20. Apply a timing label on the solution container. See Figure 25–16. The timing label may be applied at the time the IV is started. Follow agency practice.

21. Label the IV tubing with the date and time of attachment. This labeling may also be done at the time the IV is started.

    Rationale The tubing is labeled to ensure that it is changed every 48 hours or sooner.

22. Assess the patient's reaction to the setting up of the IV. If the patient expresses anxiety and fear, assist the patient to deal with his or her emotions, and record the reaction on the chart.

23. Notify the responsible nurse when the intravenous infusion has been set up.

24. Assist with starting the IV as needed.

FIGURE 25–15

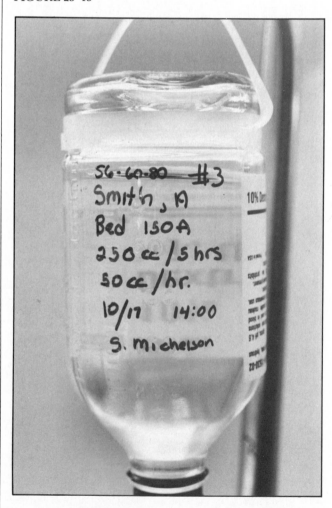

REGULATING INTRAVENOUS FLOW RATES

An important nursing function for an intravenous infusion is to regulate the flow rate of the solution. The physician usually describes in the IV order how long an infusion should last, ie, 3,000 mL over 24 hours. It is then a nursing responsibility to calculate the correct flow rate and regulate the infusion. Problems that can result from incorrectly regulated infusions are discussed in Technique 25-2.

There are a number of commercially prepared infusion sets, and each has its own type of drip chamber, so it is important to know the number of drops per mL of solution for a particular drip chamber before calculating a drip rate. This rate is called the *drop* or *drip factor* and is printed on most commercially prepared packages.

FIGURE 25-16

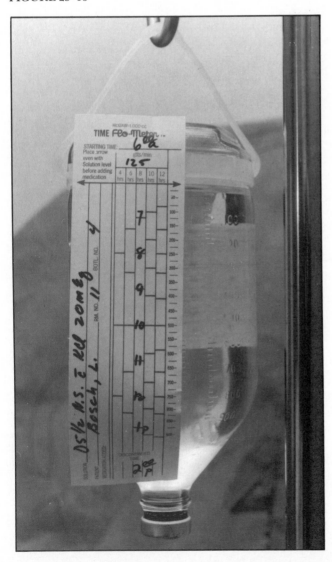

Common drop factors are 10, 15, and 20 for macrodrips and 60 for microdrips. See Technique 25-1.

There are two methods of calculating flow rates: the number of milliliters per hour and the number of drops per minute.

Milliliters per Hour

Hourly rates of infusion can be calculated by dividing the total infusion volume by the total infusion time in hours. For example, if 3,000 mL is infused in 24 hours, the number of milliliters per hour is

$$\frac{3{,}000 \text{ mL (total infusion volume)}}{24 \text{ hr (total infusion time)}} = 125 \text{ mL/hr}$$

Nurses need to check infusions at least every 30 minutes to assure that the indicated milliliters per hour have infused. A strip of adhesive marking the exact time and/or amount to be infused may be taped to the solution bottle. Some agencies make premarked labels available. See Figure 25-16.

Drops per Minute

The nurse who begins an infusion must regulate the drops per minute to ensure that the prescribed amount of solution will infuse. Drops per minute are calculated by the following formula:

Drops per minute =

$$\frac{\text{Total infusion volume} \times \text{drops/mL (or drip factor)}}{\text{Total time of infusion in } \textit{minutes}}$$

If the requirements are 1,000 mL in 8 hours (480 minutes) and the drip factor is 20 drops/mL, the drops per minute should be:

$$\frac{1{,}000 \text{ mL} \times 20 \text{ drops/mL}}{480 \text{ min}} = 41 \text{ drops/min}$$

Approximating this rate as 40 drops/min, the nurse must then regulate the drops per minute by tightening or releasing the intravenous tubing clamp and counting the drops the same way a pulse is counted. Devices such as battery-operated rate meters and infusion pumps with alarm systems facilitate a regulated flow.

Factors Influencing Flow Rates

No matter how often flow rates are regulated, several factors can change the rate of flow of an IV infusion. If an infusion is too fast or too slow, the nurse needs to consider several factors:

1. *The position of the forearm.* Sometimes having the patient change the position of the arm increases flow. Slight

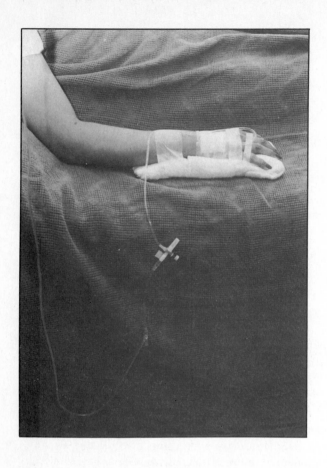

pronation, supination, extension, or elevation of the forearm on a pillow can increase flow.

2. *The position and patency of the tubing.* Not infrequently, the tubing is obstructed by the patient's weight, a kink, or a clamp closed too tightly. The flow rate also diminishes when part of the tubing dangles below the puncture site. See Figure 25-17.

3. *The height of the infusion bottle.* Elevating the height of the infusion bottle a few inches can speed the flow by creating more pressure.

4. *Possible infiltration or fluid leakage.* Swelling, a feeling of coldness, and tenderness at the venipuncture site may indicate infiltration.

FIGURE 25-17 ■ Tubing that dangles below the venipunture site can block the infusion, since the solution cannot flow against gravity.

TECHNIQUE 25-2 ■ Monitoring and Maintaining an Intravenous Infusion

An important nursing responsibility is to monitor an intravenous infusion so that the flow of the correct solution is maintained at the correct rate.

■ Assessment

1. Assess the whole infusion system regularly to ascertain problems. Common problems are fluid infiltration, phlebitis, circulatory overload, bleeding at the venipuncture site, and blockage of the infusion flow. Table 25-1 provides an assessment guide for nursing personnel responsible for intravenous infusions. For assessment of these problems, see the Intervention.

2. Assess the patient for clinical signs of fluid and electrolyte problems.

■ Planning

Nursing goals

1. To assess the correctness and the amount of solution for hydration purposes

2. To check that the system is intact, eg, that there is no leakage in the tubing or tissue infiltration

3. To check the rate of flow of the solution and whether the infusion is on schedule

4. To guard against blockage of the flow of solution

■ Intervention

1. Check the physician's order on the patient's chart to determine the type and sequence of solutions to be infused.

2. Check the nursing care plan for the rate of flow, infusion schedule, and relevant problems.

3. Inspect the patient's infusion site for fluid infiltration, ie, the escape of intravenous fluid into the interstitial tissues, usually near the intravenous site. The needle becomes dislodged from the patient's vein, and the intravenous fluid flows into the subcutaneous tissue. The clinical signs are swelling, coolness, pain, pallor at the site, and discomfort. To ascertain the presence of infiltration:

a. Palpate the surrounding tissue for edema.

b. Feel the surrounding skin for changes in temperature.

If infiltration is not evident, the following measures can determine whether the needle is dislodged from the vein:

c. If the tubing does not have a backcheck valve, lower the infusion bottle below the level of the venipuncture site to see if blood returns. Blood may indicate that the intravenous needle is still in the vein. This method is not foolproof, however, because the needle may be penetrating the vein wall partially.

d. Use a sterile syringe of saline to withdraw fluid from the rubber at the end of the tubing near the venipuncture site. If blood does not return, discontinue the intravenous infusion.

e. Try to stop the flow by applying a tourniquet 10 to 15 cm (4 to 6 in) above the insertion site and opening the roller clamp wide. If the infusion continues to flow slowly, the needle is in subcutaneous tissue (it has infiltrated).

f. If the patient is elderly or hypovolemic, it may be necessary to combine steps d and e to check for blood return before discontinuing the infusion.

4. Inspect for the presence of *phlebitis* (inflammation of a vein), which can occur with or without a blood clot. If a blood clot exists, the condition is called *thrombophlebitis*. Phlebitis can occur as a result of injury to a vein, eg, because of mechanical trauma or chemical irritation. Chemical injury to a vein can occur from intravenous electrolytes and medications. The clinical signs are redness, warmth, and swelling at the intravenous site and burning pain along the course of a vein. A new venipuncture site is usually selected, and the injured vein is not used for further infusions.

5. Be alert to signs of circulatory overload. Circulatory overload means that the circulatory system contains more fluid than normal. An adult normally has about 6 L of blood in circulation. A significant increase in this volume, eg, when an IV is administered too quickly, can cause circulatory overload, which may result in pulmonary edema and cardiac failure. The clinical signs of cardiac failure are dyspnea, reduced urine output, edema, weak and rapid pulse, and shallow, rapid respirations. The clinical signs of pulmonary edema are dyspnea, coughing, and frothy sputum.

6. Inspect for bleeding at the intravenous site. This can occur during an IV but is more likely to occur after the needle has been removed from the vein. The site of the needle or catheter insertion should always be inspected for evidence of blood, particularly in patients who bleed readily, eg, patients receiving heparin.

7. Ensure that the correct solution is being infused. If the solution is incorrect, slow the rate of flow to a minimum to maintain the patency of the needle or catheter and report the matter to the repsonsible nurse. Change the solution to the correct one. See Technique 25-3. Agencies have different policies about how and to whom to report an incident.

Rationale   If the IV is terminated, the patient will have to have another venipuncture before the new solution is administered.

8. Check that the system is intact. If there is leakage, locate the source. If the leak is at the needle connection, tighten the tubing into the needle. If the leak cannot be stopped, slow the IV as much as possible without stopping it, and replace the tubing with a new sterile set. See Technique 25-3. Report to the responsible nurse. Estimate how much solution was lost if the amount was substantial.

TABLE 25-1   ■   Checklist for an Intravenous Infusion

Component	Data
Solution container	
Name of solution	_____
Amount of solution	_____
Number of container	_____
Date and time	_____
Time of completion	_____
Next solution	
Name of solution	_____
Amount of solution	_____
Number of container	_____
Date and time	_____
Time of completion	_____
Tubing	
Intact	_____
Coiled smoothly	_____
Unobstructed	_____
Drip chamber	
Appropriately filled	_____
Dripping at correct rate	_____
Patient	
Venipuncture site	_____
Dry or wet	_____
Bleeding	_____
Swelling	_____
Skin color	_____
Skin temperature	_____
Pain	_____
Respirations	_____
Pulse	_____
Urine output	_____
Edema	_____
Sputum and cough	_____
Psychologic concerns	_____

9. Compare the rate of flow regularly, eg, every hour, against the schedule. If the rate is ahead of schedule, slow it, so that the infusion will be completed at the planned time. If it is behind schedule, check agency practice. Some agencies permit nursing personnel to adjust a rate of flow 3 mL/min or less. Adjustments above 3 mL/min require a physician's order. If the rate of flow is 150 mL/hr or more, the rate of flow must be checked more frequently, eg, every 15 to 30 minutes.

   Rationale IV infusions that are off schedule can be harmful to a patient. Solution that is administered too slowly can supply insufficient fluid, electrolytes, or medication for a patient's needs. Solution administered too quickly may cause circulatory overload and possible pulmonary edema or cardiac failure.

10. Inspect for blockages. The flow of solution can be blocked or impeded for several reasons.

    a. Check whether the tubing is kinked. Arrange the tubing so that it is lightly coiled with no pressure on it. Sometimes the tubing becomes caught under the patient's arm and the weight of the arm blocks the flow.

    b. Check whether the bevel of the needle or catheter is blocked against the wall of the vein. If it is blocked, pull back gently on the needle or catheter, and turn it slightly. Do not turn a butterfly needle; instead, raise or lower the angle of the needle slightly, using a sterile gauze pad under the wings.

       Rationale Turning a butterfly needle can injure the vein. The sterile gauze pad protects the skin and changes the position of the bevel of the needle.

    c. Check the tubing clamp. If it is closed, adjust it to the open position.

    d. Check the position of the solution container. If it is less than 1 m (3 ft) above the IV site, readjust it to the correct height on the pole.

       Rationale If the container is too close in height to the IV site, the solution may not flow into the vein because there is insufficient gravitational pressure of the fluid to overcome the pressure of the blood within the vein.

    e. Check the position of the tubing. If it is dangling below the venipuncture, coil it carefully on the surface of the bed.

       Rationale The solution cannot flow upward into the vein against the force of gravity. See Figure 25–17 earlier.

11. Check the drip chamber. If it is less than half full, squeeze the chamber to allow the correct amount of fluid to flow in.

12. Implement corrective measures for problems, as outlined or recommended by the agency.

13. If the patient is able, teach him or her when to call for assistance, eg, if the solution stops dripping or the venipuncture site becomes swollen. In addition, to help the patient maintain an intravenous infusion, instruct her or him to:

    a. Avoid sudden twisting or turning movements of the arm with the infusion.

    b. Avoid stretching or placing tension on the tubing.

    c. Try to keep the tubing from dangling below the level of the needle.

    d. Notify a nurse if the patient notices:

       ■ A sudden change in the flow rate.

       ■ The solution container becoming nearly empty.

       ■ Blood in the IV tubing.

       ■ Discomfort at the IV site.

■ Evaluation

Expected outcomes

1. IV infusion on schedule
2. IV system intact
3. IV site intact
4. Absence of tissue infiltration
5. Absence of complaints by patient
6. Urinary output adequate for fluid intake
7. Good skin turgor
8. Normal specific gravity of urine

Unexpected outcomes

1. IV infusion behind or ahead of schedule
2. Signs of tissue infiltration
3. Bleeding at IV site
4. Signs of IV system blockage
5. Signs of circulatory overload
6. Signs of phlebitis
7. Signs of IV system leakage
8. Complaints of IV site discomfort
9. Inadequate urine output
10. Increased or decreased specific gravity of urine
11. Poor skin turgor

Upon obtaining an unexpected outcome:

1. Implement corrective measures where possible.
2. Report your findings to the responsible nurse and/or physician.

TECHNIQUE 25–3   ■   Changing an Intravenous Container and Tubing

Intravenous solution containers are changed when only a small amount of fluid remains in the neck of the container and fluid still remains in the drip chamber. The Centers for Disease Control (CDC) recommend that tubing be changed every 48 hours to decrease the incidence of phlebitis. Usually the tubing is changed at a time when the container is being changed.

It is important to know agency practices regarding the frequency of changing infusion tubing and cleaning venipuncture sites.

■ Assessment

1. Assess the patient for signs of IV infiltration, circulatory overload, and phlebitis.
2. Assess the IV system for blockage of the infusion flow.

Other data include:

1. Whether the patient is allergic to tape
2. The physician's order for the kind, amount, and rate of solution to be infused

■ Planning

Nursing goals

1. To maintain the patient's hydration status and the continuity of an intravenous infusion by adding a new container
2. To reduce the possibility of problems, eg, phlebitis, by changing the tubing

Equipment

To change the container

1. A container with the correct kind and amount of sterile solution.

To change the tubing

2. An administration set with sterile tubing, drip chamber, etc.
3. Tape for taping the needle and new tubing.
4. A sterile gauze square for positioning the needle.
5. Antiseptic solution and/or ointment for cleaning the site. Check agency practice.
6. Sterile swabs.
7. A receptacle (eg, a kidney basin) for discarded fluid.

Place the equipment within reach at the bedside.

■ Intervention

1. Explain the procedure to the patient and reassure him or her as needed. Neither change should be painful. Some patients may be anxious, but as long as sterile technique is maintained there is no danger. Changing the solution container and tubing takes only a couple of minutes.
2. Compare the number of the new container against the number of the used container. Read the label of the new container.
3. Inspect the labels on the patient's IV tubing and the needle for date and time for changing.

Changing a container

4. Remove the cover from the new container so that it is ready for spiking. Maintain the sterility of the container top. Follow the manufacturer's directions in setting up the container. Sometimes it is hung on the IV pole before inserting the spike, sometimes it is placed on a table.
5. Close the clamp on the tubing to stop the flow of solution.
6. Take the used solution container off the pole, and invert it.
7. Remove the spike from the container, maintaining its sterility.
8. Hold the new container with one hand so it will not slip, and insert the spike into the container with the other. Do not twist the tubing.
   Rationale   Twisting could break the connections of the tubing.
9. Hang the container on the pole if it is not already hung.
10. Adjust the clamp, and regulate the rate of flow of the solution according to the order on the chart.
11. Label the solution container if this was not done prior to changing the container. Go to step 24.

Changing a container and tubing

12. Follow steps 1–4.
13. Open the administration set, and attach it to the container, using sterile technique.
14. Tighten the clamp and hang the container on the pole if it is not already hung.
15. Remove the protective cap from the end of the tubing, and prime the tubing as in Technique 25–1, step 16, on page 552. Clamp the tubing, and replace the protective cap.

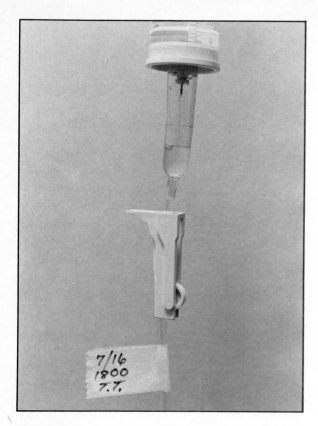

FIGURE 25-18

Rationale Replacing the cap maintains the sterility of the end of the tubing.

16. Remove the tape and the dressing carefully from around the needle. Take care not to dislodge the needle in the vein.

17. Place a sterile swab under the hub of the catheter to absorb any leakage that might occur when the tubing is disconnected. Clamp the old tubing.

18. Holding the hub of the needle with the fingers of one hand, remove the tubing with the other hand, using a twisting, pulling motion. Place the end of the tubing in the kidney basin or other receptacle.

Rationale Holding the needle firmly but gently maintains its position in the vein.

19. Continue to hold the needle, and grasp the new tubing with the other hand. Remove the protective cap, and, maintaining sterility, insert the tubing end tightly into the needle hub.

20. Open the clamp to start the solution flowing.

21. Clean the venipuncture site, working from the insertion point outward in a circular manner. Iodine or ethyl alcohol is frequently used. Some agencies also place water-soluble iodine ointment, eg, Betadine, at the site.

22. Apply a sterile dressing over the site and tape the needle in place. See Technique 25–5, step 15, on page 561. Apply a labeled tape over the dressing. The label should include: the date and time the dressing is applied; the original date and time of the venipuncture; the size of the catheter or needle; and your initials, as the nurse who changed the dressing. Tape a label on the new tubing with the date and time of the change and your initials. See Figure 25–18.

23. Regulate the rate of flow of the solution according to the order on the chart.

24. Record the change of the solution container and/or tubing in the appropriate place on the patient's chart. Also record the fluid intake according to agency practice. Some agencies have special flow sheets or intake and output records for recording IVs. Record the number of the container if the containers are numbered at the agency.

25. Record the response of the patient, your assessment of the IV site, and whether the dressing was changed.

■ **Evaluation** See Technique 25–2 on page 556.

TECHNIQUE 25-4 ■ Discontinuing an Intravenous Infusion

Discontinuing an infusion is not an uncomfortable procedure; in fact, it is usually a relief for the patient and takes only a couple of minutes. IVs are usually discontinued for one of two reasons:

1. The patient's oral fluid intake and hydration status are satisfactory, so that no further intravenous solutions are ordered.

2. There is a problem with the infusion that cannot be fixed. Consult with the responsible nurse before discontinuing an IV because of such a difficulty.

■ **Assessment**

See Technique 25–1 on page 546. Other data include: the physician's order. Check it against the number of the solution container to confirm that all fluid ordered for the patient has indeed infused.

■ Planning

Nursing goals

1. To ensure that the patient's hydration status is satisfactory
2. To ensure that the patient's oral fluid intake is adequate
3. To discontinue an intravenous infusion safely

Equipment

1. A small sterile dressing and tape to cover the site temporarily
2. Dry or antiseptic-soaked swabs, according to agency practice

■ Intervention

1. Clamp the infusion tubing.
   Rationale   Clamping the tubing will prevent the fluid from flowing out of the needle onto the patient or bed.
2. Loosen the tape at the venipuncture site while holding the needle firmly and applying countertraction to the skin.
   Rationale   Movement of the needle can injure the vein and cause discomfort to the patient. Countertraction prevents pulling the skin and causing discomfort.
3. Hold a swab above the venipuncture site.
4. Withdraw the needle or catheter by pulling it out along the line of the vein.
   Rationale   Pulling out in line with the vein avoids injury to the vein.
5. Apply firm pressure immediately to the site, using the swab, for 2 to 3 minutes.
   Rationale   Pressure helps stop the bleeding and prevents hematoma formation.
6. Hold the patient's arm or leg above his or her body if any bleeding persists.
   Rationale   Raising the limb decreases blood flow to the area.
7. Check the needle or catheter to make sure it is intact. Report a broken needle or catheter to the responsible nurse immediately.
   Rationale   If a piece of needle or tubing remains in the patient's vein it could move centrally (toward the heart or lungs) and cause serious problems.
8. Apply the sterile dressing.
   Rationale   The dressing continues the pressure and covers the open area in the skin, preventing infection.
9. Assess the patient's response to the IV in terms of the appearance of the venipuncture site (see Table 25–1, earlier); the patient's pulse, respirations, color, edema, sputum, cough, and urine output; and how the patient feels physically and psychologically.
10. Discard the IV solution container, if infusions are being discontinued, and discard the used supplies appropriately.
11. Record the amount of fluid infused on the intake and output record and on the patient's chart, according to agency practice. Include the container number, type of solution used, time of discontinuing the infusion, and patient's response.

■ **Evaluation**   See Technique 25–2 on page 556.

TECHNIQUE 25–5   ■   Starting an Intravenous Infusion Using a Butterfly Needle or Over-the-Needle Angiocatheter 🏠

Agency practices vary about which nurses perform venipunctures and start intravenous infusions. In many settings nurses must be supervised and approved before they are permitted to start infusions on their own. Some agencies have teams of specially prepared nurses who initiate all intravenous infusions.

■ Assessment

Assess the patient for:

1. Veins that would be satisfactory venipuncture sites.

Veins that are continually distended with blood, that have been damaged due to previous venipunctures, or that have become knotted and tortuous are normally not used. Veins that are easily palpated are often easier to enter than veins that are highly visible or deeply buried under adipose tissue. Highly visible veins tend to roll away from the needle.

2. Tendency to bleed easily. Such patients require special observation after a venipuncture.
3. Injury to the extremity selected. Intravenous infusions are normally not started on injured limbs

because of possible impaired circulation, discomfort for the patient, and obstruction of the site by dressings etc.

4. Any abrasions in the skin area chosen for the venipuncture. If an abraded area must be used, record the abrasions.

5. Hydration status for baseline data. See Technique 25–1.

Other data include:

1. Whether the patient has any allergies, eg, to tape or povidone-iodine.

2. The order for the type and amount of solution and the length of time the infusion is to run.

3. Agency policy about shaving the area before a venipuncture. Some agencies do not permit shaving because of the possibility of nicking the skin and subsequent infection.

■ Planning

Nursing goals

1. To start an intravenous infusion of fluid safely.

2. To maintain or enhance the patient's hydration status.

Equipment

1. A sterile butterfly (wing-tipped) needle. A 2.5-cm (1-in) needle, #21 or #23 gauge, is used for most infusions; a #19 needle is used for whole blood.
   or
   An over-the-needle angiocatheter (ONC) of suitable size, eg, #22 gauge for clear liquid infusions, #20 gauge for infusing drug boluses or peripheral fat solutions.

2. Antiseptic swabs.

3. A tourniquet.

4. A receptacle for discarded fluid.

5. Adhesive or nonallergenic tape.

6. Skin preparation materials if the skin at the site will have to be shaved.

7. A container of sterile parenteral solution. (Discolored or cloudy solution may be contaminated.)

8. An intravenous administration set.

9. An intravenous stand (pole).

10. A towel or pad to place under the patient's arm.

11. An arm splint, if required.

12. Gauze squares or other appropriate dressings.

13. Antiseptic ointment, eg, povidone-iodine.

■ Intervention

Preparing the infusion equipment

1. Follow Technique 25–1, steps 1–21, on pages 549–552, if the equipment has not already been prepared.

Selecting and preparing the venipuncture site

2. Prepare strips of adhesive tape to stabilize the IV needle once it is inserted.

3. Select a site, starting at the distal end of the vein.
   Rationale Veins can become sclerotic from irritation by the infusion or the needle. Sclerosis may then interfere with venous flow. If so, more proximal parts of the veins can be used.

4. If necessary, shave the skin where adhesive tape will be applied. Check agency policy.

Dilating the vein

5. Place the extremity in a dependent position (lower than the patient's heart).
   Rationale Gravity slows venous return and distends the veins. Distending the veins makes it easier to insert the needle properly.

6. Apply a tourniquet firmly 15 to 20 cm (6 to 8 in) above the venipuncture site. The tourniquet must be tight enough to obstruct venous flow but not so tight that it occludes arterial flow. If a radial pulse can be palpated, the arterial flow is not obstructed.
   Rationale Obstructing arterial flow inhibits venous filling.

7. If the vein is not sufficiently dilated:
   a. Massage or stroke the vein distal to the site and in the direction of venous flow toward the heart.
      Rationale This action helps fill the vein.
   b. Encourage the patient to rapidly clench and unclench the fist.
      Rationale Contracting the muscles compresses the distal veins, forcing blood along the veins and distending them.
   c. Lightly tap the vein with your fingertips.
      Rationale Tapping may distend the vein.

8. If steps 5–7 fail to distend the vein, remove the tourniquet, and apply heat to the entire extremity for 10 to 15 minutes. Then repeat steps 5–7.
   Rationale Heat dilates superficial blood vessels, causing them to fill.

9. Clean the skin at the site of entry with a topical antiseptic swab, eg, alcohol, and then an anti-infective, eg, povidone-iodine (Betadine) solution.

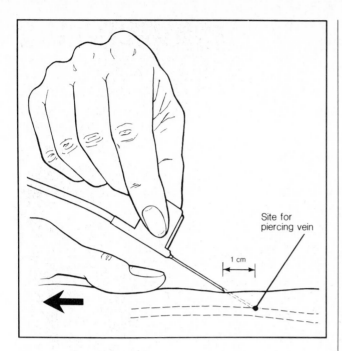

FIGURE 25-19

10. Use one thumb to pull the skin taut below the entry site.

    Rationale   This stabilizes the vein and makes the skin taut for needle entry. It can also make initial tissue penetration less painful.

Inserting a needle

11. Hold the needle, pointed in the direction of the blood flow, at a 30° angle, with the bevel up, and pierce the skin beside the vein about 1 cm (½ in) below the site planned for piercing the vein. See Figure 25-19.

12. Once the needle is through the skin, lower the needle so it is almost parallel with the skin. Follow the course of the vein and pierce one side of the vein.

    Rationale   Lowering the needle reduces the chances of puncturing both sides of the vein.

13. When blood flows back into the needle tubing, insert the needle farther up the vein 2 to 2.5 cm (¾ to 1 in) or to the hub of the butterfly needle. Sudden lack of resistance can be felt as blood enters the needle.

14. Release the tourniquet, attach the infusion, and initiate flow as quickly as possible.

    Rationale   Attaching the tubing quickly prevents the patient's blood from clotting and obstructing the needle.

15. Tape the needle securely by the H method (see Figure 25-20) or crisscross (chevron) method (see Figure 25-21). You may need to place a cotton ball

or small gauze square under the needle to keep it in position in the vein. Go to step 27.

Inserting an over-the-needle angiocatheter

16. Insert the catheter by the direct or indirect method. For the direct method, hold the catheter bevel up, at a 15° to 20° angle, and thrust the catheter through the skin and into the vein in one thrust. For the indirect method, first pierce the skin, then reduce

FIGURE 25-20

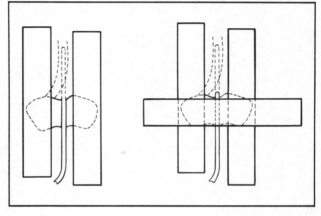

FIGURE 25-21

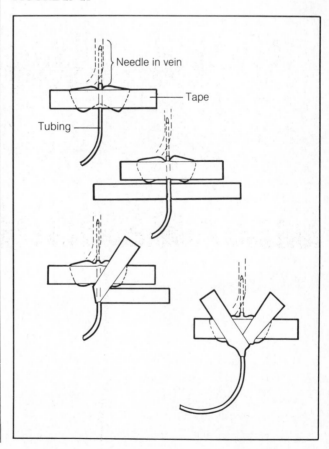

FIGURE 25-22

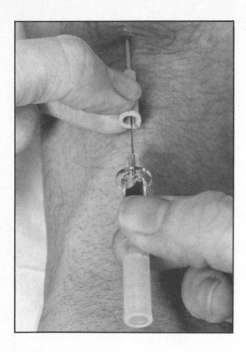

FIGURE 25-23

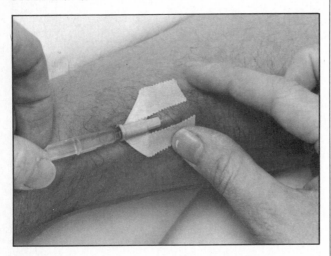

FIGURE 25-24

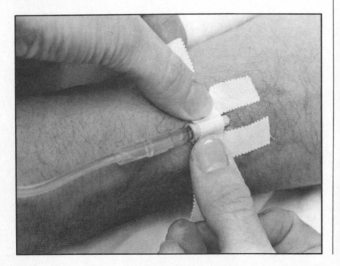

the angle, and advance the catheter into the vein. Sudden lack of resistance is felt as the catheter enters the vein.

Rationale The direct method is preferred for large veins and the indirect method for smaller veins (Peck, 1985, p 40).

17. Once blood appears in the catheter or you feel the lack of resistance, advance the catheter another 0.6 cm (¼ in).

Rationale The catheter is advanced to ensure that it, and not just the metal needle, is in the vein.

18. Release the tourniquet.

19. Remove the protective cap from the distal end of the tubing, and hold it ready to attach to the catheter, maintaining the sterility of the end.

20. Grasp the hub of the catheter with your thumb and index finger, and withdraw the needle. See Figure 25-22.

21. Advance the catheter up to the hub or until you feel resistance.

22. Attach the end of the infusion tubing to the catheter hub.

23. Initiate the infusion.

24. Inspect the insertion site for signs of infiltration, eg, swelling.

25. Tape the catheter in place.

 a. Place the first tape, sticky side up, under the catheter hub, and fold the sides as shown in Figure 25-23.

 b. Place the second strip, sticky side down, across the catheter hub. See Figure 25-24.

 c. Place the third strip, sticky side up, under the catheter hub distal to the second strip, and fold each side diagonally across the catheter. See Figure 25-25.

FIGURE 25-25

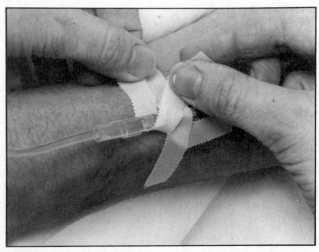

26. Dress the venipuncture site according to agency policy. In some agencies, the nurse puts a small amount of antiseptic ointment, eg, povidone-iodine, over the venipuncture site, then a gauze square. In other agencies a sterile transparent occlusive dressing is applied. This permits assessment of the site without disturbing the dressing. This type of dressing can be left on for 72 hours unless there are complications (Peck, 1985, p 32).

For a butterfly needle or angiocatheter

27. Loop the tubing, and secure it to the dressing with tape.

    Rationale Looping and securing the tubing prevents the weight of the tubing or any movement from pulling on the needle or catheter.

28. Apply a padded armboard to splint the elbow or wrist joint if needed.

29. Adjust the infusion rate of flow according to the order.

30. Label a piece of tape with the date and time of insertion, type and gauge of needle or catheter used, and your initials. Apply the tape label over the venipuncture dressing. See Figure 25–26.

31. Record starting the IV on the patient's chart. Some agencies provide a special form for this purpose. Include the date and time of the venipuncture, amount and type of solution used, including any additives (eg, kind and amount of medications), absorption time, container number, drip rate, type and gauge of the needle or catheter, venipuncture site, and patient's general response.

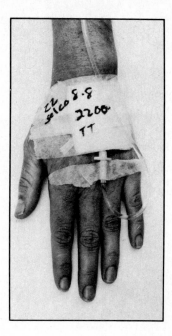

FIGURE 25–26

Sample Recording

Date	Time	Notes
6/8/86	1800	IV #1 1,000 mL D5W started in right basilic vein. BF needle #21G inserted. Drip rate 125 mL/hr. Completion time 0200 hours. IV running well. No discomfort. ———————— Dino C. Anastasio, NS

■ **Evaluation**   See Technique 25–2 on page 556.

TECHNIQUE 25–6 ■ Using an Infusion Pump or Controller

A number of kinds of pumps and controllers are used with IV infusions. Each should be set up according to the manufacturer's directions. A pump (see Figure 25–27) delivers a measured amount of IV solution or medication to the patient at a constant high pressure. A controller, on the other hand, operates by gravitational force (see Figure 25–28). The IV container must be at least 76 cm (30 in) above the venipuncture site for a controller to work. Because controllers do not provide the same pressure as pumps, they cannot be used to keep an arterial line open or to administer highly viscid fluids.

Pumps measure the flow rate in milliliters per hour. Some pumps are volumetric and are very precise. Controllers regulate the gravitational flow by counting the drops and compressing the IV tubing to obtain the desired infusion rate. Because drops vary in size, controllers are not as accurate as pumps.

Some pumps and controllers are equipped with alarm systems, which are triggered when there is a change in the flow rate, when there are air bubbles in either the drip chamber or the intravenous tubing, when battery power is low, or when an occlusion is present. If the equipment has an alarm system, explain the alarm to the patient, and let the patient hear it so that he or she will know what to expect if it comes on later.

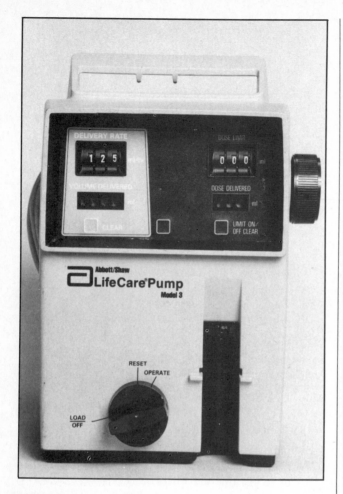

FIGURE 25–27 ■ An intravenous infusion pump.

■ **Assessment**   See Technique 25–2 on page 554.

■ **Planning**

Nursing goals

1. To administer precise amounts of specific medications intravenously, eg, cardiovascular drugs, antihypertensive drugs, and antibiotics
2. To administer precise amounts of certain intravenous infusions and maintain the patient's hydration status

Equipment

1. The controller or pump.
2. A modular unit if required. Some controllers and pumps use a modular unit to which the IV tubing and the extension tubing are attached.
3. The IV solution or medication.
4. An IV pole.
5. An IV administration set with compatible IV tubing.

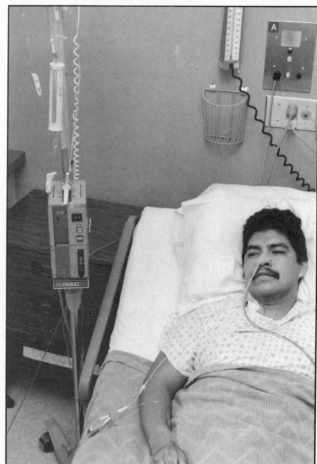

FIGURE 25–28 ■ An intravenous infusion controller.

6. Sterile peristaltic tubing or a cassette if required.
7. Alcohol swabs and tape.

■ **Intervention**

Setting up an infusion controller

1. Plug the machine into the electric outlet, unless battery power is used.
2. Attach the controller to the IV pole so that it will be below and in line with the IV container.
3. Open the IV container, maintaining the sterility of the port, and spike the container using the administration set.
4. Place the IV container on the IV pole, and position the drip chamber 76 cm (30 in) above the venipuncture site.
   Rationale This provides sufficient gravitational pressure for the fluid to flow into the patient.
5. Fill the drip chamber of the IV tubing one-third full.
   Rationale If the drip chamber is filled more than half way, the drops may be miscounted.

6. Rotate the drip chamber.

   Rationale   This removes vapor that could make the drop count inaccurate.

7. Prime the tubing, and close the clamp. Nonvolumetric controllers (regulators that measure the infusion in gtt/min) use standard tubing that is gravity primed.

   Rationale   Priming expels all the air from the tubing.

8. Attach the IV drop sensor to the drip chamber so that it is below the drop port but above the fluid level. Make sure the sensor is plugged into the controller.

   Rationale   This placement ensures an accurate drop count.

9. Insert the tubing into the controller according to the manufacturer's instructions.

10. Perform a venipuncture or connect the tubing to the primary IV tubing or catheter.

11. Open the IV control clamp completely.

12. Set the dials on the front of the controller to the appropriate infusion rate and volume. Set the volume at 50 mL less than the required amount, if the controller counts the volume infused.

    Rationale   This will give the nurse time to attach a new container before the present one runs out completely.

13. Press the power button and the start button. Turn on the alarm switch.

14. Count the drops for a full minute.

    Rationale   The nurse verifies that the rate has been correctly set and the controller is operating accurately.

15. Some agencies recommend that all connections be taped. Count the drop rate again after the taping.

    Rationale   Taping could change the drop rate.

16. Record starting the IV with the controller, giving the data required for an intravenous infusion.

Setting up an infusion pump

17. Plug the machine into the electric outlet, unless battery power is used.

18. Attach the pump to the IV pole, usually at eye level.

    Rationale   Because the pump does not depend on gravity pressure it can be placed at any level. Eye level is convenient for checking its functioning.

19. Open the IV container, maintaining the sterility of the port, and spike the container with the administration set.

20. Place the IV container on the IV pole above the pump.

21. Follow steps 5–6.

22. Prime the tubing, and close the clamp. Most volumetric chamber pumps, ie, pumps calibrated to infuse a specific volume of fluid at a specific rate (mL/hr), have a cassette that must also be primed. Manufacturers give instructions for doing this. Often the cassette must be inverted or tilted to be filled with fluid. Some volumetric pumps use special tubing, which is gravity primed.

23. Position the drop sensor, if required, on the drip chamber. See step 8.

24. Load the machine according to the manufacturer's instructions.

25. Follow steps 10–16.

Monitoring an infusion pump or controller

26. Monitor the drop rate and the patient's response every half hour. Check the infusion, eg, for infiltration at the venipuncture site or leakage. See Technique 25–2.

27. If the alarm sounds, check that:

    a. The drip chamber is correctly filled.

    b. The IV tubing clamp is fully open.

    c. The container still has solution.

    d. The drop sensor is correctly placed.

    e. The IV container is correctly placed.

    f. The tubing is not pinched or kinked.

28. Discontinue the same way an intravenous infusion is terminated. See Technique 25–4.

■ **Evaluation**   See Technique 25–2 on page 556.

BLOOD TRANSFUSIONS

A *blood transfusion* is the introduction of whole blood or components of the blood, such as plasma, serum, erythrocytes, or platelets, into the venous circulation. See Table 25–2 for types of blood and blood products, and indications for their use.

Blood transfusions are given for the following reasons:

1. To restore blood volume after severe hemorrhage

2. To restore the red blood cell level after severe and chronic anemias and to maintain blood hemoglobin levels

TABLE 25–2 ■ Blood Products and Indications for Use

Type of blood product	Indications
Whole blood (Type A, B, AB, O, and/or Rh positive or negative)	To treat blood volume deficiencies, eg, in acute hemorrhage; not indicated for correction of chronic anemia
Plasma	To expand blood volume; to restore circulation and renal blood flow when plasma volume is decreased but red cell mass is adequate, as in acute dehydration or burns; to replace deficient coagulation factors in bleeding disorders
Packed red cells (high hematocrit, since approximately 80% of plasma is removed)	Used when blood volume is adequate but red cell mass is inadequate, as in chronic anemia
Platelets	For patients with severe thrombocytopenia (reduced platelets); platelets plug small vascular leaks prior to clotting
Albumin	To expand blood volume when volume is reduced in shock or burns; to increase level of albumin in patients with hypoalbuminemia
Prothrombin complex (Konyne, Proplex)—contains factors VII, IX, and XI and prothrombin	For bleeding associated with deficiencies of those factors
Factor VIII fractions	For hemophiliacs
Fibrinogen preparations	For bleeding associated particularly with congenital hypofibrinogenemia (deficiency of fibrinogen, necessary for blood coagulation)

3. To provide plasma factors, such as antihemophilic factor (AHF), or factor VIII, which controls bleeding

Blood Matching

Blood groups

Human blood is classified into four main groups (A, B, AB, and O) on the basis of polysaccharide antigens on the erythrocyte surface. These antigens, type A and type B, commonly cause antibody reactions and are called *agglutinogens.* In other words, group A blood contains type A agglutinogen, group B blood contains type B agglutinogen, group AB blood contains both A and B agglutinogens, and group O blood contains neither agglutinogen.

In addition to agglutinogens on the erythrocytes, *agglutinins* (antibodies) are present in the blood plasma. The agglutinins are referred to as *alpha (anti-A) agglutinins,* which agglutinate type A cells, and *beta (anti-B) agglutinins,* which agglutinate type B cells. No individual

can have agglutinins and agglutinogens of the same type; that person's system would attack its own cells. Thus group A blood does not contain agglutinin A but does contain agglutinin B. Group B blood does not contain agglutinin B but does contain agglutinin A. Group AB blood contains neither agglutinin, and Group O contains both anti-A and anti-B agglutinins. Blood transfusions must be matched to the recipient's blood type in terms of compatible agglutinogens. Mismatched blood will cause a hemolytic reaction. The most common blood types are A and O. Type B blood is found in 20% of the Black population and only 9% of the White population. Almost 50% of both populations have type O blood. See Table 25–3.

Rhesus (Rh) groups

Rh antigens, also on the surface of erythrocytes, are present in about 85% of the population and can be a major cause of hemolytic reactions. Persons who possess the Rh factor are referred to as *Rh positive;* those who do

TABLE 25–3 ■ Survey of Information on Blood Groups

Blood type (red blood cell agglutinogens)	Agglutinins in plasma	Possible donors	Percentage of White population	Percentage of Black population
A	Anti-B (beta)	Types A and O	41	30
B	Anti-A (alpha)	Types B and O	9	20
AB	None	Types AB, A, B, and O	3	3
O (no agglutinogen)	Anti-A and anti-B	Type O	47	47

TABLE 25–4 ■ Transfusion Reactions: Clinical Signs and Nursing Interventions

Reaction	Clinical signs	Nursing interventions
Hemolytic reaction	Chills, fever, headache, back pain, hemoglobinemia, hemoglobinuria, oliguria, jaundice, dyspnea, cyanosis, chest pain, vascular collapse, hypotension	1. Observe patient closely for first 10 minutes of transfusion, since these reactions occur rapidly 2. Discontinue blood immediately when reaction is assessed 3. Notify physician of patient's symptoms and vital signs 4. Notify laboratory to type and cross-match blood and confirm diagnosis; send donor blood back to laboratory and have specimen of recipient's blood retested 5. Maintain intravenous infusion with D5W or saline 6. Monitor vital signs every 15 minutes to assess shock and temperature 7. Record fluid intake and output to assess degree of kidney functioning 8. Save first voided specimen for laboratory analysis 9. Implement treatment as prescribed by physician
Febrile reaction	Fever, shaking, chills, warm flushed skin, headache, backache, nausea, hematemesis, diarrhea, red shock, confusion or delirium	For mild reaction: 1. Observe patient closely for first 30 minutes of transfusion For severe reaction: 1. Stop transfusion 2. Maintain intravenous infusion with saline or D5W 3. Monitor patient's vital signs every 30 minutes 4. Notify physician 5. Notify laboratory to take culture of patient's and donor's blood 6. Implement therapy as prescribed by physician 7. Apply alcohol sponges for fever if necessary
Allergic reaction	Urticaria, occasional wheezing, arthralgia, generalized itching, nasal congestion, bronchospasm, severe dyspnea, circulatory collapse	For mild reaction: 1. Slow transfusion 2. Implement therapy as prescribed by physician For severe reaction: 1. Stop transfusion 2. Notify physician immediately 3. Maintain intravenous infusion with saline or D5W 4. Monitor vital signs frequently

not are referred to as *Rh negative.* Some other blood factors are the Hr, Kell, Lewis M, N, and P factors. These rarely cause major reactions because their antigenic properties are poor.

The Rh factor differs from the A and B agglutinogens in that it cannot cause a hemolytic reaction on the first exposure to mismatched blood. This is because the Rh antibody is *not* normally present in the plasma of persons who are Rh negative.

Transfusion Reactions

Transfusion reactions can be categorized as hemolytic, febrile, and allergic. The signs, symptoms, and nursing actions for each type of reaction are outlined in Table 25–4. The *hemolytic reaction,* a fatal response, occurs when agglutinins and agglutinogens of the same type come in contact; eg, type A agglutinogen and anti-A agglutinin,

or type B agglutinogen and anti-B agglutinin. *Agglutination* (clumping) and *hemolysis* (rupture) of the red cells result from such contact. It is essential, therefore, to match the donor's blood type to the recipient's. Otherwise the agglutinins present in the recipient's plasma will agglutinate the red cells donated. Because type O blood has neither A nor B agglutinogens, it can be donated to recipients with any of the four types of blood; this type is called the *universal donor.* Type AB blood, because it has neither anti-A nor anti-B agglutinins in plasma, is referred to as a *universal recipient,* able to receive any of the four blood types. Table 24–3 summarizes compatibility among blood groups.

Febrile reactions (bacterial reactions) are rare. They occur as a result of contaminated blood or sensitivity to the donor's white blood cells. *Allergic reactions* are relatively common and are thought to be due to allergenic substances or antibodies in the donor's plasma.

TECHNIQUE 25–7 ■ Initiating, Maintaining, and Terminating a Blood Transfusion

■ Assessment

1. Obtain baseline data on the patient's blood pressure, pulse, temperature, and respirations, if data are not already available.

2. Determine whether the patient has known allergies or has had previous adverse reactions to blood.

3. Note specific signs related to the patient's pathology and reason for needing the transfusion. For example, for an anemic patient note the hemoglobin level.

4. During the transfusion, assess the patient for clinical signs of transfusion reaction. See Table 25–4 earlier.

■ Planning

Nursing goal

To administer a blood transfusion safely and with minimal discomfort.

Equipment

1. A unit of whole blood. Blood is usually provided in plastic bags by the blood bank. One unit of whole blood is 500 mL of blood in a container.

2. A blood administration set. There are two types: a straight line and a Y-set. The Y-set is preferred because the infusion can be maintained with saline if any adverse effects arise from the transfusion. The infusion tubing has a filter inside the drip chamber. The tubing clamp should be just under the drip chamber. A Y-set can also be used when a saline solution is needed, to run with the blood (eg, when giving packed cells) or to flush the line before the blood enters the tubing (eg, when a running IV infusion is not saline).

3. A venipuncture set containing a #18 needle or catheter, if one is not already in place, alcohol swabs, and tape. When blood is to be administered quickly, a #15 needle or a larger catheter, eg, #14, is often used.

4. A container of 250 mL of saline solution. Some agencies recommend that saline be run through the tubing before and after a blood transfusion.

5. An IV pole.

■ Intervention

1. Check that there is a signed consent form from the patient, if required by the agency. If the patient is a Jehovah's Witness, written permission is required.

2. If the patient has an IV running, check whether the needle and solution are appropriate to administer blood. The needle should be #18 gauge or larger, and the solution must be saline. If the infusion is not compatible, remove it, and cap the bottle to maintain sterility. Dextrose, Ringer's solution, medications and other additives, and hyperalimentation solutions are incompatible.

3. When obtaining the blood, check the requisition form and the blood bag label with a laboratory technician or according to agency policy. Specifically check the patient's name, identification number, blood type (A, B, AB, or O) and Rh group, the blood donor number, and the expiration date of the blood.

4. With another nurse (the agency may require an RN) compare the laboratory blood type record with:

   a. The patient's name and identification number.

   b. The number on the blood bag label.

   c. The ABO group and Rh type on the blood bag label.

5. Sign the appropriate form with the other nurse according to agency policy.

6. Make sure that the blood is not left at room temperature for more than one-half hour before starting the transfusion because red blood cells deteriorate after two hours at room temperature. Agencies may designate different times at which the blood must be returned to the blood bank if it has not been started.

Initiating a transfusion

If the patient does not have an IV running, you need to perform a venipuncture on a suitable vein and start an IV infusion of normal saline. In some agencies an IV must be running before the blood is obtained from the blood bank.

7. Obtain a Y-set for blood administration. See Figure 25–29.

8. Ensure that the attached blood filter is suitable for whole blood or the blood components to be transfused.

9. Close all the clamps on the Y-set.

10. Spike a container of 0.9% saline solution with one of the Y-set spikes, and hang the container about 1 m (36 in) above the planned venipuncture site.

11. Open the clamp on the normal saline tubing, and squeeze the drip chamber. Tap the drip chamber as needed to remove any residual air.

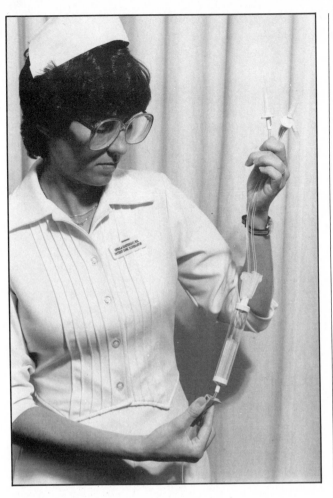

FIGURE 25–29

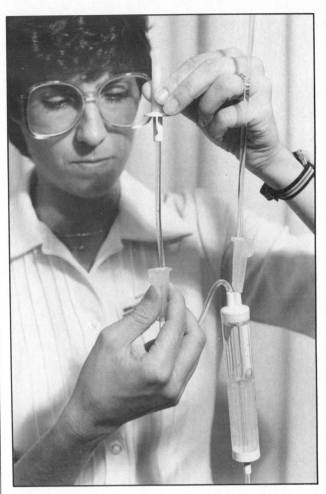

FIGURE 25–30

FIGURE 25–31

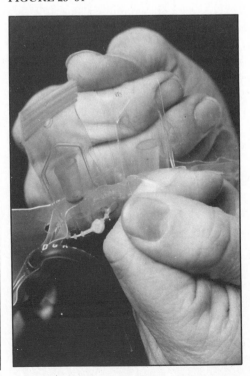

Rationale This primes the upper saline line and blood filter.

12. Open the clamp on the empty Y-set line that is to receive blood. See Figure 25–30.

    Rationale This primes the empty part of the line, because normal saline then flows up the blood line.

13. When the blood line is primed, close the clamp on it.

14. Leave the clamp on the normal saline line open.

15. Open the main roller clamp below the filter, and prime the lower tubing.

16. Close the main roller clamp.

17. Invert the blood bag gently several times to mix the cells with the plasma.

    Rationale Rough handling can damage the cells.

18. Perform a venipuncture. See Technique 25–5.

19. Expose the port on the blood bag by pulling back the tabs. See Figure 25–31.

20. Insert the remaining Y-set spike into the blood bag.

21. Hang the blood bag at the same level as the saline container.

22. Attach the primed infusion tubing to the needle, and tape it securely.

23. Close the upper roller clamp on the normal saline line, open the upper roller clamp on the blood line, and open the main roller clamp below the filter to infuse the blood.

24. Run the blood for the first 15 minutes at 20 drops per minute. Observe the patient closely for signs of adverse reactions such as chilling, nausea, vomiting, skin rash, or tachycardia.

25. If any of these reactions occur, close the clamp on the transfusion, open the clamp on the tubing with normal saline, and notify the responsible nurse or physician immediately. Follow agency procedure about obtaining urine specimens etc.

26. Record starting the blood, including vital signs, type of blood, blood unit number, sequence number (eg, #1 of three ordered units), site of the venipuncture, size of the needle, and drip rate.

Maintaining a transfusion

27. Fifteen minutes after initiating the transfusion, check the patient's vital signs. If there are no signs of a reaction, establish the required flow rate. Most adults can tolerate receiving one unit of blood in 1½ to 2 hours.

28. Assess the patient every 30 minutes, or more often, depending on the patient's condition, including vital signs.

Terminating a transfusion

29. If no infusion is to follow, clamp the blood tubing and remove the needle.

    or

    If the primary IV is to be continued, flush the line with the saline solution, attach the primary IV container, and adjust the drip to the desired rate. Often a normal saline or other solution is kept running in case of a delayed reaction to the blood.

30. Again assess the patient's vital signs.

31. On the requisition attached to the blood unit, fill in the time the transfusion was completed and the amount transfused.

32. Attach one copy of the requisition to the patient's record and another to the empty blood bag.

33. Return the blood bag and requisition to the blood bank.

34. Record completion of the transfusion, the amount of blood absorbed, the blood unit number, and the vital signs. If the primary IV infusion was continued, record connecting it.

Sample Recording

Date	Time	Notes
12/12/87	1100	1 unit whole blood administered. No adverse reactions. BP stable at 120/70, TPR 37, 88, 14. 500 mL saline started at 10 gtt/min.———— Selina L. Ward, SN

■ Evaluation

Expected outcomes

1. Positive change in clinical signs related to patient's pathology
2. Vital signs stable
3. Absence of complaints

Unexpected outcomes

1. Significant change in vital signs
2. Signs of transfusion reaction (see Table 25–4)
3. No change in clinical signs related to patient's pathology

Upon obtaining an unexpected outcome:

1. Report your findings to the responsible nurse and/or physician.
2. Implement the actions indicated in Table 25–4 on page 567.

TOTAL PARENTERAL NUTRITION (INTRAVENOUS HYPERALIMENTATION)

Total parenteral nutrition (TPN), also referred to as intravenous hyperalimentation (IVH), is the parenteral administration of solutions of dextrose, water, fat, proteins, electrolytes, vitamins, and trace elements. TPN is the provision of all needed calories. PN is the provision of nutritional solutions, with additional calories coming from other sources, eg, tube feeding. TPN is a means of achieving an anabolic state in patients who are unable to maintain a normal nitrogen balance. Such patients may include those with severe malnutrition, severe burns, bowel disease disorders (eg, ulcerative colitis or enteric fistula), acute renal failure, hepatic failure, metastatic cancer, or major surgeries where nothing may be taken by mouth for more than five days.

Many of the sepsis problems associated with conventional IV therapy are also associated with TPN. Moreover, the problems are magnified because: (a) patients receiving TPN therapy are often critically ill, may be malnourished, and are sometimes immunosuppressed, (b) TPN catheters are left in place for long periods of time, (c) the intralipids used in TPN therapy support the growth of a wide variety of microorganisms, and (d) the therapy uses the central venous system because of the osmolarity of the fluid. Infection control is therefore of utmost importance during TPN therapy. The nurse must always observe surgical aseptic technique when changing solutions, tubing, dressings, and filters.

TPN (IVH) Sites

Because TPN solutions are hypertonic (highly concentrated in comparison to the solute concentration of blood), they are injected only into high-flow central veins where they are diluted by the patient's blood. This prevents injury to the intimal layer of these blood vessels. Patients receiving TPN are thought to be predisposed to thrombophlebitis and possibly bacteremia.

Typically TPN solutions are administered through a central IV line that rests in the patient's superior vena cava. This may be a standard line or a Hickman, Broviac, or other catheter (see Types of Central Venous Lines on this page). After the catheter is inserted, it is attached to IV tubing previously primed with a solution of 5% dextrose in water or normal saline, which is infused until catheter placement is confirmed. The catheter is secured in place by suture, appropriate taping, or both. An antimicrobial ointment and a temporary dressing are then applied over the insertion site until placement of the catheter is confirmed by x-ray examination. Because an improperly placed catheter may cause a pneumothorax, the nurse must assess the patient for signs of chest pain and labored breathing and auscultate the lungs for abnormal breath sounds. If the catheter is misplaced, the physician will either manipulate it or remove it and insert another catheter. When correct catheter placement is confirmed, the nurse places a secure occlusive dressing over the insertion site (see Technique 25–11) and then commences infusion of the TPN solution.

Administering TPN (IVH) Solutions

TPN is a mixture of 10% to 50% dextrose in water, amino acids, and special additives such as vitamins (eg, B complex, C, D, K), minerals (eg, potassium, sodium, chloride, calcium, phosphate, magnesium), and trace elements (eg, cobalt, zinc, manganese). Additives are adapted to each patient's nutritional needs. Fat emulsions may be given to provide essential fatty acids to correct and/or prevent essential fatty acid deficiency or to supplement the calories for patients who, for example, have high calorie needs or cannot tolerate glucose as the only calorie source.

Because TPN solutions are high in glucose content, infusions are started gradually to prevent hyperglycemia.

The patient needs to adapt to TPN therapy by increasing his or her insulin output from the pancreas. For example an adult patient may be given 1 L/day (40 mL/hr) of TPN solution the first day, if the infusion is tolerated; the amount may be increased to 2 L (80 mL/hr) for 24 to 48 hours, and then to 3 L (120 mL/hr) within three to five days. When TPN therapy is to be discontinued, the TPN infusion rates are decreased slowly to prevent hyperinsulinemia and hypoglycemia. Weaning a patient from TPN may take up to 48 hours but can occur in 6 hours as long as the patient receives adequate carbohydrates either orally or intravenously.

CENTRAL VENOUS LINES

A central venous line is a catheter inserted into a large vein located centrally in the body. The tip of the catheter may terminate in the vein, eg, the superior vena cava, or in the right atrium of the heart. Insertion of the line may be a nonsurgical or a surgical procedure. Central venous lines are usually inserted by physicians, although some nurses who are specially prepared insert central venous lines that exit peripherally in the antecubital fossa of the arm.

Central venous lines are inserted primarily for the following reasons:

1. To administer nutritional solutions that are highly irritating to smaller veins
2. To administer irritating medications
3. To monitor central venous pressure (CVP)
4. To withdraw central venous blood

Types of Central Venous Lines

Standard central venous lines are catheters of variable length that are inserted in a nonsurgical procedure. They are usually made of polyethylene or silicone rubber and vary in size. A 20-cm long #16 gauge catheter is frequently used. The catheters are radiopaque so that they will show up on fluoroscopy or x-ray films. Short lines are used when the tip is inserted to the superior vena cava or subclavian vein; longer lines are used when the tip is inserted to the right atrium of the heart. A peripherally inserted line is a long venous catheter; two kinds are the Intrasil catheter and the Drum catheter.

Catheters are also inserted surgically. Examples are the Hickman catheter and the Broviac catheter. The Hickman is a single- or double-lumen catheter, with a 1.6-mm internal diameter of the lumen. It is therefore large enough for the passage of nutritional substances, blood, and antibiotics. The drawbacks of the single lumen Hickman catheter are that the administration of nutri-

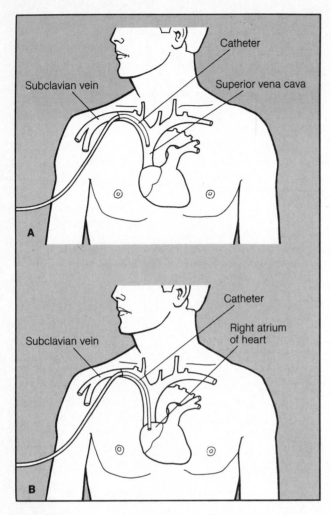

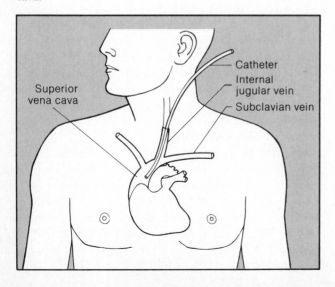

FIGURE 25-32   ■   A central venous line with the exit site on the chest below the clavicle: **A,** the tip of the catheter is in the superior vena cava; **B,** the tip of the catheter is in the right atrium.

FIGURE 25-33   ■   A central venous line inserted into the left jugular vein with the tip of the catheter in the superior vena cava.

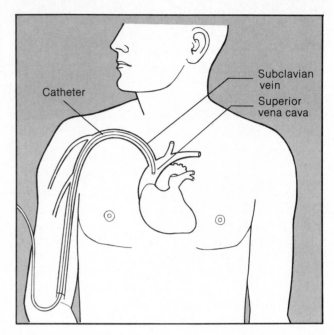

FIGURE 25-34   ■   A central venous line inserted peripherally at a point in the antecubital fossa of the right arm, with the tip of the catheter in the superior vena cava.

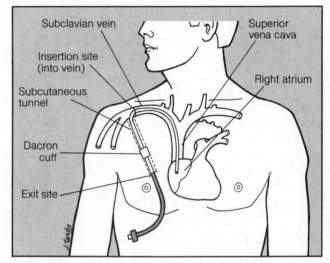

FIGURE 25-35   ■   A Hickman catheter surgically inserted into the chest wall, entering the subclavian vein, and extending into the right atrium.

tional substances must be interrupted if the catheter needs to be used for measuring central venous pressure or to administer blood, and the risk of infection is increased. A double Hickman catheter is used for this reason. It is the fusion of two Hickman catheters or a Hickman and a Broviac catheter. The Broviac line has an internal diameter of 1.0 mm, narrower than the Hickman but still large enough to administer nutritional substances. With the double lumen catheter, the administration of TPN can be continued through the smaller lumen while antibiotics, for example, can be administered through the larger lumen. The Broviac catheter used alone is like a single Hickman catheter. However, because its lumen is narrower, blood cannot be withdrawn through it. These surgically inserted lines are intended for use over an extended period.

Nonsurgical Insertion

The insertion of a standard central venous line is normally considered a nonsurgical procedure. Commonly, the line is inserted below the clavicle (the infraclavicular approach) into the right or left subclavian vein, and the tip of the catheter remains in the subclavian vein or the superior vena cava (see Figure 25–32, *A*), ie, a short line is used; it can also be extended into the atrium of the heart (see Figure 25–32, *B*), ie, a long line can be used. This site permits freedom of movement for ambulation, but a pneumothorax can occur during insertion. Another approach for a standard central venous line is through the right or left jugular vein (the supraclavicular approach). This site hinders head and neck movement somewhat but provides a straight line to the subclavian vein (and superior vena cava). See Figure 25–33. This is an especially useful approach for children.

When the infra- and supraclavicular approaches are used, a local anesthetic is usually applied to the site prior to the catheter insertion. While the physician is inserting the catheter, the nurse monitors the patient's pulse rate.

The onset of arrhythmia may indicate that the catheter tip is irritating the heart and placement requires adjustment.

Another type of central venous line, eg, the Intrasil catheter, is inserted more peripherally, eg, into a vein in the antecubital fossa of the arm, and threaded up the vein in the arm into the right atrium of the heart. The position of the catheter is verified by fluoroscopy. See Figure 25–34. This type of line can be used to administer nutritional solutions, to obtain blood specimens, and to measure pressure in the right atrium of the heart.

The exit of this catheter (at the antecubital fossa) looks like that of an intravenous line. It is important for nurses to know that the catheter extends farther into the vein and that its purpose and care differ.

Surgical Insertion

The surgical insertion of a central venous catheter (eg, a Hickman, Quinton, or Corcath catheter) involves an incision into the tissue of the chest. The catheter is inserted under the subcutaneous tissue to a centrally located vien, eg, the subclavian vein. It is then inserted into the vein and extended into the atrium of the heart. See Figure 25–35. These catheters usually have Dacron cuffs that promote growth of the subcutaneous tissue around the catheter, thus helping to prevent infection. With this type of insertion, the exit site of the catheter is on the chest some distance from its insertion site into the venous system.

TECHNIQUE 25-8 ■ Inserting and Removing a Central Venous Catheter

This procedure is usually carried out by a physician with nursing assistance. Ensure that the patient has signed a consent form before commencing.

■ Assessment

Assess the patient for:

1. Understanding of the procedure. Answer any questions, and clarify any aspects of the procedure that the patient does not understand. Continue to explain parts of the procedure while the central line is being inserted.
2. Ability to hold his or her breath, maintain the required position, and not move when requested.
3. Allergy to iodine and to the local anesthetic.
4. Hydration status for baseline data. See Assessment in Technique 25–1 on page 546.
5. Nutritional status for baseline data, eg, weight,

anthropometric measures. See Technique 24–1 on page 519.
6. Vital signs for baseline data, and other clinical signs See Table 8–1 on page 105.

Other data include:

For insertion

1. The physician's order for the central venous line and the route of insertion

For removal

2. The length of the catheter

■ Planning

Nursing goals

1. To support the patient while a central venous line is inserted or removed
2. To assist the physician during the insertion

Equipment

For insertion

1. Masks for the nurse and the physician. In some agencies the patient wears a mask also.
2. A skin preparation set, if the area needs to be shaved, or soap, water, a washcloth, and a towel, to clean the insertion site.
3. Sterile gloves for the physician and the nurse.
4. A sterile gown for the physician. In some agencies, the physician wears a clean gown.
5. Povidone-iodine sponges and ointment.
6. A sterile drape.
7. Alcohol swabs or sterile gauze squares and alcohol 70%.
8. Sterile 4 × 4 gauze squares.
9. Moisture-proof sterile dressing material.
10. Adhesive tape.
11. Skin anesthetic.
12. A sterile 3-mL syringe with a 1-in #25 gauge needle to instill the anesthetic.
13. A sterile 10-mL syringe.
14. Two radiopaque intracatheters (inside stylets or needles) of suitable size and length, eg, #16, 20 cm. Different sizes may be provided. Two intracatheters are furnished in case a second is needed, eg, because the first becomes contaminated.
15. A bath blanket.

For removal

16. Sterile gloves.
17. A mask for the nurse; one for the patient if an infection is suspected.
18. A sterile drape.
19. Alcohol sponges.
20. Povidone-iodine ointment and 4 × 4 sterile gauze squares.
21. Sterile moisture-proof dressing materials.

■ **Intervention**

Catheter insertion

1. Assist the patient to a Trendelenburg's position. If the patient cannot tolerate this position, use a supine position.
   Rationale In Trendelenburg's position, the veins will dilate, and the risk of an air embolism is reduced, because slight positive pressure is induced in the central veins.
2. Place a rolled bath blanket under the patient's back between the shoulders for a subclavian insertion.

Rationale In this position venous distention is increased.
   or
   Place a rolled bath blanket under the opposite shoulder for a jugular insertion.
   Rationale The blanket will extend the neck, making anatomic structures more visible for selecting the site.
3. Turn the patient's head to the opposite side.
   Rationale This position makes the site more visible and reduces the chance of contamination from microorganisms in the patient's respiratory tract.
4. Establish a sterile field with the sterile equipment in a convenient area for the physician.
5. Wash and dry the insertion site with soap and water; shave the skin, if necessary.
   Rationale Washing will remove dirt and reduce the number of microorganisms present.
6. Don a mask and sterile gloves.
7. Clean the site with povidone-iodine sponges. Use a circular motion, working outward.
   Rationale This reduces the number of microorganisms. Working outward prevents reintroducing microorganisms to the site.
8. Offer the physician the syringe and needle for the local anesthetic.
9. Wipe the top of the vial of anesthetic and invert it, so the physician can withdraw the anesthetic into the syringe. The physician injects the anesthetic.
10. Open the packages with the sterile catheter needles and the 10-mL syringe for the physician. The physician will insert the catheter. Explain to the patient what is going on, and provide support. Maintain the patient in position.
11. Prepare the infusion for attachment to the catheter. See Technique 25–1 on page 546.
12. After the infusion is attached, apply povidone-iodine ointment to the site, and apply a 4 × 4 sterile gauze dressing.
13. After x-ray examination or fluoroscopy confirms the position of the catheter, secure the dressing with tape.
14. Tape all connections.
    Rationale Taping prevents inadvertent separation of parts, leakage, and potential infection.
15. Establish the infusion. See Technique 25–9.
16. Label the dressing with the date and time of insertion and the length of the catheter, if it is not indicated on the catheter.
17. Record on the patient's record the time of insertion, the size and length of the catheter, the site of insertion, the name of the physician, the time of the x-ray examination and the results, the kind of

infusion, the rate of flow, and the response of the patient in terms of vital signs, color, discomfort, etc.

Sample Recording

Date	Time	Notes
12/12/86	1900	#14, 18-cm subclavian catheter inserted by Dr. R. Sullivan. 1,000 mL D5W 60 mEq KCl started at 36 mL/hr. Placement confirmed by fluoroscopy at 1850 hr. Vital signs stable. Slight pallor.————————Naomi Treasure, NS

18. Monitor the patient. See Technique 25–9, steps 13–27.

Catheter removal

19. Establish a sterile field, and open the sterile packages.
20. Place some povidone-iodine ointment on one sterile gauze square.
21. Loosen the dressing.
22. Don a mask, and put one on the patient if necessary.
23. Close the clamp on the infusion.
24. Don sterile gloves.
25. Remove any sutures that secure the catheter.

26. Grasp the catheter hub or needle, and carefully withdraw it, maintaining the direction of the vein.
27. Inspect the catheter to make sure it is intact. If it is not, notify the responsible nurse or physician immediately.

    Rationale   A piece of the catheter in a vein could cause an embolus.
28. Apply pressure over the site with sterile gauze until the bleeding stops.
29. Clean the area with an alcohol sponge.

    Rationale   The alcohol will remove any adhesive and old blood.
30. Apply the povidone-iodine ointment on the gauze, and cover it with a moisture-proof dressing.

    Rationale   The ointment will seal the site and, with the dressing, prevent exposure to the air.
31. Record on the patient's record the time of removal, the size, length, and condition of the catheter, and your assessments of the patient.

Sample Recording

Date	Time	Notes
1/6/86	0800	#14, 18-cm subclavian catheter removed intact. BP 150/90, P 62 regular, R 15.————————Rosaura Rodriguez, NS

TECHNIQUE 25–9   ■   Establishing and Monitoring TPN (IVH) Therapy

Meticulous patient monitoring is necessary to assess the patient's response to TPN and to prevent complications. Significant changes occur in the patient's fluid, electrolyte, glucose, amino acid, vitamin, and mineral levels.

■ Assessment

Assess the patient for:

1. Understanding of the procedure. Answer any questions, and clarify any aspects of the procedure that the patient does not understand. Continue to explain parts of the procedure while TPN is being established.
2. Hydration and electrolyte status for baseline data. See Assessment in Technique 25–1 on page 546.
3. Nutritional status for baseline data, eg, weight, anthropometric measurements. See Technique 24–1 on page 519 and Table 24–1 on page 519.

4. Nutritional and caloric needs.
5. Vital signs for baseline data.

Other data include:

1. The type of infusion, the hyperalimentation solution ordered, and the rate of flow
2. The site of the catheter insertion

■ Planning

Nursing goals

1. To support the patient during the procedure
2. To reduce the occurrence of infection
3. To enhance the patient's comfort
4. To facilitate the initiation of TPN therapy
5. To maintain the patient's safety

Equipment

1. A small IV solution container of 5% dextrose in water or of normal saline. This is used to maintain the patency of a newly established infusion until the TPN catheter placement is confirmed.

2. The TPN (IVH) solution ordered.

3. Sterile TPN tubing (extension tubing) including a Y-set.

4. A 0.22-micron cellulose membrane filter (optional). This air-eliminating filter reduces the risk of air embolism. The filter is attached to the distal end of the IV tubing. See Figure 25–36.

5. An infusion pump (optional).

6. Tape to secure the tubing connections if Luer-Lok connections are not available.

7. An IV pole.

See Technique 25–8 for equipment for site preparation and catheter insertion. See Technique 25–11 for additional supplies required for the permanent dressing of the TPN site.

■ Intervention

1. Assist the patient with any comfort measures, eg, using a bedpan, before starting the procedure.

2. Offer a premedication to the patient, if ordered.

Establishing the infusion

3. Remove the ordered TPN (IVH) solution from the refrigerator one hour before use, and check each ingredient and the proposed rate against the order on the chart.

   Rationale Infusion of a cold solution can cause pain, hypothermia, and venous spasm and constriction.

4. Inspect the solution for cloudiness or presence of

FIGURE 25–36 ■ An air-eliminating filter on a TPN line.

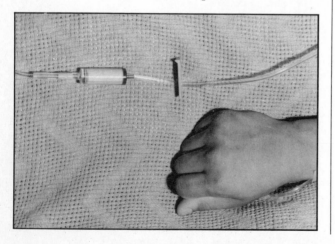

particles, and ensure that the container is free from cracks.

5. Connect:

   a. The infusion pump tubing (if a pump is used). See Technique 25–6.

   b. The filter.

   c. The extension tubing.

   Place the filter between the pump and the extension tubing to avoid disrupting the dressing.

6. Tape the tubing connections.

   Rationale This will prevent inadvertent separation, which can lead to air embolism, leakage, and contamination.

7. Insert the pump tubing spike into the port of the normal saline or 5% dextrose and water solution container, using surgical aseptic technique.

8. Start the flow of solution, and prime the tubing to remove air. If air bubbles become trapped in the Y-set tubes, gently tap the tubing.

   Rationale This dislodges air bubbles and prevents air embolism.

9. Stop the flow of solution, place the tubing protector cap on the end of the tubing, and hang the tubing on the IV pole.

   Rationale The protector cap maintains the sterility of the open-ended tubing.

10. The physician prepares the site and inserts the catheter. When the TPN catheter is inserted, attach the IV tubing, and initiate the flow of the solution.

11. After correct placement of the TPN catheter is confirmed by x-ray examination, change the solution container from the normal saline or dextrose solution to the TPN solution ordered.

12. Apply a permanent dressing over the catheter insertion site. See Technique 25–11.

Monitoring the infusion

13. Check the catheter tubing for leaks and obstructions.

14. Inspect the catheter insertion site for signs of infiltration, eg, swelling.

    Rationale Infiltration of TPN solution can cause necrosis of tissues and sloughing of the dermis and epidermis.

15. Observe the patient for signs of thrombosis or thrombophlebitis at the catheter insertion site (eg, edema or redness) and along the course of the vein (eg, pain or swelling of the arm, neck, or face). Purulent thrombolphlebitis may result in a purulent discharge, which appears at the insertion site with slight pressure. If you observe such signs, notify the physician, who may order removal of the catheter

and initiation of a heparin infusion at a peripheral vein site.

16. Observe the patient for signs of air embolism (apprehension, dyspnea, tachycardia, chest pain, hypotension, cyanosis, and loss of consciousness). If air embolism is suspected, give the patient oxygen and place the patient on the left side with the head lowered.

    Rationale   Lowering the head increases intrathoracic pressure, decreasing the flow of air into the vein during inhalation. A left side-lying position helps prevent the air from moving to the pulmonary artery.

17. Monitor the patient's vital signs every four hours. If fever or abnormal vital signs occur, notify the physician.

    Rationale   An elevated temperature is one of the earliest indications of catheter-related sepsis.

18. Inspect the dressing every four hours for intactness, cleanliness, and presence of bleeding. Change the dressing at least every 48 hours, or more often if it is moist or loose, in accordance with agency policy. See Technique 25-11.

19. Change the IV tubing every 24 hours or in accordance with agency policy. See Technique 25-10.

20. Always practice strict surgical aseptic technique when changing solutions, tubing, filters, and dressings.

21. Never use the TPN infusion line to (a) take central venous pressure (CVP) measurements, (b) take blood samples, (c) piggyback other solutions, (d) infuse blood or blood products, or (e) inject medications.

22. Before administering any TPN solution, check its expiration date. Most solutions must be used within 24 hours of preparation, unless they are refrigerated.

23. Carefully monitor the infusion flow rate and the laboratory test results to detect complications such as hyperglycemia or electrolyte imbalance. Use of an infusion pump keeps the infusion rate regular.

24. Collect double-voided urine specimens at least every six hours or in accordance with agency policy, and test the urine for specific gravity and glucose and acetone levels. If the specific gravity is abnormal, notify the physician, who may alter the constituents of the TPN solution. Also notify the physician if the glucose level is elevated to ¼% (+ +). Supplementary insulin may be ordered and given subcutaneously or added directly to the TPN solution by pharmacy personnel.

    Rationale   Glucosuria is often the first sign of catheter-related sepsis.

25. Record the patient's daily fluid intake and output and calorie intake as baseline data. Precise replacement for fluid and electrolyte deficits can then be more readily determined.

26. Weigh the patient daily, at the same time and in the same garments. A gain of more than 0.5kg (1.1 lb) per day indicates fluid excess and should be reported. Measure arm circumference and triceps skin fold thickness to assess the patient's physical changes. See Technique 24-1.

27. Monitor the results of laboratory tests (eg, serum electrolytes, blood glucose, and blood urea nitrogen) and report abnormal findings to the physician.

■ Evaluation

Expected outcomes

1. Solution infused at rate ordered
2. Solution tolerated well
3. Dressing remained intact and dry between planned changes
4. No infiltration appeared around catheter
5. Insertion site remained clean
6. No discomfort
7. Weight gain or stable weight
8. Good skin turgor

Unexpected outcomes

1. Solution did not flow at prescribed rate
2. Patient complains of weakness, nausea, etc
3. Dressing wet between changes
4. Swelling around catheter exit
5. Inflammation, swelling, odor, and/or discharge at insertion site
6. Patient restless; complains of discomfort at exit site of catheter
7. Weight loss or excessive weight gain
8. Poor skin turgor

Upon obtaining an unexpected outcome:

1. Report your findings to the responsible nurse and/or physician.
2. Adjust the nursing care plan appropriately.

TECHNIQUE 25-10 ■ Changing TPN (IVH) Tubing

The CDC recommends that TPN tubing be changed at least once every 48 hours. Some experts advise that it be changed every 24 hours. This procedure is best carried out when the TPN solution container is being changed. Strict surgical aseptic technique must be practiced.

■ Assessment

1. Assess the patient for signs of infiltration, circulatory overload, and phlebitis.
2. Assess the TPN system for disruptions to the infusion flow, eg, leaks at connections.

Other data include:

1. Whether the patient is allergic to tape or povidone-iodine
2. The physician's order for the kind, amount, and rate of solution to be infused

■ Planning

Nursing goals

1. To prevent infection
2. To prevent air embolism

Equipment

1. Sterile gloves, if agency policy dictates
2. Sterile 2 × 2 gauze squares to place under the tubing–catheter connection site and to clean the junction of the catheter and tubing, if agency practice indicates
3. A new solution container and administration set (tubing)
4. Tape to secure the tubing to the catheter
5. Antiseptic to clean the catheter and tubing junction as agency practice indicates

■ Intervention

1. Assist the patient to the supine position.
   Rationale This lowers the negative pressure in the vena cava thus decreasing the risk of air embolism when the catheter is opened.
2. Prepare the solution container, attach the new IV tubing, and prime the tubing as you would for a conventional IV.
3. Carry out a surgical hand wash.

4. Remove the tape securing the tubing to the dressing and the catheter hub connection.
5. Open the package containing the sterile gauze squares.
6. Don sterile gloves, if required by the agency.
7. Place the sterile gauze underneath the TPN catheter–IV tubing connection site. Clean the junction of the catheter and tubing.
   Rationale This prevents the transfer of microorganisms from the patient's skin to the open TPN catheter tip when it is detached; it also decreases the number of microorganisms at the catheter–tubing junction.
8. Ask the patient to perform the Valsalva maneuver (forced expiration against a closed glottis), ie, to take a breath, close his or her mouth, breathe out, and bear down.
   Rationale The Valsalva maneuver increases intrathoracic pressure, creating more pressure on the large veins entering the heart and reducing the return of blood to the heart. It therefore reduces the risk of air entering the large heart vein via the opened TPN catheter and the risk of subsequent air embolism.
9. Ask the patient to turn her or his head away while you detach the IV tubing by rotating it out of the hub. See Figure 25-37.
   Rationale Turning the head to the side reduces the chances of contaminating the equipment.
10. Quickly attach the new primed IV tubing to the TPN catheter, ensuring a tight seal.
    Rationale The tubing must be attached quickly

FIGURE 25-37

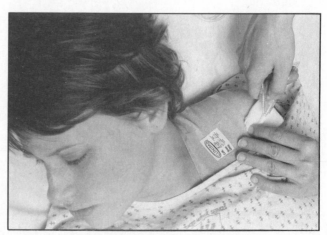

while the patient is performing the Valsalva maneuver to prevent air embolism.

11. Open the clamp on the new tubing, and adjust the flow to the rate ordered.

12. Secure the tubing to the catheter with tape if a Leur-Lok connection is not present.
    Rationale   This prevents accidental separation of the tubes and contamination of the TPN system.

13. Loop and tape the tubing over the dressing.
    Rationale   This prevents tension on the catheter and inadvertent separation of tubing and catheter.

14. Mark the date and time of the tubing change on the new IV tubing or drip chamber.

■ **Evaluation**

Expected outcomes

1. Insertion site remained clean
2. Vital signs normal

3. No clinical signs of air emboli
4. No clinical signs of thrombosis or thrombophlebitis

Unexpected outcomes

1. Inflammation, swelling, odor, and/or discharge at insertion site
2. Vital signs abnormal
3. Clinical signs of emboli, eg, apprehension, dyspnea, tachycardia, chest pain, hypotension, cyanosis
4. Clinical signs of thrombosis or thrombophlebitis, eg, edema or redness at insertion site, pain, swelling along course of vein

Upon obtaining an unexpected outcome:

1. Report your findings to the responsible nurse and/or physician.
2. Adjust the nursing care plan appropriately.

TECHNIQUE 25–11   ■   Changing a TPN (IVH) Dressing

Nurses need to change TPN dressings at least every 48 hours and more frequently if a dressing becomes wet or loose.

■ **Assessment**

Assess the patient for:

1. Allergies, especially to iodine, which is used to clean the insertion site
2. Any indications of infection at the catheter site, eg, redness, discomfort, discharge, swelling, or odor

■ **Planning**

Nursing goal

To prevent infection of the TPN site and subsequent systemic infection.

Equipment

1. A sterile dressing kit containing:
   a. Gloves (2 pairs).
   b. Some 4 × 4 gauze sponges for cleaning and dressing application.

   c. Tissue forceps (optional) for cleaning.
   d. Solution bowls for the cleaning solutions.
   e. Precut drain gauze (optional).
   f. A 2 × 2 gauze for the insertion site.

2. Two face masks (one for the nurse and one for the patient).

3. Isopropyl alcohol.

4. Antiseptic solutions. Usually 10% acetone and 1% iodine tincture or povidone-iodine solutions are used. If the patient is allergic to iodine, substitute 70% alcohol. Swabs may be prepackaged in the sterile kit.

5. Povidone-iodine ointment. If the patient is allergic to iodine, substitute a combination of antimicrobial and antifungal agents.

6. Tincture of benzoin. This may be available in a spray container.

7. Sterile scissors to cut gauze for the drain site, if precut gauze is not available.

8. Elastoplast tape or transparent occlusive dressing such as Op-site, to cover the gauze dressings.

9. Nonallergenic 2.5-cm (1-in) tape to secure the Elastoplast.

10. A waterproof bag for used dressings and supplies.

■ **Intervention**

1. Assist the patient to a supine or a semi-Fowler's position.

2. Don a mask and have the patient don a mask (if tolerated by the patient or as agency policy indicates) and turn her or his head away from the insertion site.

   Rationale This helps protect the TPN insertion site from the nurse's and patient's nasal and oral microorganisms. Turning the patient's head also makes the site more accessible.

3. Clean the patient's overbed table with isopropyl alcohol, and allow it to air dry.

4. Do a surgical hand wash and, if agency policy indicates, apply alcohol and allow the hands to air dry.

5. Open the sterile supplies on the clean overbed table, and fill the solution bowls with the required solutions, if indicated.

6. If iodine ointment is used, squeeze some of it onto a corner of a sterile gauze.

7. Remove the soiled dressing by pulling the tape slowly and gently from the skin.

   Rationale This prevents catheter displacement and skin irritation.

8. Inspect the skin for signs of irritation or infection. Inspect the catheter for signs of leakage or other problems. If infection is suspected, take a swab of the drainage for culture, label it, send it to the laboratory, and notify the physician.

9. Don sterile gloves.

10. Clean the catheter insertion site with sterile gauze sponges soaked in a solvent such as acetone 10%. Clean in a circular motion, moving from the insertion site outward to the edge of the adhesive border. Take care not to jostle or get acetone on the catheter. Take a new sponge for each wipe. Repeat until the sponge is unstained after use.

    Rationale Acetone defats the skin, destroys bacterial cell walls, and removes old adhesive tape, which would irritate the skin if left on. Cleaning from the insertion site outward and discarding sponges after each wipe avoids introducing contaminants from the uncleaned area to the site. Jostling the catheter can cause discomfort to the patient and could dislodge the catheter. Acetone is kept off the catheter because it could corrode the catheter.

11. Using the method in step 10, clean the insertion site and catheter for two minutes with povidone-iodine solution or iodine tincture. Focus on the insertion site, and allow the iodine to air dry for at least 30 seconds. If using alcohol 70% as a substitute for iodine, clean the area for five minutes.

    Rationale The iodine solution is an antiseptic with antimicrobial properties that last a long time even after drying.

12. Ensure that the connection of the catheter to the IV tubing is secure, if it is within the dressing site.

13. Remove your gloves, and put on the other sterile pair.

    Rationale The gloves used for cleaning are considered contaminated.

14. Continue to clean the skin with povidone-iodine solution for three minutes or with alcohol solution for five minutes. Follow agency practice about cleaning and drying times.

15. Apply the povidone-iodine ointment to the insertion site and to the catheter hub, taking care not to loosen the catheter–tubing connection.

16. If the catheter is taped in place, ensure that the tape is clean. If the tape is soiled, remove and replace it with sterile tape, using the crisscross (chevron) taping method. See Figure 25–21 on page 561.

17. Apply the precut sterile drain gauze around the catheter. (If precut gauze is not available, cut a 2 × 2 sterile gauze square using the sterile scissors.) Apply sufficient sterile gauze dressings to cover the catheter and skin.

    Rationale This protects the catheter and skin surrounding the insertion site from airborne contaminants.

18. If using Elastoplast dressing, apply tincture of benzoin to the skin surrounding the dressing gauzes and allow it to air dry about one minute.

    Rationale This protects the patient's skin when adhesive tape or Elastoplast is applied and promotes adhesion of the cover dressing. Appropriate drying time is essential or skin breakdown can occur when the dressing is removed.

19. Remove your gloves.

20. Have the patient abduct his or her arm and turn his or her head away from the dressing site. Tape the dressing securely to the skin with Elastoplast or transparent occlusive dressing. Make sure that the adhesive covering is occlusive. See Figure 25–42 on page 584, for example.

    Rationale Arm abduction and head rotation ensure that the patient's range of motion is not limited by the adhesive dressing and decrease the potential for skin abrasion caused by movement of the adhesive.

21. Loop and tape the IV tubing (not the filter) over the occlusive dressing.

    Rationale Looping prevents tension on the catheter and its inadvertent detachment if the tubing is pulled.

22. Seal all the dressing cover edges with nonallergenic tape.
23. Label a strip of tape with the date, time, and your initials, and apply it to the dressing.

■ Evaluation

Expected outcomes

1. Area around catheter clean
2. Evidence of healing

Unexpected outcome

Evidence of infection at site around catheter, eg, swelling, inflammation, odor, and/or discharge. Upon obtaining an unexpected outcome:

1. Report your findings to the responsible nurse and/or physician.
2. Adjust the nursing care plan appropriately.

TECHNIQUE 25–12   ■   Monitoring Central Venous Pressure (CVP)

Measurement of the central venous pressure (CVP) determines the pressure of blood in the right atrium (right atrial blood pressure), which reflects the right ventricular blood pressure. A CVP measurement enables the nurse or physician to assess blood volume and the capacity of the right side of the heart to receive and eject blood.

The CVP is measured with a manometer attached to an IV apparatus and a catheter placed in the right atrium or near the right atrium in the superior vena cava. The CVP catheter is most commonly threaded through the subclavian, jugular, or antecubital veins, generally by the physician.

Normally the CVP ranges from 5 to 15 cm H_2O; variations occur within the same patient, from changes in position and hydration status or blood volume, and from patient to patient.

■ Planning

Nursing goals

1. To assess hydration status
2. To monitor fluid replacement and determine specific fluid requirements
3. To evaluate blood volume, eg, to monitor the degree of hemorrhage in a postoperative patient
4. To maintain the patency of the CVP line
5. To prevent infection of the insertion site
6. To prevent air embolism

Equipment

1. A standard IV setup with pole. The IV tubing must not have an in-line filter, which distorts CVP readings. Some agencies use a separate line and normal saline solution for CVP measurements if the primary IV solution contains dextrose. Dextrose solutions tend to be sticky and interfere with the movement of the manometer ball and flow of solution in the manometer. The separate line with normal saline may be set up in tandem with the primary IV line. Check agency policy.
2. A CVP manometer set with stopcock and extension tubing. One type of manometer is a disposable one-piece apparatus (see Figure 25–38); other kinds have two parts: a disposable length of tubing attached to a stopcock and a reusable metal measuring scale. The measuring scale usually ranges from 0 to 30 cm of water.
3. A leveling device, if available.
4. Nonallergenic tape or an indelible marker.

■ Intervention

1. Maintain the patient in a supine position without a pillow unless this position is contraindicated. If the patient feels breathless, elevate the head of the bed slightly; note the exact position, because it must be used for all subsequent CVP readings, and the manometer level must be adjusted accordingly.
   Rationale   The patient must always be in the same position for this procedure to ensure reliable comparative readings.
2. Check that the level of the patient's right atrium (zero reference point) is aligned with the zero point on the manometer scale. To align them, use the leveling rod on the manometer or a yardstick with

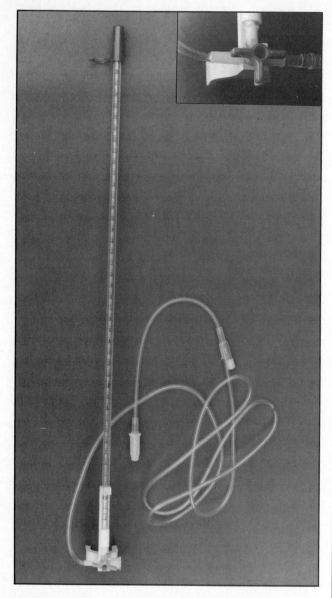

FIGURE 25-38 ■ A CVP manometer. Note the enlargement of the stopcock in the upper right-hand corner.

a level attached. See Figure 25-39. When the rod is horizontal (ie, aligned with the patient's right atrium), a bubble appears between two lines in the viewing window of the leveling device. See Figure 25-40. If an adjustment is required, first raise or lower the bed, and second readjust the manometer on the IV pole.

Rationale To ensure an accurate reading, the zero mark of the manometer must correspond with the level of the patient's right atrium, and the manometer must be vertical.

3. Temporarily increase the IV infusion rate.

Rationale This is necessary to check the patency of the CVP catheter and avoid possible release of any thrombus into the bloodstream.

4. If the line is *not* patent, notify the responsible nurse or physician. If the line is patent, proceed with CVP measurement.

5. Adjust the stopcock to the *IV-container-to-manometer* position (see Figure 25-41, *A*), and slowly fill the manometer with IV solution to about the 15-cm level or to a level just above the previous reading.

6. Adjust the stopcock to the *manometer-to-patient* setting (see Figure 25-41, *B*), and observe the fall in fluid level in the manometer tube. Note also the slight fluctuations in the fluid level with the patient's inspiration and expiration. If the fluid level does not fluctuate, ask the patient to cough.

Rationale The fluid level falls with inspiration due to a decrease in intrathoracic pressure. It rises with expiration due to an increase in intrathoracic pressure. No fluctuation may indicate that the CVP catheter is lodged against the vein wall. Coughing can change the catheter position.

7. When the fluid level stabilizes (usually between 5 and 15 cm H_2O), lightly tap the manometer tube with your index finger.

FIGURE 25-39

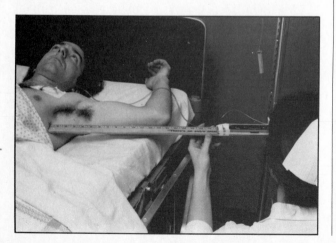

FIGURE 25-40

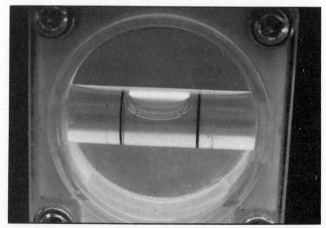

Rationale This dislodges air bubbles that can distort the reading.

8. Note the *lowest* level the fluid column reaches. Inspect the column at eye level and take the CVP reading from the base of the meniscus. If the manometer tube contains a small floating ball, take the reading from its midline.

9. Readjust the stopcock to the *IV-container-to-patient* position (see Figure 25–41, *C*), and lower the IV container below the patient's heart, to check for blood backflow.

   Rationale The backflow of blood gives a final check that the CVP catheter is patent.

10. Readjust the IV flow clamp to the appropriate infusion rate.

11. Record the date, time, and pressure reading on the appropriate record. If the patient was placed in a position other than supine, record the position used.

    Rationale To ensure consistent comparative readings, the patient must take the same position for each CVP reading.

12. Check with the physician about the degree of change in CVP at which he or she is to be notified. Report changes of 5 cm or more immediately.

■ **Evaluation**

Expected outcome

Normal CVP from 5 to 15 cm H_2O.

Unexpected outcomes

1. Higher or lower CVP than normal
2. Change of 5 cm or more from patient's baseline CVP

Upon obtaining an unexpected outcome:

1. Repeat the assessment to confirm your findings.
2. Report your findings to the responsible nurse and/or physician.

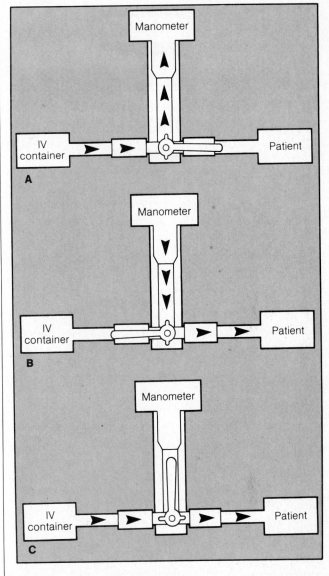

FIGURE 25–41

TECHNIQUE 25–13 ■ Changing a Dressing for a Surgically Inserted Central Venous Line

The distal end of a central venous catheter lies on the chest somewhere between the nipple and the sternum. The proximal tip lies in the right atrium of the heart.

When the catheter is newly inserted, there are two sites that require dressing: the insertion site, where the catheter enters the vein, and the exit site, where the catheter leaves the chest. See Figure 25–35 on page 572. Once the insertion site incision has healed, only the catheter exit site requires care.

The distal end of the catheter is threaded and has a male Luer-Lok cap. In some agencies the Luer-Lok cap is replaced with a special cap that has an injection port, which is also threaded. The cap is screwed onto the catheter securely. Some authorities also recommend that the cap be taped to prevent it from dislodging or allowing an air embolus to enter. See Figure 25–42. Some authorites suggest that the catheter should have a smooth clamp in place continously. The clamp must not have teeth, because they could damage the catheter. It is normally placed over tape on the line, as an added precaution against severing the catheter. The clamp is closed when the catheter is not being used.

The insertion site for the catheter is cleaned the way any surgical incision is cleaned until it is healed. See Technique 35–1 on page 828. The frequency of dressing changes varies among agencies; however, once every 24 or 48 hours is not unusual.

The exit site is also cleaned, and the dressing is changed

FIGURE 25–42 ■ Taping a cap on a central venous catheter.

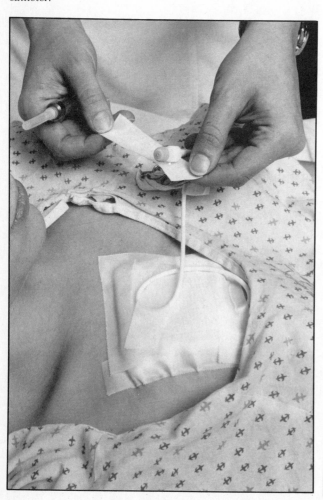

until the site is completely healed. At that time practices vary at different agencies. At some, the healed exit site is left exposed to the air and cleaned with hydrogen peroxide only when it is soiled. Agencies also vary in choice of dressing materials.

■ Assessment

Assess the patient for:

1. Any indications of infection at the dressing sites: redness, swelling, discharge, odor, or discomfort
2. The condition of the catheter
3. Any allergies, eg, to iodine

Other data include: the date and time of the previous dressing change.

■ Planning

Nursing goals

1. To promote skin healing and prevent infection
2. To assess the healing process

Equipment

Sterile technique is used, and some agencies also require sterile gloves and masks; others do not because the exit site is a considerable distance from the insertion site. Determine agency practice.

1. Sterile cotton-tipped applicators.
2. Hydrogen peroxide.
3. Antiseptic solution, eg, povidone-iodine solution.
4. Sterile precut 2 × 2 gauze squares.
5. Antiseptic ointment, eg, povidone-iodine ointment.
6. Tape. Some agencies use air-occlusive tape to make the dressing airtight.

Where the catheter has a Luer-Lok cap, some agencies change the cap at the time the dressing is changed.

■ Intervention

1. Assist the patient to a supine position, and expose the dressing site.
2. Open the sterile supplies.
3. Remove the old dressing, and inspect it for any discharge.
4. Clean the site using a sterile applicator and hydrogen peroxide.
   Rationale Hydrogen peroxide will remove any crusts and has an antiseptic action.
5. Use a new sterile applicator each time you apply more hydrogen peroxide.

Rationale Remoistening a used applicator would contaminate the hydrogen peroxide.

6. Clean the site in a circular pattern moving outward from the catheter to about 8 cm (3 in).

   Rationale Moving outward prevents introducing microorganisms from the skin to the catheter site.

7. Permit the area to air dry.

8. Repeat steps 4–6 using povidone-iodine solution.

9. Permit the area to air dry.

   Rationale This leaves a film of antiseptic on the skin.

10. Clean the catheter with the antiseptic solution, working from the site to the connection. Some agencies use alcohol for this purpose.

    Rationale Moving from the site to the connection prevents the introduction of microorganisms at the site. The antiseptic solution reduces the number of microorganisms on the catheter.

11. Apply the antiseptic ointment directly on the opening around the catheter.

    Rationale The ointment provides a physical as well as a chemical barrier to the entrance of microorganisms.

12. Apply a sterile precut 4 × 4 gauze around the catheter and over the site (see Figure 25–43) and another sterile 4 × 4 gauze completely over the exit site and catheter.

    Rationale The precut 4 × 4 gauze around the catheter protects the skin from irritation from the catheter. Both gauzes serve as a barrier to microorganisms entering the site.

13. Tape the gauze in place so that all edges are secured. Some authorities suggest completely covering the gauze with tape (Munro-Black, 1984, p 56). See Figure 25–42 on page 584.

14. Loop the catheter and tape it to the patient.

    Rationale A secured looped catheter will prevent direct pulling on the site.

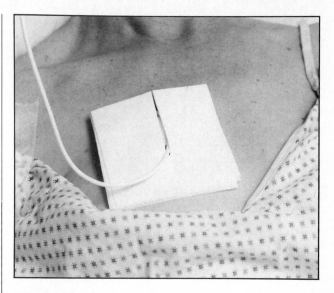

FIGURE 25–43

15. Label the dressing with the date, the time, and your initials.

16. Record your assessments and the dressing change on the patient's chart.

■ **Evaluation**

Expected outcomes

1. Incision clean
2. Dressing dry
3. Some serosanguineous drainage initially

Unexpected outcomes

1. Discharge at incision sites
2. Redness around incision sites
3. Pain at incision sites

Upon obtaining an unexpected outcome: Report your findings to the responsible nurse and/or physician.

TECHNIQUE 25–14 ■ Flushing and Administering a Medication through a Central Venous Catheter

When a central venous catheter is not in continous use, it is necessary to flush it with heparin to prevent the formation of blood clots and thus maintain its patency. Heparin flushes are ordered by a physician. They are usually performed:

1. After the insertion of the catheter
2. When a continuous infusion is discontinued
3. After the administration of a medication
4. After withdrawing a blood specimen

5. Periodically as ordered by the physician, eg, every 8 to 12 hours

Medications can be administered through a central venous catheter either continously or intermittently, in an infusion or directly with a syringe. For continuous administration, the medication can be injected into the infusion solution and the flow rate regulated by the drip chamber of the infusion. For intermittent administration, the medication can be instilled in a second infusion set (see Technique 25–1) and infused at designated intervals.

When the central venous catheter is not attached to an infusion, medications can be administered directly into the catheter using a syringe and needle.

■ **Assessment**

1. Assess the system for blockages to the flow of fluid in the catheter.
2. Assess the flow rate, if an infusion is running.
3. Assess the patient's response to the particular medication, eg, body temperature if the patient has an elevated temperature and is receiving an antibiotic.
4. Inspect the catheter and tubing for any leaks.

Other data include:

1. Whether the medication is compatible with heparin
2. The physician's order for the medication, including the rate of infusion
3. The agency's recommended practice for flushing the catheter

■ **Planning**

Nursing goals

1. To maintain the patency of the catheter
2. To administer ordered medications accurately and safely

Equipment

For a heparin flush

1. A sterile injection cap (heparin lock) to fit on the distal end of the catheter, if one is not already in place (ie, if an infusion is running). The cap may be a screw type, or a male Luer-Lok cap.
2. A sterile syringe of heparinized normal saline and a ⅝-in to 1-in needle. The concentration and amount are ordered by a physician. A solution of 0.3 mL of heparin (1,000 units per/mL) in 30 mL of normal saline is often used. The Hickman catheter has an internal volume of 2 mL. Agencies differ in the amount of solution and heparin injected.
   Rationale A ⅝-in to 1-in needle is not likely to

penetrate much beyond the cap and therefore is not likely to damage the catheter.

3. A rubber-shod clamp or tape and a cannula clamp.
4. Swabs with an antiseptic, eg, alcohol or povidone-iodine.

For administering a medication

5. A medication of the required strength in a syringe with a ⅝-in to 1-in needle. Determine whether the medication is compatible with heparin.
6. A sterile syringe with 5 mL of saline solution for flushing before and after a medication that is incompatible with heparin.

■ **Intervention**

Heparin flush with an infusion running

1. Place tape for the clamp around the catheter if a clamp is not there already.
   Rationale The tape protects the catheter from damage by the clamp.
2. Close the stopcock to stop the infusion.
3. Apply the rubber-shod clamp or the cannula clamp over the tape on the catheter. See Figure 25–44.
   Rationale The clamp closes the catheter.

FIGURE 25–44

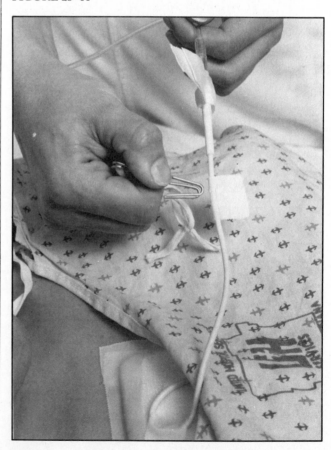

4. Clean the area where the catheter and the infusion tubing join with antiseptic, and allow it to dry.

    Rationale The antiseptic reduces the number of microorganisms in the area.

5. Open the package or container with the sterile cap.

6. Detach the infusion tubing, and insert the sterile cap, making sure not to touch the end that is inserted into the catheter or the end into which the needle will be inserted. Screw the cap securely into the catheter.

    Rationale The ends must remain sterile so as not to contaminate the inside of the catheter or the needle.

7. Insert the needle of the syringe into the center of the cap. See Figure 25–45. If the distal portion of the cap was contaminated, wipe it with antiseptic before inserting the needle.

    a. First insert the needle of the syringe containing saline, if the infusion contained a medication that is incompatible with heparin.

    b. Insert the needle of the syringe containing heparinized saline only, if incompatibility is not a problem.

8. Open the clamp on the catheter.

9. Inject the saline or the heparinized saline. In some agencies, all but 0.5 mL of solution is injected, and the clamp is closed as the last 0.5 mL is injected.

    Rationale Instilling the last 0.5 mL while the clamp is closing slightly increases the pressure in the catheter, preventing a backflow of blood into the tip of the catheter and subsequent clot formation at that point.

10. Remove the needle and syringe from the cap.

11. Repeat steps 7–10 for the heparinized saline injection if saline was injected first.

12. Record discontinuation of the infusion, installation of the cap (heparin lock) on the catheter, injection of the heparin flush, and your assessments, on the patient's chart. In some agencies this is recorded on the IV flow sheet.

Sample Recording

Date	Time	Notes
6/9/86	1210	IV #8 discontinued, 1,000 mL infused. Heparin lock placed on Hickman catheter. 2.5 mL heparinized saline injected. No leaks observed from catheter. ———— Michelle R. Splane, NS

Heparin flush without an infusion

13. Clean the distal portion of the cap (where the needle will be inserted) with an antiseptic swab.

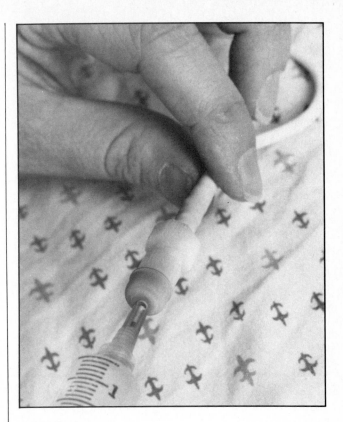

FIGURE 25–45

14. Insert the needle of the syringe into the center of the cap.

15. Inject the heparinized saline. See step 9 above.

16. Follow steps 10 and 12.

17. Record the heparin flush and your assessments on the patient's record.

Administering a medication

18. Clean the end of the cap on the catheter with an antiseptic swab.

19. If the medication to be administered is incompatible with heparin:

    a. Insert the needle of the syringe with 2.5 mL of saline solution into the catheter cap.

    b. Inject the saline. See step 9.

    Rationale The saline will clear the catheter of heparin. If the medication is compatible with heparin, or after steps a–b, insert the needle of the syringe with the medication into the catheter cap.

20. Inject the medication at the rate ordered by the physician.

21. Remove the needle and syringe.

22. Clean the cap with an antiseptic swab.

23. If the medication is incompatible with heparin, repeat step 19, a–b. After that, or if the medication is compatible with heparin, insert the needle of the

syrinage with the heparinized saline into the catheter cap.

24. Inject the heparinized saline solution, and close the clamp. See step 9.
25. Remove the syringe and needle.
26. Inspect the catheter for leaks.
27. Record the medication, the flush, and your assessments on the patient's chart.

■ Evaluation

Expected outcomes

1. Heparinized saline injected easily
2. Medication injected easily
3. No discomfort reported by the patient

Unexpected outcomes

1. Resistance encountered to injection
2. Solution could not be injected
3. Injection caused patient pain

Upon obtaining an unexpected outcome:

1. Ask the patient to turn, to take deep breaths, to cough, or to raise his or her hands above the head. Then try to inject the solution again. If the tip of the catheter was against the wall of a vein, these measures may move it.
2. If the solution cannot be injected on the second try, notify the responsible nurse and/or physician.

TECHNIQUE 25–15 ■ Withdrawing Blood through a Central Venous Catheter

Because of its viscosity, blood can be obtained only through a relatively large lumen catheter, eg, the larger lumen of a double-lumen Hickman catheter. Blood cannot be drawn through a Broviac catheter or a standard subclavian or peripheral line.

■ Assessment

1. Determine the reason for the blood specimen.
2. Check existing laboratory records for baseline data about the blood constituents to be measured.

Other data include: the order from the physician to obtain a blood specimen from the catheter.

■ Planning

Nursing goal

To obtain a blood specimen for laboratory analysis.

Equipment

1. The apropriate test tubes for the amount of blood needed. Mark each tube beforehand with the amount required.
2. Tape to secure connections if Luer-Lok connections are not used.
3. Povidone-iodine or alcohol swabs to clean the catheter cap.

4. One sterile syringe large enough to obtain the amount of blood required.
5. One sterile syringe of sufficient size for an initial collection of heparinized blood, which is discarded. Determine agency policy about how much blood to discard.
6. Sterile 2 × 2 gauzes to hold the catheter cap if its sterility is to be maintained for reinsertion.
7. A sterile cap if a new one is to be applied to the catheter.
8. One syringe and needle filled with heparinized saline solution (for a catheter with a heparin lock).
9. Two 10-mL syringes filled with sterile normal saline (for a catheter with a multiport adapter and a continuous infusion).
10. A rubber-shod clamp or tape and a cannula clamp.

■ Intervention

From a catheter with a heparin lock

1. Clean the junction of the cap and the catheter with an antiseptic swab. Permit it to air dry.
   Rationale   Cleaning with an antiseptic swab reduces the number of microorganisms by friction and chemical means.
2. Open the package of sterile 2 × 2 gauze.

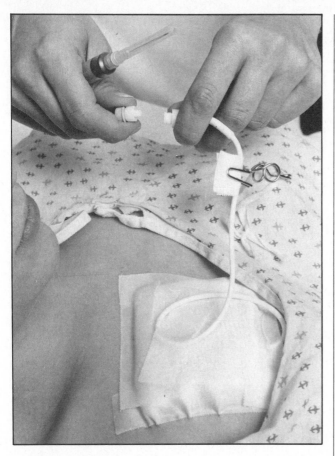

FIGURE 25–46

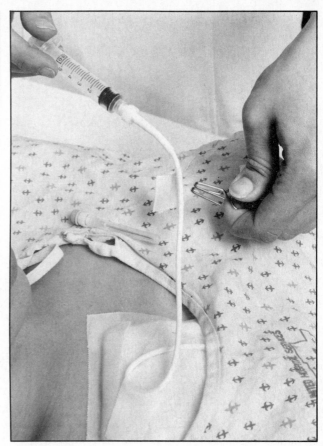

FIGURE 25–47

3. Open the package with the sterile cap if the cap is to be replaced.

4. Ensure that the clamp on the catheter is closed and secure.

5. Remove the cap from the catheter. See Figure 25–46. If the cap is to be reapplied, maintain the sterility of the part inserted into the catheter, and place the cap on the sterile gauze.

6. Attach the empty syringe for discardable blood to the catheter.

7. Release the clamp and aspirate the amount of fluid (blood and heparinized saline) to be discarded.

8. Close the clamp.

   Rationale   The clamp must always be closed *before* the cap or syringe is removed from the catheter, so that air cannot enter and form an air embolus.

9. Remove the syringe and set it aside.

10. Attach the syringe to be used to collect the specimen.

11. Open the clamp. See Figure 25–47.

12. Aspirate the amount of blood required.

13. Clamp the catheter.

14. Remove the syringe from the catheter.

15. Lay the syringe with the blood aside, but only for a minute because the blood will clot. If you will take

longer, ask another person to put the blood into the test tubes.

16. Put the cap on the catheter, maintaining the sterility of the inside of the catheter and the part of the cap inserted in the catheter. Use the cap that was removed or a new sterile cap.

17. Insert the needle of the syringe with the heparinized saline into the catheter cap.

18. Unclamp the catheter.

19. Inject the heparinized saline. See Technique 25–14, step 9.

20. Clamp the catheter.

21. Remove the syringe and needle.

22. Transfer the blood sample from the syringe to the test tubes.

23. Tape the cap on the catheter. Go to step 35.

From a multiport adapter with an infusion

24. Remove the tape from the port to be used if it was taped.

25. Follow steps 1–4.

26. Close the clamp on the port connected to the infusion.

27. Attach the syringe with sterile saline to the port, and unclamp the catheter line.
28. Instill the saline, then reclamp the catheter.
29. Follow steps 6–15.
30. Attach the second syringe with sterile saline to the port, unclamp the catheter, and instill the saline.
31. Clamp the catheter.
32. Remove the syringe.
33. Attach the cap to the port, maintaining the sterility of the inside of the port and the cap. Tape the cap.
34. Open the clamp on the port attached to the infusion, and monitor the infusion rate.
35. Record your assessments, the blood volume aspirated, any medications injected, the disposition of the specimens, and the tests ordered.
36. Arrange for the specimens to be sent to the laboratory.

■ Evaluation

Expected outcome

Obtained blood specimen required.

Unexpected outcome

Could not obtain blood specimen. Upon obtaining an unexpected outcome:

1. Ask the patient to turn, to take deep breaths, to cough, or to raise hands above the head. Then repeat the technique.
2. If blood cannot be obtained on a second try, notify the responsible nurse and/or physician.

References

Anderson MA, Aker SN, Hickman RO: The double-lumen Hickman catheter. *Am J Nurs* (February) 1982; 82:272–273.

Beaumont E: The new IV infusion pumps. *Nursing 77* (July) 1977; 7:31–35.

Huey FL: Setting up and troubleshooting. *Am J Nurs* (July) 1983; 83:1026–1028.

Karrei I: Hickman catheters: Your guide to troublefree use. *Can Nurse* (December) 1982; 78:25–27.

Keithley JK, Fraulini KE: What's behind that I.V. line? *Nursing 82* (March) 1982; 12:32–42.

Munro-Black J: The ABC's of total parenteral nutrition. *Nursing 84* (February) 1984; 14:50–56.

Nursing 80 Photobook Series: *Managing IV Therapy.* Intermed Communications, 1980.

Peck N: Perfecting your I.V. therapy techniques. (3 parts.) *Nursing 85* (May) 1985; 15:38–43, (June) 1985; 15:48–51, and (July) 1985; 15:32–35.

Swearingen PL: *The Addison-Wesley Photo-Atlas of Nursing Procedures.* Addison-Wesley, 1984.

Ungvarski PJ: Parenteral therapy. *Am J Nurs* (December) 1976; 76:1974–1977.

Wittig P, Semmler-Bertanzi DJ: Pumps and controllers—a nurse's assessment guide. *Am J Nurs* (July) 1983; 83:1022–1025.

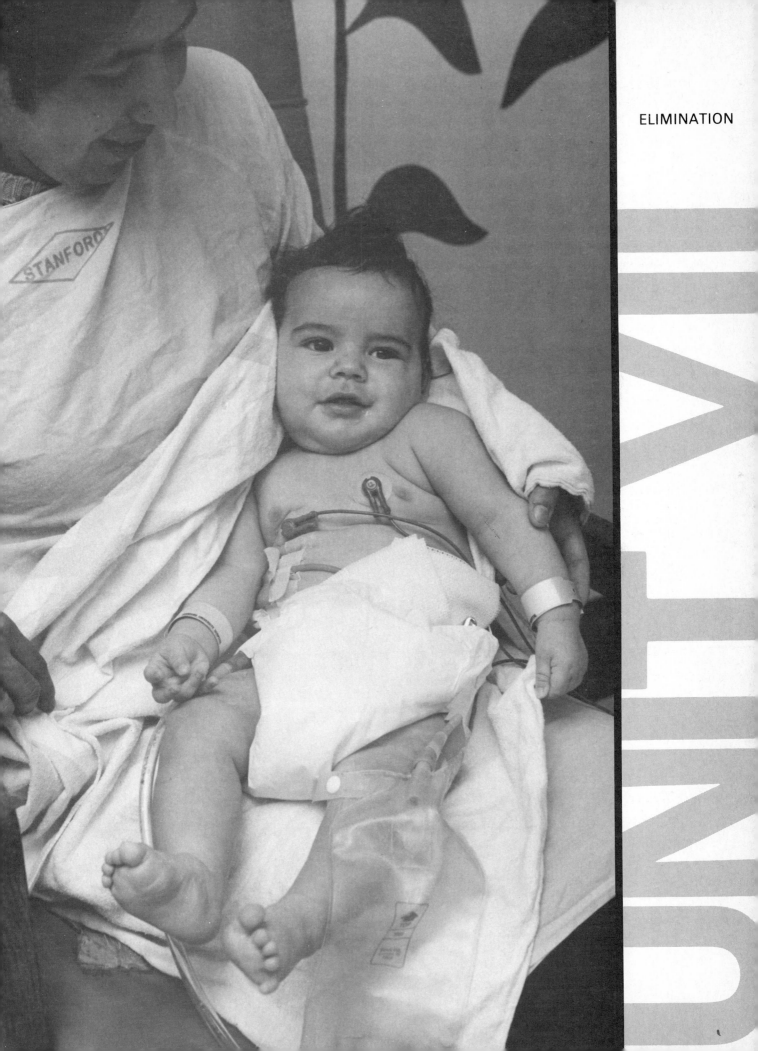

ELIMINATION

UNIT VII

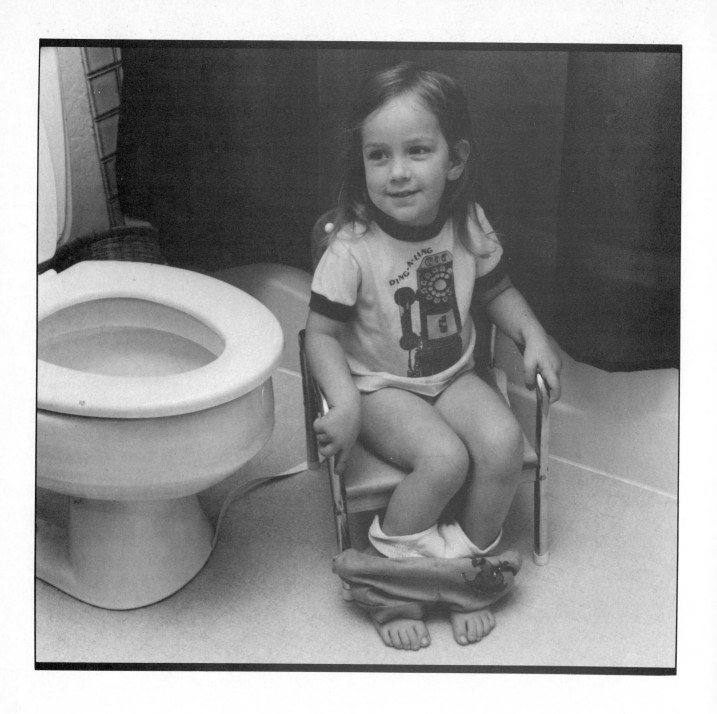

FECAL ELIMINATION

26

Elimination of the waste products of digestion is essential to health. Adequate elimination depends on the correct functioning of the small and large intestines, the nervous system, and the urinary system, as well as factors such as diet, exercise, fluid intake, and regularity.

Nurses are involved frequently in assisting patients with a variety of bowel and urinary problems brought about by illness, diagnostic tests, age, or faulty health habits. Common elimination aids include the use of bedpans and urinals, the administration of enemas, and the ɩ of rectal tubes or rectal suppositories. Urinary s and urinary elimination aids other than the urinal are discussed in chapter 27. This chapter deals with elimination of fecal matter and flatulence.

Chapter Outline

The Large Intestine

Bedpans and Urinals

- Technique 26–1 Giving and Removing a Bedpan
- Technique 26–2 Giving and Removing a Urinal

Enemas

- Technique 26–3 Administering an Enema
- Technique 26–4 Siphoning an Enema

- Technique 26–5 Inserting a Rectal Tube to Relieve Flatulence
- Technique 26–6 Removing a Fecal Impaction Digitally
- Technique 26–7 Inserting a Rectal Suppository
- Technique 26–8 Obtaining and Testing a Specimen of Feces

Objectives

Upon completion of this chapter, the student will:

1. Know specific terms and facts about feces, fecal elimination, bedpans, urinals, and enemas
   1.1 Define selected terms
   1.2 Identify the structures of the large intestine
   1.3 Identify essential aspects of defecation
   1.4 Identify common characteristics of normal and abnormal urine and feces
   1.5 Identify various types of bedpans and urinals
   1.6 Identify specific guidelines for the care of bedpans and urinals
   1.7 Compare cleansing, carminative, retention, and return flow enemas
   1.8 Identify types of solutions commonly used for enemas
2. Understand specific facts about techniques used to promote or maintain fecal elimination
   2.1 Identify relevant assessment data
   2.2 Identify nursing diagnoses for which the technique may be implemented
   2.3 Identify nursing goals related to the technique
   2.4 Identify expected and unexpected outcomes from assessment data
   2.5 Identify reasons underlying selected steps of the technique

3. Perform techniques that safely and effectively promote and maintain fecal elimination
   3.1 Assess the patient adequately
   3.2 Collect additional data from appropriate sources
   3.3 Select pertinent nursing goal(s) for the patient
   3.4 Establish relevant outcome criteria for the patient following the technique
   3.5 Collect necessary equipment before the technique
   3.6 Implement interventions to enhance both the effectiveness of the technique and the patient's comfort and safety
   3.7 Communicate relevant information about the patient to the appropriate persons through records or reports
   3.8 Evaluate the outcomes of the technique
4. Evaluate own performance of specific techniques in a laboratory or clinical setting with the assistance of another
   4.1 Use the performance checklists provided
   4.2 Identify areas of strength and weakness
   4.3 Alter performance in response to own evaluation and that of another

Terms

- anal canal   the distal portion of the rectum, which opens onto the body surface distally
- anus   the opening of the anal canal on the body surface
- bedpan   a receptacle used to collect urine and feces

- carminative   an agent that assists in the passage of flatus from the colon
- cecum   the dilated pouch that constitutes the first part of the large intestine adjoining the small intestine
- chyme   semifluid material produced by the digestion

of food in the stomach; it is found in the small and large intestines

■ colitis   inflammation of the colon

■ colon   that part of the large intestine that extends from the cecum to the rectum; sometimes used interchangeably with large intestine

■ constipation   defecation of small, dry, hard stools or passage of no stool for an abnormal period of time

■ defecation   the expulsion of feces from the anus

■ diarrhea   defacation of liquid feces and increased frequency of defecation

■ distention (tympanites)   excessive flatus in the intestines or peritoneal cavity

■ electrolyte   a compound that is able to conduct an electrical impulse in an aqueous (water) solution

■ enema   a solution that is injected into the rectum and the sigmoid colon

■ eructation   ejection of gas from the stomach through the mouth; belching

■ fecal impaction   a mass of hardened feces in the folds of the rectum

■ fecal incontinence   inability to control the passage of feces through the anus

■ feces   the body wastes and undigested food eliminated from the rectum

■ flatulence   the presence of excessive amounts of gas in the stomach or intestines

■ flatus   gas or air normally present in the stomach or intestines

■ frequency   voiding at frequent intervals

■ gastrocolic reflex   increased peristalsis of the colon after food has entered the stomach

■ haustrum   a saclike formation of a part of the colon produced by contraction of the longitudinal and circular muscles (plural: haustra)

■ hemorrhoid   a distended vein in the rectum

■ hypertonic   possessing a greater osmotic pressure than another fluid, eg, blood; increased tension, eg, of a muscle

■ hypotonic   possessing a lesser osmotic pressure than another fluid, eg, blood; decreased tension, eg, of a muscle

■ ileocecal valve   membranous folds between the distal ileum and the cecum (entrance to the large intestine)

■ ileum   small intestine

■ incontinence   the inability to control the elimination of urine or feces

■ micturate   pass urine from the body (urinate, void)

■ nocturia   increased urinary frequency at night

■ occult   hidden

■ osmosis   the passage of a solvent (eg, water) through a semipermeable membrane from an area of lesser concentration to an area of greater concentration

■ parasite   plant or animal that lives on or within another living organism

■ perineum   the surface area between the vagina and the anus in females and between the scrotum and the anus in males

■ peristalsis   wavelike movement produced by circular and longitudinal muscle fibers of the intestines to propel contents onward

■ rectum   the distal portion of the large intestine

■ sacrum   the triangular bone at the base of the spine

■ sigmoid colon   the distal portion, shaped like the letter S, of the colon

■ sphincter   a circular, ringlike muscle that opens and closes an orifice when it relaxes and contracts

■ suppository   a solid, cone-shaped, medicated substance
inserted into the rectum, vagina, or urethra

■ tonicity   the effective osmotic pressure equivalent of a fluid; normal condition of tensity or tone of a muscle

■ urgency   the feeling one must void immediately

■ urinal   a receptacle used to collect urine

■ urine   the fluid of water and waste products excreted by the kidney

■ void   urinate, micturate

THE LARGE INTESTINE

The large intestine is responsible for the formation of feces (waste products) and their elimination from the body. Extending from the ileocecal valve to the anus, the large intestine in an adult is 125 to 150 cm (50 to 60 in) in length. The first section of it after the valve is the cecum, to which the appendix is attached. See Figure 26–1. The cecum is also attached to the ascending colon. The transverse colon crosses the abdomen at about the level of the umbilicus. It then joins the descending colon, which is attached to the sigmoid colon in the lower left quadrant of the abdomen. The sigmoid colon is attached to the rectum, the most distal portion of which is the anal canal. See Figure 26–2.

FIGURE 26–1 ■ Parts of the large intestine.

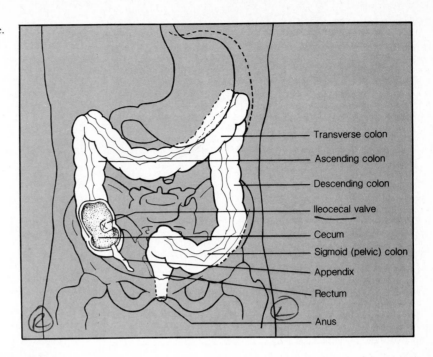

- Transverse colon
- Ascending colon
- Descending colon
- Ileocecal valve
- Cecum
- Sigmoid (pelvic) colon
- Appendix
- Rectum
- Anus

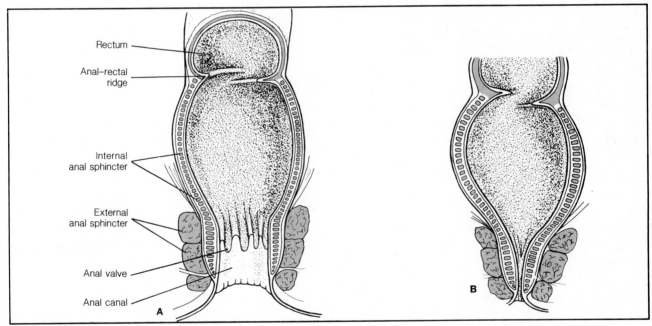

Rectum
Anal–rectal ridge
Internal anal sphincter
External anal sphincter
Anal valve
Anal canal
A
B

FIGURE 26–2 ■ The rectum, anal canal, and anal sphincters: **A,** open; **B,** closed.

The large intestine is a muscular tube lined with mucous membrane. The muscle fibers are both circular and longitudinal, thus permitting the intestine to enlarge and contract in both width and length. The longitudinal muscles are shorter than the colon and therefore cause the large intestine to form pouches, or haustra. See Figure 26–3.

Defecation

The frequency of defecation is highly individual, varying from several times per day to two or three times per week.

The amount defecated also varies from person to person. When peristaltic waves move the feces into the sigmoid colon and the rectum, the sensory nerves in the rectum are stimulated, and the individual becomes aware of the need to defecate. The *internal* anal sphincter relaxes, and feces move into the anal canal. After the individual is seated on a toilet or bedpan, the *external* anal sphincter is relaxed voluntarily. Expulsion of the feces is assisted by contraction of the abdominal muscles and the diaphragm, which increases abdominal pressure, and by contraction of the levator ani muscles of the pelvic floor, which moves the feces through the anal canal. See Figures

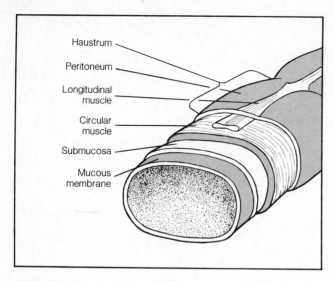

FIGURE 26–3 ■ The layers of the wall of the large intestine.

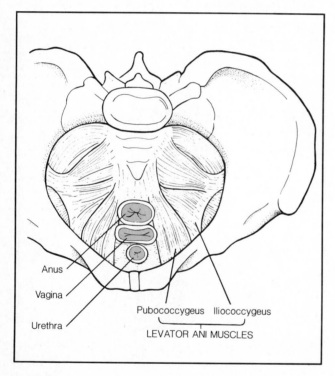

FIGURE 26–4 ■ The levator ani muscles of the pelvic floor aid in expulsion of the feces.

26–2 and 26–4. The feces are then expelled through the anus.

Normal defecation is facilitated by (a) thigh flexion, which increases the pressure within the abdomen, and (b) a sitting position, which increases the downward pressure on the rectum.

If the defecation reflex is ignored, or if defecation is consciously inhibited by contracting the external sphincter muscle, the urge to defecate normally disap-

pears for a few hours before occurring again, Repeated inhibition of the urge to defecate can result in expansion of the rectum to accommodate accumulated feces and eventual loss of sensitivity to the need to defecate. Constipation can be the ultimate result.

Feces

Normal feces are made of about 75% water and 25% solid materials. They are soft but formed. If the feces are propelled very quickly along the large intestine, so that there is not time for most of the water in the chyme to be reabsorbed, the feces will be more fluid, perhaps containing 95% water. This is called *diarrhea*. Normal feces require a normal fluid intake (see Chapter 23); feces that contain less water may be hard and difficult to expel. This condition is known as *constipation*.

Feces are normally brown, chiefly due to the presence of stercobilin and urobilin, which are derived from bilirubin (a red pigment in bile). Another factor that affects fecal color is the action of bacteria such as Escherichia coli or staphylococci, which are normally present in the large intestine. The action of microorganisms on the chyme is also responsible for the odor of feces.

Flatus

An adult usually forms 7 to 10 L of flatus in the large intestine every 24 hours. The gases include carbon dioxide, methane, hydrogen, oxygen, and nitrogen. Some are swallowed with food and fluids taken by mouth, and others are formed through the action of bacteria on the chyme in the large intestine.

The gases that are swallowed are mostly expelled through the mouth, by eructation. The gases formed in the large intestine are chiefly absorbed through the intestinal capillaries into the circulation. Excessive gas, or flatulence, can form in the colon, however, from a variety of causes, such as abdominal surgery, anesthetics, and narcotics. If this gas cannot be expelled through the anus, it may be necessary to insert a rectal tube or provide a return flow enema to remove it. See Techniques 26–4 and 26–5.

BEDPANS AND URINALS

Although the focus of this chapter is fecal elimination, both bedpans and urinals are discussed in this section and in Techniques 26–1 and 26–2.

There are two main types of bedpans: the regular high back pan (see Figure 26–5, *A*) and the slipper or fracture pan (see Figure 26–5, *B*). The slipper pan has a low back and is used for patients who are unable to elevate their buttocks because of physical problems or therapy that contraindicates such movement.

A *urinal* is a receptacle for urine only. Several designs are available: one is used primarily for male patients (see Figure 26–6, *A*) and one for female patients (see Figure 26–6, *B*). Female patients often use a bedpan for both urine and feces, while male patients generally use a urinal for urine and a bedpan for feces.

A *commode* is sometimes used instead of a bedpan when the patient can get out of bed but is unable to go to a bathroom. A commode is like an armchair with an open seat (like a toilet seat) with a receptacle under it to receive the urine and feces. The receptacle may be a special one that fits the commode or simply a bedpan that fits under the toiletlike seat. A commode may or may not be on wheels and freely movable. Some commodes have a plain seat as well, thus doubling as regular chairs.

Guidelines for the Care of Bedpans and Urinals

The care of bedpans and urinals relates largely to medical aseptic practices and to the feelings people attach to elimination.

1. In order to maintain medical asepsis, each patient is provided with her or his own bedpan or urinal.

2. Bedpans and urinals are stored in an appropriate place out of sight. Bedside units are often designed to provide a specific place for bedpans and urinals that is not visible to others and is separate from the patient's personal possessions. It is usually also separated from other equipment used by the patient for hygienic care. Medical aseptic practice prohibits the placing of a bedpan on the floor under the patient's bed or on overbed tables. Some bedside tables have a hook on which the urinal can hang so that it is accessible to the patient.

3. A clean bedpan cover is placed over the bedpan after use and for transporting it to and from the patient's bedside. Covers are also available for covering and transporting urinals.

4. Bedpans and urinals should always be handled from the outside. Urinals and the slipper (fracture) pan have handles that the nurse can use to carry them. The high back bedpan needs to be supported with both hands on its base for transport.

5. Elimination equipment is thoroughly cleaned and dried after use. Disposable equipment is discarded. Rinsing devices, cleaning brushes, and disinfectant solutions are generally located in the patients' bathrooms or unit utility rooms. Bedpans and urinals periodically need to be recycled through a central supply area for comprehensive cleaning, which includes resterilization.

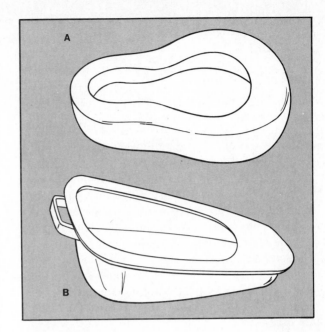

FIGURE 26–5   ■   Two types of bedpans: **A,** the high back or regular pan; **B,** the slipper or fracture pan.

FIGURE 26–6   ■   Two types of urinals: **A,** male urinal; **B,** female urinal.

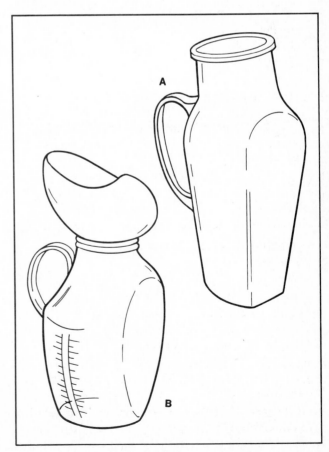

TECHNIQUE 26–1 ■ Giving and Removing a Bedpan

Many patients confined to bed are able to use a bedpan or urinal independently, provided the equipment is placed within safe and easy reach. Some patients, however, require varying degrees of assistance from a nurse. For example, some patients are incontinent (that is, they lack the ability to control their elimination). These patients require assistance to establish a regular schedule for using the bedpan or urinal. Others may have physical impairments, such as paralysis, that prevent them from manipulating the equipment independently. Still others, such as those who have lost the ability to speak due to a stroke, are unable to communicate their needs to the nurse. In such situations the nurse has to determine the patient's needs and provide the appropriate assistance.

Using a bedpan or urinal can be embarrassing to many patients. For the elderly, physically impaired, or critically ill it can also be a tiring procedure.

■ Assessment

For patients unable to communicate verbally, observe any behaviors that might indicate the need to eliminate. For example, many such patients become agitated or restless when they need to void or defecate. Other data include:

1. When the patient last voided and/or defecated.
2. How much assistance the patient requires. For example, can the patient reach the bedpan from the bed? Can the patient lift himself or herself on and off a bedpan? What position is the patient able to assume? Can the patient clean himself or herself after elimination?
3. The position that best facilitates voiding. For example, male patients often find it easier to void when standing by the bedside.
4. Whether a specimen of the feces or urine is required for testing.
5. Whether any problems exist in the patient's urine or feces, as indicated in the patient's chart, for which specific progress assessments need to be made.
6. Whether the patient is receiving medications, such as a diuretic or an "iron pill," that alter the color, consistency, or amount of urine or feces.

■ Nursing Diagnosis

Nursing diagnoses that may indicate the need to assist a patient to use a bedpan include:

1. Impaired physical ability, related to:
   a. neuromuscular impairment
   b. musculoskeletal impairment
   c. trauma
   d. surgical procedure
   e. imposed medical restrictions

■ Planning

Nursing goals

1. To provide a receptacle for elimination of waste material for patients confined to bed
2. To obtain a specimen of urine or stool for laboratory examination
3. To obtain an accurate measurement and assessment of the patient's urine or stool

Equipment

1. A clean bedpan and bedpan cover
2. Toilet tissue
3. A basin of water, soap, washcloth, and towel, so that the patient can wash his or her hands after using the bedpan
4. An aerosol freshener to remove odors in the room after defecation (optional)
5. Equipment for a specimen as required (see Technique 26–8)
6. A bag or receptacle to discard the toilet tissue, if a specimen of urine or feces is required

■ Intervention

Giving the bedpan

1. Tuck the bedpan cover under the mattress at the side of the bed. Warm the bedpan by running water inside the rim of the pan or over the pan. Dry the outside of the pan, and place it on the foot of the bed or on an adjacent chair.

   Rationale A cold bedpan may make the patient tense and thus hinder elimination. When warming a metal pan, which retains heat, take care not to burn the patient.

2. For patients who can assist by raising their buttocks:
   a. Fold down the top bed linen on the near side to expose the patient's hip, and adjust the patient's gown so that it will not fall into the bedpan.

   Rationale A pie fold at the top bedclothes exposes

the patient minimally and facilitates placement of the bedpan. See Figure 26–7.

b. Ask the patient to flex the knees, rest the weight on the back and the heels, and then raise the buttocks. Assist the patient to lift the buttocks by placing the hand nearest the patient's head palm up under the patient's lower back, resting the elbow on the mattress, and using the forearm as a lever. See Figure 26–7.

Rationale Use of appropriate body mechanics by both patient and nurse prevents unnecessary strain and exertion.

c. Place a regular bedpan under the patient's buttocks with the narrow end toward the foot of the bed and the patient's buttocks resting on the smooth, rounded rim. Place a slipper (fracture) pan with the flat end under the patient's buttocks.

Rationale Improper placement of the bedpan can cause skin abrasion to the sacral area and spillage of the bedpan's contents.

d. Replace the top bed linen and the side rail as needed.

Rationale It is important to reduce undue exposure and to prevent falls.

e. Provide the patient with toilet tissue, and ensure that the call light is readily accessible. Ask the patient to signal when finished. Leave the patient only when, in your judgment, it is safe to do so.

Rationale Having necessary items within reach prevents falls.

3. For helpless patients who cannot raise their buttocks on and off a bedpan:

a. Assist the patient to a side-lying position with the back toward you.

b. Place the bedpan against the patient's buttocks with the open rim toward the foot of the bed. See Figure 26–8.

c. Hold the far hip with one hand and the bedpan with the other. Smoothly roll the patient toward you and onto his or her back with the bedpan in place (see Figure 26–9). Assume a wide stance and move your weight from the front leg to the back leg when moving the patient.

Rationale Use of appropriate body mechanics prevents undue muscle exertion and strain.

d. Elevate the head of the bed to a semi-Fowler's position.

Rationale This position relieves strain on the patient's back and permits a more normal position for elimination.

e. If the patient is unable to assume a semi-Fowler's position, place a small pillow under the patient's back.

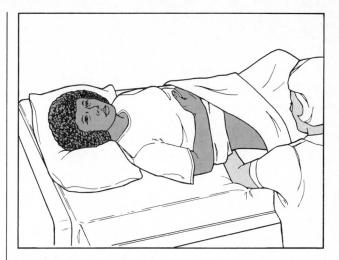

FIGURE 26–7

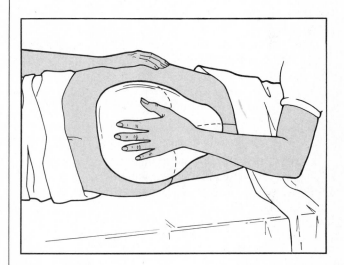

FIGURE 26–8

FIGURE 26–9

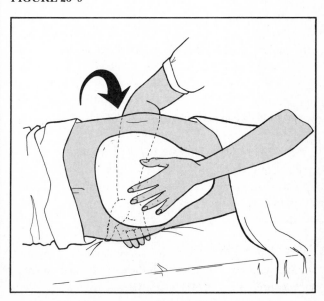

f. Provide the patient with a call light.

Removing the bedpan

4. For patients who can raise their buttocks:

   a. Elevate the bed to the high position, and then remove the bedpan by again pie-folding the top linen back and having the patient raise her or his buttocks.

   b. Cover the bedpan, and place it on an adjacent chair or at the foot of the bed.

   Rationale Covering the bedpan reduces offensive odors and reduces the patient's embarrassment.

   c. If the patient requires assistance to clean the perineal area:

   ■ Wrap toilet tissue several times around the hand, and wipe the patient from the pubic area to the anal area, using one stroke for each piece of tissue.

   Rationale Cleaning in this direction—from the less soiled area to the more soiled area—helps prevent the spread of microorganisms.

   ■ Turn the patient on the side, spread the buttocks, and clean the anal area in the same manner.

   ■ Place the soiled tissue in the bedpan.

   ■ Wash the anal area with soap and water as indicated and thoroughly dry the area.

   Rationale Adequate washing and drying prevents skin abrasion and excessive accumulation of microorganisms.

   ■ Replace the drawsheet if it is soiled.

5. For helpless patients:

   a. Return the bed to the flat position if needed.

   b. Fold the top bed linen down to the patient's thighs.

   c. Holding the bedpan securely with one hand, gently roll the patient to a side-lying position either facing you or away from you. If you are alone and the patient is helpless, it is safer and easier to roll the patient toward you rather than away from you. If you are planning to turn the patient away from you, raise the side rail or have another nurse present to prevent a fall.

   d. Remove and cover the bedpan, and place it safely on an adjacent chair or at the foot of the bed.

   e. Clean the anal area as in step 4c.

6. Offer the patient materials to wash and dry the hands.

   Rationale Hand washing following elimination is a sanitary practice that prevents the spread of microorganisms.

7. Spray the air with an air freshener if there is an unpleasant odor unless contraindicated for the pa-

tient with respiratory problems or offensive to the patient.

Rationale Elimination odor can be embarrassing to patients and visitors alike. However, sprays may be harmful to patients with respiratory problems, and some perfume sprays are offensive to some people.

8. Acquire a specimen if required. Place it in the appropriately labeled container. Specimen collection is described in Techniques 26–8 and 27–10.

9. Empty and clean the bedpan. Provide a clean bedpan cover, if necessary, before returning it to the patient's unit.

10. Record on the patient's chart any significant data about the urine or bowel movement according to agency procedure.

Sample Recording

Date	Time	Notes
4/23/86	1300	Large, dark brown, liquid stool. Complained of cramplike pain in lower abdomen before defecation. Pain relieved on defecation.————— Annette S. Cohen, NS

11. Refer to the patient's chart or nursing care plan for any nursing or medical orders related to elimination problems. For example, the physician may have ordered "Kaopectate 60 mL following each loose bowel movement."

■ Evaluation

1. Assess the color, odor, amount, and consistency of the stool. See Table 26–1 for some characteristics of normal and abnormal feces.

2. Assess the color, odor, amount, and consistency of the urine. Chapter 27 provides information about characteristics of normal and abnormal urine and about urinary problems. See Table 27–1 on page 622.

3. Examine the perineal-anal area for any redness or excoriation.

4. Assess the patient's ability to control urine or bowel elimination. For incontinent patients, a routine schedule of offering a urinal or bedpan on awakening in the morning, before or after meals, and at bedtime may alleviate the problem. For patients who have *urgency* or *frequency*, a bedpan can be placed within easy reach of the patient at all times. Patients with *nocturia* may need a bedpan for nighttime use only.

Expected outcomes

1. Normal brown, formed, moist stool

2. Defecation at usual time

TABLE 26–1 ■ Characteristics of Normal and Abnormal Feces

Characteristic	Normal	Abnormal	Possible cause
Color	Adult: brown	Clay or white	Bile obstruction
	Infant: yellow	Black; tarry	Drug, eg, iron; upper gastro-intestinal bleeding
		Red	Lower gastrointestinal bleeding; some foods, eg, beets
		Pale	Malabsorption of fat
Consistency	Formed; moist	Hard	Constipation
		Watery	Diarrhea, eg, intestinal irritation
Odor	Aromatic: affected by ingested food	Pungent	Infection, blood
Frequency	Adult: varies from 1–3 movements per day to once every 3 days	More than 3 movements per day; fewer than 1 movement per week	
	Infant: 1–6 movements per day	More than 6 movements per day; fewer than 1 movement every 2 days	
Shape	Cylindrical (contour of rectum)	Narrow	Obstruction
Amount	100–400 g per day (varies with diet)		

3. Normal transparent straw- or amber-colored urine
4. Clear consistency of urine
5. Faint aromatic odor of urine
6. 1,200–1,500 mL urine output in 24 hours for an adult

Unexpected outcomes

1. Clay-colored or black, tarry stools
2. Solid, dry, or watery stools
3. Pungent odor of stools
4. Absence of defecation

5. Abnormal color of urine, eg, dark amber, red, or dark brown
6. Viscid thick urine
7. Mucous plugs in urine
8. Offensive odor of urine
9. Increased or decreased urine output
10. Pain or difficulty voiding
11. Incontinence

Upon obtaining an unexpected outcome: Report your findings to the responsible nurse and/or physician.

TECHNIQUE 26–2 ■ Giving and Removing a Urinal 🏠

Most male patients will be familiar with a male urinal. Some female patients, however, may not be familiar with female urinals (see Figure 26–6 on page 597) and may require instruction about their use. Note that some female patients find it easier to void using a bedpan rather than a urinal.

■ **Assessment**   See Technique 26–1 on page 598.

■ **Nursing Diagnosis**   See Technique 26–1 on page 598.

■ **Planning**

Nursing goals   See Technique 26–1 on page 598.

Equipment

1. A clean urinal and urinal cover or bag
2. Toilet tissue for females
3. A dampened washcloth or a basin of water, soap, and towel so that the patient can wash hands after using the urinal
4. Specimen equipment
5. A bag or receptacle to discard the toilet tissue, if a specimen is required

■ Intervention

1. Assist the patient to an appropriate position, such as a semi-Fowler's position or, for the male patient, standing at the side of the bed.

Giving the urinal

2. Offer the urinal to the patient so that he or she can position it independently.
    or
3. Place the urinal between the patient's legs with the handle uppermost so that urine will flow into it.
4. Tuck the urinal cover under the mattress at the side of the bed.
5. Leave the signal cord within reach of the patient.
    Rationale This can prevent a fall if a patient who is standing to void feels weak and needs assistance.
6. Leave the patient for two or three minutes or until the patient signals.
    or
7. Remain, if the patient needs support to stand at the bedside or other assistance.

Removing the urinal

8. Remove and cover the urinal or place it in a urinal bag.
9. If wet, wipe the area around the urethral orifice with a tissue.
10. Make sure the patient's perineum is dry.
11. Offer the patient a dampened washcloth or water, soap, and a towel to wash and dry hands.
12. Change the drawsheet if it is wet.

13. Measure the urine if the patient is on intake and output, and provide a specimen if required. See Technique 27–10 on page 657.
14. Empty and rinse out the urinal, and return it to the patient's bedside unit.
15. Record the amount of urine, if it was measured, and assessment data, eg, cloudiness, redness. See Table 27–1 on page 622.

Sample Recording

Date	Time	Notes
8/15/86	0900	Voided 275 mL (9 fl oz) of cloudy dark orange urine. ———— Arnold S. Shaw, NS

16. Refer to the patient's chart for any orders, such as: "Increase fluid intake to 3,000 mL."

■ Evaluation

1. Assess the color, odor, amount, and consistency of the urine. See Table 27–1 for normal and abnormal constituents of urine.
2. Examine the perineum of the female and the genitals of the male for any redness or excoriation.
3. Assess the patient's ability to control urination.

Expected outcomes

1. Normal transparent straw- or amber-colored urine
2. Clear consistency of urine
3. Faint aromatic odor
4. Output of 1,200–1,500 mL in 24 hours

Unexpected outcomes

1. Abnormal color, eg, dark amber, red, or dark brown
2. Viscid thick urine
3. Mucous plugs in urine
4. Offensive odor
5. Increased or decreased output
6. Pain or difficulty voiding

Upon obtaining an unexpected outcome: Report your findings to the responsible nurse and/or physician.

ENEMAS

Types of Enemas

Enemas are classified into four groups, according to their action: cleansing, carminative, retention, and return flow.

A *cleansing enema* stimulates peristalsis by irritating the colon and rectum and/or by distending the intestine with the volume of fluid introduced. Two kinds of cleansing enemas are the *high enema* and the *low enema*. The high enema is given to clean as much of the colon as possible. Often about 1,000 mL (1 L) of solution is administered to an adult, and the patient changes from the left lateral to the dorsal recumbent position and then to the right lateral position during the administration, so that the fluid can follow the large intestine. See Figure 26–1 on page 595. The fluid is administered at a higher pressure than for a low enema; that is, the container of solution is held higher. Cleansing enemas are most effective if held for five to ten minutes. The low enema is used to clean the rectum and the sigmoid colon only. About 500 mL (0.5 L) of solution is administered to an adult, and the patient maintains the left side-lying position during its administration.

A *carminative enema* is given primarily to expel flatus. The solution instilled into the rectum releases gas, which in turn distends the rectum and the colon, thus stimulating peristalsis. For an adult, 60 to 180 mL of fluid is instilled.

A *retention enema* introduces oil into the rectum and sigmoid colon. The oil is retained for a relatively long period of time (eg, one to three hours). It acts to soften the feces and to lubricate the rectum and anal canal, thus facilitating passage of the feces.

A *return flow enema*, sometimes referred to as the *Harris flush* or *colonic irrigation*, is used to expel flatus. It is discussed in Technique 26–4.

Various solutions are used for enemas. The specific solution may be ordered by the physician or dictated by agency practice. Table 26–2 lists some of these solutions, giving the quantity and proportions frequently used.

An enema is a relatively safe procedure for the patient. The chief dangers are irritation of the rectal mucosa by too much soap or an irritating soap and negative effects of a *hypertonic* (possessing a greater tonicity than blood) or *hypotonic solution* (possessing a lesser tonicity than blood) on the body fluid and electrolytes. A hypertonic solution, such as the phosphate solutions of some commercially prepared enemas, is slightly irritating to the mucous membrane, and it causes fluid to be drawn into the colon from the surrounding tissues. The process by which this happens is called *osmosis*. Because only a small amount of fluid is normally administered, the advantages of comfort, retention for only five to seven minutes, and convenience generally outweigh these disadvantages. However, electrolyte and fluid imbalances can occur, particularly in infants under 2 years of age. The solution can cause hypocalcemia (a decreased amount of calcium in the blood serum) and hyperphosphatemia (an excessive amount of phosphate in the blood).

The repeated administration of hypotonic solutions, such as tap water enemas, can result in absorption of the water from the colon into the bloodstream. This increases the blood volume and can produce water intoxication. For this reason, some health agencies limit the number of tap water enemas given consecutively to three. This is of particular concern when the order is "enemas until returns are clear"—for example, prior to a visual examina-

TABLE 26–2 ■ Types of Enemas Commonly Used for Adults

Name	Constituents
Commercially prepared enema	90–120 mL of a hypertonic solution such as sodium phosphate (see directions on the package)
Saline	9 mL of sodium chloride to 1,000 mL of water
Tap water	1,000 mL of tap water
Soap	5 mL of white bland soap to 1,000 mL of water
Oil, eg, olive oil	90–120 mL of oil (commercially prepared): mineral, olive, or cottonseed

tion of the large intestine. Hypotonic solutions can also be unsafe for patients with decreased kidney function or acute heart failure.

Guidelines for Administering Enemas

1. The appropriate size rectal tube needs to be used. For adults this is usually #22 to #30 Fr. Children use a smaller tube, such as a #12 Fr. for an infant and a #14 to #18 Fr. for the toddler and school-age child.

2. Rectal tubes must be smooth and flexible with one or two openings at the end through which the solution flows. They are usually made of rubber or plastic. Any tube with a sharp or ragged edge should not be used because of the possibility of damaging the mucous membrane of the rectum. The rectal tube is lubricated with a water-soluble lubricant to facilitate insertion and decrease irritation of the rectal mucosa.

3. Enemas for adults are usually given at 40.5 to 43 °C (105 to 110 °F); those for children are given at 37.7 °C (100 °F), unless otherwise specified. Some oil retention enemas are given at 33 °C (91 °F). High temperatures can be injurious to the bowel mucosa; cold temperatures are uncomfortable for the patient and may create spasm of the sphincter muscles.

4. The amount of solution to be administered depends on the kind of enema, the age and size of the person, and the amount of fluid that can be retained.

   a. Infant, 250 mL or less

   b. Toddler or preschooler, 250 to 350 mL or less

   c. School-age child, 300 to 500 mL

   d. Adolescent, 500 to 750 mL

   e. Adult, 750 to 1000 mL

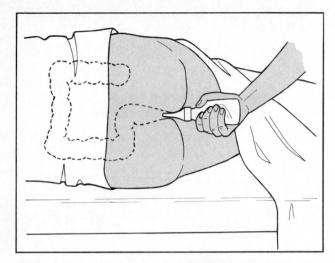

FIGURE 26-10 ■ The left lateral position is assumed for an enema. Note the commercially prepared enema.

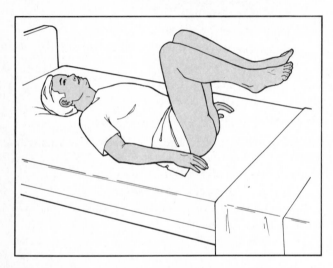

FIGURE 26-11 ■ A back-lying position for self-administration of an enema.

FIGURE 26-12 ■ An infant's legs are immobilized for an enema by placing a diaper under the bedpan and over the thighs.

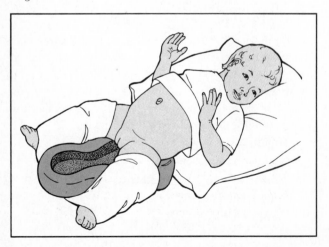

5. When an enema is administered, the patient usually assumes the left lateral position (see Figure 26-10), so that the sigmoid colon is below the rectum, thus facilitating instillation of the fluid. During a high cleansing enema, the patient changes position from left lateral to dorsal recumbent and then to right lateral. In this way the entire colon is reached by the fluid.

6. The distance to which the tube is inserted depends on the age and size of the patient. In adults, it is normally inserted 7.5 to 10 cm (3 to 4 in). In children it is inserted 5 to 7.5 cm (2 to 3 in) and in infants only 2.5 to 3.75 cm (1 to 1.5 in). If any obstruction is encountered when the tube is inserted, the tube should be withdrawn and the obstruction reported.

7. The force of flow of the solution is governed by:

   a. Height of the solution container

   b. Size of the tubing

   c. Viscosity of the fluid

   d. Resistance of the rectum

The higher the solution container is held above the rectum, the faster the flow and the greater the force (pressure) in the rectum. During most adult enemas, the solution container should be no higher than 30 cm (12 in) above the rectum. During a high cleansing enema, the solution container is usually held 30 to 45 cm (12 to 18 in) above the rectum, because the fluid is instilled farther to clean the entire bowel. For an infant, the solution container is held no more than 7.5 cm (3 in) above the rectum.

8. The time it takes to administer an enema largely depends on the amount of fluid to be instilled and the patient's tolerance. Large volumes, such as 1,000 mL, may take 10 to 15 minutes to instill; small volumes require less time.

9. The length of time that the enema solution is retained depends on the purpose of the enema and the ability of the patient to contract the external sphincter to retain the solution. Oil retention enemas are usually retained two to three hours. Other enemas are normally retained five to ten minutes. To assist an incontinent person to retain the solution, the nurse can press the buttocks together, providing pressure over the anal area.

10. While the enema solution is in the body, the patient may have a feeling of fullness and some abdominal discomfort.

11. When it is time for the patient to defecate, the nurse may assist her or him to a commode or toilet, depending upon the patient's preference and physical condition.

12. For self-administration of an enema, an adult can assume a back-lying position (see Figure 26-11).

13. When administering an enema to an infant, the infant's legs can be immobilized by a diaper (see Figure 26-12).

TECHNIQUE 26–3 ■ Administering an Enema

Before administering an enema, determine if a physician's order is required. At some agencies, a physician must order the kind of enema and sometimes the temperature of the enema and the time to give it, eg, the evening before surgery or the morning of the examination. When the patient has rectal pathology the physician may also specify the size of the rectal tube to use. At other agencies, enemas are given at the nurses' discretion, ie, as necessary on a p.r.n. order.

It is important that the nurse be aware that prepackaged enemas have their own instructions, which should be followed unless there are other instructions from the physician or the agency.

■ Assessment

1. Assess the patient for abdominal distention by palpating the patient's abdomen. The distended abdomen appears swollen and feels firm rather than soft when palpated. The patient may experience cramps.
2. Determine when the patient last had a bowel movement and the amount, color, and consistency of the feces.
3. Determine the sphincter control by asking the patient about his or her control of fecal elimination.

Other data include:

1. The purpose of the enema. Knowing why the enema is prescribed will help you determine the type and amount of solution to administer, if not specified by the physician's order.
2. Whether the patient can use a toilet or commode or must remain in bed and use a bedpan.

■ Nursing Diagnosis

Nursing diagnoses that may indicate the need to administer an enema include:

1. Alteration in bowel elimination: constipation, related to:
   a. Immobility
   b. Surgery
   c. Lack of exercise
   d. Lack of roughage in the diet
   e. Retention of barium

■ Planning

Nursing goals

1. To stimulate peristalsis and remove feces or flatus
2. To soften feces and lubricate the rectum and colon
3. To clean the rectum and colon in preparation for an examination
4. To remove feces prior to a surgical procedure or a delivery, thereby preventing inadvertent defecation and subsequent contamination
5. To reduce body temperature
6. To relieve a specific problem by administering a medication rectally

Equipment

1. A disposable enema unit (see Figure 26–13).
   or
2. An enema set containing:
   a. A container to hold the solution.
   b. Tubing to connect the container to the rectal tube.
   c. A clamp to compress the tubing, to control the flow of solution into the patient.
   d. A rectal tube of the correct size. See Guideline 1 on page 603.
   e. Lubricant to apply to the rectal tube before it is inserted.
   f. A bath thermometer to check the temperature of the solution.
   g. Soap, salt, or other ingredients as required.
   h. The prescribed amount of solution at the correct temperature. The nurse places the solution in the container, checks that the temperature and amount of solution are correct, and then adds the soap, salt, or other ingredients as needed.
3. A bath blanket to drape the patient.
4. A waterproof absorbent pad to protect the bed.
5. Tissue wipes.
6. A bedpan or commode if the patient is unable to reach the bathroom.

■ Intervention

1. Explain the procedure to the patient. Indicate that the patient may experience a feeling of fullness while the solution is being administered.
2. Assist adult and school-aged patients to a left lateral position, with the right leg acutely flexed, and drape them with the bath blanket.

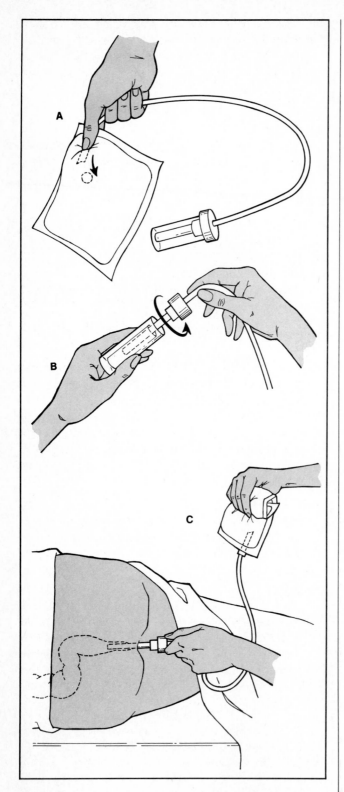

FIGURE 26–13 ■ One type of commercially prepared disposable enema: **A,** the bead that seals the tube is expelled from the tube into the bag so that the solution can flow through the tubing; **B,** the protector cover of the insertion tip is rotated to distribute the lubricant on the tip before the cover is removed; **C,** after the tube has been inserted, the bag is inverted and compressed.

Rationale This position facilitates the flow of solution by gravity into the sigmoid and descending colon, which are on the left side. See Figure 26–1 on page 595. Having the right leg acutely flexed provides for adequate exposure of the anus.

For infants and small children, the dorsal recumbent position is frequently used. Position them on a small padded bedpan with support for the back and head. Secure the legs by placing a diaper under the bedpan and pinning it around the thighs. See Figure 26–12 earlier.

3. Place the waterproof pad under the patient's buttocks to protect the bed linen.

4. Lubricate 5 cm (2 in) of the rectal tube if the enema is for an adult and 2.5 cm (1 in) if it is for a child. Some commercially prepared enema sets already have lubricated nozzles.

Rationale Lubrication facilitates insertion through the sphincters and minimizes trauma.

5. Open the clamp, and run some solution through the connecting tubing and the rectal tube; then close the clamp.

Rationale The tubes are filled with solution to expel any air in them. Air instilled into the rectum causes unnecessary distention.

6. Inspect the anal area for the presence of hemorrhoids.

7. Insert the rectal tube smoothly and slowly into the rectum, directing it toward the umbilicus. See Figure 26–14. Insert the tube an appropriate distance. See guideline 6 on page 604. Note any sign of discomfort on inserting the tube and any obstruction to the passage.

Rationale Inserting the tube toward the umbilicus guides the tube along the length of the rectum. The rectum of the average adult is 10 to 20 cm (4 to 6 in) long, but the size varies with age. See the illustrations of the rectum and anal canal in Figures 26–1 and 26–2 on page 595. The rectal tube is inserted beyond the internal sphincter.

8. If resistance is encountered at the internal sphincter, ask the patient to take a deep breath, and run a small amount of solution through the tube. If the resistance persists, withdraw the tube and report the resistance to the responsible nurse.

Rationale Deep breathing and inserting a small amount of solution may relax the sphincter.

9. If there is no resistance, open the clamp, and raise the solution container to the appropriate height above the rectum: 30 to 45 cm (12 to 18 in) for an adult, 7.5 cm (3 in) for an infant.

Rationale At this height, the solution does not exert enough pressure to damage the lining of the rectum.

or

10. Compress a pliable commercial container by hand.

11. Administer the fluid slowly. If the patient complains of fullness or pain, use the clamp to stop the flow for 30 seconds and then restart the flow at a slower rate. If you are using a plastic commercial container, roll it up as the fluid is instilled.

    Rationale Administering the enema slowly and stopping the flow momentarily decreases the likelihood of intestinal spasm and premature ejection of the solution. Rolling up the container prevents subsequent suctioning of the solution.

12. Assess the patient for skin color, perspiration, and dyspnea.

13. After all the solution has been instilled, or when the patient cannot hold any more and wants to defecate, close the clamp, and remove the rectal tube from the anus.

    Rationale The urge to defecate usually indicates that sufficient fluid has been administered.

14. Apply firm pressure over the anus with tissue wipes or press the buttocks together to assist retention of the enema. Have the patient remain lying down. Encourage the patient to hold the enema.

    Rationale Some enemas are more effective if they are retained from five to ten minutes. The time depends on the type of enema. It is easier for the patient to retain the enema when lying down than when sitting or standing because gravity promotes drainage and peristalsis.

FIGURE 26–14

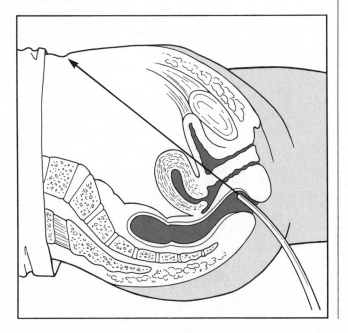

15. Assist the patient to a sitting position on the bedpan, commode, or toilet. If a specimen of feces is required, have the patient use a bedpan or commode.

    Rationale A sitting position is preferred because it promotes defecation.

16. Ask the patient not to flush the toilet if he or she is using one.

    Rationale The nurse needs to observe the feces.

17. Record administration of the enema; the amount, color, and consistency of returns; and the relief of flatus and abdominal distention.

Sample Recording

Date	Time	Notes
6/29/86	2100	1,000 mL saline enema given. Returned large amount of hard, white stool and large amount of flatus. Abdomen soft and less distended. P 72. ————————————— Roxy-Ann B. Stanley, NS

18. Teach the patient practices that develop regular and normal defecation, such as:

    a. Eating a balanced diet containing adequate bulk (roughage and fiber content). Bulk is found primarily in unrefined breakfast cereals, whole wheat flour, raw fruits, and raw vegetables.

    b. Maintaining an adequate fluid intake, eg, 1,500 mL daily.

    c. Eating regular meals.

    d. Establishing a regular time for defecation and allowing adequate time to defecate.

    e. Doing regular and sufficient amounts of exercise.

■ Evaluation

Assess the patient's response to the enema, in terms of feces and flatus passed, pulse rate, fatigue, and discomfort. Observe the feces for color, odor, and consistency. Feces may be black (tarry feces) due to the presence of old blood; clay-colored (acholic) due to absence of bile; green or orange due to the presence of an infection. Food, such as beets, can also affect the stool color. Hard stools may indicate constipation, whereas string-shaped stools may indicate disease of the rectum. A putrid, rotten odor may indicate a digestive problem. See Table 26–1. The patient may be able to tell you whether a large, moderate, or small amount of flatus was passed or whether no flatus was expelled.

Expected outcomes

1. Decreased abdominal distention

2. Return of all the solution and feces

3. Clear returns, indicating all feces have been removed, eg, in preparation for examination of the large intestine
4. Decreased abdominal discomfort

Unexpected outcomes

1. Unchanged abdominal distention
2. Enema solution is not expelled

3. No feces expelled with solution
4. Unchanged abdominal discomfort

Upon obtaining an unexpected outcome:

1. Report your findings to the responsible nurse.
2. Siphon enema solution if it cannot be expelled. Determine if a physician's order is required. See Technique 26–4.
3. Adjust the nursing care plan appropriately.

Administering an Enema to an Incontinent Patient

Occasionally a nurse needs to administer an enema to a patient who is unable to control his or her external sphincter muscle and thus cannot retain the enema solution for even a few minutes. In that case the patient assumes a supine position on a bedpan. The head of the bed can be elevated slightly, eg, to 30° if necessary, and the patient's head and back are supported by pillows. The nurse wears a glove over the hand that holds the rectal tube, to prevent direct contact with the solution and feces that are expelled over the hand into the bedpan during administration of the enema.

TECHNIQUE 26–4 ■ Siphoning an Enema

When a patient is unable to expel the solution following administration of an enema, the solution needs to be siphoned out. To *siphon* means to draw off by means of pressure and gravity. Siphoning an enema may require a physician's order.

■ **Assessment**

1. Inspect and palpate the patient's abdomen for distention.
2. Determine whether the patient is experiencing any abdominal pain or feeling of fullness.
3. Determine the rate and the quality of the respirations.

Other data include: the amount of enema solution that was instilled into the patient.

■ **Nursing Diagnosis**   See Technique 26–3 on page 605.

■ **Planning**

Nursing goal

To remove the enema solution safely and comfortably.

Equipment

1. A bedpan
2. A rectal tube
3. A funnel
4. Lubricant for the tip of the rectal tube
5. A container of water at 40 °C (105 °F)

■ **Intervention**

1. Assist the patient to a right side-lying position.
   Rationale In this position, the sigmoid colon is uppermost, thus facilitating drainage of the solution from it by gravity.
2. Place the bedpan on a chair at the side of the bed near the patient's hips.
3. Attach the open end of the rectal tube to the base of the funnel.
4. Lubricate the rectal tube. See Technique 26–3, step 4, on page 606.
5. Fill half of the funnel and the entire rectal tube with water.
   Rationale Filling the funnel and rectal tube will expel the air.

6. Pinch the tube and gently insert it into the rectum. See guideline 6 on page 604, for how far to insert the tube.

7. Hold the funnel about 10 cm (4 in) above the level of the anus. Release the pinched rectal tube, and quickly lower and invert the funnel over the bedpan. *Rationale* This action initiates siphoning, which draws the enema fluid out of the rectum and colon, through the rectal tube and funnel, and into the bedpan.

8. Record the technique and your assessments on the patient's chart.

■ Evaluation

Note the amount of fluid siphoned off; the presence of feces; the color and consistency of the feces; and other pertinent data.

Expected outcome

All the enema fluid was siphoned off.

Unexpected outcome

None or part of the enema fluid was siphoned off. Upon obtaining an unexpected outcome:

1. Report your findings to the responsible nurse.
2. Adjust the nursing care plan appropriately.

Administering a Return Flow Enema

The return flow enema (Harris flush or colonic irrigation) is a repetitive instillation and drainage of fluid to and from the rectum. It is similar to Techniques 26–3 and 26–4. Initially, the solution (100 to 200 mL for an adult) is instilled into the patient's rectum and sigmoid colon. Then the solution container is lowered so that the fluid flows back out through the rectal tube into the container. This alternating flow of fluid into and out of the large intestine stimulates peristalsis and the expulsion of flatus. The inflow-outflow process is repeated five or six times, and the solution is replaced several times during the procedure as it becomes thick with feces. A total of about 1,000 mL of solution is usually used for an adult.

Till ∅ more Bubbles   Dr's order

TECHNIQUE 26–5   ■   Inserting a Rectal Tube to Relieve Flatulence

Rectal tubes are left in the rectum for varying lengths of time. Generally it is recommended that a tube remain in the rectum for no longer than 30 minutes, to prevent undue irritation of the rectal lining. The tube is then reinserted as needed every two or three hours. Some agencies advocate attaching the open end of the rectal tube to a connecting tube that is attached to a collecting receptacle containing water. The passage of flatus can then be assessed by noting gas bubbles in the water.

■ Assessment

1. Palpate the patient's abdomen to determine the amount of distention.
2. Auscultate the abdomen for bowel sounds.
3. Determine whether the patient is experiencing any abdominal discomfort.
4. Assess respiratory rate. Flatulence can cause pressure upward on the diaphragm, resulting in difficult respirations.
5. Assess signs associated with flatulence, such as eructations and their frequency and the passage of flatus by rectum.

Other data include:

1. Factors contributing to the patient's flatulence, such as:

   a. The patient's patholgoy with specific reference to gastrointestinal problems

   b. Medications the patient is receiving

   c. The patient's activity schedule, to determine whether inactivity is a contributing factor

   d. The patient's dietary intake, to determine if gas-forming foods are being ingested

2. Baseline data regarding pulse and respirations

■ **Nursing Diagnosis** See Technique 26–3 on page 605.

■ **Planning**

Nursing goals

1. To relieve the patient's discomfort from flatulence and intestinal distention
2. To relieve difficult respirations

Equipment

1. A rectal tube (#22 to #30 Fr. for adults; #14 to #18 Fr. for children, according to their age)
2. Lubricant for the tip of the rectal tube
3. A paper towel in which to carry the lubricant and rectal tube to the bedside
4. Tape to attach the rectal tube to the buttock (optional)
5. Either a waterproof absorbent pad (eg, an abdominal or incontinence pad) to wrap around the open end of the rectal tube, or a connecting tube and a receptacle containing water

■ **Intervention**

1. Assist the patient to a left lateral position, and fold back the bedclothes to expose the anus.
2. Lubricate the insertion tip of the rectal tube liberally for 5 cm (2 in).
   Rationale Lubrication reduces resistance to passage of the tube through the anal sphincters.
3. Gently insert the rectal tube into the rectum 10 to 15 cm (4 to 6 in) for an adult. Insert the tube 5 to 10 cm (2 to 4 in depending on the patient's age) for a child.
   Rationale The rectal tube can be inserted farther for this procedure than is recommended for an enema, since fluid will not be administered.
4. Tape the rectal tube to the patient's buttock.
   Rationale Taping prevents dislodging of the tube.
5. Place the open end of the rectal tube in a folded absorbent pad.
   Rationale The folded absorbent pad will catch any liquid fecal material that seeps through the tube.
   or
6. Attach the open end of the rectal tube to a connecting tube and a drainage receptacle filled with water. Place the distal end of the tubing below the level of the water in the collecting receptacle.

Rationale Gas bubbles can be noted only if the tubing is below the water level.

7. Leave the patient in a comfortable lateral position.
8. After 30 minutes, remove the rectal tube.
9. Determine whether flatus has been expelled.
10. Record insertion and removal of the rectal tube and other pertinent data on the patient's record.

Sample Recording

Date	Time	Notes
8/2/86	1310	Rectal tube 22 Fr. inserted for flatulence and abdominal distention. P 82, R 24. ——————————— Sarah P. Stein, NS
8/2/86	1340	Rectal tube removed. States feels some relief; much flatus expelled. P 82, R 20. ——————————— Sarah P. Stein, NS

11. Assist the patient to take measures that will prevent flatulence and distention. These measures depend on the cause. For example, an anxious patient who is hyperventilating and swallowing large amounts of air may need to learn appropriate breathing patterns and ways to relax. Others may need to reduce their ingestion of carbonated beverages. Most patients will achieve more effective elimination of flatus with increased ambulation.

■ **Evaluation**

1. Inspect and palpate the abdomen for changes in abdominal distention.
2. Determine if any abdominal discomfort has been relieved.

Expected outcomes

1. Abdominal distention reduced
2. Abdominal discomfort relieved
3. Bowel sounds normal
4. Respiratory rate normal, difficult respirations relieved

Unexpected outcomes

1. Abdominal distention unchanged
2. Abdominal discomfort unchanged
3. Bowel sounds hypoactive
4. Dyspnea unchanged

Upon obtaining an unexpected outcome:

1. Report your findings to the responsible nurse.
2. Adjust the nursing care plan appropriately, eg, for reinsertion of the rectal tube.

TECHNIQUE 26–6 ■ Removing a Fecal Impaction Digitally

Fecal impaction is indicated by the passage of no stools, seepage of liquid feces, rectal pain, desire to defecate to no avail, and a general feeling of malaise. The nurse can confirm the presence of an impaction through digital examination of the rectum.

Although fecal impaction can generally be prevented, digital removal of impacted feces is sometimes necessary. When fecal impaction is suspected, the patient is often given an oil retention enema, a cleansing enema two to four hours later, and daily additional cleansing enemas, suppositories, or stool softeners. If these measures fail, manual removal is necessary. This process involves breaking up the fecal mass digitally and removing it in portions. Because the bowel mucosa can be injured during this procedure, some agencies restrict and specify the personnel permitted to conduct digital disimpactions. Rectal stimulation is also contraindicated for some patients, since it may cause an excessive vagal response resulting in cardiac arrhythmia.

After a disimpaction, various interventions can be used to remove remaining feces, eg, a cleansing enema or the insertion of a suppository.

■ Assessment

1. Determine the patient's pattern of defecation and any indications of an impaction. This information may be obtained from the patient and/or the patient's record.
2. Assess the presence of fecal impaction by digital examination of the rectum.
3. Determine if the patient is experiencing nausea, headache, abdominal pain, malaise.

Other data include:

1. Whether the patient's medications could be contributing to the problem
2. The patient's activity schedule (inadequate exercise predisposes to constipation and fecal impaction)
3. The patient's dietary intake, with particular reference to roughage and fluids

■ Nursing Diagnosis   See Technique 26–3 on page 605.

■ Planning

Nursing goals

1. To relieve pain and discomfort caused by blockage of impacted feces
2. To reestablish normal defecation

Equipment

1. A moisture-resistant bedpad
2. A bedpan and cover
3. Toilet tissue
4. A pair of disposable plastic gloves
5. Lubricant

■ Intervention

1. Explain to the patient what you plan to do and why. This procedure is distressing, tiring, and uncomfortable, so the patient may desire the presence of another nurse or support person.
2. Assist the patient to a right lateral or Sims's position with the patient's back toward you.
   Rationale When the patient is lying on the right side, the sigmoid colon is uppermost; thus gravity can aid removal of the feces.
3. Place the disposable bedpad under the patient's hips, and arrange the top bedclothing so that it falls obliquely over the patient's hips, exposing only the buttocks.
4. Place the bedpan and toilet tissue nearby on the bed or a bedside chair.
5. Put on the gloves.
6. Lubricate the gloved index finger.
   Rationale Lubricant reduces resistance by the anal sphincter as the finger is inserted.
7. Gently insert the index finger into the rectum, moving toward the umbilicus.
8. Gently massage around the stool.
   Rationale Gentle action prevents damage to the rectal mucosa and dislodges the stool.
9. Work the finger into the hardened mass of stool to break it up.
10. Work the stool down to the anus, remove it in small pieces, and place them in the bedpan.
11. Carefully continue to remove as much fecal material as possible; at the same time, note the patient's response.
    Rationale Manual stimulation could result in excessive vagal nerve stimulation and subsequent cardiac arrhythmia.
12. Assist the patient to a position on a clean bedpan, commode, or toilet.
    Rationale Digital stimulation of the rectum may induce the urge to defecate.
13. Record the removal of a fecal impaction and

pertinent data about the stool and the patient's response, eg, decreased abdominal pain, on the patient's record.

Sample Recording

Date	Time	Notes
9/28/86	1000	Rectal examination for fecal impaction. Moderate amount dark brown feces removed digitally. Abdominal pain unchanged. Unable to defecate following procedure. ———— Bruce L. Ching, NS

■ Evaluation

1. Assess the stool for amount, color, and consistency.
2. Determine if any abdominal discomfort has been relieved.
3. Inspect and palpate the patient's abdomen for any changes in distention one hour after removal of the impaction.

Expected outcomes

1. Elimination of feces
2. Decreased headache, abdominal pain, nausea, malaise

Unexpected outcomes

1. No feces expelled
2. Headache, abdominal pain, nausea, malaise unchanged

Upon obtaining an unexpected outcome:

1. Report your findings to the responsible nurse and/or physician.
2. Adjust the nursing care plan appropriately, eg, increase fluid intake and activity if the patient's condition warrants.

TECHNIQUE 26–7 ■ Inserting a Rectal Suppository

Insertion of medications into the rectum in the form of suppositories is a frequent practice. Rectal administration is a convenient and safe method of giving certain medications. Its advantages include:

1. It avoids irritation of the upper gastrointestinal tract in patients who encounter this problem.
2. It is advantageous when the medication has an objectionable taste or odor.
3. The drug is released at a slow but steady rate.
4. Rectal suppositories are thought to provide higher bloodstream levels (titers) of medication, since the venous blood from the lower rectum is not transported through the liver (Hahn, Barkin, Oestreich, 1982, p 99).

■ Assessment

1. Assess the patient's need for the medication, eg, abdominal distention and/or discomfort if the suppository is intended to stimulate defecation.
2. Determine whether the patient desires to defecate or when she or he last defecated. Suppositories that are given for a systemic effect should be given when the rectum is free of feces, since this will enhance absorption of the drug.

Other data include:

1. Whether the rectal route is suitable for the patient, eg, whether the patient has had recent rectal surgery or has rectal pathology.
2. The specific suppository ordered, its dosage, the time of administration, and the reason for it.
3. The action of the medication and any side effects. A pharmacology reference can provide this information.

■ Planning

Nursing goals

1. To provide a local medicinal effect (eg, a laxative suppository to soften feces and stimulate defecation)
2. To provide a systemic medicinal effect (eg, an aminophylline suppository to dilate the patient's bronchi and enhance breathing)

Equipment

1. The correct suppository
2. A fingercot or glove (disposable or rubber)
3. A paper towel

4. Lubricant, placed in the paper towel, in an amount sufficient to cover the suppository tip and the nurse's index finger

■ Intervention

1. Assist the patient to a left lateral position with the upper leg acutely flexed.

   Rationale In a left lateral position, the sigmoid colon is lowermost, thereby lessening the likelihood of feces in the sigmoid expelling the suppository.

2. Fold back the top bedclothes to expose only the buttocks.

3. Inspect the anal area for hemorrhoids, bleeding, and irritation.

4. Unwrap the suppository and leave it on the opened wrapper.

5. Don the glove or fingercot on the hand to be used to insert the suppository.

   Rationale The glove or fingercot prevents contamination of the nurse's hand by rectal microorganisms and feces.

6. Lubricate the flat end of the suppository.

   Rationale This end is inserted first. Lubrication prevents anal friction and tissue damage on insertion.

7. Lubricate the gloved index finger.

8. Ask the patient to breathe through the mouth.

   Rationale This usually relaxes the external anal sphincter.

9. Insert the suppository gently into the anus, flat end first, or according to the manufacturer's instructions (Logio, 1985, p 10), and along the wall of the rectum with the gloved index finger. For an adult, insert the suppository 10 cm (4 in); for a child or infant, insert it 5 cm (2 in) or less. See Figure 26–15.

   Rationale The suppository needs to be placed along the wall of the rectum, rather than amid feces, in order to be absorbed effectively. When the flat end is inserted first the rectum is less likely to expel it.

10. Withdraw the finger. Remove the fingercot or glove by turning it inside out and placing it on the paper towel.

    Rationale Turning it inside out contains the rectal microorganisms and prevents their spread.

11. Press the patient's buttocks together for a few seconds.

    Rationale This helps to dispel any urge the patient may have to expel the suppository.

12. Ask the patient to retain the suppository as long as possible. If the patient has been given a laxative suppository, place the call light within easy reach

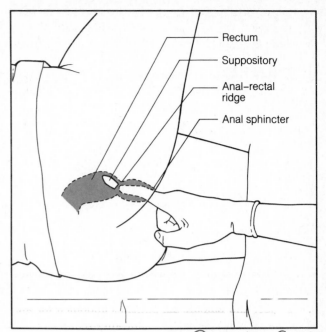

FIGURE 26–15

so the patient can summon assistance to use the bedpan or toilet.

13. Record the type of suppository given, the time it was given, the amount of time it was retained if it was expelled, and the results or effects, on the patient's record.

Sample Recordings

Date	Time	Notes
2/28/87	0900	Dulcolax suppository 10 mg inserted. ——— Eric P. Jones, NS
	0935	Large amount soft brown stool and much flatus expelled. ——— Eric P. Jones, NS

or

Date	Time	Notes
2/28/87	1025	Marked dyspnea, R 32, P 120. Aminophylline suppository 500 mg inserted. ——— Margery Smith, NS
	1055	Breathing easier. R 20, P 96. ——— Margery Smith, NS

■ Evaluation

1. Assess the stool for amount, color, and consistency if the suppository was given to stimulate defecation.

2. Assess the patient for other effects of the suppository, depending on the medication, eg, relief of pain, relief of dyspnea.

Expected outcomes

1. The medication produces the effects intended, eg, relief of dyspnea.
2. The suppository was inserted easily.
3. The anal area appeared normal: no hemorrhoids, bleeding, or irritation.

Unexpected outcomes

1. The medication did not have the intended effect.
2. The suppository could not be inserted.

3. The anal area appeared reddened; bleeding or hemorrhoids were present.

Upon obtaining an unexpected outcome:

1. Report your findings to the responsible nurse and/or physician.
2. Adjust the nursing care plan appropriately, eg, increase fluid intake if patient's condition permits.

TECHNIQUE 26-8 ■ Obtaining and Testing a Specimen of Feces

Specimens of feces are collected for a variety of tests. Often the specimen is sent to the laboratory. However, testing for occult (hidden) blood is done by a nurse on a nursing unit. Some of the reasons for testing feces are:

1. To detect the presence of occult blood. In this case only a small sample (about 1 tablespoon) of stool is required, and it need not be kept warm or examined immediately. The patient is sometimes placed on a meat-free diet for three days before specimen collection, as meat ingestion can create falsely positive results. The presence of blood in the stool may indicate bleeding from a duodenal ulcer or from other lesions elsewhere in the intestine.

2. To analyze for dietary products and digestive secretions, for example, fat content or bile. For these kinds of tests, the nurse needs to collect and send the total quantity of stool expelled at one time instead of a small sample. An excessive amount of fat in the stool (steatorrhea) can indicate faulty absorption of fat from the small intestine. A decreased amount of bile can indicate obstruction of bile flow from the liver and gallbladder into the intestine.

3. To detect the presence of parasites, such as amebae, worms, or their eggs. The stools of patients with diarrhea or dysentery are commonly analyzed for parasites. To test for parasites, the specimen must be sent to the laboratory while it is still warm.

4. To detect the presence of bacteria or viruses. Only a small amount of feces is required for this type of analysis because the specimen will be cultured. With diarrheal stools, a large sterile cotton swab may be dipped into the specimen and the swab taken to the laboratory in a sterile test tube. Stools need to be

dealt with immediately for viral or bacterial cultures. If for some reason there is a delay between the time the specimen is collected and the time the culture is started, the specimen must be kept in a cold refrigerator. Because patients receiving antibiotics or sulfonamides may produce falsely negative cultures, the nurse needs to note these medications on the requisition for the stool specimen.

■ Assessment

1. Determine from the patient when he or she expects to have a bowel movement.
2. Determine whether the patient can assist by notifying a nurse when he or she needs to defecate or by using a bedpan and then notifying a nurse.
3. Determine whether the patient experiences any abdominal discomfort before, during, or after defecation.
4. Inspect the skin around the anus for any irritation, especially if the patient defecates frequently and has liquid stools.

Other relevant data include:

1. The reason for collecting the stool specimen and the correct method of obtaining and handling it (eg, amount to be obtained, whether a preservative needs to be added to the stool, and whether it needs to be sent immediately to the laboratory). In many situations it may be necessary to confirm this information by checking with the agency laboratory.
2. Whether there are other interventions related to the specimen collection, eg, dietary or medication orders.

3. Whether any interventions (eg, medication) are ordered to follow a defecation.

■ Nursing Diagnosis

Nursing diagnoses that may indicate the need to obtain a specimen of feces and, in some instances, to test the specimen for occult blood include:

1. Alterations in bowel elimination: diarrhea, related to:
   a. nutritional disorders
   b. infectious process
   c. anxiety
   d. tube feedings
   e. allergies

■ Planning

Nursing goals

1. To obtain a specimen of feces for the ordered tests
2. To test for the presence of occult blood

Equipment

Collecting a specimen of feces

1. A clean or sterile bedpan or bedside commode. For an infant, the stool is scraped from the diaper.
2. A cardboard or plastic specimen container with a lid, or a sterile swab in a test tube, for stool culture, as policy dictates.
3. Two tongue blades to transfer the stool specimen from the bedpan to the specimen container.
4. A paper towel to wrap the used tongue blades before disposal.
5. A completed specimen identification label.
6. A completed laboratory requisition.
7. An air freshener.

Testing for occult blood in the feces

8. A clean bedpan or bedside commode
9. Two tongue blades
10. A paper towel to wrap the used tongue blades
11. Test product

■ Intervention

Collecting a specimen of feces

1. Explain to the patient that a stool specimen is required, the purpose for it, and how the patient can assist.

2. Assist ambulatory patients to use a bedpan placed on a bedside chair or under the toilet seat in the bathroom, or to use a bedside commode.
3. Instruct the patient:
   a. not to contaminate the specimen, if possible, by urine or menstrual discharge
   b. to notify the nurse as soon as possible after defecation, particularly for specimens that need to be sent to the laboratory immediately
4. After the patient has defecated, cover the bedpan or commode.
   Rationale Covering the bedpan reduces odor and embarrassment to the patient.
5. Clean the patient as required, and inspect the skin around the anus for any irritation, especially if the patient defecates frequently and has liquid stools. Assist him or her to a comfortable, safe position.
6. Take the pan to the bathroom or utility room.
7. Assess the feces for color, odor, consistency, amount, and the presence of abnormal constituents, such as blood or mucus. See Table 26–1 on page 601.
8. Using one or two tongue blades, transfer some or all of the stool to the specimen container, taking care not to contaminate the outside of the container. The amount of stool to be sent depends on the purpose for which the specimen is collected. For a culture, dip a sterile swab into the specimen, preferably where purulent fecal matter is present. Place the swab in a sterile test tube using sterile technique.
9. Wrap the used tongue blades in a paper towel before disposing of them in a waste container.
   Rationale Wrapping the used tongue blades prevents the spread of microorganisms by contact with other articles.
10. Place the lid on the container as soon as the specimen is in the container.
    Rationale Putting the lid on immediately prevents the spread of microorganisms.
11. Empty and clean the bedpan or commode and return it to its place.
12. Ensure that the specimen label and the laboratory requisition have the correct information on them and are securely attached on the specimen.
    Rationale Inappropriate identification of the specimen can lead to errors of diagnosis or therapy for the patient.
13. Provide an air freshener for any odors unless contraindicated by the patient, eg, a spray may increase dyspnea.
14. Arrange for the specimen to be taken to the laboratory. Specimens to be cultured or tested for parasites need to be sent immediately.

15. Record the collection of the specimen on the patient's chart and on the nursing care plan. Include in the recording the date and time of the collection; the color, odor, and consistency of the feces; and any other clinical signs.

Testing for occult blood

16. Because positive results of occult blood may occur if the patient has eaten meat within three days, some physicians order a red-meat-free diet for the patient for three days before the test. Oral iron preparations may also be discontinued, since undigested portions of them may mask the presence of occult blood in the stools.

17. Obtain a stool specimen.

18. Select a test product, and follow its directions. For example: ↑ occult Bld

   a. For a Guaiac test, smear a thin layer of feces on a paper towel or filter paper with a tongue blade, and drop reagents onto the smear as directed.

   b. For a Hematest, smear a thin layer of feces on filter paper, place a tablet in the middle of the specimen, and add two drops of water as directed.

   c. For a Hemoccult slide, smear a thin layer of feces over the circle inside the envelope, and drop reagent solution onto the smear.

19. Note the reaction and record it on the patient's chart. For all tests, a blue color indicates a positive result, ie, the presence of occult blood.

■ Evaluation

Expected outcomes

1. Feces appeared normal: color, amount, consistency, and odor.
2. No abdominal discomfort before, during, or after defecation.
3. Skin around anus normal.

Unexpected outcomes

1. Feces appeared abnormal. See Table 26–1 on page 601.
2. Increased abdominal discomfort.
3. Bleeding from the anus after defecation.
4. Skin around anus reddened.

References

Aman RA: Treating the patient, not the constipation. *Am J Nurs* (September) 1980; 80:1634–1635.

Blackwell AK, Blackwell W: Relieving gas pains. *Am J Nurs* (January) 1975; 75:66–67.

Hahn, AB, Barkin, RL, Oestreich, SJK: *Pharmacology in Nursing,* 15th ed. Mosby, 1982.

Hogstel M: How to give a safe successful cleansing enema. *Am J Nurs* (May) 1977; 77:816–817.

Lewin D: Care of the constipated patient. *Nurs Times* (March 25) 1976; 72:444–446.

Logio T: Suppository insertion—which end is first? *Nursing 85* (February) 1985; 15:10.

Mager-O'Connor E: How to identify and remove fecal impactions. *Geriatr Nurs* (May/June) 1984; 5:158–161.

Miller J: Helping the aged manage bowel function. *J Gerontol Nurs* (February) 1985; 11:37–41.

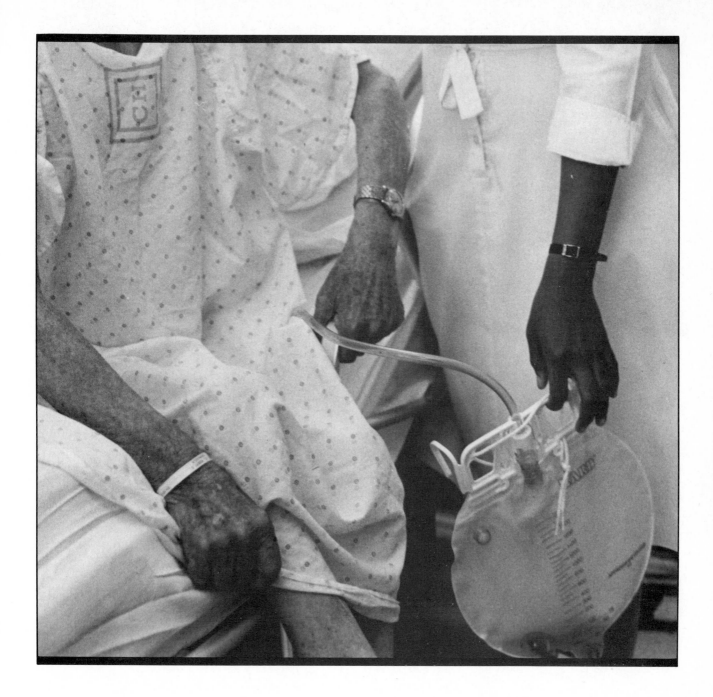

URINARY ELIMINATION

27

The urinary system extends interiorly from the urinary meatus, along the urethra, into the urinary bladder, through the ureters, to the kidneys. This system normally does not contain microorganisms except at the urinary meatus; therefore, any techniques that introduce equipment into the urinary tract must be sterile. A urinary catheterization introduces a catheter into the urinary bladder, and a bladder irrigation also introduces fluid into the bladder. Peritoneal dialysis also requires surgical aseptic technique, although in this instance a catheter and solution (dialysate) are introduced into the peritoneal cavity to remove waste products normally excreted through the urinary system. Specimens of urine are collected routinely from hospital patients for a variety of tests.

Chapter Outline

The Urinary System

Urethral Catheters

Suprapubic Catheters

Urinary Catheterization

■ Technique 27–1 Female Urinary Catheterization Using a Straight Catheter

■ Technique 27–2 Male Urinary Catheterization Using a Straight Catheter

■ Technique 27–3 Inserting a Retention Catheter

■ Technique 27–4 Providing Catheter Care

■ Technique 27–5 Removing a Retention Catheter

■ Technique 27–6 Irrigating a Catheter or a Bladder and Instilling Medication into a Bladder

■ Technique 27–7 Applying and Removing a Drainage Condom

■ Technique 27–8 Suprapubic Catheter Care

Kidney Impairment and Peritoneal Dialysis

■ Technique 27–9 Peritoneal Dialysis

Urine Specimens and Tests

■ Technique 27–10 Collecting a Urine Specimen from an Adult or a Child Who Has Urinary Control

■ Technique 27–11 Collecting a Urine Specimen from an Infant

■ Technique 27–12 Collecting a Timed Urine Specimen

■ Technique 27–13 Collecting a Urine Specimen for Culture and Sensitivity by Clean Catch

■ Technique 27–14 Testing Urine for Specific Gravity, pH, Glucose, Ketones, and Occult Blood

Objectives

Upon completion of this chapter, the student will:

1. Know essential terms and facts about urinary elimination, urethral and suprapubic catheterization, methods to promote or maintain urinary drainage systems, peritoneal dialysis, and collecting and testing urine
   1.1 Define selected terms
   1.2 Identify various types of urinary catheters
   1.3 Identify essential parts of suprapubic catheters
   1.4 Identify various types of urinary drainage systems (eg, open, closed, straight, continuous, intermittent)
   1.5 Identify reasons for using various types of catheters or drainage systems
   1.6 Give the rationale for using sterile technique for catheterization
   1.7 Identify advantages of a suprapubic catheter
   1.8 Identify advantages of an external urinary device (condom)
   1.9 Identify essential aspects of peritoneal dialysis
2. Understand facts about urinary elimination techniques
   2.1 Identify relevant assessment data
   2.2 Identify nursing diagnoses for which the technique may be implemented
   2.3 Identify nursing goals related to the technique
   2.4 Identify anticipated and unanticipated outcomes from assessment data
   2.5 Identify reasons underlying selected steps of the technique
3. Perform urinary elimination techniques safely
   3.1 Assess the patient adequately
   3.2 Collect additional data from appropriate sources
   3.3 Select pertinent nursing goals for the patient
   3.4 Establish relevant outcome criteria for the patient following the technique
   3.5 Collect necessary equipment before the technique
   3.6 Implement interventions to enhance the effectiveness of the technique and enhance the patient's comfort and safety
   3.7 Communicate relevant information to the appropriate persons
   3.8 Determine the evaluative outcomes of the technique
4. Evaluate own performance of specific techniques in a laboratory or clinical setting with the assistance of another
   4.1 Use the performance checklists provided
   4.2 Identify areas of strength and weakness
   4.3 Alter performance in response to own evaluation and that of another

Terms

- **albuminuria** the presence of serum albumin in the urine
- **anuria** failure of the kidneys to produce urine, resulting in total lack of urination
- **catheter** a tube of plastic, rubber, metal, or other material, used to remove or instill fluids into a cavity such as the bladder
- **condom** a rubber or plastic sheathlike device applied externally to the penis that can be used to catch urine and direct it to a drainage bag
- **dialysate** the water-based solution instilled into the peritoneal cavity during peritoneal dialysis; it contains glucose, normal serum electrolytes, and no body waste products
- **dysuria** painful urination
- **enuresis** involuntary urination, particularly at night, after the age of 4 years; bedwetting
- **frequency** voiding more often than usual
- **glycosuria** abnormally high amounts of glucose in the urine
- **hematuria** blood in the urine
- **incontinence** inability to retain urine (urinary incontinence) or feces (anal incontinence)
- **meatus** an opening, such as the opening of the urethra through which urine is excreted
- **micturition** voluntary discharge of urine; voiding; urination
- **nocturia (nycturia)** increased frequency of urination at night

- **oliguria** production of abnormally small amounts of urine by the kidneys
- **orifice** the external opening of a body cavity, such as the urethra or the anus
- **peritoneal dialysis** instillation and removal of a solution from the peritoneal cavity
- **polyuria** production of abnormally large amounts of urine by the kidneys; diuresis
- **proteinuria** protein in the urine
- **pyuria** pus in the urine
- **residual urine** the amount of urine remaining in the bladder after voiding
- **retention** accumulation of urine in the bladder
- **retroperitoneal space** a space behind the peritoneum
- **specific gravity** the weight of a substance compared with the weight of an equal amount of another substance used as a standard (eg, water used as a standard has a specific gravity of 1, while urine has a specific gravity of 1.010 to 1.025)
- **sphincter** a ringlike muscle that closes or constricts a natural orifice such as the urethra
- **suppression** the sudden stoppage of a secretion or an excretion, such as urine
- **suprapubic** above the symphysis pubis
- **trigone** a triangular area at the base of the bladder
- **urgency** a feeling that one *must* void
- **urinalysis** laboratory analysis of the urine
- **void** urinate; micturate

THE URINARY SYSTEM

The urinary tract is one of four routes in the body by which wastes are eliminated. Urine is formed in the kidneys, which are situated in the retroperitoneal space within the body. The kidneys filter from the blood products for which the body has no use. The functional unit of the kidney that carries out this filtration is the nephron. See Figure 27–1. Once urine is formed within the kidney, it is carried into the kidney pelvis, a funnel-shaped tube, and the ureter. The ureters of an adult are about 25 cm (10 in) long. They extend from the kidneys to the urinary bladder and enter the bladder on the posterior aspect of the base. See Figure 27–2.

The urinary bladder is a hollow, muscular organ that lies behind the symphysis pubis. In the male it lies in front of the rectum and above the prostate gland (see Figure 27–3); in the female it lies in front of the uterus and vagina (see Figure 27–4). The base of the bladder is called the *trigone* with the ureter openings marking the posterior corners of the trigone and the opening of the urethra marking the apex. The urethra of the adult female is approximately 4 cm (1.5 in) in length. In the adult male it is about 20 cm (8 in) long. The urethra extends from the bladder to the external surface of the body. This external opening is called the *urinary meatus*. In the female it is located between the labia minora, in front of the vagina and below the clitoris (see Figure 27–5); in the male it is located at the distal end of the penis (see Figure 27–6).

The urethra, in both males and females, has a continuous mucous membrane lining with the bladder and the ureters. Thus an infection of the urethra can readily extend through the urinary tract to the kidneys.

Both male and female urethras have two sphincter

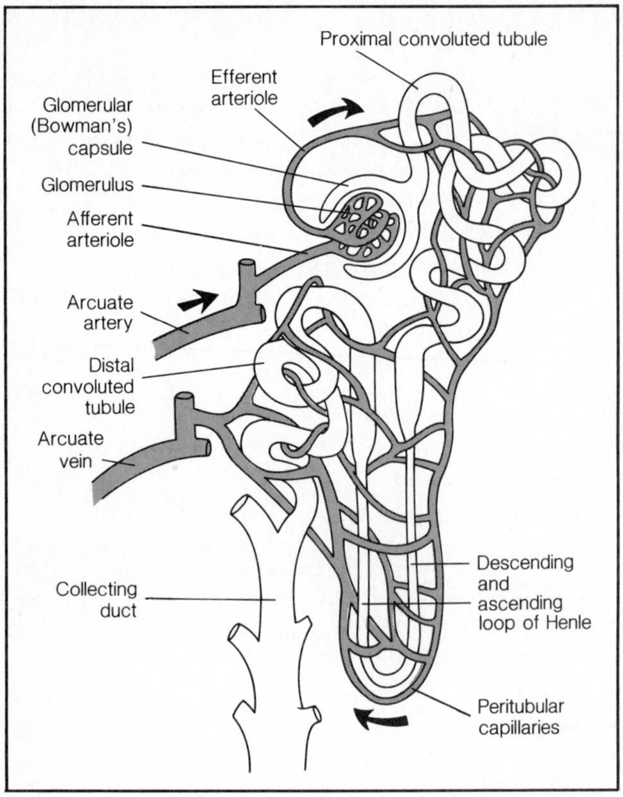

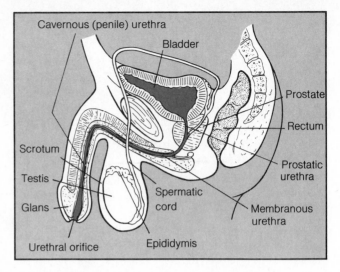

FIGURE 27-3 ■ The male urogenital system.

FIGURE 27-1 ■ The nephron unit of the kidney.

muscles. The internal sphincter muscle is situated at the base of the urinary bladder and is involuntary. The second sphincter muscle is under voluntary control; in the female, it is situated at about the midpoint of the urethra, and, in the male, it is distal to the prostatic portion of the urethra.

Urine collects in the urinary bladder until the individual becomes aware of the urine and consciously releases it, or voids. Babies have no conscious control, and the urine is released after a small amount accumulates in the bladder.

For a description of some of the normal and abnormal characteristics of urine, see Table 27-1.

FIGURE 27-4 ■ The female urogenital system.

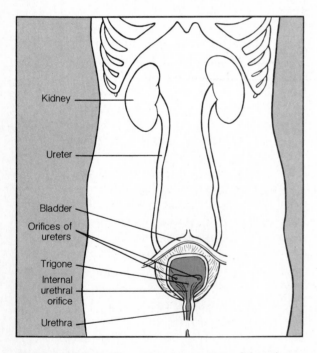

FIGURE 27-2 ■ The anatomic structures of the urinary tract.

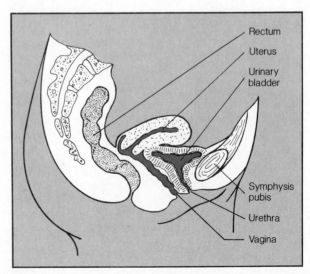

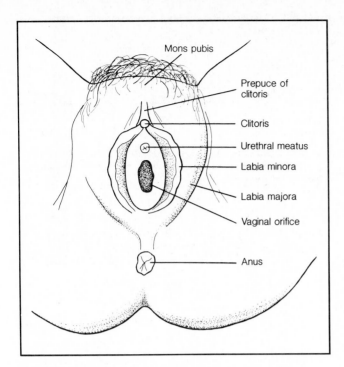

FIGURE 27–5 ■ Location of the female urinary meatus in relation to surrounding structures.

FIGURE 27–6 ■ Location of the male urethral meatus in relation to surrounding structures: **A,** an uncircumcised penis; **B,** a circumcised penis.

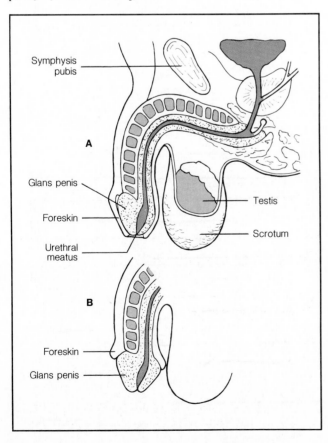

Developmental Variables

Only with maturation of the central nervous system and the body muscles can urinary control be established. This normally takes place between 2 and 4½ years of age. Boys are usually slower than girls in developing this control. Once individuals develop control, they normally maintain it through life unless disease processes occur.

The volume of urine output in a 24-hour period normally increases from the time of birth to adulthood. See Table 27–2. The output of an elderly person, however, may decrease from that of the normal adult. This can be due to the deterioration of the kidneys that comes with age.

Common Problems

Common urinary problems are urinary retention, urinary incontinence, enuresis, and other altered urinary patterns, such as frequency, urgency, polyuria, and urinary suppression.

Retention

Urinary retention is the accumulation of urine in the bladder and inability of the bladder to empty itself. Because urine production continues, retention results in distention of the bladder. An adult urinary bladder normally holds 250 to 450 mL of urine when the micturition reflex is initiated. With urinary retention, some adult bladders may distend to hold 3,000 to 4,000 mL of urine.

Occasionally a patient will have *urinary retention with overflow.* In this situation, the bladder is holding urine, and only the overflow urine is excreted when the pressure of the urine becomes too great for sphincter control. The patient then voids small amounts of urine frequently or dribbles urine, while the bladder remains distended.

Retention can be identified by several clinical signs: discomfort in the pubic area, bladder distention, inability to void or frequent voiding of small volumes (25 to 50 mL), a disproportionately small amount of fluid output in relation to intake, and increasing restlessness and need to void. Bladder distention can be assessed by palpation and percussion above the symphysis pubis.

Incontinence

Urinary incontinence is a temporary or permanent inability of the external sphincter muscles to control the flow of urine from the bladder. It is the opposite of retention. If the bladder is totally emptied during incontinence, it is referred to as *complete incontinence;* if it is not totally emptied, it is referred to as *partial incontinence* (eg, dribbling).

Incontinence is commonly seen in elderly patients as part of the aging process. It is also seen in patients who have enlarged prostate glands, spinal cord injuries,

TABLE 27-1 ■ Characteristics of Normal and Abnormal Urine

Characteristic	Normal	Abnormal	Possible causes
Amount in 24 hours (adult) (see Table 27–2)	1,200–1,500 mL	Under 1,200 mL	Decreased fluid intake
			Kidney failure
		Over 1,500 mL	Diabetes
			Diuretics
			Increased fluid intake
Color	Straw, amber	Dark amber	Concentrated urine, eg, as result of insufficient fluid intake
	Transparent	Cloudy	Infectious process
		Dark orange	Drugs, eg, pyridium
		Red or dark brown	Disease process causing blood in urine
Consistency	Clear liquid	Mucous plugs, viscid, thick	Infectious process
Odor	Faint aromatic	Offensive	Infectious process
Sterility	No microorganisms present	Microorganisms present	Infection of the urinary tract
pH	4.5 to 8	Under 4.5	Urinary tract infections
		Over 8	Uncontrolled diabetes
			Starvation
			Dehydration
Specific gravity	1.010 to 1.025	Under 1.010	Diabetes mellitus
			Nephrosis
			Excessive water loss
		Over 1.025	Diabetes insipidus
			Severe renal damage
Glucose	Not present	Present	Diabetes mellitus
			Brain injury
			Myocardial infarction
Ketone bodies (acetone)	Not present	Present	Diabetic coma
			Starvation
			Prolonged vomiting
Blood	Not present	Occult	Kidney disease
		Bright red	Hemorrhage

TABLE 27-2 ■ Average Daily Excretion of Urine by Age

Age	Amount (mL)
1–2 days	15–60
3–10 days	100–300
10 days–2 months	250–450
2 months–1 year	400–500
1–3 years	500–600
3–5 years	600–700
5–8 years	700–1,000
8–14 years	800–1,400
14 years through adulthood	1,500
Older adulthood	1,500 or less

urinary tract infections, bladder spasms, or loss of consciousness, or who are taking medications that interfere with sphincter control, eg, narcotics and sedatives. Two specific kinds of incontinence are distinguished:

1. *Stress incontinence* is the inability to control urine flow at a time when the intraabdominal pressure increases, for example, when coughing, sneezing, or even laughing. It is generally caused by inability of the external sphincter muscle to close. It is seen in children who have not yet learned to control the external sphincter and in adults who have a disease process interfering with the sphincter action.

2. *Urge incontinence* occurs when the patient's need to void is so urgent that he or she cannot get to the toilet in time.

This kind of incontinence is commonly caused by lower urinary tract infections or bladder spasms.

Enuresis

Enuresis (bedwetting) occurs most often in children. When wetting occurs in a child over the age of 4, it generally occurs at night and is referred to as *nocturnal enuresis*. It may happen once or several times during the night. Some children may wet in the daytime during periods of excitement or when absorbed with play, particularly on cold, damp days. Other children may wet because they have not yet learned complete bladder control. In school-age children, wetting rarely occurs during the school hours but sometimes occurs during play at recess, during the lunch hour, or after school. Because of absorption in play, the child does not realize the need to urinate until it is too late to reach a toilet.

Other altered urinary patterns

Frequency and nocturia Frequency is generally considered voiding at frequent intervals, that is, more often than usual. The frequency of voiding normally increases with an increase in fluids. Frequency without an increase in fluid intake may be the result of *cystitis* (an acutely inflamed bladder), stress, or pressure on the bladder, eg, because of pregnancy. The total amount of urine voided may be normal, since the amounts voided each time are small, such as 50 to 100mL.

Nocturia or nycturia is increased frequency at night that is not a result of increased fluid intake. Like frequency, it is usually expressed in number of times the person voids, for example, "nocturia × 4."

Urgency Urgency is the feeling that the person *must* void. There may or may not be a great deal of urine in the bladder, but the person feels a need to void immediately. Often the person hurries to the toilet in fear of being incontinent if he or she does not urinate. Urgency accompanies psychologic stress and irritation of the trigone and urethra. It is also common in young children who have poor external sphincter control.

Dysuria Dysuria is either painful or difficult voiding. It can accompany a *stricture* (decrease in caliber) of the urethra, urinary infections, and injury to the bladder and/or urethra. Often patients will say that they have to push to void or that burning accompanies or follows voiding. Burning during micturition is often due to an irritated urethra; burning following urination may be the result of a bladder infection when the irritated rugae (ridges) of the trigone rub together. The burning may be described as severe, like a hot poker, or more subdued, like a sunburn.

Polyuria Polyuria or diuresis is the production of abnormally large amounts of urine by the kidneys, such as 2,500 mL/day, without an increased fluid intake. This can happen as a result of diabetes mellitus, hormone imbalances (eg, deficiency of antidiuretic hormone, or ADH), and chronic kidney disease.

URETHRAL CATHETERS

Catheters are tubes commonly made of rubber or plastic, although certain types are made of woven silk or metal. Two categories of urinary catheters are straight catheters and retention catheters. The *straight* or *Robinson catheter* is a single-lumen tube with a small eye or opening about 1¼ cm (½ in) from the insertion tip. See Figure 27–7, *A*.

The *retention* or *Foley catheter* contains a second, smaller tube throughout its length on the inside. This tube is connected to a balloon near the insertion tip. After catheter insertion, the balloon is inflated to hold the catheter in place within the bladder. The outside end of the retention catheter is bifurcated, that is, it has two openings, one to drain the urine, the other to inflate the balloon. See Figure 27–7, *B*.

FIGURE 27–7 ■ Two types of commonly used catheters: **A,** a straight (Robinson) catheter; **B,** a retention (Foley) catheter with the balloon inflated.

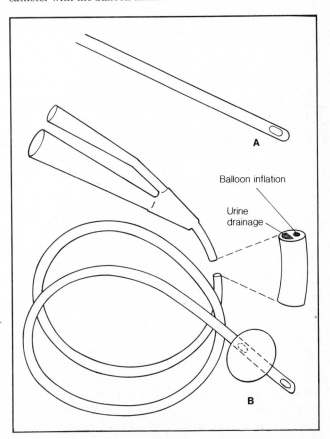

Balloon inflation

Urine drainage

A

B

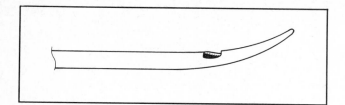

FIGURE 27–8 ■ The catheter coudé, a urethral catheter with a curved tip.

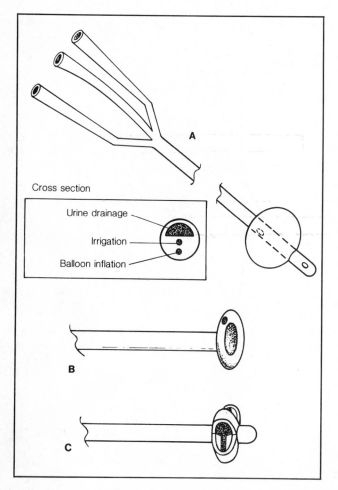

Cross section

Urine drainage

Irrigation

Balloon inflation

FIGURE 27–9 ■ Three types of retention catheters: **A,** a three-way Foley; **B,** a de Pezzer (mushroom); **C,** a Malecot.

Another type of straight catheter is the *catheter coudé* (elbowed catheter), which has a curved tip. See Figure 27–8. This is sometimes used for elderly men who have a hypertrophied prostate, because its passage is often less traumatic to the gland than other types of straight catheters. It is somewhat stiff and is more readily controlled.

There are several other types of retention catheters. One that is frequently used for a patient requiring continual or periodic bladder irrigations is the *three-way Foley catheter.* It is similar to the two-way Foley catheter described earlier, except that it has a third channel through which sterile fluid can flow into the urinary bladder. From the bladder, the fluid then flows through a second channel into a receptacle. Other types are the *de Pezzer* or *mushroom catheter,* which has a single channel and a noncollapsible mushroom tip, and the *Malecot catheter,* which has a single channel and a tip with two or four wings. The wings collapse when traction is applied, for example, when the catheter is removed from the urinary bladder. See Figure 27–9.

Catheters are sized by the diameter of the lumen and are graded on a French scale of numbers; the larger the number, the larger the lumen. Small sizes, such as #8 or #10, are used for children; #14, #16, and #18 are commonly used for adults. Men frequently require a larger size than women. Only even numbers are available.

The balloons of retention catheters are sized by the volume of fluid or air used to inflate them. The two commonly used sizes are 5 mL and 30 mL balloons. The size of the balloon is indicated on the catheter along with the diameter, eg, "#18 Fr.—5 mL."

SUPRAPUBIC CATHETERS

A suprapubic catheter is inserted through the abdominal wall above the symphysis pubis into the urinary bladder. See Figure 27–10. The physician inserts the catheter using local anesthesia, in the patient's bed unit, or using general anesthesia in conjunction with bladder or vaginal surgery, in the operating room. The catheter may be secured in place either with sutures or with a commercial retention body seal, or with both sutures and a body seal. It is then attached to a closed drainage system. When the catheter is removed, the muscle layers of the bladder contract over the insertion site to seal off the opening. See Technique 27–8 on page 646 for care of a suprapubic catheter.

URINARY CATHETERIZATION

Urinary catheterization is the introduction of a catheter through the urethra into the urinary bladder. This is usually performed only when absolutely necessary, since certain hazards are incurred. Because the urinary structures are normally sterile except at the end of the urethra, the danger exists of introducing microorganisms into the bladder. This hazard is greatest for patients who have lowered resistance due to disease processes. Once an infection is introduced into the bladder, it can ascend the ureters and eventually involve the kidneys. Even after the catheter has been inserted and left in place for a time, the hazard of infection remains, since pathogens can be introduced through the catheter lumen. Thus, strict surgical aseptic technique is used for catheterizations.

Another hazard is trauma, particularly in the male

FIGURE 27–10 ■ A suprapubic catheter in place.

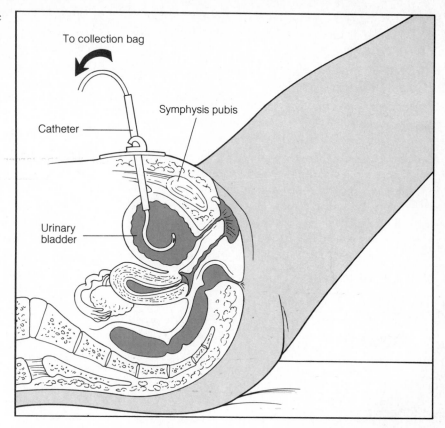

patient, whose urethra is longer and more tortuous. It is important to insert a catheter along the normal contour of the urethra. Damage to the urethra can occur if the catheter is forced through strictures or at an incorrect angle. For females, the urethra lies posteriorly, then takes a slightly anterior direction toward the bladder. See Figure 27–4 on page 620. For males, the urethra is normally curved (see Figure 27–3 on page 620), but it can be straightened by elevating the penis to a position perpendicular to the body.

TECHNIQUE 27–1 ■ Female Urinary Catheterization Using a Straight Catheter 🏠

■ Assessment

1. Determine when the patient last voided and the amount. Volumes of less than 30 mL or more than 500 mL per hour must be reported immediately to the responsible nurse.

2. Assess for urinary retention, which is indicated by:

   a. A distended urinary bladder. Palpate or percuss the bladder just above the symphysis pubis. To palpate the bladder, indent the skin more than 1.3 cm (0.5 in) by pressing the fingers of one hand upon the fingers of the other. See Figure 27–11. This increases the pressure for palpation. To percuss the bladder, place the middle finger of one hand against the skin, and strike it sharply with

FIGURE 27–11

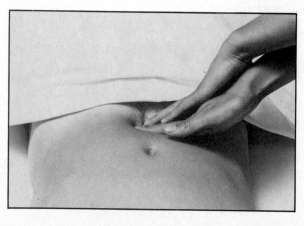

the middle finger of the other hand. The resulting sound when the bladder is full will be duller than normal.

b. The voiding of only small amounts, eg, 30 to 50 mL each hour.

c. Restlessness or abdominal discomfort.

3. Assess for evidence of urinary infection, eg, fever, urgency, lower back pain, or frequency.

4. Determine whether the patient can lie quietly and maintain the appropriate position during the catheterization so that you can maintain the sterility of the equipment during exposure of the urinary meatus (particularly in females). Assistance may be required for a restless patient. See also Technique 10–15 on page 225.

Other data include:

1. The physician's order for the catheterization.

2. If the patient is retaining urine, whether the order specifies a maximum amount of urine to be removed during the catheterization. Usually no more than 750 mL is removed at one time, to avoid redirection of the blood supply to the pelvic blood vessels, leading to hypovolemic shock.

3. Any direction on the patient's chart about the type of catheter to use.

4. The size of catheter to use. Consult the nursing care plan.

5. Relevant information on the patient's chart, such as an unusual placement of the urethral orifice. This is particularly important for patients who have had vaginal repairs.

■ Nursing Diagnosis

Nursing diagnoses that may indicate the need for a urinary catheterization include:

1. Alteration in pattersn of urinary elimination (retention) related to:
   a. Obstruction at the bladder neck
   b. Infection
   c. Inflammatory process
   d. Loss of muscle tone

■ Planning

Nursing goals

1. To relieve discomfort due to bladder distention and to provide gradual decompression of a distended bladder

2. To assess the amount of residual urine if the bladder is emptied incompletely

3. To obtain a urine specimen to assess the presence of abnormal constituents and the characteristics of the urine

4. To empty the bladder completely prior to surgery, to prevent inadvertent injury to adjacent organs such as the rectum or vagina

Equipment

1. A sterile catheterization kit containing:
   a. Gloves.
   b. Drapes to protect the bed and to provide a sterile field.
   c. A fenestrated drape (optional) to place over the perineum.
   d. An antiseptic solution recommended by agency policy, eg, aqueous benzalkonium chloride (Zephiran Chloride) 1:750, to clean the labia and urinary meatus.
   e. Cotton balls or gauze squares to apply the antiseptic.
   f. Forceps to apply the antiseptic.
   g. A water-soluble lubricant for the insertion tip of the catheter to facilitate insertion and reduce the chance of trauma to the mucous membrane lining the urethra.
   h. A catheter of appropriate size (#14 or #16).
   i. A receptacle for the urine. Often the base of the kit serves this purpose.
   j. A specimen container if a specimen is to be acquired.

2. A bag or receptacle for disposal of the cotton balls.

3. A flashlight or lamp to provide light on the genital area.

4. A mask, clean gown, and cap, if required by agency policy.

5. A bath blanket.

6. Soap, a basin of warm water, a washcloth, and a towel.

7. Disposable gloves (optional).

■ Intervention

1. Obtain assistance if the patient requires help to maintain the required position.

2. Explain the technique to the patient, and provide support as needed. Some patients fear pain and need to learn that they will experience no pain, only a slight sensation of pressure.

3. Provide privacy. Exposure of the genitals is embarrassing to most patients.

   Rationale Relieving the patient's tension can facilitate insertion of the catheter, because the urinary sphincters are more likely to be relaxed.

4. Assist the patient to a supine position with knees flexed and thighs externally rotated. Pillows can be used to support the knees and elevate the buttocks.

   Rationale Raising the patient's pelvis gives the nurse a better view of the urinary meatus.

5. Drape the patient. Use a bath blanket to cover the patient's chest and abdomen. Pull the patient's gown up over her hips. Cover her legs and feet with the bed sheet or another blanket. Place it diagonally on the patient with a corner around each foot. See Figure 27–12.

6. Wash the perineal–genital area with warm water and soap; rinse and dry. Disposable gloves may be used.

   Rationale Cleanliness reduces the possibility of introducing microorganisms with the catheter. Appropriate rinsing removes soap that could inhibit the action of the antiseptic used later.

7. Adjust the light for vision of the urinary meatus. It may be necessary to use a flashlight or to place a gooseneck lamp at the foot of the bed, so that it focuses on the perineal area.

8. Put on a mask if required by agency policy. Some agencies also advocate the use of a clean gown and a surgical cap if the nurse's hair is long.

9. At the patient's bedside, open the sterile kit and the catheter, if it is packaged separately, and don the sterile gloves (see Technique 7–6). The kit can be placed between the patient's thighs.

10. Drape the patient with the sterile drapes, being careful to protect the sterility of your gloves. Use the first drape as an underpad, and place it under the buttocks. Keep the underpad edges cuffed over your gloves to prevent contamination of the gloves against the patient's buttocks. If the other drape is fenestrated, place it over the perineal area exposing only the labia. Place thigh drapes from the side farthest to the side nearest you. If an underpad is not available, place the two thigh drapes so that they overlap between the patient's thighs.

11. Pour the antiseptic solution over the cotton balls, if they are not already prepared.

12. Lubricate the insertion tip of the catheter liberally. Place it aside in the sterile container ready for use.

    Rationale Water-soluble lubricant facilitates insertion of the catheter by reducing friction. It is important to lubricate at this point, because the nurse will subsequently have only one sterile hand available.

13. Separate the labia majora with the thumb and index or other finger of one hand, and clean the labia minora on each side using forceps and cotton balls soaked in antiseptic. Use a new swab for each stroke, and move downward from the pubic area to the

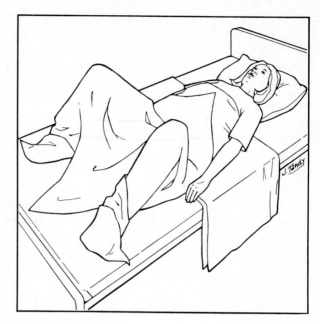

FIGURE 27–12

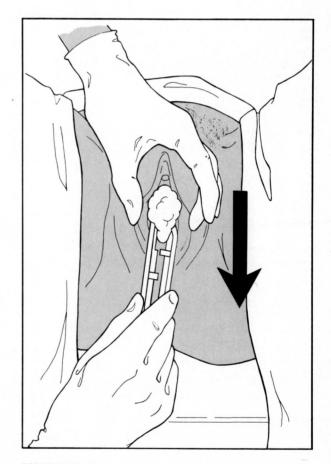

FIGURE 27–13

anus. See Figure 27–13. Then separate the labia minora with two other fingers, still using the same hand. See Figure 27–14.

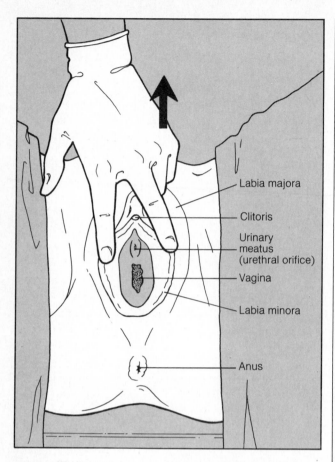

FIGURE 27–14

Rationale The hand that touches the patient becomes contaminated. It remains in position exposing the urinary meatus, while the other hand remains sterile holding the sterile forceps. Cleaning from anterior to posterior cleans from the area of least contamination to the area of greatest contamination.

14. Expose the urinary meatus adequately by retracting the tissue of the labia minora in an upward (anterior) direction. See Figure 27–14. Clean first from the meatus downward and then on either side, using a new swab for each stroke. Once the meatus is cleaned, do not allow the labia to close over it.

    Rationale Keeping the labia apart prevents the risk of contaminating the urinary meatus.

15. Assess any signs, such as excoriation of the tissues surrounding the urinary meatus, swelling of the urinary meatus, or the presence of discharge around the urinary meatus.

16. Place the drainage end of the catheter in the urine receptacle. Then pick up the insertion end of the catheter with your uncontaminated, sterile, gloved hand, holding it 5 to 8 cm (2 to 3 in) from the insertion tip for an adult and 2 to 3 cm (1 in) for

1½ – 2" ♀

an infant or small child. If agency policy requires, use sterile forceps to pick up the catheter.

Rationale The adult female urethra is approximately 4 cm (1.5 in) long. The nurse holds the catheter far enough from the end to allow full insertion into the bladder and to maintain control of the tip of the catheter so it will not accidentally become contaminated.

17. Gently insert the catheter into the urinary meatus about 5 cm (2 in) for an adult, 2.5 cm (1 in) for a small child, or until urine flows. Insert the catheter in the direction of the urethra. If the catheter meets resistance during insertion, do not force it. Ask the patient to take deep breaths. If this does not relieve the resistance, discontinue the procedure, and report the problem to the responsible nurse. Exercise caution to prevent the catheter tip from becoming contaminated. If it becomes contaminated, discard it.

    Rationale Forceful pressure exerted against the urethra can produce trauma. Deep breaths by the patient may relax the external sphincter.

18. When the urine flows, transfer your hand from the labia to the catheter to hold it in place at the meatus.

19. Collect a urine specimen. Pinch the catheter, and transfer the drainage end of it into the sterile specimen bottle. Usually 30 mL of urine is sufficient for a specimen.

20. Empty the bladder or drain the amount of urine specified in the order. For adult patients experiencing urinary retention, it is recommended that no more than 750 mL be removed at one time. Remove the catheter slowly.

    Rationale Removing large amounts of urine too quickly can induce engorgement of the pelvic blood vessels and hypovolemic shock. Usually the physician prescribes the amount to be removed and times at which the remaining urine is to be withdrawn.

21. Dry the patient's perineum with a towel or drape.

22. Assess the urine for color, clarity, odor, and the presence of any abnormal constituents, such as blood. Measure the amount of urine.

23. Send the specimen to the laboratory.

24. Record the catheterization, the reason for it, any pertinent observations, and whether a specimen was taken and sent to the laboratory.

Sample Recording

Date	Time	Notes
1/26/87	1900	C/o pubic discomfort. Has not voided since surgery. Bladder palpable above symphysis pubis. Is restless. Catheterized for 650 mL clear amber urine. Discomfort relieved. Less restless.———Sylvia F. Tompkins, RN

Size of cath used States

■ Evaluation

Expected outcomes

1. Normal color, odor, and consistency of urine
2. Residual urine of 30 mL
3. Decreased bladder distention

Unexpected outcomes

1. Abnormal color, odor, or consistency of urine
2. Residual urine over 50 mL

3. Bladder distention unchanged
4. Restlessness
5. Pubic discomfort

Upon obtaining an unexpected outcome:

1. Report your findings to the responsible nurse and/or physician.
2. Adjust the nursing care plan appropriately, eg, reassess abdominal discomfort in 15 minutes.

TECHNIQUE 27–2   ■   Male Urinary Catheterization Using a Straight Catheter 🏠

■ **Assessment**   See Technique 27–1 on page 625.

■ **Nursing Diagnosis**   See Technique 27–1 on page 626.

■ **Planning**

Nursing goals   See Technique 27–1 on page 626.

Equipment

See Technique 27–1 on page 626. A #16 or #18 catheter is usually used for an adult male.

■ **Intervention**

1. Follow Technique 27–1, steps 1–3.
2. Assist the patient to a supine position with the knees slightly flexed and the thighs slightly apart.
   Rationale This allows greater relaxation of the adbominal and perineal muscles and permits easier insertion of the catheter.
3. Drape the patient by folding the top bedclothes down so that the penis is exposed and the thighs are covered. Use a bath blanket to cover the patient's chest and abdomen.
4. Follow Technique 27–1, steps 6–8.
5. Open the sterile tray, and don the sterile gloves (see Technique 7–6). Place the tray directly on the patient's thighs, if he is not restless.
6. Place a drape under the penis and a second drape

above the penis over the pubic area. See Figure 27–15. If a fenestrated drape is available, place it over the penis and pubic area, exposing only the penis.

7. Pour the antiseptic solution over the cotton balls if they are not already prepared.
8. Lubricate the insertion tip of the catheter liberally for about 5 to 7 cm (2 to 3 in). Place it aside on the sterile tray ready for insertion.
   Rationale Water-soluble lubricant facilitates insertion of the catheter by reducing friction. It is important to do this step before cleaning, since the nurse will subsequently have only one sterile hand available.

FIGURE 27–15

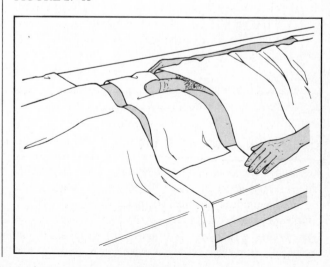

9. Clean the urinary meatus with antiseptic swabs. Grasp the penis firmly behind the glans, and spread the meatus between the thumb and forefinger. Retract the foreskin of an uncircumcised male. The hand holding the penis is now considered contaminated. With the other hand, use sterile forceps to pick up a swab. Clean the meatus first, and then wipe the tissue surrounding the meatus in a circular fashion. Discard each swab after only one wipe.

Rationale To avoid stimulating an erection, firm pressure rather than light pressure is used to grasp the penis. Using forceps maintains the sterility of the nurse's glove. *Use @ least 3 cotton Balls*

10. Place the drainage end of the catheter in the urine receptacle. Then pick up the insertion end of the catheter with your uncontaminated, sterile, gloved hand, holding it about 8 to 10 cm (3 to 4 in) from the insertion tip for an adult or about 2.5 cm (1 in) for a baby or small boy. In some agencies the catheter is picked up with forceps.

FIGURE 27–16

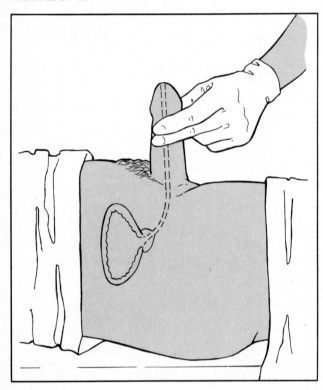

Rationale The male urethra is approximately 20 cm (8 in) long. The nurse holds the catheter far enough from the end to maintain control of the tip of the catheter so it will not accidentally become contaminated.

11. To insert the catheter, lift the penis to a position perpendicular to the body (90° angle) and exert slight traction (pulling or tension upward). See Figure 27–16. Insert the catheter steadily about 20 cm (8 in) or until urine begins to flow. To bypass slight resistance at the sphincters, twist the catheter or wait until the sphincter relaxes. Have the patient take deep breaths or try to void. If difficult resistance is met, discontinue the procedure, and report the problem to the responsible nurse.

Rationale Lifting the penis perpendicular to the body straightens the downward curvature of the urethra. Slight resistance is normally encountered at the external and internal urethral sphincters. Deep breaths by the patient can help to relax the external sphincter. Forceful pressure exerted against a major resistance can traumatize the urethra.

12. While the urine flows, lower the penis and transfer your hand to hold the catheter in place at the meatus.

13. Collect a urine specimen (if required) after the urine has flowed for a few seconds. Pinch the catheter, and transfer the drainage end of the catheter into the sterile specimen bottle. Usually 30 mL of urine is sufficient for a specimen.

14. Empty the bladder or drain the amount of urine specified in the order. For adult patients experiencing urinary retention, it is recommended that no more than 750 mL be removed at one time. Remove the catheter slowly.

Rationale Removing large amounts of urine too quickly can induce engorgement of the pelvic blood vessels and hypovolemic shock. Usually the physician prescribes the amount to be removed and times at which the remaining urine is to be withdrawn.

15. Dry the patient's penis with a towel or drape.

16. Follow Technique 27–1, steps 22–24.

■ **Evaluation** See Technique 27–1 on page 629.

Measuring Residual Urine

Residual urine is normally nil or only a few milliliters. However, whenever there is a bladder outlet obstruction (eg, enlargement of the prostate gland) or loss of bladder muscle tone, there can be large amounts of residual urine. Loss of bladder tone may be the result of spinal or cranial neurologic disorders affecting the nerve and muscle regulation of the bladder, following pelvic surgery, or prolonged indwelling catheterization of the bladder. The consequence of incomplete emptying of the bladder is urinary stasis and, ultimately, infection.

Measurement of residual urine may be prescribed by the physician or responsible nurse in accordance with agency policy. Incomplete emptying of the bladder may be suspected when the patient experiences frequency and when only small amounts of urine are voided at a time (eg, 100 mL in an adult). The purposes of measuring the residual urine are: (a) to determine the degree to which the bladder is emptying, and (b) to assess the need to establish therapy that will empty the bladder (eg, insertion of a retention catheter).

To measure the residual urine, the nurse asks the patient to void and then immediately catheterizes the patient (see Techniques 27–1 and 27–2). Both the amount of urine voided and the amount of residual urine are measured and recorded. Generally, if the amount of residual urine exceeds 50 mL, an indwelling catheter is inserted.

TECHNIQUE 27–3 ■ Inserting a Retention Catheter

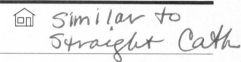 *Similar to Straight Cath*

The procedure for inserting a urinary retention catheter is similar to the basic catheterization procedure, with differences occurring primarily after the catheter is inserted. Prior to insertion of the catheter, the nurse needs to test the balloon of the retention catheter to see that it is intact, and following the insertion, the nurse inflates the balloon and attaches a urinary drainage system.

■ **Assessment** See Technique 27–1 on page 625.

■ **Nursing Diagnosis** See Technique 27–1 on page 626.

■ **Planning**

Nursing goals

1. To manage incontinence when all other measures have failed
2. To provide for intermittent or continuous bladder drainage and irrigation
3. To prevent urine from contacting an incision after perineal surgery
4. To facilitate accurate measurement of urinary output for critically ill patients whose output needs to be monitored hourly

Equipment

1. A sterile retention catheter set containing:
   a. Gloves.
   b. Drapes to protect the bed and to provide a sterile field.
   c. Antiseptic solution to clean the labia minora or glans penis and the urinary meatus.
   d. Cotton balls or gauze squares.
   e. Forceps.
   f. A water-soluble lubricant for the catheter.

   g. A retention catheter, #14 or #16 for adults, #8 or #10 for children. The catheter may be supplied separately from the sterile set in some agencies. The catheter may be attached to sterile tubing and a receptacle for the urine (closed drainage system). See Figure 27–17. If these are not in the set, acquire a drainage bag and tubing.
   h. A prefilled syringe to inflate the balloon of the catheter. Sterile water is often used.
   i. A receptacle for the urine, generally the base of the set.
   j. A specimen container and label.
2. Nonallergenic tape to secure the catheter to the patient.
3. A safety pin or clip to attach the catheter tubing to the bedding.
4. Two bath blankets or other coverings.
5. Soap, a basin of warm water, a washcloth, and a towel.
6. A flashlight or gooseneck lamp (optional)
7. A gown, mask, and cap, if required by agency policy.

between legs on BED

■ **Intervention**

1. Explain to the patient the reason for inserting the retention catheter, how long it will be in place, and the ways in which the urinary drainage equipment needs to be handled to maintain and facilitate the drainage of urine. Reassure the patient that the procedure is painless. Some patients fear spillage of urine when they experience the urge to void during insertion of the catheter and for a short period of time after the catheter is in place. Reassure these patients that the catheter drains the urine and that the urge to void will disappear.
2. Follow Technique 27–1, steps 3–7, for the female patient, or Technique 27–2, steps 1–4, for the male patient.

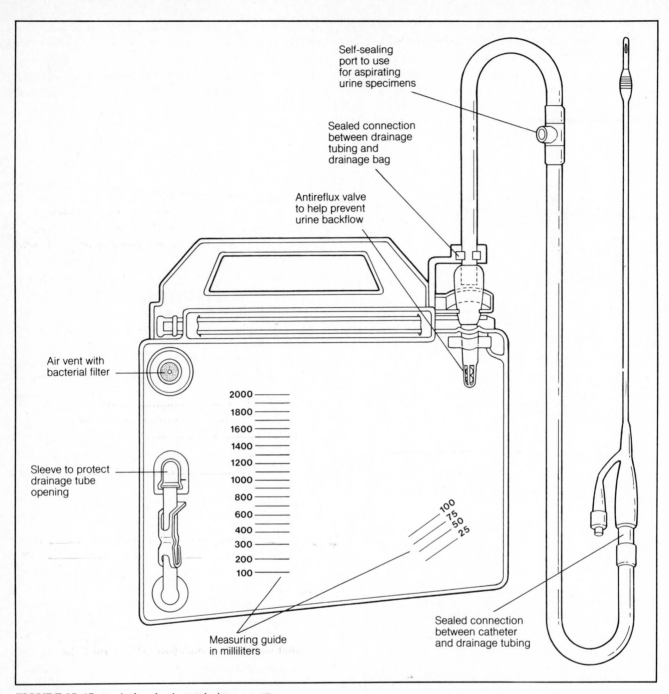

FIGURE 27-17 ■ A closed urinary drainage system.

3. Don a cap (if required) and mask. Wash your hands, using surgical aseptic technique. In some agencies, gowns are required and are donned after the hand wash.

For a female patient

4. Open the sterile equipment, and don the sterile gloves. Place the tray between the patient's thighs if she can assume the position comfortably.

5. Drape the patient with the sterile drapes, being careful to protect the sterility of the gloves. Use the

first drape as an underpad, placing it under the patient's buttocks with the edges cuffed over your gloves to prevent contamination of the gloves. If an underpad is not available, place two drapes over the thighs so that they overlap between the thighs. If the other drape is fenestrated, place it over the pubic area exposing only the patient's labia.

6. Test the catheter balloon by attaching the prefilled syringe to the balloon valve and injecting the fluid. The balloon should inflate appropriately and should not leak. Withdraw the fluid, and set aside the catheter with the syringe attached for later use. If

the balloon leaks or does not inflate adequately, replace the catheter. In such a case, withdraw the fluid, and detach the syringe for later use. Ask another nurse to obtain a second catheter and open the package for you, then test the new balloon.

or

Remove the equipment and obtain another catheter. Then start the Intervention over with the new sterile equipment.

7. Pour the antiseptic solution over the cotton balls or gauzes if they are not already prepared.

8. Lubricate the insertion tip of the catheter liberally. Place it aside on the sterile tray ready for insertion. Remove the cap from the specimen container, if needed.

Rationale Water-soluble lubricant facilitates insertion of the catheter by reducing friction. It is important to do this step before cleaning the perineum, since the nurse will subsequently have only one sterile hand available.

9. Separate the labia majora with the thumb and fourth finger of one hand. Clean the labia minora on each side with antiseptic, using forceps and cotton balls or gauzes. Use a swab only once, and move downward. Then separate the labia minora with your index and middle fingers, still using the same hand. Expose the urinary meatus adequately by retracting the tissue of the labia minora in an upward (anterior) direction. See Figure 27-14 earlier. Clean first from the meatus downward and then on either side. Once the meatus is cleaned, do not allow the labia to close over it.

Rationale This cleans from the area of least contamination to the area of greatest contamination. The hand that touches the patient becomes contaminated. It remains in position exposing the urinary meatus while the other hand remains sterile. Keeping the labia apart prevents contamination of the urinary meatus.

10. Place the drainage end of the catheter in the urine receptacle. Pick up the insertion end of the catheter with the sterile, gloved hand (or forceps, if that is agency practice), holding it approximately 5 to 8 cm (2 to 3 in) from the tip for an adult, or 2 to 3 cm (1 in) for an infant or small child.

Rationale The adult female urethra is approximately 4 cm (1.5 in) long.

11. Gently insert the catheter into the urinary meatus about 5 cm (2 in) for an adult, 2.5 cm (1 in) for a small child, or until urine flows. Insert the catheter in the direction of the urethra. If the catheter meets resistance during insertion, do not force it. Ask the patient to take deep breaths. If this does not relieve the resistance, discontinue the procedure, and report the problem to the responsible nurse.

Rationale Pressure exerted against the urethra can produce trauma. Deep breaths may help relax the external sphincter.

12. When the urine flows, transfer your hand from the labia to the catheter, 5 cm (2 in) from the urethral orifice, to hold it in place.

13. After the urine has flowed for a few seconds, collect a urine specimen (usually 30 mL), if required. Pinch the catheter, and transfer the drainage end of it into the sterile specimen bottle.

14. Insert the catheter an additional 2.5 to 5 cm (1 to 2 in) beyond the point at which urine began to flow.

Rationale The balloon of the catheter is located behind the opening at the insertion tip, and sufficient space needs to be provided to inflate the balloon. This ensures that the balloon is inflated inside the bladder and not in the urethra, where it could produce trauma.

15. Inflate the balloon by injecting the contents of the prefilled syringe into the valve of the catheter. See Figure 27-18, *A*. Placement of the catheter and balloon in a male patient is shown in Figure 27-18, *B*. If the patient complains of discomfort or pain during the balloon inflation, withdraw the fluid, insert the catheter a little farther, and inflate the balloon again. Insert no more fluid than the balloon size indicates (eg, 5 mL or 30 mL), and remove the syringe. A special valve prevents backflow of the fluid out of the catheter. When 30-mL balloons are used, some agency policies state that only 15 mL of fluid is injected for inflation.

16. When the balloon is safely inflated, apply slight tension on the catheter until you feel resistance. Then move the catheter slightly back into the bladder.

Rationale Resistance indicates that the catheter balloon is inflated appropriately, and the catheter is well anchored in the bladder. Moving the catheter slightly back into the bladder keeps the balloon from exerting undue pressure on the neck of the bladder.

17. If the drainage bag and tubing are not already attached to the end of the catheter, remove the protective cap or plug from the tubing, and attach the catheter. Handle the ends of both the catheter and the drainage tube at least 2.5 cm (1 in) away from their tips.

Rationale The sterility of the tips of both the catheter and the drainage tube must be maintained so that microorganisms do not enter the system and move to the bladder.

18. Ensure that the emptying base of the drainage bag is closed. Secure the drainage bag to the bed frame using the hook or strap provided. Suspend the bag off the floor, but keep it below the level of the patient's bladder. See Figure 27-19.

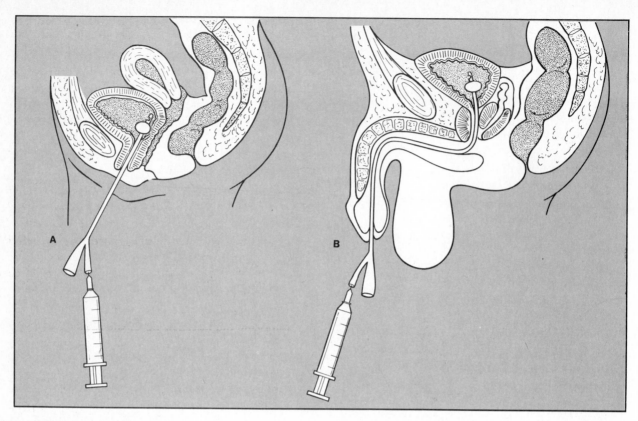

FIGURE 27–18

Rationale Urine flows by gravity from the bladder to the drainage bag. The bag should be off the floor so that the emptying portion does not become grossly contaminated.

19. Anchor the catheter with nonallergenic tape to the inside of the patient's thigh. See Figure 27–19.

Rationale Taping restricts the movement of the catheter, thus reducing friction and irritation in the urethra when the patient moves.

20. Coil the drainage tubing beside the patient so that the tubing runs in a straight line down to the drainage bag, and fasten it to the bedclothes with tape, a tubing clamp, or a safety pin. See Figure 27–19.

Rationale The drainage tubing should not loop below its entry into the drainage bag, since this impedes the flow of urine by gravity.

21. Dry the patient's perineum with a towel or drape.

22. Record the time and date of the catheterization; the reason; pertinent observations, such as the color and amount of urine; whether a specimen was taken and sent to the laboratory; whether all urine was emptied from the bladder; and the patient's response.

size #16

23. Adjust the nursing care plan to include the following care in relation to the retention catheter:

 a. Measure fluid intake and output, and compare the two. Empty the drainage bag regularly. Apply povidone-iodine to the end of the drainage tube before replacing it in the spout.

 b. Encourage the patient to take large amounts of fluids orally, as much as 3,000 mL daily if permitted.

 c. Provide perineal–genital and catheter care twice daily or as needed (eg, 0900 and 2100 hours). Avoid using powders or lotions. If the meatus is excoriated, an antibacterial ointment may be applied.

 d. Teach the patient about care of the tubing, fluid intake, and perineal–genital care.

24. Observe the flow of urine every two or three hours, and note color, odor, and any abnormal constituents. If blood clots are present, check the catheter more frequently to ascertain whether it is plugged.

25. Frequently observe the patency of the drainage system:

 a. Ensure that there are no obstructions in the drainage. For example, check that there are no kinks in the tubing, the patient is not lying on the tubing, and the tubing is not clogged with mucus or blood.

 b. Check that there is no tension on the catheter or tubing, that the catheter is securely taped to the patient's thigh or abdomen, and that the tubing is fastened appropriately to the bedclothes.

 c. Ensure that gravity drainage is maintained. For example, check that there are no loops in the tubing below its entry to the drainage receptacle

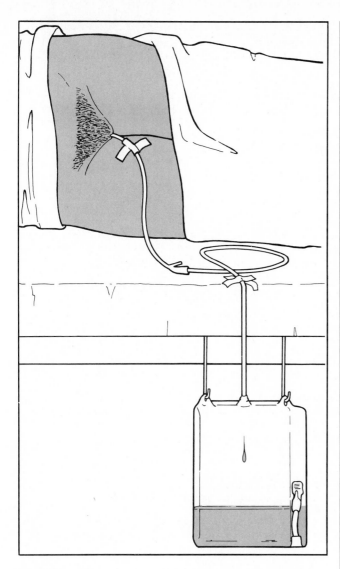

FIGURE 27–19

and that the drainage receptacle is below the level of the patient's bladder.

    d. Ensure that the drainage system is well sealed or closed. For example, check that there are no leaks at the connection sites in open systems. You may apply waterproof tape around the connection site of the catheter and tubing to ensure closure.

26. Ascertain the agency's policies about changing catheters and drainage systems. Some agencies advocate changes weekly or every other week. Others change the catheter only when sediment accumulates at the distal end. Sediment is present if you feel sandy particles when rolling the end of the catheter between your thumb and fingers. The drainage bag and tubing are generally changed along with the catheter but need to be changed more frequently if sediment accumulates, if leakage occurs, or if a strong odor is evident. Clean the catheter–tubing junction with an antiseptic solution prior to the change.

27. Assess the patient for signs of a possible urinary infection, eg, cloudy urine, strong odor, urethral burning, and fever or chills.

28. Determine the agency's practices about prophylactic measures to acidify the patient's urine and prevent urinary infection. For example, some agencies advocate a diet high in meat, eggs, poultry, and fish.

For a male patient

29. Open the sterile equipment, and don the sterile gloves. Place the tray directly on the patient's thighs if he is not restless.

30. Drape the patient with the sterile drapes, being careful to protect the sterility of your gloves. Place a drape under the penis and a second drape above the penis over the pubic area.

31. Follow steps 6–7.

32. Lubricate the insertion tip of the catheter liberally for about 5 to 7 cm (2 to 3 in). Place it aside on the sterile tray ready for insertion.

    Rationale Water-soluble lubricant facilitates insertion of the catheter by reducing friction. It is important to do this step before cleaning, since the nurse will subsequently have only one sterile hand available.

33. Clean the urinary meatus with antiseptic swabs. Grasp the penis firmly behind the glans, and spread the meatus between the thumb and forefinger. Retract the foreskin of an uncircumcised male. The gloved hand holding the penis is now considered contaminated. With the other hand, use sterile forceps to pick up a swab. Clean the meatus first, and then wipe the tissue surrounding the meatus in a circular fashion. Discard each swab after only one wipe.

    Rationale Using forceps maintains the sterility of one glove.

34. Place the drainage end of the catheter in the sterile receptacle. Coil excess tubing in your hand. Pick up the insertion end of the catheter with the sterile gloved hand (or forceps, if that is agency policy), holding it about 10 cm (4 in) from the tip for an adult, about 2.5 cm (1 in) for an infant or small child.

    Rationale The adult male urethra is approximately 20 cm (8 in) long. The catheter is held far enough from the end to maintain control and sterility of the tip.

35. To insert the catheter, lift the penis perpendicular to the body (90° angle) and exert slight traction upward. Insert the catheter steadily about 20 cm (8 in) or until urine begins to flow. Twist the catheter to bypass slight resistance at the sphincters or wait until the sphincter relaxes. Have the patient take deep breaths or try to void. If difficult resistance is

met, discontinue the procedure, and report the problem to the responsible nurse.

Rationale Slight resistance is normally encountered at the external and internal urethral sphincters. Deep breaths can help relax the sphincters. If forceful pressure is exerted against major resistance, the urethra can be traumatized.

36. When the urine flows, lower the penis, and transfer your hand to the catheter 5 cm (2 in) from the urethral orifice to hold it in place.

37. Follow steps 13–18.

38. Anchor the catheter with nonallergenic tape to the patient's thigh or abdomen.

Rationale This prevents skin excoriation at the penile–scrotal junction and restricts movement of the catheter, thus reducing friction and irritation of the urethra.

FIGURE 27–20

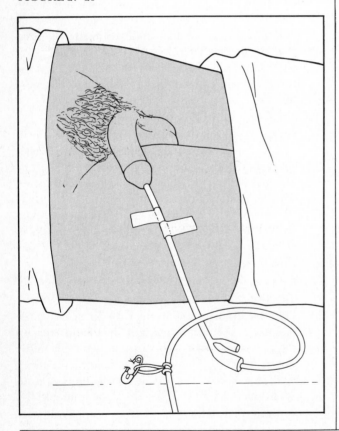

39. Coil the drainage tubing beside the patient so that the tubing runs in a straight line to the drainage bag, and fasten it to the bedclothes with a tubing clamp, safety pin, or tape. See Figure 27–20.

Rationale Letting the tubing loop below the level of entry into the bag can impede the flow of urine.

40. Dry the patient's penis with a towel or drape.

41. Follow steps 22–28.

Sample Recording

Date	Time	Notes
7/12/87	2000	#18 5-mL Foley catheter inserted and connected. 750 mL clear amber urine drained, and catheter clamped. Stated burning pain over pubic area relieved. Instructed about I & O. Dr. Bradley notified, and bladder decompression regimen established q.2h.————Ron J. Randall, SN

■ Evaluation

Expected outcomes

1. Normal color, odor, and consistency of urine
2. Decreased bladder distention
3. Balance between fluid intake and output
4. Patent drainage system
5. Skin around urinary meatus intact

Unexpected outcomes

1. Blood clots in urine
2. Hematuria
3. Cloudy urine
4. Strong, pungent urine odor
5. Fever, chills
6. Excoriation of urinary meatus
7. Imbalance between fluid intake and output

Upon obtaining an unexpected outcome:

1. Report your findings to the responsible nurse and/or physician.
2. Adjust the patient's nursing care plan appropriately.

Obtaining a Urine Specimen from a Retention Catheter

Sterile urine specimens can be acquired from closed drainage systems by inserting a sterile 1-in needle (#21 to #25 gauge), attached to a 3-mL syringe, into the end of the catheter or through a drainage port in the tubing.

See Figure 27–21. Note that aspiration of urine from catheters can be done only with self-sealing rubber catheters, not plastic, silicone, or silastic catheters.

First the nurse cleans the entry point of the needle with a disinfectant swab. The needle is then inserted at an angle, to facilitate self-sealing of the rubber, and at a place where it will not puncture the tube leading to the balloon. If the urine is not readily available, the drainage tubing is elevated slightly to return urine to the area or the catheter is pinched or clamped about 5 to 7 cm (3 in) from its tip for a short period until urine appears.

After the urine is drawn into the syringe, the nurse transfers it to a *sterile* specimen container, caps the container, labels it, and sends it to the laboratory immediately for analysis or refrigeration. See Technique 27–10 later.

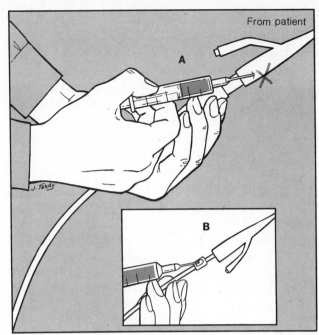

FIGURE 27–21 ■ Obtaining a urine specimen from a retention catheter: **A,** from a specific area, sometimes designated by a patch, near the end of the catheter; **B,** from a drainage port in the tubing.

TECHNIQUE 27–4   ■   Providing Catheter Care

Patients with retention catheters require special catheter care in addition to the perineal–genital care described in chapter 14, since the presence of a retention catheter can predispose the patient to a urinary infection. Catheter care is usually given directly after perineal–genital care. Because catheter care varies considerably from agency to agency, check agency practice.

■ Assessment

Assess the patient for: complaints of perineal irritation or discomfort. Other data include: agency practices regarding catheter care. Agencies provide different types of equipment and solutions for cleaning patients who have catheters. Some agencies require that patients with indwelling catheters receive sterile catheter care once or twice a day.

■ Nursing Diagnosis   See Technique 27–1 on page 626.

■ Planning

Nursing goals

1. To remove normal secretions and odors
2. To prevent infection

Equipment

1. A sterile catheter care kit containing:
   a. A drape to cover the legs and perineal area around the catheter and the urinary meatus
   b. Gloves to wear during the procedure
   c. An antiseptic solution, such as a water-soluble iodine solution
   d. Cotton balls or applicator swabs
   e. An antibiotic ointment, such as neomycin, or hydrocortisone
   f. Sterile forceps
   g. A small receptacle for the discarded balls or swabs
2. A bath blanket (optional)

BID   Soap & water

■ Intervention

1. Discuss the possibility that the patient may provide his or her own care. Because of exposure of the genital area, some patients find this procedure embarrassing and often prefer to learn to do it themselves.
2. Arrange the bedclothes or bath blanket so that only the perineal area is exposed.
3. Open the sterile catheter care kit using surgical aseptic technique.

4. Don the sterile gloves.

5. Drape the patient.

6. Pour antiseptic on the cotton balls or swabs.

7. Put some sterile ointment on one cotton ball or swab.

8. Assess the area around the urinary meatus for inflammation, swelling, and discharge. Determine the color, amount, and consistency of any discharge. Note any odor from the area.

9. Clean the perineal–genital area, using forceps and cotton balls or swabs. Use each swab only once.

   a. For a female patient, clean the labia majora, moving downward. Then separate the labia majora with your thumb and fourth finger, and clean the labia minora. Then separate them with the index and middle fingers of the same hand. Expose the urinary meatus adequately by retracting the tissue of the labia minora in an upward (anterior) direction. Clean first from the meatus and catheter downward and then on either side.

   b. For a male patient, clean the meatus by grasping the penis behind the glans and spreading the urinary meatus between your thumb and forefinger. Retract the foreskin of an uncircumcised male. Clean the meatus around the catheter first, and then wipe the tissue surrounding the meatus in a circular fashion.

10. Assess the area around the urinary meatus for:

    a. Discomfort experienced by the patient.

    b. Inflammation or swelling.

    c. Discharge (note the color, amount, and consistency).

    d. Odor.

11. Using a new swab, clean along the catheter for about 10 cm (4 in). Use a circular motion to ensure that all sides of the catheter are cleaned.

12. Apply antiseptic ointment around the base and along about 2.5 cm (1 in) of the catheter.

    Rationale This protects the urethra from infection.

13. Inspect the patency of the drainage system. See Technique 27–3, step 25, on page 634.

14. Follow Technique 27–3, steps 26–27, on page 635.

15. Record on the patient's chart the technique, the time, and pertinent assessment data. Report any problems to the responsible nurse.

Sample Recording

Date	Time	Notes
4/30/87	0900	Catheter care given. No apparent urethral redness or swelling. Small amount of thick white discharge around base of catheter. No complaints of discomfort. ——————— ——————— Yvonne A. Able, NS

16. Check and adjust the nursing care plan, if necessary, to include regular catheter care.

■ Evaluation

Expected outcome

Skin around urethra intact.

Unexpected outcomes

1. Complaints of perineal irritation

2. Reddened and swollen urinary meatus

3. Discharge from urinary meatus

4. Pungent odor emanating from urethral meatus

Upon obtaining an unexpected outcome: Report your findings to the responsible nurse and/or physician.

TECHNIQUE 27–5 ■ Removing a Retention Catheter

Retention catheters are removed after their purpose has been achieved, usually on the order of the physician. A few days prior to removal the catheter may be clamped for specified periods of time (eg, two to four hours) and then released. This causes some distention of the bladder and stimulation of the bladder musculature.

■ Assessment

Assess the urine in the drainage bag in terms of amount, color, and consistency. Other data include:

1. The medical or nursing order and the time for removal of the catheter.

2. The size of the Foley catheter balloon. Either inspect the catheter or check the nursing care plan.

■ Planning

Nursing goal

To prevent trauma to the urethra when removing the catheter.

Equipment

1. A receptacle for the catheter after its removal, eg, a kidney basin.
2. A syringe to deflate the balloon. A needle may also be required to deflate some types of balloons.
3. Cotton balls to dry the genital area.
4. Disposable gloves, if desired, to protect the nurse.

■ Intervention

1. Clamp the catheter.

   Rationale   This prevents spillage of urine that might remain in the catheter.

2. Insert the syringe into the balloon inflation tube of the catheter and draw out all the fluid.

   Rationale   The balloon needs to be completely deflated to prevent trauma to the urethra when the catheter is withdrawn.

3. Gently withdraw the catheter from the urethra.

4. Place the catheter in the kidney basin or other receptacle.

5. Dry the genital area with cotton balls.

6. Measure the urine in the drainage bag.

7. Record the time the catheter was removed and the amount, color, and consistency of the urine in the drainage bag.

8. Adjust the nursing care plan to:

   a. Encourage the patient to drink up to 3,000 mL of fluid daily if not contraindicated.

[handwritten: Reinsert if have not voided in 8°]

Rationale   If the urethra has been irritated by the catheter, the patient may experience some burning when voiding. This problem is minimized by diluting the urine with an increased fluid intake.

   b. Monitor the patient's fluid intake and output.

■ Evaluation

1. Assess the frequency of voiding, or any unusual symptoms related to voiding following the technique.
2. Assess fluid intake and output following the technique.

Expected outcomes

1. Urine clear, light amber
2. Able to void adequate amounts following catheter removal
3. Adequate 24-hour fluid intake

Unexpected outcomes

1. Urine abnormal in color or consistency
2. Unable to void adequate amounts following catheter removal
3. Inadequate 24-hour fluid intake

Upon obtaining an unexpected outcome: Report your findings to the responsible nurse and/or physician.

TECHNIQUE 27–6   ■   Irrigating a Catheter or a Bladder and Instilling Medication into a Bladder

An *irrigation* is a flushing or washing out using a specified solution. Irrigations can be carried out on several body parts, such as the eye, ear, throat, vagina, or urinary bladder, and on drains connected to the body, such as urinary catheters. A *plain irrigation* is the introduction of a solution to the bladder or catheter and its immediate removal. Catheter irrigations are carried out chiefly to clear a catheter that has become blocked.

In a bladder *instillation,* a small amount of liquid is placed in the bladder and allowed to remain there for a specific period of time. For example, an antiseptic solution may be instilled through a catheter, which is then clamped for 30 minutes so that the antiseptic will remain in contact with the walls of the bladder. Bladder instillations and irrigations are rarely performed because of the danger of transmitting microorganisms into the urinary bladder.

A simple urinary drainage system consists of a retention catheter, tubing, and a receptacle (collecting bag) for the urine. This is called a *straight drainage system,* and it depends on the force of gravity to move the urine from the urinary bladder to the collecting bag. When this system is not or cannot be opened anywhere along it from the catheter to the bag, it is referred to as a *closed system.* Closed systems are being used increasingly, because of the danger of pathogenic microorganisms entering the urinary tract whenever the system is opened. The more traditional type of system is the *open system,* in which the

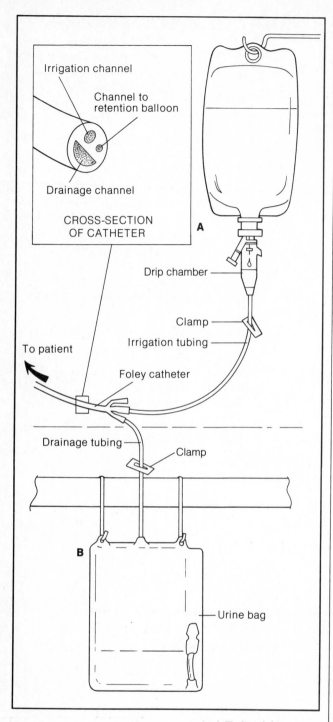

Irrigation channel

Channel to retention balloon

Drainage channel

CROSS-SECTION OF CATHETER

A

Drip chamber

Clamp

Irrigation tubing

To patient

Foley catheter

Drainage tubing

Clamp

B

Urine bag

FIGURE 27–22 ■ An intermittent bladder irrigation system.

tubing may be separated from the catheter to perform such techniques as a bladder irrigation.

A number of variations of the straight drainage system permit irrigation of the urinary bladder. The simplest is the plain irrigation system, which requires a two-way or preferably three-way Foley catheter. A variation of the plain irrigation is the intermittent irrigation, in which one lumen of a three-way catheter is connected by tubing

to a drip chamber and then to a container of sterile solution. The second lumen is attached to tubing and then to a urine receptacle. See Figure 27–22. There are clamps on both tubes. The clamp from the solution container (*A*) is released while the clamp to the urine bag (*B*) is closed. The fluid enters and remains in the bladder. The container tubing is then reclamped, and the urine receptacle tubing is unclamped, permitting the solution to flow out of the bladder. This process is carried out regularly. The same system can be used for continuous irrigations by carefully regulating the flow of fluid leaving the solution container and permitting it to flow freely out of the bladder into the urine bag.

There are several variations of this irrigation system. One requires a specific fluid pressure to build up in the urinary bladder before the irrigation system "trips," allowing the solution to flow out of the bladder into a receptacle. These systems are usually set up by a physician and monitored by nurses.

■ Assessment

1. Assess whether the catheter and tubing are indeed blocked. Compare the amount of urine in the bag with the drainage on the previous shift or with the patient's fluid intake (see chapter 23). If urine does not appear to be running freely, "milk" the catheter and tubing, working from the patient toward the drainage bag. See Figure 27–23. This can dislodge an obstruction, avoiding the necessity of an irriga-

FIGURE 27–23 ■ Milking the catheter tubing to remove an obstruction such as a blood clot.

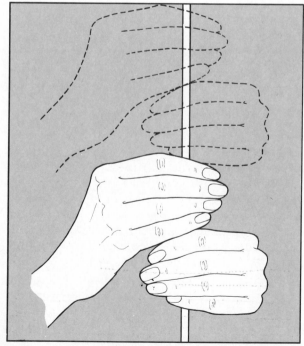

tion to remove it. It is important to milk away from the patient so that the obstruction, eg, a blood clot, is forced into the drainage bag and not into the urinary bladder.

2. Assess the patient for distress. If the urine flow is obstructed, the patient may experience a feeling of fullness just above the pubic symphysis. If the bladder has been the site of recent surgery, the patient may report severe pain due to acute bladder spasms. Determine when the pain began.

3. Assess the color and clarity of the urine drainage and the presence of any abnormal constituents, such as blood.

Other data include:

1. The physician's order for a bladder irrigation or instillation. In most agencies, a physician's order is required.

2. The type of solution, amount, and strength to be used for the instillation or irrigation. If the physician has not specified these on the patient's chart, check agency policies. Some agencies recommend the use of sterile normal saline at room temperature for both catheter and bladder irrigations. To irrigate an adult bladder, 1,000 mL is commonly used; for a catheter irrigation, 200 mL is normally required. The strength, amount, and kind of medication for a bladder instillation are specified by the physician.

C - Clamp

■ Planning

Nursing goals

1. To maintain the patency of a urethral catheter, eg, to remove pus or blood clots that have formed in the bladder and are blocking the catheter

2. To treat a bladder infection by irrigating the bladder with a sterile medicated solution

Equipment

For using a syringe with a closed drainage system

1. A sterile irrigation or instillation set containing:

   a. A sterile container for the solution. Check that the container is large enough to hold the amount of fluid to be used.

   b. Absorbent cotton balls or gauze squares with a disinfectant.

   c. A drape to protect the bedding and provide a sterile field

   d. A standard syringe (30 or 50 mL) with a #18 or #19 gauge needle. *Catheter*

2. The sterile irrigating solution or medication to be instilled into the bladder. The solution is generally room temperature, although warming it to body

temperature makes it more comfortable for the patient.

3. A tubing clamp.

4. A bath blanket.

For using a syringe with an open drainage system

The following additional equipment is required:

5. A sterile drainage tube protector. The inside of a sterile foil package can be used if a protector is not available.

6. A sterile Asepto or catheter syringe to instill the solution. The Asepto (or bulb) syringe is a plastic or glass syringe with a rubber bulb. See Figure 27–24, *A.* Bulb syringes come in different sizes, eg, 2 oz, 4 oz. The bulb pushes the solution into the catheter and can also be used to create suction for withdrawing the solution. A second type of syringe is the catheter syringe with an adapter tip. See Figure 27–24, *B.*

7. A sterile drainage receptacle, if an irrigation is being performed.

For intermittent irrigations using a Y-connector and a two-way Foley catheter

8. A container of sterile irrigating solution.

9. A sterile Y-connector, with sterile tubing to connect to the solution container, a drip chamber, and a clamp.

10. An IV pole.

FIGURE 27–24 ■ Two types of irrigating syringes: **A,** an Asepto syringe; **B,** a catheter syringe with an adapter tip.

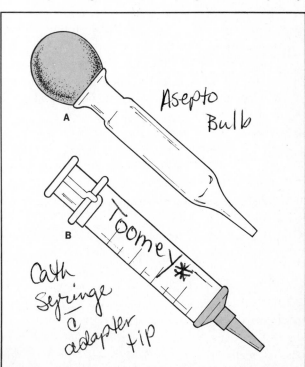

11. A two-way Foley catheter inserted into the patient's bladder.

12. Sterile drainage tubing, a clamp, and a drainage receptacle. The tubing connects the catheter to the receptacle.

13. A bath blanket.

For continuous irrigations using a three-way Foley catheter

14. A container of sterile irrigating solution.

15. Sterile irrigation tubing, a drip chamber, and a clamp.

16. An IV pole.

17. A three-way Foley catheter inserted into the patient's bladder.

18. Sterile drainage tubing and a drainage bag. The tubing connects the catheter to the bag.

19. A bath blanket.

■ Intervention

1. Determine the amount of urine in the urine bag.

   Rationale This amount has to be deducted from subsequent measurements of the irrigating fluid returns.

2. Assist the patient to a dorsal recumbent position, to facilitate the flow of the irrigating fluid into the bladder.

3. Fold back the top bedclothes to expose the retention catheter. Place a bath blanket across the patient's chest and abdomen to prevent undue exposure.

For a closed drainage system

4. Open the sterile set beside or between the patient's thighs, using sterile technique.

5. Place the drape under the end of the catheter.

6. Clamp the drainage tubing for a bladder irrigation or bladder instillation. Leave it unclamped for a catheter irrigation.

   Rationale Clamping prevents the urine and solution from draining through the tubing.

7. Draw the irrigation solution into the syringe, maintaining the sterility of the syringe and the solution.

8. Attach the needle to the syringe, maintaining the sterility of the needle.

9. Using a disinfectant swab, wipe the place on the catheter lumen or the port on the drainage tubing through which the solution is to be instilled. The correct place on the catheter lumen is usually marked.

10. Insert the needle into the port. See Figure 27–21, earlier.

11. Infuse the solution gently into the catheter. For a catheter irrigation, instill about 30 to 40 mL of fluid for an adult; for a bladder irrigation, instill about 100 to 200 mL. Use smaller amounts for children. For a bladder instillation, instill the amount of medication specified in the order.

    Rationale Gentle instillation avoids injury to the lining of the bladder and bladder spasms.

12. Remove the needle from the port.

13. For a *catheter irrigation,* immediately lower the catheter so that the fluid will run toward the distal end of the catheter into the drainage tubing.

    or

    For a *bladder instillation,* leave the catheter clamped so the fluid will remain in the bladder.

    or

    For a *bladder irrigation,* unclamp the drainage tubing so the solution will run out of the bladder through the catheter and tubing.

14. For an irrigation, repeat steps 6–13 until all the solution has been used or until the purpose of the irrigation has been accomplished.

15. Empty the urine bag. Record on the appropriate records (eg, the bedside output record) the amount of urine drained by subtracting the amount of solution used from the volume of fluid in the bag.

16. Assess the response of the patient to the irrigation or instillation in terms of discomfort and the color and clarity of the irrigating fluid and the urine flow.

17. Record on the patient's chart the technique, the time, the color and clarity of the irrigation returns, the presence of any abnormal constituents, and any discomfort experienced by the patient. Add the amount of fluid instilled to the intake and output record.

For an open drainage system

18. Follow steps 4–5.

19. After disinfecting the ends, separate the catheter from the drainage tubing, and place the tubing protector over the end of the tubing. Hold the catheter and the tubing at least 2.5 cm (1 in) from their ends.

    Rationale This distance avoids contaminating the ends of the catheter and tubing.

20. Draw the fluid into the syringe, then gently inject it into the catheter, maintaining the sterility of the end of the catheter, the syringe, and the solution. See Figure 27–25.

21. For a *bladder or catheter irrigation:*

    a. Remove the syringe, and allow the fluid to return through the catheter into the drainage receptacle.

    b. Repeat steps 20–21a until the catheter is running freely or until the purpose of the irrigation has been accomplished.

22. For a *bladder instillation,* clamp the catheter after instilling the solution. Leave the clamp in place for the time ordered.

    Rationale   The solution will remain in the bladder for the designated time.

23. Reattach the catheter to the tubing, maintaining the sterility of the ends of the tubing and the catheter. For a bladder instillation, open the catheter clamp at the designated time, and drain the bladder contents into the receptacle.

24. Coil the drainage tubing carefully on the bed so that the urine can flow through it freely.

25. Empty the irrigation drainage receptacle.

26. Follow steps 16–17.

For an intermittent irrigation using a Y-connector

This system uses a two-way catheter with a Y-connector attached to the catheter end. See Figure 27–26.

27. Insert the sterile irrigation tubing into the sterile solution bag.

28. Close the clamp on the irrigation solution, and hang the container on the IV pole.

29. Attach the stem of the sterile Y-connector to the catheter, maintaining the sterility of the inside of the catheter.

30. Open the clamp, permit some solution to run through the tubing, then close the clamp.

    Rationale   The solution expels the air from the tubing.

31. Attach one arm of the Y-connector to the irrigation tubing.

32. Attach the other arm of the Y-connector to the sterile drainage tubing.

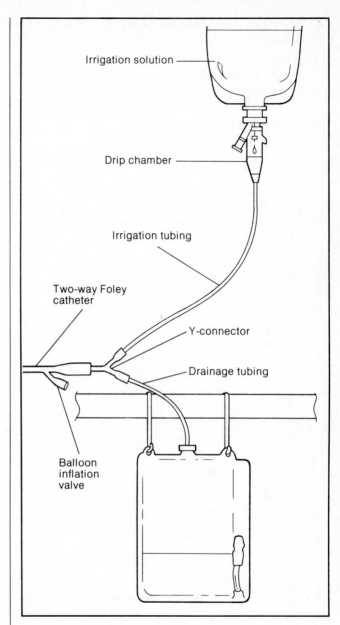

FIGURE 27–26

FIGURE 27–25

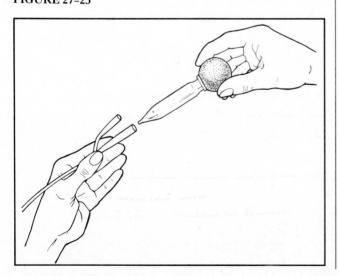

33. Clamp the drainage tubing.

    Rationale   Urine and irrigating solution then cannot flow out of the bladder.

34. Open the clamp on the tubing from the solution container, and let the prescribed amount of fluid run into the bladder at the prescribed rate. If the amount is not specified by the physician, instill about 100 mL for an adult.

35. Close the irrigation clamp.

36. Open the drainage clamp, and permit the fluid and urine to flow into the receptacle.

37. Repeat steps 33–36 until the returning fluid is clear or as ordered by the physician.

38. Assess the response of the patient in terms of any discomfort and the color and clarity of the return flow.

39. Record the technique on the patient's chart including your assessments.

For a continuous irrigation using a three-way Foley catheter

40. Using sterile technique, assemble the equipment as for an intermittent irrigation, except that one port of the three-way catheter is connected to the irrigation tubing and the other is connected to the drainage tubing. See Figure 27–22 on page 640. In some closed systems, the tubings are already connected to the catheter.

41. Open the flow clamp on the drainage tubing.

42. Adjust the flow rate, using the clamp on the irrigation tubing, as specified by the physician. If the order does not specify, the rate should be 40 to 60 drops per minute.

43. Inspect the fluid returns for amount, color, and clarity. The amount of returning fluid should correspond to the amount of fluid entering the bladder.

44. Record the technique and your assessments on the patient's chart.

Sample Recording

Date	Time	Notes
4/24/87	1400	Catheter irrigated with 200 mL normal saline at room temperature. Returns slightly blood-tinged with some small blood clots. Catheter running freely. No discomfort. ———————————— Sandi R. Bailey, NS

■ Evaluation

Expected outcomes

1. Clear irrigation returns
2. Patent catheter

Unexpected outcomes

1. Blood clots or sediment in irrigation returns
2. Suprapubic discomfort
3. Inadequate urine output

Upon obtaining an unexpected outcome:

1. Repeat the technique.
2. Report your findings to the responsible nurse and/or physician.

TECHNIQUE 27–7 ■ Applying and Removing a Drainage Condom

The application of a *condom*, also referred to as a *urinary sheath* or *external catheter*, and attachment of its base to a urinary drainage system are commonly prescribed for males who experience incontinence. Use of a condom appliance is preferable to insertion of a retention catheter, because it avoids entrance into the urethra and bladder and minimizes the risk of urethral or bladder infection.

Methods of applying condoms vary with the length of time the condom is to be worn. Condoms that are to be worn for short periods are generally applied with elastic tape only; condoms that are to be worn for longer periods (eg, a few days) require additional measures to protect the foreskin and to ensure secure attachment. Follow the manufacturer's instructions when applying a condom.

■ Assessment

Assess when the patient experiences incontinence. Some patients may require a condom appliance at night only, others continuously.

■ Nursing Diagnosis

Nursing diagnoses that may indicate the need for a condom include: Alteration in patterns of urinary elimination related to incontinence.

■ Planning

Nursing goals

1. To collect urine and control urinary incontinence
2. To permit the patient physical activity without fear of embarrassment because of leaking urine
3. To prevent skin irritation as a result of urine incontinence

Equipment

1. A condom drainage kit containing:
   a. A drainage condom made of plastic or rubber.

b. Elastic tape. Ordinary tape is contraindicated because it is not flexible and can stop blood flow.

c. Skin paste or tincture of benzoin. A plasticized skin spray may also be used; it is more readily removed and less likely to irritate the skin.

d. Skin bonding cement, also called *skin prep*.

e. Applicator swabs or tongue depressors.

f. A razor.

g. Extension tubing.

h. A leg drainage bag and straps.

2. Soap, a basin of warm water, a washcloth, and a towel.

Some commercially prepared appliances (eg, Texas Catheter Navy drainage) are equipped with an adhesive foam strip. For these, skin spray, skin bonding cement, and elastic tape are not used. Instead, the adhesive foam or plastic strip is attached below the rolled edge of the condom and not against the skin. The following equipment is then required in addition to item 2:

3. The condom

4. A skin protector

5. A leg drainage bag and straps

6. Extension tubing

■ **Intervention**

Applying the condom

1. Position the patient in either a supine or a bed-sitting position, and cover the patient's body with the bedclothes, exposing only the penis.

2. Inspect the penis for skin irritation (contact dermatitis), excoriation, swelling, or discoloration.

3. Clean the genital area, and dry it thoroughly, to minimize skin irritation and excoriation after the condom is applied.

4. Shave or trim any hair on the base of the penis unless a skin protector is being applied.

   Rationale Hair will adhere to the condom and cause discomfort when the condom is removed.

5. Remove the protective film from the underside of the plastic skin protector and apply the protector to the base of the penis. Then remove the protective film from the anterior surface of the skin protector.

   or

   Apply skin paste, tincture of benzoin, or plasticized skin spray around the base of the penis where the elasticized tape is to be applied. After the paste, tincture, or spray feels dry, apply a thin layer of skin bonding cement.

6. Roll the condom smoothly over the penis, leaving 2.5 cm (1 in) between the end of the penis and the

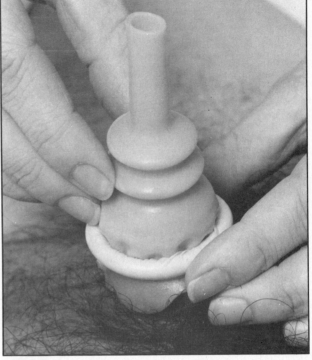

FIGURE 27–27

FIGURE 27–28

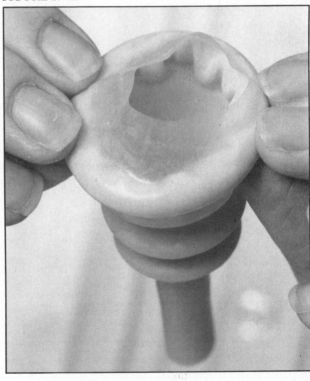

rubber or plastic connecting tube. See Figure 27–27. Make sure that no pubic hair is caught in the condom. On some models the condom is rolled first, so that the inner flap is exposed, which is applied around the urinary meatus to prevent the reflux of urine. See Figure 27–28.

7. Optional (depending on the kind of condom): Secure the condom firmly but not too tightly to the penis by wrapping a strip of elastic tape spirally around two-thirds the length of the penis, making sure that the spirals do not overlap.

   Rationale Overlapping spirals prevent the tape from stretching and could impede the blood circulation in the penis.

8. Attach the urinary drainage system securely to the condom. Make sure that the tip of the penis is not touching the condom and that the condom is not twisted.

   Rationale The condom could irritate the tip of the penis, and a twisted condom could obstruct the flow of urine.

9. Attach the urinary drainage bag to the bed frame, if the patient is to remain in bed, or to the patient's leg, if he is ambulatory. See Figure 27–29.

   Rationale Attaching the drainage bag to the leg helps control the movement of the tubing and prevents twisting of the thin material of the condom appliance at the tip of the penis.

10. Teach the patient about attaching the drainage system to his leg, keeping the drainage bag below the level of the condom, and avoiding loops or kinks in the tubing.

FIGURE 27–29

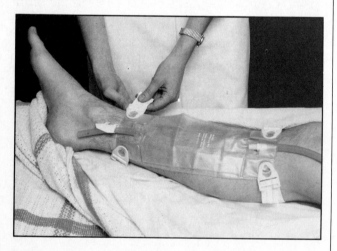

11. Assess the urine for color and characteristics, eg, clarity, odor.

12. Record the application of the condom, the time, and pertinent observations, such as irritated areas on the penis.

13. Observe the penis for swelling and discoloration 30 minutes following the application of the condom. Also check urine flow.

    Rationale Swelling and discoloration could indicate that the condom is too tight. Normally some urine will be present in the tube if the flow is not obstructed.

Removing the condom

14. Remove the tape, if it was applied, and roll off the condom. Remove the plasticized skin spray (it peels off readily) or the skin protector every one or two days to provide skin care to the penis. Wash the penis with soapy water, rinse, and dry it thoroughly.

15. Change the condom daily, and assess the foreskin for signs of irritation, swelling, and discoloration.

■ Evaluation

Expected outcomes

1. Normal color, odor, and consistency of urine
2. No discomfort associated with condom
3. Skin under condom intact
4. Urinary meatus normal
5. Urine draining well

Unexpected outcomes

1. Abnormal color, odor, or consistency of urine
2. Discomfort associated with condom
3. Skin irritation under condom
4. Urinary meatus reddened
5. Urine not draining
6. Condom leaking

Upon obtaining an unexpected outcome:

1. Report your findings to the responsible nurse.
2. Adjust the nursing care plan appropriately.

TECHNIQUE 27–8 ■ Suprapubic Catheter Care

Suprapubic catheters (see Figure 27–10 on page 625) are advantageous over urethral catheters because:

1. They are associated with a lower rate of urinary tract infections.

2. They are more comfortable for the patient.

3. They allow the opportunity to evaluate the patient's ability to void normally; the patient is asked to void normally when the suprapubic catheter is clamped. To assess the patient's ability to void normally with a urethral catheter, you must first remove the catheter.

4. They facilitate evaluation of the patient's residual urine.

Two commonly used suprapubic catheters are the *Cystocath* and the *Bonanno catheter*. See Figure 27–30. These are narrow-lumen catheters with a curl at the distal end that prevents the catheter from being expelled by the bladder through the urethra. The Cystocath has a disc that holds the catheter in place on the abdominal wall; the Bonanno catheter has wings for that purpose. Attachments of the catheter to the drainage system tubing also vary: The Cystocath is joined with a stopcock; the Bonanno with a Luer-Lok adapter.

The most common problem with the suprapubic catheter is blockage of drainage due to sediment, clots, or the bladder wall itself obstructing the catheter or catheter tip. Dislodgement of the catheter and hematuria following the use of a large-bore catheter are less common problems. Care of suprapubic catheters includes maintenance of a patent drainage system, skin care around the insertion site, periodic clamping of the catheter preparatory to removing it, and measurement of residual urine. The physician's order about management of the catheter is followed. Orders generally include: leaving the catheter open to drainage for 48 to 72 hours, then clamping the catheter for three- to four-hour periods during the day until the patient can void satisfactory amounts. Satisfactory voiding is determined by measuring the patient's residual urine after voiding.

■ Assessment

Assess the patient for:

1. Color, consistency, clarity, and amount of urine drained, hourly for the first 24 hours and then at least three times daily.

2. Fluid intake, to ensure it is adequate to maintain a satisfactory urine output.

3. Bladder discomfort. Bladder spasms may occur during the first 24 to 48 hours. Spasms are identified by the presence of intermittent pain that does not affect the amount of urinary output.

4. Indications of an obstruction in the drainage system. Obstruction is identified by distention and tenderness of the bladder (assessed by palpation), feelings of fullness, pubic pain, and a reduction in urinary output.

5. Amount of residual urine after voiding. See Intervention, steps 18–20.

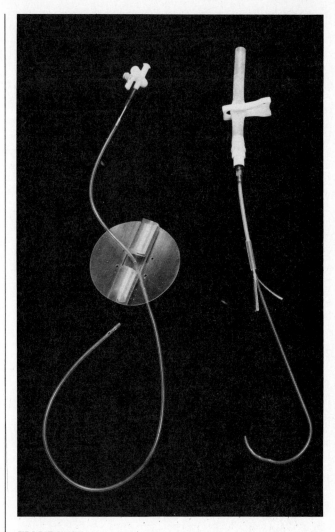

FIGURE 27–30 ■ Two types of suprapubic catheters: a Cystocath (left) and a Bonanno (right).

6. Redness and discharge at the skin around the insertion site.

7. Vital signs, to compare to baseline data.

■ Planning

Nursing goals

1. To maintain the patency of the drainage system

2. To prevent infection of the insertion site and urinary bladder

3. To ensure a satisfactory fluid intake and output

Equipment

For maintaining drainage

1. A sterile syringe (30 to 50 mL) with a #22 gauge needle (optional)

2. Sterile saline solution or urinary irrigant (optional)

3. Sterile alcohol swabs or povidone-iodine applicators

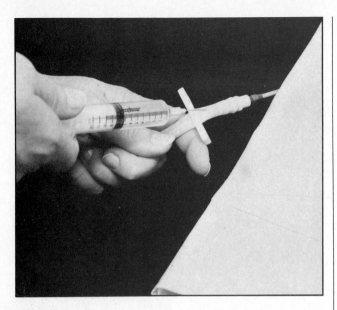

FIGURE 27–31

For a dressing change

4. A sterile dressing set containing:

    a. 4 × 4 gauzes

    b. Precut 4 × 4 drain sponges (eg, Telfa pads)

    c. Povidone-iodine or hydrogen peroxide solution

    d. Applicator swabs

    e. A container for the solution

    f. Povidone-iodine ointment

    g. Forceps

    h. Gloves

    i. Nonallergenic tape

5. A moisture-resistant line-saver pad

6. A moisture-resistant bag for the soiled dressing

For removal of the catheter

7. A 3-mL syringe with a #22 gauge needle if a urine specimen is required

8. Alcohol wipes

9. A sterile dressing set (see item 4) with suture scissors

10. 2 × 2 gauzes

11. An Elastoplast bandage

12. A moisture-resistant bag

■ Intervention

Maintaining the catheter

1. Make sure the catheter and drainage tubes are securely connected. Tape these connections to avoid separation of the tubes.

2. If the catheter is not connected to drainage:

    a. Connect the catheter to a closed urinary drainage

bag, maintaining the sterility of the ends of the tubes.

    b. Initiate drainage by removing all air from the tubing. To remove air, clean the soft rubber connecting tubing of a Bonanno catheter or the marked injection port on the stopcock of the Cystocath with an alcohol swab or povidone-iodine applicator, insert a sterile syringe with a #22 gauge needle, pull back on the plunger, and aspirate until urine flows past the Luer-Lok connection (see Figure 27–31) or the stopcock (see Figure 27–32). Make sure the Cystocath stopcock arrow is turned toward the collection bag and is open for drainage.

    Rationale   The catheter drains by siphonage. Removing the air creates a mild suction.

3. Ensure that the tubing is not kinked, that it runs straight up from the collection bag, and that excess tubing is coiled appropriately and taped to the patient's abdomen or leg. After emptying the bag, clean the drainage port with povidone-iodine solution before replacing it in the sleeve.

4. Make sure the Cystocath stopcock arrow is turned toward the part of the system to be turned off:

    a. For urine to drain, turn the arrow toward the rubber injection port on the stopcock. See Figure 27–33.

    b. For irrigating the catheter, turn the arrow toward

FIGURE 27–32

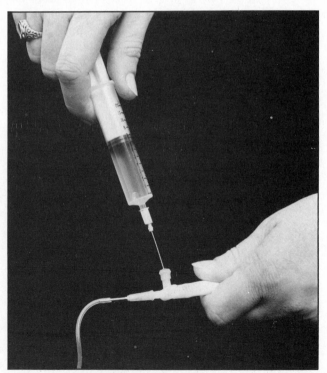

the drainage bag so that fluid will flow into the patient's bladder, not the bag. See Figure 27–34.

c. For clamping the catheter, turn the arrow toward the catheter insertion site. See Figure 27–35.

5. If urine does not drain well, implement the following steps in order:

a. Have the patient turn from side to side.

Rationale Movement may dislodge obstruction of the tip of the catheter by the bladder wall.

b. Milk the catheter tubing from the insertion site toward the drainage bag. See Figure 27–23 earlier.

Rationale This can dislodge clots or sediment.

c. Irrigate the tubing as a last alternative and only if there is a physician's order to do so:

- Fill a sterile syringe with sterile normal saline or other urinary irrigant supplied by the agency, and attach a #22 needle, maintaining sterility.

- Clean the injection port of the catheter with an alcohol swab or povidone-iodine applicator.

- Insert the #22 needle and syringe as in step 2b.

- Slowly inject 30 mL of the irrigant.

- Observe the return flow of fluid by gravity.

- If fluid does not return, aspirate one-half the irrigant to dislodge a blood clot.

- Remove the needle.

- If a stopcock is present, turn the arrow toward the rubber injection site.

  Rationale This allows urine to drain from the catheter into the drainage bag.

d. If the above actions fail:

- Disconnect the catheter from the tubing, using strict surgical aseptic technique.

- Clean the end of the catheter with an alcohol swab or povidone-iodine applicator.

- Insert the syringe, filled with irrigant and without the needle, into the end of the catheter.

- Instill the solution to irrigate the catheter, and then aspirate the clot.

- Again clean the end of the catheter with the alcohol or iodine.

- Reconnect the catheter to the drainage tubing.

Go to step 29.

Changing the dressing

6. Assist the patient to lie on the side opposite the drainage tube.

Rationale This position exposes the tube more clearly.

7. Place the moisture-resistant pad under the patient's hip below the drain.

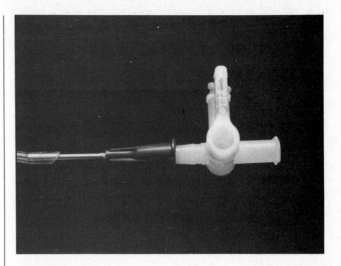

FIGURE 27–33

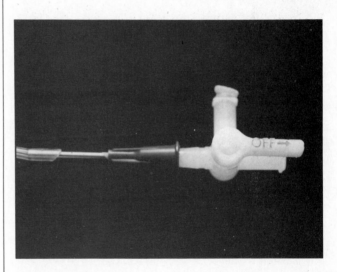

FIGURE 27–34

FIGURE 27–35

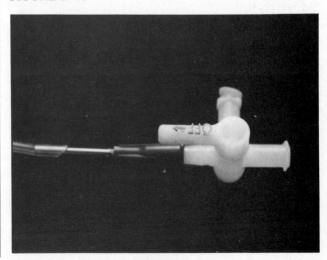

8. Open the sterile dressing kit. Open the waste bag, roll its top edges outward, and place it away from the sterile field.

   Rationale Rolling the edges outward keeps the top of the bag open for use. Placing it away from the sterile field prevents contamination of the sterile field.

9. Carefully remove the tape from the suprapubic tube dressing. Using forceps, remove the soiled dressings, and discard them in the bag. A Cystocath may or may not have a dressing over the disc.

   Rationale Forceps are used to keep the nurse's hands clean.

10. When removing the tape and dressings, be careful not to jar the catheter.

    Rationale Jarring the catheter can cause bladder spasms.

11. Don sterile gloves.

12. Clean the catheter insertion site, using the sterile forceps.

    Rationale Forceps keep the gloves sterile for handling the dressings.

    a. Clean around the drain, moving from the insertion site outward. See Figure 35–7 on page 836. Use a new swab for each wipe.

       Rationale Moving from the insertion site outward prevents wiping contaminants into the wound.

    b. Discard each used swab in the bag, being careful not to contaminate the forcep tips on the edge of the bag.

13. Apply a small amount of povidone-iodine ointment around the insertion site.

14. Place a precut 4 × 4 Telfa drain gauze around the suprapubic catheter over the insertion site.

    Rationale The Telfa dressing does not stick to the skin when it becomes soiled, and thus its removal is facilitated.

15. Place several uncut 4 × 4 gauzes over the Telfa gauze and catheter.

    Rationale These gauzes absorb drainage and support and stabilize the catheter.

16. Apply nonallergenic tape over the 4 × 4 gauzes to hold them in place.

17. Gently loop the catheter on the patient's abdomen, and tape it in place. Go to step 29.

    Rationale Looping prevents the catheter from pulling on the bladder.

Measuring residual urine

After the first few days of catheter insertion, the physician will order periodic catheter clamping, eg, every three to four hours, to determine how well the patient can void

normally. After the patient voids, measure the patient's residual urine.

18. When the catheter is clamped or closed by a stopcock, have the patient notify you of feelings of suprapubic discomfort or feelings of fullness.

    Rationale These feelings indicate a distended bladder, which can be confirmed by palpation.

19. Ask the patient to void normally, and measure the amount voided.

    Rationale Measurement indicates whether the patient can void a satisfactory amount. Normally a person voids 150 to 350 mL of urine.

20. a. Empty the drainage bag attached to the catheter.

       Rationale This clears it for the residual urine measurement.

    b. Unclamp the catheter or open the stopcock for about five minutes.

    c. Allow the residual urine to drain from the bladder through the catheter into the bag. After five minutes, measure it.

       Rationale Improper emptying of the bladder after voiding leaves larger than normal amounts of urine in the bladder. The physician may order removal of the catheter when the amount of residual urine is 100 mL or less.

    d. If ordered, obtain a sterile specimen of the residual urine from the emptying spout of the bag.

       Rationale A sterile specimen of the first residual urine sample is often ordered for culture and sensitivity, to ensure that the urine and the bladder are free of microorganisms.

Removing the catheter

21. Obtain a urine specimen (2 to 2.5 mL) while the catheter is clamped, using the syringe and needle as in step 2b.

22. Unclamp the catheter or open the stopcock for drainage, and drain the patient's urine for 15 to 20 minutes.

23. Remove the dressing, and dispose of it in the moisture-resistant bag. The Cystocath may or may not have a dressing over the disc.

24. Loosen the Cystocath disc.

25. Inspect the insertion site, and remove any sutures. See Figure 27–36. For removing sutures, see Technique 35–5 on page 839.

26. Remove the catheter with a steady, continous pull.

27. Apply pressure over the insertion site with gauze squares.

28. Clean the site with antiseptic solution or swabs. Apply povidone-iodine ointment and an Elastoplast bandage.

29. Ensure that the patient's fluid intake is satisfactory, eg, 3,000 mL/day or as ordered by the physician.

30. Record the technique and your assessments on the appropriate records.

FIGURE 27–36

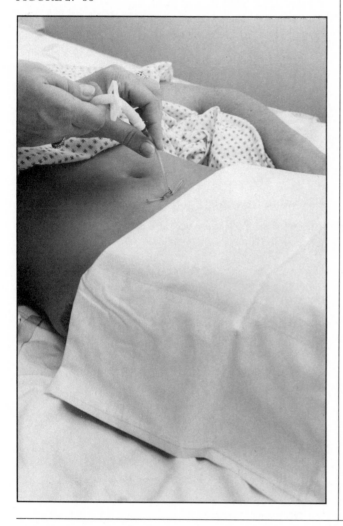

Sample Recording

Date	Time	Notes
6/7/87	1400	SP catheter draining well. Urine slightly pink. SP dressing dry and intact.
6/8/87	0600	SP catheter clamped.
	0900	Tolerated SP clamping for 3-hr period. Voided 90 mL urine. Residual urine 240 mL. Dressing changed. Small amount serosanguineous drainage. Insertion site appears clean.————— Sally M. Sharp, RN

■ Evaluation

Expected outcomes

1. Adequate urine drainage
2. Clear, light amber urine (may be slightly pink for first 24 hours)
3. Slight serosanguineous drainage on initial dressings
4. Satisfactory fluid intake
5. Stable vital signs

Unexpected outcomes

1. Inadequate urine drainage
2. Urine containing blood clots or heavy sediment
3. Dark amber or bright red urine
4. Bleeding at insertion site
5. Inadequate fluid intake
6. Unstable vital signs

Upon obtaining an unexpected outcome:

1. Report your findings to the responsible nurse and/or physician.
2. Adjust the patient's nursing care plan appropriately, eg, to increase fluid intake or inspect drainage on the dressing.

KIDNEY IMPAIRMENT AND PERITONEAL DIALYSIS

Normally the kidneys produce urine continously at the rate of 60 to 120 mL/hr (720 to 1,440 mL/day) in the adult. Newborns need to start micturition within 24 to 36 hours after birth. *Suppression* is the sudden stoppage of urine production. A situation in which the kidneys are producing no urine, or less than 100 mL/day, is called *anuria.* The terms *complete kidney shutdown* or *renal failure* have the same meaning. *Oliguria* is the production of abnormally small amounts of urine by the kidneys, eg, 100 to 500 mL/day.

Both anuria and oliguria can occur as a result of kidney disease, severe heart failure, burns, and shock. These signs can be fatal if some other means, such as an artificial kidney, is not used to remove the body wastes. Other critical signs of renal failure are the presence of uremic frost (urea crystals) on the skin, an elevated blood urea nitrogen (BUN) level, an aromatic odor to the skin, and signs of fluid and electrolyte imbalances.

Peritoneal dialysis, also referred to as *peritoneal exchange,* is used as a temporary or permanent measure when kidney function is impaired. It is the instillation and drainage of a solution (a dialysate) from the peritoneal cavity. Its purpose is to remove impurities, excess fluid, and electrolytes from the blood that would normally be excreted through the kidneys.

The dialysate solution contains water, glucose, and normal serum electrolytes but no body waste products. When it is instilled into the peritoneal cavity, the body's waste products and excess electrolytes pass across the semipermeable peritoneal membrane by diffusion (moving from an area of high concentration to an area of low concentration) to the dialysate. The dialysate containing these waste products is then removed from the peritoneal cavity and replaced with fresh dialysate. This process replaces kidney function and permits the kidneys to rest. Because the dialysate contains glucose in higher concentrations than the blood, it also draws fluid from the blood across the peritoneal membrane by the process of osmosis. In osmosis, fluids move from an area of lower concentration to one of higher concentration.

TECHNIQUE 27-9 ■ Peritoneal Dialysis

For peritoneal dialysis, a physician inserts a catheter into the peritoneal cavity. This may be done at the bedside or in the operating room. Nurses assist with insertion of the catheter, change the dressing at the catheter site, perform fluid exchanges, and assist with removal of the catheter. The peritoneal dialysis system and basic components are shown in Figure 27–37.

Some patients go home with a peritoneal catheter in place and perform the exchange on themselves. Often they need to do this three to six times a day in order to eliminate waste products from the body. Continuous ambulatory peritoneal dialysis (CAPD) necessitates a catheter (a Tenchkoff catheter) sutured into the peritoneal cavity. The patient is ambulatory and free to resume normal activities between exchanges.

■ Assessment

Assess the patient for:

1. Vital signs, for baseline data. These are monitored closely (every 15 minutes) during the first fluid exchange and every hour with subsequent exchanges. Too rapid or excessive fluid loss can cause hypovolemic shock.
2. Weight, for baseline data. The patient is also weighed daily to give an indication of how much fluid is being removed.
3. Abdominal girth, as an indication of fluid retention.
4. Edema.

Other data include: the physician's order, specifying the amount and type of solution for each peritoneal exchange, the number of exchanges, the length of time the fluid is to remain in the peritoneal cavity, and the amount of fluid to be withdrawn from the peritoneal cavity.

■ Nursing Diagnosis

Nursing diagnoses that may indicate the need for peritoneal dialysis include:

1. Urinary suppression related to chronic kidney disease
2. Risk of elevated BUN related to oliguria
3. Risk of fluid overload and peripheral and pulmonary edema related to oliguria
4. Risk of hyperkalemia (elevated serum potassium) related to oliguria

■ Planning

Nursing goal

To remove by-products of metabolism from the blood.

Equipment

For inserting a peritoneal catheter

1. A sterile peritoneal dialysis set containing:
   a. A peritoneal catheter. These are usually made of nylon and have many holes.
   b. A local anesthetic, eg, lidocaine, a #25 gauge ⅝-in needle, and a 3-mL syringe.
   c. Alcohol sponges.
   d. A scalpel with a blade.
   e. A precut gauze to place around the catheter.
   f. Tubing and a clamp.
   g. A drape.
   h. Sutures, needles, and a needle driver.
   i. A trocar.
   j. A connector.
   k. 4 × 4 gauze.

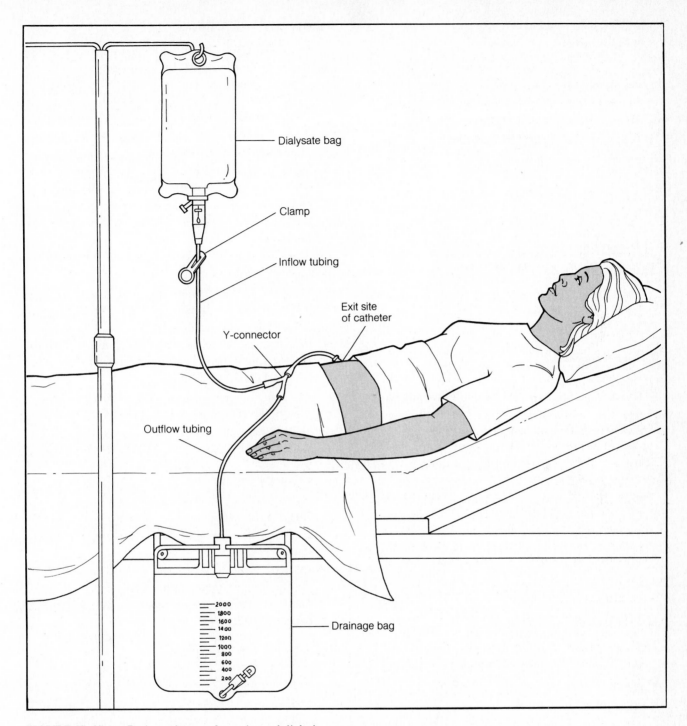

FIGURE 27–37 ■ Basic equipment for peritoneal dialysis.

l. A specimen container.

m. Antiseptic ointment, eg, povidone-iodine.

n. A protective catheter cap.

o. A 10-mL syringe and a 1½-in needle.

p. Scissors.

2. A skin preparation set containing:

a. Povidone-iodine solution.

b. A razor and blade.

c. Gauze sponges.

3. Nonallergenic tape.

4. Sterile gloves, masks, caps, and gowns, depending on agency practice.

For infusing the dialysate

5. A 1,000-mL container of peritoneal solution at body temperature, 37 °C (98.6 °F), or the amount and kind ordered by the physician. When the solution is at body temperature, patient discomfort is decreased.

6. An IV pole.
7. A drainage bag.
8. A sterile peritoneal dialysis administration set.

For changing the catheter site dressing

9. Sterile gloves.
10. Sterile cotton-tipped applicators.
11. Hydrogen peroxide to clean around the catheter.
12. Povidone-iodine solution.
13. Povidone-iodine ointment.
14. A precut sterile 2 × 2 gauze.
15. Nonallergenic tape.

■ Intervention

Inserting a peritoneal catheter

1. Explain the technique to the patient. Inserting the trocar (which is the physician's responsibility) may be uncomfortable. If the patient tenses the abdominal muscles as if for a bowel movement, discomfort can be reduced.
2. Ask the patient to urinate before the technique.
   Rationale Emptying the bladder lessens the danger that it will be punctured by the trocar.
3. Assist the patient to a supine position, and arrange the bedding to expose the area around the umbilicus.
   Rationale The insertion site is usually in the midline just below the umbilicus.
4. Add any prescribed medication to the dialysate solution. Heparin is sometimes added to prevent the accumulation of fibrin in the catheter; povidone-iodine solution is added to prevent the growth of microorganisms.
5. Check the label on the solution container and the solution itself. The solution should be clear and the seals unbroken.
6. Spike the solution container, close the clamp, and hang the container on the IV pole.
7. Prime the tubing. See Technique 25–1, step 16, on page 552. Close the tubing clamp.
8. Open the sterile supplies.
9. Assist the physician as needed. The physician prepares the skin first, then injects the local anesthetic. After making a small incision, the physician inserts the catheter into the cavity, using the trocar to guide it.
10. Connect the end of the tubing from the solution to the catheter.
11. Connect the drainage receptacle to the outflow tubing. Close the tubing clamp.
12. Cover the catheter site with the precut sterile gauze and tape the dressing in place.

Infusing peritoneal dialysate

13. Open the clamp on the inflow tubing so that the dialysate can flow into the peritoneal cavity for the period specified in the physician's order (usually 5 to 10 minutes).
14. Clamp the inflow tubing.
    Rationale With the tubing clamped, air will not enter the peritoneal cavity.
15. Leave the fluid in the cavity for the designated time. This may range from, eg, 10 minutes to 4 hours.
16. Assess the patient's vital signs every 15 minutes for the first exchange and hourly on subsequent exchanges.

Removing the fluid

17. Unclamp the outflow tubing, permitting the fluid to drain into the drainage bag by gravity.
18. If the fluid does not drain freely, assist the patient to change position or raise the head of the bed. Drain only the amount specified in the physician's order.
19. Clamp the outflow tubing.
20. Measure the amount of outflow fluid, and compare it with the amount of solution infused.
21. Calculate the fluid balance. If more fluid was infused than removed, the patient's fluid balance is negative (–); if more fluid was removed than infused, the fluid balance is positive (+).
22. Repeat steps 13–21 for each exchange.
23. Check the dressing at the catheter site.
    Rationale The dressing should remain dry during the dialysis.
24. Disconnect the catheter from the tubing, and cover the end of the catheter with a sterile cap.
    Rationale The catheter may remain in place between exchanges.

Changing the catheter site dressing

25. Follow Technique 25–11 on page 579.

■ Evaluation

Expected outcomes

1. Decreased abdominal girth
2. Decreased weight
3. Vital signs within normal range
4. Site around catheter clean and dry, with no signs of infection
5. Returned dialysate clear or slightly yellow
6. Fluid balance positive

Unexpected outcomes

1. No change in abdominal girth
2. Increased or no change in weight
3. Vital signs abnormal
4. Site around catheter inflamed or moist
5. Returned dialysate red, green, cloudy, or milky
6. Fluid balance negative

Upon obtaining an unexpected outcome:

1. Report your findings to the responsible nurse and/or physician.
2. Adjust the nursing care plan appropriately.

URINE SPECIMENS AND TESTS

Urine specimens are collected for a number of types of tests. Routine urine examination is usually done on the first voided specimen in the morning, because it tends to have a higher, more uniform concentration and a more acid pH than specimens later in the day (Byrne et al, 1986, p 5). A clean voided specimen is usually adequate for routine examination; a clean-catch specimen is needed for bacteriologic culture.

Timed Urine Specimens

Several urine tests require timed specimens. Urine specimens are collected at timed intervals, for short periods (1 to 2 hours) or long periods (12 to 24 hours). All timed urine specimens need to be refrigerated, to prevent bacterial growth and decomposition of the urine components, which can affect the findings. For some timed specimens, large collection containers are kept in a refrigerator, often in the laboratory, not at the bedside. Each voiding of urine is collected in a small clean container and then emptied immediately into the large refrigerated bottle. In most instances the entire amount of urine voided is collected.

For some tests, a chemical urine preservative, eg, toluene or acetic acid, is added to the large collection container. Other tests require different preservatives, since certain additives invalidate the results for certain tests. It is wise to contact the laboratory prior to the specimen collection to confirm the additive for a test.

Tests using timed urine specimens

Some of the tests performed on timed urine specimens include:

1. Quantitative albumin test (24 hours) to determine the daily amount of albumin lost in the urine in such conditions as kidney disease, hypertension, drug toxicity, or severe heart failure involving kidney damage.

2. Amino acid tests (24 hours) to determine acquired or congenital disease of the kidneys.

3. Amylase test (2, 12, or 24 hours). Amylase is a pancreatic enzyme that may be excreted in the urine in certain diseases of the pancreas.

4. Quantitative chlorides test (24 hours) to determine the total excretion of chloride. This test may be performed in the management of cardiac patients who are on low-salt diets.

5. Concentration and dilution tests to determine disorders of the kidney tubules in concentrating and diluting urine. These specimens are collected over varying periods of time. Specimens are commonly collected at hourly intervals for two to four hours after the patient has been given a specified amount of clear fluid to drink. Check agency procedures.

6. Creatinine test or creatinine clearance test (24 hours) to reflect the degree of kidney impairment. Creatinine is formed in the muscles from creatine in relatively constant daily amounts and is excreted in the urine. Elevated creatinine content indicates a disturbance in kidney function.

7. Estriol determination test (24 hours) to measure the level of this hormone in the urine of high-risk pregnant women such as those with toxemia or diabetes. Estriol is the major form in which estrogen is excreted in the urine. Low levels can indicate inadequate function of the placenta and possible fetal distress.

8. Glucose tolerance test (24 hours) to determine disorders of glucose metabolism that may arise from malfunction of the liver or pancreas. Tests are performed on both the blood and the urine after the patient is given a large amount of glucose orally or intravenously.

9. 17-hydroxycorticosteroid test (24 hours) to assess the functioning of the adrenal cortex. Corticosteroids are hormones that are produced in the adrenal cortex, altered, and then excreted in the urine.

10. Urobilinogen test (random times or 2 hours) to determine obstruction of the biliary tract, excessive destruction of red blood cells, or liver damage. These

specimens are collected in brown bottles because they need to be protected from light.

Clean-Catch Specimens

In the past, catheterization was the preferred method of acquiring specimens for culture that were free from contamination, particularly from females. The trend today is to use the clean voided midstream (CVMS) method. Even though the specimen may be somewhat contaminated by skin bacteria, it is better to have a contaminated specimen than to cause infection to the patient's urinary tract. A bacterial count can generally reveal whether the bacteria in CVMS specimens came from the skin or from a urinary infection. Bacterial counts below 10,000/mL of urine generally mean skin contamination of the specimen and not a true urinary tract infection. Counts above 100,000/mL generally indicate a true infection of the urinary tract. Analyses showing counts between 10,000 and 100,000 are usually repeated.

It is obvious that a CVMS specimen cannot be obtained from patients with indwelling catheters. If a patient has an indwelling catheter, the aspiration method is used. This involves inserting a sterile needle with a syringe into a disinfected port on the catheter, withdrawing urine, and transferring the urine into a sterile specimen container.

Guidelines for obtaining urine specimens for culture and sensitivity

1. Use medical and surgical aseptic technique to keep all specimens as free as possible from external contamination by microorganisms residing near the urethral opening.

2. Clean external skin surfaces surrounding the urinary meatus with an antiseptic, and rinse with sterile water, prior to specimen collection.

3. Use sterile specimen containers and lids.

4. Send all specimens to the laboratory immediately. Bacterial cultures need to be started promptly before contaminating organisms that may have been introduced have a chance to grow, multiply, and produce false results in the tests.

Routine Urine Testing

Several urine tests are simple to perform and are often done by nurses on the nursing units or are taught to patients, who perform them on their own urine. Tests commonly performed on urine include those for specific gravity, pH, presence of glucose and ketone bodies, and presence of occult blood.

Specific gravity

The specific gravity is the weight or degree of concentration of a substance compared with that of an equal volume of another, such as distilled water, taken as a standard. The speicific gravity of distilled water is 1.00 g/mL (in other words, 1 mL of water weighs 1 g). The specific gravity of urine is measured by a urinometer (hydrometer), calibrated in units of 0.001. The instrument is placed in a glass cylinder containing the urine. The scale on the urinometer progresses from 1.000 at the top to 1.060 at the bottom. The specific gravity of urine is normally about 1.010 to 1.025 g/mL. A low specific gravity is often the result of overhydration or a disease that affects the kidneys' ability to concentrate solutes in the urine. A high specific gravity is often the result of dehydration or a disease that increases water reabsorption by the kidneys, causing concentrated urine. False positive results are caused by drugs such as dextran and radiopaque materials used in x-ray examination of the urinary tract.

pH (acid–base)

The pH is a measurement of the concentration of hydrogen ions, which indicates the acidity or alkalinity of a substance. Discrete measurements of pH are made on a scale of 1 to 14 in which the value 7 is neutral, below 7 is acid, and above 7 is alkaline (base). Such quantitative measurements, however, are conducted in the agency laboratory, where specific reactive agents are used.

Urine becomes increasingly acidic when increasing amounts of sodium and excess acid are retained in the body. Ingestion of various foods also affects urinary pH. A diet rich in animal protein and cranberry juice decreases the pH and produces an acid urine. A diet high in citrus fruits, most vegetables, milk, and other dairy products increases the pH and produces an alkaline urine.

Control of the urine pH is an important factor in certain medical therapies. For example, the formation of renal stones is partially dependent on the urinary pH; therefore, patients being treated for stones are often given diets or medications to alter the pH and prevent stone formation. Certain medications, eg, streptomycin, neomycin, and kanamycin, are more effective for treating urinary tract infections provided the urine is alkaline.

Presence of glucose

Urine is tested for glucose to screen patients for diabetes mellitus or to follow the progress of a known diabetic. Normally the amount of glucose in the urine is negligible, although individuals who have ingested large amounts of sugar may show small amounts of glucose in their urine.

Several commercial products are commonly used to test for the presence of glucose, eg, Clinitest tablets and Clinistix, Diastix, and Tes-Tape reagent strips. Each uses a color scale to measure the quantity of glucose in the urine, but the scales are not interchangeable from one product to the other. The scales grade the results as negative, trace, one plus (1+ or +), two plus (2+ or ++), three plus (3+ or +++), etc. Each grade reflects a specific percentage of glucose, which varies from one testing product to another. For example, a 2+ result from a Clinitest reaction indicates 75% glucose in the urine, whereas a 2+ result from a Tes-Tape strip indicates 25% glucose.

False readings can arise from medications a patient is receiving, depending on the type of chemical product used to test the urine for glucose. For example, tetracycline and large doses of ascorbic acid and chloral hydrate can generate false positive results from Clinitest tablets. For this reason, many agencies stock more than one testing product. Nurses need to compare the medications a patient is receiving with the literature about each product, and choose the appropriate product for the test.

Presence of ketone bodies

Ketone bodies are products of incomplete fat metabolism and appear in the urine in instances of fasting, very low intake of carbohydrates, and uncontrolled diabetes mellitus. Usually the urine is tested for ketone bodies at the same time it is tested for glucose. Tablets or reagent strips are used.

Presence of occult blood

Normal urine is free of blood. When blood is present, it may be clearly visible or not visible (occult). Commercial reagent strips are used to test for occult blood in the urine.

TECHNIQUE 27–10 ■ Collecting a Urine Specimen from an Adult or a Child Who Has Urinary Control

■ Assessment

Determine if the patient can assist with the technique. Other data include: any special directions for collecting the specimen.

■ Planning

Nursing goal

To obtain a urine specimen of sufficient quantity.

Equipment

1. A wide-mouthed specimen container with a lid
2. A clean bedpan, urinal, or commode for patients who are unable to void directly into the specimen container
3. A completed specimen identification label
4. A completed laboratory requisition
5. Disinfectant and swabs

■ Intervention

1. Inform the patient that a urine specimen is required, the purpose of it, and how he or she can assist. Often the patient is able to provide the specimen independently. Male patients generally have little difficulty, but female patients usually need to stand over a toilet bowl and hold the container between their legs during the process of voiding. About 14 mL (4 oz) of urine is generally required. Check agency policy.

2. Provide the assistance required by patients who are seriously ill, physically incapacitated, or disoriented. Some may need to use a bedpan or urinal in bed; others may require supervision and/or assistance in the bathroom. Whatever the situation, give explicit directions.

3. Explain that all specimens must be free of fecal contamination, so voiding needs to occur at a different time from defecation. Instruct female patients to discard the toilet tissue in the toilet or in a waste bag rather than in the bedpan, since tissue in the specimen makes laboratory analysis more difficult.

4. Give the patient the specimen container and direct him or her to the bathroom to void 14 mL (4 oz) into it.
   or
   Assist the patient to void into a bedpan or urinal. Transfer about 14 mL (4 oz) of the urine from the bedpan, urinal, or commode to the specimen container.

5. Assess the characteristics and amount of urine. See Table 27–1 at the beginning of this chapter.

6. Put the lid tightly on the container.
   Rationale This prevents spillage of the urine and contamination of other objects.

7. If the outside of the container has been contaminated by urine, clean it with a disinfectant.
   Rationale This prevents the spread of microorganisms.

8. Empty the bedpan or urinal.

9. Ensure that the specimen label and the laboratory requisition have the correct information on them. Attach them securely to the specimen.

   Rationale Inappropriate identification of the specimen can lead to errors of diagnosis or therapy for the patient.

10. Arrange for the specimen to be taken immediately to the laboratory or placed in a refrigerator.

    Rationale Urine deteriorates relatively rapidly from bacterial contamination, when left at room temperature; specimens should be analyzed immediately after collection.

11. Record collection of the specimen on the patient's chart. Include the date and time of collection and the appearance and odor of the urine.

■ Evaluation

Expected outcomes

1. Urine characteristics normal. See Table 27–1 on page 622.
2. No evidence of skin irritation around perineum.

Unexpected outcomes

1. Urine characteristics abnormal. See Table 27–1.
2. Skin area around perineum irritated.

Upon obtaining an unexpected outcome:

1. Report your findings to the responsible nurse and/or physician.
2. Adjust the nursing care plan appropriately.

TECHNIQUE 27–11 ■ Collecting a Urine Specimen from an Infant

■ Assessment

Determine whether there are any special directions about collecting the specimen.

■ Planning

Nursing goal

To obtain a urine specimen of the correct amount at the correct time.

Equipment

1. A plastic, disposable, urine collection bag. This is a specially designed clear plastic bag with an adhesive backing and an opening that is applied over the infant's urethral meatus or penis. See Figure 27–38.
2. Sterile cotton balls to clean and dry the perineal area.
3. Soap and a basin of water.
4. Antiseptic solution.
5. Sterile water.
6. A diaper.
7. A specimen container.
8. A disinfectant.
9. A completed specimen label.
10. A completed laboratory requisition form.

■ Intervention

1. If parents are present, explain why a urine specimen is being taken and the method of obtaining it.

2. Before and throughout the procedure, handle the infant gently, and talk in soothing tones.
3. Remove the infant's diaper and clean the perineal–genital area with soap and water and then with an antiseptic.

FIGURE 27–38

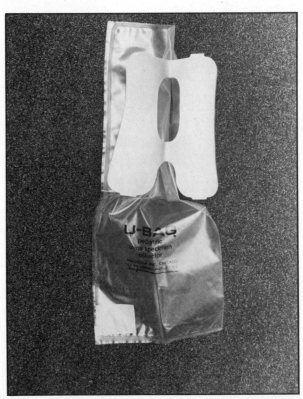

Rationale Cleaning is necessary to remove powder, baby oil, lotions, secretions, and fecal matter from the genitals. It also reduces the number of microorganisms on the skin and subsequent contamination of the voided urine.

a. For girls, separate the labia and wash, rinse, and dry the perineal area from the front to the back (clitoris to anus) on each side of the urinary meatus, and then over the meatus. See Figure 27–39. Repeat this procedure, using the antiseptic solution to clean, the sterile water to rinse, and some dry cotton balls to dry.

b. For boys, clean and disinfect both the penis and the scrotum in the manner described above. Wash the penis in a circular motion from the tip toward the scrotum, and wash the scrotum last. See Figure 27–40. Retract the foreskin of an uncircumcised boy.

Rationale Freeing the skin of all moisture and secretions facilitates proper adhesion of the urine collection bag and prevents leakage of urine.

4. Inspect the infant's perineum for signs of irritation.

5. Remove the protective paper from the bottom half of the adhesive backing of the collection bag. See Figure 27–41.

6. Spread the infant's legs apart as much as possible.

FIGURE 27–39

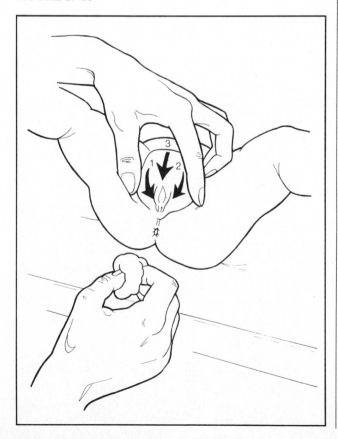

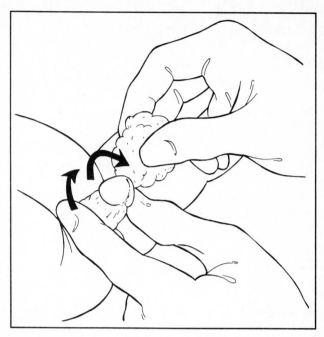

FIGURE 27–40

FIGURE 27–41

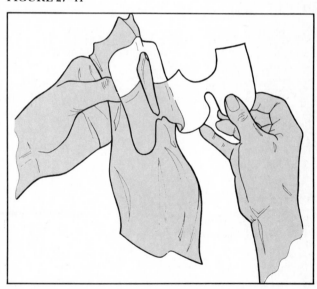

Rationale Spreading the legs separates and flattens the folds of the skin.

7. Place the opening of the collection bag over the urethra or the penis and scrotum. The base of the opening needs to cover the vagina or to fit well up under the scrotum. See Figure 27–42.

8. Press the adhesive portion firmly against the infant's skin, starting at the perineum (the area between the anus and the genitals) and working outward.

Rationale This method prevents wrinkles, which could cause leakage of urine.

9. Remove the protective paper from the top half of the adhesive backing, and press it firmly in place, working from the top center outward.

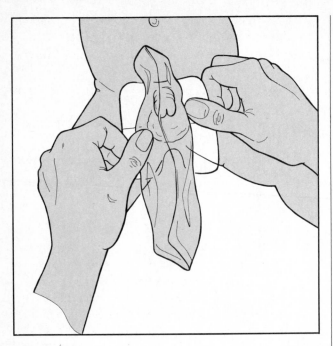

FIGURE 27-42

10. Apply a loose-fitting diaper.

    Rationale A diaper helps keep the urine bag in place.

11. Elevate the head of the crib mattress to semi-Fowler's position.

    Rationale Semi-Fowler's position aids the flow of urine by gravity into the collection portion of the urine bag.

12. After the child has voided a desired amount, gently remove the bag from the skin.

13. Empty the urine from the bag through the opening at its base into the specimen container. Discard the urine bag.

14. Measure the urine, and assess its characteristics. See Table 27-1.

15. Tightly apply the lid to the specimen container.

    Rationale The lid will prevent spillage of urine from the container and contamination of other objects.

16. If the outside of the specimen container has been contaminated, clean it with a disinfectant.

    Rationale Cleaning the outside of the container prevents the spread of microorganisms.

17. Apply the infant's diaper, and leave him or her in a comfortable and safe position held by a parent or in a crib.

18. Ensure that the specimen label and the laboratory requisition have the correct information on them. Attach them securely to the specimen.

    Rationale Incorrect identification of the specimen can lead to subsequent errors of diagnosis or therapy for the infant.

19. Arrange for the specimen to be sent to the laboratory immediately or refrigerate it.

20. Record collection of the urine specimen and your assessments.

■ **Evaluation** See Technique 27-10 on page 658.

TECHNIQUE 27-12 ■ Collecting a Timed Urine Specimen

■ **Assessment** See Technique 27-10 on page 657 and Table 27-1 on page 622.

■ **Planning**

Nursing goal

To elicit the patient's cooperation and to collect all urine at the correct times.

Equipment

1. Appropriate specimen containers with or without preservative in accordance with the specific test. These are generally obtained from the laboratory and placed in the patient's bathroom or in the utility room.

2. Completed specimen identification labels. The labels need to indicate the date and time of each voiding in addition to the usual identification information. They may also be numbered sequentially, eg, 1st specimen, 2nd specimen, 3rd specimen.

3. A completed laboratory requisition.

4. A bedpan or urinal.

5. An alert card indicating the specific times for urine collection. This is placed in the patient's room, on or near the bed. It reminds all nursing staff that the test is in progress.

6. A disinfectant.

■ Intervention

1. Give the patient explicit instructions about the purpose of the test and how she or he can assist. Tell the patient when the specimen collection will begin and end; for example, a 24-hour urine test commonly begins at 0700 hours and ends at the same hour the next day. Instructions should include the following facts:

   a. All urine must be saved and placed in the specimen containers once the test starts.

   b. The urine must be free of fecal contamination and toilet tissue.

   c. Each specimen must be given to the nursing staff immediately so that it can be placed in the appropriate specimen bottle.

2. Start the collection period by having the patient void in the toilet or bedpan or urinal. Discard this urine. (Check agency procedure.) Collect all subsequent urine specimens, including the one at the end of the period.

3. Have the patient ingest the required amount of liquid for certain tests.

4. Measure the urine, and inspect each specimen for color, odor, and chracteristics.

5. Record the starting time of the test on the patient's chart.

6. Instruct the patient to void all subsequent urine into the bedpan or urinal and to notify the nursing staff when each specimen is provided. Some tests require that the patient void at specified times.

7. Place each specimen into the appropriately labeled container. For some tests each specimen is not kept separately but is poured into a large bottle in the laboratory refrigerator. Note assessment data for each specimen, if indicated for the specific test.

8. If the outside of the specimen container is contaminated with urine, clean it with a disinfectant.
   Rationale Cleaning prevents the transfer of microorganisms to others.

9. Ensure that each specimen is refrigerated throughout the timed collection period.
   Rationale Refrigeration prevents bacterial decomposition of the urine.

10. Have the patient provide the last specimen five to ten minutes before the end of the collection period.

11. Assess the color, odor, and clarity of the patient's urine.

12. Inform the patient that the test is completed.

13. Remove the alert signs and specimen equipment from the patient's unit and bathroom.

14. Record completion of the specimen collection on the patient's chart. Include the date and specific time. In addition, if indicated for the specific test, note the time each urine specimen was collected, the volume of each specimen, the appearance of the urine, and other relevant data such as fluid intake or restrictions.

■ Evaluation

Expected outcome

Urine appears normal. See Table 27–1 on page 622.

Unexpected outcome

Urine has abnormal characteristics. See Table 27–1. Upon obtaining an unexpected outcome:

1. Report your findings to the responsible nurse and/or physician.

2. Adjust the nursing care plan appropriately.

TECHNIQUE 27–13   ■   Collecting a Urine Specimen for Culture and Sensitivity by Clean Catch

■ Assessment

Assess the patient's ability to carry out the technique.

■ Planning

Nursing goals

1. To identify an infecting microorganism in the urine

2. To monitor the progress of a patient being treated for a known infection of the urinary tract

Equipment

The equipment used varies from agency to agency. Some agencies use commercially prepared disposable clean-catch kits. See Figure 27–43. Others use agency-prepared

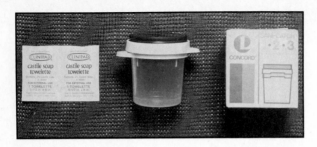

FIGURE 27-43

sterile trays. Both prepared trays and kits generally contain the following items:

1. Sterile cotton balls in a container, to clean and dry the genitals and perineal area.
2. An antiseptic, such as aqueous Zephiran 1:700. The antiseptic may need to be added to an agency-prepared tray.
3. A container of sterile water to rinse the perineal area after cleaning.
4. Sterile gloves to wear when swabbing and cleaning.
5. A urine receptacle.
6. A sterile specimen container for the urine specimen.
7. A specimen identification label.

Additional supplies:

8. A completed laboratory requisition form.
9. A bath blanket, if the patient is not ambulatory.
10. A disinfectant.

■ Intervention

1. Inform the patient that a urine specimen is required; give the reason for it, and explain the method to be used to collect it.
2. Ask the patient to wash and dry his or her genitals and perineum thoroughly with soap and water. A clean perineum is essential, to reduce the number of skin bacteria and to minimize contamination of the specimen.
3. Assist the ambulatory patient to the bathroom. The preferred method to collect the specimen from ambulatory patients is to have them provide the specimen while standing over the toilet in the bathroom.
4. Assist nonambulatory patients to an upright sitting position on a urine receptacle. Provide appropriate covers for the patient: Fold back the top bed linen to the bottom of the bed and drape the patient in a bath blanket, exposing only the perineal area.
5. Assist female patients to spread their legs apart enough to ensure that the urine will not touch the legs.

6. Open the sterile kit or tray, using sterile technique.
   Rationale Sterile technique is essential to maintain the sterility of the specimen container.
7. Put on the sterile gloves.
8. Pour the antiseptic solution over the cotton balls.
9. Clean the patient's vulvar area or the tip of the penis with the antiseptic.
   Rationale The antiseptic reduces the number of bacteria near the urethral opening and minimizes contamination of the urine specimens.
10. For female patients:
    a. Swab the labia minora from front to back, using one swab for each wipe.
       Rationale Swabbing from front to back cleans from the area of least contamination to the area of greatest contamination.
    b. Spread the labia minora well apart, using the thumb and another finger, eg, the third finger, of one hand.
    c. Swab between the labia minora over the urethra from front to back.
       Rationale The urethra is considered less contaminated than the vagina and anus.
    d. Rinse the area with sterile water.
       Rationale Rinsing removes the antiseptic and other external contaminants.
    e. Dry the area with sterile cotton balls.
11. For male patients:
    a. Hold the penis with one hand and clean the urinary meatus using a circular motion. Retract the foreskin of an uncircumcised male.
    b. Wash outward from the meatus in a circular motion, using one swab for each wipe.
       Rationale This cleans from the area of least contamination to the area of greatest contamination.
    c. Rinse the area with sterile water.
    d. Dry the area with cotton balls, in the same manner used for cleaning.
12. Ask the patient to start voiding.
    Rationale Initial voiding clears additional external contaminants at the urethral opening.
13. After the patient has begun to void, place the specimen container under the stream of urine to collect 30 to 60 mL of midstream urine. Handle only the outside of the container.
    Rationale Handling only the outside protects the sterility of the inside.
14. Put the sterile cap tightly on the specimen container, touching only the outside of the cap.
    Rationale Capping the container prevents spillage of urine and contamination of other objects. Touch-

ing only the outside of the cap retains the sterility of the inside of the cap.

15. Inspect the urine for normal and abnormal characteristics. See Table 27-1 earlier.

16. Clean the outer surface of the container with a disinfectant.

    Rationale Cleaning the outer surface prevents the transfer of microorganisms to others.

17. Remove your gloves and wash hands.

18. Ensure that the specimen label and the laboratory requisition have the correct information on them. Attach them securely to the specimen.

    Rationale Inaccurate identification and/or information on the specimen container can lead to errors of diagnosis or therapy.

19. Arrange for the specimen to be sent to the laboratory immediately.

    Rationale Bacterial cultures must be started immediately, before any contaminating organisms can grow and multiply.

20. Record collection of the specimen, any pertinent observations of the urine in terms of color, odor, or consistency, and any difficulty in voiding that the patient experienced.

■ Evaluation

Expected outcomes

1. Able to provide an uncontaminated urine specimen.
2. Urine appears normal. See Table 27-1 on page 622.

Unexpected outcomes

1. Unable to provide a clean-catch specimen.
2. Urine has abnormal characteristics. See Table 27-1.

Upon obtaining an unexpected outcome:

1. Report your findings to the responsible nurse.
2. Adjust the nursing care plan appropriately, eg, obtain another specimen.

TECHNIQUE 27–14 ■ Testing Urine for Specific Gravity, pH, Glucose, Ketones, and Occult Blood

■ Planning

Nursing goals

1. To determine the patient's hydration status from a specific gravity measurement
2. To determine the acidity or alkalinity of the patient's urine
3. To determine the presence of glucose and ketone bodies in the urine
4. To determine the presence of occult blood in the urine

Equipment

For specific gravity

1. A urinometer (hydrometer) and a glass cylinder for the urine
   or
2. A spectrometer or refractometer

For urine pH

3. Litmus paper (red or blue)

For glucose

4. A reagent tablet or reagent test strip

5. The appropriate color scale
6. A clean test tube and a dropper if a tablet is used

For ketone bodies

7. A reagent tablet or test strip

For occult blood

8. A reagent strip

■ Intervention

Measuring specific gravity

1. Have the patient fast for 12 hours prior to the specimen collection, if required by the agency.
2. To measure with a urinometer:

   a. Pour at least 20 mL of a fresh urine sample in the glass cylinder, or fill the cylinder three-quarters full.

   b. Place the urinometer into the cylinder and give it a gentle spin to prevent it from adhering to the sides of the cylinder.

   c. Hold the urinometer at eye level, and read the measurement at the base of the meniscus at the surface of the urine. See Figure 27–44.

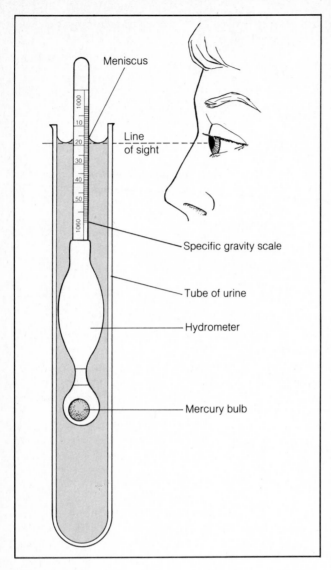

Meniscus

1000
10
20
30
40
50
1060

Line of sight

Specific gravity scale

Tube of urine

Hydrometer

Mercury bulb

FIGURE 27–44

Rationale The concentration of the urine affects the degree to which the urinometer will float. The depth to which it sinks indicates the specific gravity.

    d. Discard the urine, clean the equipment with soap and water, wash hands, and record the measurement on the patient's chart.

3. To measure with a spectrometer or refractometer:

    a. Be sure to follow the manufacturer's directions.

    b. Place one or two drops of urine on the slide.

    c. Turn on the instrument light, and look into the instrument. The specific gravity will appear on a scope.

    d. Write down the number, then turn off the instrument.

    e. Remove the urine with a damp towel or gauze.

Measuring pH

4. Dip a strip of either red or blue litmus paper into the urine specimen

5. Observe the color of the litmus paper, and compare it to a standardized color chart on the bottle. The blue litmus paper, more commonly used, remains blue if the urine is alkaline and turns red if it is acidic. The red litmus paper remains red in the presence of acid urine and turns blue if the urine is alkaline. Whichever litmus strip is used, red always indicates acid urine and blue alkaline urine.

Testing for glucose

6. Obtain a freshly voided specimen. Most agencies require a *second-voided specimen:* Have the patient void, and in 30 minutes have the patient void again, providing a specimen for the test this time.

    Rationale A second-voided specimen more accurately reflects the present condition of the body. Urine that has accumulated in the bladder, eg, overnight, reflects the condition of the body at the time the urine was produced, eg, 0300 hours.

7. Select the appropriate equipment and testing product for the patient. If Clinitest tablets are used, obtain a clean test tube and dropper.

8. Follow the directions specified by the manufacturer to carry out the test. If Clinitest tablets are used, be careful not to touch the bottom of the test tube, because this becomes extremely hot when the tablet boils in the presence of urine and water.

9. Compare the results with the appropriate color chart, and record them on the patient's chart. Most agencies now record the findings in percentage of glucose in the urine rather than 2+ or 3+.

Testing for ketone bodies

10. Place one or two drops of urine on a reagent tablet (eg, an Acetest tablet), or dip a reagent test strip (eg, Ketostix) into the urine.

11. Observe and compare the results with the appropriate color chart, to determine the quantity of ketones present.

12. Record the results in accordance with the product used and agency practice. The results may be graded as negative, small, moderate, or large amounts, or as negative, positive, or strongly positive.

Testing for occult blood

13. Dip the reagent strip (eg, Hemastix) into a sample of urine.

14. Compare the color change with a color chart in the same manner as for other reagent strips.

15. Record the results on the appropriate record.

■ Evaluation

Expected outcomes

1. Specific gravity of 1.010 to 1.025
2. Urine pH of 4.5 to 8
3. Negative result for glucose and ketone bodies
4. Negative result for occult blood

Unexpected outcomes

1. Specific gravity above 1.025 or below 1.010
2. Urine pH above 8 or below 4.5

3. Presence of glucose
4. Presence of ketone bodies
5. Presence of occult blood

Upon obtaining an unanticipated outcome: Report your findings to the responsible nurse and/or physician.

References

Baum ME: "I want to be dry": The (almost) carefree way to conquer urinary incontinence. *Nursing 78* (February) 1978; 8:75–76, 78.

Beaumont E: Urinary drainage systems. *Nursing 74* (January) 1974; 4:52–60.

Beber R: Freedom for the incontinent. *Am J Nurs* (March) 1980; 80:482–484.

Byrne CJ et al: *Laboratory Tests: Implications for Nursing Care.* Addison-Wesley, 1986.

Davis V, Lavandero R: Caring for the catheter carefully . . . before, during and after peritoneal dialysis, part 2. *Nursing 80* (December) 1980; 10:23–27.

Demmerle B, Bartol MA: Nursing care for the incontinent person. *Geriatr Nurs* (November/December) 1980; 1:246–250.

DeGroot J: Catheter-induced urinary tract infections: Can we prevent them? *Nursing 76* (August) 1976; 6:34–37.

DeGroot J: Urethral catheterization: Observing "niceties" prevents infections. *Nursing 76* (December) 1976; 6:51–55.

DeGroot J, Kunin CM: Indwelling catheters. *Am J Nurs* (March) 1975; 75:448–449.

Fischbach F: *A Manual of Laboratory Diagnostic Tests.* Lippincott, 1980.

Garner J: Urinary catheter care: Doing it better. *Nursing 74* (February) 1974; 4:54–56.

Killon A: Reducing the risk of infection from indwelling urethral catheters. *Nursing 82* (May) 1982; 12:84–88.

Kinney AB, Blount M, Dowell M: Urethral catheterization: Pros and cons of an invasive but sometimes essential procedure. *Geriatr Nurs* (November/December) 1980; 1:258–263.

Musial EM: Peritoneal dialysis. In: *Nurses Reference Library: Procedures.* Intermed Communications, 1983.

Swearingen PL: *The Addison-Wesley Photo-Atlas of Nursing Procedures.* Addison-Wesley, 1984.

Whyte JF, Thistle NA: Male incontinence: The inside story on external collection. *Nursing 76* (September) 1976; 6:66–67.

Woodrow M: Suprapubic catheters, part 1: A direct line to better drainage. *Nursing 76* (October) 1976; 6:40–45.

Woodrow M: Suprapubic catheters, part 2: A direct line to better drainage. *Nursing 76* (November) 1976; 6:40–42.

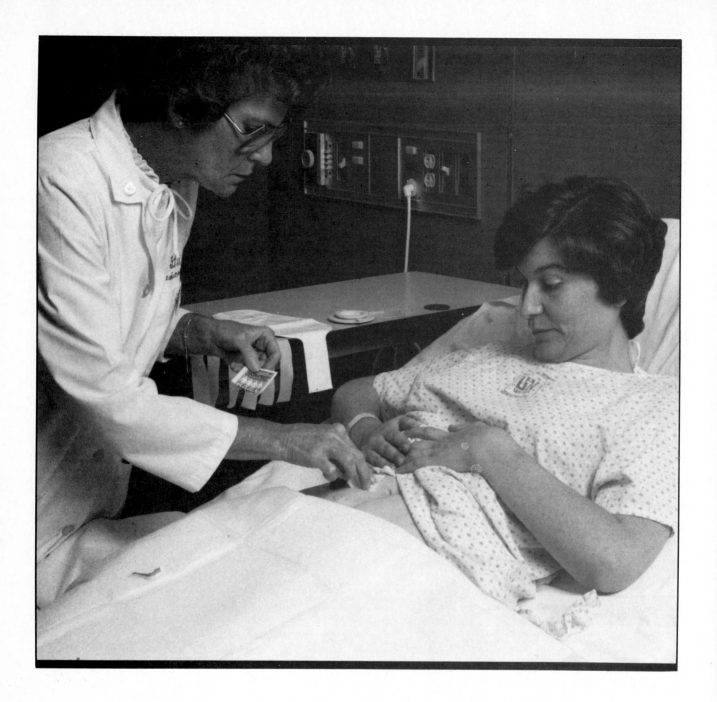

OSTOMY CARE

28

An "ostomy" is an opening on the abdominal wall for the elimination of feces or urine. There are many types, depending on which organ is involved—the stomach, small intestine, large intestine, or ureter.

Adjusting to the creation of an ostomy is difficult for most patients. They must learn skills to deal with a new elimination process, to care for the stoma, and to prevent elimination problems. In addition, patients often have to overcome negative reactions to the problem that necessitated this traumatic surgery and come to accept their condition.

Chapter Outline

Objectives

Upon completion of this chapter, the student will:

1. Know essential terms and facts about ostomies and
ostomy care
   1.1 Define selected terms
   1.2 Identify various types of ostomies
   1.3 Describe major ways ostomies are constructed
   1.4 Identify selected nursing interventions for bowel
   diversion ostomy patients
   1.5 Differentiate between distal and proximal stomas
   of bowel diversion ostomies
   1.6 Explain how and why the character of drainage
   differs among selected colostomy sites
   1.7 Identify various types of urinary diversion
   ostomies
2. Understand facts about ostomy techniques
   2.1 Identify relevant assessment data
   2.2 Identify nursing diagnoses for which the
   technique may be implemented
   2.3 Identify nursing goals related to the technique
   2.4 Identify expected and unexpected outcomes from
   assessment data
   2.5 Identify reasons underlying selected steps of the
   technique

3. Perform ostomy techniques safely
   3.1 Assess the patient adequately
   3.2 Collect additional data from appropriate sources
   3.3 Select pertinent nursing goals for the patient
   3.4 Establish relevant outcome criteria for the patient
   following the technique
   3.5 Collect necessary equipment before the technique
   3.6 Implement interventions to enhance the effectiveness of the technique and enhance the patient's
   comfort and safety
   3.7 Communicate relevant information about the
   patient to the appropriate persons through
   records or reports
   3.8 Evaluate the outcomes of the technique
4. Evaluate own performance of specific techniques
   in a laboratory or clinical setting with the assistance
   of another
   4.1 Use the performance checklists provided
   4.2 Identify areas of strength and weakness
   4.3 Alter performance in response to own evaluation
   and that of another

Terms

■ **appliance**   a device or bag that is secured to the abdomen to collect either urine or feces through an ostomy

■ **barrier (of the skin)**   a protective covering for the skin, eg, a liquid, spray, or material such as karaya

■ **colostomy**   a surgically created opening of the colon on the abdomen

■ **cystectomy**   removal of the bladder

■ **effluent**   urine or feces discharged through a stoma

■ **enterostomal therapy (ET) nurse**   a person who specializes in ostomy care

■ **ileostomy**   a surgically created opening of the small intestine on the abdomen

■ **irrigation**   the washing out of an organ or body cavity

■ **-ostomy**   a suffix referring to an opening or outlet

■ **peristomal**   the skin area that surrounds a stoma

■ **stoma**   a surgically created opening in the abdominal wall; it may be permanent or temporary

■ **ureterostomy**   a specific type of urostomy in which the ureter opens onto the abdominal wall

■ **urostomy (urinary diversion)**   a surgically created opening into the urinary tract that permits the drainage of urine through the abdomen

■ **vesicostomy**   a surgically created opening of the bladder on the abdomen

BOWEL DIVERSION OSTOMIES

There are many types of ostomies, depending on the organs involved. A gastrostomy is an opening through the abdominal wall into the stomach. A jejunostomy is an opening through the abdominal wall into the jejunum. An ileostomy is an opening into the ileum (small bowel). A colostomy is an opening into the colon (large bowel). See Figure 28–1, which shows a colostomy stoma with the surgical incision to the right and retention sutures supporting the incision. A ureterostomy is an opening into the ureter. Gastrostomies and jejunostomies are generally performed to provide an alternate feeding route. The purpose of bowel and urinary ostomies is to divert and drain fecal or urinary material. Urinary diversion ostomies are discussed later in this chapter. Bowel diversion ostomies are often classified according to (a) whether they are permanent or temporary, (b) their anatomic location, and (c) the construction of the stoma.

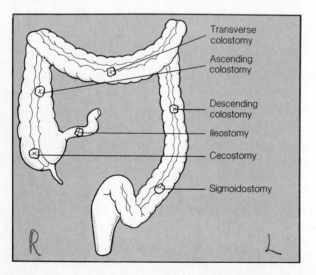

FIGURE 28–1 ■ A colostomy stoma, with the surgical incision to the right. Note the retention sutures supporting the incision.

FIGURE 28–2 ■ The locations of bowel diversion ostomies.

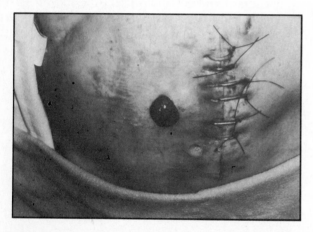

Permanence

Colostomies can be either temporary or permanent. Temporary colostomies are generally performed for traumatic injuries or inflammatory conditions of the bowel. They allow the distal diseased portion of the bowel to rest and heal. Permanent colostomies are performed to provide a means of elimination when the rectum or anus is nonfunctional as a result of disease or birth defect. They are commonly performed for diseases such as cancer of the bowel. The diseased portion may or may not be removed.

Anatomic Location

An ileostomy generally empties from the distal end of the small intestine. A cecostomy empties from the cecum (the first part of the ascending colon). An ascending colostomy empties from the ascending colon. A transverse colostomy empties from the transverse colon. A descending colostomy empties from the descending colon. A sigmoidostomy empties from the sigmoid colon. See Figure 28–2.

The location of the ostomy influences the character and management of the fecal drainage. The farther along the bowel, the more formed the stool, since the large bowel reabsorbs water from the fecal mass. In addition, more control over the frequency of stomal discharge can be established. For example:

1. An ileostomy produces liquid fecal drainage and drains constantly and it cannot be regulated. Ileostomy drainage contains some digestive enzymes, which are damaging to the skin. Ileostomy patients must wear an appliance continuously and take special precautions to prevent skin breakdown. Odor is minimal, however, compared to colostomies because fewer bacteria are present.

2. An ascending colostomy is similar to an ileostomy in that the drainage is liquid and cannot be regulated. However, digestive enzymes are not present, and odor is a problem requiring control (eg, a deodorant inside the appliance).

3. A transverse colostomy produces a malodorous, mushy drainage because some of the liquid has been reabsorbed. There is usually no control.

4. A descending colostomy produces increasingly solid fecal drainage. Stools from a sigmoidostomy are of normal consistency, and the frequency of discharge can be regulated. Patients with a sigmoidostomy may not have to wear an appliance at all times, and odors can usually be controlled.

The length of time that an ostomy is in place also helps to determine the consistency of the stool, particularly with transverse and descending colostomies. Over time, the stool becomes more formed because the remaining functioning portions of the colon tend to increase water reabsorption in compensation.

Construction

There are three major types of stoma constructions: the loop colostomy, the double-barreled colostomy, and the end colostomy. See Figure 28–3.

1. For a loop colostomy (Figure 28–3, *A*), a loop of bowel is brought out onto the abdomen. To keep the bowel from slipping back, a plastic rod may be placed underneath the bowel loop, opened (unfolded) so that it lies flat against the abdomen, and sutured to the skin. The rod holds the bowel in place until the underlying abdominal incision heals (seven to ten days). During surgery or two or three days after surgery, one or two openings are made into the bowel loop by cautery or by incision. If two openings are made the proximal or functioning opening discharges fecal material. The other opening is the distal or nonfunctioning end. It discharges only mucus unless emergency surgery was performed without the usual bowel preparation. In this instance some fecal matter may be discharged. When only one opening is made, it connects to both proximal and distal parts of the bowel. The loop colostomy is relatively large and cumbersome. It is created generally for an emergency, eg, an acute bowel obstruction or bowel injury. Complete diversion of fecal matter is not achieved with this procedure because the bowel is not separated.

2. In the double-barreled colostomy (Figure 28–3, *B*), two separate stomas are constructed. One is the proximal or functioning stoma, and the other is the distal or resting stoma. The stomas are generally adjacent to one another —one above the other or side by side.

3. An end colostomy has only one stoma (Figure 28–3, *C*), which arises from the end of the proximal portion of the bowel. The distal end of the bowel and rectum is either resected by an abdominoperineal resection (removal through abdominal and perineal incisions) or is closed off by sutures and remains in the abdominal space. The latter is often referred to as an "end colostomy and Hartmann pouch," the pouch referring to the remaining distal portion of the bowel.

NURSING INTERVENTIONS FOR BOWEL DIVERSION OSTOMY PATIENTS

A patient who has a stoma usually requires nursing assistance in four major areas: psychosocial factors, diet, stoma and skin care, and odor control. Enterostomal therapy nurses are recognized specialists for these patients.

Psychosocial Factors

A person who undergoes surgery that results in a stoma is likely to have strong reactions to the operation. In some instances the ostomy is palliative treatment for an

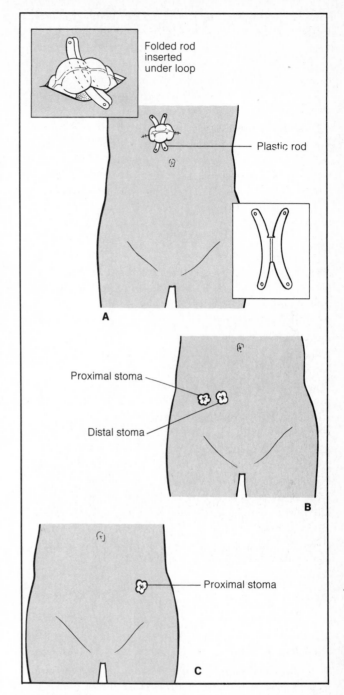

FIGURE 28–3   ■   Three types of colostomies: **A,** the loop colostomy using a plastic rod; **B,** the double-barreled colostomy; **C,** the end colostomy.

underlying disease, eg, a malignancy of the rectum. Here the patient faces not only adjustment to the stoma but also adjustment to a disease process that may not be cured. The patient may feel that health is lost and that his or her life-style must change. Some patients and family members go through a process of grieving before accepting the ostomy and learning to deal with it.

A stoma means changes in both the method and pattern of defecation, which is a highly personal function.

The patient will be very aware of other people's reactions to the stoma and particularly sensitive to any negative behavior that could be interpreted as meaning that she or he is offensive. It is important for nurses to communicate acceptance and understanding and to provide the same privacy during care that is normally provided for elimination.

In some instances an ostomy brings relief from pain. For example, for a person who has experienced years of discomfort and difficulty due to ulcerative colitis, the creation of an ileostomy may mean that he or she will be able to lead a more normal life than has been possible in the past.

Diet

The patient who has had intestinal surgery will usually be on nothing by mouth until bowel function returns and then a liquid and low residue diet until the bowel has healed or as tolerated. After that the patient can ingest most or all pre-illness foods and fluids and should maintain a well-balanced diet. Patients are generally encouraged not to restrict their diets but rather to use discretion. For example, if gas or odor production are of concern before a specific social engagement, gas- and odor-forming foods can be avoided prior to the event. In addition, a gas-filtering pouch can be used. Odor-forming foods do not need to be restricted because an intact appliance will contain odor. Often patients are concerned about gas formation because they believe the excessive gas formation that occurs postoperatively when bowel function returns will become their usual pattern. They need to be assured that this is temporary.

The following guidelines may be helpful in controlling gas and odor by dietary means:

1. Certain foods, eg, cheese, onions, and cucumbers, are known to produce a definite odor in feces.
2. Cabbage, brussels sprouts, garlic, onions, sauerkraut, broccoli, corn, cauliflower, and legumes are known to be gas-forming foods.
3. Sucking carbonated drinks through a straw can result in the ingestion of air, which will cause gas.
4. Certain foods, eg, parsley and yogurt, are thought to reduce the odor of feces.

The patient with an ileostomy may encounter two problems that can usually be prevented by diet: (a) blockage near the stoma due to the accumulation of cellulose, and (b) fluid and electrolyte imbalance. Cellulose (fiber, roughage) is normally not digested but passes along the gastrointestinal tract for expulsion through the anus. Prior to defecation, cellulose and other waste products accumulate in the sigmoid colon and rectum, which expand to accommodate them. However, with an ileostomy, the accumulated waste products can block the ileum, often at the point where it passes through the abdominal wall. Blockage is best prevented by teaching the patient to chew potentially obstructing foods well and introducing them one at a time, so that if a problem results the offending food can be avoided. Examples of potentially obstructing foods are corn, celery, and whole grains.

Fluid and electrolyte imbalance can occur because the patient is without a functioning colon. The colon normally functions to allow water and sodium to be reabsorbed through its wall into the blood circulation. Patients who have ileostomies tend to lose excessive amounts of sodium and fluid through the ileal effluent. Therefore, their diet should be high in fluids, sodium, and potassium, especially when diarrhea is present or if losses are significant from other routes, such as a high sodium loss from excessive perspiration. Patients need to be taught to respond to thirst and the signs and symptoms of fluid and electrolyte imbalance. Major sources of sodium and potassium are listed in Table 23–4 on page 511.

Stoma and Skin Care

Care of the stoma and skin is important for all patients who have ostomies. With a colostomy or ileostomy, the fecal material is irritating to the peristomal skin. This is particularly true of ileal effluent, which contains digestive enzymes. With a urostomy, the urine is irritating to the skin and can cause skin breakdown.

It is important that the peristomal skin be assessed for irritation each time the appliance is changed. Any irritations or skin breaks need to be treated immediately. The skin is kept clean by washing off any excretion, then drying it thoroughly. A barrier, eg, karaya, is applied over the skin around the stoma, to prevent the skin from coming into direct contact with any excretion. An appliance (bag) is then fitted to the stoma so that there is no leakage around it. It is exceedingly important that the skin be dry before the appliance is attached, because the pouch will not adhere to moist skin and will cause effluent to leak onto the skin.

Odor Control

Because fecal odor is generally considered socially unacceptable, odor control is essential. As soon as the patient is out of bed, he or she can learn to work with the ostomy in the bathroom, so that the odor of feces remains there and not at the bed.

For odor control, it is necessary to use the appropriate kind of appliance. An intact appliance is odorproof and will contain odor within it. The appliance should be rinsed thoroughly when it is emptied. Deodorizers can be placed in the pouch of the appliance, or pouches with charcoal filter discs are available. Oral intake of charcoal or bismuth subcarbonate are thought by some to help and can be taken with the physician's approval.

TECHNIQUE 28-1   ■   Changing a Bowel Diversion Ostomy Appliance

Disposable ostomy appliances can be applied for up to seven days. They need to be changed whenever the effluent leaks onto peristomal skin or when it cannot be rinsed completely away. Many people prefer to change them daily or whenever they become soiled, but this practice can be detrimental to the integrity of the peristomal skin and is expensive. Check agency practice in this regard.

Many types of appliances are available commercially. See Figure 28–4. All appliances have three things in common: a pouch to collect the effluent, an outlet at the bottom for easy emptying, and a faceplate. Temporary disposable pouches are tranparent plastic and have a peel-off adhesive square into which a hole the size of the stoma is cut. Permanent pouches are an opaque rubber or vinyl and have a solid ring faceplate that fits around the stoma.

It is important to select an appliance designed for the particular type of stoma. Some agencies employ an enterostomal therapy nurse who can assist in selecting the appliance. An appliance should have the following characteristics:

1. The appliance needs to be odor-resistant.
2. The opening needs to be just large enough to fit closely around the stoma.
3. If the bag has an adhesive-backed disc, it must be nonallergenic.
4. If the appliance has a belt, it should fit comfortably around the patient's waist (this depends on the model used). Many patients do not use belts unless it is absolutely necessary.

Disposable postoperative pouches should be:

1. Transparent to enable assessment of the stoma
2. Odorproof to enhance patient acceptability
3. Drainable so that the pouch can be emptied without removing it
4. Adjustable so that the size of the opening can be altered to accommodate changes in stoma shape and size as edema resolves

■ Assessment

Assessment of the stoma, peristomal skin, and effluent is usually done when the appliance is changed, unless the pouch is transparent and the stoma and effluent are visible. See Intervention, steps 6, 11, and 12. Assess:

1. The color of the stoma. It should appear red and similar in color to the mucosal lining of the inner

cheek. Very pale or darker-colored stomas with a bluish or purplish hue indicate impaired blood circulation to the area.

2. The stoma for swelling. Most stomas protrude slightly from the abdomen. New stomas normally appear swollen, but this generally decreases postoperatively over two or three weeks. Changes may occur for as long as six weeks postoperatively. The size of the stoma varies with the kind and location. For example, a loop colostomy of the

FIGURE 28-4 ■ Ostomy appliances: **A,** temporary disposable; **B,** permanent reusable.

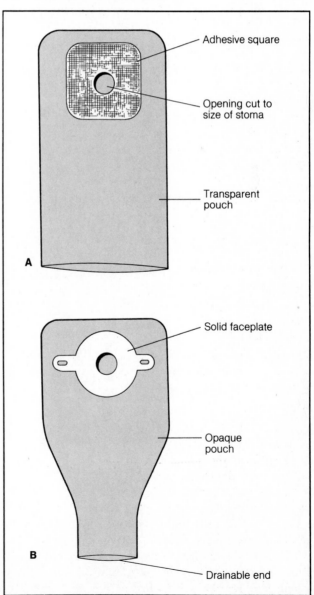

transverse colon can be expected to be larger than an end colostomy of the sigmoid colon. Lack of decrease in the size of a stoma may indicate a problem, eg, blockage.

3. The peristomal skin for any redness and irritation. Peristomal skin is the 5 to 13 cm (2 to 5 in) of skin surrounding the stoma.

4. The amount and type of feces. For ileal effluent and feces (colostomy effluent), assess the amount, color, and consistency. Note abnormalities, such as pus or blood.

5. Whether the patient is allergic to tape that may be used to secure the ostomy appliance to the abdomen. If the patient has a documented reaction to adhesives, do a 24-hour tape patch test. To do a tape patch test, experiment with at least three or four different types of tape (silk, paper, and foam). Cut strips of each type, label them with a marking pen, and place them on the patient's abdomen. See Figure 28–5. A 24-hour tape patch test is best done before the patient has surgery and on the patient's nonoperative side. The abdomen, rather than the inner arm,

is used since abdominal skin is more sensitive. Abdominal hair may first need to be removed using scissors or an electric razor or clippers. During the next 24 hours, note complaints of itching or burning by the patient, and at the end of the period remove the tape and inspect the abdomen for redness and swelling. Document the specific allergies, if present, on the patient's chart, and provide the patient with an allergic alert arm band.

Other data include:

1. The kind of ostomy and its placement on the abdomen. Surgeons often draw diagrams when there are two stomas. It is important to confirm which is the functioning stoma and any orders about the care of the stomas.

2. The size of the stoma, the type and amount of effluent, and the condition of the peristomal skin as baseline data.

3. The teaching plan for the learning needs of the patient and family members regarding the ostomy and self-care.

FIGURE 28–5 ■ A 24-hour tape patch allergy test.

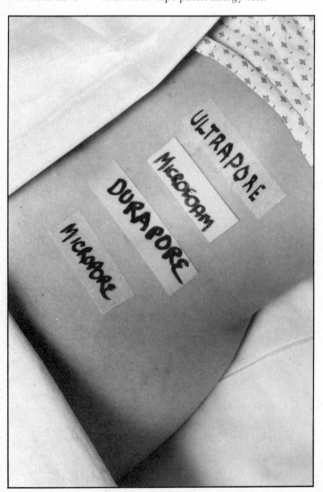

■ Planning

Nursing goals

1. To apply a clean appliance and minimize odors for the patient's comfort and self-esteem

2. To assess and care for the peristomal skin

3. To collect effluent for assessment of the amount and type of output

4. To keep the patient's clothing clean

Equipment

1. Solvent (presaturated sponges or liquid) for removing the appliance. This is not needed in most cases and should be used only when absolutely necessary.

2. A receptacle for the soiled appliance. To minimize odor, a waterproof bag can be used to wrap the bag prior to disposal. If the agency uses plastic bags to line the wastebaskets, this receptacle can be used and then removed after the procedure.

3. Cleaning materials, including tissues (to wipe away the stool), warm water, mild soap (optional), a washcloth or cotton balls, and a towel.

4. Tissue or gauze pad to cover the stoma.

5. A skin barrier for the skin. Some agencies use liquid protective coverings or a peristomal skin barrier in the form of a disc or sheet.

6. A measuring guide to measure the stoma.

7. Pen or pencil to trace the stoma size on the skin barrier disc and appliance faceplate.

8. Scissors to cut out the circle from the skin barrier and the appliance.

9. Tail closure or an elastic band for the spout of the appliance.

10. Special adhesive, with a brush to apply it to the bag, if needed. Additional adhesives are rarely necessary with currently available pouches.

11. A stoma guidestrip for centering opaque appliances around the stoma to prevent pressure or irritation to the stoma by the appliance. Guidestrips are 6-in (15.2-cm) strips of ½-in (1.3-cm) wide paper. They may be commercially made or made out of regular bond paper.

12. A deodorant (liquid or tablet) for a nonodorproof colostomy bag.

13. Tape to secure a detachable faceplate as necessary.

■ Intervention

1. Explain the procedure to the patient and family member if present. Changing an ostomy appliance should not cause discomfort, but it may be distasteful to the patient.

   Rationale Family members can be supportive and helpful to the patient if properly informed.

2. Communicate acceptance and support of the patient. Colostomy effluent may have an unpleasant odor, and the patient may feel "dirty." It is important to change the appliance competently and quickly and not to convey disgust. Timing is also an important factor. Avoid times close to meal hours whenever possible.

3. Provide privacy, preferably in the bathroom, where the patient can learn to deal with the ostomy as he or she would at home.

4. Assist the patient to a comfortable sitting or lying position, and expose only the stoma area.

5. Unfasten the belt if one is being worn.

6. Empty the pouch when it is one-third to one-half full. Assess the consistency and amount of effluent.

   Rationale When the fluid level in the bag becomes too high, the weight of it may loosen the faceplate and separate it from the skin, causing the effluent to leak and irritate the peristomal skin.

7. Remove the appliance. Apply solvent with an applicator if needed. Peel the bag off slowly while holding the patient's skin taut.

   Rationale Occasionally adhesives require the application of a solvent before removing. Holding the skin taut minimizes patient discomfort and prevents skin abrasion.

8. If the appliance is disposable, discard it in a moistureproof bag.

9. Using warm water and mild soap, clean the peristomal skin and the stoma. Check agency practice on the use of soap.

   Rationale Soap is sometimes not advised because it can be irritating to the skin.

10. Dry the area thoroughly by patting with a towel or cotton swabs.

   Rationale Excessive rubbing can abrade the skin.

11. Assess the stoma for color and size.

12. Assess the peristomal skin for any redness, ulceration, or irritation. Transient redness is normal after the removal of adhesive.

13. Place a piece of tissue or gauze pad over the stoma, and change it as needed.

   Rationale The tissue will absorb any seepage from the stoma.

There are two methods for preparing and applying the skin barrier (peristomal seal) and ostomy appliance. One method is described in steps 14–15; the other is described in step 16.

14. Prepare and apply the skin barrier. There are many types of skin barriers, so read the manufacturer's directions as well as the steps below. If using a sheet or disc type, such as Stomahesive, Reliaseal, Colly-Seel ring, HolliHesive, Crixiline, or Premium Barrier:

   a. Use the stoma measuring guide to measure the size of the stoma. See Figure 28–6.

FIGURE 28–6

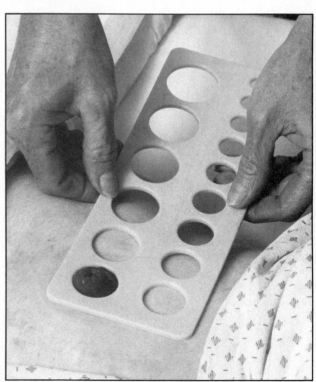

b. Trace a circle on the backing of the skin barrier the same size as the stomal opening.

c. Make a template of the stoma pattern.

Rationale A template aids other nurses and the patient with future appliance changes but will need to be adjusted as the stoma size decreases.

d. Cut out the traced stoma pattern to make an opening in the skin barrier.

e. Remove the backing to expose the sticky adhesive side on certain products, such as Stomahesive or Reliaseal. Moisten and rub a Colly-Seel ring with tap water until the ring becomes sticky; knead the ring to make it more flexible.

f. Center the skin barrier over the stoma and gently press it onto the patient's skin, smoothing out any wrinkles or bubbles. See Figure 28–7.

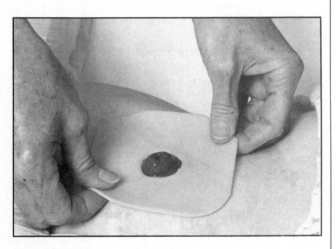

FIGURE 28–7

FIGURE 28–8

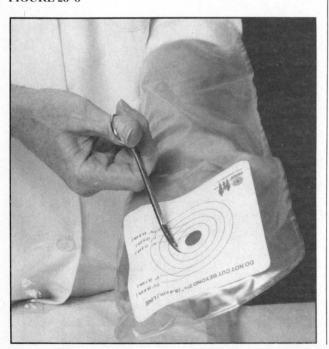

If using Skin Prep liquid or wipes or a similar product, eg, Stomahesive:

g. Cover the stoma with a gauze pad to avoid getting the Skin Prep on the stoma.

h. Either wipe the product evenly around the peristomal skin or use a brush to apply a thin layer of the liquid plastic coating to the same area.

i. Allow the skin barrier to dry, until it no longer feels tacky.

If applying a karaya ring seal:

j. Select a seal with an opening that is the same size as the stoma.

k. Place the ring around the stoma, ensuring that it fits snugly around its base.

l. Gently press the seal to the skin.

15. Prepare and apply the clean appliance. Remove the tissue over the stoma before applying the pouch. To apply a *disposable pouch* with *adhesive square*:

a. If the appliance does not have a precut opening, trace a circle one-eighth to one-sixth inch larger than the stoma size on the appliance's adhesive square.

Rationale The opening is made slightly larger than the stoma to prevent rubbing, cutting, or trauma to the stoma.

b. Cut out a circle in the adhesive. Take care not to cut any portion of the pouch. See Figure 28–8.

c. Peel off the backing from the adhesive seal.

d. Center the opening of the pouch over the patient's stoma and apply it directly onto the skin barrier. See Figure 28–9.

FIGURE 28–9

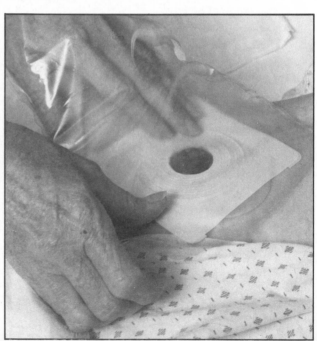

e. Gently press the adhesive backing onto the skin and smooth out any wrinkles, working from the stoma outward.

Rationale Wrinkles allow seepage of effluent, which can irritate the skin or soil clothing.

f. Remove the air from the pouch.

Rationale Removing the air helps the pouch lie flat against the abdomen.

g. Place a deodorant in the pouch (optional).

h. Close the pouch by turning up the bottom a few times, fanfolding its end lengthwise, and securing it with a rubber band or tail closure clamp.

To apply a *reusable pouch* with *faceplate attached:*

i. Apply either adhesive cement or a double-faced adhesive disc to the faceplate of the appliance, depending on the type of appliance being used. Follow the manufacturer's directions.

j. Insert a coiled paper guidestrip into the faceplate opening. The strip should protrude slightly from the opening and expand to fit it. See Figure 28–10.

Rationale The guidestrip helps you center the appliance over the stoma and prevents pressure or irritation to the stoma by an ill-fitting appliance.

k. Using the guidestrip, center the faceplate over the stoma.

l. Firmly press the adhesive seal to the peristomal skin. The guidestrip will fall into the pouch; commercially prepared guidestrips will dissolve in the pouch.

m. Place a deodorant in the bag if the bag is not odorproof. Most pouches are odorproof.

n. Close the end of the pouch with the designated clamp. See Figure 28–11.

o. Attach the pouch belt and fasten it around the patient's waist (optional).

To apply a *reusable pouch* with *detachable faceplate:*

p. Apply a skin sealant (eg, Skin Prep) to the faceplate.

Rationale This makes it easier to remove the adhesive disc from the faceplate.

q. Remove the protective paper strip from one side of the double-faced adhesive disc.

r. Apply the sticky side to the back of the faceplate.

s. Remove the remaining protective paper strip from the other side of the adhesive disc.

t. Center the faceplate over the stoma and skin barrier, then press and hold the faceplate against the patient's skin for a few minutes to secure the seal. See Figure 28–12.

u. Press the adhesive around the circumference of the adhesive disc.

v. Tape the faceplate to the patient's abdomen using

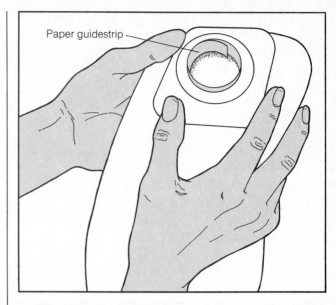

FIGURE 28–10

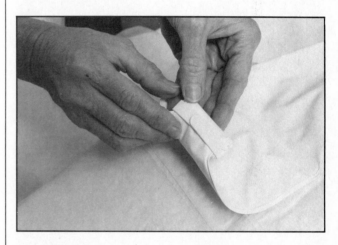

FIGURE 28–11

FIGURE 28–12

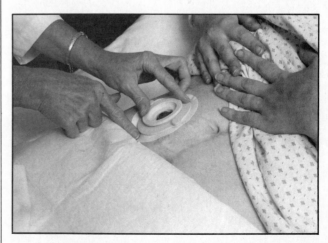

four or eight 7.5-cm (3-in) strips of tape. Place the strips around the faceplate in a "picture-framing" manner, one strip down each side, one across the top, and one across the bottom. See

Figure 28–13. The additional four strips can be placed diagonally over the other tapes to secure the seal.

w. Stretch the opening on the back of the pouch and position it over the base of the faceplate. Ease it over the faceplate flange.

x. Place the lock ring or "bead-o-ring" (see Figure 28–14) between the pouch and the faceplate flange (see Figure 28–15) to seal the pouch against the faceplate.

y. Close the base of the pouch with the appropriate clamp.

z. Attach the pouch belt and fasten it around the patient's waist (optional).

16. If a disc or wafer-type skin barrier is used, an alternate method can be used to replace steps 14 and

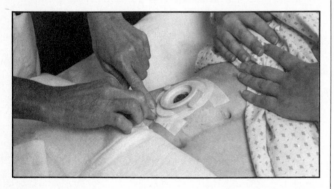

FIGURE 28–13

FIGURE 28–14

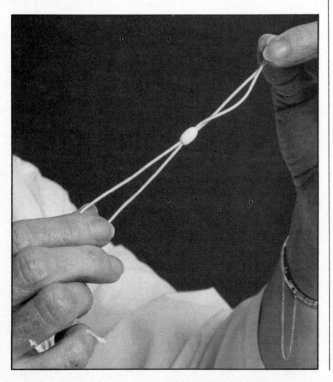

15. For this method, the ostomy appliance is put onto the skin barrier and then applied in one assembled unit to the patient's skin.

Rationale Applying the skin barrier and the appliance together is not only quicker but thought by some to reduce the chance of wrinkles. It also is easier for the patient to apply without help.

To apply *skin barrier and appliance as one unit:*

a. Prepare the skin barrier as in steps 14a–14d.

b. Prepare the appliance as in steps 15a–15c.

c. Center the opening of the pouch over the skin barrier.

d. Remove the backing to expose the sticky adhesive side on the skin barrier.

e. Center the skin barrier and appliance over the stoma, and press it onto the patient's skin.

17. Assess the patient's response to the technique in terms of skills learned; the amount, color, and consistency of the drainage; the condition of the skin; and the patient's fatigue, discomfort, and behavior about the ostomy.

18. Discard the bag, or clean it if it is to be used again. Measure liquid feces, then empty the feces into a toilet or hopper. If the bag is to be reused, wash it with cool water and mild soap, rinse, and dry.

19. Wash a soiled belt with warm water and mild soap, rinse, and dry.

20. Report to the responsible nurse any increase in stoma size or skin irritation.

FIGURE 28–15

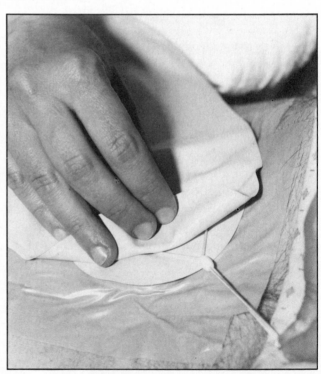

21. Record on the patient's chart any discoloration of the stoma; the appearance of the peristomal skin; the amount and type of drainage; and the patient's fatigue, discomfort, and significant behavior about the ostomy.

22. Adjust the patient's teaching plan and nursing care plan as needed. Include on the teaching plan the equipment and procedure used.

    Rationale Learning to care for the ostomy is facilitated for the patient if procedures implemented by nurses are consistent.

Sample Recording

Date	Time	Notes
10/5/87	1400	Colostomy appliance changed. 350 mL dark brown liquid feces. Stoma pink, 8 cm. Peristomal skin intact. No discomfort. Helped to clean the peristomal skin. ——————————— Ramona L. de Santo, NS

■ Evaluation

Expected outcomes

1. Stoma is a healthy red color.
2. Peristomal skin is normal, with no signs of redness or irritation.

Unexpected outcomes

1. Stoma appears very pale or dark red with a purplish cast.
2. Peristomal skin is reddened.

Upon obtaining an unexpected outcome:

1. Notify the responsible nurse and/or physician.
2. Adjust the nursing care plan appropriately.

TECHNIQUE 28–2   ■   Irrigating a Colostomy

A colostomy irrigation is similar to an enema. The purpose of irrigation is to distend the bowel sufficiently to stimulate peristalsis, which causes evacuation to occur.

The physician initially is responsible for determining whether a colostomy should be irrigated, what solution should be used, and the type of irrigation to be given. The last may be preestablished by agency policy, however.

Routine daily irrigations done to control the time of elimination ultimately become the patient's decision. Some patients prefer to control the time of elimination by rigid dietary regulation and not be bothered with irrigations, which can take up to one hour to complete. When regulation by irrigation is chosen, it should be done at the same time each day. Control by irrigations also necessitates some control of the diet. For example, laxative foods that might cause an unexpected evacuation need to be avoided.

In most patients, a relatively small amount of fluid (300 to 500 mL) stimulates evacuation. In others, up to 1,000 mL may be needed, since a colostomy has no sphincter and the fluid tends to return as it is instilled. This problem is reduced by the use of a cone on the irrigating catheter. The cone helps to hold the fluid within the bowel during the irrigation.

Irrigations are commonly used for end colostomies and descending colostomies; they are not advised for ascending colostomies or ileostomies, where the effluent is liquid in nature.

■ Assessment

1. See Technique 28–1.
2. Assess the patient's readiness to select and use the equipment. Because many types of irrigation sets are available, patients should begin with a "starter set" until they are familiar with the colostomy and the problems of irrigating it. Later, with the help of an enterostomal therapy nurse or a qualified person from a surgical supply house, the patient can select the set most appropriate for his or her needs.
3. Auscultate the abdomen for bowel sounds.
4. Palpate the abdomen for distention.

Other data include:

1. The type and amount of solution to be used and whether the stoma needs to be dilated.
2. Which is the distal stoma and which is the proximal stoma, if the colostomy is not an end colostomy.

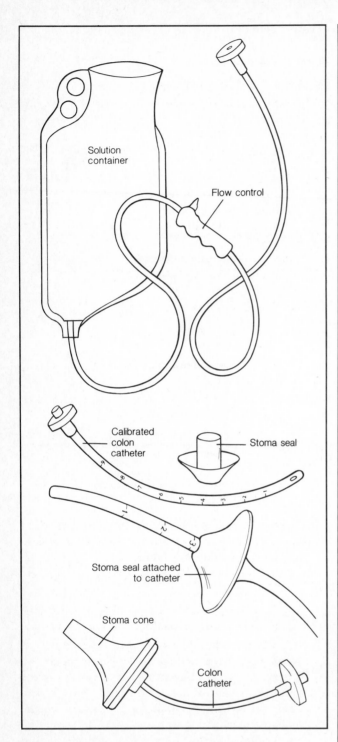

Solution
container

Flow control

Calibrated
colon
catheter

Stoma seal

Stoma seal attached
to catheter

Stoma cone

Colon
catheter

FIGURE 28–16 ■ Colostomy irrigation equipment.

Confirm the purpose of the irrigation and which stoma is to be irrigated. Usually the proximal stoma is irrigated, to stimulate the bowel to evacuate. However, the physician may want the distal stoma irrigated as well in preparation for diagnostic procedures (eg, roentgenography).

3. Whether the patient is to remain in bed or is able to walk to the bathroom, how much the patient is

participating in colostomy care, and any specific problems.

4. An appropriate time for the irrigation. If the patient has had a colostomy for a long time, the irrigation needs to be given at her or his scheduled time to maintain regularity. For a newly established colostomy, select a time based on the patient's previous bowel habits and one that will allow the patient to participate in usual daily activities. Encourage the patient to select the time and to maintain it.

■ **Planning**

Nursing goals

1. To empty the colon of feces and prevent obstruction or constipation

2. To regulate a sigmoid or end colostomy and reduce the number of colostomy movements, so that the patient can carry out daily activities without fear of fecal drainage

3. To expel gas

4. To clean the colon in preparation for tests or surgery

Equipment

A variety of equipment is available for colostomy irrigation, but the basic components are similar. The following equipment is usually needed:

1. A moisture-resistant bag for the soiled colostomy bag or dressings.

2. A clean colostomy appliance or dressings.

3. Irrigation equipment. See Figures 28–16 and 28–17.
   a. A bag to hold the solution. For routine irrigations for regulation, the bag is usually filled with 500 mL of warm (body temperature) tap water, or other solution as ordered. For a bowel preparation, 1,000 mL of solution is needed.
   b. Tubing attached to the bag.
   c. A tubing clamp or flow regulator.
   d. A #28 rubber colon catheter, calibrated in either centimeters or inches, with a stoma cone or seal.
   e. A disposable stoma irrigation drainage sleeve with belt to direct the fecal contents into the toilet or bedpan.

4. Lubricant.

5. Clean rubber gloves (optional) to protect the nurse's hands from contamination, and one glove to dilate the stoma if ordered by the physician.

6. A bath blanket to cover the patient as required.

7. An IV pole as required to suspend the irrigation bag.

8. A disposable bedpad, bedpan, and cover, if the patient is to remain in bed.

■ **Intervention**

1. Explain the procedure and its purpose to the patient. The total irrigation process usually takes about one hour.

2. If the patient is to remain in bed, assist him or her to a side-lying position, and place a disposable bedpad on the bed in front of the patient. Place the bedpan on top of the disposable pad, beneath the stoma. If the patient is ambulatory, assist him or her to sit on the toilet or on a commode in the bathroom.

3. Ensure that the patient's gown or pajamas are moved out of the way to prevent soiling, and drape the patient appropriately with the bath blanket to prevent undue exposure. Throughout the technique provide explanations, and encourage the patient to participate as much as the patient desires.

4. Hang the solution bag on an IV pole so that the bottom of the container is at the level of the patient's shoulder, or 30 to 45 cm (12 to 18 in) above the stoma.

   Rationale This height provides a pressure gradient that allows fluid to flow into the colon. The rate of flow can be regulated by the tubing clamp.

5. Attach the colon catheter securely to the tubing.

6. Open the regulator clamp, and run fluid through the tubing to expel all air from it. Close the clamp until ready for the irrigation.

   Rationale Air distends the bowel and can cause cramps.

7. Remove the soiled colostomy bag, and place it in the moisture-resistant bag.

   Rationale Placing the colostomy bag in such a container prevents the transmission of microorganisms and helps reduce odor.

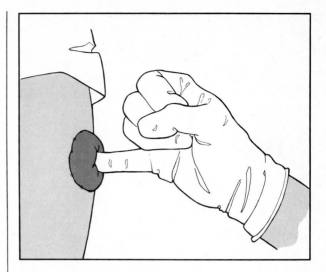

FIGURE 28–18

8. Center the irrigation drainage sleeve over the stoma, and attach it snugly.

   Rationale This prevents seepage of the fluid onto the skin.

9. Direct the lower open end of the drainage sleeve into the bedpan or between the patient's legs into the toilet.

10. If ordered by the physician, dilate the stoma:

    a. Put on a glove.

    b. Lubricate the tip of the little finger.

    c. Gently insert the finger into the stoma, using a massaging motion. See Figure 28–18.

       Rationale A massaging motion relaxes the intestinal muscles.

    d. Repeat steps b and c above, using progressively larger fingers until maximum dilation is achieved.

       Rationale Stoma dilation is performed to stretch and relax the stomal sphincter and to assess the direction of the proximal colon prior to an irrigation.

11. Lubricate the tip of the stoma cone or colon catheter.

    Rationale Lubricating the tip of the cone or catheter eases insertion and prevents injury to the stoma.

12. Using a rotating motion, insert the catheter or stoma cone through the opening in the top of the irrigation drainage sleeve and gently through the stoma. See Figure 28–19. Insert a catheter only 7 cm (3 in); insert a stoma cone just until it fits snugly. Many practitioners prefer using a cone to avoid the risk of perforating the bowel. If you have difficulty inserting the catheter or cone, do not apply force.

    Rationale A rotating motion on insertion helps to

FIGURE 28–17 ■ A commercially prepared colostomy irrigation set. The irrigation solution bag is on the left and the collecting bag (irrigation drainage sleeve) on the right; the stoma cone is fitted to the catheter.

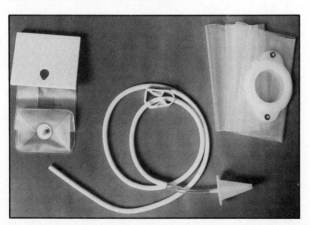

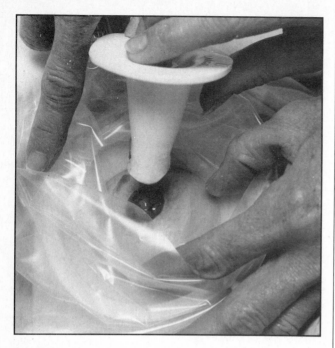

FIGURE 28-19

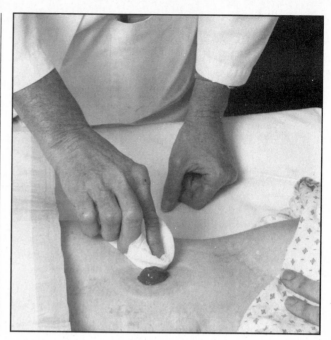

FIGURE 28-20

open the stoma. Forcing the cone or catheter may traumatize or perforate the bowel.

13. Open the tubing clamp, and allow the fluid to flow into the bowel. If cramping occurs, stop the flow until the cramps subside and then resume the flow.

    Rationale Fluid that is administered too quickly or is too cold may cause cramps.

    If the fluid flows out as fast as you put it in, press the stoma cone or seal more firmly against the stoma to occlude it. If a stoma cone or seal is not available, press around the stoma with your fingers to close the stoma against the catheter.

14. After all the fluid is instilled, remove the catheter or cone and allow the colon to empty. In some agencies the stoma cone is left in place for 10 to 15 minutes before it is removed. Although not always indicated, you may ask the patient to gently massage the abdomen and sit quietly for 10 to 15 minutes until initial emptying has occurred.

    Rationale Massaging the abdomen encourages initial emptying.

15. Clean the base of the irrigation drainage sleeve, and seal the top and bottom with a drainage clamp, following the manufacturer's instructions.

16. Encourage an ambulatory patient to move around for about 30 minutes.

    Rationale Complete emptying of the colon takes up to half an hour. Moving around facilitates peristalsis.

17. Empty the irrigator drainage sleeve, and remove it.

18. Clean the area around the stoma, and dry it thoroughly. See Figure 28-20.

19. Put a colostomy appliance on the patient as needed. See Technique 28-1.

20. Promptly report to the responsible nurse any problems, such as no fluid or stool returns, difficulties inserting the tube, peristomal skin redness or irritation, and stomal discoloration.

21. Record the irrigation on the patient's chart. Include the time of the irrigation, the type and amount of fluid instilled, the returns, and the patient's response.

Sample Recording

Date	Time	Notes
12/5/86	0900	Colostomy irrigated with 750 mL warm tap water. Water and large amount soft brown stool expelled. Stoma is pink, and tube inserted without difficulty. Peristomal skin intact. Asked questions about irrigation, looked at stoma for first time. Observed stoma care and pouch application. ———————— Chung-Hao Jen, NS

22. Adjust the nursing care plan according to the patient's learning needs, problems encountered, etc.

■ **Evaluation**

Expected outcomes

1. Feces evacuated through the stoma

2. Irrigating solution expelled

3. Abdomen less distended

4. Bowel sounds normal

Unexpected outcomes

1. No fecal returns
2. Absence of or partial returns of irrigating solution
3. Abdominal distention unchanged
4. Bowel sounds absent
5. Excessive bleeding from stoma

Upon obtaining an unexpected outcome:

1. Report your findings to the responsible nurse and/or physician.
2. Adjust the nursing care plan appropriately.

URINARY DIVERSION OSTOMIES

There are four main types of urinary diversion ostomies:

1. Cutaneous ureterostomy
2. Ileal conduit
3. Vesicostomy
4. Ureterosigmoidostomy or ureteroileosigmoidostomy

Permanent urinary diversion stomas are indicated for any condition that requires a total cystectomy, eg, cancer of the bladder. Temporary urinary diversion stomas are indicated for any condition requiring partial cystectomy, trauma to the lower urinary tract, or severe chronic urinary tract infections.

Ureterostomy

In cutaneous ureterostomy, the ureters are diverted to the abdominal wall or flank, and a ureteral stoma is formed. Ureterostomies are small compared to colostomies (about 0.5 mm or 1/4 in in diameter) and drain continously. They may involve the right or left ureter (*unilateral ureterostomy,* Figure 28–21, *A*) or both ureters (*bilateral ureterostomy,* Figure 28–21, *B*), in which case each one is covered by a separate appliance, unless they are placed close to each other.

Variations of the bilateral ureterostomy include:

1. The *double-barreled ureterostomy,* in which both ureters are brought to the skin surface to form side-by-side stomas. See Figure 28–21, *C.*

2. The *loop ureterostomy,* in which the ureters are looped out to the skin surface of each flank to form the stomas. See Figure 28–21, *D.*

3. The *transureteroureterostomy,* in which one ureter is first connected to the other, and then the receiving ureter is brought to the skin surface to form a stoma. See Figure 28–21, *E.*

Ileal Conduit

The ileal (ileo) conduit is also referred to as *ileal (ileo) loop, ileal (ileo) bladder, ureteroileostomy,* or *Bricker's loop.* See Figure 28–22. In this procedure, a segment of the ileum

FIGURE 28–21 ▪ Five types of ureterostomies: **A,** right unilateral ureterostomy; **B,** bilateral ureterostomy; **C,** double-barreled ureterostomy; **D,** flank loop ureterostomy; **E,** transureteroureterostomy.

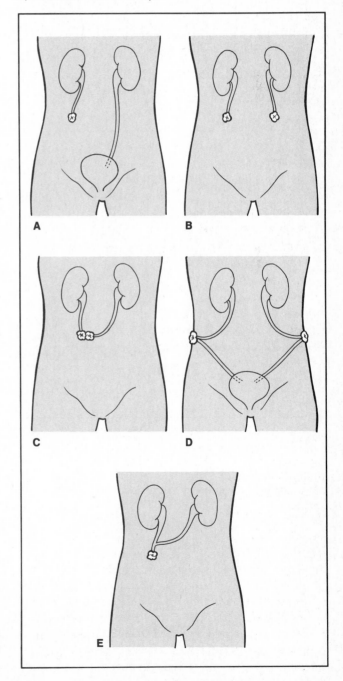

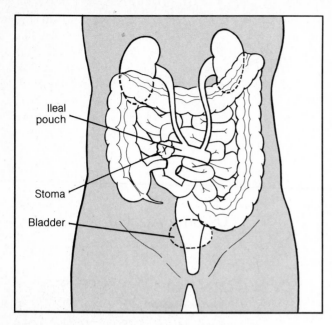

FIGURE 28–22 ■ An ileal conduit.

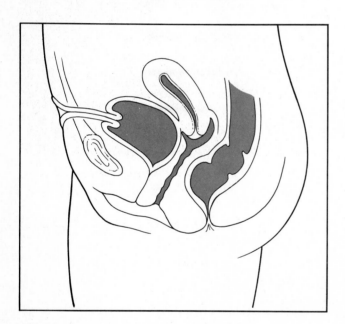

FIGURE 28–23 ■ A continent vesicostomy.

is removed, and the intestinal ends are reattached. One end of the portion removed is closed with sutures to create an ileal pouch, and the other end is brought out through the abdominal wall to create a stoma. The ureters are implanted into the ileal pouch, and the bladder is usually removed. The advantages of this procedure over ureterostomies are that the ileal stoma is larger and more readily fitted with an appliance; there is less chance of an ascending kidney infection, since the mucous membrane lining of the ileum acts as a barrier to microorganisms; and the stoma is less likely to stenose, a major problem with ureterostomy stomas. For these reasons, the ileal conduit is one of the most commonly used urinary diversion procedures.

Vesicostomy

In vesicostomy, the anterior wall of the bladder is sutured to the abdominal wall, and a stoma is formed from the bladder wall. The urethral neck is sutured closed so that urine from the bladder empties directly through the stoma. To provide urinary control, a *continent vesicostomy* is usually performed. See Figure 28–23. In this procedure a tube is formed from part of the bladder wall. A stoma is formed at one end of the tube. A nipplelike valve is created from the bladder wall at the internal end. Urine drains through this type of vesicostomy only after a catheter is inserted through the stoma into the bladder pouch.

Ureterosigmoidostomy

Ureterosigmoidostomy and ureteroileosigmoidostomy are two urinary diversion procedures that result in urine

Figure 28–24 ■ **A,** Ureterosigmoidostomy; **B,** ureteroileosigmoidostomy.

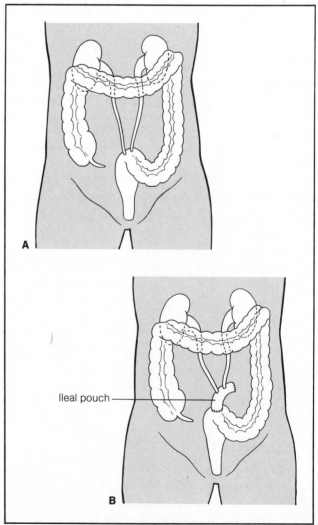

being excreted through the rectum. In ureterosigmoidostomy, the more common procedure, the ureters are implanted into the sigmoid colon. See Figure 28–24, *A*. One major complication with this type of procedure is pyelonephritis (infection of the kidney pelvis) from reflux of fecal material and intestinal microorganisms into the ureters and kidney pelvis. In ureteroileosigmoidostomy, a segment of the ileum is resected and connected to the sigmoid colon. The ureters are then implanted into this ileal pouch. See Figure 28–24, *B*. This procedure is thought to reduce the incidence of pyelonephritis. In both of these procedures, urine mixes with fecal material, resulting in very liquid stools and possible anal leakage of urine.

TECHNIQUE 28–3   ■   Changing a Urinary Diversion Ostomy Appliance

Various types of vinyl urinary stoma appliances are available (see Figure 28–25). The disposable one-piece pouch may be attached either to a nonallergenic adhesive-backed faceplate, which may or may not be precut, or to a semipermeable skin barrier, which is permeable to vapor and oxygen but impermeable to liquid. The latter attachment maintains skin integrity more effectively. Reusable pouches have opaque faceplates, which may or may not be attached to the pouch. Some have belt attachments, and one type has an adaptable insert that can be adjusted to stoma size. The enterostomal therapy nurse selects the pouch that best suits the patient by considering the type of ostomy, the stoma location and shape, and the peristomal skin surface, as well as the patient's body size and contour, physical and mental abilities, skin allergies, financial status, and life-style.

Generally a urinary diversion appliance adheres to the patient's skin for two to five days. They are usually changed twice a week. The nurse's responsibilities include stoma and peristomal care.

■ Assessment

Assess:

1. The stoma size, shape, and color for baseline data. Stoma size and shape vary. Ureterostomy stomas are generally flush with the skin; ileal conduit stomas usually protrude like a bud. The color should be bright red. A dark red or blue can indicate impaired circulation and must be reported.
2. The stoma for bleeding. Slight bleeding when the stoma is touched is normal, but other bleeding should be reported.
3. The peristomal skin for any redness and irritation.
4. Complaints of burning sensation under the faceplate. This may indicate skin breakdown.
5. The amount, color, clarity, and odor of the urine.
6. The patient's allergies to tape. See Assessment in Technique 28–1 on page 671.

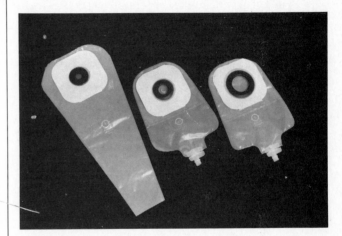

FIGURE 28–25 ■ Examples of urinary appliances used for management of urinary diversion ostomies.

7. The patient's and family members' learning needs regarding the ostomy and self-care.
8. The patient's emotional status.

Other data include:

1. The surgeon's orders about care of the stoma(s)
2. The agency's practices regarding the procedure for changing this type of ostomy appliance and what types of appliances are stocked by the agency
3. The size of the stoma(s), the type and amount of urine, and the condition of the peristomal skin, according to the patient's chart
4. The type and size of appliance currently used and what special barrier substance is applied to the skin, according to the nursing care plan

■ Planning

Nursing goals

1. To prevent peristomal skin irritation due to urine leakage

2. To monitor the amount, color, clarity, and odor of urine

3. To minimize odors

Equipment

If a commercially prepared stoma care kit is not available, the following supplies need to be assembled:

1. Ostomy pouch with adhesive-backed faceplate
2. Ostomy pouch belt (optional)
3. Graduated pitcher or receptacle for the urine
4. Basin filled with warm water, soap (optional), cotton balls, and towel
5. Gauze pads
6. Skin barrier (Skin Prep liquid or wipes or similar product, eg, Stomahesive, or ready-made wafer-type or disc-type barrier) for the peristomal skin
7. Stoma measuring guide
8. Adhesive solvent in the form of presaturated sponges or liquid (optional)
9. Adhesive cement (optional) for reusable pouches if double-faced adhesive disc is not used
10. Scissors or electric razor
11. Waterproof bag for the soiled appliance

■ Intervention

1. Communicate acceptance and support of the patient throughout the technique.

   Rationale This procedure often evokes negative emotional and psychologic responses from the patient.

2. Assist the patient to a supine position in bed or to stand if able.

   Rationale A back-lying or standing position helps to separate abdominal skin folds that interfere with appliance application.

3. Unfasten the belt if one is being worn.

4. Empty the urine from the pouch, when it is one-third to one-half full, into the graduated receptacle. It may be necessary to detach the pouch from a collection bag and tubing if the pouch is attached to a drainage system during the night.

   Rationale The pouch is emptied when only one-third to one-half full because the weight of more urine may loosen the adhesive faceplate seal and separate the appliance from the skin. Pouches are often attached to a drainage sytem during the night to prevent accumulation and stagnation of urine in the appliance.

5. Remove the appliance. Apply solvent, if needed, and peel the bag off slowly while holding the patient's skin taut. Avoid touching the stoma with adhesive solvent.

   Rationale Holding the skin taut minimizes patient discomfort and prevents skin abrasion. Adhesive solvent is irritating and may burn the stoma.

6. Discard a disposable appliance in a waterproof bag. If the appliance is reusable, wash it with lukewarm water and soap, and then air dry it to prevent it from becoming brittle.

7. Using cotton balls, carefully wash the peristomal skin with warm water and soap, if needed, and thoroughly rinse the soap from the area.

   Rationale Washing the area will remove stagnant urine, which has a strong odor. The oily residue of soap can prevent proper adherence of the appliance.

8. Dry the area thoroughly by patting with a towel or with cotton balls.

   Rationale Excessive rubbing can abrade the skin.

9. Assess the stoma for color, swelling, and retraction. Remember that ileal conduit stomas may protrude slightly from the abdomen (about ½ to ¾ in); ureterostomy stomas are usually flush with the skin. New stomas will appear swollen, but this decreases postoperatively over two to three weeks. The size of the stoma varies with the kind and location. For example, the stoma of an ileal conduit will be larger than a ureterostomy stoma.

   Rationale A lack of decrease in the size of the stoma or change in color may indicate circulatory problems. Retraction may create leakage problems and subsequent skin irritation.

10. Assess the peristomal skin for any redness, ulceration, or irritation. Place a gauze pad over the stoma, and change it as needed.

    Rationale The gauze pad will absorb the constant seepage of urine and prevent it from contacting the skin.

11. Remove excessive peristomal skin hair using scissors or an electric razor. Do not use a straight-edged razor.

    Rationale This will prevent discomfort and irritation of the hair follicles when the appliance is removed. It is easy to inadvertently damage the skin with a straight-edged razor.

12. Prepare and apply the skin barrier (peristomal seal). If using *Skin Prep liquid or wipes* or other similar product:

    a. Cover the stoma with a gauze pad to avoid getting the Skin Prep on the stoma.

    b. Either wipe the Prep evenly around the peristomal skin, or use an applicator to apply a thin layer of the liquid plastic coating to the area.

    c. Allow the Skin Prep to dry until it no longer feels tacky.

If using a *wafer* or *disc-type* barrier, read the manufacturer's directions as well as the steps below. (Note that the karaya ring seal, although effective in protecting the skin, is less effective with urinary ostomies than with bowel ostomies because urine tends to melt the product.)

    d. Use the stoma measuring guide to measure the size of the stoma.

    e. Trace a circle on the backing of the skin barrier the same size as the stomal opening.

    f. Make a template of the stoma pattern.

      Rationale A template aids other nurses and the patient with future appliance changes.

    g. Cut out the traced stoma pattern to make an opening in the skin barrier.

    h. Remove the backing on one side of the skin barrier to expose the sticky adhesive.

    i. Attach the skin barrier to the faceplate of the ostomy appliance when it is prepared.

      Rationale Assembling the skin barrier and the appliance before application enhances the speed of application, an important consideration for constantly draining urostomies.

13. Prepare the clean appliance. To prepare a *disposable pouch* with adhesive square:

    a. If the appliance does not have the precut opening, trace a circle no more than 2 to 3 mm (⅛ in) larger than the stoma size on the appliance's adhesive square.

      Rationale The opening is made slightly larger than the stoma to prevent rubbing, cutting, or trauma to the stoma.

    b. Cut out the traced circle in the adhesive. Take care not to cut any portion of the pouch.

    c. Peel off the backing from the adhesive seal, and attach the seal to a disc-type skin barrier or, if a liquid product was used, to the patient's peristomal skin.

To prepare a *reusable pouch* with *faceplate attached:*

    d. Depending on the type of appliance, apply either adhesive cement or a double-faced adhesive disc to the faceplate. Follow the manufacturer's directions.

To prepare a *reusable pouch* with *detachable faceplate:*

    e. Remove the protective paper strip from one side of the double-faced adhesive disc.

    f. Apply the sticky side of the disc to the back of the faceplate.

    g. Remove the remaining protective paper strip from the other side of the adhesive disc.

    h. Attach the faceplate to a disc-type skin barrier or, if a liquid product was used, to the patient's peristomal skin.

14. Apply the clean appliance with disc-type skin barrier, if used, as follows:

    a. Remove the gauze pad over the stoma before applying the pouch.

For a *disposable pouch:*

    b. Gently press the adhesive backing onto the skin and smooth out any wrinkles, working from the stoma outward.

      Rationale Wrinkles allow seepage of urine, which can irritate the skin and soil clothing.

    c. Remove the air from the pouch.

      Rationale Removing the air helps the pouch lie flat against the abdomen.

    d. Attach the spout of the pouch to a urinary drainage system or cap the spout. Temporary disposable pouches are often attached to drainage systems.

For a *reusable pouch* with *faceplate attached:*

    e. Insert a coiled paper guidestrip into the faceplate opening. The strip should protrude slightly from the opening and expand to fit it.

      Rationale The guidestrip helps in centering the appliance over the stoma and prevents pressure or irritation to the stoma by the appliance.

    f. Using the guidestrip, center the faceplate over the stoma.

    g. Firmly press the adhesive seal to the peristomal skin. The guidestrip will fall into the pouch; commercially prepared guidestrips will dissolve in the pouch.

    h. Place a deodorant in the bag (optional).

    i. Close the spout of the pouch with the designated cap.

    j. Optional: Attach the pouch belt and fasten it around the patient's waist. Wash a soiled belt with warm water and mild soap, rinse, and dry if needed.

For a *reusable pouch* with *detachable faceplate:*

    k. Press and hold the faceplate against the patient's skin for a few minutes to enhance the seal.

    l. Press the adhesive around the circumference of the adhesive disc.

    m. Tape the faceplate to the patient's abdomen using four or eight 7.5-cm (3-in) strips of tape. Place the strips around the faceplate in a "picture-framing" manner, one strip down each side, one across the top, and one across the bottom. The additional four strips can be placed diagonally over the other tapes to enhance the seal.

    n. Stretch the opening on the back of the pouch, and position it over the base of the faceplate. Ease it over the faceplate flange.

    o. Place the lock ring or "bead-o-ring" between the

pouch and the faceplate flange to secure the pouch against the faceplate.

p. Close the spout of the pouch with the appropriate cap.

q. Optional: Attach the pouch belt and fasten it around the patient's waist.

15. Assess the amount, color, and consistency of the drainage; the condition of the skin; and the patient's response to the technique in terms of fatigue, discomfort, behavior about the ostomy, and skills learned.

16. Record on the patient's chart the color of the stoma; the appearance of the peristomal skin; the amount and type of drainage; and the patient's fatigue, discomfort, and significant behavior about the ostomy.

17. Adjust the patient's teaching plan and nursing care plan as needed. Include on the teaching plan the equipment and procedure used.

Rationale Learning to care for the ostomy is facilitated for the patient if procedures implemented by nurses are consistent.

The patient will also need to learn self-care and ways to reduce odor. Use of deodorant tablets in the appliance, soaking a reusable pouch in dilute vinegar solution, a diet that makes the urine more acid, and drinking plenty of fluids all help to control odor.

Rationale A high fluid intake dilutes the urine, making it less odorous. Ascorbic acid and cranberry juice increase the acidity of urine, which in turn inhibits bacterial action and odor.

Information about ostomy clubs and other community services available should also be included.

■ Evaluation

Expected outcomes

1. Normal color and odor of urine (initially after surgery urine will be sanguineous)
2. Some mucus in the urine if an ileal conduit was performed; absence of mucus for ureterostomy
3. Red stoma
4. Peristomal skin intact
5. No complaints of discomfort under appliance

Unexpected outcomes

1. Abnormal color, odor, and consistency of urine
2. Pale or dark red- or blue-colored stoma
3. Swelling or retraction of stoma
4. Peristomal skin irritation
5. Complaints of burning around stoma
6. Excessive bleeding from stoma

Upon obtaining an unexpected outcome: Report your findings to the responsible nurse and/or physician.

References

Broadwell DC, Jackson BS, eds. *Principles of Ostomy Care.* Mosby, 1982.

Ritter M: Karaya reconsidered . . . the original skin barrier for persons with an ostomy. *J Enterost Ther* (January/February) 1983; 10:35–36.

Smith DB: Colostomy irrigations—so simple . . . irrigation takes on complex variables and requires individualization in each situation. *J Enterost Ther* (January/February) 1983; 10:22–23.

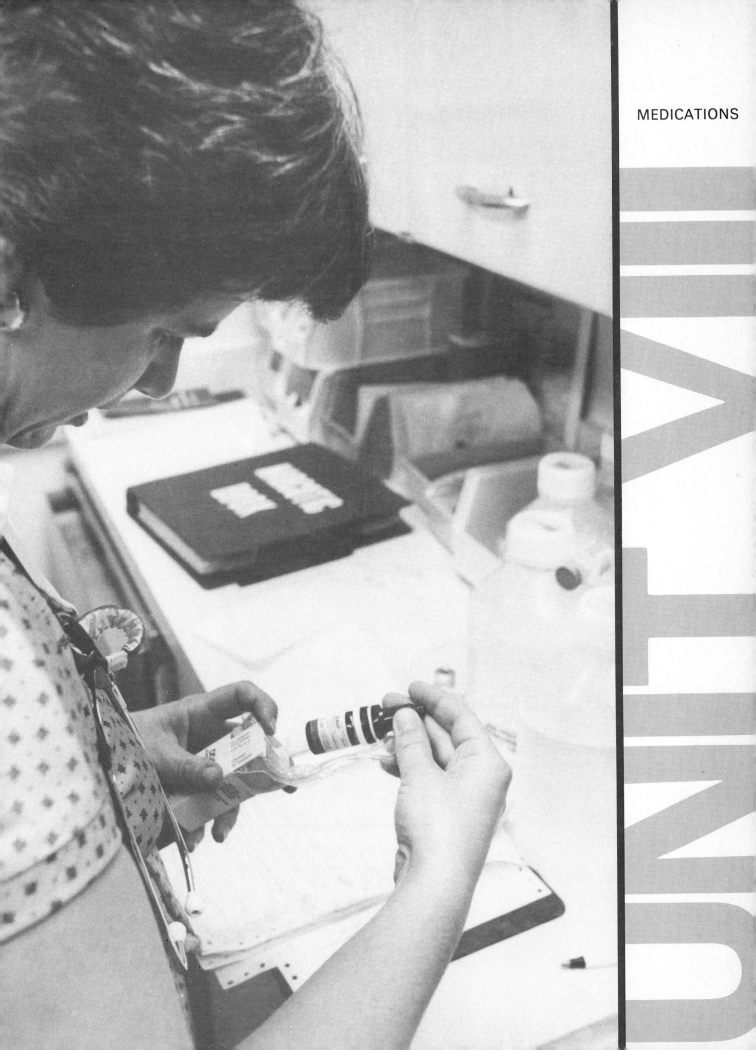

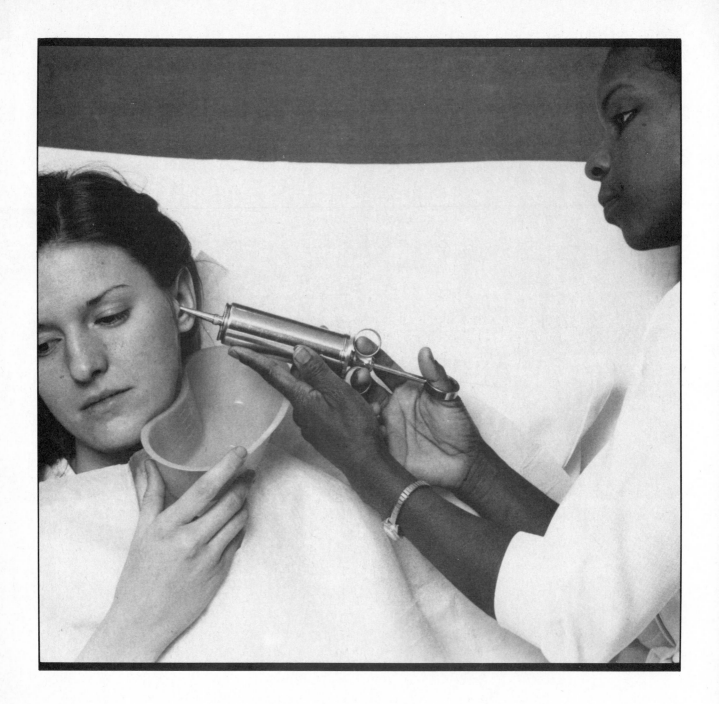

ORAL MEDICATIONS, TOPICAL MEDICATIONS, AND IRRIGATIONS

29

The preparation and administration of medications is a vital nursing function. Medications are administered by a variety of routes. Although this chapter focuses on oral and topical routes of administration, the concepts basic to the safe administration of drugs for all routes of administration are also discussed.

The nurse's responsibility requires knowledge not only about how to prepare and administer drugs but also about the organs being treated, how medications act on the body, their usual dosages, their desired effects, and their undesired effects. Such knowledge is gradually and continuously achieved, enhanced by directed and independent study using available resource materials. An irrigation, or lavage, is washing or flushing out of a part of the body, eg, an organ, cavity, or wound. The purpose of most irrigations is to clean. There are, however, other purposes, which are indicated in the techniques later in the chapter.

Chapter Outline

Types of Medications

Medication Policies and Practices

Routes of Administration

Medication Orders

Systems of Measurement

Variables Influencing Drug Action

Administering Medications

■ Technique 29–1 Administering Oral Medications

■ Technique 29–2 Administering Dermatologic Medications

■ Technique 29–3 Administering Ophthalmic Irrigations and Instillations

■ Technique 29–4 Administering Otic Irrigations and Instillations

■ Technique 29–5 Administering Nasal Instillations

■ Technique 29–6 Administering Vaginal Irrigations and Instillations

Objectives

Upon completion of this chapter, the student will:

1. Know essential terms, abbreviations, and facts about the administration of oral and topical medications and irrigations

   1.1 Define selected terms

   1.2 Identify commonly used abbreviations associated with medication orders

   1.3 Identify five main routes of drug administration

   1.4 Identify the essential parts of a medication order

   1.5 Identify basic units of weight and volume within the metric, apothecaries', and household systems of measurement

   1.6 Identify approximate equivalents within each system of measurement and between systems

   1.7 Identify essential aspects of administering medications

2. Understand facts about medications and irrigations

   2.1 Identify relevant assessment data

   2.2 Identify nursing diagnoses for which the technique may be implemented

   2.3 Identify nursing goals related to the technique

   2.4 Identify expected and unexpected outcomes from assessment data

   2.5 Identify reasons underlying selected steps of the technique

3. Perform medication and irrigation techniques safely

   3.1 Assess the patient adequately

   3.2 Collect additional data from appropriate sources

   3.3 Select pertinent nursing goals for the patient

   3.4 Establish relevant outcome criteria for the patient following the technique

   3.5 Collect necessary equipment before the technique

   3.6 Implement interventions to enhance the effectiveness of the technique and enhance the patient's comfort and safety

   3.7 Communicate relevant information about the patient to the appropriate persons

   3.7 Evaluate the outcomes of the technique

4. Evaluate own performance of specific techniques in a laboratory or clinical setting with the assistance of another

   4.1 Use the performance checklists provided

   4.2 Identify areas of strength and weakness

   4.3 Alter performance in response to own evaluation and that of another

Terms

■ analgesic   a medication used to relieve pain

■ biotransformation   the process of deactivating or detoxifying the biologically active chemicals in drugs to more easily excreted forms

■ cohesive   sticking together

■ dermatologic   relating to the skin

■ emulsion   a liquid that contains another liquid with which it will not mix and in which it will not dissolve

■ excoriation   loss of the superficial layers of the skin

■ gelatinous   like jelly

■ instillation   insertion of a medication into a body cavity

- ■ irrigation   the washing of a body cavity by a stream of water or other fluid
- ■ medication (medicine, drug)   a chemical or biologic compound administered to humans or animals for disease prevention, cure, or relief, or to affect the structure or function of the body
- ■ narcotic   a drug that induces insensibility while relieving pain
- ■ ophthalmic   relating to the eye

- ■ otic   relating to the ear
- ■ pruritus   itching
- ■ rubefacient   a substance that reddens the skin
- ■ scored   marked with a line or groove
- ■ suspension   a preparation of a finely divided, undissolved substance dispersed in a liquid vehicle
- ■ volatile   evaporating readily

TYPES OF MEDICATIONS

Medications are manufactured as different types of preparations. The type of preparation can determine the method of administration, eg, an elixir is taken by mouth, an ointment is applied to the skin or mucous membrane.

Some medications are prepared in more than one form. Penicillin, for example, is prepared as a tablet and as an aqueous suspension. It is very important that a nurse obtain the correct preparation of the medication for the route that has been ordered. The different types of preparations are briefly described in Table 29–1.

TABLE 29–1 ■ Types of Drug Preparations

Type	Description	Type	Description
Aqueous solution	One or more drugs dissolved in water		more drugs used for application to the skin and mucous membrane
Aerosol spray or foam	A liquid, powder, or foam deposited in a thin layer on the skin by air pressure	Paste	A preparation like an ointment but thicker and stiffer, which penetrates the skin less than an ointment
Aqueous suspension	One or more drugs finely divided in a liquid such as water	Pill	One or more drugs mixed with a cohesive material, in oval, round, or flattened shapes
Capsule	A gelatinous container to hold a drug in powder, liquid, or oil form		
Cream	A nongreasy, semisolid preparation used on the skin	Powder	A finely ground drug or drugs; some are used internally, others externally
Elixir	A sweetened and aromatic solution of alcohol used as a vehicle for medicinal agents	Spirit	A concentrated alcoholic solution of a volatile substance
Extract	A concentrated form of a drug made from vegetables or animals	Suppository	One or several drugs mixed with a firm base such as gelatin and shaped for insertion into the body; the base dissolves gradually at body temperature, releasing the drug
Fluid extract	An alcoholic solution of a drug from a vegetable source; the most concentrated of all fluid preparations		
Gel or jelly	A clear or translucent semisolid that liquefies when applied to the skin	Syrup	An aqueous solution of sugar often used to disguise unpleasant-tasting drugs
Liniment	An oily liquid used on the skin		
Lotion	An emollient liquid that may be a clear solution, suspension, or emulsion used on the skin	Tablet	A powdered drug compressed into a hard small disc; some are readily broken along a scored line; others are enteric-coated to prevent them from dissolving in the stomach
Lozenge (troche)	A flat, round, or oval preparation that dissolves and releases a drug when held in the mouth		
Ointment	A semisolid preparation of one or	Tincture	An alcoholic or water-and-alcohol solution prepared from drugs derived from plants

MEDICATION POLICIES AND PRACTICES

Dispensing medications is the responsibility of pharmacists. The pharmacist may dispense directly to the patient or to a person who will administer the drug. In some agencies, a senior nurse may be delegated the responsibility of dispensing drugs in the absence of a pharmacist, eg, on the night shift or on a holiday.

In most agencies, graduate nurses are permitted to administer all types of medications (oral, topical, and parenteral), unless the unit-dose system is used and pharmacy personnel are delegated this function. Agency practice determines who is permitted to administer intravenous medications; agency practices vary. Licensed vocational nurses are often permitted to administer oral medications only, while registered nurse students who have demonstrated competence are generally allowed to administer all types of medications. It is essential that the nursing student check agency policies and practices governing medications before administering them.

ROUTES OF ADMINISTRATION

Pharmaceutical preparations are designed for a specific route of administration. Normally, the route of administration is specified when the drug is ordered. When a nurse is administering the drug, it is essential that the pharmaceutical preparation be appropriate to the route ordered. For example, phenobarbital is taken orally; phenobarbital sodium may be taken parenterally.

Oral

Most commonly, drugs are administered orally. Oral administration is usually least expensive and most convenient for most patients. It is also a safe method of administration in that the skin is not broken as it is for an injection.

The major disadvantages of oral administration are that the drugs may have an unpleasant taste or be difficult to swallow, irritate the gastric mucosa, be absorbed irregularly from the gastrointestinal tract, be absorbed slowly, and in some cases harm the teeth.

Sublingual

A drug may be given sublingually, that is, placed under the tongue, where it dissolves. See Figure 29–1. The drug is largely absorbed into the blood vessels on the underside of the tongue in relatively short time. The medication should not be swallowed. Drugs such as nitroglycerine are commonly given in this manner.

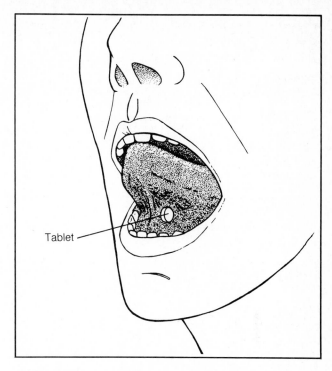

FIGURE 29–1 ■ Sublingual administration of a tablet.

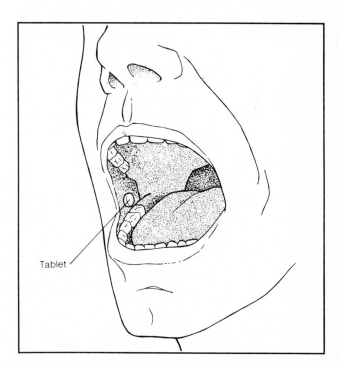

FIGURE 29–2 ■ Buccal administration of a tablet.

Buccal

Buccal means pertaining to the cheek. In buccal administration, a medication (eg, a tablet) is held in the mouth against the mucous membranes of the cheek until the drug dissolves. See Figure 29–2. The drug may act locally on the mucous membranes of the mouth or systemically when it is absorbed through the buccal mucosa or swallowed in the saliva.

Parenteral

Administration other than through the alimentary tract, ie, by needle, is called *parenteral* administration. Some of the more common routes for parenteral administration are:

1. *Subcutaneous* (hypodermic): into the subcutaneous tissue, just below the skin
2. *Intramuscular:* into a muscle
3. *Intradermal:* under the epidermis (into the dermis)
4. *Intravenous:* into a vein

Some of the less commonly used routes for parenteral administration are *intraarterial* (into an artery), *intracardiac* (into the heart muscle), *intraosseous* (into a bone), and *intrathecal* or *intraspinal* (into the spinal canal). These less common injections are normally carried out by physicians. All parenteral therapy utilizes sterile equipment and sterile drug solutions. Parenteral therapy has the primary advantage of fast absorption of a measured amount of drug. Its primary disadvantage is that it allows little or no margin for error because after administration it is irretrievable.

Topical

Topical applications are those applied to a circumscribed surface area of the body. They are designed to affect only the area to which they are applied, but some systemic absorption may occur. Topical applications include:

1. *Dermatologic preparations,* medications applied to the skin.
2. *Instillations,* medications applied into body cavities or orifices, such as the urinary bladder, eyes, ears, nose, rectum, or vagina.
3. *Inhalations,* medications administered into the respiratory tract by nebulizers or positive pressure breathing apparatuses. Air, oxygen, and vapor are generally used to carry the drug into the lungs.

MEDICATION ORDERS

A physician is the person who usually determines the patients' medications needs and orders medications, although in some settings nurse practitioners now order some drugs. Usually, the order is written, although telephone and verbal orders are acceptable in a number of agencies. Nursing students need to know the agency's policies about medication orders. In many hospitals, for example, only graduate nurses are permitted to accept telephone and verbal orders.

Types of Medication Orders

Four common medication orders are the stat order, the single order, the standing order, and the p.r.n order.

1. A stat order indicates that the medication is to be given immediately and only once, eg, Demerol 100 mg IM stat.
2. The single order is for a medication to be given once at a specified time, eg, Seconal 100 mg h.s. before surgery.
3. The standing order may or may not have a termination date. A standing order may be carried out indefinitely (eg, multiple vitamins daily) until an order is written to cancel it, or it may be carried out for a specified number of days (eg, Demerol 100 mg IM q.4h. × 5 days). In some agencies, standing orders are automatically canceled after a specified number of days and must be reordered.
4. A p.r.n. order permits the nurse to give a medication when in her or his judgment the patient requires it, eg, Amphojel 15 mL p.r.n. The nurse must use good judgment as to when the medication is needed and when it can be safely administered. Another type of p.r.n. order, eg, Demerol 75 mg IM q.3h. p.r.n., places a time constraint on when the medication can be given. It is important for the nurse who administers a p.r.n. medication to clearly document the need for the medication, the time it is given, and the patient's response to it.

Policies about physicians' orders vary considerably from agency to agency. Generally, there is an order as to which medicines are to be given to a patient by nurses and which medications a patient can keep at the hospital bedside to self-administer. Hospitals also have varying policies regarding orders. It is not unusual for a patient's orders to be automatically canceled after surgery or an examination involving an anesthetic. New orders must then be written. This policy is a safety measure to ensure that physicians are aware of their patients' conditions, particularly at critical times. Most agencies also have lists of abbreviations officially accepted for use in the agency. Both nurses and physicians may need to refer to these lists if they have been working in a different agency. These abbreviations can be used on legal documents, such as patients' charts. See Table 29–2 for abbreviations commonly used in medication orders.

Essential Parts of the Drug Order

The drug order has six essential parts: the full name of the patient, the date the order is written, the name of the drug to be administered, the dosage of the drug, the method of administration, and the signature of the physician or nurse practitioner. In addition, unless it is a standing order, it should state the number of doses or the number of days the drug is to be administered.

Full name of the patient

A patient's full name, that is, the first and last names and middle initials or names, should always be used to avoid confusion between two patients who have the same last name. In some agencies, the patient's admission number is put on the order as further identification.

Some hospitals imprint the patient's name and hospital number on all forms. This imprinter is on the nursing unit; it is much like the credit card imprinters used in shops.

Date

Shown on an order are the day, the month, and the year the order was written; some agencies also require that the time of day be written. Writing the time of day on the order can eliminate errors when nursing shifts change and help to clarify whether a change in the patient's condition occurred before or after the physician last wrote orders. Putting the time of day on the order also makes it clear when certain orders automatically terminate. For example, in some settings, narcotics can be ordered for only 48 hours after surgery. Therefore a drug that is ordered at 1600 hours February 1, 1987, is automatically canceled at 1600 hours February 3, 1987.

Many agencies use the 24-hour clock, which eliminates confusion between morning and afternoon times. Time with the 24-hour clock starts at midnight, which is 0000 hours. See Figure 4–2 on page 38.

Name of the drug

The name of the drug ordered must be clearly written. In some settings, only generic names are permitted; however, trade names are widely used in hospitals and health agencies. In most settings where drug orders are written, nurses and physicians can refer to the *Hospital Formulary* (most hospitals provide their own formulary, listing all drugs stocked in the hospital) or to other drug reference books available. A nurse who is unsure about a drug that is ordered needs to look it up in a suitable reference before preparing or administering the drug.

In some situations, hospital patients may continue to take medications prescribed before they were admitted. To know what drug the patient is taking, the nurse needs to check the drug label or check with the physician or the pharmacy if the bottle is unlabeled.

Dosage

The dosage of the drug includes the amount, the times or frequency of administration, and in many instances the strength; for example, tetracycline *250 mg* (amount)

four times a day (frequency); hydrochloric acid *10%* (strength) *5 mL* (amount) *three times a day with meals* (time and frequency).

Dosages can be written in apothecaries' or metric systems, but the metric system is being used increasingly in North America.

TABLE 29–2 ■ Common Abbreviations Used in Medication Orders

Abbreviation	Explanation	Example of administration time
a.c.	before meals	0700, 1100, and 1700 hours
ad lib	freely, as desired	
agit	shake, stir	
aq	water	
aq dest	distilled water	
b.i.d.	twice a day	0900 and 2100 hours
c̄	with	
cap	capsule	
comp	compound	
dil	dissolve, dilute	
elix	elixir	
h.	an hour	
h.s.	at bedtime	
M. or m.	mix	
no.	number	
non rep	do not repeat	
OD	right eye	
OS or o.l.	left eye	
OU	both eyes	
p.c.	after meals	0900, 1300, and 1900 hours
p.o.	by mouth	
p.r.n.	when needed	
q.	every	
q.d.	every day	
q.AM (o.m.)	every morning	1000 hours
q.h. (q.1h.)	every hour	
q.2h.	every 2 hours	0800, 1000, 1200 hours, etc
q.3h.	every 3 hours	0900, 1200, 1500 hours, etc
q.4h.	every 4 hours	1000, 1400, 1800 hours, etc
q.6h.	every 6 hours	0600, 1200, 1800, 2400 hours
q.h.s.	every night at bedtime	
q.i.d.	four times a day	1000, 1400, 1800, 2200 hours
q.o.d.	every other day	0900 hours on odd dates
q.s.	sufficient quantity	
rept	may be repeated	
Rx	take	
s̄	without	
Sig. or S.	label	
s.o.s.	if it is needed	
ss or s̄s̄	one half	
stat	at once	
sup or supp	suppository	
susp	suspension	
t.i.d.	three times a day	1000, 1400, and 1800 hours
Tr. or tinct	tincture	

Method of administration

Also included in the order is the method of administering the drug. This part of the order, like other parts, is frequently abbreviated, eg, IM for intramuscular, s.c. for subcutaneous, and p.o. for by mouth. It is not unusual for a drug to have several possible routes of administration; therefore, it is important that the route be included in the order. If the nurse believes the patient's condition makes the ordered route of administration inappropriate, the nurse must notify the physician to change the order. Changes in a patient's condition sometimes make it impossible to carry out a standing order. For example, if a patient becomes unconscious, a standing order for an oral medication must be changed.

Signature

The signature of the ordering physician or nurse makes the drug order a legal request. An unsigned order has no validity, and the ordering physician or nurse needs to be notified if her or his order is unsigned.

In agencies where telephone orders are taken, the nurse taking the order usually indicates on the written order the name of the person who phoned it in. The nurse signs the order, but usually the person who ordered the drug must also sign at a later date. Some hospitals have policies that those who give orders by telephone must sign those orders within a certain time, for example, 48 hours after they have communicated the order.

Communicating a Medication Order

A drug order is usually written on the patient's chart or in a special book designed for that purpose. From there, it is usually transcribed by a nurse or clerk to the Kardex and to a medication card (see Figure 29–3) or to a medication list.

Medication cards vary in form but include the patient's name, room and bed number, name of the drug, dose, times, and method of administration. In some agencies, the date that the order was prescribed and the date the order expires are also included, along with the signature of the person transcribing the order. The responsibility for transcribing medication orders is the nurse's; however, it may be delegated to a clerk.

SYSTEMS OF MEASUREMENT

Three systems of measurement are used in North America: the metric system, the apothecaries' system, and the household system, which is similar to the apothecaries' system. It would be much simpler for everyone if one system were universally accepted; however, because all systems are in current use, it is necessary for nurses to become familiar with the three systems and to be able to convert from one to the other as it is necessary. In recent years, Canada has officially adopted the metric system, and it is being used increasingly in the United States.

Metric System

The metric system, devised by the French in the latter part of the 18th century, is the system prescribed by law in most European countries. The metric system is very logically organized into units of ten; it is a decimal system. Basic units can be multiplied or divided by ten to form secondary units. Multiples are calculated by moving the decimal point to the right, and divisions by moving the decimal point to the left.

Basic units of measurement are the meter, the liter, and the gram. Prefixes derived from Latin designate subdivi-

FIGURE 29–3 ■ A sample medication card containing essential information.

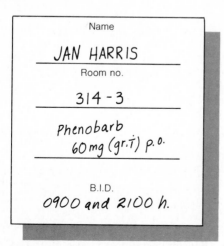

FIGURE 29–4 ■ Basic metric measurements of volume and weight.

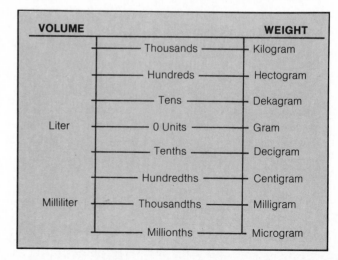

sions of the basic unit: deci (1/10 or 0.1), centi (1/100 or 0.01), milli (1/1,000 or 0.001), and micro (1/1,000,000 or 0.000001). Multiples of the basic unit are designated by prefixes derived from Greek: deka (10), hecto (100), and kilo (1,000). Only the measurements of volume (the liter) and of weight (the gram) are discussed in this chapter. These are the measures used in medication administration. See Figure 29–4. In medical and nursing practice the kilogram (kg) is the only multiple of the gram (g) used, and the milligram (mg) and microgram (mcg) the only subdivisions. Fractional parts of the liter (L) are usually expressed in milliliters (mL), for example, 600 mL; and multiples of the liter are usually expressed, for example, as 2.5 L or 2,500 mL.

Apothecaries' System

The apothecaries' system, older than the metric system, was brought to the United States from England during the colonial period. North Americans are familiar with most units of measure in the apothecaries' system, since they have been used in everyday life. For example, milk is bought in pints or quarts, gasoline is purchased by the gallon, people weigh themselves in pounds, and distances are measured in feet, inches, or miles.

The basic unit of weight in the apothecaries' system is the grain, likened to a grain of wheat, and the basic unit of volume is the minim, a volume of water equal in weight to a grain of wheat. The word *minim* means "the least." In ascending order the other units of weight are the scruple, the dram, the ounce, and the pound. Today the scruple is seldom used. The units of volume are, in ascending order, the fluid dram, the fluid ounce, the pint, the quart, and the gallon.

Quantities in the apothecaries' system are often expressed by lowercase Roman numerals, particularly when the unit of measure is abbreviated. The Roman numeral follows rather than precedes the unit of measure. For example, a fluid ounce is abbreviated as f℥. Two fluid ounces are written as f℥ii, and four fluid ounces are written as f℥iv. One-half fluid ounce is written as f℥ss, and one and one-half fluid ounces as f℥iss.

Household System

Household measures may be used when more accurate systems of measure are not required. Included in household measures are drops, teaspoons, tablespoons, cups, and glasses. Although pints and quarts are often found in homes, they are defined as apothecaries' measures.

Converting Units of Weight and Volume

Sometimes drugs are dispensed by a pharmacy in grams when the dosage was ordered in milligrams, or they are dispensed in milligrams but ordered in grains. Or a nurse

TABLE 29–3   ■   Approximate Volume Equivalents: Metric, Apothecaries', and Household Systems

Metric		Apothecaries'		Household
1 mL	=	15 minims (min or m)	=	15 drops (gtt)
15 mL	=	4 fluid drams (f℥)	=	1 tablespoon (Tbsp)
30 mL	=	1 fluid ounce (f℥)	=	same
500 mL	=	1 pint (pt)	=	same
1,000 mL	=	1 quart (qt)	=	same
4,000 mL	=	1 gallon (gal)	=	same

TABLE 29–4   ■   Approximate Weight Equivalents: Metric and Apothecaries' Systems

Metric		Apothecaries'
1 mg	=	1/60 grain (gr)
60 mg	=	1 gr
1 g	=	15 gr
4 g	=	1 dram (dr)
30 g	=	1 ounce
500 g	=	1.1 pound (lb)
1,000 g (1 kg)	=	2.2 lb

may find that the doctor has ordered a medicated irrigation in an apothecaries' unit of volume (for example, a quart), while the solution is dispensed only in metric (liter) containers. In all situations, it is the nurse's responsibility to convert the units of measure or weight; thus nurses must be aware of approximate equivalents within each system of measurement and between systems. See Tables 29–3 and 29–4.

ADMINISTERING MEDICATIONS

Steps in Administering Medications

When administering any drug, regardless of the route of administration, the nurse follows five steps:

1. Identification of the patient
2. Administration of the drug
3. Provision of adjunctive nursing care as indicated
4. Recording
5. Evaluation of the patient's response to the drug

Identifying the patient

Identifying a patient sounds simple and usually is, but errors can and do occur, and a patient may get a drug intended for another. In hospitals, most patients wear some means of identification, such as wristbands with their names and hospital identification numbers. To prevent mistakes, nurses also ask the patient's name or state the name clearly and then listen to the patient's response before administering any medication.

Administering the drug

Equally important is giving the correct drug. Medication orders and cards or lists need to be read carefully and checked against the name on the medication envelope or on the drawer in which the patient's medications are kept if a medication cart is used. The medication is then administered in the dosage and by the route ordered.

Adjunctive nursing intervention

Patients may need help when receiving medications. They may require physical assistance, eg, in assuming positions for intramuscular injections; or they may need explanations about the medications and guidance about measures to enhance drug effectiveness and prevent complications, eg, drinking fluids. Some patients convey fear about their medications. The nurse can allay fears by listening carefully to patients' concerns and giving correct information. Patients may give the nurse information regarding their drugs. A patient may say that an analgesic is effective for only 10 or 15 minutes, another patient may feel nauseated about 20 minutes after ingesting a drug, a third patient may feel dizzy each afternoon at about the same time, and a fourth may have pain in the right leg. This type of information needs to be recorded and, when appropriate, relayed to the physician. In some cases, simple nursing measures can relieve the problem, eg, the nurse can provide food with certain medications to help prevent nausea; in other instances, it may be necessary for the physician to reassess the needs of the patient.

Recording

Once complete, the intervention is recorded on the patient's record. The facts recorded are name of the drug; dosage; method of administration; specific relevant data, such as pulse rate (taken in most settings prior to the administration of digitalis); and any other pertinent information. The record should include the exact time of administration and in most agencies the signature of the nurse providing the medication. Often medications that are given regularly are recorded on a special flow record; p.r.n. or stat medications are recorded on the flow record as well as on the nurse's notes.

Evaluating patient response

The response of the patient to a medication can often be detected directly after intravenous administration, 10

to 20 minutes after an intramuscular or subcutaneous injection, and anywhere from immediately to several days after oral administration. For example, the ingestion of aluminum hydroxide gel (Amphojel) often provides almost immediate relief to a patient with epigastric pain; on the other hand, the effects of an antibiotic may not be noticeable for three or four days.

The kinds of behavior that reflect the action or lack of action of a drug are as variable as the purposes of the drugs themselves. The anxious patient may show the effects of a tranquilizer by behavior reflecting a lowered stress level, for example, slower speech or fewer random movements. The effectiveness of a sedative can often be measured by how well a patient slept; the effectiveness of an antispasmodic, by how much pain the patient feels. In all nursing activities, nurses need to be aware of the medications that a patient is taking and record their effectiveness as assessed by the patient and the nurse on the patient's chart. If appropriate, the nurse may also report the response of the patient to the senior nurse and to the physician directly.

Guidelines for Administering Medications

1. Although medications are prescribed chiefly by physicians, the nurses who administer them are responsible for their own actions. Therefore you should question any order you consider incorrect. The physician's order should include the name of the medication, the dosage, and the method and frequency of administration. The order may include additional directions, eg, "Withhold dosage if pulse is below 60."

2. Before administering a medication, make sure that you are knowledgeable about the drug. Most nursing units have drug reference books.

3. Federal laws govern the use of narcotics and barbiturates. Narcotics and barbiturates are kept in a drawer or cupboard with a double lock. Special forms are used for recording them. The data usually required are the name of the patient, drug, and physician; date; time of administration; dosage; and signature of the person who prepared and administered the drug.

4. Medication cards are used in some agencies as guides for preparing medications. A card normally includes the patient's name, room and bed number, name of the drug, dosage, and times and method of administration. In some agencies, the date on which the order was prescribed and the date on which it expires are also included.

5. To avoid errors while preparing and giving medications, concentrate on the task. Use the "five rights" as a guide: right drug, right dose, right route, right patient, right time.

6. To prevent an error when preparing medications, read the label on the container three times: before taking it off the shelf, while pouring the medication, and after placing it back on the shelf.

7. Ensure that the drug preparation is appropriate to the route prescribed.

8. If you prepare medications, you must also administer and chart them. You are the only person who can confirm the medication.

9. When preparing medications, do not use the following:

a. Medications from unmarked containers or containers with illegible labels—even though you think you can identify the drug.

b. Medications that are cloudy or have changed color.

c. Medications that have a sediment at the bottom unless the medication normally requires shaking before use.

Return such medications to the pharmacy. Write the reason for their return on the label.

10. Never return a medication to a container or transfer a medication from one container to another. This practice avoids mixing drugs or placing a drug in the wrong container.

11. Identify the patient correctly and carefully, using the appropriate means of identification, eg, the identification bracelet.

12. With rare exceptions, patients have the right to know the name and the action of the drug they are taking, and they have the right to refuse a medication. Medications that are refused must be discarded and the reason for refusal recorded.

13. Provide the correct adjunctive nursing measures with the medication, eg, measure a pulse rate before giving a digitalis preparation or notify the physician before giving the drug if the apical pulse is below 60.

14. Medications should not be left at the bedside, with the exception of antacids, nonnarcotic cough syrups, nitroglycerin, lotions or ointments, certain eye medications, and inhalants. Check agency policies about each of these. When medications are left at the bedside, determine from the patient when she or he takes or applies them.

15. Give medications within 30 minutes of the time ordered, except for preoperative medications, which must be given at the exact time ordered, or medications that are ordered to be given hourly or every two hours (eg, eye medications prior to surgery).

16. If a patient vomits after taking an oral medication, report the fact to the responsible nurse, and state the names of all medications given. Withhold the medication(s). Often the physician will reorder the same drug by a different route, eg, subcutaneously or intramuscularly.

17. Special precautions must be observed for certain drugs. Most agencies require that two qualified nurses double-check the dosages of anticoagulants, insulin, digitalis preparations, and certain IV medications. Check agency policies.

18. After a medication has been administered, record it on the patient's chart. The recording should include the time, the name of the drug, the dosage, the route of administration, and any related data.

19. Most agencies have an official list of abbreviations used in medication orders and in recording. See Table 29–2 for commonly used abbreviations.

20. Evaluate the effectiveness of a medication a suitable time after its administration. For example, the initial effectiveness of an intramuscularly injected analgesic can be evaluated 10 to 20 minutes after administration. The duration of its effectiveness must also be evaluated.

21. Medications are usually discontinued before surgery, and the physician writes new orders after the surgery. New orders are generally given for drugs a newly admitted patient takes at home or when a patient is transferred to another service within an agency or outside the agency. Check agency policies.

22. When medications are intentionally omitted, eg, before surgery or a diagnostic test, record the omission and the reason on the patient's chart. It may also be necessary to notify the prescriber.

23. Medication errors sometimes occur. When an error is made, report it immediately to the responsible nurse so that corrective measures can be implemented promptly. Errors are usually documented on an unusual incident form that becomes a part of the agency's file. Check the policies and practices of the agency.

TECHNIQUE 29–1 ■ Administering Oral Medications

Oral medications are generally the most easily taken of all drugs. Adjustments may be necessary for the very young, the very old, or for those who have difficulty swallowing solids. For easier ingestion, tablets can be crushed and mixed with a small amount of liquid or soft food, such as jelly or applesauce. It is preferable, however, to obtain a more suitable dosage form, eg, a liquid medication. Enteric-coated tablets and capsules should not be broken, because the coating is intended to prevent the medicine from being activated and absorbed in the stomach.

Arrange a time when you will not be interrupted to

prepare medications. Quietness and concentration are necessary to prevent drug errors. Once prepared, medications should not be out of your sight unless they are stored with appropriate precautions.

■ Assessment

Intelligent assessment of the patient requires knowledge of the patient's diagnosis, the plan of care, the expected actions of the drug, undesirable side effects, and signs of toxicity. Before administering medications, it is necessary that you learn about each patient and the drug to be given from available sources. Assess:

1. Clinical signs indicating a need for the medication, eg, pain before giving an analgesic.
2. The patient's ability to swallow the medication. If the patient does have difficulty swallowing, obtain a liquid dosage form, if available. If not available, crush a tablet or open a capsule, and then monitor the patient carefully for variations in therapeutic response or adverse effects.

Other data include: the adjunctive interventions required for specific drugs, eg, pulse measurement.

■ Planning

Nursing goals

1. To administer the correct medication and dose ordered by the physician at the correct time
2. To monitor the therapeutic effects of the medication

Equipment

1. A medication tray or cart.
2. Medication cards or list. To save time and avoid retracing steps, arrange the cards in the order in which you will give the medications. Plan to give medications first to patients who do not require assistance and last to those who do.
3. Disposable medication cups. Small paper cups are needed for tablets and capsules; for liquids, waxed or plastic calibrated medication cups are needed.

■ Intervention

1. Check the date on the medication order, and verify the order for accuracy. It should contain the following:
   a. Patient's name.
   b. Name of the drug and dosage.
   c. Time for administration.
   d. Route of administration, eg, oral (p.o.), subcutaneous or hypodermic (s.c. or H), intramuscular (IM), or intravenous (IV).

Records of medication orders include the physician's order, which is usually on the patient's chart, the Kardex record, and the medication card. The surest check is to compare the medication card against the physician's order. In some settings a medication Kardex or computer printout is used instead of medication cards. This Kardex or printout is usually kept in the medications room or in the medication cart. Any discrepancies in the order should be brought to the notice of the responsible nurse or the physician, whichever is appropriate in the agency.

2. Read the medication card, and take the appropriate medication from the shelf, drawer, or refrigerator. The medication may be dispensed in a bottle, box, or envelope.

3. Compare the label of the medication container against the order on the medication card. If these are not identical, recheck the patient's chart. If there is still a discrepancy, check with the responsible nurse.

4. Prepare the correct amount of medication for the required dose, without contaminating the medication.
   a. If administering tablets or capsules from a bottle, pour the required number into the bottle cap, and then transfer the medication to the paper cup. See Figure 29–5. Usually all tablets or capsules to be given to the patient are placed in the same paper cup. Medications that require specific assessments, eg, pulse measurements, respiratory rate or depth, or blood pressure, must be kept separate from the others.
   b. If administering a liquid medication, remove the cap, and place it upside down on the countertop to avoid contaminating it. Hold the bottle with the label next to your palm so that if any spills, the label will not become soiled and illegible. See Figure 29–6. Hold the medication cup at eye level and fill it to the desired level, using the bottom of the *meniscus* (crescent-shaped upper surface of a column of liquid) as the measurement guide. See Figure 29–7.
   c. If administering an oral narcotic from a narcotic dispenser, expose the tablet by turning the dial or sliding out the numbered dose, and drop it into the cup. These containers are sectioned and numbered. See Figure 29–8. After removing a tablet, you must record the fact on the appropriate narcotic control record and sign it.
   d. Open unit-dose medications at the patient's bedside.

5. Place the prepared medication and medication card together on the tray or cart.

6. Check the label on the container again, and return the bottle, box, or envelope to its storage place.

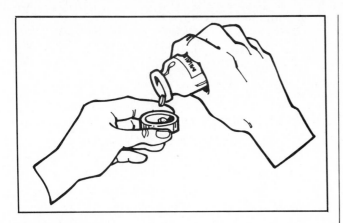

FIGURE 29–5

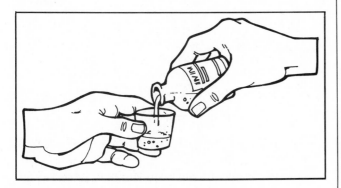

FIGURE 29–6

7. Identify the patient by comparing the name on the medication card with the name on the patient's identification bracelet or by asking the patient to tell you his or her name.

8. Explain to the patient the purpose of the medication and how it will help, using language that she or he can understand. Include relevant information about effects, eg, tell the patient receiving a diuretic that she or he can expect an increase in urine.

9. Assist the patient to a sitting position or, if not possible, to a lateral position.

   Rationale These positions facilitate swallowing and prevent aspiration.

10. Take the required assessment measures, eg, pulse and respiratory rates or blood pressure. The pulse rate is taken before administering digitalis preparations. Blood pressure is taken before giving hypotensive drugs. The respiratory rate is taken prior to administering narcotics, since narcotics depress the respiratory center. If the rate is below 12, the responsible nurse should be consulted.

11. Give the patient sufficient water or juice to swallow the medication if appropriate.

    Rationale Fluids ease swallowing and facilitate absorption from the gastrointestinal tract. Liquid medications are generally diluted with 15 mL (½ oz) of water to facilitate absorption.

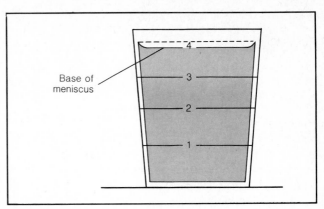

FIGURE 29–7

FIGURE 29–8

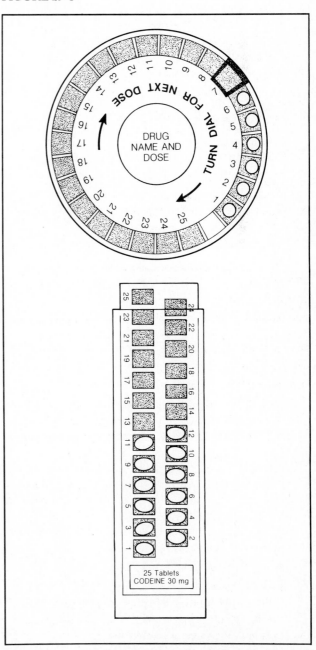

12. If the patient is unable to hold the pill cup, use the pill cup to introduce the medication into the patient's mouth.

    Rationale Putting the cup to the patient's mouth avoids contamination of the medication and of the nurse's hands.

13. If the patient has difficulty swallowing, have him or her place the medication on the back of the tongue before taking the water.

    Rationale Stimulation of the back of the tongue produces the swallowing reflex.

14. If the medication is harmful to tooth enamel or irritating to the oral mucous membrane, eg, liquid iron preparations, have the patient use a glass straw and drink water following the medication.

15. If the patient says that the medication you are about to give is different from what she or he has been receiving, do not give the medication without checking the original order.

16. If the medication has an objectionable taste, have the patient suck a few ice chips beforehand, or give the medication with juice, applesauce, or bread.

    Rationale The cold will desensitize the taste buds, and juices, bread, etc, can mask the taste of the medication.

17. Stay with the patient until all medications have been swallowed.

18. Record the medication given, dosage, time, any complaints of the patient, and your signature. If there are other patients who require medications, give these out before charting.

19. Return the medication card to the slot of the next time it is due.

20. Return to the patient within 30 minutes to evaluate the effects of the medication, eg, relief of pain.

■ Evaluation

Expected outcomes

1. Medication was swallowed and tolerated.
2. Medication had desired effect, eg, an analgesic decreased a patient's pain.

Unexpected outcomes

1. Medication induced nausea and/or vomiting.
2. Medication had no effect or undesired effect.

Upon obtaining an unexpected outcome:

1. Report your findings to the responsible nurse and/or physician.
2. Adjust the nursing care plan appropriately.

TECHNIQUE 29–2 ■ Administering Dermatologic Medications

Dermatologic preparations include lotions, liniments, ointments, pastes, powders, creams, gels and jellies, and aerosol sprays and foams.

1. Lotions are liquids that have varying viscosities. They may be clear solutions, suspensions, or emulsions that contain water, alcohol and/or other solvents. Some (eg, calamine lotion) contain an insoluble powder and need to be shaken before use. Lotions may have an emollient (soothing and softening) effect on the skin, or they may be mildly acid or alkaline. They are generally applied when large skin areas are involved, when hairy portions of the body need treatment, or when the preparation is to be applied without rubbing.

2. Liniments are oily, soapy, or alcoholic liquids that usually contain a rubefacient. They are rubbed on the skin.

3. Ointments are greasy semisolid preparations of a medication in some type of base, eg, petrolatum.

They are often applied to dry skin lesions. Some ointments are soothing; others are antimicrobial or astringent. Ointments that are applied to the eye or around an open wound need to be sterile so as not to transmit microorganisms.

4. Pastes are similar to ointments but contain a higher powder content, are stiff in consistency, and may be useful in absorbing secretions from skin lesions. Pastes penetrate the skin less than do ointments. An example is zinc oxide paste, which is used on babies to protect excoriated areas from urine and feces.

5. Powders are nonabsorbable finely ground medications, usually applied to the skin as a protective. They are useful for reducing friction, eg, between thighs, beneath the breasts, or between toes. Examples are talcum powder and cornstarch. The disadvantages of powders are that they do not adhere to dry skin surfaces and tend to cake on moist surfaces.

6. Creams are generally nongreasy, white, semisolid preparations that contain water and can usually be removed with water. An example is hydrocortisone cream. They are usually applied on areas where cosmetic appeal is desired or on moist areas.

7. Gels and jellies are usually clear or translucent semisolids that liquefy when applied to the skin. They may contain water or alcohol and are easily removed. An example is K-Y jelly. These preparations are useful when lubrication and cosmetic appeal are desirable.

8. Aerosol sprays deposit a thin layer of liquid or powder onto the designated area. Examples are Kenalog or Solarcaine spray and Desenex aerosol powder. Aerosol sprays are generally used when large skin areas need to be treated and when manual application is painful, eg, when treating burns.

9. Aerosol foams are generally used on hairy areas of the body or in body cavities, such as the rectum or vagina. Examples are Epifoam and ProctoFoam.

■ Assessment

Assess any discomfort experienced by the patient, eg, pruritis, and the need for medication. Other data include:

1. The physician's order for the name of the preparation, the strength, the frequency or timing of the application, and the site of application

2. Whether sterile technique is required

3. The purpose of the application and the reactions that can be anticipated

■ Planning

Nursing goals

1. To protect the skin and/or mucous membrane

2. To treat localized infectious lesions, eg, with antibiotic or antifungal agent

3. To apply an antiseptic when normal skin protective mechanisms are broken down

4. To provide heat or relieve pain

5. To soothe irritated skin, eg, from pruritus

Equipment

Use sterile supplies and technique for all open skin lesions.

1. Warm water or other specified solution, clean towel, or sterile gauze squares or cotton balls to clean the area to be treated.

2. The ordered preparation at the correct strength.

3. Tongue blades for applying ointments and creams.

4. Gloves (optional) to use instead of tongue blades or

when the nurse's hands need to be protected from infection.

5. Sterile gauze to hold the medication, if it is taken from a stock jar, or for applying liquids. A stock jar is not taken to the bedside because it must remain free of the patient's microorganisms.

6. Sterile dressings and tape, if necessary, to place over the application. Check the physician's order.

7. The patient's medication card or treatment sheet.

8. A clean gown or pajamas (optional).

■ Intervention

1. Check that the part to be treated is clean; if not, wash it with warm water or other solution as directed, and pat it dry with a clean towel or sterile gauze squares or cotton balls. Assess the affected area for redness, rashes, swelling, and discharge.

2. Place a small amount of cream (eg, emollient), on the tongue blade, and spread it evenly on the skin.
   or

3. Pour some lotion on the gauze and pat the skin area with it.
   or

4. If a liniment is used, rub it into the skin with the hands using long, smooth strokes.

5. Repeat the application until the area is completely covered. No skin should show through cream or ointment.

6. Apply a sterile dressing as necessary.

7. Provide an agency gown or pajamas for the patient to wear after the application if the medication will come in contact with the patient's clothing.
   Rationale Agency clothes can be washed more easily.

8. Record on the patient's chart the type of preparation used, the site to which it was applied, the time, and the response of the patient, including data about the appearance of the site, discomfort, itching, etc. Return 15 to 30 minutes after the application to assess the response of the patient, eg, redness (for a rubefacient), and/or relief of itching, burning, swelling, or discomfort.

9. Adjust the nursing care plan as necessary for the next application.

Sample Recording

Date	Time	Notes
12/5/86	1200	Calamine lotion applied to dorsal surfaces of both hands. Left hand appears red but dry. Itchiness relieved. ———— Hilaria D. Maciel, NS
12/5/86	1215	No discomfort.———— Hilaria D. Maciel, NS

■ Evaluation

Expected outcome

Positive change in clinical signs.

Unexpected outcome

Absence of change or negative change in clinical signs, eg, redness unchanged, increased discharge, increased discomfort. Upon obtaining an unexpected outcome:

1. Report your findings to the responsible nurse and/or physician.
2. Adjust the nursing care plan appropriately.

TECHNIQUE 29–3 ■ Administering Ophthalmic Irrigations and Instillations

An eye irrigation is administered to wash out the conjunctival sac of the eye. In a hospital, sterile equipment is usually used; however, clean supplies are normally satisfactory in a home. For an eye irrigation in the home, an eyecup is frequently used. The nurse ascertains that the eyecup is clean and that it has no chips along the edge, which could injure the skin.

Medications for the eyes are instilled in the form of liquids or ointments. Usually sterile preparations are used, but sterile technique is not always indicated. Prescribed liquids are usually dilute, eg, less than 1% strength.

For information about the anatomic structure of the eye, see chapter 13, Figures 13–13 and 13–14 on pages 306 and 307.

■ Assessment

See Intervention, step 5. Other data include:

1. The physician's order for the preparation, strength, and number of drops if it is a liquid instillation; the frequency of the instillation; and which eye is to be treated. Abbreviations are frequently used to identify the eye: OD (right eye), OS (left eye), OU (both eyes).
2. For an irrigation, the type, amount, temperature, and strength of the solution, and the frequency of the irrigation.

■ Planning

Nursing goals

For an irrigation

1. To treat an inflammatory process of the conjunctiva
2. To apply an antiseptic solution
3. To remove a foreign object or an irritating chemical

4. To apply heat or cold to the eye
5. To prepare an eye for surgery

For an instillation

6. To anesthetize the eye
7. To dilate the pupil for retinal examination
8. To soothe irritated conjunctival tissue
9. To decrease intraocular pressure
10. To relieve an eye infection

Equipment

For an irrigation

1. A sterile container for the irrigating solution.
2. Irrigating solution. Usually 60 to 235 mL (2 to 8 oz) of solution at 37 °C (98.6 °F) is appropriate.
3. A sterile eye syringe or eye irrigator. An eyedropper can be used if only small amounts of solution are required.
4. A sterile kidney basin to catch the irrigating solution.
5. Sterile cotton balls to clean the eyelid and lashes before the procedure and to dry around the eye after the irrigation.
6. Sterile normal saline (optional) to clean the eyelids and lashes.
7. A moisture-proof drape to protect the patient and the bedclothes.
8. Sterile gloves (optional) to protect the nurse from contamination if the eye is infected.

For an instillation

9. The medication. Some eye medications are packaged in plastic containers that are also used to administer the preparation. Ointments are usually supplied in small tubes.
10. A sterile eyedropper, if needed.
11. Sterile absorbent sponges. Soak some sponges in

sterile normal saline for cleaning the eyelid and eyelashes.

12. The patient's medication card or treatment sheet.

13. A sterile eye dressing (pad) as needed and paper eye tape to secure it.

■ Intervention

1. Explain the technique to the patient. The administration of an ophthalmic irrigating solution or medication is not usually painful. Ointments are often soothing to the eye, but some liquid preparations may sting initially.

2. Assist the patient to a comfortable position either sitting or lying. Tilt the patient's head toward the affected eye, and ensure that the light source does not shine into the patient's eyes. See Figure 29–9.

   Rationale   The patient's head is tilted so that the solution will run from the eye to the basin at the side, not to the other eye. The light source is directed slightly away from the eye, particularly if the patient is photophobic.

3. Place the drape to protect the patient and the bedclothes, and position the basin against the patient's cheek below the eye on the affected side.

4. Clean the eyelid and lashes with sterile cotton balls, moistened with sterile irrigating solution or sterile normal saline, wiping from the inner canthus to the outer canthus. Don gloves before handling the eye structures if they are infected.

   Rationale   If not removed, material on the eyelid and lashes can be washed into the eye. Cleaning toward the outer canthus prevents contamination of the other eye and the lacrimal duct.

5. Assess:

   a. The eye for redness, the location and nature of any discharge, lacrimation, and swelling of the eyelids or of the lacrimal gland.

   b. Any complaints of the patient, eg, itching, burning, pain, blurring of vision, and photophobia.

   c. The patient's behavior, eg, squinting, blinking excessively, frowning, or rubbing the eyes.

For an irrigation

6. Expose the lower conjunctival sac by separating the lids with the thumb and forefinger (see Figure 29–10). Or, to irrigate in stages, first hold the lower lid down, then hold the upper lid up. Exert pressure on the bony prominences of the cheekbone and beneath the eyebrow when holding the eyelids.

   Rationale   Separating the lids prevents reflex blinking. Exerting pressure on the bony prominences minimizes the possibility of pressing the eyeball and causing discomfort.

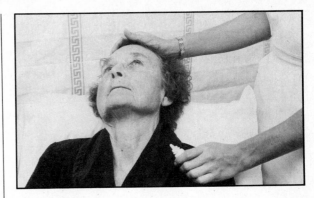

FIGURE 29–9

7. Fill and hold the eye irrigator about 2.5 cm (1 in) above the eye.

   Rationale   At this height the pressure of the solution will not damage the eye tissue, and the irrigator will not touch the eye.

8. Irrigate the eye, directing the solution onto the lower conjunctival sac and from the inner canthus to the outer canthus.

   Rationale   Directing the solution in this way prevents possible injury to the cornea and prevents fluid and contaminants from flowing down the nasolacrimal duct.

9. Irrigate until the solution leaving the eye is clear (no discharge is present) or until all the solution has been used.

10. Instruct the patient to close and move the eye periodically.

    Rationale   Eye closure and movement help to move secretions from the upper to the lower conjunctival sac.

11. Dry around the eye with cotton balls.

FIGURE 29–10

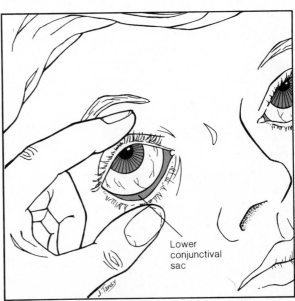

Lower conjunctival sac

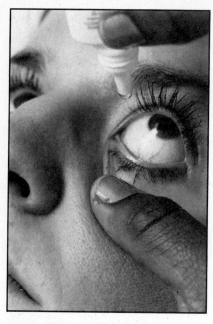

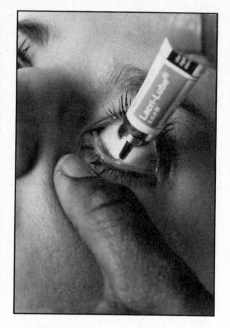

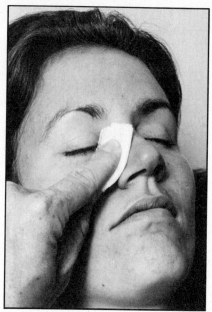

FIGURE 29–11

FIGURE 29–12

FIGURE 29–13

For an instillation

12. Check the ophthalmic preparation as to name, strength, and number of drops if a liquid is used. Draw the correct number of drops into the dropper if a dropper is used. If ointment is used, discard the first bead.

    Rationale Checking medication data is essential to prevent a medication error. The first bead of ointment from a tube is considered to be contaminated.

13. Instruct the patient to look up to the ceiling and give him or her a piece of tissue.

    Rationale The patient is less likely to blink if he or she is looking up and the cornea is partially protected by the top eyelid. A tissue is needed to press on the nasolacrimal duct after a liquid instillation (see step 18) or to wipe excess ointment from the eyelashes after an ointment is instilled.

14. Expose the lower conjunctival sac by placing the thumb or fingers of your nondominant hand on the patient's cheekbone just below the eye and gently drawing the skin on the cheek down. If the tissues are edematous, handle the tissues carefully to avoid damaging them. See Figure 29–11.

    Rationale Placing the fingers on the patient's cheekbone minimizes the possibility of touching the cornea, avoids putting any pressure on the eyeball, and prevents the patient from blinking or squinting.

15. Using a side approach, instill the correct number of drops onto the outer third of the lower conjunctival sac. Hold the dropper 1 to 2 cm (0.4 to 0.8 in) above the sac. See Figure 29–11.

    Rationale The patient is less likely to blink if a side approach is used. When instilled into the conjunctival sac, drops will not harm the cornea as they might if dropped directly on it. The dropper must not touch the sac or the cornea.

    or

16. Holding the tube above the lower conjunctival sac, squeeze 3 cm (0.8 in) of ointment from the tube into the lower conjunctival sac from the inner canthus outward. See Figure 29–12.

17. Instruct the patient to close the eyelids but not to squeeze them shut.

    Rationale Closing the eye spreads the medication over the eyeball. Squeezing can injure the eye and push out the medication.

18. For liquid medications, press firmly or have the patient press firmly on the lasolacrimal duct for at least 30 seconds. See Figure 29–13. Check agency practice.

    Rationale Pressing on the nasolacrimal duct prevents the medication from running out of the eye down the duct.

19. Wipe the eyelids gently from the inner to the outer canthus, to collect excess medication.

20. Apply an eye pad if needed, and secure it with paper eye tape.

For an irrigation and instillation

21. Assess the patient's response in terms of the character and amount of any discharge, the appearance of the eye, and any discomfort, burning, etc. Assess any

changes immediately after the instillation or irrigation and again 15 to 30 minutes later.

22. Record on the patient's chart the instillation or irrigation, the name of the drug, the strength, the number of drops if a liquid, the time, and the response of the patient.

23. Adjust the nursing care plan as needed for the next instillation or irrigation, and include any necessary patient education about rubbing the eyes, etc.

Sample Recording

Date	Time	Notes
12/5/86	0900	C/o⁄ burning sensation OD. Moderate amount yellow purulent discharge at inner canthus and on eyelashes. Conjunctiva red. OD irrigated with 90 mL normal saline at 38 °C. Returns cloudy. Stated "eye feels better" following irrigation. ———————— Deborah M. Mondeau, NS

■ Evaluation

Expected outcomes

1. Normal color of conjunctiva
2. Absence of discharge and lacrimation
3. Absence of itching or burning

Unexpected outcomes

1. Conjunctiva reddened
2. Swelling of eyelids
3. Discharge at inner canthus
4. Complaints of blurred vision or photophobia
5. Complaints of burning or itchiness
6. Frequent blinking, frowning, or rubbing of eyes

Upon obtaining an unexpected outcome:

1. Report your findings to the responsible nurse.
2. Adjust the nursing care plan appropriately.

TECHNIQUE 29–4 ■ Administering Otic Irrigations and Instillations

Irrigations of the external auditory canal are generally carried out for cleaning purposes, although applications of heat and of antiseptic solutions are sometimes prescribed. Irrigations are usually performed in a hospital, using sterile supplies and equipment so that microorganisms will not be introduced into the ear. If done at home, sterile supplies are not ususaly necessary because the patient is accustomed to the microorganisms in the home environment. Medical aseptic technique is used to instill medications to the ear unless the tympanic membrane is damaged, in which case sterile technique is used. For information about the structures of the ear see chapter 13, Figures 13–27 and 13–28 on pages 317 and 318.

The position of the external auditory canal varies with age. In the child under three years of age, it is directed upward on the inside. In the adult, the external auditory canal is an S-shaped structure about 2.5 cm (1 in) long. Hairs grow along the outer third of the canal.

■ Assessment

This assessment may be carried out after Intervention, steps 5 and 17.

1. Assess the pinna of the ear and the meatus of the external auditory canal for signs of redness and abrasions and the type and amount of any discharge.

2. Assess the patient for complaints of discomfort.

3. If indicated, use an otoscope (see Technique 10–9 on page 194) to assess:

    a. The external canal for any foreign bodies.

    b. The color and amount of cerumen in the canal.

    c. The external canal for swelling, redness, and discharge. The lining should be intact, pink, and without lesions.

    d. The state of the tympanic membrane. See Figure 10–43 on page 197. Report any tears or abrasions to the responsible nurse and/or the physician before proceeding with the irrigation or instillation.

Other data include:

1. The physician's order stating the kind of medication or irrigation; the time, amount, and dosage (if it is an instillation) or strength (if it is an irrigation); and the temperature (if it is an irrigation).

2. Which ear is to be treated.

3. The reason for the irrigation or instillation.

4. Whether the technique should be sterile.

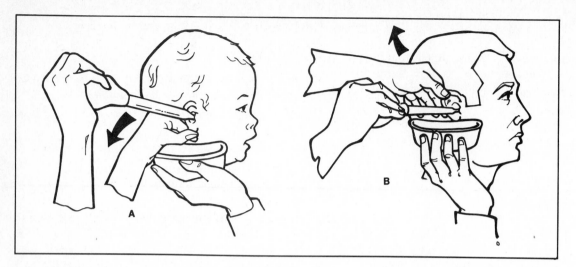

FIGURE 29-14

■ Planning

Nursing goals

For an irrigation

1. To clean the canal, eg, to remove cerumen or pus
2. To apply heat
3. To remove a foreign object, eg, an insect

For an instillation

4. To soften earwax so that it can be readily removed at a later time
5. To obtain a specific therapeutic effect for a disease process
6. To relieve pain

Equipment

For an irrigation

1. A container for the irrigating solution.
2. Irrigating solution. About 500 mL (16 oz) of solution is required. Normal saline is frequently used. The temperature is body temperature: for an adult, 37.0 °C (98.6 °F). Use a thermometer to make sure the temperature of the solution is appropriate.
3. A syringe. A rubber bulb or Asepto syringe is frequently used.
4. A basin to receive the irrigating solution. A kidney basin is often used because the small curve will fit closely against the head.
5. A moisture-resistant towel to protect the patient (and the bed) from the solution.
6. Applicator swabs for cleaning the external ear.
7. Absorbent cotton balls to dry the pinna of the ear after the irrigation.

For an instillation

8. The correct medication bottle with a dropper. To make the instillation more comfortable for the patient, warm the container in your hand or place it in warm water for a short time.
9. The patient's medicine card or treatment sheet.
10. A cotton-tipped applicator to wipe the auditory meatus.
11. A flexible rubber tip (optional) for the end of the dropper, which prevents injury from sudden motion, eg, by a child or disoriented patient.
12. A cotton fluff to cover the auditory meatus following the installation.

■ Intervention

For an irrigation

1. Explain to the patient what you plan to do. Adjust the explanation to the patient's needs. The patient may experience a feeling of fullness, warmth, and occasionally dizziness and discomfort when the fluid comes in contact with the tympanic membrane.
2. Assist the patient to a sitting or lying position with head turned toward the affected ear.
   Rationale The solution can then flow from the ear canal to a basin.
3. Place the moisture-resistant towel around the patient's shoulder under the ear.
4. Place the basin under the ear to be irrigated.
5. Clean the pinna of the ear and the meatus of the ear canal with applicator swabs and solution.
   Rationale Any discharge is removed, so that it will not be washed into the ear canal.
6. Fill the syringe with solution.
   or
7. Hang up the irrigating container, and run solution through the tubing and the nozzle.
   Rationale Solution is run through to remove air from the tubing and nozzle.

8. Straighten the patient's auditory canal. For an infant, gently pull the pinna downward. See Figure 29–14, *A*. For an adult, pull the pinna upward and backward. See Figure 29–14, *B*.

   Rationale The auditory canal is straightened so that the solution can flow the entire length of the canal.

9. Insert the tip of the syringe or nozzle into the auditory meatus, and direct the solution gently upward against the top of the canal.

   Rationale The solution will flow around the entire canal and out at the bottom. The solution is instilled gently because strong pressure from the fluid can cause discomfort and damage the tympanic membrane.

10. Continue instilling the fluid until all the solution is used or until the canal is cleaned, depending on the purpose of the irrigation. Take care not to block the outward flow of the solution with the syringe or nozzle.

11. Dry the outside of the ear with absorbent cotton balls. Place a cotton fluff in the auditory meatus, to absorb the excess fluid.

12. Assist the patient to a side-lying position on the affected side.

    Rationale Lying with the affected side down helps drain the excess fluid by gravity.

13. Assess the patient's response to the irrigation in terms of discomfort, dizziness, and the appearance and odor of the fluid returns.

14. Record the irrigation; the type, concentration, amount, and temperature of the solution used; the appearance of the returns; and the patient's response in terms of discomfort and dizziness. Go to step 27.

Sample Recording

Date	Time	Notes
12/5/86	1100	Irrigated left ear with 60 mL normal saline at 40 °C. Returns clear with several dark brown flecks. No discomfort, no dizziness.———————————Josephine A. deSanto, NS

For an instillation

15. Assist the patient to a side-lying position with the ear being treated uppermost. See Figure 29–15.

16. Apply a mummy restraint to an infant unless a support person or another nurse is available to hold the baby.

17. Wipe the auditory meatus with a cotton-tipped applicator.

    Rationale The auditory meatus is cleaned to remove any drainage.

18. Partially fill the ear dropper with medication.

19. Straighten the patient's ear canal. See step 8 and Figure 29–14.

20. Instill the correct number of drops along the side of the ear canal.

21. Press gently but firmly a few times on the tragus of the ear.

    Rationale Pressing on the tragus assists the flow of medication into the ear canal.

22. Have the patient remain in the side-lying position for about five minutes.

    Rationale This prevents the drops from escaping and allows the medication to reach all sides of the canal cavity.

23. Insert a small piece of cotton fluff loosely at the meatus of the auditory canal for 15 to 20 minutes. Do not press it into the canal.

    Rationale The cotton helps retain the medication when the patient is up. If pressed tightly into the canal the cotton would interfere with the action of the drug and the outward movement of normal secretions.

24. Assess the patient's response in terms of the character and amount of discharge, appearance of the canal, discomfort, etc, after the instillation and again 15 to 30 minutes later.

25. Record on the appropriate record the instillation, the time, the dose, any complaints of the patient, and observations made. Many agencies use flow sheets that require only the nurse's signature; others may require that a notation be made on the nurse's notes.

Sample Recording

Date	Time	Notes
12/5/86	0900	Auralgan gtt ꭕꭕꭕ instilled into left ear. States ear less painful. No discharge present.——————————————— Margaret N. Kerr, NS

FIGURE 29–15

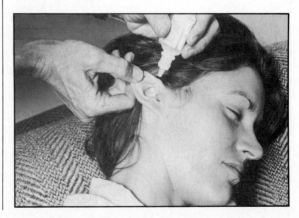

26. Return in 15 minutes to assess the drainage on the absorbent cotton ball. Remove the cotton ball if drainage appears complete, and assist the patient to a comfortable position.

■ Evaluation

Expected outcomes

1. No discomfort in ear
2. Pinna of ears appear normal
3. No discharge in the external auditory canals
4. Both tympanic membranes intact and pink

Unexpected outcomes

1. Large amount of black cerumen in external auditory canal
2. Tympanic membrane appears swollen, with yellow discharge

Upon obtaining an unexpected outcome:

1. Report your findings to the responsible nurse.
2. Adjust the nursing care plan appropriately.

TECHNIQUE 29–5 ■ Administering Nasal Instillations

A nasal instillation is given in the form of nose drops or a nasal spray. For a nasal spray the medication is dissolved in water. It is sprayed into one nostril while the patient inhales with the other nostril occluded. The second nostril is then sprayed in the same manner. The instillation of nasal medications is usually not a sterile procedure unless it is carried out postoperatively.

Nasal instillations are sometimes intended for the nasal sinuses, which are hollow cavities in the facial bones. There are four groups of sinuses: sphenoid, ethmoid, frontal, and maxillary. See Figure 29–16, A, for a lateral view, 29–16, B, for a frontal view. the sinuses are lined with mucous membrane, which is continuous with the mucous membrane of the nasal passage.

■ Assessment

Some of this assessment may be carried out during the Intervention. Assess:

1. The amount and character (color, thickness, odor) of any nasal discharge.
2. Congestion of the mucous membranes and any obstruction to breathing. Ask the patient to hold one nostril closed and blow out gently through the other nostril. Listen for the sound of any obstruction to the air. Repeat for the other nostril.
3. Facial discomfort. An infected or congested sinus can cause an aching, full feeling over the area of the sinus and facial tenderness on palpation.
4. Any crusting, redness, bleeding, or discharge of the mucous membranes of the nostrils. Use a nasal speculum. The membrane normally appears moist, pink, and shiny.

FIGURE 29–16 ■ The four groups of facial sinuses: **A,** lateral view; **B,** frontal view.

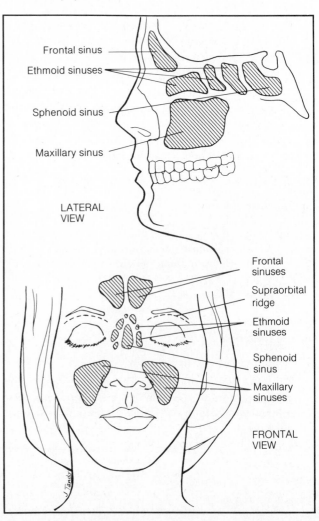

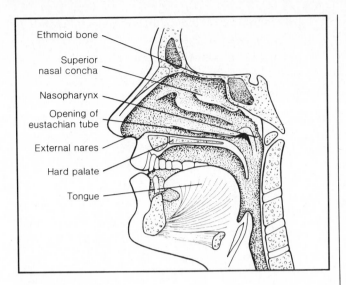

FIGURE 29-17

Other data include:

1. The physician's order for the solution to be used, its strength, the number of drops, and the frequency of the instillation.
2. The physician's order for the area to receive the instillation, eg, the eustachian (auditory) tube or specific sinuses. The position the patient is to assume depends on where the solution is to run.

■ Planning

Nursing goals

1. To relieve nasal congestion
2. To relieve infections of the nasal passages and/or the sinuses

Equipment

1. The solution ordered by the physician.
2. A dropper for administering the solution. Some solution containers come with a dropper.
3. Disposable tissues.

■ Intervention

1. Ask the patient to blow his or her nose to clear the nasal passages.
2. To treat the opening of the eustachian tube, have the patient assume a back-lying position; the drops will flow into the nasopharynx, where the eustachian tube opens. See Figure 29–17. To treat the ethmoid and sphenoid sinuses, have the patient take a back-lying position with the head over the edge of the bed or a pillow under the shoulders so that the head is tipped backward. This is called the Proetz position. See Figure 29–18. To treat the maxillary

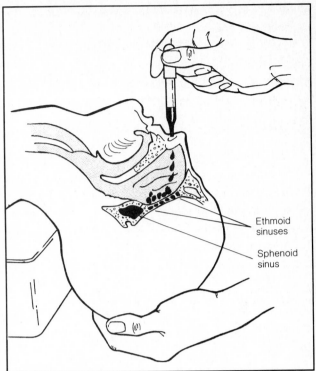

FIGURE 29-18

and frontal sinuses, have the patient assume the same back-lying position, with the head turned toward the side to be treated. This is called the Parkinson position. See Figure 29–19. If only one side is to be treated, be sure the patient is positioned so that the correct side is accessible. If the patient's head is over the edge of the bed, support it with your hand so that the neck muscles are not strained.

FIGURE 29-19

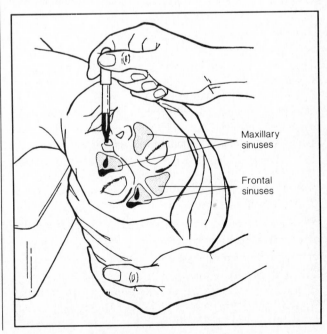

3. Confirm that you have the correct solution at the correct strength.

4. Draw up the required amount of solution into the dropper.

5. Hold the tip of the dropper just above the nostril, and direct the solution laterally toward the midline of the superior concha of the ethmoid bone as the patient breathes through his or her mouth. Do not touch the mucous membrane of the nares.

   Rationale If the solution is directed toward the base of the nasal cavity it will run down the eustachian tube. Touching the mucous membrane with the dropper could damage the membrane and cause the patient to sneeze.

6. Repeat for the other nostril if indicated.

7. Ask the patient to remain in the position for five or ten minutes.

   Rationale The patient remains in the same position to help the solution flow into the desired area.

8. Discard any remaining solution in the dropper.

9. Assess the patient's response to the instillation in terms of reduction in congestion, ease of breathing through the nose, and discomfort. The patient may need to be assessed 15 to 30 minutes after the instillation, when the medication has taken effect, as well as when it is administered.

10. Record in the patient's chart the instillation, the time, and the response of the patient.

■ Evaluation

Expected outcomes

1. No nasal discharge
2. No obstruction to breathing
3. No facial discomfort
4. Mucous membranes appear normal

Unexpected outcomes

1. Nasal congestion in both nostrils
2. Serous nasal discharge
3. Discomfort over maxillary area
4. Mucous membranes reddened

Upon obtaining an unexpected outcome:

1. Report your findings to the responsible nurse.
2. Adjust the nursing care plan appropriately.

TECHNIQUE 29–6 ■ Administering Vaginal Irrigations and Instillations

A vaginal irrigation (douche) is the washing of the vagina by a liquid at a low pressure. It is similar to the irrigation of the external auditory canal in that the fluid returns immediately after being inserted. Vaginal irrigations are not necessary for ordinary female hygiene but are used to treat specific problems. See Nursing Goals.

Vaginal medications, or instillations, are inserted as creams, jellies, foams, suppositories, or irrigations (douches). Medical aseptic technique is usually used. Vaginal creams, jellies, and foams are applied by using a tubular applicator with a plunger. Suppositories are inserted with the index finger of a gloved hand.

■ Assessment

This assessment may be carried out after Intervention, steps 5 and 20. Assess:

1. Any odor and discharge from the vagina
2. Complaints of vaginal discomfort
3. Clinical signs of generalized infection, eg, elevated body temperature, rapid pulse

Other data include:

1. The specific medication, its dosage, and the time of administration. Carefully check the medication order.
2. The reason for the vaginal instillation.

■ Planning

Nursing goals

For a vaginal irrigation

1. To prevent infection by applying an antimicrobial solution that discourages the growth of microorganisms
2. To remove an offensive or irritating discharge
3. To reduce inflammation or prevent hemorrhage by the application of heat or cold

For a vaginal instillation

4. To relieve vaginal discomfort, eg, itching or pain
5. To relieve infection

Equipment

For a vaginal irrigation

In hospitals, sterile supplies and equipment are used; in a home, sterility is not usually necessary because patients are accustomed to the microorganisms in their environments. Sterile technique is indicated if there is an open wound.

1. A vaginal irrigation set (these are often disposable) containing:

   a. A nozzle

   b. Tubing and a clamp

   c. A container for the solution

   d. A moisture-resistant drape

2. Irrigating solution. Usually 1,000 to 2,000 mL at 40.5 °C (105 °F) is required. Check agency practice. Normal saline, tap water, sodium bicarbonate solution (8 mL of sodium bicarbonate to 1,000 mL of water), and vinegar solution (8 mL of vinegar to 1,000 mL of water) are commonly used.

3. A thermometer to check the temperature of the solution. This is usually measured before the equipment is taken to the patient.

4. A moisture-proof pad to protect the bedding and a drape to cover the patient's legs.

5. A bedpan to receive the irrigation returns.

6. Tissues to dry the perineum.

7. Gloves (optional). They may be required to protect the nurse from infection.

8. An IV pole on which to hang the solution container.

For a vaginal instillation

9. The patient's medicine card or treatment sheet.

10. The correct vaginal suppository or cream. Suppositories are designed to melt at body temperature, so they are generally stored in the refrigerator to keep them firm for insertion.

11. Disposable gloves: one to insert a suppository and the other to expose the vaginal orifice. Only one glove is needed if an applicator is used.

12. Lubricant for a suppository.

13. An applicator for vaginal cream.

14. A paper towel.

15. A clean perineal pad and T-binder or sanitary belt.

■ Intervention

1. Explain the technique to the patient. A vaginal irrigation or instillation is normally a painless procedure and in fact may bring relief from itching and burning if an infection is present. It usually takes about ten minutes. Many patients feel embarrassed about these procedures, and some may prefer to

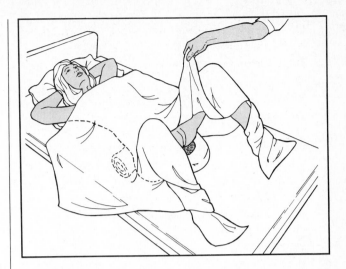

FIGURE 29–20

perform the procedure themselves if instruction is provided.

2. Carefully check the physician's order for the specific medication or solution ordered, its dosage, and the time of administration. Ensure that the medication card agrees with the medication order.

3. Provide privacy, and ask the patient to void.

   Rationale The patient will have less discomfort during the treatment, and the possibility of injuring the vaginal lining is decreased, if the bladder is empty.

Vaginal irrigation

4. Assist the patient to a back-lying position with the hips higher than the shoulders so that the solution will flow into the posterior fornix of the vagina. Position the patient on a bedpan, and provide comfortable support for the lumbar region of the back with a roll or pillow. Place the waterproof drape under the bedpan to protect the bedding. Provide a drape for the legs so that only the perineal area is exposed. See Figure 29–20.

5. Provide perineal care to remove microorganisms.

   Rationale This decreases the chance of flushing microorganisms into the vagina.

6. Clamp the tubing. Hang the irrigating container on the IV pole so that the base is about 30 cm (12 in) above the vagina.

   Rationale At this height the pressure of the solution should not be great enough to injure the vaginal lining.

7. Run fluid through the tubing and nozzle into the bedpan.

   Rationale Fluid is run through the tubing to remove air and to moisten the nozzle.

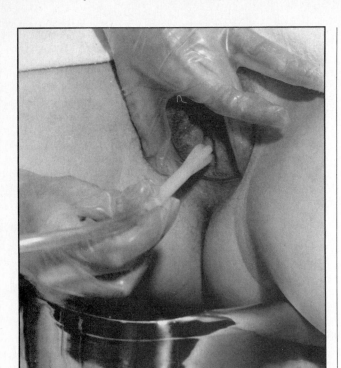

FIGURE 29–21

8. Run some fluid over the perineal area, then insert the nozzle carefully into the vagina. See Figure 29–21. Direct the nozzle toward the sacrum, following the direction of the vagina.

9. Insert the nozzle about 7 to 10 cm (3 to 4 in), and rotate it several times.

   Rationale Rotating the nozzle irrigates all parts of the vagina.

10. Use all the irrigating solution, permitting it to flow out freely into the bedpan.

    Rationale Obstructing the flow of the returns could result in injury to the tissues from pressure.

11. Remove the nozzle from the vagina.

12. Assist the patient to a sitting position on the bedpan.

    Rationale Sitting on the bedpan will help drain the remaining fluid by gravity.

13. Dry the perineum with tissues.

14. Remove the bedpan.

15. Assess the response of the patient in terms of the color of the fluid returns and the presence of any flecks, discomfort, redness of the vagina, and odor from the vagina.

16. Remove the moisture-resistant pad and the drape.

17. Apply a dressing if indicated.

18. On the patient's chart, record the irrigation; the amount, type, strength, and temperature of the irrigating solution; any discomfort, etc; and the response of the patient to the irrigation.

Vaginal instillation (suppository, cream, foam, jelly)

19. Assist the patient to a back-lying position with the knees flexed and the hips rotated laterally. Drape the patient as shown in Figure 29–20.

20. Ensure that the perineal area is clean.

Vaginal suppository

21. Unwrap the suppository and put it on the opened wrapper.

22. Don gloves.

    Rationale Gloves prevent contamination of the nurse's hands from vaginal and perineal microorganisms.

23. Lubricate the rounded (smooth) end of the suppository. The rounded end is inserted first.

    Rationale Lubrication facilitates insertion.

24. Lubricate your gloved index finger.

25. Expose the vaginal orifice by separating the labia with your nondominant hand.

26. Insert the suppository about 8 to 10 cm (3 to 4 in) along the posterior wall of the vagina, or as far as it will go. The posterior wall of the vagina is about 2.5 cm (1 in) longer than the anterior wall since the cervix protrudes into the uppermost portion of the anterior wall. The anterior wall is usually about 6 to 7.5 cm (2½ to 3 in).

27. Withdraw the finger and remove the gloves, turning them inside out and placing them on a paper towel.

    Rationale Turning the gloves inside out prevents the spread of microorganisms.

28. Have the patient remain lying in the supine position for five to ten minutes following insertion. The hips may also be elevated on a pillow.

    Rationale The patient remains lying down to allow the medication to flow into the posterior fornix after it has melted.

Vaginal cream, jelly, foam

29. Fill the applicator with the prescribed cream, jelly, or foam. Directions are provided with the manufacturer's applicator.

30. Put a glove on your nondominant hand and expose the vaginal orifice. A second glove may also be worn to protect your hands from microorganisms.

31. Gently insert the applicator about 5 cm (2 in).

32. Slowly push the plunger until the applicator is empty.

33. Remove the applicator and place it on the paper towel.

    Rationale The applicator is put on a paper towel to prevent the spread of microorganisms.

34. Remove the glove, turning it inside out, and place it on the paper towel.

35. Have the patient remain in bed in the supine position for five to ten minutes following the instillation.
36. Apply a clean perineal pad and a T-binder if there is excessive drainage.
37. Report to the responsible nurse pertinent data, eg, excessive drainage or discomfort, and record the instillation as you would other medications and instillations.
38. Assess the patient's response to the instillation in terms of discharge, discomfort, etc.

■ Evaluation

Expected outcomes

1. Absence of vaginal discharge or odor
2. No complaints of vaginal discomfort

Unexpected outcomes

1. Large amount of thick white vaginal discharge
2. Complaints of vaginal burning or itchiness
3. Temperature 39 °C (102.2 °F), pulse 96 beats per minute

Upon obtaining an unexpected outcome:

1. Report your findings to the responsible nurse and/or physician.
2. Adjust the nursing care plan appropriately.

References

Budd R: We changed to unit-dose system. *Nurs Outlook* (February) 1971; 19:116–117.

Galton L: Drugs and the elderly: What you should know about them. *Nursing 76* (August) 1976; 6:39–43.

Lambert ML: Drug and diet interactions. *Am J Nurs* (March) 1975; 75:402–406.

Matus NR (consultant): Topical therapy: Choosing and using the proper vehicle. *Nursing 77* (November) 1977; 7:8–10.

Reiss BS, Melick ME: *Pharmacological Aspects of Nursing Care.* Delmar, 1984.

Sklar CL: You and the law: Accidents, imponderables, what is foreseeable and what is not: What constitutes nursing negligence in the administration of medications? *Can Nurse* (December) 1981; 77:48, 50.

Stewart DY, Kelly J, Dinel BA: Unit-dose medication: A nursing perspective. *Am J Nurs* (August) 1976; 76:1308–1310.

Todd B: Drugs and the elderly: Using eye drops and ointments safely. *Geriatr Nurs* (January/February) 1983; 4(1):53–56.

Todd B: Drugs and the elderly: Topical analgesics. *Geriatr Nurs* (May/June) 1983; 4(3):152, 192, 196.

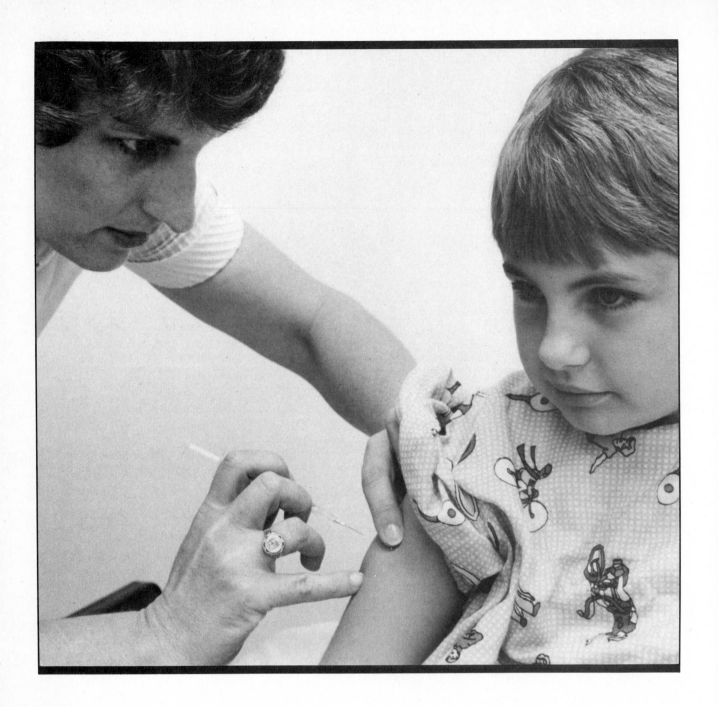

PARENTERAL MEDICATIONS

30

Parenteral medications are medications that are administered by a route other than the alimentary canal. They are given subcutaneously, intramuscularly, intradermally, and intravenously. Because parenteral medications are absorbed more quickly than oral medications and are irretrievable once injected, it is essential that the nurse prepare and administer them carefully and accurately. Administering parenteral drugs requires all the nursing knowledge for oral and topical drugs plus considerable manual dexterity and the use of sterile technique.

Chapter Outline

Objectives

Upon completion of this chapter, the student will:

1. Know essential terms and facts about the administration of parenteral medications
   1.1 Define selected terms
   1.2 Identify equipment used for administering parenteral medications
   1.3 Identify essential aspects of preparing medications from ampules and vials
   1.4 Identify sites commonly used to administer parenteral medications
   1.5 Identify methods used to locate specific sites for subcutaneous and intramuscular injections
   1.6 Identify reasons for using various parenteral routes
2. Understand facts about the administration of parenteral medications
   2.1 Identify relevant assessment data
   2.2 Identify nursing diagnoses for which the technique may be implemented
   2.3 Identify nursing goals related to the technique
   2.4 Identify expected and unexpected outcomes from assessment data
   2.5 Identify reasons underlying selected steps of the technique

3. Administer parenteral medications safely
   3.1 Assess the patient adequately
   3.2 Collect additional data from appropriate sources
   3.3 Select pertinent nursing goals for the patient
   3.4 Establish relevant outcome criteria for the patient following the technique
   3.5 Collect necessary equipment before the technique
   3.6 Implement interventions to enhance the effectiveness of the technique and enhance the patient's comfort and safety
   3.7 Communicate relevant information about the patient to the appropriate persons through records or reports
   3.8 Evaluate the outcomes of the technique
4. Evaluate own performance of specific techniques in a laboratory or clinical setting with the assistance of another
   4.1 Use the performance checklists provided
   4.2 Identify areas of strength and weakness
   4.3 Alter performance in response to own evaluation and that of another

Terms

▪ **ampule** a small, sealed, glass flask containing a medication or solution
▪ **bevel** a slanting edge; the slanted part at the tip of a needle
▪ **bleb** a small, smooth, slightly raised area on the skin, usually filled with fluid; wheal
▪ **gauge** the diameter of the shaft of a needle
▪ **hematoma** a collection of blood in a tissue, organ, or space due to a break in the wall of a blood vessel
▪ **heparin** a substance that slows coagulation of blood
▪ **incompatibility (of medications)** an undesired chemical or physical reaction between a drug and an infusion solution, between two or more drugs, or between a drug and the container or tubing
▪ **infiltration** the diffusion or accumulation of substances in tissues or cells
▪ **injection point** a site on tubing for the insertion of a needle
▪ **insulin** a hormone normally formed by the islands of Langerhans in the pancreas; also a preparation for administration
▪ **intradermal** within the skin (intracutaneous)

- intramuscular   within or inside muscle tissue
- intravenous   within a vein
- subcutaneous   beneath the layers of the skin (hypodermic)

- syringe   an instrument used to inject or withdraw liquids
- vial   a small glass bottle with a rubber stopper
- viscous   thick, sticky

EQUIPMENT FOR INJECTIONS

Syringes

All syringes have three parts: the tip, which connects with the needle; the barrel, or outside part, on which the scales are printed; and the plunger, which fits inside the barrel. See Figure 30–1. Most syringes used today are made of plastic and are individually packaged for sterility in a paper wrapper or a rigid plastic container. They may be prefitted with needles. These syringes and needles may be disposable or nondisposable.

Types of syringes

There are several kinds of syringes, differing in size, shape, and material. The three most commonly used types are the standard hypodermic syringe, the insulin syringe, and the tuberculin syringe. See Figure 30–2.

Hypodermic syringes come in 2, 2.5, and 3 mL sizes. They usually have two scales marked on them: the minim and the milliliter. The milliliter scale is the one normally used; the minim scale is used for very small dosages, such as "epinephrine minims iii H."

Insulin syringes are similar to hypodermic syringes, except that they have a scale especially designed for insulin: a 100-unit calibrated scale intended for use with U-100 insulin. This scale is replacing the U-40 and U-80 scale used for 40-unit and 80-unit insulins.

The *tuberculin syringe* was designed to administer tuberculin. It is a narrow syringe, calibrated in tenths and hundredths of a milliliter (up to 1 mL) on one scale and in sixteenths of a minim (up to 1 min) on the other scale. This type of syringe can also be useful in administering other drugs, particularly when small or precise measurement is indicated, for example, for pediatric dosages.

Syringes are made in other sizes as well, for example, 5, 10, 20, and 50 milliliters. These are not generally used to administer drugs directly to patients but can be useful for adding sterile solutions to intravenous flasks or for irrigating wounds.

Glass syringes

Nondisposable glass syringes are less widely used now that disposable plastic syringes are available. However, because glass syringes can be sterilized, they are often placed in sterile treatment sets for special procedures, eg, administering a local anesthetic. Glass syringes, like disposable syringes, can be fitted with special Luer-Lok tips. These have threaded seals, so that the needle connects more securely to the syringe than on a standard type of syringe. See Figure 30–3. The Luer-Lok tips can be attached to devices other than needles, eg, irrigators.

Disposable plastic syringes

Most frequently used today is the disposable plastic syringe. The syringe is supplied with a needle, which may

FIGURE 30–1 ■ The three parts of a syringe.

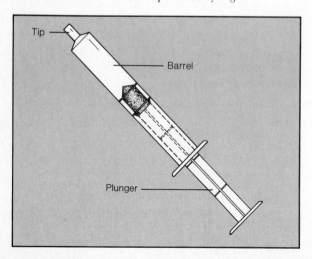

FIGURE 30–2 ■ Three kinds of syringes: **A,** hypodermic; **B,** insulin; **C,** tuberculin.

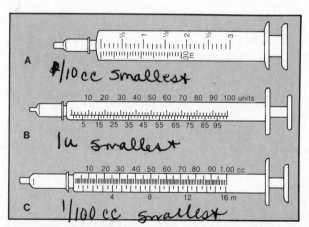

have a plastic cap over it. The syringe and needle may be packaged together or separately in a paper wrapper or in a rigid plastic container. See Figure 30–4.

Disposable prefilled syringes and cartridges

Injectable medications are frequently supplied in prefilled unit-dose syringes with needles or cartridge-needle units. These prefilled syringes and cartridge-needle units are disposable. The cartridge-needle units, however, require special metal or plastic cartridge holders or syringes for administration. These syringes and cartridges come with manufacturer's directions for use.

Needles

Needles are made of stainless steel and may or may not be disposable. Reusable needles need to be sharpened periodically before resterilization, because the points become dull with use and are occasionally damaged or acquire burrs on the tips. A dull or damaged needle should never be used.

A needle has three discernible parts: the hub, which fits onto the syringe; the cannula, or shaft, which is attached to the hub; and the bevel, which is the slanted part at the tip of the needle. See Figure 30–5. A disposable needle has a plastic hub.

Needles used for injections have three variables: the slant or length of the bevel, the length of the shaft, and the gauge (or diameter) of the shaft. The bevel of the needle may be short or long. Longer bevels provide the

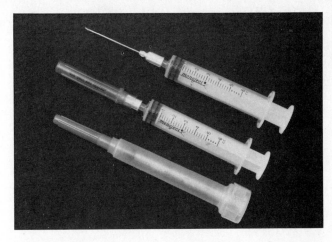

FIGURE 30–4   ■   Disposable plastic syringe and needle: **top,** with syringe and needle exposed; **middle,** with plastic cap over the needle; **bottom,** with plastic case over the needle and syringe.

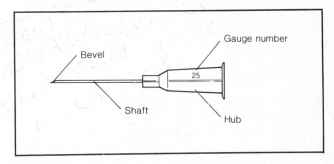

FIGURE 30–5   ■   The parts of a needle.

FIGURE 30–3   ■   Glass syringes: **A,** with a glass tip; **B,** with a metal tip; **C,** with a Luer-Lok.

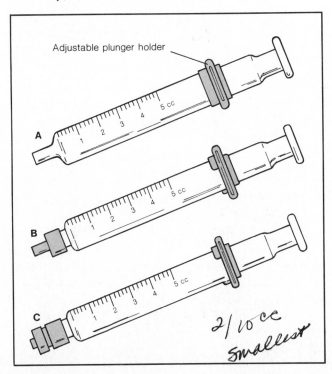

sharpest needle and are commonly used for subcutaneous and intramuscular injections. Short bevels are used for intradermal and intravenous injections, because a long bevel can become occluded if it rests against the side of a blood vessel.

The shaft length of commonly used needles varies from ¼ to 5 in, and the gauge varies from 14 to 27. The larger the gauge number, the smaller the diameter of the shaft. Smaller gauges produce less tissue trauma, but larger gauges are necessary for viscous medications, such as penicillin. For subcutaneous injections, it is usual to use a needle of 24 to 26 gauge and ⅜ to ⅝ in long. Obese patients may require a 1-in needle. For intramuscular injections, a longer needle, eg, 1 to 1½ in, with a larger gauge, eg, gauge 20 to 22, is used. See Figure 30–6.

Ampules and Vials

Ampules and vials are frequently used to package sterile parenteral medications. See Figure 30–7. An ampule is a glass container usually designed to hold a single dose of a drug. It is made of clear glass and has a particular shape with a constricted neck. Some ampule necks have colored marks around them, and some are scored for easy

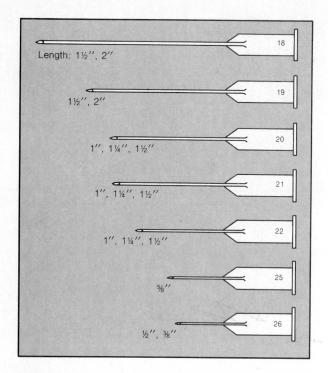

FIGURE 30-6 ■ The sizes of needles commonly used for injections.

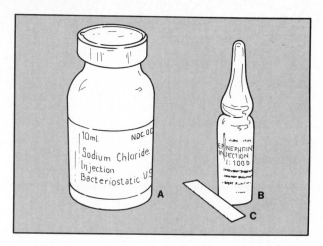

FIGURE 30-7 ■ **A,** vial; **B,** ampule; **C,** ampule file.

opening. If the neck is not scored, it is filed with a small file, then broken off at the neck.

Vials are small glass bottles with sealed rubber caps. They come in different sizes, from single to multidose vials. Vials usually have a metal cap that protects the rubber seal; it is easily removed.

TECHNIQUE 30-1 ■ Preparing Medications from Ampules and Vials

■ Planning

Nursing goal

To maintain sterile technique while withdrawing the required amount of medication from a vial or ampule.

Equipment

1. The vial or ampule of sterile medication.
2. Sterile gauze.
3. A needle and syringe.
4. Special filter needle (optional) for withdrawing premixed liquid medications from multidose vials.
5. Antiseptic solution.
6. Sterile water, if neccessary. Some vials contain only a powder, and it is necessary to instill a liquid such as sterile water to prepare the medication. The manufacturer specifies preparation directions.
7. File if required to open the ampule.
8. Medication card if one is used.

■ Intervention

1. Check the label on the ampule or vial carefully against the medication card or the patient's chart to make sure that the correct medication is being prepared.
2. Follow the three checks for administering medications. Read the label on the medication before it is taken off the shelf, before pouring the medication, and after placing it back on the shelf.

Ampules

3. Flick the upper stem of the ampule several times with a fingernail or, holding the upper stem of the ampule, make a large circle with the arm extended.
   Rationale This will bring all the medication down to the main portion of the ampule. See Figure 30-8.
4. Partially file the neck of the ampule if necessary to start a clean break.
5. Place a piece of sterile gauze on the far side of the

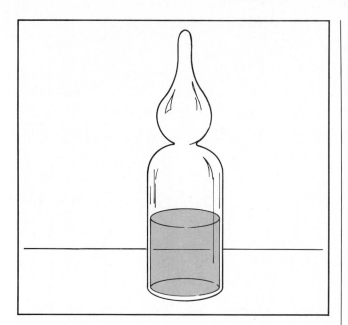

FIGURE 30–8

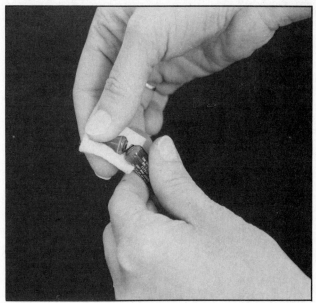

FIGURE 30–9

ampule neck, and break off the top by bending it toward the gauze. See Figure 30–9.

Rationale The sterile gauze protects the nurse's fingers from the broken glass.

6. Assemble the syringe and needle, if not preassembled. Hold the barrel of the syringe in the middle, and insert the plunger, maintaining the sterility of the plunger except at its uppermost end (which you are holding). Attach the needle to the barrel by holding the hub of the needle and maintaining the sterility of the remainder of the needle and the tip of the syringe. Many needles have protective caps to help maintain their sterility.

7. Remove the cap from the needle, insert the needle in the ampule, and withdraw the amount of drug required for the dosage. See Figure 30–10. With a single-dose ampule, hold the ampule slightly on its side, if necessary, to obtain all the medication.

Vials

8. Mix the solution, if necessary, by rotating the vial between the palms of the hands, not by shaking.

Rationale Some vials contain aqueous suspensions, which settle when they stand. In some instances shaking is contraindicated, because it may cause the mixture to foam.

9. Remove the protective metal cap, and clean the rubber cap with an antiseptic, such as 70% alcohol, on a sterile gauze, rubbing in a rotary motion.

Rationale The antiseptic cleans the cap so that the needle will not be contaminated when it is inserted.

10. Remove the cap from the needle; then draw up into the syringe the amount of air equal to the volume of the medication to be withdrawn. In some agencies, a special filter needle is used to draw up premixed liquid medications from multidose vials. The filter needle is then replaced by a regular needle to inject the medication into the patient. The filter prevents any solid material from being drawn up through the needle.

11. Carefully insert the needle into the vial through the center of the rubber cap, maintaining the sterility of the needle.

12. Inject the air into the vial, keeping the bevel of the

FIGURE 30–10

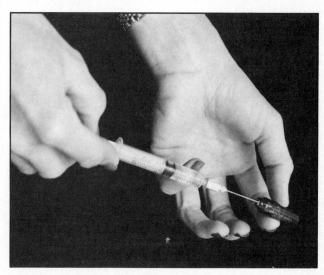

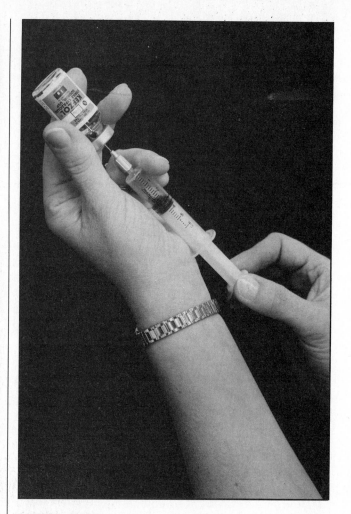

FIGURE 30–11

FIGURE 30–12

needle above the surface of the medication. See Figure 30–11.

Rationale The air will allow the medication to be drawn out easily, since negative pressure is not created inside the vial. The bevel is kept above the medication to avoid creating bubbles in the medication.

13. Invert the vial and hold it at eye level while withdrawing the correct dosage of the drug into the syringe. See Figure 30–12.

14. Withdraw the needle from the vial, and replace the cap over the needle, thus maintaining its sterility. If a filter needle was used to withdraw the medication, replace it with a regular needle before injecting the patient.

Preparing powdered drugs

Several drugs (eg, penicillin) are dispensed as powders in vials. A liquid (solvent or diluent) must be added to a powdered medication before it can be injected. The technique of adding a solvent to a powdered drug to prepare it for administration is called *reconstitution*. Powdered drugs usually have printed instructions (enclosed with each packaged vial) that describe the amount and kind of solvent to be added. Commonly used solvents are sterile water or sterile normal saline. Some preparations are supplied in individual-dose vials; others come in multidose vials.

15. Read the manufacturer's directions. The following are two examples of the preparation of powdered drugs:

a. *Single-dose vial:* Instructions for preparing a single-dose vial direct that 1.5 mL of sterile water be added to the sterile dry powder, thus providing a single dose of 2 mL. The volume of the drug powder was 0.5 mL.

b. *Multidose vial:* A dose of 750 mg of a certain drug is ordered for a patient. On hand is a 10-g multidose vial. The directions for preparation read: "Add 8.5 mL of sterile water, and each milliliter will contain 1.0 g or 1,000 mg." Thus, after adding the solvent, the nurse will give 750/1,000 or ¾ mL (0.75 mL) of the medication.

16. Withdraw an equivalent amount of air from the vial before adding the solvent, unless otherwise indicated by the directions.

17. Add the amount of sterile water or saline indicated in the directions.

18. If a multidose vial is reconstituted, label the vial with the date it was prepared, the amount of drug contained in each milliliter of solution, and your initials. Time is an important factor to consider in the expiration of these medications.

19. Once reconstituted, store the medication in the vial in a refrigerator, if indicated.

TECHNIQUE 30–2   ■   Mixing Two Types of Insulin or Other Medications

Frequently patients need more than one drug injected at the same time. To spare the patient the experience of being injected twice, two drugs (if compatible) are often mixed together in one syringe and given as one injection. It is common, for instance, to combine two types of insulin in this manner or to combine injectable preoperative medications, such as morphine or meperidine (Demerol) with atropine or scopolamine. Drugs may be mixed from two vials, from two ampules, or from one vial and one ampule. Drugs may also be mixed in intravenous solutions. When uncertain about drug compatibilities, the nurse should consult a pharmacist before mixing the drugs.

Although there are several types of insulin available, all have the same basic action; however, they vary in their time of action. Some act within 2 hours and last for 8 to 10 hours, whereas others act within 6 hours and last for 24 to 36 hours. Often patients are given two types of insulin, short- and long-acting; these two types vary in content. Chemically, insulin is a protein, which, when hydrolyzed in the body, yields a number of amino acids. Some insulin preparations contain an additional modifying protein, such as globulin or protamine, that slows absorption. This fact is relevant to the mixing of two insulin preparations for injection. A vial of insulin that does *not* have the added protein should never be contaminated with insulin that does have the added protein. For example, regular insulin (crystalline zinc insulin, CZ) should never be adulterated with protamine zinc, globin zinc, or isophane (NPH), which all have added protein.

■ Planning

Nursing goals

1. To prevent contaminating the medication in one vial (or ampule) with medication from the other vial (or ampule)

2. To maintain the sterility of each drug and of the syringe and needle

Equipment

1. The patient's medication cards. Confirm that they correspond with the physician's order.

2. Two vials of medication, or one vial and one ampule, or one vial and one cartridge. Note that insulin is prepared in units rather than milligrams or grains. It is available in 40, 80, and 100 units per milliliter of solution. It is essential when preparing insulin that the appropriate calibrations on the syringe be used; for example, the 40-unit scale on the syringe is used only when administering 40-unit insulin and the 80-unit scale only for 80-unit insulin. In the hospital, insulin may be stored in the refrigerator to prevent deterioration.

3. Sterile hypodermic or insulin syringe and needle. If insulin is being given, use a small hypodermic needle gauge (26 gauge).

4. Additional sterile subcutaneous or intramuscular needle (optional).

5. Sterile disinfectant-soaked swabs.

■ Intervention

Mixing medications from two vials

1. Inspect the appearance of the medication for clarity.
   Rationale Preparations that have changed in appearance should not be used.

2. If using insulin, thoroughly mix the solution in each vial prior to administration. Rotate the vials between the palms of the hands and invert the vials.
   Rationale Mixing ensures an adequate concentration and thus an accurate dose. Shaking insulin vials can make the medication frothy, making precise measurement difficult.

3. Clean the tops of the vials with disinfectant swabs.

4. Inject a volume of air equal to the volume of medication to be withdrawn into vial *A* or into the

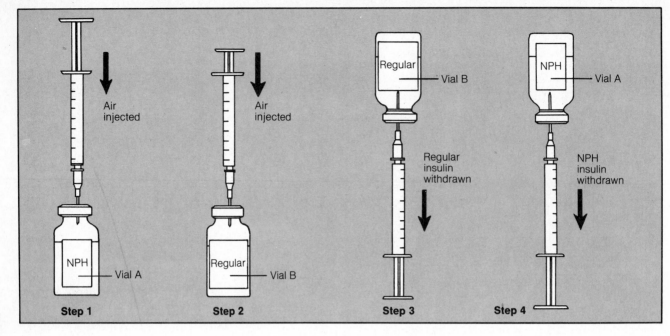

FIGURE 30–13

vial of insulin with added protein, eg, NPH insulin. See Figure 30–13, step 1.

Rationale The same needle is used to inject air into and withdraw medication from the second vial. It must not be contaminated with the medication in vial *A*.

5. Withdraw the needle from vial *A*, and inject the prescribed amount of air into vial *B* or into the vial of insulin without added protein (eg, regular or crystalline zinc insulin). See Figure 30–13, step 2.

6. Withdraw the required amount of medication from vial *B*. See Figure 30–13, step 3.

7. Using a newly attached sterile needle, withdraw the required amount of medication from vial *A*. See Figure 30–13, step 4. The syringe now contains a mixture of medications from vials *A* and *B*.

Rationale With this method, neither vial is contaminated by microorganisms or by medication from the other vial.

Mixing medications from one vial and one ampule

8. First prepare the medication from the vial.

Rationale Ampules do not require the addition of air prior to withdrawal of the drug.

9. Then withdraw the required amount of medication from the ampule.

Mixing medications from a vial or ampule and a cartridge

10. Make sure that you have the correct dosage in the cartridge. Withdraw and discard any excess medication.

11. Draw up the required amount of medication from the vial or ampule and add this to the medication in the cartridge.

TECHNIQUE 30–3 ■ Administering a Subcutaneous Injection

A subcutaneous injection is the introduction of a medication into the subcutaneous tissues. It is also referred to as a hypodermic injection. Among the many kinds of drugs administered subcutaneously are vaccines, pre-operative medications, narcotics, insulin, and heparin.

Common sites for subcutaneous injections are the outer aspect of the upper arms and the anterior aspects of the thighs. These areas are convenient and normally have good blood circulation. Other areas that can be used are the abdomen, the scapular areas of the upper back and the upper ventro/dorsal gluteal areas. See Figure 30–14. Patients who administer their own injections, such as diabetics who require insulin, usually use the abdomen and anterior thigh sites.

Subcutaneous sites need to be rotated in an orderly fashion to minimize tissue damage, aid absorption, and avoid discomfort. This is especially important for patients who must receive repeated injections, eg, diabetics. To accomplish this, the nurse or patient can prepare a diagram indicating the sites to be used and after each injection mark its location on the diagram. See Figure 30–15.

■ Assessment

Assess the patient's need for the medication if it is provided p.r.n. (eg, an analgesic).

■ Planning

Nursing goals

1. To provide medications to patients who are unable to ingest oral medications, eg, unconscious patients or those who are nauseated, vomiting, or fasting
2. To administer drugs that are destroyed by digestive

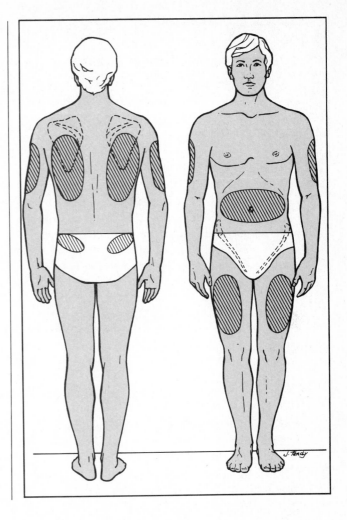

FIGURE 30–14 ■ The sites of the body commonly used for subcutaneous injections.

FIGURE 30–15 ■ A system of rotating injection sites on the body, commonly used for the administration of insulin: **A,** sites used by the nurse; **B,** sites used by the patient.

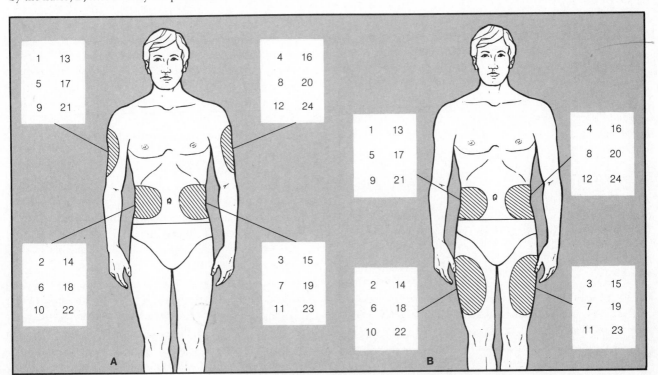

enzymes (eg, insulin) or are inactive orally (eg, heparin)

3. To provide more rapid absorption and action of a drug than can be achieved by the oral route

Equipment

1. The patient's medication card or order.

2. A vial or ampule of the correct sterile medication.

3. A sterile syringe and needle. Generally a 2-mL syringe and a #25 gauge needle are used for subcutaneous injections. The length of the needle depends on the amount of adipose tissue at the site and the angle used to administer the injection. Generally, a ⅝-in needle is used for adults when the injection is administered at a 45° angle; a ½-in needle is used at a 90° angle. Shorter needles, eg, ⅜ in, may be used for children, and longer ones, eg, 1 in, may be necessary for very obese adults. To determine the appropriate length of the needle for a 90° angle injection, pinch a fold of skin between your thumb and forefinger at the injection site, then measure the width of the skin fold by placing a needle that will not be used for the injection against the skin surface. The appropriate needle length is one-half the width of the skin fold (Pitel, 1971, p 78). When this method of measuring is used, the needle is inserted without pinching the skin.

4. Sterile antiseptic-soaked swabs to clean the top of a medication vial and the injection site.

5. Dry sterile gauze for opening an ampule.

■ Intervention

1. Check the medication order. See Technique 30–1, steps 1 and 2, on page 718.

FIGURE 30–16

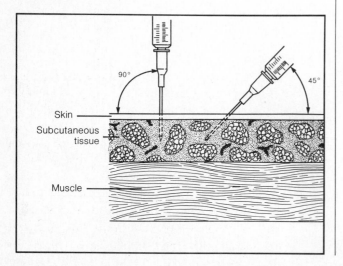

2. Prepare the drug dosage from a vial or ampule. See Technique 30–1, on page 718.

3. Select a site free of tenderness, hardness, swelling, scarring, itching, burning, or localized inflammation. Select a site that has not been used frequently.

Rationale These conditions could hinder the absorption of the medication and also increase the likelihood of an infection at the injection site.

4. As agency policy indicates, clean the site with an antiseptic swab. Start at the center of the site and clean in a widening circle. Allow the area to dry thoroughly. Place the swab between the third and fourth fingers of the nondominant hand for later use.

Rationale Recommendations differ about the necessity of cleaning the skin prior to injections. Some believe that the antiseptic lessens the number of microorganisms on the skin; others (Dann, 1966, p 1121; Lacey, 1968, p 212) think that cleaning destroys the normal antibacterial properties of the skin. The swab's mechanical action does remove skin secretions, which contain microorganisms.

5. Remove the needle cap while waiting for the antiseptic to dry. Pull the cap straight off to avoid contaminating the needle by the outside edge of the cap.

Rationale The needle will become contaminated if it touches anything but the inside of the cap, which is sterile.

6. Expel any air bubbles from the syringe by inverting the syringe and gently pushing on the plunger until a drop of solution can be seen in the needle bevel. If air bubbles still remain, flick the side of the syringe barrel.

or

7. When it is important that the entire amount of medication be administered, Wong (1982, p 1237) recommends leaving 0.2 mL of air in the syringe. This is referred to as the *air-bubble technique.* Others (Chaplin, Shull, Welk, 1985, p 59) do not recommend this technique.

Rationale Users of the air-bubble technique believe that this small amount of air ensures that only air remains in the needle bore and that all the medication is injected into the patient. Nonusers believe that the risk of medication error is increased when the "dead-space volume" (residual amount of drug in the syringe hub and needle) is expelled during injection, since it is *not* part of the syringe barrel calibration.

8. Grasp the syringe in your dominant hand by holding it between your thumb and fingers with palm facing upward for a 45° angle insertion or with the palm downward for a 90° angle insertion. See Figure 30–16.

⋆ 9. Using the nondominant hand, [pinch] or spread the
? skin at the site, and insert the needle, using a firm
. steady push. See Figure 30–17.

Rationale Recommendations vary about whether
to pinch or spread the skin. Pinching the skin is
thought to desensitize the area somewhat and thus
lessen the sensation of needle insertion. Spreading
the skin can make it firmer and facilitate needle
insertion. Some recommend neither pinching nor
spreading the skin (Pitel, 1971, p 79). The nurse
needs to judge which method to use depending on
the patient's tissue firmness.

10. When the needle is inserted, move your nondominant hand to the barrel of the syringe and your
dominant hand to the end of the plunger.

11. Aspirate by pulling back on the plunger. If blood
appears in the syringe, withdraw the needle, discard
the syringe, and prepare a new injection. If blood
does not appear, continue to administer the medication.

Rationale This step determines whether the needle
has entered a blood vessel. Subcutaneous medications may be dangerous if placed directly into the
bloodstream; they are intended for the subcutaneous
tissues, where they are absorbed more slowly.

12. Inject the medication by holding the syringe steady
and depressing the plunger with a slow, even
pressure.

Rationale Holding the syringe steady and injecting
the medication at an even pressure minimizes discomfort for the patient.

13. Remove the needle quickly, pulling along the line
of insertion while depressing the skin with your
nondominant hand.

Rationale Depressing the skin places countertraction on it and minimizes the patient's discomfort
when the needle is withdrawn.

14. Massage the site lightly with a sterile antiseptic-
soaked swab, or apply slight pressure.

Rationale Massage is thought to disperse the medication in the tissues and facilitate its absorption.
Massaging is omitted with heparin injections.

15. If bleeding occurs, apply pressure to the site until
it stops. Bleeding rarely occurs after subcutaneous
injection.

16. Dispose of supplies according to agency procedure.

Rationale Proper disposal protects the nurse and
others from injury and contamination.

17. Record the medication given, dosage, time, route,
any complaints of the patient, and your signature.

18. Assess the effectiveness of the medication 15 to 30
minutes after the injection or as appropriate, depending on the medication.

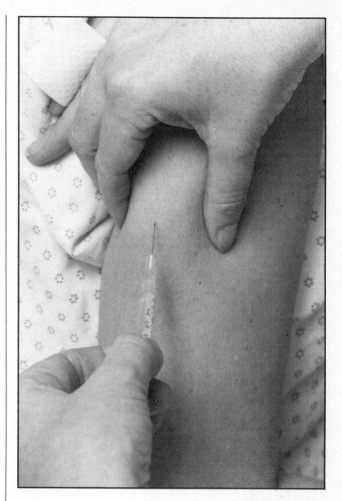

FIGURE 30–17

Variations for a heparin injection

The subcutaneous administration of heparin requires
special precautions because of the drug's anticoagulant
properties.

19. Select a site on the abdomen above the level of the
iliac crests.

Rationale These areas are away from major muscles
and are not involved in muscular activity, as the
arms and legs are; thus, the possibility of hematoma
is reduced.

20. Use a ½-in, #25 or #26 gauge needle, and insert it at
a 90° angle. Draw 0.1 mL of air into the syringe when
preparing the heparin, and inject it after the heparin.

Rationale This step fills the needle with air and
prevents any leakage of heparin into the intradermal
layers when the needle is inserted and when the
needle is withdrawn, thus minimizing the possibility
of a hematoma.

21. Check agency practices regarding aspiration. ⋆

Rationale Some agencies recommend that the nurse
not aspirate to determine needle placement because

this can cause the needle to move, possibly damaging tissue and rupturing small blood vessels, causing bleeding and severe bruising.

22. Do not massage the site after the injection.

Rationale Massaging could cause bleeding and ecchymoses.

23. Alternate sites of subsequent injections.

▪ Evaluation

Expected outcomes

1. Absence of bruises, tenderness, swelling, scarring, itching, hardness, burning, or localized inflammation at the injection site

2. Clinical signs indicating effectiveness of the medication, eg, dry mouth after the administration of atropine.

Unexpected outcomes

1. Presence of bruises, tenderness, swelling, scarring, itching, hardness, burning, or localized inflammation at the injection site

2. No change in clinical signs

Upon obtaining an unexpected outcome:

1. Report your findings to the responsible nurse.

2. Adjust the nursing care plan appropriately; eg, for a patient having pain, employ other measures to treat the pain if not already carried out.

TECHNIQUE 30–4 ▪ Administering an Intramuscular Injection

The intramuscular (IM) injection route is ordered for the following reasons:

1. Medications that irritate subcutaneous tissue, for example, penicillin and paraldehyde, may safely be given by intramuscular injection.

2. The speed of absorption is faster than by the subcutaneous route because of the greater blood supply to the body muscles.

3. Muscles can usually take a larger volume of fluid without discomfort than subcutaneous tissues, although the amount varies among people, chiefly with muscle size and condition.

Sites

A number of body sites are used for intramuscular injections. Frequently used sites are the dorsogluteal, ventrogluteal, vastus lateralis, rectus femoris, deltoid, and triceps muscles. Only healthy muscles should be used for injections.

The dorsogluteal site

The dorsogluteal site is composed of the thick gluteal muscles of the buttocks. See Figure 30–18. The injection site must be chosen carefully to avoid striking the sciatic nerve, major blood vessels, or bone. There are two methods of establishing the exact site, which is the upper

FIGURE 30–18 ▪ Lateral view of the right buttock showing the three gluteal muscles used for intramuscular injections.

FIGURE 30–19 ▪ One method to establish the dorsogluteal site for an intramuscular injection.

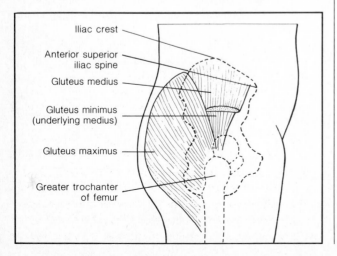

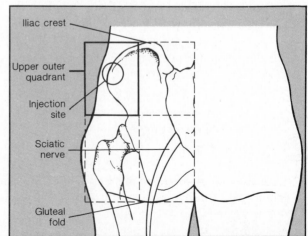

outer aspect of the upper outer quadrant of the buttock, about 5 to 8 cm (2 to 3 in) below the crest of the ilium:

1. Divide the buttock by imaginary lines as in Figure 30–19. The vertical line extends from the crest of the ilium to the gluteal fold. The horizontal line extends from the medial fold to the lateral aspect of the buttock. From these landmarks, the upper outer aspect of the upper outer quadrant is established. See Figure 30–19. It is important to palpate the crest of the ilium so that the chosen site is high enough. Visual calculations alone can result in an injection that is placed too low and injures other structures.

2. Palpate the posterior superior iliac spine, then draw an imaginary line to the greater trochanter of the femur. This line will be lateral to and parallel to the sciatic nerve. The injection site is then lateral and superior to this line. See Figure 30–20.

In the past, the dorsogluteal site was most commonly used for intramuscular injections. However, because of the problems caused by inaccurately locating the site, it is losing favor as the best intramuscular site.

The dorsogluteal site can be used for adults and for children with well-developed gluteal muscles. Because these muscles are developed by walking, it is generally not used for infants under 3 years.

To administer an injection into this site, have the patient assume a prone position with the toes pointing medially. See Figure 30–21, A. A side-lying position can also be used, with the upper leg flexed at the thigh and the knee and placed in front of the lower leg. See Figure 30–21, B. Both positions promote relaxation of the gluteal muscles.

The ventrogluteal site

The ventrogluteal site, also known as von Hochstetter's site, uses the gluteus medius muscle, which lies over the

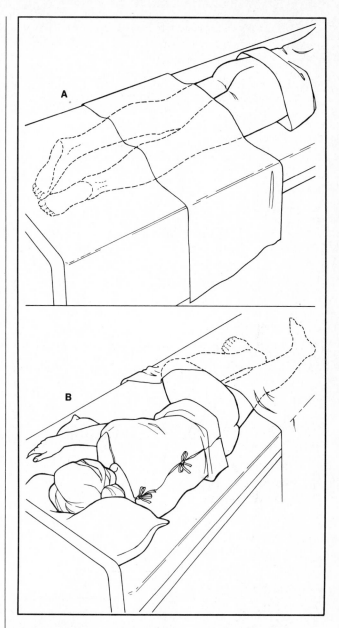

FIGURE 30–21 ■ Two positions for an intramuscular injection into the gluteal muscles: **A,** prone position with the toes pointed inward; **B,** lateral position with the upper leg acutely flexed.

FIGURE 30–20 ■ A second method for establishing the dorsogluteal site for an intramuscular injection.

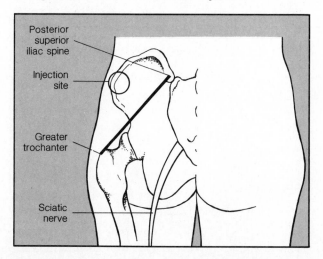

gluteus minimus. See Figure 30–18. Use of this site is gaining in favor because there are no large nerves or blood vessels in the area and less fat than in the buttock area. It is also farther from the rectal area and tends to be less contaminated, which is a consideration when giving injections to infants and incontinent adults.

To establish the exact site, the heel of the nurse's hand is placed on the greater trochanter with the fingers pointing toward the patient's head. The right hand is used for the left hip, and the left hand for the right hip. With the index finger on the anterior superior iliac spine, the middle finger is stretched dorsally, palpating the crest of the ilium and then pressing below it. The triangle

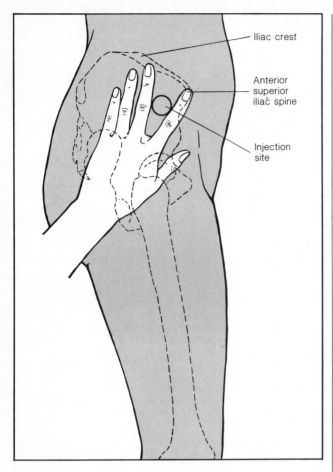

FIGURE 30–22 ■ The ventrogluteal site for an intramuscular injection.

FIGURE 30–23 ■ The vastus lateralis muscle of the upper thigh, used for intramuscular injections.

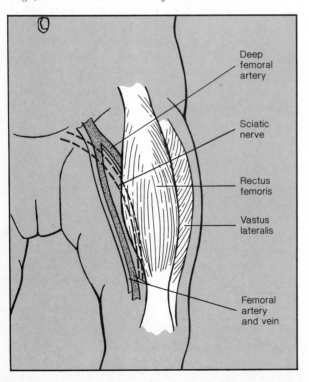

formed by the index finger, the third finger, and the crest of the ilium is the injection site. See Figure 30–22.

This site is suitable for infants, children, and adults. The patient position for the injection can be a back- or side-lying position with the knee and hip flexed to relax the gluteal muscles.

The vastus lateralis site

The vastus lateralis muscle is usually thick and well-developed in both adults and children. It is increasingly recommended as the site of choice for intramuscular injections because there are no major blood vessels or nerves in the area. It is situated on the anterior lateral aspect of the thigh. See Figure 30–23. The middle third of the muscle is suggested as the site. It is established by dividing the area between the greater trochanter of the femur and the lateral femoral condyle into thirds and selecting the middle third. See Figure 30–24. The patient can assume a back-lying or a sitting position for an injection into this site.

The rectus femoris site

The rectus femoris muscle, which belongs to the quadriceps muscle group, can also be used for intramuscular injections. It is situated on the anterior aspect of the thigh. See Figure 30–25. This site can be used for infants and children generally and for adults when other sites are contraindicated. Its chief advantage is that the patient who administers his or her own injections can reach this site easily. Its main disadvantage is that an injection here

FIGURE 30–24 ■ The vastus lateralis site for an intramuscular injection.

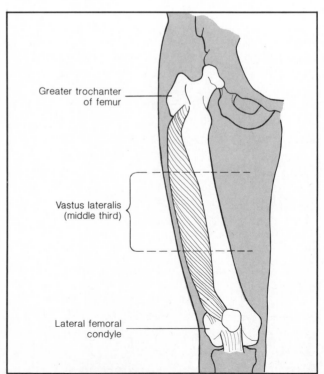

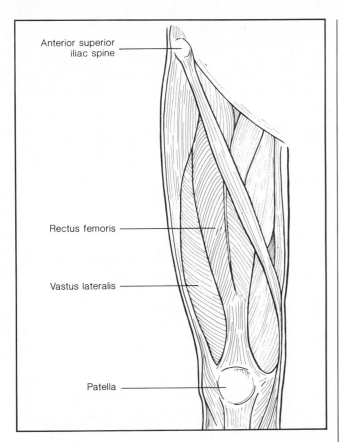

FIGURE 30–25 ■ The rectus femoris muscle of the upper right thigh, used for intramuscular injections.

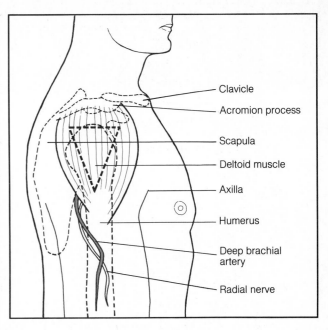

FIGURE 30–26 ■ The deltoid muscle of the upper arm, used for intramuscular injections.

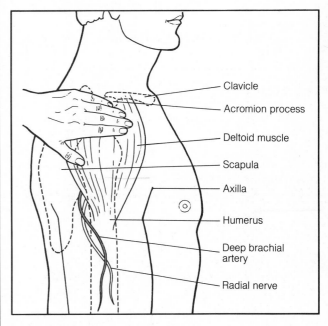

FIGURE 30–27 ■ A method for establishing the deltoid muscle site for intramuscular injection.

may cause considerable discomfort for some people. The patient assumes a sitting or back-lying position for an injection at this site.

The deltoid and triceps sites

The deltoid muscle is found on the lateral aspect of the upper arm. It is not used often for intramuscular injections because it is a relatively small muscle and is very close to the radial nerve and radial artery. To locate the densest part of the muscle, the nurse palpates the lower edge of the acromial process and the midpoint on the lateral aspect of the arm that is in line with the axilla. A triangle within these boundaries indicates the deltoid muscle about 5 cm (2 in) below the acromion process. See Figure 30–26. Another method of establishing the deltoid site is to place four fingers across the deltoid muscle with the first finger on the acromion process, ie, the site is three finger breadths below the acromion process. See Figure 30–27.

The lateral head of the triceps muscle on the posterior aspect of the upper arm can also be used as an injection site. The site of choice is about midway between the acromion process and the olecranon process of the ulna (the elbow). See Figure 30–28. This site is not often used unless other sites are contraindicated.

Sitting or lying positions can be assumed for injections using the deltoid and triceps sites.

■ Assessment

Assess the patient's need for the medication if it is a p.r.n. order, eg, Demerol 75 mg IM p.r.n. for pain.

■ Planning

Nursing goals

1.   To administer a prescribed medication by injection into a muscle.

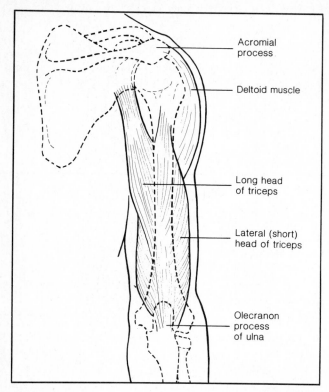

FIGURE 30-28 ■ Posterior view of the upper right arm showing the triceps muscle, used for intramuscular injections.

2. To provide a medication when the intramuscular route is the route of choice:

   a. When more rapid absorption of a medication is required than can be attained by the oral route

   b. When a systemic action is required from a drug that is irritating to subcutaneous tissues

   c. When the volume of the dose is between 1.5 and 5 mL of solution

Equipment

1. The medication card or the patient's chart.
2. The sterile medication. This is usually provided in an ampule or vial.
3. A sterile syringe and needle. Choose the size of syringe appropriate for the amount of solution to be administered. Usually a 2- to 5-mL syringe is needed. Some medications, such as paraldehyde, require a glass syringe, because the medication interacts with plastic. The size and length of the needle are determined by the muscle to be used, the type of solution, the amount of adipose tissue covering the muscle, and the age of the patient. A large muscle, such as the gluteus medius, usually requires a #20 to #23 gauge needle, 1½ to 3 in long, whereas the deltoid muscle requires a smaller, #23 to #25 gauge needle, ⅝ to 1 in long. Oily solutions such as paraldehyde require a thicker needle, eg, #21 gauge instead of

#23 gauge. Also, the greater the amount of adipose tissue over the muscle, the longer the needle must be to reach the muscle. Therefore, 3-in needles may be needed for obese patients, whereas 1½-in needles are used for thinner people. Infants and young children usually require smaller, shorter needles such as #22 to #25 gauge, ⅝ to 1 in long.

4. A swab saturated in an antiseptic solution for cleaning the site.
5. Dry sterile gauze, if an ampule must be opened.

■ Intervention

1. Check the medication order. See Technique 30-1, steps 1 and 2 on page 718.
2. Prepare the correct dosage of the drug from a vial or ampule. See Technique 30-1, steps 2-19.
3. If the medication is particularly irritating to subcutaneous tissue, change the needle on the syringe before the injection.

   Rationale Because the outside of the new needle is free of medication, it does not irritate subcutaneous tissues as it passes into the muscle.

4. Select the intramuscular site for adequate muscle mass. The skin surface over the site should be free of bruises, abrasions, and infection. Determine if the size of the muscle is appropriate to the amount of medication to be injected. An average adult's deltoid muscle can usually absorb 0.5 mL of medication, although some authorities believe 2 mL can be absorbed by a well-developed deltoid muscle, and the gluteus medius muscle can absorb 1 to 5 mL (Newton, Newton, 1979, p 19), although 5 mL may be very painful. The site should not have been used frequently. If injections are to be frequent, sites should be alternated. If necessary discuss an alternate method of providing the medication with the person prescribing it.

5. Establish the exact site for the injection and assist the patient to an appropriate position. See Sites earlier in this technique.

6. Clean the site with an antiseptic swab. Using a circular motion, start at the center and move outward about 5 cm (2 in).

7. Remove the needle cover. See Technique 30-3, step 5.

8. Invert the syringe and expel any excess air that may have accidentally entered the syringe, leaving only 0.2 mL of air if the air-bubble technique is being used. It may be necessary to flick the syringe to move the bubbles out. The remaining air will rise to the plunger end when the needle is pointed downward. See Figure 30-29.

Rationale   Users of the air-bubble technique for IM injections believe that, in addition to clearing the medication from the bore of the needle, this technique prevents medication from leaking into subcutaneous tissue and onto the skin surface, where it can cause pain and tissue damage (Wong, 1982, p 1237). Nonusers believe that the best way to prevent leakage is to use the Z-track method described below. However, if the nurse is administering (a) Wyeth's vaccines of diphtheria and tetanus toxoids prepared with aluminum adjuvant, or (b) diphtheria and tetanus toxoids and pertussis vaccine, or (c) tetanus toxoid, it is recommended that the air-bubble technique be used to prevent abscess formation (Chaplin, Shull, Welk, 1985, p 59).

9. Use the nondominant hand to spread the skin at the site.

   Rationale   Spreading the skin makes it firmer and facilitates needle insertion. Under some circumstances, eg, when the patient is emaciated or an infant, the muscle may be bunched.

10. Holding the syringe between the thumb and forefinger, pierce the skin quickly at a 90° angle (see Figure 30–30), and insert the needle into the muscle (see Figure 30–31).

    Rationale   Using a quick motion lessens the patient's discomfort.

11. Aspirate by holding the barrel of the syringe steady with your nondominant hand and by pulling back

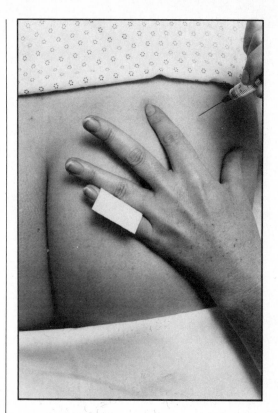

FIGURE 30–30

FIGURE 30–31

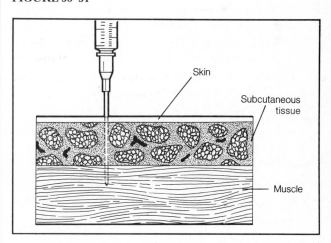

on the plunger with your dominant hand. If blood appears in the syringe, withdraw the needle, discard the syringe, and prepare a new injection.

Rationale   This step determines whether the needle is in a blood vessel.

12. If blood does not appear, inject the medication steadily and slowly, holding the syringe steady.

    Rationale   Injecting medication slowly permits it to disperse into the muscle tissue, thus decreasing the patient's discomfort. Holding the syringe steady minimizes discomfort.

FIGURE 30–29

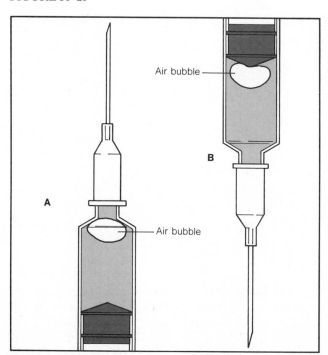

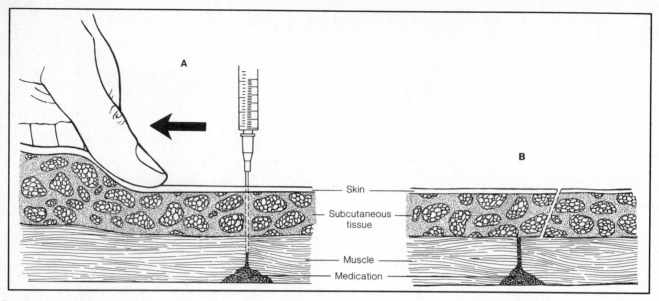

FIGURE 30–32

13. See Technique 30–3, steps 12–18, for withdrawing the needle, massaging the site, disposing of supplies, recording, and conducting follow-up assessment.

Sample Recording

Date	Time	Notes
12/5/86	0800	Penicillin G 500 mg IM into left vastus lateralis. No discomfort, moving well. ———————— Rebecca I. Feinstein, NS

Variation for a Z-track injection

This is a variation of the standard intramuscular technique used to administer intramuscular medications that are highly irritating to subcutaneous and skin tissues.

14. Follow steps 1–8.
15. Attach a clean sterile needle to the syringe.
    Rationale A new needle will not have any medication adhering to the outside that could be irritating to tissues.
16. With the nondominant hand, pull the skin and subcutaneous tissue about 2.5 to 3.5 cm (1 to 1½ in) to one side at the injection site (see Figure 30–32, *A*).
17. Insert the syringe and medication as in steps 10–12.
18. Maintain the traction for 10 seconds; then remove the needle and permit the skin to return to its normal position.
    Rationale During this time, muscle tissues relax and begin to absorb the medication. When the skin

returns to its normal position, the needle track is interrupted, and the medication does not seep into the needle track or subcutaneous tissue. See Figure 30–32, *B*.

19. Do not massage.
    Rationale Massage might cause seepage into delicate tissue.

■ Evaluation

Expected outcomes

1. Intact skin surface at the site of the injection
2. Absence of infection at the injection site
3. No muscle tenderness when palpated
4. Clinical signs indicating effectiveness of medication, eg, decreased pain following administration of an analgesic

Unexpected outcomes

1. Presence of bruising or abrasions at injection site
2. Injection site reddened, hard, hot to touch
3. Discomfort when palpating the muscle
4. No change in clinical signs

Upon obtaining an unexpected outcome:

1. Report your findings to the responsible nurse.
2. Adjust the nursing care plan appropriately.

TECHNIQUE 30–5 ■ Administering an Intradermal Injection

An intradermal (intracutaneous) injection is the administration of a drug into the dermal layer of the skin just beneath the epidermis. Usually only a small amount of liquid is used, for example, 0.1 mL. This method of administration is frequently indicated for allergy and tuberculin tests and for vaccinations. Common sites for intradermal injections are the inner lower arm, the upper chest, and the back beneath the scapulae. See Figure 30–33.

■ Planning

Nursing goals

1. To aid in diagnosing allergies and sensitivities
2. To administer some types of immunizations

Equipment

1. The patient's medication card. Check that it corresponds with the order on the patient's record.
2. A vial or ampule of the correct sterile medication.
3. A sterile syringe and needle. A ½-in, #25 gauge needle is generally used.
4. Acetone and 2 × 2 sterile gauze square (optional).
5. Alcohol swab. A colorless antiseptic that will not hinder the reading of the test is used.
6. A dry sterile gauze pad.

■ Intervention

1. Check the physician's orders carefully for the medication, dosage, and route.
2. Determine the agency's practices about how to prepare the injection site. Some agencies defat the skin with acetone before disinfecting the area with alcohol.
3. Prepare the medication. See Technique 30–1 or 30–2.
4. Explain to the patient that the medication will produce a small bleb like a blister. The patient will feel a slight prick as the needle enters the skin. Some medications are absorbed slowly through the capillaries into the general circulation, and the bleb gradually disappears. Other drugs remain in the area and interact with the body tissues to produce redness and induration (hardening), which will need to be interpreted at a particular time, eg, in 24 or 48 hours. This reaction will also gradually disappear.

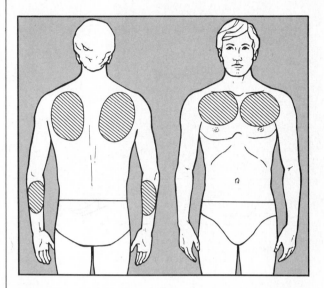

FIGURE 30–33 ■ Sites of the body commonly used for intradermal injections.

5. Assist the patient to either a sitting or lying position in case he or she feels faint.
6. Inspect the skin at the injection site for abrasions, localized inflammation, redness, tenderness, hardness, swelling, scarring, itching, or burning. Avoid using such sites.
7. Defat the skin with acetone if agency policy dictates, using a gauze square or swab moistened with acetone. Start at the center and widen the circle outward.
8. Clean the site with an antiseptic swab using the same method. Allow the area to dry thoroughly.
   Rationale Recommendations differ about the necessity of cleaning the skin prior to injections. Some believe that the antiseptic lessens the number of microorganisms on the skin; others (Dann, 1966, p 1121; Lacey, 1968, p 212) think that cleaning destroys the normal antibacterial properties of the skin.
9. Remove the needle cap while waiting for the antiseptic to dry. Take care to pull the cap straight off, to avoid contaminating the needle by the outside edge of the cap. The needle should touch only the inside of the cap, which is sterile.
10. Expel any air bubbles from the syringe by inverting the syringe and gently pushing on the plunger until a drop of solution can be seen in the needle bevel. For some air bubbles it may be necessary to flick the barrel of the syringe. Small bubbles that adhere

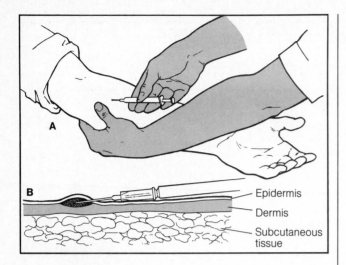

FIGURE 30–34

to the plunger are of no consequence, since a small amount of air will not harm the tissues.

11. Grasp the syringe in your dominant hand, holding it between thumb and four fingers, with your palm upward. Hold the needle at a 15° angle to the skin surface, with the bevel of the needle up.

12. With your nondominant hand, pull the skin at the site until it is taut, and thrust the tip of the needle firmly through the epidermis into the dermis. See Figure 30–34, *A*. Do not aspirate.

13. Inject the medication carefully so that it produces a small bleb on the skin. See Figure 30-34, *B*.

14. Withdraw the needle quickly while providing countertraction on the skin, and wipe the injection site gently with a dry sterile gauze pad. Do not massage the area.

Rationale A dry sterile gauze is used since alcohol interferes with some diagnostic skin tests. Massage can disperse the medication into the tissue or out through the needle insertion site.

15. Reapply the needle cover and dispose of the supplies according to agency procedures. Generally the needle and its cover are separated from the syringe, and both are placed in a special container for safety reasons.

16. Assess the patient's response to the injection in terms of discomfort, faintness, etc.

17. Record the medication given, in accordance with agency practice, including the time, dosage, route, site, and patient response.

■ Evaluation

Expected outcomes

1. A small wheal on the skin surface
2. Clinical signs indicating the action of the medication

Unexpected outcomes

1. No wheal appears on the skin.
2. Site bleeds after needle is withdrawn. Medication may have been injected into the subcutaneous tissue.
3. Immediate redness appears. This could indicate incorrect injection technique.
4. Site is immediately painful.

Upon obtaining an unexpected outcome:

1. Report your findings to the responsible nurse and/or physician.
2. Assess the patient for adverse clinical signs depending upon the medication injected.

INTRAVENOUS MEDICATIONS

Medications are administered intravenously via:

1. Intravenous bottle or bag
2. Volume-control administration set
3. Additional intravenous container
4. Intravenous push (bolus)

Because intravenous (IV) medications enter the patient's bloodstream directly, they are appropriate when a rapid effect is required (eg, in a life-threatening situation such as a cardiac arrest). The IV route is also appropriate when medications are too irritating to tissues to be given by other routes, eg, levarterenol bitartrate (Levophed) for acute hypotension. When an IV line is already established, this route is desirable because it avoids the discomfort of other parenteral routes. See Technique 25–5, on page 559.

There are, however, potential hazards in giving IV medications: infection and rapid, severe reactions to the medication. To prevent infection, sterile technique is used during all aspects of IV medication techniques. To safeguard the patient against severe reactions, the nurse must administer the drug slowly, following the manufacturer's recommendations. The patient is assessed closely during the administration, and the medication is discontinued immediately if an untoward reaction occurs.

TECHNIQUE 30-6   ■   Adding an IV Medication to an IV Bottle or Bag

IV medications can be added to a new fluid container prior to hanging it or to a fluid container that is already attached and running. Electrolytes (eg, potassium chloride) and vitamins (eg, Solu-B) are commonly administered by this method.

■ Assessment

1. Before administering the medication, inspect and palpate the intravenous insertion site for signs of infection, infiltration, or a dislocated needle. Inspect the surrounding skin for redness, pallor, or swelling. Palpate the surrounding tissues for coldness and presence of edema.
2. Take the vital signs for baseline data.

Other data include:

1. The specific medication and dosage.
2. Which infusions are to be used with the medication. For example, the order may say to infuse the medication with 1,000 mL of 5% dextrose and water rather than with normal saline.
3. The compatibility of the drugs and solutions being mixed. You may need to consult a pharmacist for this information. An incompatibility is an undesired chemical or physical reaction between a drug and an infusion solution, between two or more drugs, or between a drug and the container or tubing.

■ Planning

Nursing goals

1. To provide and maintain a constant level of a medication in the blood
2. To administer well-diluted medications at a continuous and slow rate
3. To maintain sterile technique while adding the IV medication to the IV container

Equipment

1. The correct solution container, if a new one is to be attached. Confirm its sterility by ensuring that there are no container cracks or leaks, fluid discoloration, or seal damage.
2. The physician's order or the medication card.
3. The correct sterile medication. If the medication is in a powdered form, a diluent (eg, sterile saline solution or water) will also be necessary.

4. Antiseptic swabs.
5. A sterile syringe of appropriate size (eg, 5 or 10 mL) and a 1- to 1½-in, #20 or #21 gauge sterile needle.
6. A medication label to attach to the IV solution container.

■ Intervention

1. Prepare the medication from a vial or ampule as described in Technique 30-1 on page 718. Check the agency's practice about whether a special filter needle is to be used when withdrawing the medication. A filter needle may be used to draw up premixed liquid medications from multidose vials. The filter prevents any solid material from being drawn up. If a filter needle is used, replace it with a regular needle to inject the medication into the solution container.
2. Compare the name on the medication card with the patient's identification band.
3. For a glass IV container, remove the metal cap and the rubber disc, if the bottle is vented. Locate the injection port.
   or
4. For a plastic container, locate the separate, self-sealing, soft rubber injection port. An injection port may be designated in several ways, eg, by a triangular indentation or by the word *add* . It is important not to inject medication through the port for the administration spike or through an air vent port if there is an injection port. (See chapter 25 for further information about infusion equipment.)
5. Clean the injection port with an antiseptic swab.
6. Remove the needle cover from the medication syringe, and inject the medication into the port. See Figure 30-35.
7. Remove the needle. For a glass container, cover the top immediately either with:
   a. An antiseptic swab with the metal IV cap taped over it.
      or
   b. The special sterile cap provided by the manufacturer.
8. Gently rotate the solution container to mix the drug with the solution.
9. Attach the medication label upside down to the fluid container. See Figure 30-36 for the information to be included on the medication label.

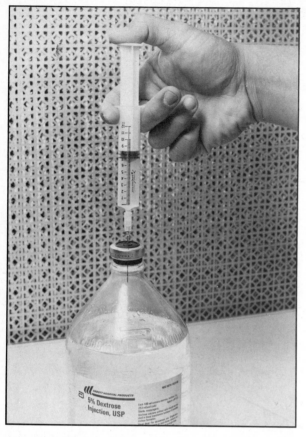

FIGURE 30–35

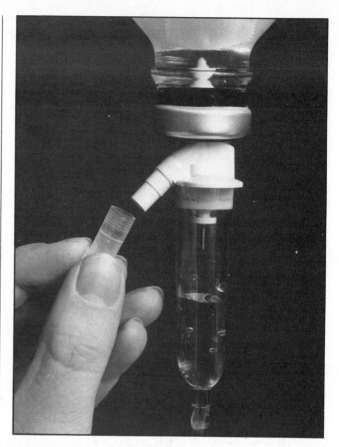

FIGURE 30–37

Rationale This makes the label easy to read when the container is hanging.

10. Spike and hang the container, and regulate the flow rate according to the dosage required when the medication is to be administered. See Technique 25–1, step 13, on page 551, for the procedure for spiking a container.

11. Record the IV infusion and medication.

12. Carefully monitor the IV infusion to maintain

FIGURE 30–36

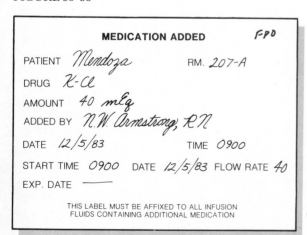

MEDICATION ADDED   FPD

PATIENT *Mendoza*   RM. *207-A*

DRUG *K-Cl*

AMOUNT *40 mEq*

ADDED BY *N.W. Armstrong, RN*

DATE *12/5/83*   TIME *0900*

START TIME *0900*   DATE *12/5/83* FLOW RATE *40*

EXP. DATE ——

THIS LABEL MUST BE AFFIXED TO ALL INFUSION
FLUIDS CONTAINING ADDITIONAL MEDICATION

delivery of the medication and IV fluid at the specified rate.

13. During the administration, observe the patient for signs of an adverse reaction, such as noisy respirations, changes in pulse rate, chills, nausea, or headache. If any adverse sign occurs, notify the physician or responsible nurse. Also monitor the patient for signs of the intended action of the medication.

Variations for adding medications to an infusing container

See chapter 25 for additional information about intravenous infusion equipment.

14. For an IV bottle with a vented administration set:

a. Make sure there is sufficient solution in the bottle to ensure proper dilution of the drug.

b. Close the IV flow clamp.

Rationale Closing the clamp is essential to prevent the medication from infusing to the patient before it is properly diluted with the solution. Undiluted medication can produce a severe reaction.

c. Detach the air vent cap, taking care not to contaminate the end. See Figure 30–37.

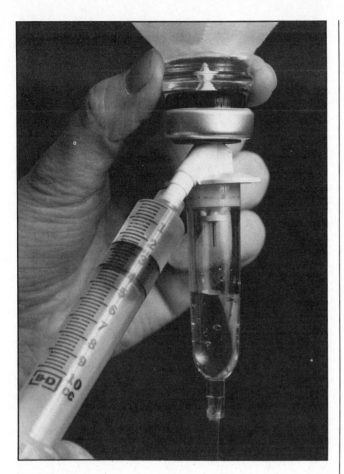

FIGURE 30–38

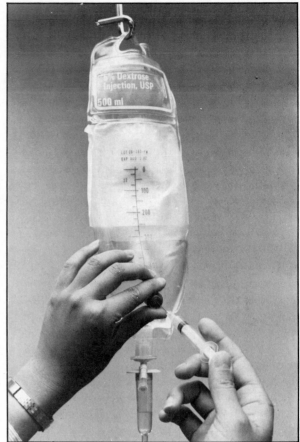

FIGURE 30–39

d. Insert the tip of the medication syringe *without the needle* into the air vent port. See Figure 30–38.

e. Instill the medication.

f. Reattach the air vent.

or

For a vented IV bottle:

g. After ensuring that there is sufficient solution in the bottle, close the IV flow clamp.

h. Clean the medication port with an antiseptic swab.

i. Insert the syringe needle through the port and instill the medication. The medication port is usually marked by a triangular imprint.

or

For a plastic IV bag:

j. After ensuring that there is sufficient solution in the bag, close the IV flow clamp.

k. Clean the medication port with an antiseptic swab.

l. While supporting and stabilizing the bag with your thumb and forefinger, carefully insert the syringe needle through the port and inject the medication. See Figure 30–39.

Rationale The bag is supported while injecting the medication to avoid puncturing the bag.

15. Gently lift and rotate the container.

Rationale This mixes the solution and medication.

16. Open the IV flow clamp and regulate the rate as ordered.

17. Attach a medication label to the IV container.

18. Follow steps 10–12 above.

■ Evaluation

Expected outcomes

1. Stable vital signs

2. Absence of side effects or clinical signs of allergy

3. Skin at IV site intact

Unexpected outcomes

1. Significant change in vital signs

2. Complaints of headache, nausea, or chills or untoward reactions

3. Infiltration at IV site

Upon obtaining an unexpected outcome:

1. Report your findings to the responsible nurse and/or physician and to the pharmacy if appropriate.

2. Discontinue the infusion of the medication if a severe reaction occurs.

3. Adjust the patient's nursing care plan appropriately, eg, treat an untoward reaction according to orders.

TECHNIQUE 30–7 ■ Adding an IV Medication to a Volume-Control Administration Set

Controlled volume administration sets have different names, depending on the manufacturer, eg, Buretrol, Soluset, Volutrol, Pediatrol. They are small fluid containers (100 to 150 mL in size) attached below the primary infusion container. Volume-control sets are equipped with either a stationary membrane filter or a floating valve filter at the base of the container and are designed to finely control the amount of infusing fluid. See Figure 30–40.

■ **Assessment**   See Technique 30–6 on page 735.

■ **Planning**

Nursing goals

1. To administer IV medications (such as some antibiotics) that do not remain stable for the length of time it takes an entire solution container to infuse

2. To administer medications intermittently

3. To avoid mixing medications that are incompatible

4. To dilute a drug so that it is less irritating to the veins than if given by direct intravenous push

5. To deliver medications diluted in precise amounts of fluid

Equipment

1. The correct solution container

2. A volume-control administration set

3. The physician's order or the medication card

4. The correct sterile medication

5. Antiseptic swabs

6. A sterile syringe of appropriate size (eg, 5 or 10 mL); a 1-to 1½-in, #20 or #21 gauge, sterile needle; and a sterile filter needle if needed to withdraw the medication

7. A medication label for the volume-control set

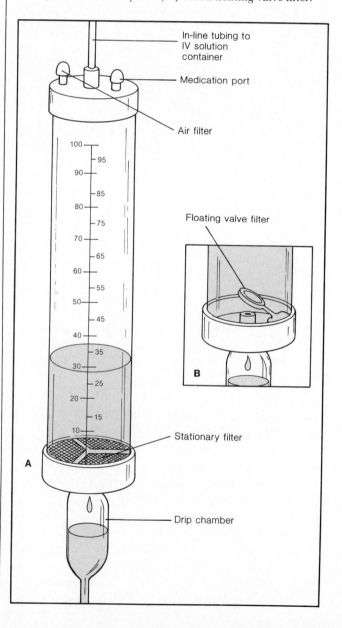

FIGURE 30–40 ■ A volume-control intravenous infusion set: **A,** with a stationary filter; **B,** with a floating valve filter.

Attaching and filling a volume-control set is similar to setting up a regular intravenous infusion but differs in the priming procedure, ie, the way in which the volume-control set is filled. The priming procedure also varies in accordance with the specific type of filter (membrane or floating valve) of the volume-control set. Assemble the equipment according to the manufacturer's instructions.

■ **Intervention**

1. Prepare the medication from a vial or ampule as described in Technique 30–1 on page 718. Check the agency's practice about whether a special filter needle is used when withdrawing the medication.

2. Compare the name on the medication card with the patient's identification band.

3. Ensure that there is sufficient fluid in the volume-control fluid chamber to dilute the medication. Generally 50 to 100 mL of fluid is used. Check the directions from the drug manufacturer.

4. Close the inflow to the fluid chamber by adjusting the upper roller or side clamp above the fluid chamber; also ensure that the clamp on the air vent of the chamber is open.

5. Clean the medication port on the volume-control fluid chamber with an antiseptic swab.

6. Insert the needle of the medication syringe into the port. See Figure 30–41.

7. Inject the medication.

8. Gently rotate the fluid chamber until the fluid is well mixed.

9. Regulate the flow by adjusting the lower roller or slide clamp below the fluid chamber.

10. Attach a medication label to the volume control fluid chamber.

11. Record the IV infusion and medication.

12. Carefully monitor the IV infusion to maintain

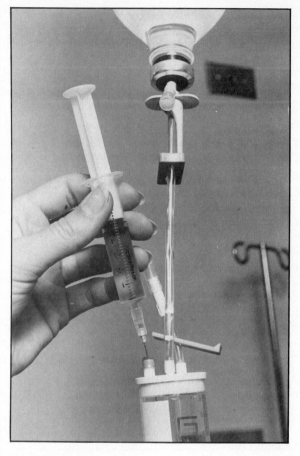

FIGURE 30–41

delivery of the medication and IV fluid at the specified rate.

13. Assess the patient's response to the medication in terms of the intended action of the medication, adverse reactions to it, discomfort, etc.

■ **Evaluation**   See Technique 30–6 on page 737.

TECHNIQUE 30–8   ■   Administering an IV Medication Using Additional Containers

Additional fluid containers and sets are sometimes attached to a primary infusion set to administer IV medications. They may be used to administer IV drugs intermittently that cannot be mixed with the primary solution for reason of incompatibility, or to maintain peak levels of a medication in the patient's bloodstream and at the same time maintain a constant total infusion rate by simultaneous infusion of the primary line. Examples of two medications commonly administered in this manner are the bronchodilator aminophylline and antibiotic cephalothin sodium (Keflin).

There are two methods of attaching additional containers: the piggyback set and the secondary set. The piggyback set (see Figure 25–10, *B* on page 550) consists of a small IV bottle (minibottle) and a short tubing line that is connected to the upper Y-port (the piggyback port) of the primary line. Either a macrodrip or a microdrip system may be used. The term *piggyback* refers to the positioning of the additive bottle, which is higher than the primary infusion bottle. Manufacturers provide an extension hook to position the primary bottle below the piggyback bottle. The piggyback set is used for intermittent IV drug administration.

The secondary set (see Figure 25–10, *A* on page 550) uses a second microdrip or macrodrip bottle of any size and a long tubing line that is attached to the lower Y-port (secondary port) of the primary line. The primary and secondary bottles are positioned at the same height. This system is used to administer IV drugs intermittently or continuously with the primary IV solution.

■ Assessment

See Technique 30–6 on page 735. Additional data include:

FIGURE 30–42

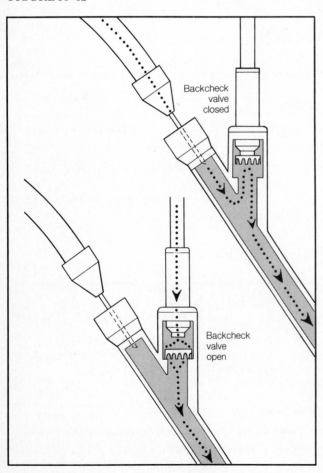

Backcheck valve closed

Backcheck valve open

1. The medication, the dosage, and how the additive set is to be attached
2. Whether the medication is compatible with the primary infusion and with any other medications that are to be added
3. If a secondary set is used, whether it is to run simultaneously with the primary infusion or if the primary infusion is to be clamped off at the time

■ Planning

Nursing goals

1. To administer IV drugs intermittently that cannot be mixed with the primary solution for reasons of incompatibility
2. To administer different IV drugs at different times
3. To maintain peak levels of a medication in the patient's bloodstream by simultaneous infusion

Equipment

1. The appropriate additive set.
2. The physician's order or the medication card.
3. The correct sterile medication.
4. A sterile syringe and needle. Generally a #20 gauge, 1-in needle is used, because longer needles can puncture the tubing and cause leakage of IV fluid.
5. A medication label.
6. An antiseptic swab.
7. Adhesive tape.

■ Intervention

1. Prepare the medication according to Technique 30–1 on page 718.
2. Compare the patient's identification band with the medication card.
3. Insert the medication into the secondary bottle. See Technique 30–6 on page 735.
4. If the medication is not compatible with the primary infusion, flush the primary line with a sterile saline solution before attaching the secondary set. To flush the line, wipe the port with an antiseptic swab, clamp the primary line, and, using a sterile needle and syringe, instill a few milliliters of sterile saline through the port to wash any primary infusion fluid out of the infusion tubing.
5. Wipe the port with an antiseptic swab.
6. Insert the needle of the secondary set into the port on the primary line, and secure it with adhesive tape. Some agencies recommend that a needle guard be taped alongside the needle to support the needle

placement and keep the needle guard handy for use when discontinuing the secondary attachment.

7. Open the clamp on the secondary line, and regulate it in accordance with the recommended rate for that medication.

8. If a secondary set is used, clamp off the primary infusion, if necessary. When a piggyback set is used, a backcheck valve in the port automatically stops the flow of the primary infusion so that only the additive set infuses. See Figure 30–42. After the piggyback solution has infused and the level of the solution is below the level of the primary infusion drip chamber, the backcheck valve is released, and the primary infusion automatically starts running.

9. Record the IV infusion and medication.

10. Carefully monitor the IV infusion to maintain delivery of the medication and the IV fluid at the specified rate.

11. Assess the patient's response to the medication in terms of the intended action of the medication, adverse reactions to it, discomfort, etc.

12. When the medication has infused, readjust the flow of the primary line at the correct rate.

13. Either retain the secondary line for subsequent use, or detach it and dispose of the equipment.

■ **Evaluation** See Technique 30–6 on page 737.

TECHNIQUE 30–9 ■ Administering an IV Medication by Intravenous Push (Bolus)

An IV push is the intravenous administration of a medication that cannot be diluted or that is needed in an emergency. Also, some drugs are administered this way to achieve maximum effect. It is important to remember that the medication is administered rapidly with an IV push, and this could be dangerous for the patient. Some agencies allow only physicians or specially trained nurses to administer IV push medications. Check agency policy.

An IV push can be administered directly into a vein through venipuncture, into an existing intravenous apparatus through an injection port (see Figure 30–43 on page 742.), or through an intermittent infusion set (heparin lock) when the patient does not have an IV running but does have a heparin lock in place. The heparin lock, also referred to as a male adapter plug (MAP), is primarily used for patients who require regular intermittent IV medications but not the fluid volume of an intravenous infusion. The set usually consists of an indwelling needle or catheter attached to a plastic tube with a sealed injection tip. See Figure 30–45 later in this chapter. It is called a *heparin lock* because small amounts of heparin are injected into it to maintain its patency. The infusion set is generally inserted into a patient's arm or hand.

■ **Assessment**

1. See Technique 30–6 on page 735.

2. Assess the patency of a heparin lock every 8 to 12 hours. See Intervention, step 19.

■ **Planning**

Nursing goals

1. To achieve immediate and maximum effects of a medication

2. To maintain the patency of a heparin lock, if present

Equipment

1. The physician's order or the medication card

2. The correct sterile medication

3. A sterile syringe of the appropriate size for the volume of medication and a sterile 2.5-cm (1-in) #25 gauge needle to prevent large puncture holes in the injection port

4. Alcohol swabs

In addition for a heparin lock,

5. A sterile syringe and needle with a heparin flush solution. Check agency practice. Many hospitals advocate the use of 100 units per milliliter of solution, and 0.5 mL is generally used. Prepackaged heparin syringes and needles are available.

6. A sterile syringe and needle with 4mL (or amount prescribed by the agency) of normal saline.

■ **Intervention**

1. Prepare the medication according to Technique 30–1 on page 718. Label the syringe with the name of the medication and the dosage.

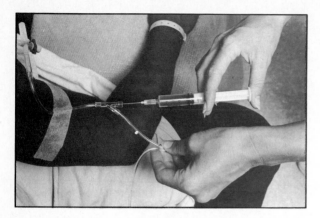

FIGURE 30-43

2. In a separate syringe, prepare the heparin solution according to agency policy, if needed. Label this syringe.

3. In another syringe, prepare the saline solution. Label this syringe.

4. Compare the name on the patient's identification band with the name on the medication card.

FIGURE 30-44

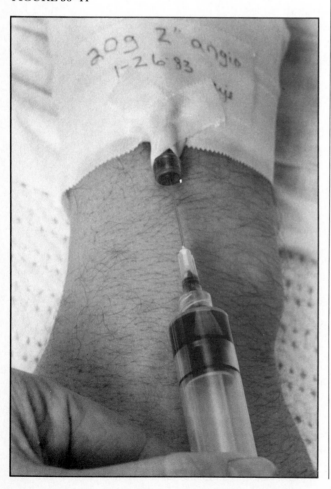

IV push into an existing IV

5. Identify an injection port nearest the patient. Some ports have a circle indicating the site for the needle insertion.

   Rationale An injection port must be used because it is self-sealing. Any puncture to the plastic tubing will leak.

6. Clean the port with an antiseptic swab.

7. Stop the IV flow by closing the clamp or pinching the tubing above the injection port (see Figure 30–43).

8. While holding the port steady, insert the needle into the port.

9. Draw back on the plunger to withdraw some blood into the IV tubing (not into the syringe).

   Rationale This shows that the needle is in the vein.

10. Inject the medication at the correct rate, withdraw the needle, reopen the clamp, and reestablish the intravenous infusion at the correct rate. If the medication is particularly irritating to the veins, run the IV rapidly for about a minute to dilute the medication, and then adjust the rate.

IV push into an intermittent infusion set

11. Swab the injection port with an antiseptic swab.

12. Insert the needle with the normal saline into the port and aspirate for blood return. See Figure 30–44.

    Rationale This ensures that the heparin lock catheter is in the vein. In some situations blood will not return even though the heparin lock is patent.

13. Inject 2 mL of the normal saline solution. This step is optional. Check agency practice.

    Rationale This is done to flush the heparin from the catheter.

    If the patient experiences burning or stinging sensations, it may be that the needle or catheter is not in the vein and the fluid is infiltrating the tissue. In this case withhold the medication until the heparin lock is replaced.

14. Remove the saline-filled syringe, and cap the needle to maintain its sterility.

    Rationale This syringe is used again, so it must be kept sterile.

15. Insert the needle attached to the medication syringe.

16. Inject the medication slowly at the recommended rate of infusion. Observe the patient closely for adverse reactions. Remove the needle and syringe when all medication is administered.

17. Reattach the saline syringe, and inject the recommended amount of saline.

Rationale   The saline injection flushes the medication through the catheter and prepares the lock for the heparin.

18. Insert the heparin syringe, and inject the heparin slowly into the set. See Figure 30–45 for a prepackaged heparin syringe.

19. Check the patency of the heparin lock at least every eight hours or according to agency practice.

   a. Aspirate for return blood flow.

   b. Flush the catheter with 2 to 3 mL of normal saline.

   c. Refill the heparin lock with heparin solution.

20. Check agency practice about recommended times for changing the heparin lock. Some agencies advocate a change every 48 to 72 hours.

IV push directly in vein

21. Perform a venipuncture. See Technique 25–5 on page 559.

22. Slowly inject the medication into the vein. The rate of the injection will vary according to the medication, the physician's order, and/or the manufacturer's directions. Many medications are injected slowly over a period of several minutes. Check drug reference information.

23. Withdraw the needle, and apply pressure to the site to prevent bleeding.

For all types of intravenous medications

24. Record the medication given, dosage, time, route, any complaints of the patient, and your signature.

25. Carefully assess the patient's response to the medica-

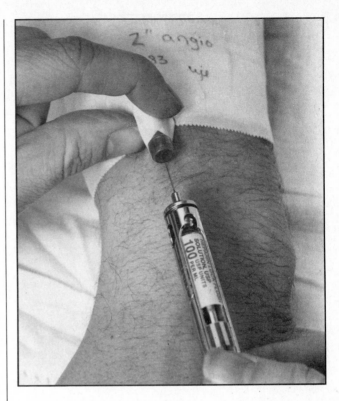

FIGURE 30–45

tion in terms of the intended action of the medication, adverse reactions to it, discomfort, etc. Because the medication is administered relatively quickly and directly into the bloodstream, it can produce sudden and severe reactions.

■ **Evaluation**   See Technique 30–6 on page 737.

References

Burke EL: Insulin injection: The site and the technique. *Am J Nurs* (December) 1972; 72:2194–2196.

Chaplin G, Shull H, Welk PC: How safe is the air-bubble technique for I.M. injections? *Nursing 85* (September) 1985; 15:59.

Chezem JL: Consultation: Aspirating before IM injections. *Nursing 74* (September) 1974; 4:87.

Dann TC: Routine skin preparation before injection—is it necessary? *Nurs Times* (August) 1966; 62:1121–1122.

Geolot DH, McKinney NP: Administering parenteral drugs. *Am J Nurs* (May) 1975; 75:788–793.

Hays D: Do it yourself the Z-track way. *Am J Nurs* (June) 1974; 74:1070–1071.

Hayter J: Why response to medication changes with age. *Geriatr Nurs* (November/December) 1981; 2:411–416.

Lacey RW: Antibacterial action of human skin. *Br J Exp Pathol* (April) 1968; 49:209–215.

Lang SH, Zawacki AM, Johnson JE: Reducing discomfort from IM injections. *Am J Nurs* (May) 1976; 76:800–801.

Motz-Harding E, Good F: The right solution: Mixing I.V. drugs thoroughly. *Nursing 85* (February) 1985; 15:62–64.

Newton DW, Newton M: Route, site, and technique: Three key decisions in giving parenteral medication. *Nursing 79* (July) 1979; 9:18–21, 23, 25.

Nursing 80 Photobook Series: *Giving Medications.* Intermed Communications, 1980a.

Nursing 80 Photobook Series: *Managing IV Therapy.* Intermed Communications, 1980b.

Peck N: Perfecting your I.V. techniques, part I. *Nursing 85* (May) 1985; 15:38–43.

Peck N: Perfecting your I.V. techniques, part II. *Nursing 85* (June) 1985;15:48–51.

Pitel M: The subcutaneous injection. *Am J Nurs* (January) 1971; 71:76–79.

Swearingen PL: *The Addison-Wesley Photo-Atlas of Nursing Procedures.* Addison-Wesley, 1984.

Winfrey A: Single-dose I.M. injections: How much is too much? *Nursing 85* (July) 1985; 15:38–39.

Wong DL: Significance of dead space in syringes. *Am J Nurs* (August) 1982; 82:1237.

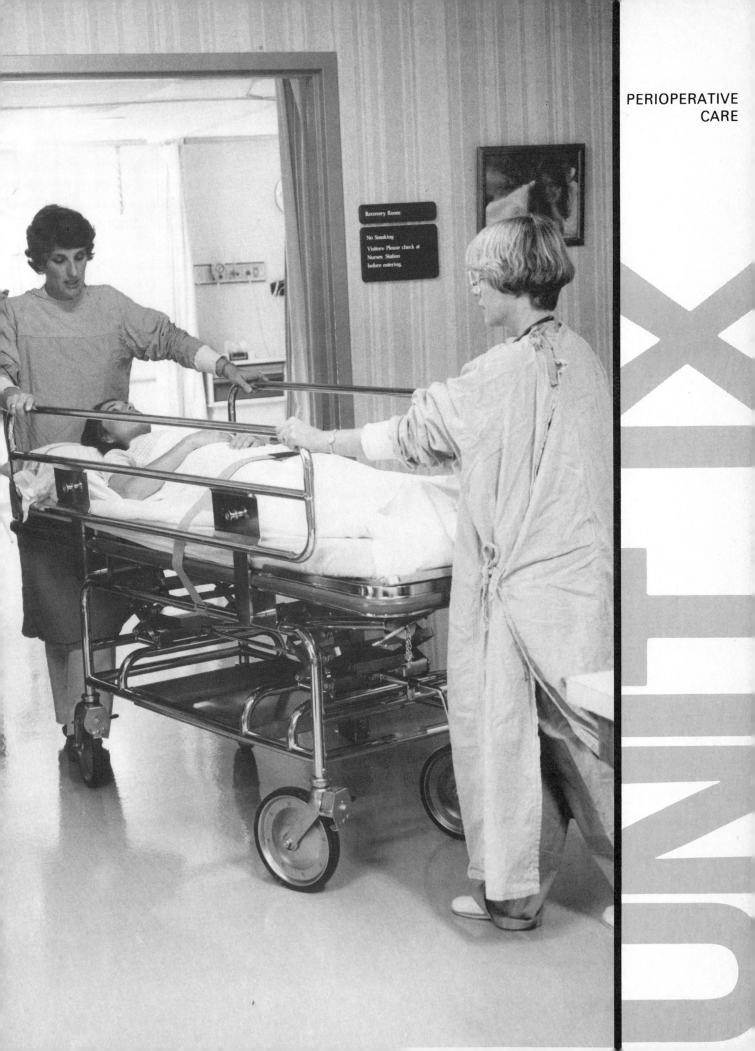

UNIT IX

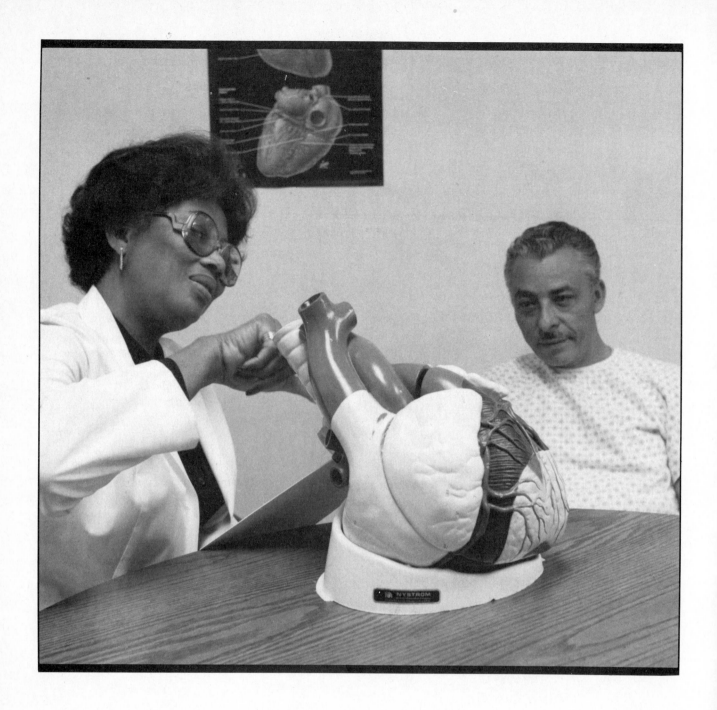

PREOPERATIVE NURSING

31

Preoperative care is care given before an operation or before a special examination if an anesthetic is to be administered. Most people are anxious about surgery and about receiving an anesthetic. An operation implies that the body will be traumatized (injured), and an anesthetic means, to many patients, lack of control over their bodies and over what happens to them.

During the preoperative period the patient is given important psychologic and physical preparation for the forthcoming surgery or examination.

Chapter Outline

Objectives

Upon completion of this chapter, the student will:

1. Know essential terms and facts about surgery, anesthesia, and preoperative care
   1.1 Define selected terms
   1.2 Identify factors that increase surgical risk
   1.3 Identify common health problems that increase surgical risk
   1.4 Identify essential information required in the nursing history of a patient having surgery
   1.5 Identify common screening tests or examinations performed prior to surgery and the reasons for them
2. Understand essential information about preoperative nursing interventions
   2.1 Identify routine interventions carried out preoperatively and the reasons for them
   2.2 Identify essentials of teaching patients to move and to carry out leg, coughing, and deep-breathing exercises
   2.3 Identify the nurse's responsibilities for preparing the patient on the day before surgery
   2.4 Identify essential steps of preoperative skin preparation and the reasons for these steps
   2.5 Identify the nurse's responsibilities for preparing the patient on the day of surgery
   2.6 Identify essential steps for inserting a nasogastric tube and the reasons for these steps
3. Understand facts about preoperative techniques
   3.1 Identify relevant assessment data
   3.2 Identify nursing diagnoses for which the technique may be implemented
   3.3 Identify nursing goals related to the technique
   3.4 Identify expected and unexpected outcomes from assessment data
   3.5 Identify reasons underlying selected steps of the technique
4. Perform techniques to prepare a patient physically and psychologically for surgery
   4.1 Assess the patient adequately
   4.2 Collect additional data from appropriate sources
   4.3 Select pertinent nursing goals for the patient
   4.4 Establish relevant outcome criteria for the patient following the technique
   4.5 Collect necessary equipment before the technique
   4.6 Implement interventions to enhance the effectiveness of the technique and enhance the patient's comfort and safety
   4.7 Communicate relevant information about the patient to the appropriate persons through records or reports
   4.8 Evaluate the outcomes of the technique
5. Evaluate own performance of specific techniques in a laboratory or clinical setting with the assistance of another
   5.1 Use the performance checklists provided
   5.2 Identify areas of strength and weakness
   5.3 Alter performance in response to own evaluation and that of another

Terms

■ ablative surgery   surgery to remove a diseased organ or other tissue

■ aeration   the process by which the blood exchanges carbon dioxide for oxygen in the lungs

■ anemia   a condition in which the blood is deficient in red blood cells or hemoglobin

■ anesthesia   loss of sensation with or without loss of consciousness

■ anesthesiologist   a physician specializing in the administration of anesthetics

■ anesthetic   a substance that produces anesthesia

■ anesthetist   a person, such as a nurse, who specializes in administering anesthetics

■ Cantor tube   a single-lumen tube inserted through the mouth into the intestines

■ caudal anesthetic   an anesthetic injected into the caudal canal, below the spinal cord

■ cilia   hairlike projections of the mucous membrane of the respiratory tract

■ coagulate   to clot

■ constructive surgery   surgery to repair a malformed organ or tissue

■ cyanosis   a bluish tinge of the skin and mucous membranes due to excessive concentration of reduced hemoglobin (hemoglobin without oxygen) in the blood

■ diagnostic surgery   surgery performed to confirm a diagnosis

■ elective surgery   surgery performed for a person's well-being but not absolutely necessary for life

■ embolus   a blood clot that has moved from its place of origin and is obstructing the circulation in a blood vessel (plural: emboli)

■ epidural block   injection of an anesthetic through a lumbar interspace into the spinal canal (external to the dura mater)

■ excise   to cut off or out

■ exploratory surgery   surgery performed to confirm the extent of a pathologic process and sometimes to confirm a diagnosis

■ Harris tube   a single-lumen tube with a metal tip that is inserted through the mouth into the intestines

■ hematocrit   the percentage of red blood cell mass in proportion to whole blood

■ hemoglobin   the red pigment in red blood cells, which carries oxygen

■ hemorrhage   bleeding, the escape of blood from the vessels

■ ischemia   the lack of blood supply to a body part

■ Levin tube   a single-lumen nasogastric tube

■ Miller-Abbott tube   a double-lumen tube inserted through the nose or mouth into the intestine

■ nasogastric tube   a plastic or rubber tube inserted through the nose into the stomach

■ nerve block   chemical interruption of a nerve pathway efected by injecting an anesthetic

■ optional surgery   surgery requested by the patient but not necessary for health

■ palliative surgery   surgery to relieve the symptoms of a disease process

■ preoperative   before an operation

■ plexus   a network (of nerves, veins, etc)

■ reconstructive surgery   surgery to repair tissues whose function or appearance is damaged

■ Salem sump tube   a double-lumen nasogastric tube

■ sedative   an agent or drug that tends to calm or tranquilize

■ thrombophlebitis   inflammation of a vein followed by formation of a blood clot

■ thrombus   a solid mass of blood constituents; a clot (plural: thrombi)

■ umbilicus   the navel; the site where the umbilical cord was attached to the fetus

■ spinal anesthesia   the introduction of an anesthetic into the subarachnoid space of the spinal canal

■ urgent surgery   surgery necessary for the patient's health

■ venous stasis   diminished flow of blood in the veins

PREOPERATIVE ASSESSMENT

Assessing Surgical Risk

The degree of risk involved in a surgical procedure is affected by the patient's (a) age, (b) nutritional status, (c) fluid and electrolyte balance, (d) general health, (e) use of medications, and (f) mental health, including attitude.

Age

Very young and elderly patients are greater surgical risks than children and adults. The neonate's physiologic response to surgery is substantially different from an adult's. Factors that affect the risk are the neonate's circulation, which is largely central, and renal function, which is not fully developed until about 6 months of age.

The neonate can respond to an additional need for oxygen only by an increased respiratory rate, and limited blood volume results in a limited fluid reserve.

Elderly persons are also at additional risk from surgery. Elderly patients often have impaired circulation due to arteriosclerosis and limited cardiac function. Energy reserves are frequently limited, and hydration and the nutritional status may be poor. In addition, elderly people can be highly sensitive to medications such as morphine sulfate and barbiturates, frequently used preoperatively and postoperatively.

Nutritional status

Two nutritional problems that can increase surgical risk are obesity and malnutrition due to protein, iron, and vitamin deficiencies. Surgery of obese patients is often deferred except in emergencies. Obese patients have overtaxed hearts and elevated blood pressures. In addition, incisions in overly fatty tissue are difficult to suture and prone to infection. Nutritional deficiencies are seen particularly among elderly and chronically ill patients. Protein and vitamins are needed for wound healing; vitamin K is essential for blood clotting.

Fluid and electrolyte balance

Dehydration and hypovolemia predispose a patient to problems during surgery. Electrolyte imbalances often accompany fluid imbalances. Imbalances in calcium, magnesium, potassium, and hydrogen ions are of particular concern during surgery. See chapter 23.

General health

Operations are least risky when the patient is in general good health. Any infection or pathophysiology increases the risk. Of particular concern are upper respiratory tract infections, which, together with a general anesthetic, can have an adverse effect on respiratory function.

Recent myocardial infarction or any cardiovascular disease also can make surgery more dangerous than usual. Renal function is essential for the excretion of body wastes. In addition, the kidneys help regulate the body's fluids and electrolytes. Any renal impairment can affect the patient's blood pressure and the ability of the body to respond to the additional stress of surgery. Metabolic and liver function affect healing and the detoxification and elimination of medications. When liver function is impaired, the liver cannot detoxify drugs and metabolize carbohydrates, proteins, and fats efficiently. Untreated diabetes mellitus predisposes to infection and impaired healing. A person whose blood does not coagulate normally may bleed more than is normal or even hemorrhage and go into shock.

Medications

The regular use of certain medications can increase risk of operations. Some of these medications are:

1. Anticoagulants, which increase blood coagulation time
2. Tranquilizers, which can cause hypotension and thus contribute to shock
3. Heroin and other depressants, which decrease central nervous system responses
4. Antibiotics that are incompatible with anesthetic agents, resulting in untoward reactions
5. Diuretics, which can create electrolyte (especially potassium) imbalances

In addition, some medications interact adversely with other medications and with anesthetic agents.

Mental health and attitude

Extreme anxiety can increase surgical risk. A person's anxiety does not always correspond to the seriousness of the surgical procedure. The surgeon needs to know if a person believes he or she will die during surgery. In some instances, professional counseling and a delay in the surgery are indicated.

Patients who have been poorly adjusted for some time may not be able to cope with the additional stress of surgery. People who cope only minimally in a stable, familiar environment can develop emotional problems postoperatively.

Physical Examination

If surgery is elective or optional, the physical examination is usually done in the physician's office prior to admission to the agency, but it is done on admission before emergency surgery. In some settings, nurses perform the physical examination. For information about physical examinations, see chapter 10. Knowledge of the patient's overall health is essential in preventing complications and reducing surgical risk.

Common health problems that increase surgical risk and may lead to the decision to postpone or cancel surgery include:

1. Certain conditions, such as angina pectoris, recent myocardial infarction, severe hypertension, or severe congestive heart failure. Well-controlled cardiac problems generally pose minimal operative risk.
2. Blood coagulation problems that may lead to severe bleeding, hemorrhage, and subsequent shock.
3. Upper respiratory tract infections or chronic obstructive lung diseases, such as emphysema. These conditions, especially when exacerbated by the effects of a general anesthetic, adversely affect pulmonary function. They also predispose the patient to postoperative lung infections.
4. Renal disease that impairs the regulation of the body's fluids and electrolytes, eg, renal insufficiency.
5. Diabetes mellitus, which predisposes the patient to wound infection and delayed healing.
6. Liver disease, such as cirrhosis, which impairs the liver's ability to detoxify medications used during surgery, to produce the prothrombin necessary for blood clotting, and to metabolize nutrients essential for healing.
7. Uncontrolled neurologic disease, such as epilepsy.

Nursing History

The nursing history required on admission provides patient data that helps the nurse to plan preoperative and postoperative care. Although forms vary considerably among agencies, essential preoperative information includes:

1. Physical condition. The patient's general appearance—color, weight, hydration status, and energy level—is noted. Problems such as obesity, malnutrition, dehydra-

tion, or marked fatigue may indicate the need for therapy prior to surgery. For instance, the dehydrated patient may need fluids administered intravenously.

2. Mental attitude. Anxiety is a normal response to surgery. However, extreme anxiety can increase the surgical risk and needs to be reported to the physician.

3. Understanding of the surgery. Determining the patient's knowledge about the surgery helps the nurse plan appropriate instruction. A well-informed patient knows what to expect and in general accepts and copes more effectively with surgery and convalescence.

4. Experience with previous surgeries. Some previous experiences may influence the patient's physical and psychologic responses to the planned surgery. For example, a patient who developed a wound infection that caused a gape in a previous incision may demonstrate acute anxiety when sutures are removed and may be unwilling to move, believing that movement will cause the wound to gape.

5. Expected outcomes of surgery. Surgery alters patient's body images and life-styles to varying degrees. A middle-aged woman about to have a hysterectomy may feel she will no longer be valued or adequate as a wife and mother; a young man having a hernia repair may worry that he will miss his chance to play in a championship football game. To provide the necessary support for adjustments, nurses need to determine each patient's concerns.

6. Use of medications. Because some medications react with anesthetics or other drugs, the nurse needs to list all medications (birth control pills, diuretics, vitamins, anticonvulsants, insulin, etc) the patient takes. Certain medications, such as anticonvulsants or insulin, must be continued throughout the operative period to prevent adverse effects. A physician's order to this effect is required, however.

7. Smoking habits. The lung tissue of a person who smokes is chronically irritated, and a general anesthetic irritates it further. When possible, nurses discourage patients from smoking on the day of surgery and are alert for respiratory complications following surgery.

8. Use of alcohol. Moderate use of alcohol does not usually present a surgical hazard, but heavy, consistent use can lead to problems during anesthesia, surgery, and recovery.

9. Names of family members and/or friends. Family members and friends provide considerable support to the surgical patient. They need to be recognized and often included in health instruction or follow-up care given to the patient.

Screening Tests

The physician is responsible for ordering all the radiologic and laboratory tests and examinations the patient needs. The nurse's responsibility is to check the orders carefully, to see that they are carried out, and to ensure that the results are obtained prior to surgery. Some screening tests conducted prior to surgery are:

1. Chest roentgenography, to determine the condition of the patient's lungs and in some situations heart size and location. The results may influence the physician's choice of both the preoperative sedation and the anesthetic.

2. Blood analysis, on the day before surgery when possible. Analysis may include: red blood cell count (RBC), hemoglobin (Hb or Hgb), and hematocrit (Hct). If substantial blood loss is anticipated during surgery, the physician may order a blood typing and cross-match and sufficient units of blood for a replacement transfusion. When the physician anticipates bleeding problems, an analysis of bleeding time, clotting time, or prothrombin time may also be ordered. The results of blood tests are important in ruling out many problems that could increase the surgical risk. For example, a high white blood cell count (WBC) may signal an infection; a low red blood cell count (RBC) or low hemoglobin may indicate anemia. Both conditions can delay healing. Other blood tests usually routinely included are fasting blood sugar, blood urea nitrogen, and creatinine.

3. Urine analysis for all patients before surgery. The results may indicate urinary infection, diabetes, or other abnormalities that warrant treatment prior to surgery. See Table 31–1 for routine preoperative screening tests.

TABLE 31–1 ■ Routine Preoperative Screening Tests

Test	Rationale
Urinalysis	To detect urinary tract infections and glucose in the urine
Chest roentgenography	To identify lung pathology and heart size and location
Electrocardiography (usual for patients who have cardiac pathology)	To determine cardiac pathology
Complete blood count (CBC)	To determine Hgb, Hct, RBC (ie, the blood's ability to carry oxygen), and WBC, which signals infection when elevated
Blood grouping and cross-matching	To establish blood type for possible blood transfusion
Serum electrolytes (Na^+, K^+, Mg^{2+}, Ca^{2+}, H^+)	To determine electrolyte imbalances
Fasting blood sugar	To detect the presence of a glucose in the blood, which may indicate metabolic disorders, eg, diabetes mellitus
Blood urea nitrogen (BUN) or creatinine	To assess urinary excretion

4. Electrocardiogram for all middle-aged and elderly patients and for patients suspected of having cardiac disease (LeMaitre, Finnegan, 1980, p 54).

In addition to these routine tests, diagnostic tests directly related to the patient's pathology are usually appropriate (eg, stomach roentgenography to clarify the pathology before gastric surgery). See chapter 11.

TECHNIQUE 31–1 ■ Preoperative Preparation and Teaching

The goal of preoperative preparation and teaching is to promote optimal physical and psychologic health, thereby minimizing surgical risk. Potential problems associated with anesthesia are also prevented.

■ Assessment

See Preoperative Assessment on page 748. Additional data include:

1. The type of surgery. The surgeon usually indicates the type of surgery in the preoperative order on the patient's chart. From this information, the nurse can determine the kind and extent of skin preparation required, if it has not been specified on the order. Agencies usually have standard directions for the skin preparations for various surgical procedures.

2. The time of the surgery. The surgeon usually arranges the date for the surgery and may specify this in the order. The exact time often is not known until the surgical schedule for the hospital is distributed.

3. The name of the surgeon. The surgeon is specified in the preoperative order.

4. The preoperative orders. Special arrangements may be ordered, such as skin preparation, enema, or insertion of a catheter or Levin tube. Some agencies maintain a Kardex file in which the surgeon's preferences are noted (eg, "Saline enema the night before surgery").

5. The agency's practices for preoperative care. Many agencies outline the nursing responsibilities for preoperative care.

6. The learning needs of the patient. The surgeon is usually responsible for explaining the surgical procedure to the patient. However, nurses are often asked to explain aspects of care. If the patient is anxious about the procedure or has questions that the nurse is unable to answer, the surgeon should be notified.

   The patient may have specific learning needs in regard to his or her postoperative condition. Learning to attend to a colostomy or the like requires some preparation *before* surgery.

   Pain is common postoperatively, and patients are reassured to learn beforehand ways in which they can minimize it, eg, holding a pillow against the abdomen when moving after abdominal surgery or when carrying out coughing and deep-breathing exercises. It is important for most patients to know that they can receive analgesics postoperatively and therefore should experience only minimal discomfort.

   Most patients who undergo operations also need to learn skills for moving, deep breathing, coughing, and various exercises. These are discussed in Intervention, steps 16–27.

7. Verification that the physician has completed the medical history and physical examination. Most hospitals require that these be completed before surgery, except in emergency situations. Nurses need to check agency policy in this regard.

8. Verification that the consent form has been signed by the patient or the family. Prior to any surgical procedure patients must sign a surgical consent form. See Figure 31–1. This requirement protects patients from having any surgical procedure they do not want or do not know about. It also protects the hospital and the health personnel from a claim by patients or family that permission was not granted. The consent form becomes a part of the patient's record and goes to the operating room with the patient.

   Obtaining legal, informed consent to perform surgery is the responsibility of the surgeon. Informed consent is possible only when the patient is told in advance of the character and importance of the surgery, its probable consequences, the chances for success, and alternative measures. Often the responsibility for obtaining consent is delegated to a nurse. The nurse must be aware of his or her responsibilities regarding consents and be aware of the particular hospital's policies.

   Adults sign their own forms unless they are mentally incompetent or unconscious, in which cases a

EL CAMINO HOSPITAL DISTRICT

Pt. Name
Hosp. No.
Rm. No.

AUTHORIZATION AND CONSENT TO SURGERY, ANESTHESIA, DIAGNOSTIC OR THERAPEUTIC PROCEDURES

YOUR DOCTOR IS _____

THE OPERATION(S) OR PROCEDURE(S) TO BE PERFORMED IS/ARE:

_____

(MEDICAL TERMINOLOGY)

_____

(LAY TERMINOLOGY)

1. The hospital maintains personnel and facilities to assist your doctor in his performance of various surgical operations and other special diagnostic and therapeutic procedures. These operations and procedures may all involve risks of unsuccessful results, complications, injury, or even death, from both known and unforeseen causes, and no warranty or guarantee is made as to result or cure. You have the right to be informed of such risks as well as the nature and purpose of the operation(s) or procedure(s) and the available alternative methods of treatment and this form is not a substitute for such explanations which are provided by the above named physician. Except in cases of emergency, the operation(s) or procedure(s) is/are not performed until the patient has had the opportunity to receive such explanations. You may refuse any proposed operation or procedure anytime prior to its performance.

2. Your doctor has recommended the operation(s) or procedure(s) set forth above. Upon your authorization and consent, such operation(s) or procedure(s), together with any different or further procedure(s) which in the opinion of your doctor may be indicated due to any emergency, will be performed on you. The operation(s) or procedure(s) will be performed by the doctor named above together with associates and assistants, including anesthesiologists and radiologists from the medical staff of El Camino Hospital. Your attending physician, surgeon, assistant surgeon, anesthesiologist, and other physicians are not agents, servants or employees of the hospital or your doctor but are independent contractors, and therefore your agents.

3. Your signature below authorizes the hospital pathologist to use his or her discretion in disposition of any member, organ or other tissue removed from your person during the above-named procedure(s).

4. Your signature below constitutes your acknowledgement (1) that you have read and agree to the foregoing; (2) that the operation(s) or procedure(s) set forth above has/have been adequately explained to you by your doctor and that you have received all of the information you desire concerning such operation(s) or procedure(s); (3) that you authorize and consent to the performance of the operation(s) or procedure(s); (4) and that you acknowledge receipt of a copy of this authorization.

SIGNATURE:_____   _____
              PATIENT/PARENT/LEGAL GUARDIAN   DATE AND TIME

_____   _____
RELATIONSHIP   WITNESS (NOT PATIENT'S DOCTOR)

_____
REASON PATIENT UNABLE TO SIGN

FIGURE 31-1 ■ A sample consent form for sugery and treatment. (Courtesy of El Camino Hospital, Mountain View, California.)

spouse or next of kin signs for them. Children 19 or younger (18 or younger in some jurisdictions) cannot sign consent forms. A parent or guardian must sign instead. However, some jurisdictions allow teenagers to give consent. In Ontario, a 16-year-old can give consent for surgery. In Quebec, a minor of 14 years can give consent (and be operated on without the parents' knowledge), provided the minor is not hospitalized longer than 12 hours and treatment is not prolonged (Creighton, 1981, p 274). If a minor's parents cannot be found, a court order can be obtained to permit surgery.

9. Results of blood, urine, and other screening tests.

■ Planning

Nursing goals

1. To identify and meet the learning needs of the patient and support persons
2. To promote the patient's peace of mind
3. To maintain fluid and nutritional needs or correct nutritional deficiencies
4. To promote rest
5. To reduce the number of skin microorganisms and thus the potential for postoperative infection
6. To prevent aspiration of vomitus and respiratory obstruction by oral prostheses during anesthesia
7. To prevent physical trauma to the patient during anesthesia
8. To protect the patient's personal property during the intraoperative period (during surgery)
9. To ensure that the patient's physical status (eg, circulation) can be assessed appropriately during the intraoperative period

■ Intervention

Preparing the patient the day before surgery

Psychologic support

1. Listen attentively and carefully to the patient to help him or her identify specific concerns or fears and talk them through. Typical questions are: What will happen during surgery? How will I feel after the operation? What will the surgeon find? How long will the hospital stay be? Some patients may be worrying about finances. Others, whose surgery involves disfigurement of some kind, may be having problems with self-image.
2. Clarify any misconceptions the patient may have. Provide accurate information and act supportively to help the patient deal with identified concerns. Do not dismiss the patient's concerns by saying, "Everything will be all right."
   Rationale Unknowns or misconceptions can produce unrealistic fears and anxiety.
3. Provide explanations to children in a language they can understand. Give children information at a rate that keeps their attention and does not overwhelm them. Show the child the anesthetic equipment and the postanesthesia room ("wake-up room") before the surgery. Explain all postoperative care and

discomfort clearly and simply, for example, "You will have a sore tummy." Confirm when the parents will visit, because this is the most important fact to the child (Luciano, 1974, p 65).

Nutritional and hydration status

4. Assess and record any sign of malnutrition. See Assessing Nutritional Status in chapter 24 on page 518.
5. Measure the patient's weight.
6. Measure the patient's fluid intake and output.
   Rationale Adequate hydration and nutrition promote healing.

Fasting six to eight hours before surgery

7. Remove food and fluids from the bedside.
8. Place a fasting sign at the bed the evening before surgery.
9. Provide the patient with a mouthwash and encourage use of it if the mouth feels dry.
10. If the patient ingests food or fluids during the fasting period, notify the surgeon.
    Rationale The patient fasts at least six to eight hours before surgery because anesthetics depress gastrointestinal functioning and because there is a danger the patient may vomit and aspirate vomitus during administration of a general anesthetic.

Special elimination care

11. Determine and provide special elimination care as ordered. Depending on the patient's condition, the type of surgery, the physician's order, and agency practice, an enema may be given the evening before surgery. Sometimes a rectal suppository is given instead of an enema, or the enema may be administered the day of surgery. In some instances, a urinary catheter is inserted the day before or the day of surgery, depending on the surgeon's order and agency practice. In other instances, no special elimination care is given.
    Rationale An enema or suppository may be given to empty the bowel because anesthesia and abdominal surgery decrease bowel activity for a few days postoperatively. A series of enemas may be given if surgery on the bowel is planned. A urinary catheter may be inserted for pelvic surgery to prevent inadvertent injury to the bladder.

Surgical skin preparation

12. See Technique 31–2 on page 759.

Hygienic care

13. Ensure that appropriate hygienic care is implemented. In many settings, patients are encouraged to bathe or shower with an antimicrobial agent the evening or the morning before surgery (or both). The bath includes a shampoo whenever possible. The patient's nails should be trimmed and free of polish.

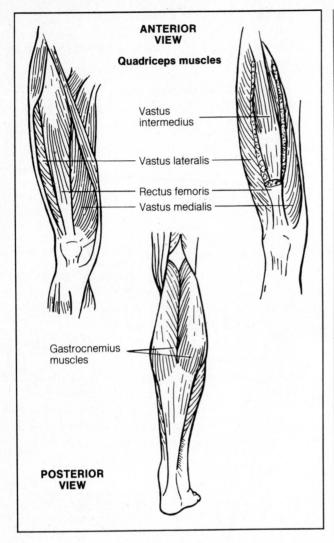

ANTERIOR VIEW

Quadriceps muscles

Vastus intermedius

Vastus lateralis

Rectus femoris
Vastus medialis

Gastrocnemius muscles

POSTERIOR VIEW

FIGURE 31–2

Rationale Nail beds need to be assessed during surgery for cyanosis and pallor, which are indications of inadequate oxygenation of the blood. Bathing with antimicrobial agents reduces the risk of post-operative incisional infections.

Rest and medications

14. Ensure that the patient rests well prior to surgery.

    Rationale Rest helps the patient manage the stress of surgery.

15. Inform the patient that the anesthetist or anesthesiologist will visit the patient preoperatively to discuss the anesthetic and order the preoperative medications. Usually a sedative is ordered the night before surgery to ensure that the patient sleeps well. Preoperative medications are discussed on page 757.

Teaching postoperative exercises

Leg exercises, coughing, deep breathing, and moving are important skills for preoperative patients to learn to speed convalescence and help prevent complications.

Leg exercises

16. Teach the patient the following three exercises, which contract and relax the quadriceps muscles (vastus intermedius, vastus lateralis, rectus femoris, and vastus medialis) and the gastrocnemius muscles (see Figure 31–2):

    a. Alternate dorsiflexion and plantar flexion of the feet. This exercise is sometimes referred to as *calf pumping*, since it alternately contracts and relaxes the calf muscles, including the gastrocnemius muscles.

    b. Flex and extend the knees, and press the backs of the knees into the bed. See Figure 31–3. Patients who cannot raise their legs can do isometric exercises that contract and relax the muscles (see chapter 19, page 430).

    c. Raise and lower the legs alternately from the surface of the bed. Extend the knee of the moving

FIGURE 31–3

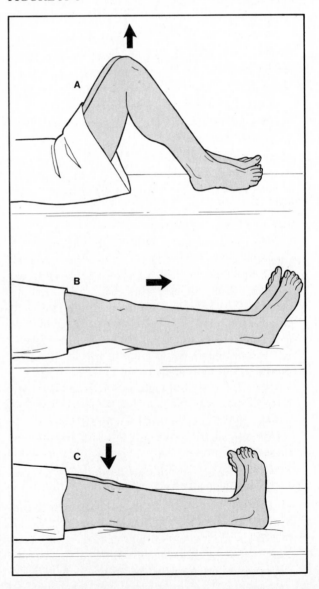

leg. See Figure 31–4. This exercise contracts and relaxes the quadriceps muscles.

Rationale Leg exercises help prevent thrombophlebitis due to slowed venous circulation (venous stasis). The major danger of thrombophlebitis is that thrombi can become emboli and lodge in the arteries of the heart, brain, or lungs, causing serious injury or death.

17. Instruct the patient to start exercising as soon after surgery as she or he is able.

18. Encourage the patient to do exercises at least once every waking hour. Note, however, that the frequency of exercising depends on the patient's condition and the agency's practices.

19. Explain to the patient that these muscle contractions will compress the veins and promote venous circulation.

Coughing and deep-breathing exercises

20. Demonstrate deep (diaphragmatic) breathing exercises as follows:

    a. Place your hands palm down on the border of your rib cage, and inhale slowly and evenly through the nose until the greatest chest expansion is achieved. See Figure 31–5.

    b. Hold your breath for 2 to 3 seconds.

    c. Exhale slowly through the mouth.

    d. Continue exhalation until maximum chest contraction is achieved.

21. Have the patient assume a sitting position and perform deep-breathing exercises while placing the palms of your hands on the border of the patient's rib cage.

    Rationale Deep-breathing exercises help remove mucus, which can form and remain in the lungs due to the effects of a general anesthetic and analgesics. These drugs depress the action of both the cilia of the mucous membranes lining the respiratory tract and the respiratory center in the brain. Deep breathing also aerates lung tissue and thereby helps prevent pneumonia, which may result from stagnation of fluid in the lungs.

22. Have the patient voluntarily cough after a few deep inhalations. Have the patient inhale deeply, hold the breath for a few seconds, and then cough one or two times. Ensure that the patient coughs deeply and does not just clear the throat. Splinting the abdomen with clasped hands and a pillow held against the abdomen helps coughing be effective.

    Rationale Deep breathing frequently initiates the coughing reflex. Voluntary coughing in conjunction with deep breathing facilitates the movement and expectoration of respiratory tract secretions.

23. If the patient will have an incision that will be painful when coughing, demonstrate how the nurse

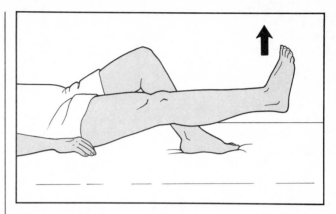

FIGURE 31–4

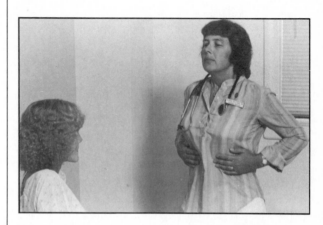

FIGURE 31–5

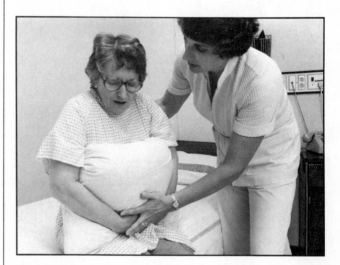

FIGURE 31–6

or patient can support (splint) it as the patient coughs. Place the palms of your hands on either side of the incision or directly over the incision, holding the palm of one hand over the other. Also instruct the patient with an abdominal incision how to splint the incision independently with a firmly rolled pillow. See Figure 31–6.

Rationale Coughing uses the abdominal and other accessory respiratory muscles. Splinting the incision may reduce pain while coughing if the incision is near any of these muscles.

24. Instruct the patient to start the exercises as soon after surgery as he or she is able.

25. Encourage patients with abdominal or chest surgery to carry out deep breathing and coughing at least three or four times daily and at each session to take a minimum of five breaths. Note, however, that the number of breaths and frequency of deep breathing varies with the patient's condition. Patients who are susceptible to pulmonary problems may need deep-breathing exercises every hour. Patients with chronic respiratory disease may need special breathing exercises, eg, pursed-lip breathing, abdominal breathing, exercises using blow bottles and various kinds of incentive spirometers. See Techniques 36–1 and 36–2 on pages 853 and 856.

26. Explain to the patient that deep-breathing and coughing exercises will increase lung expansion and prevent the accumulation of secretions, which may occur after anesthesia.

Moving

After surgery, turning in bed and early ambulation are encouraged to help patients maintain blood circulation, stimulate respiratory functions, and decrease the stasis of gas in the intestines (and its resulting discomfort). Patients who practice turning before surgery usually find it easier to do postoperatively.

27. Show the patient ways to turn in bed and to get out of bed. Have the patient start from the supine position.

   a. Instruct a patient who will have a right abdominal incision or a right-sided chest incision to turn to the left side of the bed and sit up as follows:

      ■ Flex the knees.

      ■ Hold the left arm and hand or a small pillow against the incision to splint the wound.

      ■ Turn to the left while pushing with the right foot and grasping the side rail on the left side of the bed with the right hand.

      ■ Raise himself or herself to a sitting position on the side of the bed by using the right arm and hand to push down against the mattress.

   b. For a patient with a left abdominal or left-sided chest incision, reverse the procedure.

   c. For patients with orthopedic surgery (eg, hip surgery), use special aids, such as a trapeze to assist with movement.

Preparation the day of surgery

Vital signs

28. Take vital signs to obtain comparative baseline data against which to assess the patient's responses during and following surgery. Report promptly any abnormalities, eg, an elevated temperature, to the responsible nurse and to the physician.

   Rationale Any abnormality can cause surgery to be postponed.

Fasting and oral care

29. Ensure that the patient fasts for the prescribed time.

30. Provide mouthwash, and instruct the patient not to swallow water during oral care but just to rinse out the mouth.

   Rationale The fasting patient may feel thirsty and have a dry mouth.

Hygiene and gowns

31. Assist the patient with a complete or partial bath, as required. Have the patient put on a clean hospital gown, fastened only at the neck or not at all, in accordance with agency policy. In some agencies, patients wear surgical caps or stockings for added warmth or protection. Also, antiemboli stockings are ordered for patients in some agencies. See Technique 32–4 on page 787.

   Rationale An untied gown can be readily removed during the operative and immediate postoperative period. Antiemboli stockings compress the peripheral veins and increase the venous return during the inactive period, thus preventing the formation of thrombi or emboli.

Hair and cosmetics

32. Remove or have the patient remove hairpins or clips. Long hair can be braided and fastened with elastic bands to keep it in place. All cosmetics (lipstick, rouge, nail polish, etc) must be removed. Check agency practice for the removal of nail polish if the patient does not have nail polish remover.

   Rationale Hairpins or clips may cause pressure or accidental damage to the scalp when the patient is unconscious. Cosmetics are removed so that the color of the skin, lips, and nail beds are visible to nurses and physicians when assessing circulation during and after surgery.

Valuables

33. Label jewelry, money, and other valuables, and place them in safekeeping to avoid loss or damage and subsequent legal problems. In most agencies, valuables are kept in special envelopes and locked in a storage area on the unit. If a patient does not want to remove a wedding band, tape it in place. Wedding bands must be removed, however, if there is danger of the fingers swelling after surgery. Situations warranting removal of a wedding band include surgery of or cast application to an arm and mastectomy that involves removal of the lymph nodes. Mastectomies may cause edema of the arm and hand.

Prostheses

34. Ensure that all prostheses (artificial body parts, such as partial or complete dentures, contact lenses, artificial eyes, or limbs), as well as eyeglasses, wigs, false eyelashes, and hearing aids, are removed. Also check for gum and loose teeth, a common problem with 5- or 6-year-old patients having tonsils removed. Check agency policy for the handling of prostheses. In some agencies they are placed in a locked storage area; in others they are kept at the patient's bedside.

    Rationale Partial dentures can become dislodged and obstruct an unconscious patient's breathing. Loose teeth can become dislodged and be aspirated during anesthesia. Other prostheses may become damaged.

Bowel and bladder

35. Check that the patient empties the bowel and bladder before surgery. If an enema is ordered, administer it soon enough on the day of surgery so that the patient has time to expel it. If the patient cannot void, note this on the patient's record.

    Rationale Voiding and emptying the large bowel prevent obstruction to surgery by a distended bowel or bladder, minimize risk of injury to the bowel and bladder, and minimize contamination of the peritoneal cavity if the bladder or bowel is the site of surgery.

36. Insert a retention (Foley) catheter if ordered. See chapter 27.

Special orders

37. Check the physician's orders for special requirements, such as the insertion of a nasogastric tube prior to surgery or the administration of medications, eg, insulin.

Preoperative medications

38. Check the orders for preoperative medications carefully before administering them. Usually a narcotic (eg, morphine) and a medication to dry the secretions of the mouth and respiratory tract (eg, atropine) are given by injection. Sometimes the surgeon orders that oral sedatives (eg, secobarbital) or tranquilizers be administered before the injectable medications are given. A newer trend is *not* to give any preoperative medications. It is essential to administer preoperative medications, if ordered, exactly at the time specified.

    Rationale A narcotic, sedative, or tranquilizer calms the patient before general anesthesia and enhances a smooth anesthesia induction. Atropine or a similar drying drug minimizes the danger that the patient will aspirate secretions into the lungs. Giving preoperative medications on time is essential because of their desired effect with the anesthetic.

39. After giving the preoperative medications, tell the patient that the medication will cause drowsiness and to remain quietly in bed. Raise the side rails and lower the bed for safety. Place the call light within reach. Also tell the patient that scopalomine or atropine may cause thirst and that he or she may use a mouthwash.

Recording

40. In most agencies, personnel use a preoperative checklist to record interventions. See Figure 31–7. Check the agency's forms, and follow appropriate recording procedures. It is essential that all pertinent records (laboratory records, x-ray films, consents, etc) be assembled and completed so that the operating and recovery room personnel can refer to them.

Transfer of the patient to surgery

41. When the operating room transport person arrives for the patient, carefully check the patient's identification bracelet against the patient's chart. Generally, one staff member reads the identifying data from the bracelet while another checks it against the patient's record. Do not rely on a drowsy patient to identify himself or herself.

Preparation for postoperative care

42. Prepare the patient's bed and room for the postoperative period.

    a. Make a surgical bed. See Technique 15–4 on page 368. In some agencies, the patient is brought back to the unit on a stretcher and transferred to the bed in her or his room. At other agencies, the surgical bed is taken to the recovery room (RR), and the patient is transferred there. If the latter occurs, the surgical bed needs to be made as soon as the patient goes to the operating room so that it can be taken to the RR at any time.

    b. Obtain and set up special equipment as needed, such as an intravenous pole, suction, oxygen equipment, and orthopedic appliances (traction, etc). If these are not requested on the patient's record, consult with the responsible nurse. Some surgeons have postoperative routines requiring certain equipment. In some instances, nursing personnel in the RR will notify the nursing unit before the patient arrives if special equipment is required.

    c. Obtain an emesis basin and tissues.

    d. Have available a sphygmomanometer and cuff and a stethoscope. Some agencies have sphygmomanometers attached to the wall at the head of the bed.

    e. Place an intake and output record nearby.

    f. When the patient is returned to the unit, carefully assist or lift him or her into the bed, if the patient is not already in it.

Form NS-68

ST. PAUL'S HOSPITAL
Vancouver, B.C.

PRE-OPERATIVE PREPARATION

EVENING PRIOR TO SURGERY—CHECK	Yes	Not Applicable
1. History—completed with signature		
2. Consultation (when necessary) on chart		
3. Treatment and operative consents—signed and witnessed		
4. Telephone no. of next of kin or friend:		
5. Identaband on wrist		
6. Allergy sign on chart and wristband		
7. Operative area prepared		
8. Pre-op bath or shower		
9. Pre-op teaching: a. Attended "Operation Tomorrow"		
b. Demonstrated deep breathing, coughing, and leg exercises		
c. Stated approximate time to OR and return to ward		
d. Stated expectations: • surgery planned		
• incision and dressing area		
• activity progression		
• pain and effect of analgesic		
• NPO, intravenous, diet progression		
• pre-op urine specimen		
e. Verbalized probable discharge plans		
10. H.S. sedation administered or refused—charted on anesthetic record		
11. Fasting sign posted		

DATE _____ SIGNATURE _____

IMMEDIATELY PRIOR TO SURGERY	Yes	Not Applicable
1. Pre-operative urine specimen sent		
2. Reports attached to chart—Lab, X-ray, ECG		
3. Old chart		
4. Addressograph plate attached		
5. Contact lens, wig, jewelry, make-up removed, prosthesis off		
6. Dentures and partial plates removed		
7. Voided _____ Catheterized—time _____ amount _____		
8. Patient in hospital gown		
9. Blood pressure, pulse and respirations taken at least an hour prior to pre-op medication—charted on clinical record		
10. Pre-medication administered and charted on the anesthetic record		
11. Notation made in nurses notes of time to surgery		

DATE _____ SIGNATURE _____

OPERATING ROOM	Yes	Not Applicable
1. Patient identified by circulating nurse		
2. Site of surgery checked by circulating nurse a. Left side _____ Right side _____		
b. Slate _____ Surgeon _____ History _____ Consent _____		

SIGNATURE _____

FIGURE 31-7 ■ A sample preoperative checklist. (Courtesy of St. Paul's Hospital, Nursing Department, Vancouver, British Columbia.)

■ Evaluation

Expected outcomes

1. Mild anxiety
2. Asks and answers questions about surgery
3. Expresses specific concerns about surgery and its outcomes
4. Adequate hydration status
5. Adequate nutritional status
6. Satisfactory vital signs
7. Normal serum electrolyte levels
8. Normal blood reports, eg, CBC, Hgb, Hct
9. Normal urinalysis

Unexpected outcomes

1. Extreme anxiety (eg, inappropriate or absence of verbalization, purposeless activity, withdrawal, increased muscle tension, hyperventilation, dilated pupils, pallor)
2. Dehydration
3. Obesity or emaciation
4. Elevated vital signs
5. Abnormal serum electrolyte levels
6. Abnormal blood reports
7. Abnormal urinalysis

Upon obtaining an unexpected outcome:

1. Report your findings to the responsible nurse and/or physician.
2. Adjust the nursing care plan accordingly.

TECHNIQUE 31–2   ■   Surgical Skin Preparation

The purpose of preparing the skin before surgery (preoperative skin preparation) is to destroy microorganisms and thus reduce the chance of an infection.

The skin is shaved the day of surgery, or as agency policy dictates. In some agencies the patient's skin is "prepped" in a special room just before surgery. The Centers for Disease Control recommend that the skin be prepared, ie, hair removed, and cleansed with antiseptics just before surgery (Simmons, 1983, p 133).

The area prepared is generally larger than the incision area. See Table 31–2. This practice minimizes the number of microorganisms in the areas adjacent to the incision. Hospital policy describes how the skin is prepared before various operations. In some settings, patients are shaved with electric clippers rather than razors.

TABLE 31–2   ■   Skin Preparation Areas

Area	Description	Indications	
Lower extremities			
Hip and thigh	Prepare from waistline to 15 cm (6 in) below knee; from 5 cm (2 in) past midbuttock to 5 cm (2 in) past midabdomen. Include complete perineal shave. See Figure 31–8.	Fractured femur Any upper leg or thigh surgery past	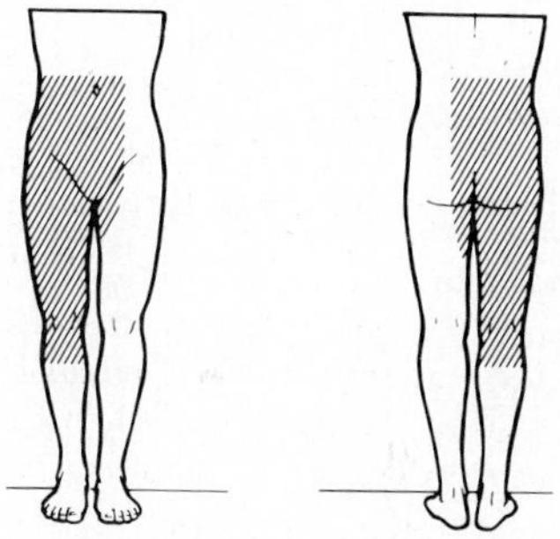 FIGURE 31–8
Knee	Prepare entire leg from ankle to groin. See Figure 31–9.	Meniscectomy Knee prosthesis	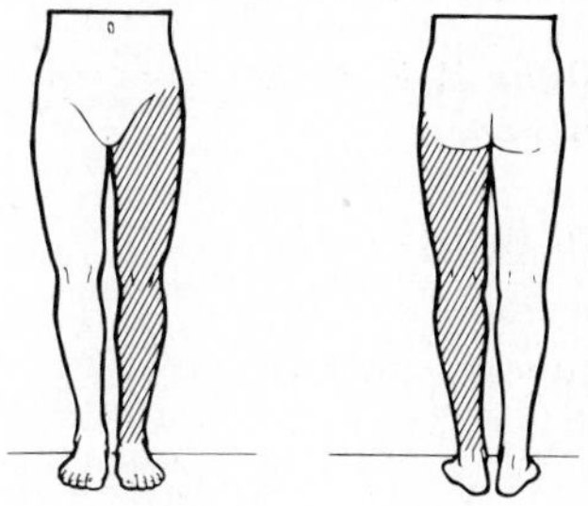 FIGURE 31–9
Lower leg or foot	Prepare entire foot and leg to 20 cm (8 in) above knee. Clean and trim toenails, and remove nail polish. See Figure 31–10.	Open reductions of tibia and fibula Ankle surgery	FIGURE 31–10 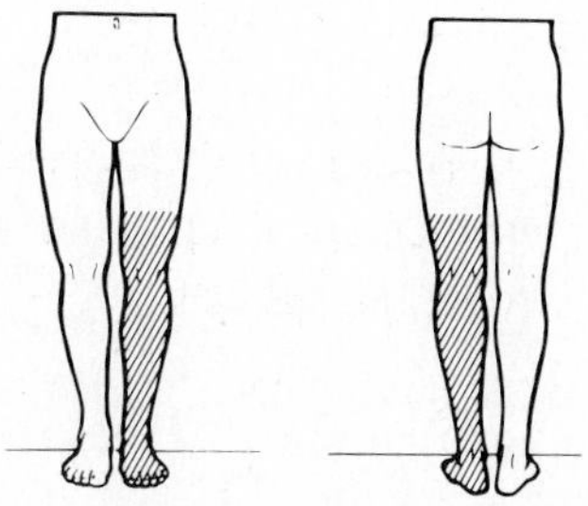

TABLE 31–2 ■ continued

Area	Description	Indications	
Foot	Prepare entire foot and leg to mid-calf. Clean and trim toenails, and remove nail polish. See Figure 31–11.	Bunions Ingrown toenails	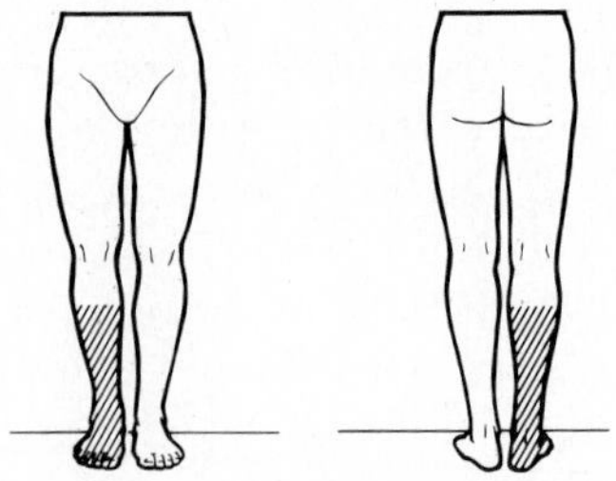 **FIGURE 31–11**
Complete lower extremity	Prepare entire foot and leg, extending up above the umbilicus. Include complete perineal shave. See Figure 31–12.	Femoral arterial graft. Ligation and stripping of varicose veins	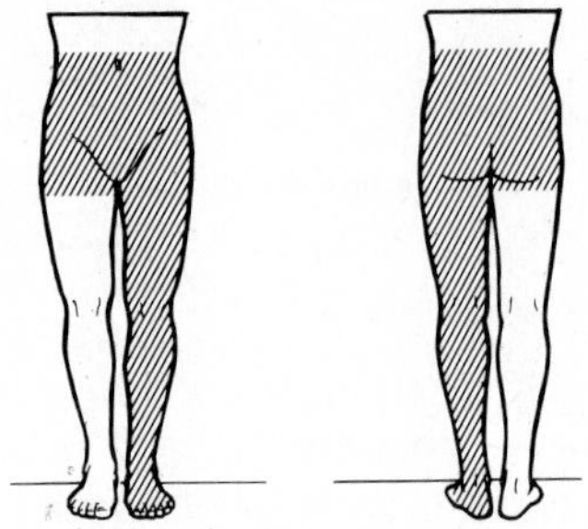 **FIGURE 31–12**
Abdomen and leg	Prepare entire abdomen to the bedline on patient's sides and from axillary margins extending down affected side to below knee and on other leg to midthigh. On the back, include buttocks, backs of legs as far down as on fronts, and a complete perineal preparation. See Figure 31–13.	Femoral popliteal artery surgery Common iliac artery surgery	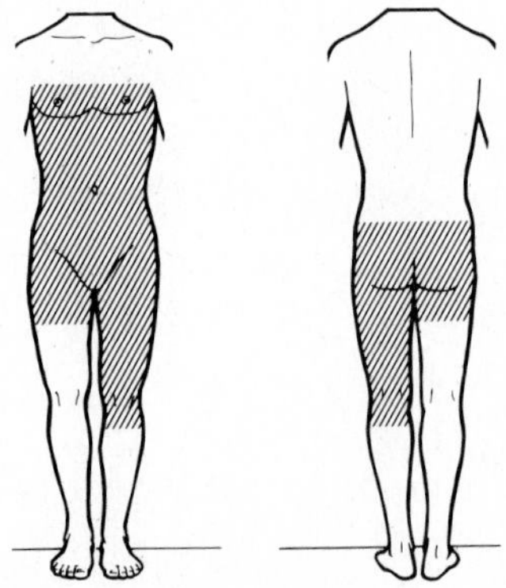 **FIGURE 31–13**
Abdomen Incision above the umbilicus	Prepare entire abdomen from axillary margins to tops of thighs, including all visible pubic hair, and to the bedline on patient's sides. See Figure 31–14.	Cholecystectomy Gastrectomy	**FIGURE 31–14**
Incision below the umbilicus	Prepare entire abdomen from nipple line to midthigh. Include all visible pubic hair when legs are together. Prepare to the bedline on each side. See Figure 31–15.	Appendectomy Hernia repair	**FIGURE 31–15** 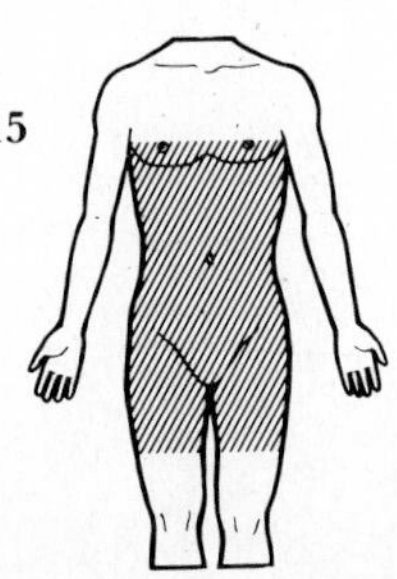

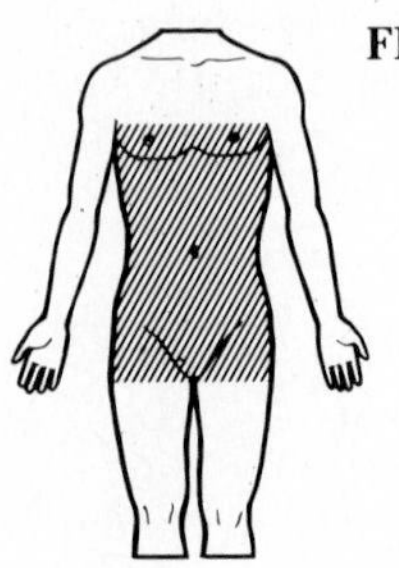

TABLE 31–2   ■   continued

Area	Description	Indications	
Perineal	Prepare pubic area (pubes), perineum, and inner side of thighs and buttocks. See Figure 31–16.	Rectal surgery Vaginal surgery Prostatectomy	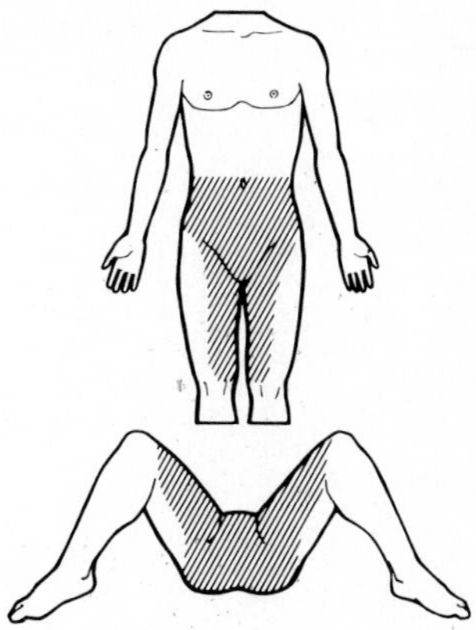 FIGURE 31–16
Kidney	Prepare from 5 cm (2 in) past midline of abdomen to 5 cm (2 in) past midline of back, from nipple line to pubes, including visible pubic hair when legs are together. Include axillary shave. See Figure 31–17.	Nephrectomy Removal of kidney stones in kidney or high in ureter	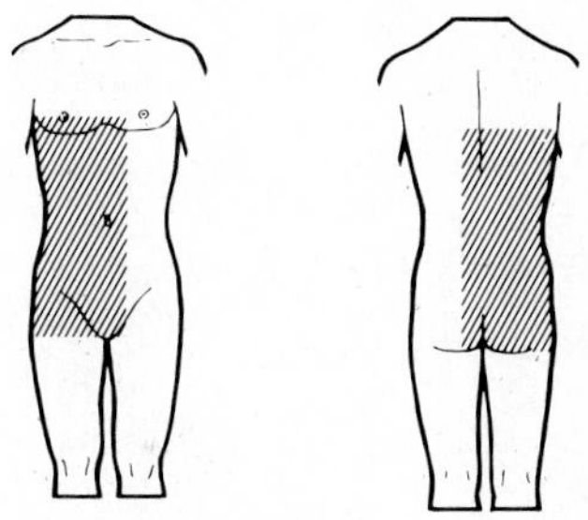 FIGURE 31–17
Back Cervical spine	Prepare from 2.5 cm (1 in) above external occipital protuberance to midlumbar area of back and to the bedline on both sides. See Figure 31–18.	Cervical spine surgery (posterior)	FIGURE 31–18
Posterior thoracic and lumbar spine	Prepare from hairline to bottom of buttocks and to the bedline on both sides. See Figure 31–19.	Thoracic spine surgery Lumbar spine surgery	FIGURE 31–19 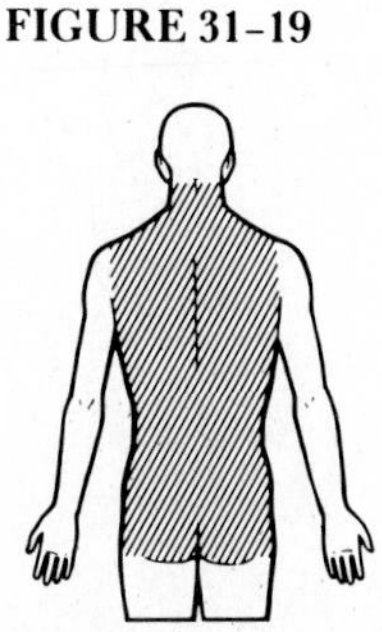

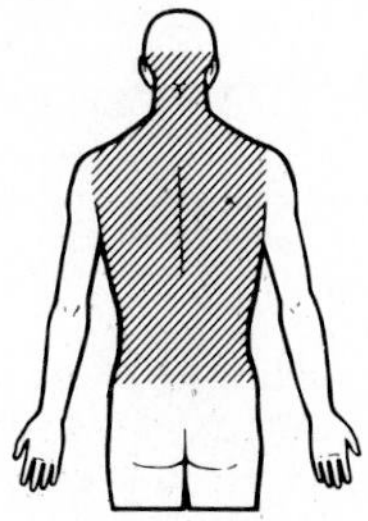

TABLE 31-2 ■ continued

Area	Description	Indications	
Spinal surgery	Prepare the back from the axillary line to midthigh and to the bedline on each side. See Figure 31-20.	Intractable pain Spinal tumor Spina bifida	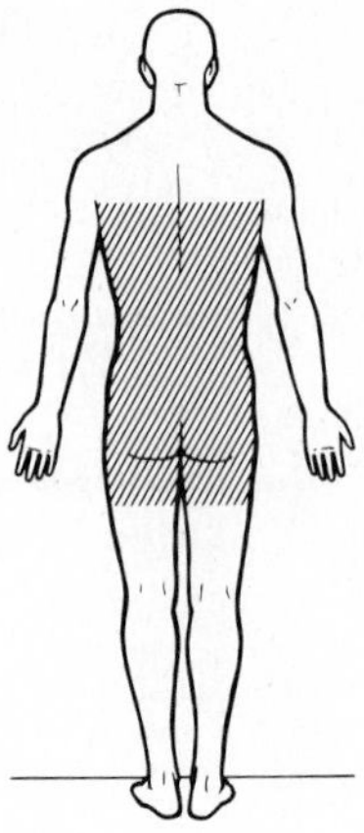 **FIGURE 31-20**
Chest			
Chest and closed heart surgery	Prepare from nipple line of opposite breast over affected breast to midline of back, from shoulder to umbilicus, and whole arm from shoulder to 2.5 cm (1 in) below elbow. Include axillary shave. It may be necessary to prepare complete chest (both sides and both shoulders). See Figure 31-21.	Breast surgery Lung surgery	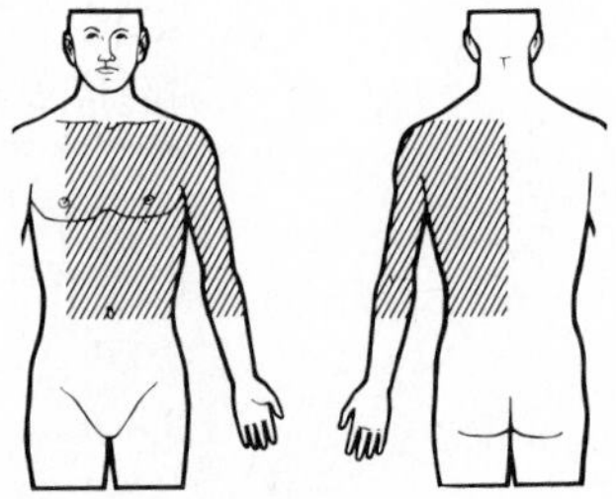 **FIGURE 31-21**
Open heart surgery	Prepare from chin to midthigh and to the bedline on each side. Include both axillae, upper arms to elbows, and visible pubic hair when legs are together. Preparation of thighs is necessary because "pump oxygenator" is used during surgery. See Figure 31-22.	Open heart surgery	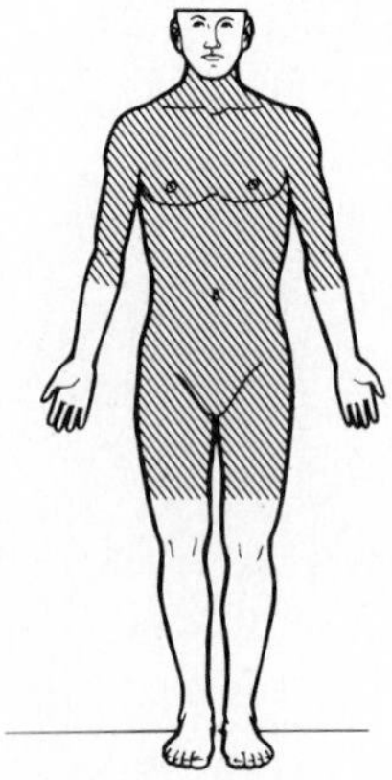 **FIGURE 31-22**
Neck	Prepare from chin to nipple line and from right shoulder to left shoulder. See Figure 31-23.	Thyroid surgery	**FIGURE 31-23** 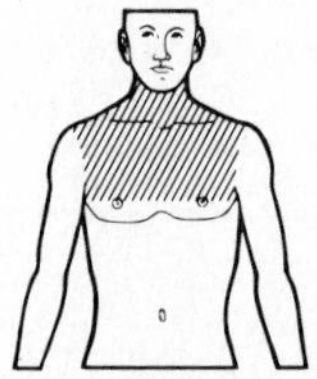

TABLE 31-2 ■ continued

Area	Description	Indications
Upper extremities		
Lower arm	Remove rings, clean and trim nails, and remove nail polish. Check that identification bracelet is on unaffected arm. Prepare entire affected hand and arm up to shoulder. See Figure 31–24.	Forearm surgery Hand surgery

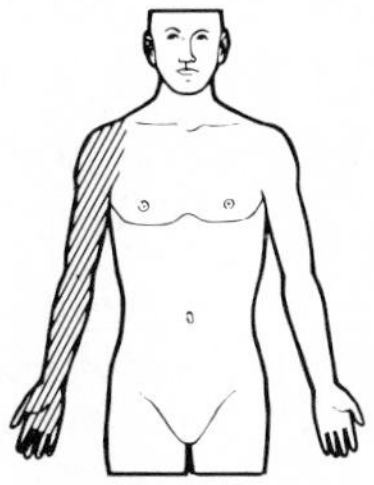

FIGURE 31–24

Upper arm	Prepare from 5 cm (2 in) past midline on back to 5 cm (2 in) past midline of chest. Include shoulder, axilla, and arm to 5 cm (2 in) below elbow. See Figure 31–25.	Shoulder surgery

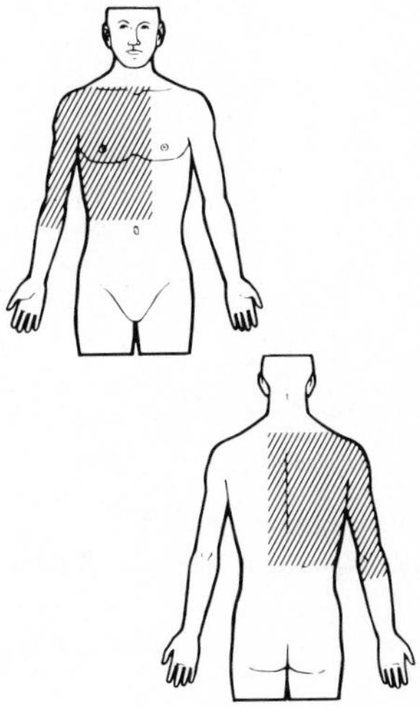

FIGURE 31–25

Elbow	Prepare entire arm, including shoulder and hand. Include axillary shave. See Figure 31–26.	

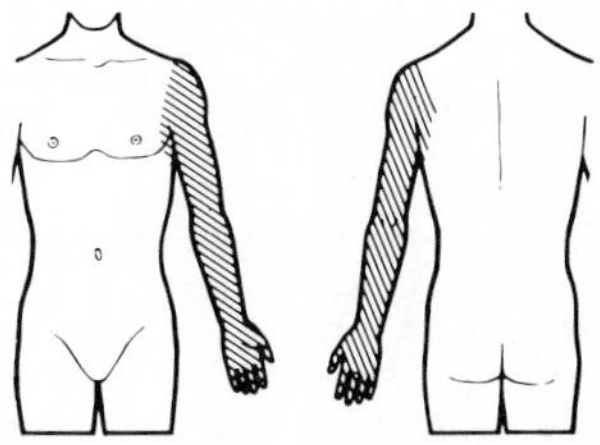

FIGURE 31–26

Upper extremity (entire)	Prepare from 5 cm (2 in) past midline on back to 5 cm (2 in) past midline on chest. Include complete shoulder, axilla, arm, and hand. See Figure 31–27.	Fracture of humerus

FIGURE 31–27

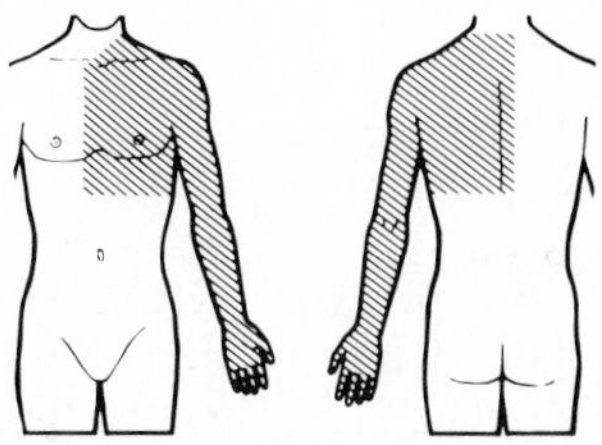

TABLE 31–2 ■ continued

Area	Description	Indications	
Head			
Cranium	Determine exact area to be prepared. Cut long hair with scissors. Shaving may be done in operating room before operation, after patient is anesthetized. Save hair, which is patient's property, to give to patient upon discharge. See Figure 31–28.	Craniotomy	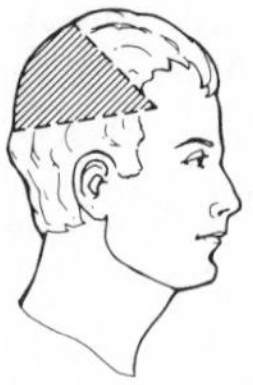 **FIGURE 31–28**
Nasal area	Have male patients shave themselves, including mustache, on morning of surgery. Prepare from bridge of nose on both sides of face to ears and under the chin. With blunt-tipped scissors, cut hairs as far up nares as possible. See Figure 31–29.	Submucous resection Removal of polyp	**FIGURE 31–29** 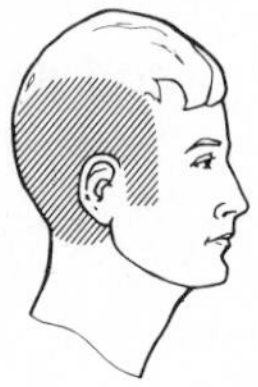
Mastoid and ear	Prepare 5 to 8 cm (2 to 3 in) behind hear. Clip all visible hair around external auditory meatus. Comb lacquer into long hair to midline on operative side; hold hair away from area with bobby pins. Repeat on morning of surgery and remove pins. See Figure 31–30.	Myringotomy (incision of tympanic membrane) Mastoidectomy Stapedectomy	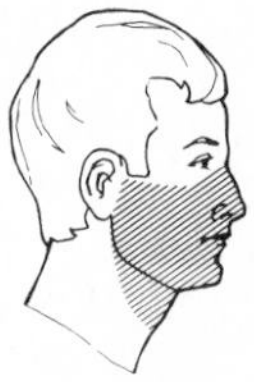 **FIGURE 31–30**
Skin	Determine exact area to be prepared from physician's order.	Skin graft Bone graft	

■ Assessment

Assess the skin preparation area for:

1. Growths, moles, etc
2. The presence of rashes, pustules, irritations, or exudate
3. Abrasions, bruises, broken or ischemic areas

Other data include:

1. The order for the "skin prep"
2. The kind of surgery to be performed and any special orders about the skin preparation, including the area to be prepared
3. The patient's allergies to solutions used in skin preparation, such as the antiseptic applied to the skin

■ Planning

Nursing goals

1. To remove the hair from a defined skin area
2. To clean the area, reducing the number of microorganisms, which could cause a wound infection postoperatively

Equipment

1. Adequate lighting for clear visibility of the hair on the skin
2. A bath blanket to drape the patient

Dry shave

3. Electric clippers with sharp heads and unbroken teeth
4. Scissors for long hair, if needed
5. Antiseptic solution and applicators, if needed

Wet shave

6. Skin preparation set, which contains a disposable razor, compartmentalized basin for solutions, moisture-proof drape to protect the bedding, soap solution, sponges for applying the soap solution, and cotton-tipped applicators for cleaning areas such as the umbilicus
7. Warm water to make the soap solution

■ Intervention

Before shaving

1. Drape the patient. Expose only the area to be shaved at one time. You will shave about 15 cm (6 in) at a time.

Dry shaving

2. Make sure the area is dry.
3. Shave with clippers; do not apply pressure.
   Rationale Pressure can cause abrasions, particularly over bony prominences.
4. Move the drape, and repeat steps 2 and 3 until entire area to be prepared is shaved. If applying antiseptic solution, follow the steps in the section below on cleaning and disinfecting.

Wet shaving

5. Place the moisture-proof towel under the area to be prepared.
6. Lather the skin well with the soap solution.
7. Stretch the skin taut and hold the razor at about a 45° angle to the skin. Shave in the direction that the hair grows. See Figure 31–31. Use short strokes and rinse the razor frequently.
   Rationale Rinsing removes hairs and lather that can obstruct the blade.
8. Wipe excess hair off the skin with the sponges.
9. Move drape and repeat steps 6–8 until entire area to be prepared is shaved.

Cleaning and disinfecting

10. Clean any body crevices, such as the umbilicus, nails, or ear canals, with applicators and solutions. Dry with swabs.
11. If an antiseptic solution is used, apply it to the area immediately after it is shaved. Leave it the designated time, then dry the area with clean swabs. Agency policy will guide you on whether to use an antiseptic and, if so, which to use and how long to leave it on.

After shaving

12. After shaving, report completion of the skin preparation to the responsible nurse. At some agencies, the skin preparation must be checked by the responsible nurse. Male perineal preparations may be checked by a male nurse if the responsible nurse is female. Report to the responsible nurse any abrasions, including those made by the clippers or razor.

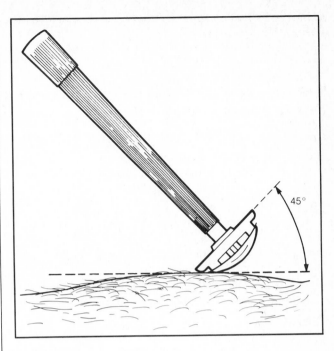

FIGURE 31-31

13. Remove the waterproof towel and bath blanket carefully so as not to spill the shaved hairs onto the bed.
14. Record the skin preparation on the patient's chart. Include an assessment of the preparation area (eg, whether or not abrasions are present) and relevant responses of the patient.

Sample Recording

Date	Time	Notes
12/5/86	0830	Wet skin prep done on left lower extremity. Skin intact. Appeared tense. Stated: "I hope the scar won't show much." ———— Eunice L. Lentz, NS

■ Evaluation

Expected outcomes

1. Absence of growths, moles, etc
2. Absence of rashes, abrasions, broken or ischemic areas

Unexpected outcomes

1. Presence of broken area
2. Presence of abraded area and bruises

Upon obtaining an unexpected outcome: Report your findings to the responsible nurse and/or physician.

GASTRIC INTUBATION

Gastric intubation is the insertion of a tube into the stomach, through either the nose, the mouth, or a gastrostomy opening. *Nasogastric tubes* can be passed through either the mouth or the nose; however, the nose is preferred because there is less discomfort from the gag reflex. A tube passed through the mouth is often called an *orogastric tube.*

Several types of nasogastric tubes are used for irrigation and gastric decompression. Gastric decompression is the reduction of the pressure within the stomach, eg, by removal of the gastric contents. The *Levin tube* is commonly used for nasogastric intubation. It is a flexible, rubber or plastic, single-lumen tube with holes near the tip. See Figure 31–32, *A.* Inserting a Levin tube is often the nurse's responsibility. The *Salem sump tube,* which is also frequently used, is a nasogastric tube with a double lumen.

Some tubes pass through the patient's mouth or nose and through the stomach into the intestines. Physicians and nurse specialists usually insert such tubes. The *Miller-Abbott tube* is a double-lumen tube; one lumen leads to a balloon near the tip, and the other lumen leads to the end of the tube opening into the intestine. See Figure 31–32, *B.* This tube is inserted into the small intestine, usually (a) to obtain secretions for diagnostic study or (b) for irrigation. The external end of the tube has a metal adapter with two openings. One inflates or deflates the balloon; the other drains intestinal secretions. The *Cantor tube* is a single-lumen tube with an inflatable bag at the tip and several holes along the distal end. See Figure 31–32, *C.* The bag is filled with mercury before the tube is inserted. The weight of the mercury causes the tube to move into the intestines. The *Harris tube* is a single-lumen tube with a metal tip. The Harris tube is used for irrigations and suctions of the small intestines. See Figure 31–32, *D.*

FIGURE 31–32 ■ Four types of tubes used for gastric and intestinal suction and irrigation: **A,** Levin; **B,** Miller-Abbott; **C,** Cantor; **D,** Harris.

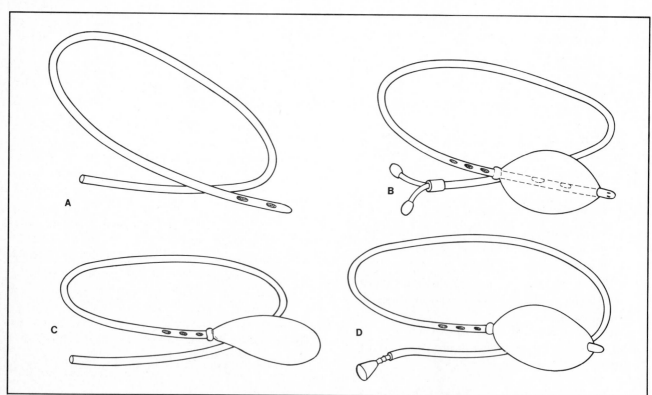

TECHNIQUE 31–3 ■ Inserting and Removing a Nasogastric Tube

Some patients, for instance, those having gastric or duodenal surgery, require the insertion of a Levin (gastric) tube preoperatively. The tube removes fluid and flatus from the stomach, thereby preventing nausea, vomiting, and distention due to reduced peristaltic action after surgery. In many agencies, insertion of a nasogastric tube is done by a registered nurse or a student with supervision. However, the passing of the tube is the responsibility of the physician for the following patients:

1. All unconscious patients
2. Confused or delirious patients
3. Patients who have abnormalities of or have undergone surgery of the mouth or esophagus
4. Patients with gastric hemorrhage
5. Pre- or postoperative gastric surgery patients

■ Assessment

Assess for:

1. Any obstructions or deformities of the nostrils. Ask the patient to hyperextend the head, and observe the nares, either by using a flashlight or by asking the patient to breathe through one nostril while occluding the other. Select the nostril that has the greatest air flow.
2. Intactness of the tissues of the nostrils, including any irritations or abrasions.
3. Abdominal distention. Palpate the abdomen for hardness and swelling.

Other data include:

1. Whether the tube is to be attached to suction
2. The size of tube to be inserted

■ Planning

Nursing goals

1. To prevent nausea, vomiting, and gastric distention
2. To provide a route for feeding the patient
3. To remove stomach contents for laboratory analysis
4. To lavage the stomach in cases of poisoning or overdose of medications

Equipment

1. A gastric tube (plastic or rubber).
2. A solution basin filled with warm water or ice. Rubber tubes are placed on ice to stiffen them for easier insertion. Plastic tubes are placed in warm water to make them more flexible for insertion.
3. A water-soluble lubricant.
4. A 20- to 50-mL syringe with an adapter to attach to the tube. It is used to withdraw stomach contents.
5. A basin in which to collect gastric contents.
6. Nonallergenic adhesive tape, 2.5 cm (1 in) wide, to secure the tube to the face.
7. A clamp (optional) to close the tube after insertion.
8. Suction apparatus, if ordered.
9. A gauze square or a plastic specimen bag and an elastic band to cover the end of the tube.
10. A safety pin and an elastic band to secure the nasogastric tube to the patient's gown.
11. A bib or towel to protect the patient's gown.
12. A glass of water and drinking straw to help the patient swallow the tube.
13. Facial tissues in case the patient's eyes water during the procedure.
14. A stethoscope to assess placement of the tube.

■ Intervention

Inserting a nasogastric tube

1. Explain to the patient what you plan to do. Adjust the explanation to the patient's needs.

   Rationale A short explanation reassures the patient and allows the nurse to confirm the patient's identity. The passage of a gastric tube is not painful, but it is unpleasant because the gag reflex is activated during insertion.

2. Assist the patient to a high Fowlers's position, and support the patient's head on a pillow.

   Rationale It is often easier for the patient to swallow in this position, and gravity helps the passage of the tube.

3. Hyperextend the patient's head to examine the patient's nostrils. Have the patient breathe through each nostril while compressing the other nostril, to select the more patent one.

   Rationale The tube is inserted through the nostril that is more patent.

4. Determine how far to insert the tube in this manner: Use the tube to mark off the distance from the tip of the patient's nose to the tip of the earlobe and then from the tip of the earlobe to the tip of the sternum. See Figure 31–33. Mark this length with adhesive tape if the tube does not have markings.

   Rationale This length approximates the distance from the nares to the stomach. The distance varies among individuals.

5. Lubricate the tip of the tube well with water-soluble lubricant to ease insertion.

   Rationale A water-soluble lubricant dissolves if the tube accidentally enters the lungs. An oil-based lubricant, such as petroleum jelly, will not dissolve and could cause respiratory complications if it enters the lungs.

6. Insert the tube, with its natural curve toward the patient, into the selected nostril.

FIGURE 31-33

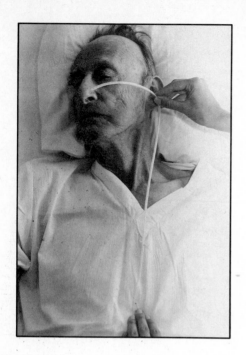

FIGURE 31-34

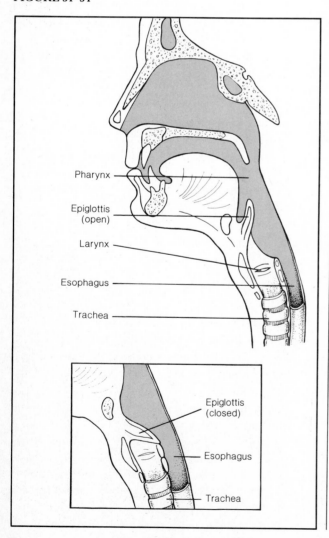

Pharynx

Epiglottis
(open)

Larynx

Esophagus

Trachea

Epiglottis
(closed)

Esophagus

Trachea

7. Have the patient hyperextend the neck, and gently advance the tube toward the nasopharynx. Direct the tube along the floor of the nostril and toward the ear on that side. Provide tissues if the patient's eyes water. If the tube meets resistance, withdraw it, relubricate it, and insert it in the other nostril.

   Rationale Hyperextension reduces the curvature of the nasopharyngeal junction. Directing the tube along the floor avoids the projections (turbinates) along the lateral wall. Slight pressure is sometimes required to pass the tube into the nasopharynx, and some patients' eyes may water at this point. Tears are a natural body response. The tube should never be forced against resistance because of the danger of injuring the patient.

8. Once the tube reaches the oropharynx (throat), have the patient tilt the head forward and encourage him or her to drink and swallow. If the patient gags, stop passing the tube momentarily. Have the patient rest, take a few breaths, and take sips of water to calm the gag reflex.

   Rationale The patient will feel the tube in the throat and may gag and retch. Tilting the head forward facilitates passage of the tube into the posterior pharynx and esophagus rather than into the larynx; swallowing moves the epiglottis over the opening to the larynx. See Figure 31-34.

9. In cooperation with the patient, pass the tube 5 to 10 cm (2 to 4 in) with each swallow, until the indicated length is inserted. If the patient continues to gag and the tube does not advance with each swallow, withdraw it slightly and inspect the patient's throat by looking through the mouth.

   Rationale The tube may be coiled. If so, it is withdrawn until it is straight, and the nurse tries again to insert it.

10. Aspirate the stomach contents with a syringe to determine placement of tube. See Table 31-3 for other methods.

    Rationale If fluid is removed, the assumption is that the tube is in the stomach. (Stomach contents are usually clear or yellow with mucus.)

11. If the signs do not indicate placement in the stomach, advance the tube 5 cm (2 in) and repeat the tests.

12. Secure the tube by taping it to the bridge of the patient's nose.

    a. Cut 7.5 cm (3 in) of tape and split it at one end, leaving a 2.5-cm (1-in) tab at the end.

    b. Place the tape over the bridge of the patient's nose, and bring the split ends under the tubing and back up over the nose. See Figure 31-35.

    Rationale Taping in this manner prevents the tube from pressing against and irritating the edge of the nostril.

TABLE 31–3 ■ Placement of a Nasogastric Tube

Nurse's action	If tube is in stomach	If tube is in lungs
To assess placement Attach distal end of tube to syringe and withdraw plunger.	Some gastric contents will fill tube.	No fluid will be in tube.
Other indications of placement Using a stethoscope, listen over the epigastric area of the abdomen while injecting 10 mL of air into tube.	Air will make a rushing sound.	There will be no sound.
Listen to distal end of tube.	There will be no sound.	There will be a crackling sound.
Ask conscious patient to talk and hum	Patient will be able to talk and hum.	Patient will be unable to talk or hum and will cough and/or choke
Note unconscious patient's color.	Color will be normal.	Patient will be cyanotic.
Place end of tube in a glass of water while patient exhales.	Few, if any, bubbles will appear in water.	Steady stream of bubbles will appear.

13. Attach the end of the tubing securely to suction, if ordered (see chapter 32, page 783).

    or

14. Clamp the end of the tubing and cover it with a gauze square or plastic specimen bag and an elastic band. The tube, if inserted preoperatively, is usually clamped.

15. Attach the end of the tube to the patient's gown by one of these two methods:

    a. Loop an elastic band around the end of the tubing and attach the elastic band to the gown with a safety pin.

    or

    b. Attach a piece of adhesive tape to the tube, and pin the tape to the gown. See Figure 31–36.

    Rationale The tube is attached to prevent it from dangling and pulling.

FIGURE 31–35

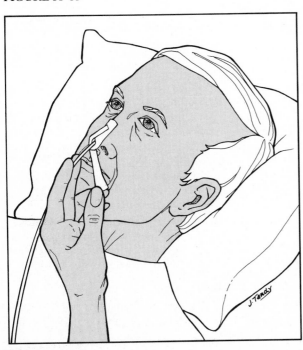

FIGURE 31–36

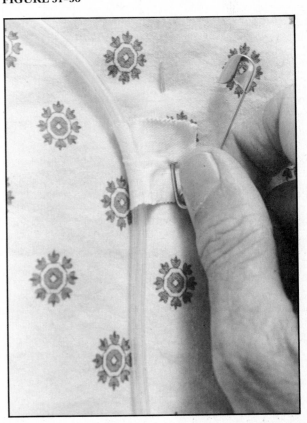

16. Record the insertion of the tube and the patient's response (discomfort, etc) .

17. Establish a plan for providing daily nasogastric tube care, including:

    a. Inspecting the nostril for discharge and irritation

    b. Cleaning the nostril and tube with moistened, cotton-tipped applicators

    c. Applying water-soluble lubricant to the nostril if it appears dry or encrusted

    d. Changing the adhesive tape as required

    e. Giving frequent mouth care, since the patient may breathe through the mouth and cannot drink

18. If suction is applied, ensure that the patency of both the nasogastric and suction tubes is maintained. Irrigations of the tube with 30 mL of normal saline may be required at regular intervals. In some agencies, irrigations must be ordered by the physician.

19. Keep accurate records of the patient's liquid intake and output, and record the amount and characteristics of the drainage.

Removing a nasogastric tube

The removal of a nasogastric tube is ordered by a physician.

20. Turn off the suction, and disconnect the tube from suction apparatus.

21. Remove the adhesive tape securing the tube to the patient's nose. Unpin the tube from the patient's gown.

22. Have the patient take a deep breath and hold it.

23. Steadily and quickly remove the tube while the patient is holding the breath.

24. Dispose of the tube in a bag.

25. Provide tissues for the patient to blow his or her nose, and offer mouthwash if desired.

26. Remove the suction apparatus from the bedside. Measure the amount of fluid drained. Then empty and clean the drainage bottle.

27. Record the removal of the tube, the patient's response, and the amount of fluid drained.

■ Evaluation

Expected outcomes

1. Tissues of the nostrils intact

2. Absence of irritation or abrasions of the tissues of the nostrils

3. Absence of obstructions or deformities of the nostrils

4. Reduced abdominal distention

Unexpected outcomes

1. Tissues of the nostrils appear reddened

2. Obstruction of the left nostril

3. Abdominal distention unchanged

Upon obtaining an unexpected outcome:

1. Report your findings to the responsible nurse.

2. Adjust the nursing care plan appropriately.

References

Creighton H: *Law Every Nurse Should Know*, 4th ed. Saunders, 1981.

Dziurbejko MM, Larkin JC: Including the family in preoperative teaching. *Am J Nurs* (November) 1978; 78:1892–1894.

Healy KM: Does preoperative instruction make a difference? *Am J Nurs* (January) 1968; 68:62–67.

Keithley JK, Tasic PW: A unified approach to assessment of the surgical patient. *Am J Nurs* (April) 1982; 82:612–614.

Laird M: Techniques for teaching pre- and postoperative patients. *Am J Nurs* (August) 1975; 75:1338–1340.

LeMaitre GD, Finnegan JA: *The Patient in Surgery: A Guide for Nurses*, 4th ed. Saunders, 1980.

Luciano K: The who, when, where, what and how of preparing children for surgery. *Nursing 74* (November) 1974; 4:64–65.

McConnell EA: All about gastrointestinal intubation. *Nursing 75* (September) 1975; 5:30–37.

McConnell EA: After surgery. *Nursing 77* (March) 1977a; 7:32–39.

McConnell EA: Ensuring safer stomach suctioning with a Salem sump tube. *Nursing 77* (September) 1977b; 7:54–57.

McConnell EA: Ten problems with nasogastric tubes . . . and how to solve them. *Nursing 79* (April) 1979; 9:78–81.

Rau J, Rau M: To breathe, or be breathed: Understanding IPPB. *Am J Nurs* (April) 1977; 77:613–617.

Simmons BP: CDC guidelines for the prevention and control of nosocomial infections: Guideline for prevention of surgical wound infections. *Am J Infect Control* (August) 1983; 11:133–141.

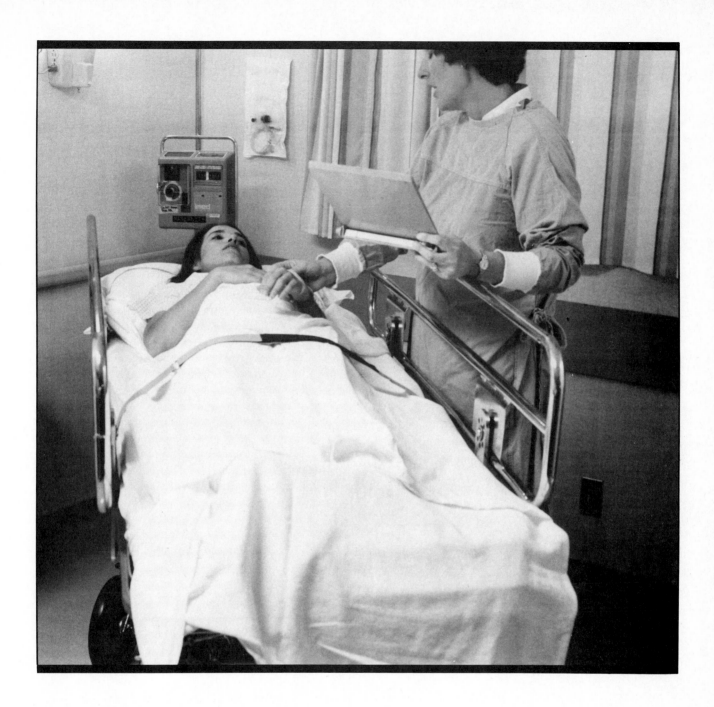

POSTOPERATIVE NURSING

32

Nursing during the postoperative period is very important for a patient's recovery. The anesthetic impairs the ability of patients to respond to environmental stimuli and to help themselves, although the degree of consciousness of patients will vary. Moreover, the surgery itself traumatizes the body, which decreases the body's resistance and energy. Nursing care includes monitoring the patient's cardiovascular, fluid balance, and neurologic status, providing comfort and safety, encouraging mobility, and preventing complications.

Chapter Outline

Recovering after Anesthesia
- Technique 32–1 Providing Postanesthetic (PAR) Care
- Technique 32–2 Providing Postoperative Nursing on the Unit

Suction
- Technique 32–3 Managing Gastrointestinal Suction
- Technique 32–4 Measuring and Applying Elastic Stockings

Objectives

Upon completion of this chapter, the student will:

1. Know essential terms and facts about postoperative nursing
   1.1 Define selected terms
   1.2 Identify assessment data required for the patient on return from the recovery room
   1.3 Identify essential information from the patient's record to plan postoperative care
   1.4 Identify general postoperative nursing interventions taken to relieve discomfort and prevent complications
   1.5 Identify postoperative complications
   1.6 Identify some causes of postoperative discomforts and complications
2. Understand facts about postoperative nursing techniques
   2.1 Identify relevant assessment data
   2.2 Identify nursing diagnoses for which the technique may be implemented
   2.3 Identify nursing goals related to the technique
   2.4 Identify expected and unexpected outcomes from assessment data
   2.5 Identify reasons underlying selected steps of the technique
3. Perform postoperative techniques safely
   3.1 Assess the patient adequately
   3.2 Collect additional data from appropriate sources
   3.3 Select pertinent nursing goals for the patient
   3.4 Establish relevant outcome criteria for the patient following the technique
   3.5 Collect necessary equipment before the technique
   3.6 Implement interventions to enhance the effectiveness of the technique and enhance the patient's comfort and safety
   3.7 Communicate relevant information about the patient to the appropriate persons
   3.8 Evaluate the outcomes of the technique
4. Evaluate own performance of specific postoperative techniques in a laboratory or clinical setting with the assistance of another
   4.1 Use the performance checklists provided
   4.2 Identify areas of strength and weakness
   4.3 Alter performance in response to own evaluation and that of another

Terms

- **affect**   feelings, emotions
- **alveolus**   a saclike dilation or cavity in the body (plural: alveoli); pulmonary alveoli are the saclike dilations in the lungs where gas exchange takes place between the lungs and pulmonary capillary blood
- **atelectasis**   collapse of the lung tissue
- **cardiac arrest**   the cessation of heart function
- **coagulate**   to clot, of blood
- **dehiscence**   a splitting open or rupture
- **edema**   excess interstitial fluid
- **embolus**   a blood clot that has moved from the site where it was formed
- **evisceration**   extrusion of the internal organs
- **hemorrhage**   bleeding internally or externally
- **hypotension**   an abnormally low blood pressure

- **hypovolemic shock**   markedly reduced volume of circulating blood
- **malignancy**   abnormal tissue having a tendency to proliferate and invade other tissues
- **phrenic**   referring to the diaphragm
- **pneumonia**   inflammation of the lung tissue
- **pulmonary embolus**   a blood clot that has moved to the lungs and is obstructing a pulmonary artery
- **purulent**   containing pus
- **singultus**   hiccups
- **stasis**   stagnation or stoppage of flow of body fluids, such as intestinal fluids, urine, or blood
- **thrombophlebitis**   inflammation of a vein, followed by formation of a blood clot
- **thrombus**   blood clot

■ tissue perfusion   passage of fluid, eg, blood, through a specific organ or body part

■ tympanites   abdominal distention

■ urinary retention   accumulation of urine in the bladder and inability to void

---

RECOVERING AFTER ANESTHESIA

Immediately following surgery, most patients are taken to a special area of the hospital referred to as the recovery room (RR), postanesthetic room (PAR), or anesthetic room (AR). Patients who have had minor surgery involving only a local anesthetic will most likely return directly to the nursing unit rather than going to the RR; or they may be sent to a day-care or short-stay unit and then be discharged to their homes. The amount of time spent in the RR will vary, depending on the patient's condition and how long it takes him or her to awaken from the general anesthetic. Patients who have had extensive surgery or whose condition is serious, may spend from one to several days in the intensive care unit (ICU).

TECHNIQUE 32–1   ■   Providing Postanesthetic (PAR) Care

Nursing intervention immediately after surgery, or postanesthetic (PAR) care, is usually carried out by recovery room nurses, who have special skills to care for patients recovering from anesthetics and surgery. Once a patient's condition has stabilized, she or he returns to a clinical nursing area; a day-surgery patient returns home.

PAR care includes regular, systematic assessment of:

1. Respiratory function
2. Cardiovascular function (circulation)
3. Neurologic status
4. Fluid and electrolyte balance
5. Dressings, tubes, and drains
6. Pain
7. Environmental safety and comfort

■ **Assessment**   See Intervention.

■ **Planning**

Nursing goals

1. To maintain or promote respiratory function
2. To maintain or promote cardiovascular function
3. To maintain fluid and electrolyte balance
4. To maintain the patient's comfort and safety

Equipment

1. Blood pressure equipment
2. Oxygen equipment
3. Suction equipment
4. Pillows for positioning
5. Emesis basin for vomitus
6. Other equipment as needed by the patient

■ **Intervention**

1. Position an unconscious patient on his or her side with the face slightly down. Do not place a pillow under the head.
   Rationale   This position keeps the tongue forward by gravity, preventing occlusion of the pharynx, and allows drainage of mucus or vomitus out of the mouth rather than down the respiratory tree.

2. Ensure maximum chest expansion by elevating the patient's upper arm on a pillow. Once the patient's reflexes return, the patient can assume a back-lying position.
   Rationale   The pressure of an arm against the chest reduces chest expansion potential.

3. Maintain an artificial airway in place, and apply suction to it until reflexes for controlling coughing and swallowing return. Generally, the patient spits out an oropharyngeal airway. Endotracheal tubes are not removed until the patient is awake and able to maintain his or her own airway. Before removing an artificial airway, apply suction to the airway and the pharynx. Then help the patient turn, cough, and take deep breaths, provided vital signs are stable.

4. Assess the rate, depth, and quality of respirations as well as the patient's chest movements. See chapter

8, page 124. Compare findings with the patient's normal respirations recorded on the chart.

5. If respirations appear extremely shallow, hold a hand in front of the patient's mouth to feel for exhaled air. If exhalations are not felt, auscultate the lungs and note bilateral air movement.

6. Supply oxygen as necessary to hypoventilating patients.

7. Assess the patient for signs of respiratory obstruction, the most common recovery room emergency. It may be due to occlusion of the pharynx by the tongue, spasm or edema of the airway, accumulation of secretions in the airway, or aspiration of regurgitated vomitus. Signs of respiratory obstruction include:

   a. Restlessness (early sign)

   b. Rapid, thready pulse (early sign)

   c. Noisy, irregular respirations

   d. Use of accessory muscles for breathing (eg, use of muscles in abdomen or neck) and intercostal retractions (indrawing between the ribs)

   e. Apprehension or anxiety

   f. Attempts to sit upright

   g. Pallor or cyanosis (late sign)

Maintaining cardiovascular function

8. Assess the patient's pulse for rate, rhythm, and quality every 15 minutes until signs stabilize and then every 30 minutes. Generally, the pulse is slightly faster after surgery, but a pulse above 110 beats per minute or below 60 beats per minute should be reported. Also, a pulse rate markedly above or below the patient's preoperative rate is abnormal; it may indicate internal hemorrhage or some other physiologic problem.

9. If the radial pulse is thready, take the apical pulse.

10. Assess the patient's blood pressure every 15 minutes until stable and then every 30 minutes.

11. Inform the physician if the patient's blood pressure falls more than 20 mm Hg after surgery or falls 5 or 10 mm Hg at each reading.

    Rationale Certain anesthetic agents and muscle relaxants may cause postoperative hypotension. It may also be a sign of hemorrhage and shock.

12. Assess the patient's skin color and condition, particularly that of the lips and nail beds.

    Rationale The color of the lips and nail beds are indicators of *tissue perfusion*(passage of blood through the vessels). Pale, cyanotic, cool, and moist skin may be a sign of circulatory problems.

13. Assess the patient for signs of common circulatory problems: hemorrhage and shock, cardiac arrest, and postoperative hypotension. Cardiac arrest is dis-

cussed in chapter 39, page 910. Disruption of sutures and insecure ligation of blood vessels can cause hemorrhage. Shock occurs as a result of massive hemorrhage or cardiac insufficiency. Signs of hemorrhage and shock include:

   a. Increase in pulse and respiratory rate

   b. Restlessness

   c. Lowered blood pressure

   d. Cold, clammy skin

   e. Thirst

   f. Pallor

14. Inspect the patient's dressings and the bedclothes underneath the patient.

    Rationale Excessive bloody drainage on dressings or on bedclothes, often appearing underneath the patient, signals hemorrhage.

15. Record the amount of drainage on dressings by describing the diameter of stains.

16. Ensure that there is adequate replacement of fluids lost during surgery to maintain the blood pressure. See steps 18–22.

17. Apply elastic (antiemboli) stockings to prevent pooling of blood in peripheral blood vessels if ordered. See Technique 32–4.

Maintaining fluid and electrolyte balance

18. Monitor and measure all of the patient's fluid intake and output.

19. Assess the patient for signs of circulatory overload. See Technique 25–2, step 5, on page 555.

    Rationale During surgery, aldosterone production increases, and as a result the body conserves sodium and fluid. Therefore, care must be taken not to overload the body with fluid.

20. Assess the patient for signs of fluid or electrolyte imbalance.

21. If the patient is receiving blood, assess for signs of adverse reactions. See chapter 25 on page 567.

22. Determine the color and consistency as well as the amount of drainage from all tubes and suction apparatuses. Make certain that all tubes are patent and that tubes and suction equipment are functioning properly.

Assessing neurologic status

After general anesthesia, patients awaken in the following sequence: respond to stimuli, ie, to loud noises or to their names spoken loudly; become drowsy; are awake but not oriented; are alert and oriented (McConnell, 1977a, p 34). The return of the patient's reflexes, such as swallowing and gagging, indicates that anesthesia is ending. Time of recovery from anesthesia varies with the kind of anesthetic used, its dosage, and the individual's response to it.

23. Arouse the patient by calling the patient by name, and in a normal tone of voice repeatedly tell the patient that the surgery is over and that she or he is in the recovery room.

Maintaining comfort and safety

24. As the patient emerges from anesthesia, assess the patient's need for analgesics and administer them as ordered. Analgesic dosages given in the RR are often reduced from normal dosages by one quarter to one third, but their effects are closely evaluated.

    Rationale Smaller dosages of analgesics are given because respiratory and cardiovascular function are depressed by anesthesia and can be impaired further by analgesic dosages that are too high.

25. Use judgment in withholding pain medications from hypotensive patients.

    Rationale Sometimes nurses in the RR withhold pain medication from hypotensive patients; however, pain may be the cause of hypotension (McConnell, 1977a, p 36).

26. Raise the patient's bed side rails, and provide warmth.

27. Notify support persons of the patient's condition.

28. Record all assessment data and care on the appropriate records.

■ **Evaluation**

Expected outcomes

1. Stable vital signs
2. Baseline rate, depth, and quality of respirations
3. Baseline rate, rhythm, and quality of pulse
4. Pink nail beds and lips
5. Dry dressings and bedclothes
6. Balanced fluid intake and output
7. Patient awake, alert, and oriented
8. Patient resting comfortably

Unexpected outcomes

1. Unstable vital signs
2. Shallow or noisy, irregular respirations
3. Restlessness or complaints of pain
4. Rapid, thready pulse; rate below 60; or absence of pulse
5. Pallor or cyanosis
6. Significant fall in blood pressure (10 to 20 mm Hg)
7. Cold, clammy skin
8. Bleeding on dressing or bedclothes
9. Imbalance in fluid intake and output
10. Abnormal constituents of drainage from drainage or suction tubes

Upon obtaining an unexpected outcome:

1. Report your findings to the responsible nurse and/or physician.
2. Adjust the patient's nursing care plan accordingly.

TECHNIQUE 32–2   ■   Providing Postoperative Nursing on the Unit

As soon as the patient returns to the nursing unit from the RR, the nurse conducts an initial assessment. The sequence of these activities varies with the situation. For example, the nurse may need to check the physician's stat orders before conducting the initial assessment; in such a case, nursing interventions to implement the orders can be carried out at the same time as assessment. Immediate postoperative care includes assessing the patient on return from the RR, initiating immediate nursing measures, and

planning and establishing a postoperative nursing care plan for the patient.

■ **Assessment**

See Intervention. For additional data, check:

1. From the patient's record:
   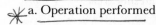 a. Operation performed

b. Presence of drains, etc, and their location

c. Anesthetic used *gas, spinal, IV*

d. Postoperative diagnosis

e. Estimated blood loss (EBL)

f. Medications administered in the RR

2. From the surgeon's postoperative orders:

a. Food and fluids permitted by mouth

b. Intravenous solutions and intravenous medications

c. Position in bed

d. Medications orders, eg, analgesics, antibiotics

e. Laboratory tests

f. Intake and output, which in some agencies are monitored for all postoperative patients

g. Activity permitted, including ambulation

In some agencies all preoperative orders are automatically canceled with surgery, and new orders are required.

■ Planning

Nursing goals

1. To provide comfort and safety for the patient
2. To closely monitor the patient's condition

FIGURE 32-1

POSTOPERATIVE INITIAL ASSESSMENT CHECKLIST

1. **Time of arrival** _____
2. **Vital signs**
   Pulse _____ Respirations _____ Blood pressure _____
3. **Skin**
   Color _____
   Condition _____
4. **Level of consciousness**
   Conscious ____ Semiconscious ____ Unconscious ____
5. **Dressing**
   Dry _____ Drainage present _____
   Blood _____ Intact _____
6. **Intravenous**
   Type of solution _____
   Amount in bottle _____ Drip rate _____
   Venipuncture site _____
7. **Drainage tubes**
   Type _____
   Attached to suction or drainage container _____
   Appearance and amount of drainage _____

8. **Patient position** _____
9. **Side rails** _____
10. **Pain**
    Type of analgesic _____
    Time last given _____
11. **Other discomforts** _____
    _____

---

3. To facilitate the patient's recovery, ie, prevent postoperative complications

Equipment

1. Blood pressure cuff and sphygmomanometer
2. Oral thermometer
3. Additional IV solution containers as necessary

■ Intervention

Initial assessment and intervention

1. Determine the time of patient's arrival at the nursing unit.

2. Obtain the vital signs—pulse, respirations, and blood pressure—and compare them with data from the RR.

3. Note the color and condition (eg, diaphoresis, coldness) of the patient's skin.

4. Assess the patient's level of consciousness. At this point, most postoperative patients are conscious but drowsy. A fully conscious patient responds verbally, is alert, and is aware of time, place, and person. A semiconscious patient has fluctuating states of awareness. An unconscious patient does not respond verbally, has variable responses to stimuli such as noise or pain, and may be incontinent of urine or feces.

5. Check dressings for moisture or bleeding. Check under the patient for pooled blood. Report blood immediately to the responsible nurse.

6. Note intravenous infusions. Record the type of solution, the amount in the bottle, the drip rate, and the venipuncture site. Obtain additional solutions as ordered.

7. Note drainage tubes, such as urinary catheters, and connect them appropriately, eg, to drainage containers or suction. Verify that fluids are draining and that tubes are not obstructed. Note the amount, color, consistency, and character of the drainage.

8. Determine what position is ordered or safe for the patient. This information is in the patient's chart, in the physician's orders, in RR records, or determined by the nurse's judgment. Patients who have had spinal anesthetics usually lie flat for 8 to 12 hours. Follow agency policy dictating how long the patient lies flat. If the patient is unconscious or semiconscious, place the patient on his or her side, if possible, or in a position that allows fluids to drain from the mouth. Otherwise, follow the patient's preference. Most patients prefer a back-lying position.

9. For the patient's safety, raise the side rails on the bed.

10. Assess the patient's pain or discomfort, and note when the patient last had an analgesic.

11. Record the patient's condition, including your assessment, on the chart. See Sample Recording later in this technique. Some agencies provide checklists for this purpose. See Figure 32–1 for a sample checklist. Many hospitals have postoperative routines for regular assessment of patients. In some agencies, assessments are made every 15 minutes until vital signs stabilize, every hour thereafter the same day, and every four hours for the next two days. It is very important that the assessments be made as frequently as the patient's condition requires.

12. Notify the patient's family or support persons of the patient's location and condition.

Ongoing postoperative assessment and intervention

Postoperative nursing interventions are designed chiefly to prevent postoperative complications. For most people who have surgery, recovery is without incident. However, although complications occur relatively rarely, nursing personnel must be aware of the possibility of complications and their clinical signs. Many of the nurse's interventions prevent more than one complication. See Table 32–1. Interventions include the so-called "stir-up regime," in which the patient is mobilized as much as possible, ie, turned, ambulated early, and encouraged frequently to do deep-breathing, coughing, and leg exercises without creating undue fatigue. See Figure 32–2 for a sample eight-hour nursing schedule for a postoperative patient. Because needs vary considerably, this sample schedule must be adapted to individual patients. Note that by grouping activities together, undisturbed rest periods can be provided. Essential steps follow.

TABLE 32–1 ■ Potential Postoperative Problems

Problem	Description	Cause	Clinical signs	Preventive interventions
Respiratory				
1. Pneumonia	Inflammation of the alveoli	Commonly the Diplococcus pneumoniae, a resident bacteria in respiratory tract	Elevated temperature, cough, expectoration of blood-tinged or purulent sputum, dyspnea, chest pain	Deep-breathing and coughing exercises, moving in bed, early ambulation
a. Lobar pneumonia	Involves one or more lobes			
b. Bronchopneumonia	Originates in bronchi and involves patches of lung tissue	Poor lung expansion and circulation, resulting in stagnation of secretions		
c. Hypostatic pneumonia	Poor or stagnant circulation causing inflammation of lung tissue			
2. Atelectasis	Collapse of the alveoli with retained secretions	Mucous plugs blocking bronchial passageways, inadequate lung expansion, analgesics, immobility	Marked dyspnea, cyanosis, pleural pain, prostration, tachycardia, increased respiratory rate, fever, productive cough, auscultatory crackling sounds	Deep-breathing and coughing exercises, turning, early ambulation, adequate fluid intake
3. Pulmonary embolism	Blood clot that has moved to the lungs and obstructs a pulmonary artery, thus inhibiting blood flow to one or more lung lobes	Stasis of venous blood from immobility, venous injury from fractures or during surgery, use of oral contraceptives high in estrogen, pre-existing coagulation or circulatory disorder	Sudden chest pain, shortness of breath, cyanosis, shock (tachycardia, low blood pressure)	Deep-breathing and coughing exercises, turning, ambulation, elastic stockings
Circulatory				
4. Hemorrhage	Bleeding internally or externally	Disruption of sutures, insecure ligation of blood vessels	Rapid weak pulse, increasing respiratory rate, restlessness, lowered blood pressure, cold clammy skin, thirst, pallor, reduced urine output	Early recognition of signs

TABLE 32–1 ■ continued

Problem	Description	Cause	Clinical signs	Preventive interventions
5. Hypovolemic shock	Markedly reduced volume of circulating blood resulting in inadequate tissue perfusion *O₂ to body*	Hemorrhage	Same as for Hemorrhage	Early recognition of signs *Warm ⅋ give O2*
6. Thrombophlebitis	Inflammation of the veins, usually of the legs and associated with a blood clot	Slowed venous blood flow due to immobility or prolonged sitting; trauma to vein, resulting in inflammation and increased blood coagulability	Aching, cramping pain; affected area is swollen, red, and hot to touch; vein feels hard; discomfort in calf when foot is dorsiflexed or when patient walks (Homan's sign)	Early ambulation, leg exercises, use of elastic stockings, adequate fluid intake
7. Thrombus	Blood clot attached to wall of vein or artery, most commonly the leg veins	Venous stasis; vein injury resulting from surgery of legs, pelvis, abdomen; factors causing increased blood coagulability, eg, use of estrogen	Same as for Pulmonary Embolism; if lodged in heart or brain, cardiac or neurologic signs	Same as for Thrombophlebitis
8. Embolus	Clot that has moved from the site where it formed to another area of the body, eg, the lungs, heart, or brain	Same as for Thrombus	Same as for Thrombus	Same as for Thrombophlebitis

Urinary

Problem	Description	Cause	Clinical signs	Preventive interventions
9. Urinary retention	Accumulation of urine in the bladder and inability of the bladder to empty itself	Depressed bladder muscle tone from narcotics and anesthetics; handling of tissues during surgery on adjacent organs (rectum, vagina)	Fluid intake larger than output; inability to void or frequent voiding of small amounts, bladder distention, suprapubic discomfort, restlessness	Monitoring of fluid intake and output, interventions to facilitate voiding
10. Urinary infection *Cause by Catheters*	Inflammation of bladder	Immobilization and limited fluid intake	Burning sensation when voiding, urgency, cloudy urine, lower abdominal pain	Adequate fluid intake, early ambulation, good perineal hygiene

Gastrointestinal

Problem	Description	Cause	Clinical signs	Preventive interventions
11. Constipation	Infrequent or no stool passage for abnormal length of time, eg, within 48 hours after solid diet started	Lack of dietary roughage, analgesics (decrease intestinal motility)	Absence of stool elimination, abdominal distention and discomfort *2-3 days*	Adequate fluid intake, high fiber diet, early ambulation
12. Singultus	Intermittent spasms of the diaphragm	Irritation of the phrenic nerve for a variety of reasons, eg, abdominal distention	Hiccups *most common p̄ ABD Surgery*	Prevent the cause
13. Tympanites *✳ give warm fluids* / *✓ Bowel Sounds*	Retention of gases within the intestines	Slowed motility of the intestines due to handling of the bowel during surgery and the effects of anesthesia	Obvious abdominal distention, abdominal discomfort (gas pains), absence of bowel sounds	Early ambulation, IV fluid progressing to clear fluids, full fluids and regular diet when peristalsis returns
14. Nausea and vomiting		Pain, abdominal distention, ingesting food or fluids before return of peristalsis, some medications, anxiety	Complaints of feeling sick to the stomach, retching or gagging	IV fluids until peristalsis returns; then clear fluids, full fluids, and regular diet; antiemetic drugs if ordered; analgesics for pain

TABLE 32–1 ■ continued

Problem	Description	Cause	Clinical signs	Preventive interventions
Wound				
15. Wound infection	Inflammation and infection of incision or drain site	Poor aseptic technique; laboratory analysis of wound swab identifies causative microorganism	Purulent exudate, redness, tenderness, elevated body temperature, wound odor	Keeping wound clean and dry, surgical aseptic technique when changing dressings
16. Wound dehiscence	Separation of a suture line before the incision heals	Malnutrition (emaciation, obesity), poor circulation, excessive strain on suture line	Increased incision drainage, tissues underlying skin become visible along parts of the incision	Adequate nutrition, appropriate incisional support and avoidance of strain
17. Wound evisceration	Extrusion of internal organs and tissues through the incision	Same as for Wound Dehiscence	Opening of incision and visible protrusion of organs	Same as for Wound Dehiscence
Psychologic				
18. Postoperative depression	See Clinical Signs	News of malignancy, severely altered body image	Anorexia, tearfulness, loss of ambition, withdrawal, rejection of others, dejected affect, sleep disturbances (insomnia, excessive sleeping)	Adequate rest, physical activity, opportunity to express anger and other negative feelings

Vital signs

13. Take the patient's vital signs at least every four hours or more frequently if they are abnormal.

    Rationale An elevated temperature along with other signs can indicate infection of the respiratory tract, urinary tract, or incision. A rapid, weak pulse and increased respiratory rate along with other signs can indicate infection, hemorrhage, or shock. A lowered blood pressure along with other signs can indicate hemorrhage, shock, or pulmonary embolism.

14. Assess the patient's respiratory rate, depth, and rhythm every four hours, or whenever the vital signs are taken. Be alert to signs of respiratory problems. See Table 32–1.

FIGURE 32–2 ■ Sample eight-hour nursing schedule for a first-day postoperative patient.

FIRST DAY POSTOPERATIVE SCHEDULE									
	0800	0900	1000	1100	1200	1300	1400	1500	1600
Take vital signs	✓				✓				✓
Assess patient's skin color and temperature	✓				✓				✓
Inspect dressing	✓		✓		✓		✓		✓
Auscultate abdomen	✓				✓				✓
Check IV infusion and site	✓	✓	✓	✓	✓	✓	✓	✓	✓
Provide analgesics	✓				✓				✓
Assist patient to deep breathe and cough	✓		✓		✓		✓		✓
Encourage patient to do leg exercises	✓	✓	✓	✓	✓	✓	✓	✓	✓
Ambulate or turn patient	✓		✓		✓		✓		✓
Provide hygienic care	✓								
Give partial assistance with bath	✓								
Provide mouth care	✓								
Rest period		✓			✓		✓		✓

Note: Measure and record fluid intake at mealtimes or when changing IV. Measure fluid output after voiding.

15. Assess the patient's skin color and temperature.

    Rationale Extreme pallor and a cold, clammy skin are signs of shock.

Deep-breathing and coughing exercises

16. Encourage the patient to do deep-breathing and coughing exercises hourly or at least every two hours during waking hours for the first few days. Assist the patient to a sitting position in bed or on the side of the bed. Have the patient splint the incision with a pillow when coughing, or splint the incision for the patient. Refer to Teaching Postoperative Exercises in Technique 31–1 on page 754.

    Rationale These exercises help prevent respiratory complications such as hypostatic pneumonia and atelectasis.

17. To assist patients who have difficulty with deep-breathing and coughing exercises, check about the use of blow bottles and incentive spirometers (see chapter 36 on page 856). For patients unable to cough up secretions, suction may be necessary (see chapter 37).

Leg exercises

18. Encourage the patient to do leg exercises every hour or at least every two hours during waking hours. See chapter 31 on page 754.

    Rationale Muscle contractions compress the veins, preventing the stasis of blood in the veins, a cause of thrombus formation and subsequent thrombophlebitis and emboli. Contractions also promote arterial blood flow.

Moving and ambulation

19. Turn the patient from side to side every two hours.

    Rationale Turning allows alternating maximum expansion of the uppermost lung.

20. Avoid placing pillows or rolls under the patient's knees.

    Rationale Pressure on the popliteal blood vessels can slow the blood circulation to and from the lower extremities.

21. Ambulate the patient as soon as possible after surgery in accordance with the physician's orders. Generally, patients begin ambulation the evening of the day of surgery or the first day after surgery, unless the surgeon orders otherwise.

    Rationale Early ambulation prevents respiratory, circulatory, urinary, and gastrointestinal complications. It also prevents general muscle weakness. See Table 32–1.

22. Schedule ambulation for periods after the patient has taken an analgesic or when the patient is comfortable.

23. Make ambulation gradual. Start by having the patient sit on the bed and dangle the feet over the side.

Assess her or his tolerance by noting color, respirations, diaphoresis, pulse rate, etc. Take the pulse before moving the patient and again after. Next, help the patient stand at the bedside and take a few steps. Increase the distance gradually as the patient's tolerance grows.

24. Provide supportive measures as required. For example, use a pillow to support an abdominal incision, or move the patient's urinary drainage bag or IV pole during ambulation. Give verbal encouragement and reassurance as necessary.

25. For patients with cardiovascular problems, apply tensor bandages up to the knees or antiemboli stockings. See Technique 32–4.

    Rationale These devices support superficial veins and prevent stasis of venous circulation.

26. If the patient cannot ambulate, periodically assist him or her to a sitting position in bed if allowed, and turn the patient frequently (see step 19).

    Rationale The sitting position permits the greatest lung expansion.

Hydration

27. Maintain IV infusions as ordered.

    Rationale IV infusions are given to balance loss of body fluids during surgery (eg, blood loss, perspiration, vomiting, and fasting).

28. Offer only small sips of water to patients who can have fluids by mouth until they establish tolerance.

    Rationale Large amounts of water can induce vomiting, since anesthetics and narcotic analgesics temporarily inhibit the motility of the stomach.

29. Offer ice chips, if permitted. The patient who cannot take fluids by mouth may be allowed to suck ice chips. Check the physician's orders.

30. Provide mouth care, and place a mouthwash at the patient's bedside.

    Rationale Postoperative patients often complain of thirst and a dry, sticky mouth. These discomforts are a result of the preoperative fasting period, preoperative medications (such as atropine or scopolamine), and loss of body fluid.

31. Measure the patient's fluid intake and output for at least two days or until fluid balance is stable without an IV.

    Rationale It is important to ensure adequate fluid balance. Sufficient fluids keep the respiratory mucous membranes and secretions moist, thus facilitating the expectoration of mucus during coughing. Also, an adequate fluid balance will prevent dehydration and the resulting concentration of the blood that, along with venous stasis, is conducive to thrombus formation.

32. Assess the patient for signs of dehydration.

Nutrition

The physician orders the patient's postoperative diet. Depending on the extent of surgery and the organs involved, some patients may be give intravenous fluids and nothing by mouth for a few days, while others may progress from a diet of clear liquids to full fluids, to a light diet, and then to a regular diet within a few days. See chapter 24.

33. Check the doctor's orders carefully regarding diet. Assess the return of peristalsis by auscultating the abdomen. Gurgling and rumbling sounds indicate peristalsis.

    Rationale Anesthetics, narcotics, handling of the intestines during abdominal surgery, changes in fluid and food intake, and inactivity all inhibit peristalsis. Oral fluids and food are usually started after the return of peristalsis.

34. Assist the patient to eat as required.

35. Observe the patient's tolerance of the food and fluids ingested.

Urinary elimination

36. Provide measures that promote urinary elimination. For example, help male patients stand at the bedside, ensure that patients are free from pain, ensure that fluid intake is adequate, and help patients walk.

37. Note any difficulties the patient has with voiding, and assess the patient for bladder distention.

38. Report promptly to the responsible nurse if a patient does not void within eight hours following surgery.

    Rationale Anesthetics temporarily depress urinary bladder tone, which usually returns within six to eight hours after surgery. Surgery in the pubic area, vagina, or rectum, during which the surgeon may manipulate the bladder, often causes urinary retention.

39. Catheterize a patient if all measures to promote voiding fail. See chapter 27. In some agencies, catheterization requires a doctor's order.

40. Measure the liquid intake and output of all patients with urinary catheters or other drainage devices. Keep I & O records for at least two days and until the patient reestablishes fluid balance without a catheter in place.

Comfort and rest

Pain is usually greatest 12 to 36 hours after surgery, decreasing on the second or third day. Analgesics are usually administered every three or four hours the first day, and by the third day most patients require only oral analgesics. Some patients may refuse to take analgesics on a regular schedule because they are not in severe pain. In this situation, assess the patient's need for analgesics (see step 42); if indicated, inform the patient that analgesics are most effective if given before pain becomes severe.

41. Provide comfort measures to relax the patient, eg, back rubs, position changes, rest periods and diverting activities.

    Rationale Tension increases pain perception and responses.

42. Administer analgesics as ordered and as required.

    Rationale Analgesics relieve pain and therefore also help the patient to do deep-breathing and coughing exercises effectively and to ambulate.

43. Observe the patient for signs of acute pain, eg, pallor, perspiration, tension, and reluctance to perform deep-breathing and coughing exercises or to move or ambulate.

44. Move and position the patient to minimize discomfort.

45. Plan to give analgesics before activities (eg, ambulation or meals) or rest periods, (eg, at bedtime).

46. Assess the effectiveness of the analgesics.

47. Listen attentively to the patient's complaints of pain; note the location, note the type of pain, and determine the cause. Do not assume that the patient's pain is caused by the incision. Often the cause can be tight dressings, irritation from drainage tubes, or muscle strains resulting from positioning on the operating table.

Fecal elimination

48. Note and report the passage of flatus.

    Rationale Abdominal distention due to reduced peristalsis is very common after surgery. Many patients who have had abdominal surgery start experiencing this discomfort about the third day after surgery. The passage of flatus indicates the return of peristalsis.

49. Auscultate the patient's abdomen to confirm the return of peristalsis.

50. Administer a rectal tube, enema, or suppository as required and if ordered.

Wound protection

51. Inspect dressings regularly to ensure that they are clean and dry.

    Rationale Excessive drainage can indicate hemorrhage, infection, or dehiscence.

52. Ensure that the dressing is fastened securely.

    Rationale An intact, secure dressing prevents infection of the wound.

53. Apply abdominal binders for support as ordered.

54. Change dressings, using sterile technique as required, when they are soiled with drainage or in accordance with the physician's or nursing orders. See chapter 35. Note that the first dressing change postoperatively may be done by the physician.

55. Inspect the wound for signs of local infection.

56. Assess the patient for signs of generalized infection, eg, elevated temperature and increased pulse and respiratory rates.
57. Report wound separations promptly.
58. If a large dehiscence or evisceration occurs, cover the wound with sterile moist saline towels or dressings and apply an abdominal binder for support of the internal organs. Notify the physician immediately.
59. Record assessment data and nursing interventions on the appropriate records.

Sample Recording: Initial Assessment on Return to Unit

Date	Time	Notes
12/22/87	1100	Transferred from PAR. Appears pale, tense, and drowsy. Is responding verbally and aware of time and surroundings. Complaining of severe abdominal pain. BP 140/70, P 88, R 18. Dressing dry and intact. IV of D5W infusing. IV site intact and dry. Foley catheter attached to closed drainage bag. Urine clear amber color.————
	1115	Demerol 75 mg IM administered. Family notified. ———— Terrence G. Fox, SN

Sample Recording: Ongoing Postoperative Intervention

Date	Time	Notes
1/26/88	1500	Vital signs stable at 125/72, T 37, P 76, R 16. Performing deep-breathing and coughing exercises well q.2h. Performing leg exercises q.1h. Ambulated first time to bathroom. Tolerated well. Voided 250 mL clear amber urine.
	1600	IV 1,000 mL D5W infused: 1,000 mL Ringer's lactate started. Tolerating sips of water and ice chips. No bowel sounds evident.————
	1630	Demerol 75 mg IM given for abdominal pain. Dressing dry and intact. ———— ————Trudy Jones, SN

■ Evaluation

Expected outcomes

1. Carries out leg exercises every one to two hours as instructed
2. Turns from side to side in bed independently
3. Coughs and does deep-breathing exercises at least every two hours as instructed
4. Walks to end of hall each morning with assistance
5. Bilateral air movement in lungs evident on auscultation
6. Vital signs normal
7. Skin color good
8. No evidence of dehydration
9. Urine output and fluid intake in balance
10. Voiding patterns normal
11. No signs of infection at site of incision
12. Dressings dry
13. Pain sufficiently controlled to enable required activity
14. Bowel activity satisfactory
15. Absence of abdominal distention
16. Absence of vomiting or complaints of nausea

Unexpected outcomes

1. Needs much encouragement and supervision to carry out leg exercises
2. Needs much assistance to turn in bed
3. Has difficulty deep breathing and coughing
4. Is tense, rigid, and bent over when walking
5. Crackles in lungs heard on auscultation
6. Absence of air movement in one lung
7. Signs of shock or hemorrhage (see Table 32–1)
8. Signs of respiratory complications (see Table 32–1)
9. Difficulty voiding; urinary retention
10. Signs of dehydration
11. Infected incision
12. Delayed return of peristalsis; abdominal distention
13. Vomiting
14. Aching, cramping pain in calf and other signs of thrombophlebitis
15. Wound dehiscence or evisceration

Upon obtaining an unexpected outcome:

1. Report your findings to the responsible nurse and/or physician.
2. Adjust the nursing care plan accordingly.

SUCTION

The manner in which suction is applied to drainage tubes depends on the type of equipment available in the agency and the amount of suction required. The following are the most commonly used:

1. *Wall suction.* In some agencies, wall suction units with piped-in negative pressure are available. See Figure 32–3.

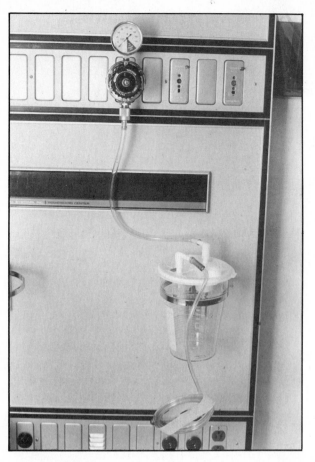

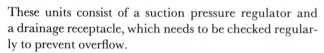

FIGURE 32–3 ■ A sample wall suction unit with piped-in negative pressure.

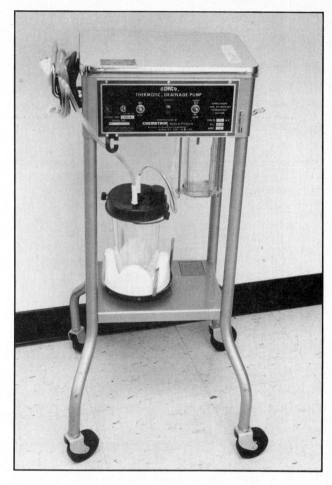

FIGURE 32–4 ■ A Gomco thermotic pump.

These units consist of a suction pressure regulator and a drainage receptacle, which needs to be checked regularly to prevent overflow.

2. Portable electric motor suction. Portable electric units are plugged into electric wall outlets. The units have an on–off switch, a motor that generates the negative pressure, and a drainage bottle. The bottle needs to be monitored regularly to prevent overflow of drainage into the motor, which can cause irreparable damage to the apparatus.

3. Gomco thermotic pump. The Gomco pump is also electrically operated but consists of a pump rather than a motor.

See Figure 32–4. It provides intermittent suction by alternating the air pressure, ie, expanding and contracting the air. As the pressure alternates, red and green lights flash on and off. The amount of suction is regulated by a "high" or "low" pressure button. The pump is commonly used to suction gastrointestinal tubes.

4. Plastic bellows wound suction. Plastic bellows suction is commonly referred to as the *Hemovac,* or portable wound suction, since it is used to suction drainage from surgical wounds. See Technique 35–6 on page 842. Suction is created by manually compressing and releasing the sides of the apparatus.

TECHNIQUE 32–3 ■ Managing Gastrointestinal Suction

Some patients return from surgery with a gastric or intestinal tube in place and orders to connect the tube to suction. The suction ordered can be continuous or

intermittent. Intermittent suctioning is less likely to harm the mucous membrane lining near the tip of the suction tube.

■ Assessment

Assess the patient for:

1. Abdominal distention by palpating the abdomen
2. Bowel sounds by auscultating the abdomen
3. Irritation of the nostril by the tube
4. Abdominal discomfort
5. Vital signs for baseline data

Other data include:

1. Whether the suction is continuous or intermittent.
2. The ordered suction pressure. A low suction pressure is between 80 and 100 mm Hg, and a high pressure is between 100 and 120 mm Hg.
3. Whether there is an order to irrigate the gastrointestinal tube and, if so, the type of solution to use.

■ Planning

Nursing goals

1. To relieve abdominal distention
2. To maintain gastric decompression after surgery
3. To remove blood and secretions from the gastrointestinal tract
4. To relieve discomfort, ie, when a patient has a bowel obstruction
5. To maintain the patency of the nasogastric tube

Equipment

Initiating and maintaining suction

1. A gastrointestinal tube in place in the patient. This may have been inserted prior to or following surgery (or prior to establishing the suction on a nonsurgical patient).
2. A suction device for either continuous or intermittent suction (see Suction on page 782).
3. A 50-mL syringe with an adapter to aspirate the stomach and the tube.
4. A basin to collect the aspirated fluid.
5. A connector to connect the gastrointestinal tube to the suction tubing.
6. Connecting tubing.
7. Cotton-tipped applicators.
8. Ointment or lubricant to decrease irritation of the nostrils.
9. A moisture-resistant pad.

Irrigating a gastrointestinal tube

10. A disposable irrigating set:
    a. A 50-mL syringe
    b. A moisture-resistant pad

c. A basin to collect the irrigating solution
d. A graduated container

11. Sterile normal saline (500 mL) or the ordered solution
12. A stethoscope

■ Intervention

Initiating suction

1. Assist the patient to the required position or to semi-Fowler's position if it is not contraindicated.
   Rationale In semi-Fowler's position the tube is not as likely to lie against the wall of the stomach and will therefore suction most efficiently. Semi-Fowler's position also prevents reflux of gastric contents, which could lead to aspiration.
2. Confirm that the tube is in the stomach by aspirating the stomach contents with the syringe and adapter. See Table 31–3 on page 769.
   Rationale The most accurate way to confirm the placement of the tube in the stomach is by withdrawing stomach contents using a syringe. Other methods listed in Table 31–3 are supplemental.
3. Connect the gastrointestinal tube to the tubing from the suction using the connector.
4. Set the suction at the recommended pressure and turn the suction on.
   a. Adjust the suction machine for the recommended suction pressure, in accordance with agency policy or the physician's order. Some suctions are preset and cannot be adjusted. If using a Gomco thermotic pump, the suction is usually set on intermittent "low" suction for a single-lumen nasogastric tube or on "high" suction for a double-lumen nasogastric tube (eg, Salem sump tube).
   b. Turn on the suction machine, and check that the suction is working. The Gomco thermotic drainage pump has a red indicator light located in the middle of the front panel; it blinks continuously when the machine is functioning. When using other suction machines, test for proper suctioning by holding the open end of the suction tube to your ear. Proper suctioning is confirmed by a sucking noise.
5. Watch the tubing for a few minutes until the gastric contents appear to be running through the tubing into the receptacle.
6. If the suction is not working properly, check that the rubber stopper in the collection bottle and all tubing connections are tightly sealed and that the tubing is not kinked.

7. Coil and pin the tubing on the bed so that it does not loop below the suction bottle.

   Rationale If the tubing falls below the suction bottle, the suction may be obstructed because of the pressure required to push the fluid against gravity.

8. If the gastrointestinal tube has an air vent, place it beside or above the patient's head. If the vent becomes blocked with gastric contents, inject 10 cc of air with a syringe to clear the vent.

   Rationale If the vent is below the patient's head, ie, in a dependent position, the gastric contents can flow into the vent and block it.

9. Assess the amount, color, odor, and consistency of the drainage. Normal gastric drainage has a mucoid consistency and is either colorless or yellow-green due to the presence of bile. A coffee-grounds color and consistency may indicate bleeding. Test the gastric drainage for pH and blood (Hematest) when indicated. A patient who has had gastrointestinal surgery can be expected to have some blood in the drainage.

10. Record initiating the suction and the time. Also record the pressure established, the color and consistency of the drainage, and assessments of the patient.

Sample Recording

Date	Time	Notes
9/18/86	1400	Suction initiated 100 mm Hg. Returns bright red. Abdomen firm and slightly distended. Bowel sounds irregular and high pitched. —————— Molly Jones, RN

Maintaining suction

11. Assess the patient regularly (every 30 minutes until the system is running well and then every two hours) to ensure that the suction is functioning properly. If the patient complains of fullness, nausea, or epigastric pain, or if the flow of gastric secretions is not evident in the tubing or the collection bottle, ineffective suctioning or blockage of the nasogastric tube is likely.

12. Inspect the suction system for patency of the system, eg, kinks or blockages in the tubing, and tightness of the connections.

    Rationale Loose connections can permit air to enter and thus decrease the effectiveness of the suction by decreasing the negative pressure.

13. To relieve blockages:
    a. Milk the suction tubing.
    b. Check the suction equipment. To do this, disconnect the nasogastric tube from the suction over a collecting basin (to collect gastric drainage), and then, with the suction on, place the end of the suction tubing in a basin of water. If water is drawn into the drainage bottle, the suction equipment is functioning properly, but the nasogastric tube is either blocked or positioned incorrectly.
    c. Reposition the patient, eg, to her or his other side if permitted. This may facilitate drainage.
    d. Rotate the nasogastric tube and reposition it. This step is contraindicated for patients with gastric surgery because moving the tube may interfere with gastric sutures.
    e. Irrigate the nasogastric tube as agency policy advocates or on the order of the physician. See steps 20–30 later in this technique.

14. Clean the patient's nostrils every three hours or as needed, using the cotton-tipped applicators and water. Apply a water-soluble lubricant or ointment.

15. Provide mouth care every three hours or as needed. See Technique 13–3 on page 304. Some postoperative patients are permitted to suck ice chips or a moist cloth to maintain the moisture of the oral mucosa.

16. Check the drainage bottle regulary to ensure that it does not overflow.

17. Empty the drainage receptacle every eight hours or whenever it becomes three quarters full. To empty:
    a. Clamp the nasogastric tube and turn off the suction.
    b. If the receptacle is graduated, determine the amount of drainage.
    c. Disconnect the receptacle.
    d. If not already measured, empty the contents into a graduated container and measure.
    e. Inspect the drainage carefully for color, consistency, and presence of substances, eg, blood clots.
    f. Rinse the receptacle with warm water.
    g. Reattach the receptacle to the suction.
    h. Turn on the suction and unclamp the nasogastric tube.
    i. Observe the system for several minutes to make sure it is functioning well.

18. Encourage the patient to turn from side to side and ambulate when permitted. To ambulate:
    a. Turn off the suction.
    b. Disconnect the gastrointestinal tube from the connector.
    c. Clamp the gastrointestinal tube, and attach it to the patient's gown. See Technique 31–3, steps 14–15, on page 769. Some agencies use a catheter plug, which is inserted into the lumen of the tube.
    d. Ambulate the patient.

e. Reestablish the suction after the patient returns to bed.

19. Record assessments of the patient, supportive care, and any problems with the suction system.

Sample Recording

Date	Time	Notes
10/7/86	800	250 mL light brown drainage. No complaints of pain. Bowel sounds hyperactive, increased pitch. Abdomen soft upon palpation. No irritation in nostrils. Nostrils cleaned with water and lubricant applied. Vital signs q.2h. BP 140/80, P 90, R 18 and stable ———— R. Woo, SN

Irrigating a gastrointestinal tube

Nasogastric tubes are generally irrigated (a) before and after the instillation of medications, (b) before and after tube feedings, and (c) as ordered to prevent clogging. Check agency policies and practices. Nasogastric irrigation may require a physician's order. Excessive irrigation can lead to metabolic alkalosis.

20. Place the moisture-resistant pad under the end of the gastrointestinal tube.

21. Turn off the suction.

22. Disconnect the gastrointestinal tube from the connector.

23. Determine that the tube is in the stomach by aspirating gastric contents using a syringe. If no contents can be aspirated, inject 10 mL of air while listening over the epigastric region using a stethoscope. See Table 31–3 on page 769.

    Rationale This ensures that the irrigating solution enters the stomach.

24. Draw up the ordered volume of irrigating solution in the syringe; 30 mL of solution per instillation is usual, but up to 60 mL may be given per instillation if ordered.

25. Attach the syringe to the nasogastric tube and *slowly* inject the solution.

26. Gently aspirate the solution.

    Rationale Forceful withdrawal could damage the gastric mucosa.

27. If you encounter difficulty in withdrawing the solution, inject 20 mL of air and aspirate again, and/or reposition the patient or the nasogastric tube.

    Rationale Air and repositioning may move the end of the tube away from the stomach wall.

    If aspirating difficulty continues, reattach the tube to

intermittent low suction and notify the responsible nurse or physician.

28. Repeat steps 23–25 until the ordered amount of solution is instilled.

29. Reconnect the nasogastric tube to suction. If a Salem sump tube is used, inject the air vent lumen with air after reconnecting the tube to suction.

30. Observe the system for several minutes to make sure it is functioning well.

31. Record verification of tube placement; the time of the irrigation; the amount and type of irrigating solution used; the amount, color, and consistency of the returns; the patency of the system following the irrigation; and assessments of the patient.

Sample Recording

Date	Time	Notes
9/19/86	1600	Tube placement confirmed by injecting 10 mL air. Tube irrigated with 30 mL normal saline × 2. 30 mL × 2 returns cloudy, pink with small clots. Suction running well. Abdomen soft, no discomfort, vital signs stable. ———— R. Woo, SN

▪ Evaluation

Expected outcomes

1. Abdomen soft upon palpation
2. Absence of abdominal distention
3. Absence of nostril irritation
4. Bowel sounds normal
5. Suction drainage about 200 mL, colorless or yellow-green or as expected for the patient, eg, pink immediately following surgery

Unexpected outcomes

1. Abdomen hard upon palpation
2. Presence of abdominal distention
3. Nostril with tube irritated
4. Suction drainage 500 mL, bright red with clots

Upon obtaining an unexpected outcome:

1. Report your findings to the responsible nurse and/or physician.
2. Adjust the nursing care plan appropriately.

TECHNIQUE 32–4 ■ Measuring and Applying Elastic Stockings

Elastic (antiemboli) stockings are indicated for patients who have problems with circulation to their feet and legs. The elastic material compresses the veins of the legs and thereby facilitates the venous blood return to the heart. These stockings are frequently applied preoperatively and/or postoperatively.

There are several types of stockings. One type extends from foot to knee and another from foot to midthigh. Women sometimes prefer to wear garters with the longer type, although garters are not necessary to hold elastic stockings in place. Another type of stocking extends to the waist and fastens with an adjustable belt and its own garters. Stockings have a partial foot that exposes either the heel or toes so that the extremity circulation can be assessed. See Figure 32–5. Elastic stockings usually come in small, medium, and large sizes.

FIGURE 32–5 ■ Two types of elastic stockings: **A,** extending to the knee with an opening above the toes; **B,** extending to midthigh with the heel exposed.

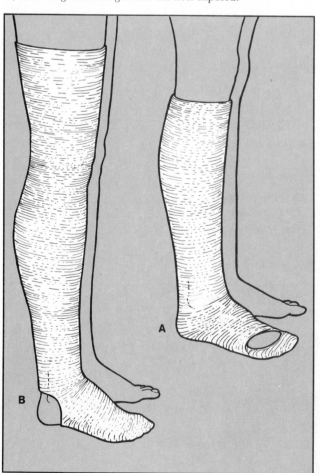

■ Assessment

Assess the patient's legs for:

1. Inadequate arterial blood circulation:
   a. Cool skin temperature in a warm environment
   b. Pallor
   c. Shiny taut skin
   d. Mild edema
2. Insufficient venous blood return:
   a. Thickening of the skin
   b. Increased pigmentation around the ankles
   c. Pitting edema (edema in which firm finger pressure on the skin produces an indentation, or pit, that remains for several seconds)
   d. Peripheral cyanosis
3. Posterior tibial (see Figure 32–6) and dorsalis pedis (see Figure 32–7) pulse rates, volumes, and rhythms.

FIGURE 32–6 ■ Assessing the posterior tibial pulse.

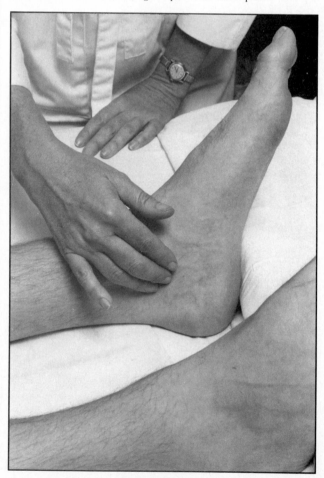

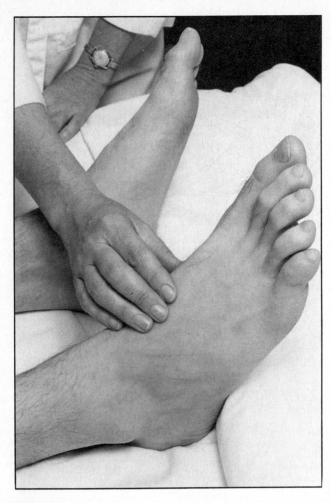

FIGURE 32–7 ■ Assessing the dorsalis pedis pulse.

4. Pain in the calf of the leg. Dorsiflex the foot abruptly and firmly while the knee is straight or slightly flexed (see Figure 32–8) to assess pain in the calf (Homan's sign). The presence of pain is a positive Homan's sign.

5. The appearance or presence of distended superficial

FIGURE 32–8 ■ Assessing Homan's sign.

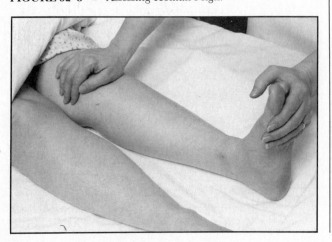

veins in the legs. Normally veins may appear distended in a dependent position but collapse when the limb is elevated.

■ Nursing Diagnosis

Nursing diagnoses that may indicate the need to apply elastic stockings include:

1. Alterations in cardiac output (decreased): related to decreased activity secondary to obesity
2. Fluid volume excess related to immobility
3. Fluid volume excess related to dependent venous pooling

■ Planning

Nursing goals

1. To assist the venous blood flow from the feet
2. To decrease or prevent edema of the feet and legs

Equipment

1. Measuring tape
2. Size chart
3. Correct size of elastic stockings

■ Intervention

1. Assist the patient to a lying position in bed. Stockings should be applied before the patient arises.

   Rationale The stockings should be donned before the veins become distended and edema occurs.

Measuring knee-length stockings

2. Measure the circumference of the calf at the widest point, ie, 15 cm (6 in) below the inferior aspect of the patella. See Figure 32–9.

FIGURE 32–9

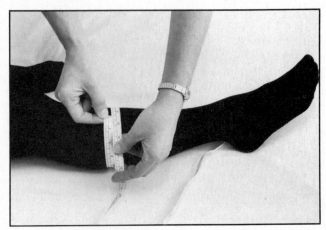

3. Measure the length of the leg from the heel to the popliteal space. See Figure 32–10.

Measuring thigh-length stockings

4. Measure the circumference of the calf as in step 2.
5. Measure the circumference of the thigh at the widest point, ie, 15 cm (6 in) above the superior aspect of the patella. See Figure 32–11.
6. Measure the length of the leg from the heel to the gluteal fold. See Figure 32–12.

Measuring waist-length stockings

7. Measure the circumference of the calf as in step 2.
8. Measure the circumference of the thigh as in step 5.
9. Measure the leg length from the bottom of the heel to the waist along the side of the body.

For all types of stockings

10. Compare the measurements to the size chart to obtain the correct size stockings.

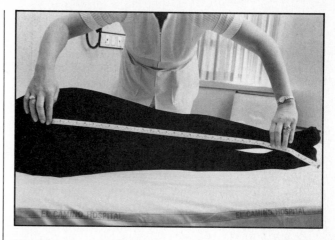

FIGURE 32–12

FIGURE 32–13

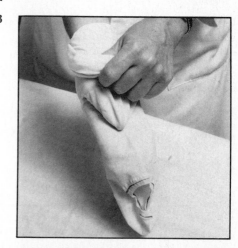

FIGURE 32–14

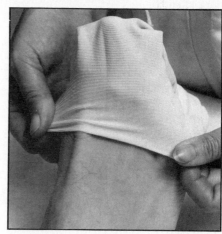

Applying elastic stockings

11. Make sure the stocking is inside out; then grasp the foot and heel of the stocking, and invert the stocking over your hand, so as to turn the leg and foot portions inside out to the heel portion. See Figure 32–13.
12. Remove your hand, and slip the foot portion of the stocking over the patient's toes, foot, and heel. See Figure 32–14. Make sure the patient's foot fits into the toe and heel portions of the stocking.

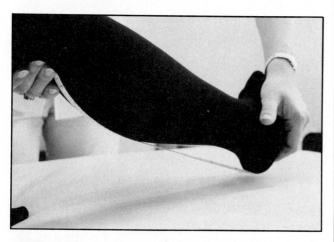

FIGURE 32–10

FIGURE 32–11

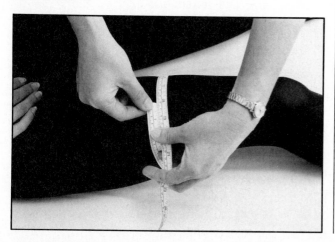

13. Pull the leg portion of the stocking over the foot and up the leg.

14. Pull the stocking up the leg evenly to its full length. Make sure there are no wrinkles or creases. Observe the lines in the material to make sure the stocking is not twisted.

    Rationale Wrinkles and creases can irritate the skin and impede blood circulation.

15. Repeat for the other leg.

16. Inspect the stocking periodically to see that the top has not rolled and that the leg above the stocking is not swollen.

Removing a stocking

17. Hold the top of the stocking with both hands and pull it down to the foot.

18. Supporting the foot at the ankle with one hand, pull the stocking over the foot and off.

19. Repeat for the other leg.

20. Record assessments and the time and application of the elastic stockings.

■ Evaluation

Expected outcomes

1. Absence of signs of poor arterial circulation
2. Absence of signs of poor venous return flow
3. Normal peripheral pulses
4. Negative Homan's sign

Unexpected outcomes

1. Cool skin temperature in a warm environment, pallor, shiny taut skin, and/or mild edema
2. Thickening of the skin, increased pigmentation around the ankles, pitting edema, and/or peripheral cyanosis
3. Peripheral pulse weak, irregular, and fast
4. Positive Homan's sign

Upon obtaining an unexpected outcome:

1. Report your findings to the responsible nurse and/or physician.
2. Adjust the nursing care plan appropriately.

References

Croushore JM: Postoperative assessment: The key to avoiding the most common nursing mistakes. *Nursing 79* (April) 1979; 9:46–50.

Dossey B, Passons JM: Pulmonary embolism: Preventing it, treating it. *Nursing 81* (March) 1981; 11:26–33.

Drain CB: Managing postoperative pain . . . It's a matter of sighs. *Nursing 84* (August) 1984; 14:52–55.

Erickson R: Tube talk principles of fluid flow in tubes. *Nursing 82* (July) 1982; 12:54–61.

Keithley JK, Tasic PW: A unified approach to assessment of the surgical patient. *Am J Nurs* (April) 1982; 82:612–614.

Laird M: Techniques for teaching pre- and postoperative patients. *Am J Nurs* (August) 1975; 75:1338-1340.

McConnell EA: All about gastrointestinal intubation. *Nursing 75* (September) 1975; 5:30–37.

McConnell EA: After surgery. *Nursing 77* (March) 1977a; 7:32–39.

McConnell EA: Ensuring safer stomach suctioning with a Salem sump tube. *Nursing 77* (September) 1977b; 7:54–57.

McConnell EA: Ten problems with nasogastric tubes . . . and how to solve them. *Nursing 79* (April) 1979; 9:78–81.

Parsons MC, Stephens GJ: Postoperative complications: Assessment and intervention. *Am J Nurs* (February) 1974; 74:240–244.

Ryan R: Thrombophlebitis: Assessment and prevention. *Am J Nurs* (October) 1976; 76:1634–1636.

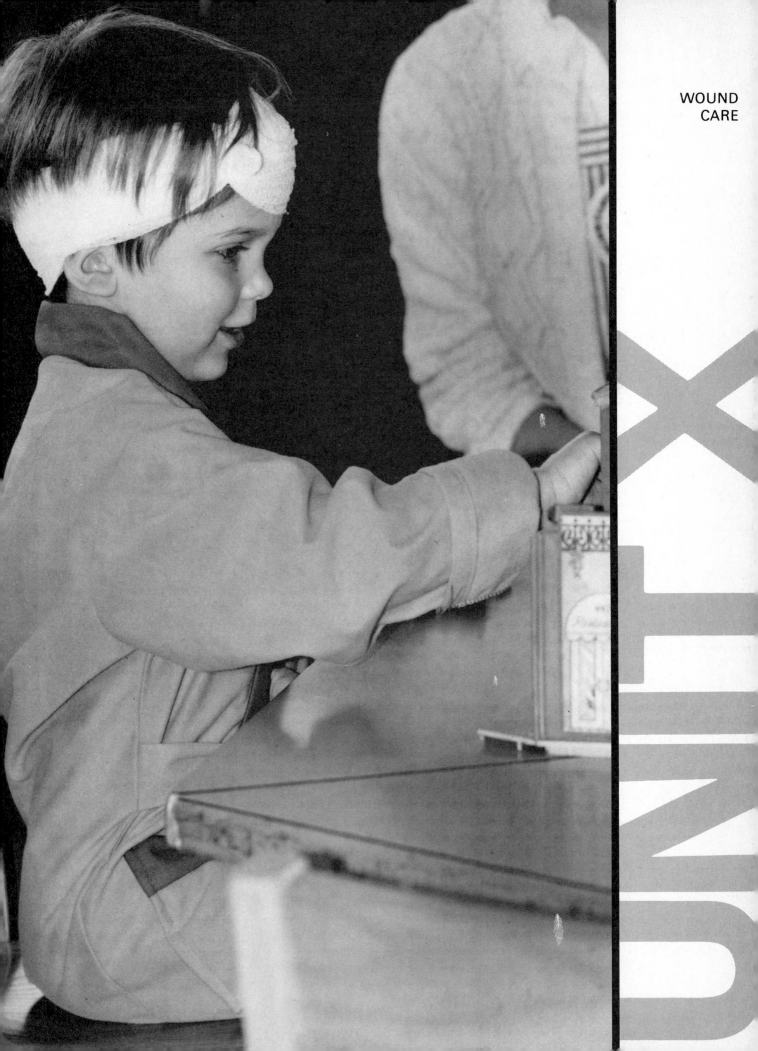

UNIT X

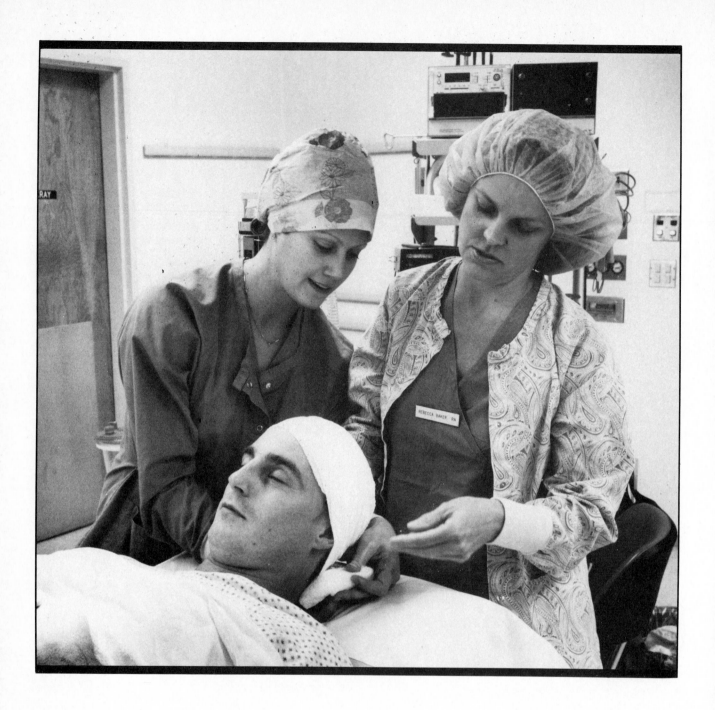

BINDERS AND BANDAGES

33 Binders and bandages are used to wrap body parts, to support injured parts of the body, to apply pressure to a wound or other area, or to hold dressings in place. A number of materials are used for binders and bandages, including gauze, flannel, and muslin. Some materials are stiff for support; others are elasticized for flexibility. There are several types of binders and bandages and several ways in which they are applied. When they are well applied, they promote healing, provide comfort and support to patients, and can prevent injury or further harm.

Chapter Outline

Binders

■ Technique 33–1 Applying Binders

Bandages

■ Technique 33–2 Basic Bandaging

■ Technique 33–3 Applying a Stump Bandage

Objectives

Upon completion of this chapter, the student will:

1. Know essential terms and facts about binders and bandages
    1.1 Define selected terms
    1.2 State purposes of binders and bandages
    1.3 Identify commonly used types of binders
    1.4 Identify methods of applying binders
    1.5 Identify common types of bandages
    1.6 Identify basic turns in bandaging
    1.7 Identify essential guidelines for bandaging
2. Understand facts about applying binders and bandages
    2.1 Identify relevant assessment data
    2.2 Identify nursing diagnoses for which the technique may be implemented
    2.3 Identify nursing goals related to the technique
    2.4 Identify expected and unexpected outcomes from assessment data
    2.5 Identify reasons underlying selected steps of the technique
3. Perform binder and bandage application techniques safely

3.1 Assess the patient adequately
3.2 Collect additional data from appropriate sources
3.3 Select pertinent nursing goals for the patient
3.4 Establish relevant outcome criteria for the patient following the technique
3.5 Collect necessary equipment before the technique
3.6 Implement interventions to enhance the effectiveness of the technique and enhance the patient's comfort and safety
3.7 Communicate relevant information about the patient to the appropriate persons
3.8 Determine the evaluative outcomes of the technique
4. Evaluate own performance of specific techniques for applying binders and bandages in a laboratory or clinical setting with the assistance of another
    4.1 Use the performance checklists provided
    4.2 Identify areas of strength and weakness
    4.3 Alter performance in response to own evaluation and that of another

Terms

■ bandage   a material used to wrap a body part

■ binder   a type of bandage applied to large body areas, eg, the abdomen or chest

■ circumference   the outer measurement of a rounded body

■ splint   a rigid bar or appliance used to stabilize a body part

BINDERS

There are five commonly used types of binders: the triangular arm binder (sling), the breast binder, the T-binder (single or double T), the straight abdominal binder, and the scultetus (many-tailed) binder. Most binders are made of muslin (plain-woven cotton fabric), flannel, or synthetic material that may or may not be elasticized. Some abdominal binders are made of an elasticized netlike material that fits the body contours and allows air to circulate around the body part.

TECHNIQUE 33-1 ■ Applying Binders

Binders are used to provide support, to apply pressure, to prevent or reduce swelling, or to retain dressings:

1. Triangular arm binder (sling): usually applied as a full triangle to support the arm, elbow, and forearm of the patient or to reduce or prevent swelling of a hand. See Figure 33-1.

2. Breast binder: to provide pressure on the breasts, for example, when drying up the milk flow after childbirth, or to support the breasts, for example, after surgery. Breast binders are pinned in the front and usually have shoulder straps to prevent the binder from slipping down. See Figure 33-2.

3. T-binder (single or double T): to retain pads, dressings, or packs in the perineal area. Single T-binders are often used for females, and double T-binders for males to prevent undue pressure on the penis. See Figure 33-3. The double T-binder can also provide greater support for large dressings on both males and females.

4. Straight abdominal binder: to provide support to the abdomen. This binder is a rectangular piece of material long enough to encircle the patient's abdomen with some overlap. See Figure 33-4. It can be made from any material, eg, a bath blanket or towel.

5. Scultetus (many-tailed) binder: to provide support to the abdomen and, in some instances, to retain dressings. See Figure 33-5.

■ Assessment

1. Assess the body area to which the binder is applied. Check for swelling, discoloration, skin abrasions, discomfort, etc.

2. Determine whether the dressing needs changing or reinforcing, depending on the physician's orders.

Other data include:

1. The type of binder and when it is to be applied (see the nursing care plan)

2. Whether adjunctive measures, eg, a cold pack, are indicated (see the patient's chart)

■ Planning

Nursing goals

1. To support or immobilize a body part
2. To provide pressure on a body part
3. To prevent or reduce swelling
4. To retain pads, dressings, or packs

Equipment

1. The appropriate binder
2. Abdominal (ABD) pads to protect bony prominences, eg, the iliac crests (for an abdominal binder), or to prevent skin surfaces from rubbing together and

FIGURE 33-1 ■ A large arm sling.

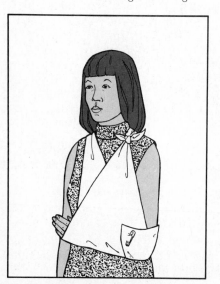

FIGURE 33-2 ■ A breast binder.

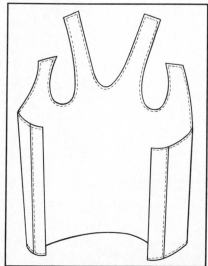

FIGURE 33-3 ■ T-binders: A, single T; B, double T.

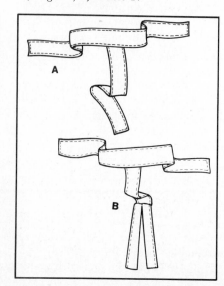

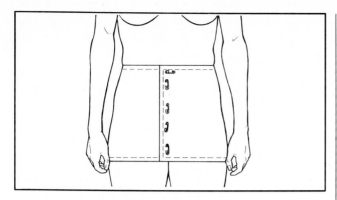

FIGURE 33-4 ■ A straight abdominal binder.

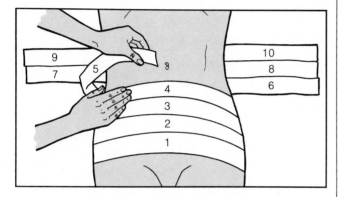

FIGURE 33-5 ■ A scultetus (many-tailed) binder.

becoming excoriated, eg, the skin beneath the breasts (for a breast binder)

3. Safety pins or tape to secure the binder

■ **Intervention**

1. If the binder is being placed directly against the skin and the area is soiled, wash and dry it.

2. Assist the patient to a comfortable lying or sitting position, supporting the area as appropriate.

Triangular arm sling

3. Have the patient flex the elbow to a 90° angle or more, depending on the purpose. The thumb should be facing upward or inward toward the body.

   Rationale A 90° angle is sufficient to support the forearm and hand and to relieve pressure on the shoulder joint (eg, to support the paralyzed arm of a stroke patient whose shoulder might otherwise become dislocated). A more acute angle is preferred if there is swelling of the hand (see step 11).

4. Place one end of the unfolded triangular binder over the shoulder of the uninjured side, so that the binder falls down the front of the patient with the point of the triangle (apex) under the elbow of the injured side. See Figure 33-6.

5. Take the upper corner and carry it around the neck

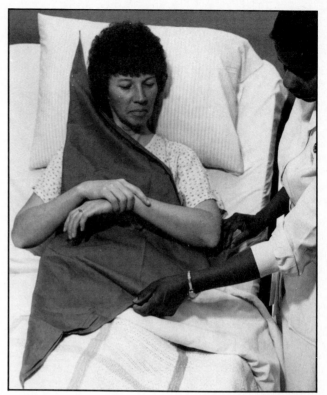

FIGURE 33-6

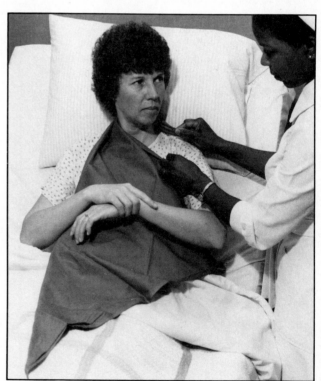

FIGURE 33-7

until it hangs over the shoulder on the injured side. See Figure 33-7.

6. Bring the lower corner of the binder up over the arm to the shoulder of the injured side. Using a reef knot,

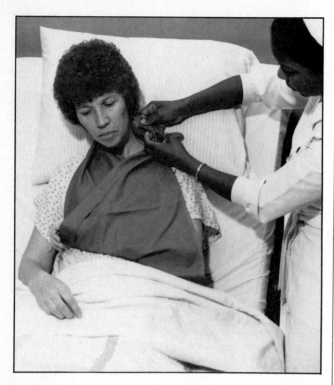

FIGURE 33-8

FIGURE 33-9 ■ **A,** Making a cravat: (1) lay the triangular bandage on a flat surface, (2) fold the point up toward the base of the bandage, (3) fold the base over on itself to make a smooth edge, (4) fold the cravat from the other side to the desired width; **B,** the cravat applied as a small arm sling.

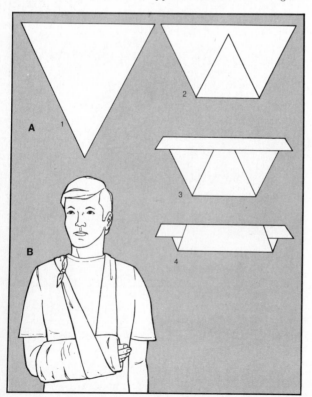

secure this corner to the upper corner at the side of the neck on the involved side. See Figure 33–8.

Rationale A reef knot will not slip. Tying the knot at the side of the neck prevents pressure on the bony prominences of the vertebral column at the back of the neck.

7. Make sure the wrist is well supported, to maintain alignment.

8. Fold the sling neatly at the elbow, and secure it with safety pins or tape. It may be folded and fastened at the front. See Figure 33–1 on page 794.

9. Remove the sling periodically to inspect the skin for indications of irritation, especially around the site of the knot.

Other uses of the triangular binder

10. *Small arm sling (cravat binder)*
    a. Make a cravat binder by folding the triangular binder in on itself, starting at the apex. See Figure 33–9, *A.*
    b. Apply the sling as in Figure 33–9, *B,* with the knot on the affected side.

11. *Triangular arm sling for maximum hand elevation*
    a. Flex the patient's arm so that the hand rests on the clavicle of the uninjured side.

    Rationale This position provides maximum elevation of the hand.

    b. Place the binder over the shoulder of the uninjured side and *over the arm* (ie, in front of the arm), so that the apex of the binder extends beyond the elbow of the injured side. See Figure 33–10, *A.*
    c. Tuck the base of the binder under the patient's arm, bring the free end across the patient's back, and, using a reef knot, tie it to the other free end at the shoulder *on the uninjured side.* The knot should rest in the hollow of the clavicle to prevent pressure on the clavicle. See Figure 33-10, *B.*
    d. Bring the apex of the sling toward the patient's back, tuck it in, and secure it with a safety pin or pins. See Figure 33–10, *C.*

12. *Hand or foot mitt*
    Apply the triangular bandage as a mitt to cover hand or foot dressings. See Figure 30–11.

Breast binder

13. Spread the binder on the bed, and have the patient lie in a supine position on top of it. Center the binder, place the lower edge at the waistline, and allow adequate armhole space.

    Rationale Adequate armhole space is needed to prevent the material from chafing the axillae.

14. If the breasts are large, place padding under each breast.

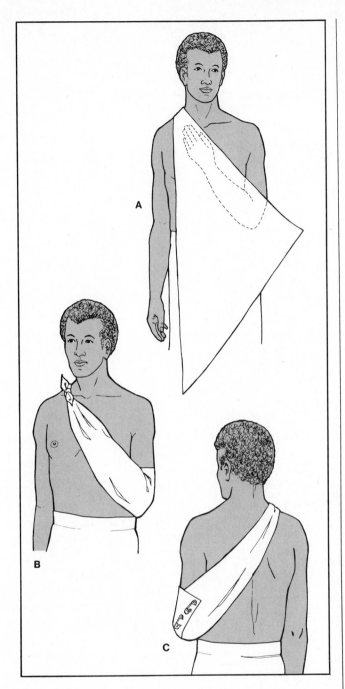

FIGURE 33-10

Rationale   This prevents skin excoriation caused by pressing the two skin surfaces tightly together.

15. Pull the binder tightly across the breast tissue at the nipple line, and fasten it at the midline with a safety pin placed vertically. Ask the patient to help by pressing the palms of her hands against the sides of the breasts.

16. While continuing to compress the breasts, pin the binder alternately above and below the first fastening. Place the pins vertically except for the lowest one, which is placed horizontally. See Figure 33-12.

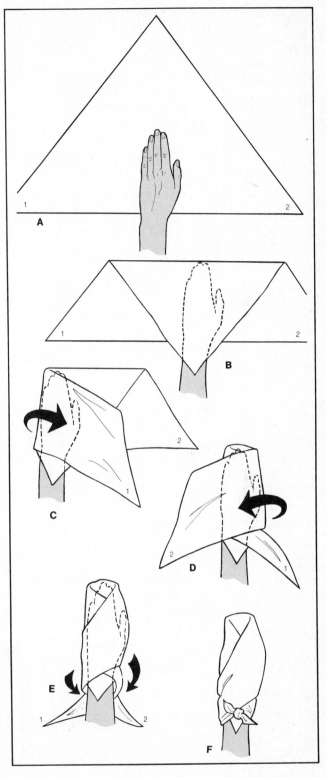

FIGURE 33-11   ■   Wrapping a hand using a triangular bandage: **A,** lay the hand in the center of the triangular bandage; **B,** fold the apex over the wrist; **C, D,** wrap the corners (1 and 2) around the hand; **E,** bring the corners around the wrist; **F,** tie a reef knot on the dorsum of the wrist.

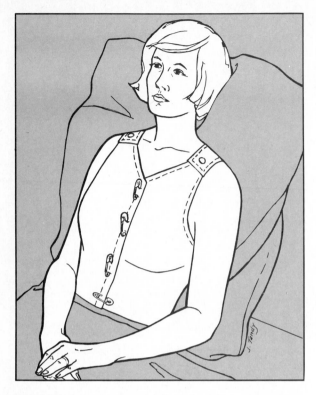

FIGURE 33-12

Rationale Fastening the pins alternately above and below distributes pressure equally, thereby providing maximum support. Placing the lowest pin horizontally allows for more comfort when moving.

17. Fasten the shoulder straps with pins if required.

T-binder

18. Select the appropriate binder for the patient, and place it smoothly under the patient with the waistband at waist level and the tails running down the midline at the back. Double T-binders may be used for females if a dressing is large (eg, after extensive surgery).

FIGURE 33-13

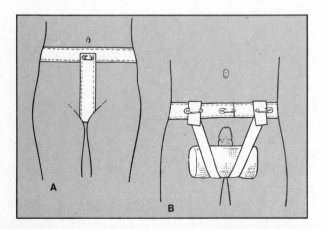

19. Bring the waist tails around the patient, overlap them, and secure them with a pin placed horizontally.
    Rationale The pins placed horizontally allow comfort when bending at the waist and moving.

20. Bring the center tail up between the patient's legs. See Figure 33–13, *A*. The two tails of the double T-binder are brought up on either side of the penis. See Figure 33–13, *B*. When dressings are in place, take care to touch only the outside of the dressings to prevent contamination of the wound or yourself.

21. Fasten the ties at the waist with a safety pin placed horizontally.

Straight abdominal or scultetus binder

22. With the patient in a supine position, place the binder smoothly under the patient with the upper border of the binder at the patient's waist and the lower border at the level of the gluteal fold.
    Rationale A binder placed above the waist interferes with respiration; one placed too low interferes with elimination and walking.

23. Apply padding over the iliac crests if the patient is thin.

24. For a straight abdominal binder, bring the ends around the patient, overlap them, and secure them with pins. See Figure 33–4 on page 795.

25. Place the top pin horizontally at the waist to allow for comfort when moving.

26. For a scultetus binder, bring the tails over to the center from alternate sides. See Figure 33–5 on page 795. The last tail is secured with a safety pin. Each tail should overlap the preceding one by about half the width of the tail for maximum support. In thin people, the tails may extend beyond the other side and require folding back.
    a. For patients who have had abdominal surgery, lace the tails from the bottom up.
       Rationale This provides maximum upward support.
    b. For the postpartum patient, lace the tails from the top down.
       Rationale This provides downward pressure on the uterus.

For all binders

27. Ensure that there are no wrinkles or creases in the binders.
    Rationale Wrinkles and creases cause pressure on the skin and subsequent excoriation.

28. Check the agency's policies on recording application of a binder. It is generally not recorded when the binder is applied to hold a dressing in place.

However, an arm sling, breast binder, or abdominal binder may be recorded, together with the assessment data and the patient's response.

Sample Recording

Date	Time	Notes
8/17/86	1000	Breast binder applied. Breasts are enlarged, hard, engorged, and painful. ————————— ————————————— Page O. Mills, NS

■ Evaluation

Expected outcomes

1. Reduced swelling
2. Absence of discomfort in affected limb or part

3. Decreased breast engorgement (breast binder)
4. Skin areas intact beneath binder

Unexpected outcomes

1. Swelling
2. Muscle strain or discomfort in affected limb or part
3. Painful breast engorgement (breast binder)
4. Skin excoriation beneath binder

Upon obtaining an unexpected outcome:

1. Report your findings to the responsible nurse and/or physician.
2. Adjust the patient's nursing care plan accordingly.

BANDAGES

Bandages are made of a number of different materials, depending on their purpose. Gauze is one of the most commonly used materials because it is light and porous and readily molds to the body. It is also relatively inexpensive, so it is generally discarded once it becomes soiled. Gauze is frequently used to retain dressings on wounds and to bandage the fingers, hands, toes, and feet. It supports dressings well and at the same time permits air to circulate, and it can be impregnated with petroleum jelly or other medications for application to wounds.

Flannel is a soft, pliable material that provides warmth to a body part. It is strong and fairly heavy and can be washed and reused.

Muslin is lighter than flannel but is also strong and supplies good support. Many binders are made of muslin. Like flannel, it can be washed and reused.

Crinoline and Kling are types of woven gauze. Kling is woven in such a manner that it will stretch and mold to the body. Crinoline is loosely woven yet strong. It is impregnated with plaster of paris for use as the base for casts.

There are many kinds of elasticized bandages that are applied to provide pressure to an area. They are commonly used as tensor bandages or as partial stockings to provide support to the legs and improve the venous circulation (see chapter 32). Some elasticized bandages have an adhesive backing and can be secured to the skin. These are most frequently used to retain dressings and at the same time provide some support to a wound.

Plastic adhesive bandages are also used to retain dressings. They are waterproof and thus retain wound drainage or keep an area dry. They have some elastic properties and therefore provide some pressure.

Guidelines for Bandaging

1. Whenever possible, bandage the part in its normal position, with the joint slightly flexed to avoid putting strain on the ligaments and the muscles of the joint.

2. Pad between skin surfaces and over bony prominences to prevent friction from the bandage and consequent abrasion of the skin.

3. Always bandage body parts by working from the distal to the proximal end, to aid the return flow of the venous blood.

4. Bandage with even pressure so as not to interfere with blood circulation.

5. Whenever possible, leave the end of the body part (eg, the finger) exposed so that you will be able to determine the adequacy of the blood circulation to the extremity.

6. Cover dressings with bandages at least 5 cm (2 in) beyond the edges of the dressing to prevent the dressing and wound from becoming contaminated.

7. Face the patient when applying a bandage to maintain uniform tension and the appropriate direction of the bandage.

TECHNIQUE 33-2 ■ Basic Bandaging 🏠

Applying bandages to various parts of the body involves one or more basic turns. For example, circular and spiral turns are used to bandage a finger. There are five basic bandaging turns: circular, spiral, spiral reverse, recurrent, and figure eight.

1. Circular turns are used to anchor bandages and to terminate them. They are also used to bandage certain areas, such as the proximal aspect of a finger or a wrist. Circular turns are not usually applied directly over a wound because of the discomfort the bandage would cause.

2. Spiral turns are used to bandage parts of the body that are fairly uniform in circumference, eg, the upper arm or upper leg.

3. Spiral reverse turns are used to bandage cylindrical parts of the body that are not uniform in circumference, eg, the lower leg or forearm.

4. Recurrent turns are used to cover distal parts of the body, eg, the end of a finger, the skull, or the stump of an amputation.

5. Figure-eight turns are used to bandage an elbow, knee, or ankle, because they permit some movement after they are applied. The *spica* bandage is a variation of the figure-eight turn.

■ Assessment

Assess the area for:

1. Any abrasions or wounds. Open areas will require dressing before a bandage is applied.

2. The color and temperature of the skin and any numbness, tingling, or pain in the area. Pale or cyanotic skin, cool temperature, tingling, and/or pain can indicate impaired circulation in the area.

Other data include:

1. The area requiring a bandage.

2. The reason for the bandage. The reason often indicates the type of bandage material required, eg, an elasticized bandage would be needed to provide pressure.

■ Planning

Nursing goals

1. To support a wound, eg, a fractured bone
2. To immobilize a wound, eg, a strained shoulder
3. To apply pressure, eg, to improve venous blood flow in the legs

4. To secure a dressing to a wound
5. To retain splints
6. To retain warmth, eg, a flannel bandage applied to a rheumatoid joint

Equipment

1. A clean bandage of the appropriate material and width. The width of the bandage depends on the size of the body part to be bandaged. For example, a 2.5-cm (1-in) bandage is used for a finger, a 5-cm (2-in) bandage for an arm, and a 7.5-cm or 10-cm (3-in or 4-in) bandage for a leg. The larger the circumference of the part, the wider the bandage.

2. Padding for bony prominences and for between skin surfaces. Abdominal dressings (ABD pads) and gauze squares are frequently used to cover bony prominences, such as the elbow, or to separate skin surfaces, such as the fingers.

3. Tape, special metal clips, or a safety pin to secure the end of the bandage.

■ Intervention

1. Provide the patient with a chair or bed, and arrange support for the area to be bandaged. For example, if a hand needs to be bandaged, have the patient place the elbow on a table, so that the hand does not have to be held up unsupported.

   Rationale Because bandaging takes a little time, holding up a body part without support can be very tiring.

2. Make sure that the area to be bandaged is clean and dry. Wash and dry the area if necessary.

   Rationale Washing and drying remove microorganisms, which flourish in warm moist areas.

3. Align the part to be bandaged with slight flexion of the joints, unless this is contraindicated.

   Rationale Slight flexion places less strain on the ligaments and muscles of the joint.

Circular turns

4. Hold the bandage in your dominant hand, with the roll uppermost (see Figure 33-14), and unroll the bandage about 8 cm (3 in).

   Rationale This length of unrolled bandage allows good control for placement and tension.

5. Apply the end of the bandage to the part of the body to be bandaged. Hold the end down with the thumb of the other hand. See Figure 33-15.

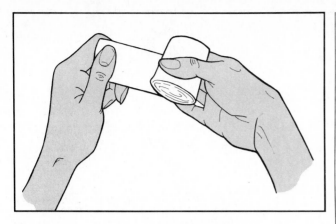

FIGURE 33–14

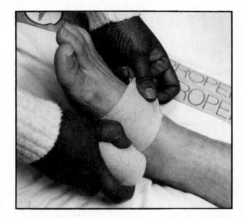

FIGURE 33–15

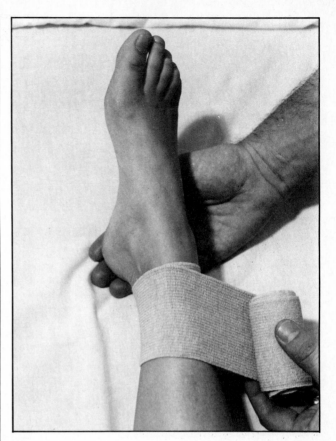

FIGURE 33–16

FIGURE 33–17

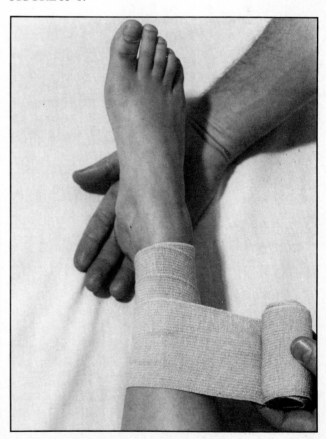

6. Encircle the body part as often as needed, each turn directly covering the previous turn. See Figure 33–16.

   Rationale This provides even support to the area.

7. Secure the end of the bandage with tape, metal clips, or a safety pin over an uninjured area.

   Rationale Clips and pins can be uncomfortable when situated over an injured area.

Spiral turns

8. See steps 1–5.

9. Make two circular turns.

   Rationale Two circular turns anchor the bandage.

10. Continue spiral turns at about a 30° angle, each turn overlapping the preceding one by two-thirds the width of the bandage. See Figure 33–17.

11. Terminate the bandage with two circular turns, and secure the end with tape, metal clips, or a safety pin over an uninjured area.

Spiral reverse turns

12. See steps 1–5.

13. Anchor the bandage with two circular turns and bring the bandage upward at about a 30° angle.

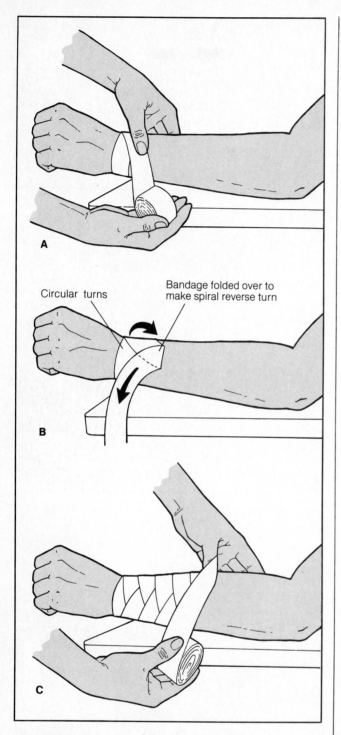

Circular turns

Bandage folded over to make spiral reverse turn

FIGURE 33–18

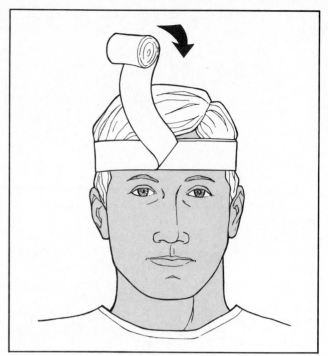

FIGURE 33–19

bandage. Make each bandage turn at the same position on the limb so that the turns of the bandage will be aligned. See Figure 33–18, *C*.

17. Terminate the bandage with two circular turns, and secure the end with tape, metal clips, or a safety pin over an uninjured area.

Recurrent turns

18. See steps 1–5.

19. Anchor the bandage with two circular turns.

20. Fold it back on itself and bring it centrally over the distal end to be bandaged. See Figure 33–19.

21. Holding it with the other hand, bring it back over the end to the right of the center bandage but overlapping it by two-thirds the width of the bandage.

22. Bring the bandage back on the left side, also overlapping the first turn by two-thirds the width of the bandage.

23. Continue this pattern of alternating right and left until the area is covered. Overlap the preceding turn by two-thirds the bandage width each time.

24. Terminate the bandage with two circular turns. See Figure 33–20. Secure the end with tape, metal clips, or a safety pin over an uninjured area.

Figure-eight turns

25. See steps 1–5 and then anchor the bandage with two circular turns.

14. Place the thumb of your free hand on the upper edge of the bandage. See Figure 33–18, *A*.

Rationale The thumb will hold the bandage while it is folded upon itself.

15. Unroll the bandage about 15 cm (6 in), then turn your hand so that the bandage falls over itself. See Figure 33–18, *B*.

16. Continue the bandage around the limb, overlapping each previous turn by two-thirds the width of the

26. Carry the bandage above the joint, around it, and then below it, making a figure eight.

27. Continue above and below the joint, overlapping the previous turn by two-thirds the width of the bandage. See Figure 33–21.

28. Terminate the bandage above the joint with two circular turns, and secure it with tape, metal clips, or a safety pin over an uninjured area.

Spica bandage

A spica bandage is a variation of the figure-eight bandage. It is commonly used to bandage the hip, groin, shoulder, breast, or thumb. This technique focuses on the thumb spica; other spica bandages are done in a similar way. A 2.5-cm (1-in) bandage is frequently used for a thumb spica, and a 7.5-cm (3-in) bandage for a hip or shoulder spica.

Thumb spica

29. See steps 1–5 above.

30. Anchor the bandage with two circular turns around the wrist.

31. Bring the bandage down to the distal aspect of the thumb and encircle the thumb. Leave the tip of the thumb exposed if possible.

    Rationale This enables the nurse to check blood circulation to the thumb.

32. Bring the bandage back up and around the wrist, then back down and around the thumb, overlapping the previous turn by two-thirds the width of the bandage.

33. Repeat steps 30 and 31, working up the thumb and hand until the thumb is covered. See Figure 33–22.

34. Anchor the bandage with two circular turns around the wrist, and secure it with safety pins, tape, or clips.

35. Record the type of bandage applied, the area to which it is applied, and any skin problems of the bandaged area or neurovascular problems of the involved extremity.

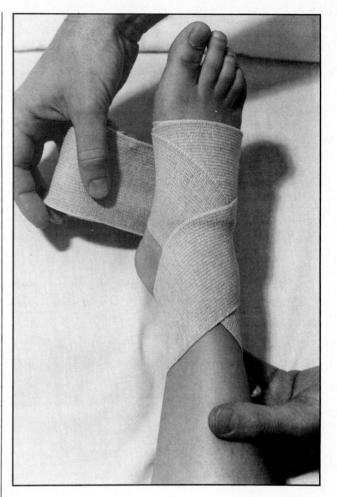

FIGURE 33–21

Sample Recording

Date	Time	Notes
4/7/86	0700	Elastic spiral bandage applied to right leg. Toes warm and pink. No numbness. ——— ——— Laura R. Stenhouse, NS

FIGURE 33–22

FIGURE 33–20

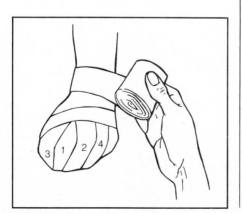

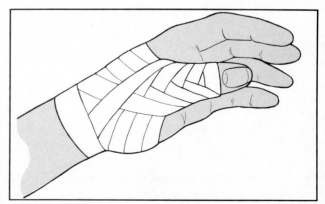

■ Evaluation

Expected outcomes

1. Absence of clinical signs of circulatory impairment, eg, extremity warm and pink
2. No complaints of pain, numbness, or tingling in the area

Unexpected outcomes

1. Extremity cyanotic and cold
2. Complaints of numbness and tingling in the area

Upon obtaining an unexpected outcome:

1. Report your findings to the responsible nurse and/or physician.
2. Adjust the nursing care plan appropriately.

TECHNIQUE 33–3 ■ Applying a Stump Bandage

When a limb is amputated, the distal portion of the limb that remains is called the *stump*. A stump bandage is usually applied after a dressing change.

■ Assessment

Assess:

1. The amount and color of any drainage that has come through the dressing.
2. The color, temperature, and swelling of the skin near the dressing. This provides baseline data for evaluating the blood circulation to and from the area after the bandage has been applied.
3. Any discomfort experienced by the patient. It is not unusual for patients who have had amputations to experience "phantom" pain, that is, pain or irritation perceived to be in the removed part of the limb.

Other data include: The surgeon's preference regarding the type of material and the kind of bandage to apply. Some surgeons may request that the stump be wrapped with a figure-eight bandage; others prefer a recurrent or a spiral bandage. Commonly the figure-eight or modified figure-eight bandages are used.

■ Planning

Nursing goals

1. To retain a dressing
2. To apply pressure, support venous return flow, and prevent swelling
3. To help shape the stump

Equipment

1. A clean bandage. The type of material will depend on the purpose of the bandage and the physician's order. An elastic bandage is often used to apply pressure. An 8-cm or 10-cm (3-in or 4-in) bandage is recommended for an adult stump.
2. Tape, safety pins, or metal clips to secure the bandage.

FIGURE 33–23

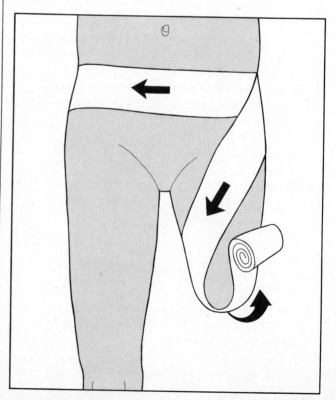

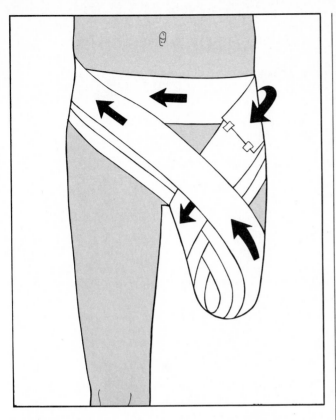

FIGURE 33–24

■ Intervention

The following interventions apply to leg amputations, but the bandaging of arm amputations is similar.

1. Assist the patient to a semi-Fowler's position in bed or to a sitting position on the edge of the bed.

2. Figure-eight bandage

  a. Anchor the bandage with two circular turns around the hips.

  b. Bring the bandage down over the stump and then back up and around the hips. See Figure 33–23.

  c. Bring the bandage down again, overlapping the previous turn, and follow a figure eight around the stump and back up around the hips.

  d. Repeat, working the bandage up the stump. See Figure 33–24.

  e. Anchor the bandage around the hips with two circular turns.

  f. Secure the bandage with adhesive tape, safety pins, or clips.

    or

  g. Place the end of the elastic bandage at the top of the anterior surface of the leg and have the patient hold it in place. Bring the bandage diagonally down toward the end of the stump.

  h. Then, applying even pressure, bring the bandage diagonally upward toward the groin area. See Figure 33–25.

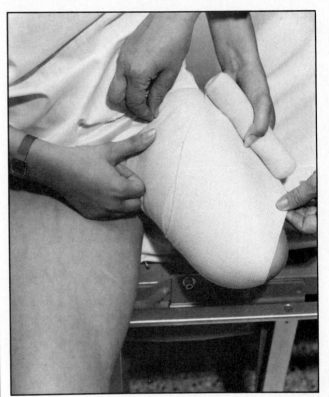

FIGURE 33–25

FIGURE 33–26

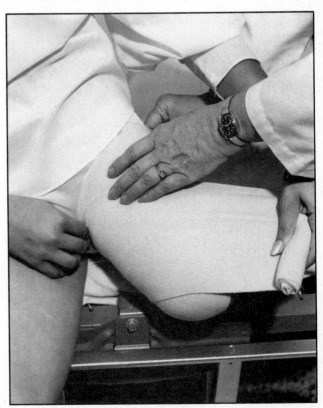

  i. Make a figure-eight turn behind the top of the leg, downward again over and under the stump, and back up to the groin area. See Figure 33–26.

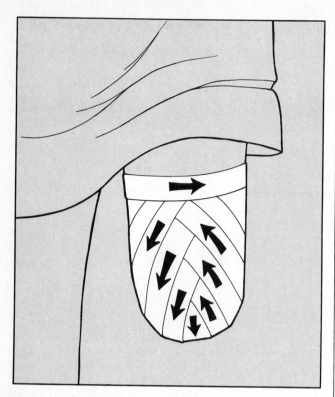

FIGURE 33–27

j. Repeat these figure-eight turns at least twice.

k. Anchor the bandage around the hips as in step 2e.

l. Secure the bandage with tape, safety pins, or clips.

3. Recurrent bandage

  a. Anchor the bandage with two circular turns around the stump.

  b. Cover the stump with recurrent turns. See Technique 33–2, steps 20–23.

  c. Anchor the recurrent bandage with two circular turns. See Figure 33–27.

  d. Secure the bandage with tape, safety pins, or clips.

4. Spiral bandage

  a. Make recurrent turns to cover the end of the stump.

  b. Apply spiral turns from the distal aspect of the stump toward the body. See Figure 33–28.

  c. Anchor the bandage with two circular turns around the hips.

  d. Secure the bandage with tape, safety pins, or clips.

■ Evaluation

Expected outcomes

1. Intact stump skin
2. Good stump skin color and temperature

Unexpected outcomes

1. Infection of stump
2. Stump skin cold and pale or cyanotic
3. Marked swelling of stump

Upon obtaining an unexpected outcome:

1. Report your findings to the responsible nurse and/or physician.
2. Adjust the patient's nursing care plan accordingly.

FIGURE 33–28

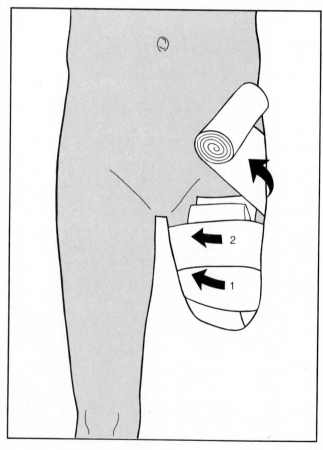

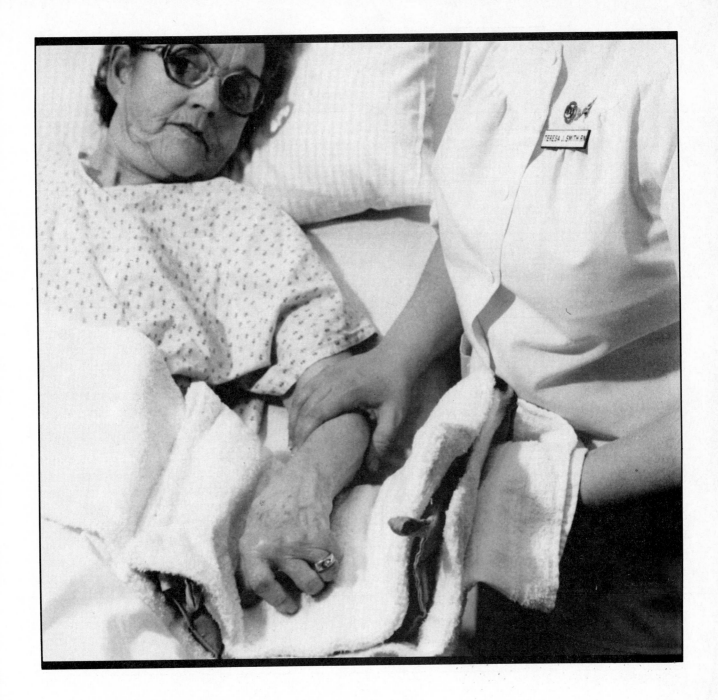

HOT AND COLD APPLICATIONS

34 Heat and cold are applied to the body to support processes involved in repairing and healing tissues. The exact form of the heat or cold applied generally depends on its purpose. Cold applied to a body part draws heat from the area, while heat, of course, adds warmth to the body part. This subtraction or addition of heat causes physiologic changes in temperature of the tissues, size of the blood vessels, capillary blood pressure, capillary surface area for exchange of fluids and electrolytes, blood viscosity, and tissue metabolism.

Chapter Outline

Objectives

Upon completion of this chapter, the student will:

1. Know essential terms and facts about hot and cold applications
   1.1 Define selected terms
   1.2 Identify essential guidelines (precautions) for applying heat and cold
   1.3 Identify recommended temperatures for hot and cold applications
   1.4 Identify methods of applying dry and moist heat
   1.5 Identify methods of applying dry and moist cold
   1.6 Identify purposes for selected methods of hot and cold applications
2. Understand facts about heat and cold applications
   2.1 Identify relevant assessment data
   2.2 Identify nursing goals related to the technique
   2.3 Identify expected and unexpected outcomes from assessment data
   2.4 Identify reasons underlying selected steps of the technique
3. Perform heat and cold application techniques safely
   3.1 Assess the patient adequately
   3.2 Collect additional data from appropriate sources
   3.3 Select pertinent nursing goals for the patient
   3.4 Establish relevant outcome criteria for the patient following the technique
   3.5 Collect necessary equipment before the technique
   3.6 Implement interventions to enhance the effectiveness of the technique and enhance the patient's comfort and safety
   3.7 Communicate relevant information about the patient to the appropriate persons
   3.8 Determine the evaluative outcomes of the technique
4. Evaluate own performance of specific heat and cold application techniques in a laboratory or clinical setting with the assistance of another
   4.1 Use the performance checklists provided
   4.2 Identify areas of strength and weakness
   4.3 Alter performance in response to own evaluation and that of another

Terms

■ **conduction** the transfer of heat from a warm object to a cooler object, or vice versa, by contact

■ **convection** transfer of heat by movement of a liquid or gas, eg, air currents

■ **exudate** material, eg, fluid and cells, that has escaped from blood vessels and is deposited in or on tissues

■ **hyperemia** increased blood flow resulting in redness of the skin

■ **ischemia** limited blood supply to an area

■ **radiation** the transfer of heat from a warm object to a cooler object by means of electromagnetic waves

■ **suppuration** the formation of pus

■ **vaporization** conversion of a solid or liquid into a gas (vapor)

■ **vasoconstriction** a decrease in the caliber (lumen) of blood vessels

■ **viscosity** the quality of being viscous (sticky or gummy)

GUIDELINES FOR APPLYING HEAT ~~KNOW~~ AND COLD

1. An individual becomes less sensitive to repeated exposure to heat and cold. The nurse who is not aware of this can inadvertently apply a cold or hot application that can damage the tissues. See Table 34–1 for recommended temperatures for hot and cold applications.

2. People vary in the ability to tolerate heat and cold. The elderly and the very young have the least tolerance.

3. Different areas of the body vary in sensitivity to temperature. For example, the back of the hand is less sensitive than the inner aspect of the wrist.

4. The larger the body area exposed to heat or cold, the less the individual's tolerance.

5. Moisture conducts heat better than air, therefore moist hot and cold applications are more likely to injure tissues.

6. Heat should not be applied when vasodilation will increase discomfort or an inflammatory process, or when the possibility of hemorrhage exists.

7. Cold should not be applied when there is evidence of impaired circulation, eg, numbness, cold feeling of the skin or mucous membranes, or a bluish tinge. Cold is also contraindicated when there is pain due to contracted muscles or when there is shivering and a lowered body temperature.

8. Whenever heat or cold is applied, the area must be checked regularly for untoward clinical signs, such as numbness, pallor or cyanosis, pain, increased swelling, or erythema (redness of the skin due to congestion of the blood). Any of these signs should be reported to the responsible nurse, and termination of the treatment should be considered. See Table 34–2.

9. Because the duration of most applications (eg, dry heat and cold, soaks, sitz baths, heat lamps, compresses, and packs) is about 15 to 20 minutes, the nurse should check the patient within 5 to 10 minutes for complaints of discomfort. If discomfort is present, the area must be

inspected for the clinical signs mentioned above. For patients who have decreased sensitivity, the skin should be observed for untoward signs.

APPLICATIONS OF HEAT AND COLD

Heat is applied to the body in both dry and moist forms. Dry heat is applied locally for heat conduction by means of a hot water bottle, electric pad, aquathermia pad, or disposable heat pack. The heat lamp and bed cradle provide dry heat by radiation. Moist heat can be provided through conduction by compress, hot pack, soak, or sitz bath.

Applications of cold may also be dry or moist. Dry cold is administered for local effect by the use of ice bags, ice

---

TABLE 34–2 ■ Effects of Hot and Cold Applications

Hot applications	Cold applications
Arteriole vasodilation (reddened skin)	Arteriole vasoconstriction (pale bluish skin)
Decreased stroke volume*	Increased stroke volume*
Increased respiratory rate	Decreased respiratory rate
Increased temperature of local tissues	Decreased temperature of local tissues
Increased amount of capillary surface	Decreased amount of capillary surface
Decreased blood viscosity	Increased blood viscosity
Increased tissue metabolism	Decreased tissue metabolism
Increased capillary blood pressure	Decreased capillary blood pressure
Muscular relaxation	Muscular contraction
Increased number of leukocytes and inflammation	Reduced inflammation

*Stroke volume is the volume of blood ejected from the ventricle of the heart with each contraction.

TABLE 34–1 ■ Recommended Temperatures for Hot and Cold Applications

Cover all of these c towel

Description	°C	°F	Application
Very cold	Below 15	Below 59	Ice bags
Cold	15–18	59–65	Cold pack
Cold	18–27	65–80	Cold compress
Tepid	27–37	80–98	Alcohol and tepid sponges
Warm	37–40	98–105	Warm bath
Hot	40–46	105–115	Aquathermia, soaks, sitz baths, irrigations, moist sterile compresses, hot water bags for debilitated or young patients *Aqua k Pads (electric)*
Very hot	Above 46	Above 115	Hot water bags for adults, heat cradles

SET 99°–100°

125°F

TABLE 34-3 ■ Reasons for Hot and Cold Applications	
Heat	Cold
Relieving muscle spasm	Decreasing and terminating bleeding
Softening exudates	
Hastening the suppuration process	Anesthetizing and reducing pain
Hastening healing	Reducing inflammation
Warming a part of the body	Controlling accumulation of fluid
Reducing congestion in an underlying organ	
Reducing pressure from accumulated fluid	
Increasing peristalsis	
Providing comfort and relaxation	

collars, ice gloves, and disposable cold packs. Moist cold is applied for either local or systemic effects. Cold moist compresses are administered to body parts for a local effect, while a tepid sponge bath is given for a systemic cooling effect. Some reasons for applying heat and cold are given in Table 34–3.

TECHNIQUE 34–1 ■ Applying a Hot Water Bottle, Electric Heating Pad, or Aquathermia Pad 🏠

A hot water bottle or bag is a common source of dry heat for local effect. It is convenient and relatively inexpensive. However, because there is a danger of burning from improper use, agencies may require the patient to sign a release that absolves the agency and its employees from any responsibility for injury incurred with the use of hot water bottles.

Electric pads have become less popular in recent years. The pad provides a constant, even heat, is lightweight, and can be molded to a body part. Electric pads, however, can burn the patient if the setting is too high. In some agencies the controls on the pads are set to a specific temperature to prevent burning.

The aquamatic or aquathermia (water-flow) pad is becoming increasingly popular. Warm water circulates inside the pad, providing a controlled temperature.

Dry heat can also be supplied by commercially prepared hot packs. See Figure 34–1. They deliver a specific amount of heat for a specific time period. To start the heat, the pack is struck sharply or kneaded, which initiates a chemical reaction. Read the manufacturer's instructions before using the pack.

■ Assessment

Assess:

1. The area to which the heat is to be applied for any signs of redness, abraded skin, swelling, or hemorrhage. Heat may be contraindicated for certain conditions.
2. Any discomfort experienced by the patient, eg, a muscle cramp.
3. The capacity of the patient to recognize when the heat is injurious. Establish whether the patient is aware of heat and cold and can discern a temperature that is too hot or too cold for the tissues.
4. The patient's degree of consciousness and general physical condition. Patients who are very young,

FIGURE 34–1 ■ Commercially prepared disposable hot packs.

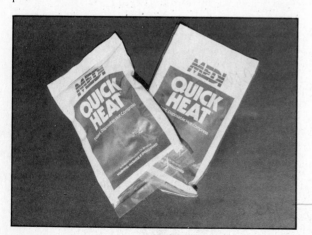

very old, unconscious, or debilitated do not tolerate heat well.

5. The blood circulation to the area. Clinical signs of impaired circulation are numbness or tingling, cyanosis, and coolness to the touch. Areas with poor blood circulation are less tolerant of heat. Report any impairment to the responsible nurse before starting the treatment.

Other data include:

1. Whether the patient is required to sign a release for the application of dry heat. If a release is required, check the patient's chart for the signed release.

2. The type of heat to be used, the temperature, and the duration and frequency of the application. Check the physician's or nursing order.

3. Agency policies or practices about the type of equipment used, the temperature recommended, and the length of heat applications.

4. At what time the heat should be applied, eg, 1000 and 1900 hours or after a surgical dressing is changed. Check the nursing care plan.

■ Planning

Nursing goals

1. To warm a body part and promote comfort, relaxation, and sleep
2. To increase blood circulation to an area
3. To reduce muscle pain

Equipment

Hot water bottle (bag)

1. A hot watter bottle with a stopper. Hot water bottles are usually made of plastic or rubber.
2. A cover for the bottle. Some agencies have special covers; others use a soft towel.
3. Hot water and a thermometer to measure the temperature of the water.

Electric heating pad **not recommended**

4. The electric pad and the control. Note whether the control is set at a specific temperature. Inspect the pad to make sure it is functioning correctly. A plastic key may be needed to set the temperature.

5. A cover. Some electric pads have waterproof covers, which should be used if there will be moisture under the pad when it is applied.

Aquathermia (water-flow) pad **Aqua K Pad**

6. The pad. Inside the pad are tubes containing distilled water.

7. The control unit, which is operated by electricity.

This unit has an opening, into which the water is poured, and a temperature gauge. The control unit is connected to the pad by tubing. See Figure 34–2.

8. Distilled water for the unit.
9. A cover for the pad.

Some aquathermia pads have an absorbent surface through which moist heat can be applied. The other surface of the pad is waterproof. These pads are disposable.

Dry heat can also be supplied by commercially prepared hot packs. Read the manufacturer's instructions before using them.

■ Intervention

1. Fold down the bedclothes to expose the area to which the heat will be applied.

Hot water bottle

2. Fill the hot water bottle about <u>two-thirds full.</u>

3. Measure the temperature of the water if this was not done before the bag was filled. Follow agency practice for the appropriate temperature. Temperatures commonly used are:
   a. 52 °C (125 °F) for a normal adult
   b. 40.5 to 46 °C (105 to 115 °F) for a debilitated or unconscious adult
   c. 40.5 to 46 °C (105 to 115 °F) for a child under two years of age

4. <u>Expel the air from the bottle.</u> ✓ For leaks
   Rationale Air remaining in the bottle prevents it from molding to the body part being treated.

5. Secure the stopper tightly.
6. Hold the bottle upside down and check for leaks.
7. Dry the bottle.
8. <u>Wrap the bottle in a towel or hot water bottle cover.</u>

FIGURE 34–2 ■ An aquathermia heating unit.

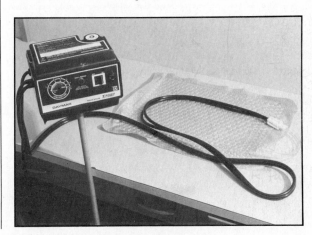

9. Apply the bottle to the patient. Support it against the body part with pillows as necessary.

10. Assess the patient's response in terms of comfort, skin reaction, and the purpose for which heat is being applied. At the first sign of pain, swelling, or excessive redness, remove the heat and report any sign to the responsible nurse. Assess the response of the patient as often as necessary for the patient's safety. Frequency of assessment depends on such factors as the patient's previous responses to applications and his or her ability to report problems. Consult the responsible nurse on frequency of assessment.

11. When the heat is applied, record on the patient's chart the application, its purpose, the time, the method used, and the site.

12. Remove the heat at the designated time. A hot water bottle will usually stay hot for 45 minutes, and then it needs to be replaced. If a disposable hot pack is used, the manufacturer's instructions state the length of time that heat is produced.

13. After removal, record the time and the response of the patient.

Electric heating pad *not recommended*

14. Ensure that the body area is dry.
    Rationale Electricity in the presence of moisture can conduct a shock.

15. Caution the patient not to insert any sharp, pointed object, eg, a pin, in the pad.
    Rationale A pin might strike a wire, damaging the pad and giving an electric shock to the patient.

16. Place the cover on the pad. Some models have waterproof covers to be used when the pad is placed over a moist dressing.

Rationale Moisture could cause the pad to short circuit and burn or shock the patient.

17. Plug the pad into the electric socket.

18. Set the control dial for the correct temperature. After the pad has heated, apply it to the body area. Follow steps 10–13.

Aquathermia pad

19. Fill the unit with distilled water until it is two-thirds full. *to top* The unit will warm the water, which circulates through the pad.

20. Remove air bubbles and secure the top.

21. *99°–100°* Regulate the temperature with the key if it has not been preset. Check the manufacturer's instructions.

22. Put the cover over the pad.

23. Plug in the unit.

24. Apply the pad to the body part. Follow steps 10–13. *Dr's. order*

▪ **Evaluation**

Expected outcomes

1. Decreased pain and muscle tension
2. Warmth of the local tissues
3. Vasodilation of the area

Unexpected outcomes

1. Increased pain
2. Excessive redness and/or swelling

Upon obtaining an unexpected outcome:

1. Report your findings to the responsible nurse.
2. Adjust the nursing care plan appropriately.

TECHNIQUE 34–2 ▪ Applying a Heat Lamp or Heat Cradle

A heat lamp is often a gooseneck lamp with a special or 60-watt bulb in it. Also used is the infrared lamp, which has an infrared element rather than a bulb. Both lamps provide dry heat to a localized area. See Figure 34–3.

A heat cradle is a metal frame that is placed on the bed over the patient. It has a row of 25-watt light bulbs and provides less localized dry heat than a heat lamp.

▪ **Assessment**

See Technique 34–1. Other data include:

1. Whether the equipment is in proper working order.
2. The type of heat to be applied, the body site, and the duration of the treatment
3. When the heat is best applied, eg, after a dressing has been removed

4. Whether the agency requires a release from the patient and, if required, whether a signed release is on the patient's chart

■ Planning

Nursing goals

Heat lamp

1. To increase circulation to an area

Heat cradle

2. To apply heat to a large body area

Equipment

1. A heat lamp or infrared lamp
   or
2. A heat cradle and bath blanket or sheet to cover the cradle

■ Intervention

Heat lamp

1. Expose the area to be treated, and drape the patient so that the body is not exposed unnecessarily.
2. Warn the patient not to touch the bulb or element of the heat lamp.
3. Dry the area with a towel to remove all moisture.
   Rationale The skin is more likely to burn if it is moist.
4. Plug in the lamp, and place it the correct distance from the area to receive the heat. Direct the lamp carefully. A 60-watt bulb is usually placed 45 to 60 cm (18 to 24 in) from the area being treated. Infrared lamps come in two sizes. Place a small lamp closer to the patient, ie, 45 to 60 cm (18 to 24 in) away. Place a large lamp 60 to 75 cm (24 to 30 in) from the patient. Do not cover the lamp.
   Rationale A cover on the lamp may catch fire.
5. Note and record the time that the treatment started. Most treatments are ordered for 15 or 20 minutes.
6. Return every five minutes to assess the patient's response.
7. Assess the patient's response in terms of discomfort, excessive redness, and any unexpected outcome. If these occur, turn off the heat and report the signs to the responsible nurse.
8. Remove the lamp at the designated time. Dress any open area as required.
9. Record on the patient's chart the treatment, the

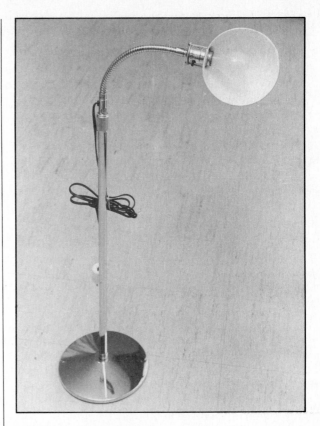

FIGURE 34–3 ■ A heat lamp used to provide dry heat.

time, the length of the treatment, and the patient's response.

Heat cradle

10. Fold the top bedclothes to the bottom of the bed to make room for the cradle.
11. Warn the patient not to touch the bulbs of the heat cradle.
12. Place the cradle carefully over the area to be heated.
13. Plug in the cradle, and check that the bulbs are on.
14. Cover the cradle with a bath blanket or sheet.
    Rationale The cover holds in the heat and prevents cooling by the circulating air.
15. Note and record the time that the treatment started. The treatment usually lasts 15 to 30 minutes.
16. Return every ten minutes to assess the patient's reaction. Follow steps 7–9.

■ Evaluation   See Technique 34–1 on page 812.

TECHNIQUE 34–3 ■ Administering Hot Soaks and Sitz Baths

A soak refers either to immersing a body part, eg, an arm, in a solution or to wrapping a part in gauze dressings and then saturating the dressing with a solution. Soaks may employ clean technique or sterile technique. Sterile technique is generally indicated for any open wounds, eg, a burn or an area that has had surgery. Dry dressings are usually applied between the soaks.

A sitz bath or hip bath is used to soak the patient's pelvic area. The patient sits in a special tub or chair, usually immersed from the midthighs to the iliac crests or umbilicus. Special tubs or chairs are preferred to the regular bathtub, which immerses the legs and results in less effective blood circulation to the perineum or pelvic area. See Figure 34–4. Disposable sitz baths are also available; they are commonly used in homes but may be used in hospitals as well.

The order usually specifies the soak, its site, the type of solution, the temperature of the solution, the length of time for the soak, the frequency, and the purpose. Whether sterile technique is used is usually a nursing judgment; if there is a break in the skin, sterile technique is indicated. The duration of soaks is generally 15 to 20 minutes.

■ Assessment

1. See Technique 34–1 on page 810.
2. Assess the appearance of the area to be soaked for redness; color, amount, and consistency of drainage; any swelling; and any break in the skin.

Other data include:

1. The site of the soak; the type and temperature of the solution to be used; the duration, frequency, and

FIGURE 34–4 ■ A sitz bath used in hospitals.

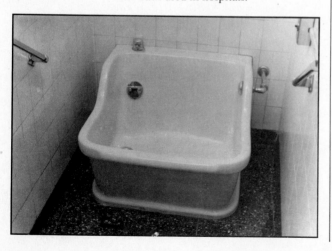

purpose of the soak, as indicated on the chart; and whether sterile technique is required.

2. The agency's practices about the temperature and the length of time recommended for soaks.

■ Planning

Nursing goals

1. To hasten suppuration, soften exudates, and enhance healing
2. To apply medications to a designated area
3. To clean a wound in which there is sloughing tissue or an exudate

Equipment

1. A container such as a small basin to soak a finger or hand, a special arm or foot bath, or a sitz tub or chair. See Figure 34–4.
2. The specified solution at the correct temperature. If a temperature is not ordered, check agency policy; 40 to 43° C (105 to 110° F) is usually indicated, as tolerated by the patient. Fill the container at least one-half full.
3. A thermometer to test the temperature of the solution. Some sitz tubs have temperature indicators attached to the water taps.
4. Towels to support the limb against the sharp edge of a basin and to dry the body part following the soak.
5. The required dressing materials. Gauze squares and roller gauze may be necessary following an extremity soak; perineal pads and a T-binder may be needed following a perineal soak.
6. A bath blanket to wrap around the shoulders of a patient who is having a sitz bath.
7. A moisture-resistant bag for discarded dressings.

■ Intervention

Hand or foot soak

1. Remove the dressings, if any, and discard in the bag. Assess the amount, color, odor, and consistency of the drainage on removed dressings.
2. Assist the patient to a well-aligned, comfortable position to prevent muscle strain; the position adopted will be maintained for 15 to 20 minutes.

3. Pad the edge of the container with a towel, and immerse the body part in the container.

   Rationale Padding is necessary to prevent pressure on the body part that rests on the edge of the container.

4. If the soak is sterile, cover the open container with a sterile drape or the container wrapper.

   Rationale Covering the open container prevents airborne contamination.

5. Assess the patient and test the temperature of the solution at least once during the soak. Assess for discomfort, need for additional support, and the response of the patient to the soak. Additional solution may be required to maintain the temperature of the soak. Report any unexpected responses to the responsible nurse immediately and terminate the soak.

6. Remove the body part from the basin at completion of the soak, and dry it thoroughly. If the soak was sterile, use a sterile towel for drying. The duration of soaks is generally 15 to 20 minutes.

7. Assess the appearance of the body part carefully, and reapply a dressing if required.

8. Record the soak, including duration, temperature, type of solution, appearance of wound, and response of the patient.

Sitz bath

9. Fill the sitz bath with water. The water level in a tub should be at the umbilicus. *umbilicus level*

10. Pad the tub or chair with towels as required. *tub*

    Rationale Padding prevents pressure on the sacrum or posterior aspects of the thighs. When a disposable sitz bath on the toilet is used, a footstool can prevent pressure on the back of the thighs.

11. Remove the patient's gown, or fasten it above the waist.

12. Remove the T-binder and perineal dressings, if present, and note the amount, color, odor, and consistency of any drainage.

13. Assess the appearance of the area to be soaked for redness, swelling, odor, breaks in the skin, and drainage.

14. Wrap the bath blanket around the patient's shoulders.

    Rationale The bath blanket will keep the patient warm.

15. Assist the patient into the bath, and provide support for the patient as needed. Leave a signal light within reach. Stay with the patient if warranted, and terminate the bath as necessary.

Rationale Some patients who have just had surgery or are weak may become faint or dizzy and need to be able to call a nurse or have the nurse remain with them.

16. Assess the response of the patient during the bath in terms of discomfort, color, and pulse rate. An accelerated pulse or extreme pallor may precede fainting. Report any unexpected or adverse responses to the responsible nurse immediately.

17. Test the temperature of the solution at least once during the bath. Adjust the temperature as needed.

18. Assist the patient out of the sitz bath, and dry the area with a towel.

19. Assess the perineal area, and reapply dressings and garments as required.

20. Record the soak, including the duration, temperature, type of solution, appearance of the wound, and response of the patient.

Sample Recording

Date	Time	Notes
12/5/86	0900	43 °C saline soak to (L) index finger × 20 min. 2 × 2 gauze saturated with purulent exudate. Finger less swollen but red. —————————— Toby N. Zacharias, NS

■ Evaluation

Expected outcomes

1. Area less reddened
2. Less drainage
3. Decreased swelling
4. Decreased discomfort

Unexpected outcomes

1. Increased discomfort
2. Large amount of seropurulent discharge
3. Swelling unchanged

Upon obtaining an unexpected outcome:

1. Report your findings to the responsible nurse and/or physician.
2. Adjust the nursing care plan appropriately.

TECHNIQUE 34–4 ■ Applying an Ice Bag, Ice Collar, Ice Glove, or Disposable Cold Pack 🏠

The ice bag, a common device used in many homes and hospitals, is a moderate-sized rubber or plastic bag, with a removable cap, into which pieces of ice can be inserted. Commercially prepared ice bags are available in some agencies. These bags are filled with an alcohol-base solution and sealed; they are kept in freezing units in a central supply area.

An ice collar is similar to an ice bag but is long and narrow. It is designed for use around the neck, though it can be used for other areas of the body.

The ice glove is simply a rubber or plastic glove that is filled with ice chips and tied at the open end. Gloves are generally used for small body parts, eg, an eye.

Disposable cold packs are similar to disposable hot packs. They come in a variety of sizes and shapes and provide a specific degree of coldness for a specified period of time, as indicated on the package. By striking, squeezing, or kneading the package, chemical reactions are activated that release the cold. The manufacturer's instructions must be followed. Most commercially prepared cold packs have soft outer coverings so they can be applied directly to the body part. See Figure 34–5.

■ Assessment

Assess:

1. The area to which the cold is to be applied. Note in particular the presence of circulatory deficiencies that may contraindicate cold therapy, eg, a bluish-purplish appearance or cold feeling of the skin, decreased sensation, numbness. Report these to the responsible nurse before applying the cold.

FIGURE 34–5 ■ A disposable ice collar provides dry cold to the neck area—for example, to control bleeding after a tonsillectomy.

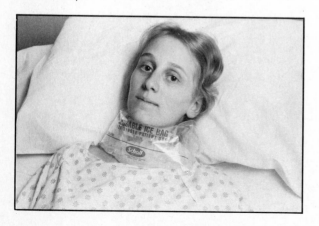

2. The patient's discomfort, eg, pain due to contracted muscles, swelling, or bleeding, to provide baseline data for comparison after the cold application. These should be reported also to the responsible nurse before applying cold.
3. The patient's body temperature. A lowered body temperature and shivering may contraindicate the application of cold.

Other data include:

1. The order for the cold application, including when, where, why, and for how long the cold is to be applied.
2. Agency practices regarding time periods for cold applications.

■ Planning

Nursing goals

1. To relieve headaches caused by vasodilation
2. To prevent swelling of tissues immediately following an injury or surgery
3. To prevent, decrease, or terminate bleeding following an injury or surgery
4. To reduce joint pain from the pressure of accumulated fluid

Equipment

1. An ice bag, collar, glove, or cold pack
2. Ice chips
3. A protective covering
4. Roller gauze, a binder, or a towel and safety pins to attach the device and keep it in place

■ Intervention

1. Assist the patient to a comfortable position, and support the body part requiring the application.
2. Expose only the area to be treated, and provide warmth to avoid chilling. Privacy may or may not be necessary, depending on the location of the application and the patient's wishes.

Ice bag, collar, or glove

3. Fill the device one-half to two-thirds full of crushed ice.

Rationale Partial filling makes the device more pliable so that it can be molded to a body part.

4. Remove excess air by bending or twisting the device.

Rationale Air inflates the device so that it cannot be molded to the body part.

5. Insert the stopper securely into an ice bag or collar or tie a knot at the open end of a glove.

Rationale This prevents leakage of fluid when the ice melts.

6. Hold the device upside down and check it for leaks.

7. Cover the device with a soft cloth cover, if it is not already equipped with one.

Rationale The cover absorbs moisture that condenses on the outside of the device. It is also more comfortable for the patient.

8. Apply the device for the time specified. The device is usually applied for 30 to 60 minutes.

9. Hold it in place with roller gauze, a binder, or a towel secured by safety pins as necessary.

10. Assess the patient's reaction in terms of comfort, the purpose of the cold application, and skin reaction (eg, pallor, mottled appearance, etc). Assess the patient's response as frequently as necessary for the patient's safety. Factors such as previous responses to applications and the patient's ability to report any problems need to be considered.

11. At the time of application, record on the patient's chart the cold application, its purpose, the method used, the site, and the patient's response.

12. Remove the cold application at the designated time.

Rationale This avoids the harmful effects of prolonged cold.

13. After removal, record the time and the patient's response.

14. Adjust the nursing care plan for the next cold application, if changes are required.

Disposable cold pack

15. Strike, squeeze, or knead the cold pack according to the manufacturer's instructions.

Rationale The action activates the chemical reaction that produces the cold.

16. Cover with a soft cloth cover if the pack does not have a cover. Most commercially prepared cold packs have soft outer coverings so they can be applied directly to the body part.

17. Follow steps 8–14.

■ Evaluation

Expected outcomes

1. Absence of clinical signs of impaired blood circulation to the area

2. Reduced temperature of the affected tissues

3. Reduced swelling and discomfort

Unexpected outcomes

1. Presence of numbness and tingling sensations

2. Presence of a bluish-purplish tinge to the skin

3. Shivering and lowered body temperature

Upon obtaining an unexpected outcome:

1. Report your findings to the responsible nurse and/or physician.

2. Adjust the nursing care plan appropriately.

TECHNIQUE 34–5   ■   Administering a Cooling Sponge Bath

The cooling sponge bath uses water or a combination of alcohol and water that is below body temperature. Alcohol evaporates at a low temperature and therefore removes body heat rapidly. However, alcohol-and-water sponge baths are less frequently used than in the past, because alcohol has a drying effect on the skin. The temperatures for cooling sponge baths range from 18 to 32 °C (65 to 90 °F). A *tepid* sponge bath generally refers to one in which the water temperature is 32 °C (90 °F) throughout the bath. For a *cool* sponge bath, the water temperature is 32 °C (90 °F) at the beginning of the bath

and is gradually lowered to 18 °C (65 °F) by adding ice chips during the bath.

■ Assessment

Assess the patient for:

1. Body temperature, pulse, and respirations if not already recorded prior to the sponge bath to provide comparative baseline data. The decision to give a tepid sponge bath is generally made only after a

marked fever is noted or a temperature increase of 1 to 2 °C or 2 to 3 °F.

2. Other signs of fever, eg, skin warmth, flushing, complaints of heat or chilling, diaphoresis, irritability, restlessness, general malaise, or delirium.

Other data include:

1. Who is responsible for ordering a sponge bath. In some agencies, a physician's order is required; others permit an order by the responsible nurse.

2. Agency practice regarding the type of bath recommended and the temperature of the solution.

■ Planning

Nursing goal

To reduce a patient's fever by promoting body heat loss through conduction and vaporization.

Equipment

1. A basin for the solution.

2. A bath thermometer to check the temperature of the solution.

3. A solution at the correct temperature. Water or equal portions of 70% alcohol and water are used.

4. Ice chips for a cool sponge bath.

5. Several washcloths and bath towels. Fewer are needed if ice bags or cold packs are used.

6. A bath blanket.

7. A thermometer to measure the patient's temperature.

A fan is sometimes used to increase air movement around the patient, which lowers the body temperature through convection. In this case, drafts are not usually eliminated during the sponge bath.

■ Intervention

1. Explain to the patient that the face, arms, legs, back, and buttocks will be sponged, but not the chest and abdomen. The procedure takes about 30 minutes.

2. Minimize drafts by closing the room door and windows as indicated.

3. Remove the patient's gown and assist him or her to a comfortable supine position. Place a bath blanket over the patient.

4. First sponge the patient's face with plain water only, and dry it. An ice bag or cold pack may be applied to the patient's head for comfort.

5. If ice bags or cold packs are not used, place bath towels under each axilla and shoulder.
   Rationale Bath towels protect the lower bed sheet from getting wet.

6. Wet three washcloths, wring them out so that they are very damp but not dripping, and place them in the axillae and groins. Or place ice bags or cold packs in these areas.
   Rationale Washcloths need to be as moist as possible to be effective. The axillae and groins contain large superficial blood vessels, which aid the transfer of heat.

7. Leave the washcloths in place for about five minutes, or until they feel warm. Rewet and replace them as required during the bath.
   Rationale Washcloths warm up relatively quickly in such vascular areas.

8. Place a bath towel under one arm. Sponge the arm slowly and gently for about five minutes or as tolerated by the patient. Or place a saturated towel over the extremity, and rewet it as necessary. Give the patient enough time to adjust to the initial reaction of chilliness and for the body to cool.
   Rationale Slow, gentle motions are indicated because firm rubbing motions increase tissue metabolism and heat production. Cool sponges given rapidly or for a short period of time tend to increase the body's heat production mechanisms by causing shivering.

9. Dry the arm, using a patting motion rather than a rubbing motion.

10. Repeat steps 8 and 9 for the other arm and the legs.

11. When sponging the extremities, hold the washcloth briefly over the wrists and ankles.
    Rationale The blood circulation is close to the skin surface in the wrists and ankles.

12. After 15 minutes check the patient's vital signs. Compare with data taken before the bath.
    Rationale The vital signs are checked to evaluate the effectiveness of the sponge bath.

13. Ask the patient to turn on his or her side, and sponge the back and buttocks for three to five minutes. Pat these areas dry.

14. Remove the washcloths from the axillae and groins, and dry these areas.

15. Recheck the patient's vital signs.

16. Record the vital signs, type of sponge bath given, and responses of the patient.

Sample Recording

Date	Time	Notes
12/5/86	1600	C/o headache, appears restless, is flushed and diaphoretic. T 104, P 110, R 24. Tepid sponge given.
	1615	T 102, P 105, R 22.
	1630	T 100, P 100, R 20. Sponge bath discontinued.————— Marya A. Shapiro, NS

■ Evaluation

Expected outcome

Reduced body temperature: either to normal or slightly above normal. If the patient's temperature has been reduced to slightly above normal, the bath can be terminated, since the body continues to cool for a period of time.

Unexpected outcome

No substantial decrease in body temperature. Upon obtaining an unexpected outcome:

1. Check with the responsible nurse about whether to continue to sponge bath or repeat it at a later time.
2. Adjust the patient's nursing care plan to include regular assessments of body temperature.

TECHNIQUE 34–6   ■   Applying Compresses and Moist Packs

Compresses and moist packs can be either hot or cold. A *compress* is a moist gauze dressing that is applied frequently to an open wound. When hot compresses are ordered, the solution is heated to the temperature indicated by the physician, eg, 40.5 °C (105 °F). When there is a break in the skin, compresses are applied using sterile technique; therefore sterile gloves or sterile forceps are needed for their application. A *hot* or *cold pack* is a hot or cold moist cloth applied to an area of the body. Hot packs are also referred to as foments. Frequently wool flannel is used because it holds heat or cold well. Packs are usually unsterile; after application, they are covered with a water-resistant material (eg, plastic wrap) to contain the moisture and prevent the transfer of airborne microorganisms to the area.

After a compress or a pack has been applied, it is advisable to apply external heat or cold, such as a hot water bottle, heating pad, or ice bag, to help maintain the temperature of the application.

■ Assessment

Assess:

1. The area to which the compress or pack is to be applied for any signs of redness, abraded skin, or discharge. If the wound is open, assess its size, appearance, and type and amount of discharge.
2. Any discomfort, swelling, or bleeding, to provide baseline data for comparison.
3. Whether the blood circulation to the area is impaired. Clinical signs of impairment are numbness or tingling, cyanosis, and coolness to the touch. Areas with poor blood circulation are less tolerant of heat and cold, so therapy may be contraindicated. Report any impairment to the responsible nurse before starting the treatment.
4. Whether the patient has a neurosensory deficiency or reduced capacity to discern skin temperature

differences. Patients who are very young, very old, unconscious, debilitated, or have neurosensory impairments are unable to effectively recognize temperature differences.

5. The patient's pulse, respirations, and blood pressure for baseline data if moist packs are to be applied over a large area of the body, eg, the posterior trunk.

Other data include:

1. The type of solution, the strength, and the temperature ordered for the compress. Check agency practice if not specified in the physician's order. Some orders require that the pack or compress be applied at as hot or cold a temperature as the patient is able to tolerate.
2. Whether sterile applications are required. Sterile compresses are needed for an open wound or a vulnerable part of the body, eg, an eye, so that microorganisms are not transmitted to the wound or body part.
3. Whether the sterile compress is to be replaced with a sterile dressing after the treatment.

■ Planning

Nursing goals

Hot compress   local – wound, site

1. To hasten the suppurative process and healing

Hot pack   larger area

2. To relieve muscle spasm or pain
3. To reduce the pressure of accumulated fluid in a tissue or joint
4. To reduce congestion in an underlying organ

Cold compress

5. To decrease or prevent bleeding
6. To reduce inflammation

Cold pack

7. To prevent swelling due to tissue trauma and inflammation

8. To anesthetize tissues and reduce pain temporarily

Equipment

Compress

1. A container for the solution

2. The solution at the strength and temperature specified by the physician or the agency

3. A thermometer to test the temperature of the solution

4. Gauze squares to soak with the solution and apply to the patient

5. Plastic to insulate the compresses, to retain the temperature and moisture

6. An insulating towel to help maintain the temperature of the compress

7. A hot water bottle (optional) to provide additional heat and maintain the heat of a hot compress

   or

8. An ice bag (optional) to maintain the cold of a cold compress

9. Ties, eg, roller gauze, to fasten the compress in place

For a sterile compress, the solution, container, thermometer, towels, and gauze squares must be sterile. In addition, sterile forceps or sterile gloves are required to maintain the sterility of the gauze when it is wrung out and applied. If a sterile thermometer is not available, pour a small amount of the solution into a clean basin, measure the temperature with a bath thermometer, and then discard the solution, since it is no longer sterile. Adjust the temperature of the solution according to your findings.

Moist pack

10. Flannel pieces or towel packs

11. A hot-pack machine for heating the packs

    or

12. A basin of water with some ice chips to cool the water

13. Plastic for insulation

14. Insulating material, eg, flannel or towels

15. A hot water bottle (optional) to provide additional heat and maintain the heat of the pack

    or

16. An ice bag (optional) to maintain the cold of the pack

17. A thermometer if a specific temperature is ordered for the pack (eg, a cold pack of 24 °C [75 °F] may be ordered)

18. Petroleum jelly to apply to surrounding skin areas if the pack tends to irritate them

19. Ties, eg, roller gauze, to fasten the pack

For a sterile moist pack, the container, solution, thermometer, and all materials must be sterile. In addition, sterile gloves or forceps are required to maintain the sterility of the pack when it is wrung out and applied.

■ Intervention

1. Assist the patient to a comfortable position, expose the area for the compress or pack, and provide support for the body part requiring the compress or pack.

Compress

2. Place the gauze in the solution.

3. Remove the wound dressing, if present. A dry, sterile dressing is often placed over open wounds between applications of moist heat or cold. To remove a sterile dressing, see Technique 35–1 on page 828.

4. Wring out the gauze so that the solution does not drip from it. For a sterile compress, use sterile forceps or sterile gloves.

5. Apply the gauze to the designated area, molding the compress close to the body.

   Rationale Air is a poor conductor of cold or heat, and molding excludes air.

6. Optional: Apply a hot water bottle or ice bag over the gauze, if the compress is not sterile. If a hot water bottle is used, the temperature of the water should be lower than usual, eg, 40 to 43 °C (105 to 110 °F), because a moist compress can burn the patient if it is too hot.

7. Cover the gauze (and hot water bottle or ice bag, if used) quickly with the plastic and the insulating material, eg, a towel.

   Rationale The compress is insulated quickly to maintain its temperature.

8. Secure the compress in place with ties.

9. Record on the patient's chart the technique, the time, the type and strength of the solution, and the appearance of the wound and surrounding skin area.

10. Assess the patient's response frequently in terms of discomfort. If the patient feels any discomfort, assess the area for erythema, numbness, etc. For applications to large areas of the body, note any change in the patient's pulse, respirations, and blood pressure. In the event of unexpected outcomes, terminate the treatment and report to the responsible nurse.

11. Remove the compress or pack at the specified time. Compresses and packs with external heat or cold usually retain their temperature anywhere from 15 minutes to one hour. Without external heat or cold, they need to be changed every five minutes.

12. Apply a sterile dressing if one is required.

13. When the compress or pack is removed, record the appearance of the area and any other responses of the patient.

Moist pack

14. Heat the flannel or towel.
15. Apply petroleum jelly to the surrounding skin, if it appears reddened.
16. Wring out the flannel. For a sterile pack, use sterile gloves.
17. Apply the flannel to the body area, molding it closely to the body part.
18. Optional: Apply a hot water bottle or ice bag over the pack, if it is an unsterile pack.
19. Cover the flannel (and ice bag or hot water bottle, if used) quickly with the plastic insulating material, eg, a towel.
20. Secure the pack in place with ties.
21. Follow steps 9–13.

Sample Recording

Date	Time	Notes
5/12/86	0910	Sterile normal saline compress with K-Matic 37.7 °C applied to sacral ulcer. Pink tissue surrounding ulcer. Small amount of serosanguineous discharge. No discomfort. —— Olga R. Resnicoff, NS
5/12/86	0940	Compress removed. No further discharge. Dry dressing applied. —— Olga R. Resnicoff, NS

■ **Evaluation**

Expected outcomes

1. Decreased discomfort
2. Decreased inflammation, swelling, or discharge
3. Decreased bleeding
4. Stable vital signs

Unexpected outcomes

1. No significant change in discomfort
2. No significant change in inflammation, swelling, or discharge
3. No significant change in bleeding
4. Increased numbness or erythema
5. Significant change in vital signs

Upon obtaining an unexpected outcome:

1. Report your findings to the responsible nurse and/or physician.
2. Adjust the patient's nursing care plan accordingly.

References

Guyton AC: *Textbook of Medical Physiology*. 6th ed. Saunders, 1981.

O'Dell AJ: Hot Packs for morning joint stiffness. *Am J Nurs* (June) 1975; 75:986–987.

Waterson M (consultant): Hot and cold therapy. *Nursing 78* (October) 1978; 8:44–49.

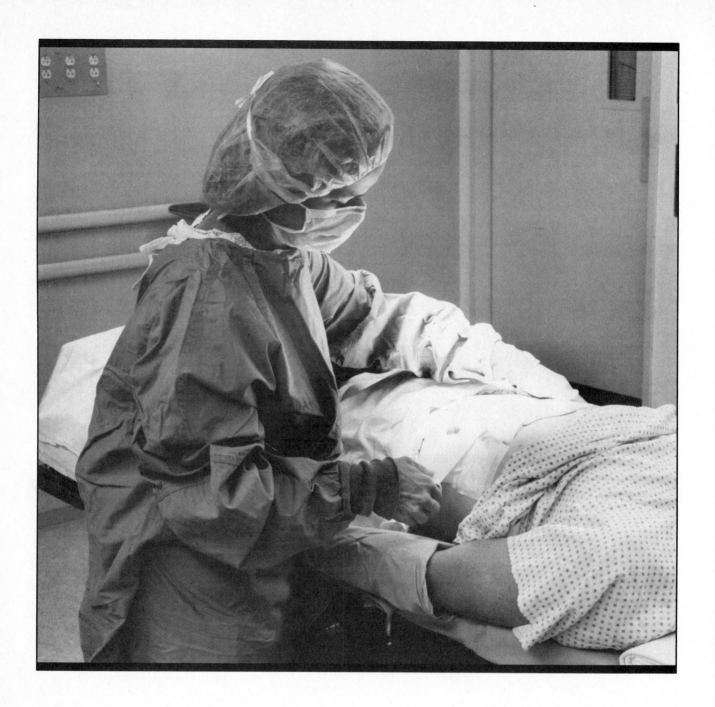

DRESSINGS, DRAINS, SUTURES, AND WOUND SUCTION

35

Although the body is remarkably protected from *trauma* (injury) by the skin and by the subcutaneous and adipose tissues, trauma does occur intentionally and unintentionally. *Intentional* trauma occurs during therapy, such as an operation, venipuncture, or radiation.

Although it is therapeutic to remove a tumor, the surgeon must cut into body tissues, thus traumatizing them.

Unintentional wounds are acquired by accident, for example, an arm may be fractured in an automobile accident. If the tissues are traumatized without a break in the skin, the result is a *closed wound.* A blow from a hard instrument causes bruising, called a *contusion,* which is considered a closed wound. An *open wound* occurs when the skin or mucous membrane surface is broken.

Wounds are further described according to the presence or absence of infection. A *clean wound* is one in which there are few or no pathogenic organisms. A *contaminated* (infected) *wound* is one in which many pathogens are present. Wounds produced intentionally are generally clean, while unintentional and other open wounds are considered contaminated. No wound is

actually sterile, because microorganisms are normally present on the skin and mucous membranes. However, the lack of virulence of the microorganisms and their limited numbers generally prevent the development of an infection.

One of the functions of nurses is to promote wound healing, which may involve changing dressings, cleaning and shortening drains, and irrigating wound sites. Surgical aseptic technique is followed for most of these measures, to prevent the introduction of pathogens into wounds.

Chapter Outline

Objectives

Upon completion of this chapter, the student will:

1. Know essential terms and facts about types of wounds, wound care, dressings, drains, and sutures
   1.1 Define selected terms
   1.2 Identify advantages of open and closed methods of wound care
   1.3 Identify commonly used dressing materials
   1.4 Identify essential aspects of taping a dressing securely
   1.5 Identify goals of wound care
   1.6 Identify types of wound drainage
   1.7 Identify essential aspects of primary intention wound healing
   1.8 Identify essential aspects of secondary intention wound healing
   1.9 Identify purposes and essential aspects of dry dressings versus wet-to-dry dressings
   1.10 Identify purposes and essential aspects of wound drains and suctions
   1.11 Identify various methods of suturing
   1.12 Identify purposes of retention sutures
2. Understand facts about techniques related to wound care
   2.1 Identify relevant assessment data
   2.2 Identify nursing goals related to the technique
   2.3 Identify expected and unexpected outcomes from assessment data
   2.4 Identify reasons underlying selected steps of the technique
3. Perform wound care techniques safely
   3.1 Assess the patient adequately
   3.2 Collect additional data from appropriate sources
   3.3 Select pertinent nursing goals for the patient
   3.4 Establish relevant outcome criteria for the patient following the technique
   3.5 Collect necessary equipment before the technique
   3.6 Implement interventions to enhance the effectiveness of the technique and enhance the patient's comfort and safety
   3.7 Communicate relevant information about the patient to the appropriate persons
   3.8 Determine the evaluative outcomes of the technique
4. Evaluate own performance of specific wound care techniques in a laboratory or clinical setting with the assistance of another
   4.1 Use the performance checklists provided
   4.2 Identify areas of strength and weakness
   4.3 Alter performance in response to own evaluation and that of another

Terms

- **abrasion** wearing away (erosion) of a structure such as the skin because of friction
- **adherent** sticking together, clinging
- **adipose** fat; of a fatty nature
- **anemia** a condition in which the blood is deficient in red blood cells or hemoglobin
- **approximate (wound edges)** to bring close together
- **cicatrix** a scar
- **collagen** a gluelike protein found in connective tissue; it is secreted by fibroblasts in granulation tissue, and it forms scar tissue
- **contusion** a closed wound that results from a blow by a blunt instrument
- **debridement** cleaning of an injured area to remove foreign debris or excessive exudate
- **dehiscence** gaping, splitting, or separating of wound edges
- **drain** a substance or appliance that assists in the discharge of drainage from a wound
- **drainage** a discharge from a wound or cavity
- **ecchymosis** a blotchy area or discoloration of the skin; a bruise
- **epithelial cells** cells that cover the surface of the body and line its cavities
- **epithelialization** the formation of skin over a wound
- **eschar** a slough produced by burning, by a corrosive application, or by death of tissue associated with loss of vascular supply, bacterial invasion, and putrefaction
- **exudate** material, eg, fluid and cells, that has escaped from blood vessels and is deposited in tissues or on tissue surfaces during the inflammatory process
- **fibrin** an insoluble protein formed from fibrinogen during the clotting of blood; it is produced by fibroblasts during healing
- **fibrinogen** a protein in blood plasma that by the action of thrombin is converted into fibrin
- **fibroblast** an immature fiber-producing cell
- **fibrous tissue** common connective tissue composed of elastic and collagen fibers
- **granulation tissue** young connective tissue with new capillaries that is formed extensively in wounds that heal by secondary intention
- **hematoma** a collection of blood in a tissue, organ, or body space, due to a break in the wall of a blood vessel
- **hemostasis** arrest of the escape of blood either by natural (clot formation) or artificial (compression or ligation) means
- **hemostat (artery forceps)** a small pair of forceps used to constrict blood vessels; also called *artery forceps*
- **incision** a cut or wound that is intentionally made, eg, during surgery
- **keloid** a rounded, hard, shiny, white or pink scarlike growth that rises above the skin surface
- **laceration** a tear, rather than a cut, of body tissue
- **leukocytosis** an abnormal increase in the number of white blood cells
- **mucin** the chief constituent of mucus
- **Penrose drain** a flexible rubber drain
- **phagocytosis** the process by which cells, eg, white blood cells, engulf microorganisms, other cells, or foreign particles
- **platelet** a disk-shaped blood element with a very fragile membrane; platelets tend to adhere to damaged or uneven surfaces and are involved in blood clotting; they are also called *thrombocytes*
- **primary intention healing** healing that occurs in a wound in which the tissue surfaces are or have been approximated and there is minimal or no tissue loss; it is characterized by the formation of minimal granulation tissue and scarring; also called *primary union* or *first intention healing*
- **purulent** containing pus
- **pus** a thick liquid associated with inflammation and composed of cells, fluid, microorganisms, and tissue debris
- **pyogenic** pus-producing
- **retention (stay) suture** a large, plain suture that attaches to underlying tissues of fat and muscle in addition to the skin; retention sutures are used to support incisions
- **sanguineous** bloody
- **secondary intention healing** healing that occurs in a wound in which the tissue surfaces are not approximated and there is extensive tissue loss; it is characterized by the formation of excessive granulation tissue and scarring; also called *secondary union*
- **suppuration** the formation of pus
- **suture** a surgical stitch used to close accidental or surgical wounds
- **tissue perfusion** passage of fluid, eg, blood through a specific organ or body part

TYPES OF WOUNDS

Wounds are frequently described according to the manner in which the wound is acquired. There are six categories of wounds by this classification: (a) incised, (b) contused, (c) abraded, (d) punctured, (e) lacerated, and (f) penetrating.

An *incised wound* or *incision* is made with a sharp instrument. It can be intentional, such as a cut made with a surgeon's scalpel, or accidental, such as a cut from a sharp knife.

A *contused wound* or *contusion* is a closed wound that occurs as the result of a blow from a blunt instrument. The skin appears bruised (*ecchymotic*) because blood from the damaged blood vessels is released into the tissues. Contused wounds are usually unintentional, although contusions may occur because of surgical manipulation.

An *abraded wound* or *abrasion* is a type of open wound that results from friction, such as a scraped knee from a fall on the road surface. It involves the skin only. Abraded wounds can also be intentional; for example, in a dermal abrasion the superficial layers of the skin are removed, either by sandpapering or by an abrasive machine, to obliterate scars and pockmarks.

A *punctured wound*, *stab wound*, or *puncture* is an open wound made by a sharp instrument that penetrates the skin and underlying tissues. Puncture wounds can be accidental, such as a wound made by stepping on a nail, or intentional, such as a wound made by a surgeon for insertion of a drain. Venipuncture and intramuscular injections are other common puncture wounds induced intentionally.

Lacerated wounds or *lacerations* occur when the tissues are torn apart, producing irregular edges. Lacerations are accidental and often result from accidents involving automobiles or machinery.

A *penetrating wound* is one in which an instrument is inserted deeply into the tissues through the skin or mucous membrane. Usually penetrating wounds are accidental, such as those from bullets or metal fragments. A bullet or other object making a penetrating wound may lodge in an internal organ.

CARE OF WOUNDS

Just as there are many types of wounds, there are many ways of caring for wounds. In general, the care varies with the type of wound, its size, the amount of exudate present, whether it is an open or closed wound, the location, the personal preference of the physician, and the presence of complicating factors.

Goals of Wound Care

1. *To prevent infection* from the entrance of microorganisms through the broken protective barriers of the skin and mucous membranes. This is accomplished by using sterile technique when caring for wounds, using antiseptic on the skin, and, on occasion, administering antibiotics as prescribed by the physician.

2. *To prevent further tissue damage.* Fragile healing wounds can be damaged by friction or injury. This is prevented by protecting the wound with dressings and by immobilizing the part with slings or binders.

3. *To promote healing.* This is accomplished by approximating wound edges with sutures (a physician's function), ensuring a good blood supply, supplying essential nutrients, and keeping the area free from body excretions.

4. *To clean wounds of foreign debris,* such as pieces of glass or excessive exudates. The former can act as irritants, and the latter can harbor microorganisms. *Debridement* is the cleaning of an injured area to remove debris, and it is usually performed by the physician. Wounds may be irrigated with water or cleaning solution such as hydrogen peroxide to clear away organic material prior to cleaning with antiseptics.

5. *To promote drainage.* Rubber or plastic tubes or drains are frequently put into wounds or ducts by the physician during surgery to promote drainage. Some of these drains, commonly referred to as *Penrose drains,* are shortened progressively throughout the healing process. They ensure removal of inflammatory exudates and blood prior to closure of the overlying skin. Other drains are placed in ducts, such as the ureter or common bile duct, to ensure patency of the duct and to prevent adhesion or closure of it during healing. Drains or tubes may be attached to suction apparatus to facilitate drainage. A portable vacuum suction (Hemovac) is sometimes used to drain blood and serous exudate from deep surgical wounds, such as those from orthopedic surgery. With this kind of suction, a vacuum is created in an evacuator bag, which gently draws the drainage out of the wound.

6. *To prevent hemorrhage.* Occlusive pressure dressings may be applied to surgical incisions for the first few days, until a dressing change is ordered by the physician. In certain body areas, such as the rectum or vagina, long strips of gauze in varying widths are packed into the orifice to apply pressure on blood capillaries and prevent bleeding. This *packing* is usually removed two to three days after surgery.

7. *To prevent skin excoriation* around draining wounds. This is accomplished by changing saturated dressings as required and by cleaning and drying wounds and surrounding skin areas. When drainage is excessive, as in some bowel (colostomy) or urinary surgery, protective ointments or pastes may be applied to surrounding skin

to prevent irritation and excoriation. The frequent removal of tape can also be irritating to the skin; thus, Montgomery straps or tie tapes (see page 827) or newer tape products that have minimal adhesive and are porous are frequently used. These cause the least skin disruption.

Open and Closed Methods of Wound Care

The closed method of wound care involves application of a dressing. The open method does not use dressings. Dressings have the following advantages:

1. They promote wound healing by absorbing drainage and debriding a wound.
2. They protect the wound from external microbial contamination.
3. They can aid in hemostasis if applied with elastic bandages.
4. They can assist in approximating wound edges.
5. They support and splint the wound site, thus reducing its mobility and trauma.
6. They cover unpleasant disfigurements.

In some situations, the physician applies a protective covering such as collodion spray instead of a gauze dressing. This spray hardens like nail polish and can be either peeled from the skin when the wound is healed or removed with a special solution. A spray covering is often preferred to a dressing, since friction is eliminated and the wound is always observable through the translucent covering. The wound is protected from external contamination because the spray is moisture-proof. For children, who are active and heal quickly, spray is frequently used. It is not advised for wounds that have drainage.

The open method is used to avoid certain disadvantages of dressings. For example, (a) dressings produce

dark, warm, moist environments in which resident and nonresident microorganisms can multiply; and (b) dressings can irritate wounds by friction. Exposing wounds to the air produces drying. This discourages the growth of microorganisms, which need moisture. The open method is frequently employed for burns.

Dressing Materials

Materials to clean wounds

Some nurses prefer cotton balls to clean wounds because of their absorbent qualities, while others prefer gauze squares, claiming that threads of cotton balls can stick to sutures. Cleaning agents vary considerably. Some of the common ones are:

Alcohol 70%

Aqueous and tincture of chlorhexidine gluconate (Hibitane)

Hydrogen peroxide

Materials to cover wounds

Several sizes of gauze are available to cover wounds. See Figure 35–1. The standard sizes are $10 \times 10\,cm$ ($4 \times 4\,in$) and $10 \times 20\,cm$ ($4 \times 8\,in$). The size and the number of pads used depend on the nature of the wound, the amount of exudate, and the location of the wound. These decisions are left to the nurse's judgment. Sometimes the gauze is precut halfway through one side to make it fit around a drain, or it is folded in a special way. See Technique 35–4, step 10.

Telfa gauze is a special type with a shiny, nonadherent surface on either one or both sides. It is applied with the shiny surface on the wound. Exudate seeps through this surface and collects on absorbent material on the other side or sandwiched between the two nonadherent surfaces. The dressing does not adhere and therefore does not cause injury to the wound when it is removed. Petrolatum gauze, another nonadherent type, is impregnated with petroleum jelly. It is placed against the wound and usually covered with gauze 4×4s.

Larger and thicker gauze dressings, called *surgipads* or *abdominal pads,* are used to cover small gauzes. They not only hold the other gauzes in place but also are absorbent and collect excessive drainage. Surgipads are more absorbent on one side, and this side is placed toward the wound; the less absorbent, more protective side is placed outward to protect the wound from external contamination. The outer side is often indicated with a blue stripe.

Materials to secure dressings

Tapes After abdominal or other types of surgery, an elastic adhesive tape may be applied over wounds because

FIGURE 35–1 ■ Some frequently used dressing materials (clockwise from bottom left): 2 × 2 gauze, 4 × 4 gauze, surgipad or abdominal pad, roller gauze, and nonadherent absorbent dressing.

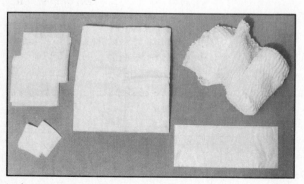

of its ability to compress, thereby controlling hemorrhage. The original tape is removed during the initial dressing change, and a lighter dressing is applied. Various tapes are available in strips to apply across a dressing, eg, nonallergenic tape and paper tape. It is important to secure the dressing at both ends and across the middle and to use tape of a sufficient width for the dressing and the wound. See Taping Dressings below.

Montgomery straps   Montgomery straps (tie tapes) are commonly used for patients who require frequent dressing changes. See Figure 35–2. These straps prevent skin irritation and discomfort caused by removing the adhesive each time the dressing is changed. Nonallergenic tie tapes are available for people who have sensitive skin. If these are not available, tincture of benzoin applied to the skin where the adhesive is to be placed protects the skin.

Bandages and binders   There are numerous types of roller bandages and binders that may be used to secure dressings, as well as to support or immobilize a wound. See chapter 33.

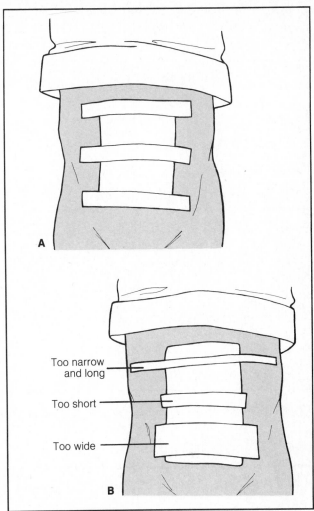

FIGURE 35–3 ▪ The strips of tape should be placed at the ends of the dressing and must be sufficiently long and wide to secure the dressing: **A**, correct taping; **B**, incorrect taping.

FIGURE 35–2 ▪ Montgomery straps, or tie tapes, are used to secure large dressings that require frequent changing.

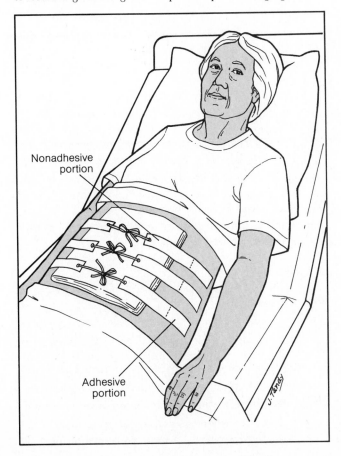

Taping dressings

It is important to tape a dressing over a wound so that (a) the dressing is maintained over the entire wound, and (b) the tape does not become dislodged. The correct type of tape must be selected for the purpose. Elastic tape can provide pressure; nonallergenic tape can be used if a patient is allergic to other tape.

1. Place the tape so that the dressing cannot fold back to expose the wound. Place strips at the ends of the dressing, and space tapes evenly in the middle. See Figure 35–3, *A*.

2. Ensure that the tape is long and wide enough to adhere to the skin but not so long or wide that it loosens with activity. See Figure 35–3.

3. Place the tape in the opposite direction from the body action, eg, across a body joint or crease, not lengthwise. See Figure 35–4.

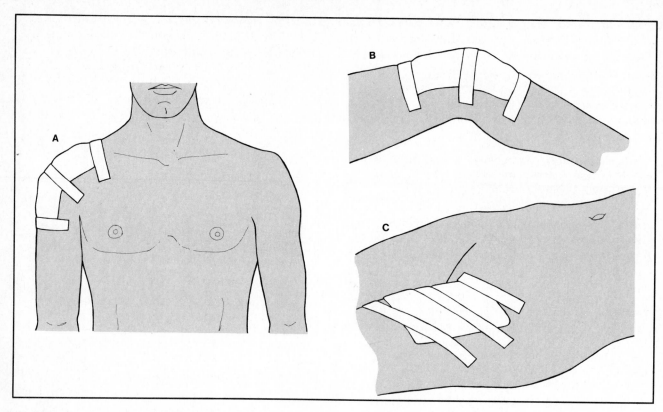

FIGURE 35–4 ■ Dressings over moving body parts must remain secure in spite of the movement.

TECHNIQUE 35–1 ■ Changing a Dry Surgical Dressing 🏠 ✳

Sterile dry dressings are used for wounds such as surgical incisions that have minimal drainage and no tissue loss and that heal by *primary intention*. For assessment of wound healing by primary intention, see Intervention, step 17. Most dressings have three layers:

1. A contact dressing that covers the incision and part of the surrounding skin and that collects fibrin, blood products, and debris from the wound

2. A gauze absorbent dressing that acts as a reservoir for excess secretions

3. A thicker outer dressing that protects the wound from external contamination

Not all surgical dressings require changing. Sometimes the surgeon applies a dressing in the operating room that remains in place until the sutures are removed, and no further dressings are required. In many situations, however, surgical dressings are changed regularly. Changing the dressing helps to prevent the growth of microorganisms that flourish in a damp, dark environment.

In some instances a patient may have a Penrose drain

inserted. The surgeon makes a stab wound to the side of the main incision and inserts the drain into the stab wound. See Technique 35–4. The main incision is considered to be cleaner than the stab wound, which usually has considerable drainage. Therefore the main incision is cleaned first, and under no circumstances are materials moved from the stab wound *to* the main incision. The main incision is kept free of the microorganisms that are around the stab wound.

■ Assessment

Assess:

1. The patient's complaints of discomfort and the location of the discomfort. Generally, incisional pain is severe for up to three days postoperatively and is relieved by narcotic analgesics. After that, milder analgesics provide relief. When patients complain of persistent severe pain, an infection or other problem may be the cause.

2. The presence of generalized symptoms of infection,

such as an elevated body temperature, diaphoresis, malaise, and leukocytosis. Infections usually occur on the fourth to sixth day.

3. The dressings for bleeding or other drainage. Inspect the bedclothes beneath the patient where drainage may collect as a result of gravity.

4. The patient's nutritional status. Good nutritional status is a significant factor in wound healing. Protein (ie, the essential amino acid cystine), and vitamins A and C are the nutrients principally involved in the healing of wounds. Protein is essential for the formation of new tissue. Vitamin A accelerates healing of skin incisions and the formation of granulation tissue. Vitamin C is thought to be necessary for collagen synthesis and the formation of capillaries in wounds. In addition, resistance to infection depends on a well-balanced diet that includes protein, carbohydrates, lipids, vitamins, and minerals.

5. The patient's weight. An obese patient is at greater risk for delayed wound healing and infection. Because adipose tissue does not have an abundant blood supply, the delivery of nutrients and cellular elements needed for healing is impaired. Adipose tissue is also more difficult for the surgeon to approximate and suture.

6. The patient's age. Many factors may inhibit wound healing in elderly patients. For example:

   a. Vascular changes associated with aging, such as atherosclerosis and atrophy of capillaries in the skin, can impair blood flow to the wound.

   b. Reduced liver function can impair the synthesis of needed blood clotting factors.

   c. Changes in the immune system may reduce the formation of antibodies and lymphocytes necessary to prevent infection.

   d. Nutritional deficiencies may reduce the numbers of red blood cells and leukocytes, thus impeding the delivery of oxygen and the inflammatory response essential for wound healing. Oxygen is needed for the synthesis of collagen and the formation of new epithelial cells.

7. Disorders such as diabetes mellitus or severe anemia that reduce tissue oxygenation or perfusion. Diabetics often have vascular changes that impair the blood supply to the area and thus tissue perfusion. Severe anemia can cause a significant reduction in the arterial pressure of oxygen that hinders its perfusion to the healing tissues.

8. Recent or current therapy with agents that suppress the immune response. Adequate immune mechanisms facilitate phagocytosis and the clearing of debris, essential aspects of the inflammatory response

that occurs during the healing process. Agents such as steroids (antiinflammatory medications) reduce the inflammatory response and delay collagen synthesis. Chemotherapeutic medications, used to treat various forms of cancer, often depress bone marrow function, decreasing the formation of leukocytes. This can impair wound healing and increase the patient's risk of infection.

■ Planning

Nursing goals

1. To promote wound healing by primary intention
2. To prevent infection
3. To assess the healing process
4. To protect the wound from mechanical trauma or external contamination

Equipment

1. A sterile dressing set that includes:

   a. A drape or towel.

   b. Cotton balls or gauze squares to clean the wound.

   c. A container for the cleaning solution.

   d. An antiseptic solution.

   e. Two pairs of forceps (thumb or artery).

   f. Gauze dressings and surgipads.

   g. Applicators or tongue blades to apply ointments.

   If a set is not available, gather these items from a central supply cart.

2. Additional supplies required for the particular dressing, eg, extra gauze dressings and ointment or powder, if ordered.

3. Disposable gloves (optional) if forceps are not used.

4. A mask.

5. A moisture-proof bag for disposal of the old dressings and the used cleaning gauzes.

6. Tape or tie tapes to secure the dressing.

7. A bath blanket, if necessary, to cover the patient and prevent undue exposure.

8. Acetone or another solution to loosen adhesive, if necessary.

■ Intervention

Preparing the patient

1. Acquire assistance for changing a dressing on an infant or young child.

   Rationale The child might move and contaminate the sterile field or the wound.

2. Assist the patient to a comfortable position, in which the wound can be readily exposed. Expose only the wound area, using a bath blanket to drape the patient, if necessary.

   Rationale Undue exposure is physically and psychologically distressing to most patients.

3. Make a cuff on the moisture-proof bag for disposal of the soiled dressings, and place the bag within reach. It can be taped to the bedclothes or bedside table.

   Rationale Making a cuff keeps the outside of the bag free from contamination by the soiled dressings and prevents subsequent contamination of the nurse's hands or of sterile instrument tips when discarding dressings or sponges. Placement of the bag within reach prevents the nurse from reaching across the sterile field and the wound and potentially contaminating these areas.

4. Don a face mask, if required, and wash your hands using surgical aseptic technique.

   Rationale Many agencies require that a mask be worn for surgical dressing changes to prevent contamination of the wound by droplet spray from the nurse's respiratory tract. The mask is donned before washing the hands because the hands will become contaminated when they touch the hair.

Removing the soiled dressing

5. Remove binders, if used, and place them aside. Untie Montgomery straps, if used.

6. If adhesive tape was used, remove it by holding down the skin and pulling the tape gently but firmly toward the wound. Use a solvent to loosen the tape, if required.

   Rationale Pressing down on the skin provides countertraction against the pulling motion. Tape is pulled toward the incision to prevent strain on the sutures or wound. Moistening the tape with acetone or a similar solvent lessens the discomfort of removal, particularly from hairy surfaces.

7. Remove the outer abdominal dressing or surgipad by <u>hand if</u> the dressing is dry, or using a disposable glove if the dressing is moist. Lift the dressing so that the underside is away from the patient's face.

   Rationale The outer surgipad is considered contaminated by the patient's clothing and linen. The appearance and odor of the drainage may be upsetting to the patient.

8. Place the soiled dressing in the waterproof bag without touching the outside of the bag.

   Rationale Contamination of the outside of the bag is avoided to prevent the spread of microorganisms to the nurse and subsequently to others.

9. Open the sterile dressing set. See Technique 7–2 on page 88.

10. Place the sterile drape beside the wound. See Technique 7–3 on page 92.

11. Remove the under dressings with tissue forceps or gloves, taking care not to dislodge any drains. If the gauze sticks to the drain, use two pairs of forceps, one to remove the gauze and one to hold the drain, or secure the drain with one hand.

    Rationale Forceps or gloves are used to prevent contamination of the patient's wound by the nurse's hands and contamination of the nurse's hands by wound drainage.

12. Assess the location, type (color, consistency), and odor of wound drainage, and the number of gauzes saturated or the diameter of drainage collected on the dressings. Three major types of exudates are serous, purulent, and sanguineous. It is important for nurses to describe an exudate accurately when assessing wound drainage.

    a. A *serous exudate* is comprised chiefly of serum (the clear portion of the blood) derived from the blood and serous membranes of the body, such as the peritoneum, pleura, pericardium, and meninges. It is watery in appearance and has few cells. An example is the fluid in a blister from a burn.

    b. A *purulent exudate* is thicker than serous exudate due to the presence of pus. It consists of leukocytes, liquefied dead tissue debris, and dead and living bacteria. The process of pus formation is referred to as *suppuration,* and the bacteria that produce pus are called *pyogenic bacteria.* Not all microorganisms are pyogenic. Purulent exudates vary in color, some acquiring tinges of blue, green, or yellow. The color may depend on the causative organism.

    c. A *sanguineous* or *hemorrhagic exudate* consists of large amounts of red blood cells, indicating damage to capillaries that is severe enough to allow the escape of red blood cells from plasma. This type of exudate is frequently seen in open wounds. Nurses often need to distinguish whether the sanguineous exudate is dark or bright. A bright sanguineous exudate indicates fresh bleeding, whereas dark sanguineous exudate denotes older bleeding.

    Mixed types of exudates are often observed. A serosanguineous exudate is commonly seen in surgical incisions; it consists of serous and sanguineous drainage.

13. Discard the soiled dressings in the bag. To avoid contaminating the forceps tips on the edge of the paper bag, hold the dressings 10 to 15 cm (4 to 6 in) above the bag, and drop the dressings into it. After the dressings are removed, discard the forceps, or set them aside from the sterile field.

grasp in ter center (handwritten)

Wash Hands before sterile (handwritten)

Rationale   These forceps are now contaminated by the wound drainage.

Cleaning and dressing the wound

14. Clean the wound, using the second pair of artery or tissue forceps and gauze swabs moistened with antiseptic solution. Keep the forceps tips lower than the handles at all times. Use a separate swab for each stroke, cleaning from the top of the incision downward. Discard each swab after use.

    Rationale   The wound is cleaned from the least to the most contaminated area, ie, from the top of the incision, which is drier, to the bottom of the incision, where any drainage will collect and which is considered more contaminated. Forceps tips are always held lower than the handle to prevent their contamination by fluid traveling up to the handle, which is contaminated by the nurse's bare hand, and back.

    a. Clean with strokes from top to bottom, starting at the center and continuing to the outside. See Figure 35–5.

       or

       Clean with strokes outward from the incision on one side and then outward on the other side. See Figure 35–6.

    b. If a drain is present, clean it after the incision. See Technique 35–4.

    c. For irregular wounds, such as a decubitus ulcer, clean from the center of the wound outward, using circular strokes.

15. Repeat the cleaning process until all drainage is removed.

16. Dry the wound with dry gauze swabs, using the strokes described in step 14.

17. Assess the overall appearance of the wound. Taylor (1983, p 44) and Bruno (1979, p 670) outline the following *sequential* signs of a primary healing wound:

    a. *Absence of bleeding and a clot* binding the wound edges together. After tissue is damaged, blood fills the area. A clot is formed from blood platelets, and the wound edges are well approximated and bound together by fibrin in the clot within the first few hours after surgical closure.

    b. *Inflammation (redness and swelling) at the wound edges* for one to three days. An inflammatory reaction begins after the clot sets, bringing white blood cells to ingest bacteria and cellular debris, and to demolish the clot.

    c. *Reduction in inflammation when the clot diminishes,* as granulation tissue starts to bridge the area. Healthy tissue at the wound edges secretes nutrients, fibroblasts, and other building materials, eg, epithelial cells, to bridge and close the

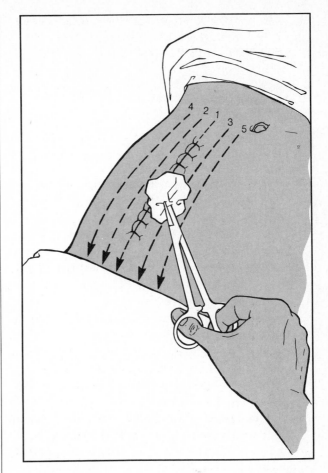

FIGURE 35–5

FIGURE 35–6

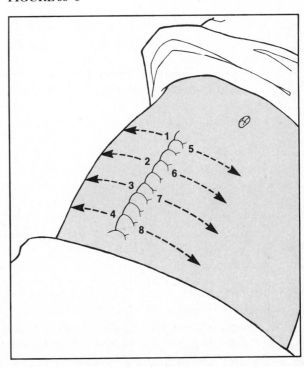

wound within seven to ten days. Increased inflammation associated with fever and drainage is indicative of wound infection; the wound edges then appear brightly inflamed and swollen.

    d. *Scar formation.* Fibroblasts in the granulation tissue secrete collagen, which forms scar tissue. Collagen synthesis starts four days after injury and continues for 6 months or longer.

    e. *Diminished scar size* over a period of months or years. Collagen fibers shorten, and wound strength increases. An increase in scar size indicates keloid formation.

18. Assess the presence of *dehiscence* (opening or gaping of the wound edges that exposes the yellow-pink subcutaneous tissue), and note its exact location. Dehiscence occurs most often on about the fifth postoperative day.

19. Apply powder or ointment if required. Shake powder directly onto the wound; use sterile applicators or tongue blades to apply ointment.

    Rationale If drainage is profuse, ointment can protect the skin from irritation. Antibiotic powders or other substances may be ordered by the physician.

20. Apply sterile dressings one at a time over the wound, using sterile forceps. Start at the center of the wound and move progressively outward. The final surgipad can be picked up by hand, touching only the outside, which is often marked by a blue line down the center.

21. Secure the dressing with tape, Montgomery straps, or a binder.

22. Record the dressing change, the wound assessment, and the patient's response.

Sample Recording

Date	Time	Notes
12/5/86	1500	Perineal dressing changed. Incision cleaned with Tr. Hibitane. Two 4 × 4 gauzes saturated with serous drainage at base of incision. Wound clean, edges closely approximated. No redness on incision line or surrounding tissue. 4 × 4 gauze and surgipads secured with T-binder. No discomfort. —————————————— Evangeline R. Puritos, RN

■ Evaluation

Expected outcome

Primary intention wound healing. See Intervention, step 17.

Unexpected outcomes

1. Wound dehiscence
2. Large amount of purulent drainage and foul odor
3. Excessive inflammation
4. Acute pain upon touching incision
5. Skin discoloration suggestive of hematoma formation

Upon obtaining an unexpected outcome:

1. Report your findings to the responsible nurse and/or physician.
2. Adjust the nursing care plan appropriately.

TECHNIQUE 35–2 ■ Applying Wet-to-Dry Dressings

Sterile wet-to-dry dressings may be prescribed for debridement of wounds with extensive tissue loss that heal by *secondary intention.* Examples of such wounds are burns, varicose ulcers, or decubitus ulcers. These wounds are not amenable to suturing. Although the basic processes of wound healing are essentially the same in primary intention and secondary intention healing, secondary intention healing is prolonged, produces extensive granulation tissue, and results in extensive scarring. In addition, the wound is more susceptible to infection because the normal skin barrier to bacterial invasion has been lost.

    Wet-to-dry dressings consist of a moistened contact dressing layer that touches the wound surface. This layer is allowed to dry between dressing changes every four to six hours. Wet-to-dry dressings are the treatment of choice for wounds requiring debridement, ie, cleaning of infected and necrotic material from the wound. The wet gauze traps necrotic material in its spaces as it dries. Dry dressings do not trap the debris as effectively. Wet dressings that do not dry out enough to trap debris promote bacterial growth in the damp environment and can cause tissue breakdown.

■ Assessment

Assess:

1. The patient's complaints of discomfort, to determine whether an analgesic is needed before wound care.
2. The presence of generalized symptoms of infection,

such as elevated body temperature, diaphoresis, malaise, and leukocytosis.

Other data include:

1. Type and strength of solution ordered by the physician for the wet-to-dry dressing.
2. Whether the wound is to be cleaned with antiseptic solution or other solution (eg, normal saline) before the wet-to-dry dressing is applied.

▪ Planning

Nursing goals

1. To promote wound healing by secondary intention
2. To prevent wound infection
3. To assess wound healing
4. To protect the wound from mechanical trauma or external contamination

Equipment

1. A sterile dressing set. See Technique 35–1 on page 829.
2. Sterile thin, fine-mesh gauze. Generally 4 × 4 non-cotton-filled gauze dressings are used. Cotton fibers are contraindicated because they can pull loose and remain in the wound, encouraging bacterial growth and contamination.
3. A sterile round or kidney-shaped container for the solution.
4. The ordered solution. The type used depends on the condition of the wound and the purpose of the dressings. Normal saline is often used to moisten necrotic tissue to help loosen and remove it. Betadine (10% solution) is often used for draining wounds infected with *Staphylococcus* or aerobic bacteria; it can cause burning and stinging, and some patients may be allergic to it. Acetic acid (0.25% solution) is often used for wounds infected with *Pseudomonas* or gram-positive and gram-negative organisms; it can be irritating to the skin surrounding the wound. Hydrogen peroxide (3% solution), not used as frequently today as in the past, is a debriding agent that facilitates removal of necrotic tissue. Sodium hypochlorite (Dakin's solution) is an antiseptic that dissolves necrotic tissue and retards *Pseudomonas* growth. Dakin's solution can cause skin breakdown, so it is used only on necrotic tissue.
5. Clean disposable gloves to remove soiled dressings.
6. Sterile gloves for cleaning the wound and applying dressings.
7. A mask.
8. A moisture-proof bag for soiled dressings.
9. Tape or tie tapes.

▪ Intervention

1. Assemble all equipment, prepare the patient, and remove the soiled dressings as in Technique 35–1, steps 1–13.
2. If the dressing adheres to underlying tissue, do not moisten it but gradually free the dressing as gently as possible.
   Rationale Wet-to-dry dressings are intended to clean wounds by debridement of the exudate or necrotic tissue.
3. Assess the character and amount of drainage on the dressings and the appearance of the wound, ie, the progress of healing by secondary intention. Observe the development and amount of granulation tissue. In wounds with extensive tissue loss, fibroblasts and capillary buds move slowly toward the center of the wound. As the capillary network develops, the tissue becomes a translucent red color. This tissue, called *granulation tissue,* is fragile, bleeds easily, may protrude above the wound margins, and may have a mucin covering. When the granulation tissue matures, marginal epithelial cells migrate and proliferate over this connective tissue base to fill the wound. If the wound does not close by epithelialization, the area becomes covered with dried plasma proteins and dead cells. This is called *eschar.* Initially, secondary intention healing wounds seep serosanguineous drainage. Later, if they are not covered by epithelial cells, they become covered with thick, gray, fibrinous tissue that is eventually converted into dense scar tissue.
4. Remove the disposable gloves and discard them in the bag.
5. Wash your hands.
6. Open the packages of the sterile dressing set, fine mesh gauze, and sterile solution container.
7. Pour the ordered solution into the solution container.
8. Don the sterile gloves.
9. Place the fine mesh gauze dressings into the solution container and thoroughly saturate them with solution.
   Rationale The entire gauze must be moistened to enhance its absorptive abilities.
10. If agency policy indicates, clean the wound gently using a circular motion. Work outward from the center of the wound to its edge and beyond. Use a separate gauze swab for each cleaning stroke.
11. Wring out excess moisture from the saturated fine mesh gauze dressings.
    Rationale Dressings that are too wet will not dry out in four to six hours.
12. Pack the moistened dressings into all depressions and grooves of the wound, ensuring that all exposed

surfaces are covered. If necessary, use forceps to feed the gauze gradually into deep depressed areas.

Rationale Necrotic tissue is usually more prevalent in depressed wound areas and needs to be covered with the wet-to-dry gauze.

13. Apply a dry 4 × 4 gauze over the wet dressings.

Rationale The dry gauze absorbs excess drainage.

14. Cover the dressings with a surgipad or abdominal pad.

Rationale The pad protects the wound from external contaminants.

15. Remove your gloves.

16. Secure the dressing at the edges only, with tape, Montgomery ties, bandage, or binder. Do not apply an airtight occlusive covering.

Rationale Occlusive dressings prevent air circulation and hinder drying of the fine mesh gauze.

17. Record the dressing change, the wound assessment, and the patient's response.

■ Evaluation

Expected outcome

Secondary intention wound healing. See Intervention, step 3.

Unexpected outcomes

1. Unabated prevalent discharge
2. Absence of granulation tissue

Upon obtaining an unexpected outcome:

1. Report your findings to the responsible nurse and/or physician.
2. Adjust the nursing care plan appropriately.

TECHNIQUE 35–3 ■ Applying a Moist Transparent Wound Barrier

Transparent wound barriers such as Op-site, Tegaderm, and Bio-occlusive are often applied to ulcerated or burned skin areas. Advantages of these dressings are:

1. They are nonporous, self-adhesive dressings that do not require changing or periodic debridement as other dressings do. They are often left in place until healing has occurred or as long as they remain intact.
2. Because they are transparent, the wound can be assessed through them.
3. Because they are occlusive, the wound remains moist and retains the serous exudate, which hastens healing and reduces the risk of infection.
4. Because they are elastic, they can be placed over a joint without disrupting the patient's mobility.
5. They adhere only to the skin area around the wound and not to the wound itself, because the wound is kept moist.
6. They allow the patient to shower or bathe without removing the dressing.

■ Assessment   See Technique 35–2 on page 832.

■ Planning

Nursing goals   See Technique 35–2 on page 833.

Equipment

1. Soap and water to clean the surrounding skin area.
2. A razor (optional) to shave the surrounding area.
3. Alcohol or acetone to defat the surrounding skin.
4. The wound barrier.
5. Sterile gauze and the wound cleaning agents specified by the physician or agency, eg, sterile saline, hydrogen peroxide, or Betadine. Check agency practice.
6. Sterile gloves to wear when cleaning the wound.
7. Scissors.
8. Paper tape.
9. A sterile #26 gauge needle and syringe to aspirate excessive drainage, if necessary.

■ Intervention

1. If the size of the wound necessitates it, acquire the assistance of a coworker to help apply the dressing.
2. Thoroughly clean the skin area around the wound with soap and water. Shave the hair within 5 cm (2 in) of the wound area if indicated. Then rub the area with alcohol or acetone, and allow it to dry.

Rationale Alcohol or acetone defats the skin. Defatted and clean, dry skin ensures better adhesion of the dressing.

3. Don gloves, and clean the wound with the prescribed solution if indicated. Remove the gloves.

4. Remove part of the paper backing on the dressing. If you have an assistant, remove all of the paper backing, and each hold the colored tabs attached to the dressing.

5. Apply the dressing at one edge of the wound site allowing at least 2.5 cm (1 in) coverage of the skin surrounding the wound.

6. Gently lay or press the barrier over the wound. Keep it free of wrinkles but avoid stretching it too tightly.
    Rationale   A stretched dressing restricts mobility.

7. Cut off the colored tabs after the wound is completely covered.

8. Reinforce the edges of the dressing with paper or other porous tape.

9. Assess the wound at least daily to determine the extent of serous fluid accumulation under the dressing, wound healing, and the need to repair the dressing. For assessment of wound healing, see Technique 35–2, Intervention, step 3, on page 833.

10. If excessive serum has accumulated, use a #26 gauge needle to aspirate the fluid. Then patch the needle hole.

11. If the dressing is leaking, remove it and apply another dressing.

■ **Evaluation**   See Technique 35–2.

TECHNIQUE 35–4   ■   Cleaning a Drain Site and Shortening a Penrose Drain

Frequently, flexible rubber drains, called *Penrose drains,* are inserted during abdominal surgery to provide drainage of excessive serosanguineous fluid and purulent material and promote healing of underlying tissues by obliterating dead space. These drains may be inserted and sutured through the incision line, but they are most commonly inserted through stab wounds a few centimeters away from the incision line, so that the incision is kept dry. Without a drain, some wounds would heal over on the surface and trap the discharge inside. Then the tissues under the skin could not heal because of the discharge, and an abscess might form.

Drains vary in length and width. The length inserted can be 25 to 35 cm (10 to 14 in), and the width 2.5 to 4 cm (0.5 to 1.5 in). To facilitate drainage and healing of tissues from the inside to the outside, or from the bottom to the top, the physician commonly orders that the drain be pulled out or shortened 2 to 5 cm (1 to 2 in) each day. When a drain is completely removed, the remaining stab wound usually heals within one to two days. In some agencies this shortening procedure is performed only by physicians; in others, it is ordered by the physician and performed by nurses. Shortening of a drain is done in conjunction with a dressing change.

■ **Assessment**

Assess any discomfort experienced by the patient and its location. Other data include:

1. Agency policies about the personnel who may shorten drains.

2. The physician's order that the drain is to be shortened by the nurse, and the length it is to be shortened, eg, 2.5 cm (1 in).

3. Whether the drain has been shortened previously. Check the nursing care plan. Drains that have not been shortened previously are often attached to the skin by a suture. If so, the suture needs to be removed before shortening the drain.

4. The location of the drain. Check the patient's chart.

5. The type and amount of discharge previously recorded on the patient's chart and previous assessments of the appearance of the wound, for baseline data.

■ **Planning**

Nursing goals

For cleaning a drain site

1. To remove any discharge from the skin, thereby reducing the danger of skin irritation

2. To reduce the number of microorganisms present and therefore reduce the possibility of infection

For shortening a drain

3. To decrease the length of the drain a designated amount, thereby encouraging healing of the wound from the inside toward the outside

Equipment

1. A sterile dressing set, including:
    a. Gauzes for cleaning the wound.

b. A container for the cleaning solution.

c. A towel or drape.

d. Surgipads and/or gauze dressings.

e. Antiseptic solution.

f. Two pairs of forceps, including at least one hemostat.

g. Cotton-tipped applicators.

2. Sterile dressing materials sufficient to cover the surgical incision and the drain site. At least two 4 × 4 gauzes are usually needed to dress the drain site; more are required if drainage is copious. A sterile precut gauze is needed to apply first around the drain site.

3. Sterile scissors to cut the drain.

4. A sterile safety pin. Add this to the sterile dressing set.

5. Sterile gloves (optional) for removing a moist outer dressing or shortening the drain if you prefer gloves to forceps.

6. A moisture-proof bag to receive the old dressings.

7. Tape, tie tapes, or other binding supplies.

8. A mask for the nurse and one for the patient, if necessary.

■ Intervention

1. Inform the patient that the drain is to be shortened and that this procedure should not be painful. Explain that the patient may feel a pulling sensation for a few seconds when the drain is being drawn out before it is shortened.

2. Ask the patient not to speak unnecessarily or touch the wound during the dressing change, so as not to

FIGURE 35-7

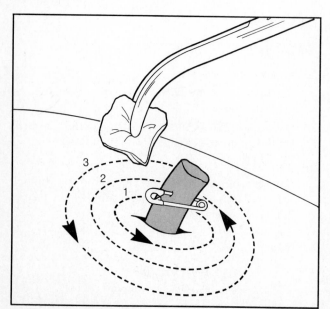

contaminate the wound. If the patient will likely want to talk, provide him or her with a mask.

3. Follow Technique 35-1, steps 1-18.

Rationale The incision is cleaned first, since it is considered cleaner than the drain site. Moist drainage facilitates the growth of resident skin bacteria around the drain.

Cleaning the drain

4. Clean the skin around the drain site by swabbing in half or full circles from around the drain site outward, using separate swabs for each wipe. See Figure 35-7. Forceps may be used in the nondominant hand to hold the drain erect while cleaning around it. Clean as many times as necessary to remove the drainage.

5. Assess the amount and character of drainage, including odor, thickness, and color.

Shortening a drain

6. If the drain has not been shortened before, cut and remove the suture. See Technique 35-5. The drain is sutured to the skin during surgery to keep it from slipping into the body cavity.

7. With a hemostat, firmly grasp the drain by its full width at the level of the skin, and pull the drain out the required length.

Rationale Grasping the full width of the drain ensures even traction.

8. Put on sterile gloves, and insert the sterile safety pin through the base of the drain as close to the skin as possible, holding the drain tightly against the skin edge and inserting the pin above your fingers. See Figure 35-8.

Rationale The pin keeps the drain from falling back into the incision. Holding the drain securely in place at the skin level and inserting the pin above the fingers prevents the nurse from pulling the drain farther out or pricking the patient during this step.

or

Use two pairs of sterile forceps instead of wearing sterile gloves to shorten the drain. This procedure requires manipulative skill.

a. After pulling the drain out, pick up the sterile safety pin at the clasp end using one pair of forceps held in the nondominant hand.

b. Securely grasp the base of the pin with the hemostat held in the dominant hand. See Figure 35-9.

c. Holding the pin securely with the hemostat, open the pin using the other forceps.

d. Use those forceps to hold the drain at the skin level while inserting the pin through the drain over the forceps.

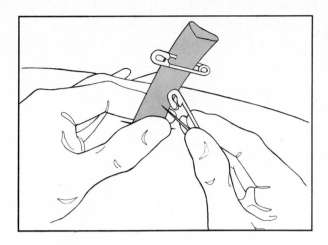

FIGURE 35–8

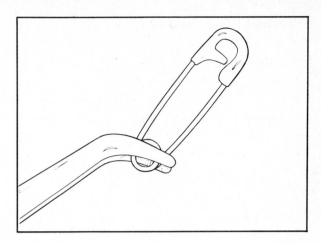

FIGURE 35–9

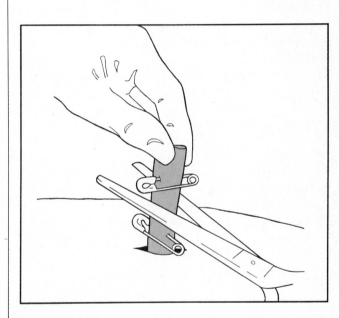

FIGURE 35–10

FIGURE 35–11

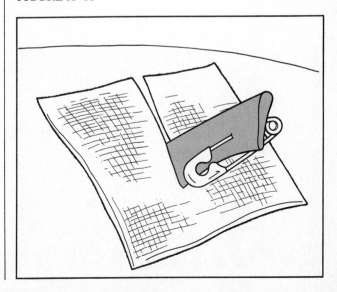

e. Close the pin using the forceps.

9. Cut off the excess drain so that about 2.5 cm (1 in) remains above the skin. See Figure 35–10. Discard the excess in the waste bag.

10. Place a precut 4 × 4 gauze snugly around the drain (see Figure 35–11) or open a 4 × 4 gauze to 4 × 8, fold it lengthwise to 2 × 8, and place the 2 × 8 around the drain so that the ends overlap.

    Rationale This dressing absorbs the drainage and helps prevent it from excoriating the skin. Using precut gauze or folding it as described, instead of cutting the gauze, prevents any threads from coming loose and getting into the wound, where they could cause inflammation and provide a site for infection.

11. Apply the sterile dressings one at a time using sterile gloved hands or sterile forceps. Take care that the dressings do not slide off and become contaminated. Place the bulk of the dressings over the drain area and below the drain, depending on the patient's usual position.

    Rationale Layers of dressings are placed for best absorption of drainage, which flows by gravity.

12. Apply the final surgipad by hand, touching only the outside unless using sterile gloves, and secure the dressing with tape or ties.

13. Record the technique on the patient's record, including the amount the drain was shortened and the type and amount of drainage present. Also see the Sample Recording in Technique 35–1.

Sample Recording

Date	Time	Notes
12/5/86	1025	Penrose drain shortened 2.5 cm. Three 4 × 4 gauzes saturated with brownish yellow drainage. Dry dressings applied. Skin intact; no redness or irritation. ——————— Maria L. Antonio, RN

■ Evaluation

Expected outcomes

1. Serosanguineous drainage at drain site
2. Decreased amount of drainage from day to day
3. Slight inflammation of skin around drain site

Unexpected outcomes

1. Purulent drainage with pungent odor
2. Copious amounts of drainage
3. Burning pain around drain site
4. Large area of inflammation around drain site

Upon obtaining an unexpected outcome:

1. Report your findings to the responsible nurse and/or physician.
2. Take a swab of the drainage for culture and sensitivity. See Technique 35–8.
3. Adjust the patient's nursing care plan appropriately.

SUTURES

Sutures are stitches used to sew body tissues together. A suture can also refer to the material used to sew the stitch. Policies vary about the personnel who may remove skin sutures. In some agencies, only physicians remove sutures; in others, registered nurses and student nurses with appropriate supervision may do so. Various suture materials are used, such as silk, cotton, linen, wire, nylon, and Dacron (polyester fiber) threads. Silver wire clips are also available. The physician prescribes the removal of sutures. Usually skin sutures are removed seven to ten days after surgery. Sterile technique and special suture scissors are used. The scissors have a short, curved cutting tip that readily slides under the suture. See Figure 35–12. Wire clips or staples are removed with a special instrument that squeezes the center of the clip to remove it from the skin. See Figure 35–13.

Retention sutures, sometimes referred to as *stay sutures,* are very large sutures made in some incisions in addition to skin sutures. See Figure 35–14. They attach underlying tissues of fat and muscle as well as skin and are used to support incisions in obese individuals or when healing may be prolonged. They are frequently left in place longer than skin sutures (14 to 21 days) but in some instances are removed at the same time as the skin sutures. Rubber tubing may be placed over them or a roll of gauze under them extending down the incision line, to prevent these large sutures from irritating the incision. Several forms of retention sutures are used, and agency policies about them may vary. The nurse should verify whether they are to be removed and which personnel may remove them.

There are various methods of suturing. Skin sutures can be broadly categorized as either (a) interrupted (each stitch is tied and knotted separately), or (b) continuous (one thread runs in a series of stitches and is tied only at the beginning and at the end of the run). Common sutures include plain interrupted (see Figure 35–15, *A*), mattress interrupted (see Figure 35–15, *B*), plain continuous (see Figure 35–15, *C*), mattress continuous (see Figure 35–15, *D*), and blanket continuous (see Figure 35–15, *E*).

FIGURE 35–12 ■ Suture scissors.

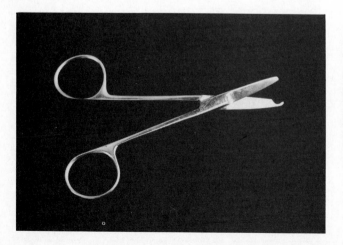

FIGURE 35–13 ■ Removing metal clips (staples) with a clip remover.

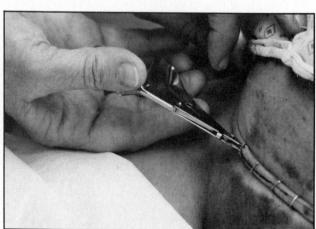

FIGURE 35–14 ■ A surgical incision with retention sutures.

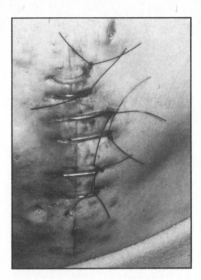

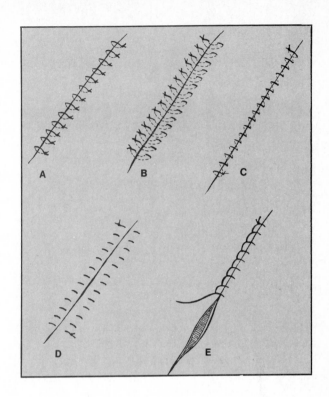

FIGURE 35–15 ■ Common methods of suturing: **A,** plain interrupted; **B,** mattress interrupted; **C,** plain continuous; **D,** mattress continuous; **E,** blanket continuous.

TECHNIQUE 35–5 ■ Removing Skin Sutures

■ Assessment

Assess the patient for any discomfort and its location. Other data include:

1. The physician's orders for suture removal. Many times only *alternate* interrupted sutures are removed one day, and the remaining sutures are removed a day or two later.
2. Whether a dressing is to be applied following the suture removal. Some physicians prefer no dressing; others prefer a small, light gauze dressing to prevent friction by clothing.

■ Planning

Nursing goals

1. To maintain the skin and the suture line intact while removing the sutures
2. To prevent microorganisms from entering the tissues under the skin while removing the sutures

Equipment

1. A sterile dressing set. See Technique 35–1 on page 829.

2. Sterile suture scissors.
3. Sterile butterfly tape (optional) to hold the wound edges together if wound dehiscence occurs.
4. A moisture-proof bag to receive used dressings and supplies.
5. A light sterile gauze pad and tape if a dressing is to be applied.

■ Intervention

1. Inform the patient that suture removal may produce slight discomfort, such as a pulling or stinging sensation, but it is not painful. Ask the patient not to touch the wound during the suture removal, so as not to contaminate the wound.
2. Remove the dressing, and clean the incision, as described in Technique 35–1. The suture line is usually cleaned with antiseptic solution before and after suture removal as a prophylactic measure to prevent infection.

Plain interrupted sutures

3. Grasp the suture at the knot with a pair of forceps.
4. Place the curved tip of the suture scissors under the

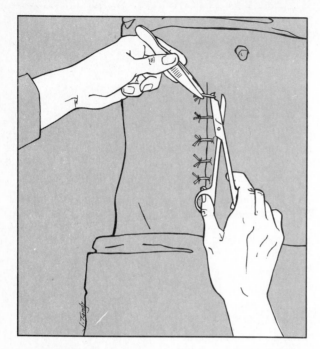

FIGURE 35-16

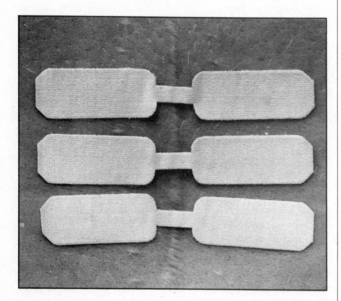

FIGURE 35-17

FIGURE 35-18

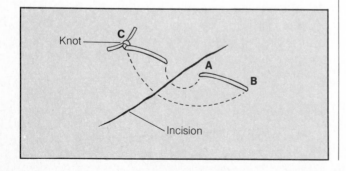

suture as close to the skin as possible, either on the side opposite the knot (see Figure 35–16) or directly under the knot. Cut the suture.

Rationale Sutures are cut as close to the skin as possible on one side of the visible part, because the suture material that is visible to the eye is in contact with resident bacteria of the skin and must not be pulled beneath the skin during removal. Suture material that is beneath the skin is considered free from bacteria.

5. With the forceps, pull the suture out in one piece. Be sure that all suture material is removed.

   Rationale Suture material left beneath the skin acts as a foreign body and causes inflammation.

6. Discard the suture onto a piece of sterile gauze or into the moisture-proof bag, being careful not to contaminate the forceps tips. Sometimes the suture sticks to the forceps and needs to be removed by wiping the tips on a sterile gauze.

7. Continue to remove *alternate* sutures, ie, the third, fifth, seventh, etc.

   Rationale Alternate sutures are removed first so that remaining sutures keep the skin edges in close approximation and prevent any dehiscence from becoming large.

8. If no dehiscence occurs, remove the remaining sutures. If dehiscence does occur, do not remove the remaining sutures, and report the dehiscence to the responsible nurse.

9. a. If a little wound dehiscence occurs, apply a sterile butterfly tape over the gap:
   ■ Attach the tape to one side of the incision.
   ■ Press the wound edges together.
   ■ Attach the tape to the other side of the incision. See Figure 35–17.

   Rationale The butterfly tape holds the wound edges as close together as possible and promotes healing.

   b. If a large dehiscence occurs, cover the wound with sterile gauze and report the problem immediately to the responsible nurse or physician.

10. Clean the incision again with skin antiseptic.

11. Apply a small, light, sterile gauze dressing, if any small dehiscence has occurred or if this is agency practice.

12. Instruct the patient about follow-up wound care. Generally, if a wound is dry and healing well, the patient can take showers in a day or two. Instruct the patient to contact the physician if wound discharge appears.

13. Record the suture removal and relevant assessment data on the appropriate records.

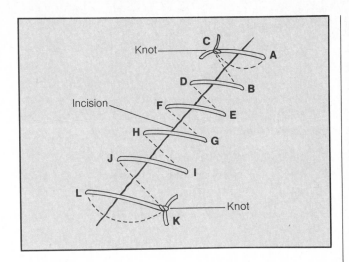

FIGURE 35–19

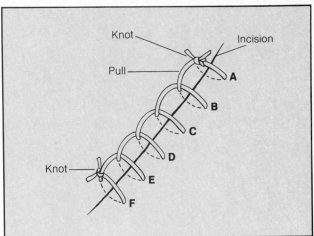

FIGURE 35–20

Sample Recording

Date	Time	Notes
12/5/86	1105	Abdominal sutures removed. Wound dry, edges approximated closely. No signs of inflammation. Gauze dressing applied. ——— ——— Gwen E. Owens, NS

Mattress interrupted sutures

See Figure 35–18. Mattress interrupted sutures do not cross the incision line outside the skin and have two threads underlying the skin.

14. When possible, cut the visible part of the suture close to the skin at *A* and *B* in Figure 35–18, opposite the knot, and remove this small visible piece. Discard it as in step 6. In some sutures, the visible part opposite the knot may be so small that it can be cut only once.

15. Grasp the knot (*C*) with forceps. Remove the remainder of the suture beneath the skin by pulling out in the direction of the knot.

16. Follow steps 7–13.

Plain continuous sutures

See Figure 35–19.

17. Cut the thread of the first suture opposite the knot at *A* in Figure 35–19. Then cut the thread of the second suture on that same side at *B*.

18. Grasp the knot (*C*) with the forceps, and pull. This removes the first stitch and the piece of thread beneath the skin, which is attached to the second stitch. Discard the sutures as in step 6.

19. Cut off the visible part of the second suture at *D*, and discard it.

20. Grasp the suture at *E*, and pull out the underlying loop between *D* and *E*.

21. Cut the visible part at *F*, and remove it.

22. Repeat steps 19–21 at *G–J*, until the last knot is reached. Note that, after the first stitch is removed, each thread is cut down the same side, below the original knot.

23. Cut the last suture at *L*, and pull out the last suture at *K*.

24. Follow steps 9–13.

Blanket continuous sutures

See Figure 35–20.

25. Cut the threads that are opposite the looped blanket edge, ie, cut at *A–F* in Figure 35–20.

26. Pull each stitch out at the looped edge, and discard it as in step 6.

27. Follow steps 9–13.

Mattress continuous sutures

See Figure 35–21.

28. Cut the visible suture at both skin edges opposite the knot (at *A* and *B* in Figure 35–21) and on the suture below opposite the knot (at *C* and *D*). Remove and discard the visible portions as in step 6.

29. Pull the first suture out by the knot at *E*.

30. Lift the second suture between *F* and *G* to pull out the underlying suture between *G* and *C*. Cut off the visible part at *F* as close to the skin edge as possible.

31. Go to the opposite side between *H* and *I*. Lift out the suture between *F* and *I*, and cut off all the visible part close to the skin at *H*.

32. Lift the suture between *J* and *K* to pull out the suture between *H* and *K*, and cut the suture close to the skin at *J*.

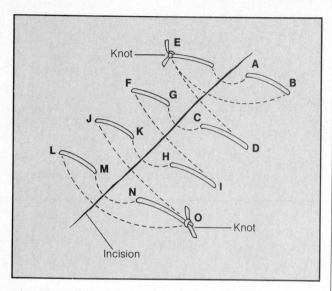

FIGURE 35-21

33. Repeat steps 31–32, working from side to side of the incision, until the last suture is reached.

34. Cut the visible suture opposite the knot at *L* and *M*. Pull out all remaining pieces of suture at *O*.

35. Follow steps 9–13.

■ **Evaluation**

Expected outcomes

1. Wound dry and clean
2. Wound edges approximated

Unexpected outcomes

1. Wound dehiscence
2. Purulent wound drainage, pronounced discomfort, swelling, and redness

Upon obtaining an unexpected outcome:

1. Report your findings to the responsible nurse and/or physician.
2. Take a swab of wound drainage for culture and sensitivity.
3. Apply butterfly tapes for dehiscence and a binder, if appropriate, to support the wound.
4. Adjust the patient's nursing care plan appropriately.

TECHNIQUE 35-6 ■ Establishing and Maintaining a Plastic Bellows Wound Suction (Hemovac, Portable Wound Suction)

The plastic bellows wound suction (Hemovac) is used to suction excessive drainage from surgical wounds. Suction is created by manually compressing and releasing the sides of the apparatus.

❋ The Hemovac is increasingly used by surgeons after various operations, eg, spinal surgery, hip surgery, radical mastectomy, head or neck surgery, and perineal surgery.

FIGURE 35-22

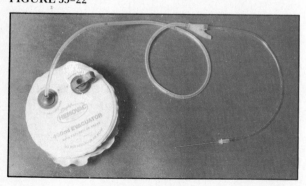

❋This type of suction is advantageous in that it exerts a *gentle,* even pressure on tissues, it is quiet, it is lightweight, and it moves easily with the patient. The unit consists of an evacuator bag, evacuator tubing with a Y-connector, and wound tubing with a needle. See Figure 35-22.

The surgeon inserts the wound drainage tube during surgery. Generally the suction is removed from three to seven days postoperatively or when the wound is free from drainage.

■ **Assessment**

1. Assess the amount, color, consistency, clarity, and odor of the drainage.
2. Assess the patient for discomfort, particularly in the area of the drain.
3. Assess the patient for clinical signs of infection, eg, elevated body temperature. See chapter 8, page 108.

Other data include: whether there is an order for irrigating the suction and, if so, the type and amount of solution to be used for the irrigation.

▪ Planning

Nursing goal

To maintain the patency of the wound suction and thereby hasten the healing process by draining excess exudate, which interferes with the formation of granulation tissue in a wound.

Equipment

To empty the evacuator bag

1. A drainage receptacle, eg, a solution basin.
2. A calibrated pitcher to measure the drainage.

To irrigate the tubing

3. A sterile 50-mL syringe.
4. A sterile #18 or #20 needle with a blunt bevel. The needle needs to fit snugly into the drainage tubing.
5. Sterile irrigating solution as ordered, eg, normal saline.
6. A sterile set with a sterile receptacle, eg, a kidney basin or solution basin and a sterile towel.

▪ Intervention

Establishing suction

Establish suction if it was not initiated by the physician.

1. Place the evacuator bag on a solid, flat surface.
2. Open the drainage plug marked *B* on top of the bag, without contaminating it.
3. Compress the bag; while it is compressed, close the drainage plug to retain the vacuum. See Figure 35–23.

Emptying the evacuator bag

4. When the drainage fluid reaches the line marked *Full,* open the drainage plug marked *B.*
5. Invert the bag, and empty it into the collecting receptacle. See Figure 35–24.
6. Reestablish suction as in steps 1–3.
7. Measure the amount of drainage, and note its characteristics.

Irrigating the evacuator and wound tubing

Because the wound tubing of a portable wound suction is siliconized and perforated with many holes, occlusions of the tubing are rare. However, when the evacuator bag is compressed and no drainage appears, either the wound

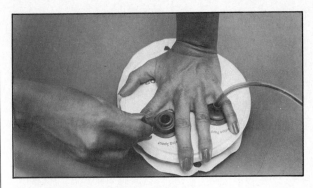

FIGURE 35–23

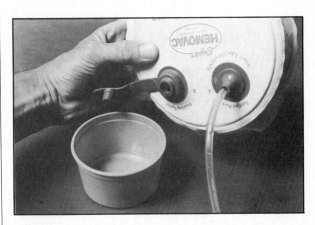

FIGURE 35–24

is free of exudate or the tubing is clogged. In the latter instance, notify the responsible nurse and/or the physician; an irrigation *may* be ordered.

8. Open the sterile set, and prepare a sterile field.
9. Fill the irrigating syringe with irrigating fluid, keeping the needle and plunger sterile.
10. Disconnect the wound tubing from the tubing connector, keeping the ends sterile to prevent contamination of the wound.
11. Insert the needle into the wound tubing, taking care not to perforate the tubing with the needle.
12. Instill the prescribed amount of irrigating fluid slowly and gently.
    Rationale Too much force could injure the tissues.
13. Detach the syringe from the tubing and place the end of the wound tubing in a sterile container.
14. Refill the syringe, if necessary, and insert the needle into the Y-connector opening. See Figure 35–25.
15. Irrigate the evacuator tubing until the fluid that runs into the evacuator bag is clear.
16. Reconnect the tubes securely, and empty the bag. Calculate the amount of drainage by subtracting the amount of irrigating fluid used.

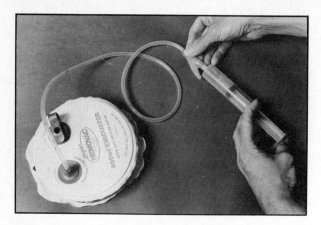

FIGURE 35–25

17. Reestablish the suction as in steps 1–3.
18. Assess the patient's response to the technique in terms of discomfort, relief from discomfort, etc.
19. Record the emptying of the evacuator bag, irrigation of the tubing, etc, on the patient's record.
20. Record the response of the patient and the amount,

appearance, etc, of the drainage on the appropriate records. For example, the amount and type of drainage should be included on the patient's intake and output record and on the nursing notes.

■ Evaluation

Expected outcomes

1. Clear, pink drainage with no odor
2. No discomfort at drain site
3. No clinical signs of infection

Unexpected outcomes

1. No drainage
2. Acute pain around drain area

Upon obtaining an unexpected outcome:

1. Report your findings to the responsible nurse and/or physician.
2. Adjust the nursing care plan appropriately.

TECHNIQUE 35–7 ■ Irrigating a Wound

An irrigation (lavage) is the washing or flushing out of an area. Sterile technique is required for a wound irrigation, because there is a break in the skin integrity.

■ Assessment

Assess the patient for:

1. Clinical signs of infection, eg, elevated body temperature
2. Discomfort, to determine the need for an analgesic before the irrigation

Other data include: the type of irrigating solution to be used, the frequency of irrigations, and the temperature of the solution. Various solutions are used, such as antibiotic solutions, antiseptic solutions, hydrogen peroxide, and Dakin's solution.

■ Planning

Nursing goals

1. To clean the area
2. To apply heat and hasten the healing process
3. To apply a medication, such as an antiseptic

Equipment

1. A sterile dressing set and dressing materials. See Technique 35–1. Arrange the set as you would for a dressing change.
2. A sterile irrigating syringe. A 50-mL piston syringe is frequently used. Piston syringes reduce the risk of aspirating drainage. For deep wounds with small openings, a sterile straight catheter may also be necessary.
3. A sterile basin for the irrigating solution.
4. A sterile basin to receive the irrigation returns.
5. Irrigating solution, usually 200 mL (6.5 oz) of solution at 32 to 35 °C (90 to 95 °F), according to the agency's or physician's choice. Sterile normal saline, Dakin's solution, hydrogen peroxide, or antibiotic solutions are frequently used.
6. Sterile gloves to wear if you will touch the wound.
7. A moisture-proof sterile drape to protect the patient and the bed.
8. Sterile petroleum jelly to protect the surrounding skin from irritation by certain solutions (eg, Dakin's solution).
9. A sterile tongue blade to apply the petroleum jelly.

■ Intervention

1. Remove the old dressing, and clean the wound. See Technique 35-1, steps 1–18.

2. Assist the patient to a position in which the irrigating solution will flow by gravity from the upper end of the wound to the lower end and then into the basin.

3. Place the waterproof drape over the patient and the bed, and position the sterile basin on it below the wound, to catch the irrigating solution.

4. If an irrigating solution, such as Dakin's solution, is being used, apply sterile petroleum jelly to the skin around the wound, using the sterile tongue blade.

5. Using the syringe, gently instill a steady stream of irrigating solution into the wound. Make sure all areas of the wound are irrigated. If you are using a catheter, insert the catheter into the wound until you feel resistance. Do not force the catheter, since this can cause tissue damage.

6. Continue irrigating until the solution becomes clear (no exudate is present) or until all the solution has been used.

   Rationale The irrigation washes away tissue debris and drainage so that later returns are clearer.

7. Using dressing forceps and sterile gauze, dry the area around the wound.

   Rationale Moisture left on the skin promotes the growth of microorganisms and can cause skin irritation.

8. Assess the appearance of the wound, noting in particular the type and amount of exudate, and the presence and extent of granulation tissue.

9. Apply a sterile dressing to the wound. See Technique 35-1, steps 20–21.

10. Record the irrigation, the solution used, the appearance of the wound, and the appearance of any exudate and sloughing tissue.

■ Evaluation

Expected outcomes

1. Drainage of an appropriate amount, color, and clarity for the particular patient

2. Decreased or no discomfort

3. No clinical signs of infection

Unexpected outcomes

1. Less or more drainage than anticipated for the patient

2. Drainage that is thick, is purulent, and/or has a foul odor

3. Increasing discomfort

Upon obtaining an unexpected outcome:

1. Report your findings to the responsible nurse and/or physician.

2. Adjust the nursing care plan appropriately.

TECHNIQUE 35-8 ■ Obtaining a Specimen of Wound Drainage

Specimens may be taken from a draining wound to identify microorganisms that are causing an infection. The specimen is often taken when the dressing is changed and before the wound is cleaned. Normal wound drainage contains few pathogens. A specimen is usually taken for culture and sensitivity when infection is suspected.

■ Assessment

Assess the patient for:

1. Pain at the wound site. A patient who has an infected wound may complain of burning pain. If the wound is painful and draining, and there is no routine for cleaning it or changing the dressing, plan to take a specimen for culture and sensitivity when the patient is comfortable, following an analgesic.

2. Clinical signs of infection, eg, fever, chills, and thirst. See chapter 8, page 108.

Other data include: whether the site from which to take the specimen is specified. If not, the specimen is normally taken at a drain site or at the site of the greatest amount of drainage.

■ Planning

Nursing goals

1. To identify the type of pathogenic microorganisms in a wound and the antibiotics to which they are sensitive

2. To evaluate the effectiveness of antibiotic therapy

Equipment

1. A sterile dressing set, including dressings, cleaning solution, scissors, swabs, medications, etc.

2. Clean gloves to protect the nurse's hands from any microorganisms in the wound drainage.

3. Sterile gloves or sterile forceps to handle the sterile supplies.

4. A moisture-proof disposal bag, to keep the microorganisms contained. Plastic or waxed paper bags are often used. A wet paper bag allows microorganisms to pass through to the outside.

5. A sterile specimen container. Usually glass tubes with secure caps are used. Two tubes will be needed if specimens are to be taken from two sites.

6. One or two sterile swabs or applicators.

7. Completed labels for each container. If specimens are being taken from more than one site, the exact site needs to be specified on the label, eg, inferior drain site or lower aspect of incision. Label each container before beginning the technique.

8. A completed requisition to accompany the specimens to the laboratory.

9. An envelope or bag in which to send the specimen tube to the laboratory.

■ Intervention

1. Explain to the patient that you plan to take a specimen of wound drainage and that it is usually a painless procedure. Listen carefully to the patient's concerns. The presence of an infection could cause the patient to worry about such matters as the date of discharge from the hospital and return to work. Communicate his or her concerns to the other members of the health team.

2. Put on clean gloves.

3. Remove the old dressing, and observe any drainage on it. Hold the dressing so that the patient does not see the drainage, unless he or she asks to. Discard the dressing in the moisture-proof bag. Handle it carefully so that the dressing does not touch the outside of the bag.

   Rationale The appearance of the drainage could upset the patient. Touching the outside of the bag will contaminate it.

4. Assess the appearance of the tissues in and around the wound and the drainage. Infection can cause reddened tissues with a thick discharge, which may be foul smelling, whitish, or colored. Determine the amount of the drainage, eg, scant or copious.

5. Remove your gloves, and dispose of them properly.

6. Open the package of sterile swabs or applicators using surgical aseptic technique.

7. Put on the sterile gloves, using surgical aseptic technique.

8. Open a specimen tube, and place the cap on a firm, dry surface so that the inside will not become contaminated. Hold the tube in one hand, and pick up a swab in the other.

9. Using the sterile swab, wipe the drainage at the designated point or where it is heaviest and nearest the wound. Absorb as much drainage as possible onto the swab. Wipe only once with one swab.

   Rationale Only one wipe is taken with each swab, to prevent contamination of the wound.

10. Insert the swab into the sterile container, taking care not to touch the top or the outside of the tube.

    Rationale The outside of the container needs to remain free of pathogenic microorganisms to prevent their spread to others.

11. Close the container securely.

12. If a specimen is required from another site, repeat steps 8–11. Specify the exact site on the label of each container, if not labeled previously. Be sure to put each swab in the tube for its own site.

13. Clean the wound as required, apply any ordered medication, and cover with sterile dressings. See Technique 35–1.

14. Assess the appearance of the tissues in and around the wound and the drainage.

15. Remove your gloves, and dispose of them appropriately.

16. Place the labeled specimen container in an envelope or bag for transportation to the laboratory. Attach the completed requisition to the container or envelope.

17. Arrange for the specimen to be transported to the laboratory. Refrigerate the specimen if it cannot be taken to the laboratory immediately.

18. Record taking the specimen, on the patient's chart and on the nursing care plan. Include the date and time; the appearance of the wound; the color, consistency, amount, and odor of any drainage; and any discomfort experienced by the patient.

Sample Recording

Date	Time	Notes
1/12/87	1100	Specimen of wound drainage from base of incision sent to laboratory. Base of incision reddened. One 4 × 4 gauze saturated with thick green drainage. No odor. C/o tenderness on movement. ———————— Sally N. Starr, NS

19. On receipt of the laboratory report, note which microorganisms were identified and the antibiotic to

which they are sensitive. Place the report in the patient's chart, and notify the physician or responsible nurse. Note if the plan of therapy is changed as a result of the report.

■ **Evaluation**

Expected outcomes

1. Positive change in wound appearance, eg, less inflammation and drainage
2. Decreased discomfort
3. Normal body temperature

4. One or more negative wound cultures

Unexpected outcomes

1. Increased inflammation of wound
2. Discomfort unchanged
3. Elevated body temperature
4. Positive wound culture

Upon obtaining an unexpected outcome:

1. Report your findings to the responsible nurse and/or physician.
2. Adjust the nursing care plan appropriately.

References

Brozenec S: Caring for the postoperative patient with an abdominal drain. *Nursing 85* (April) 1984; 15:55–57.

Brubacher LL: To heal a draining wound. *RN* (March) 1982; 45:30–35.

Bruno P: The nature of wound healing: Implications for nursing practice. *Nurs Clin North Am* (December) 1979; 14(4):667–682.

Bruno P, Craven RF: Age challenges to wound healing. *J Gerontol Nurs* (December) 1982; 8(12):686–691.

Flynn ME, Rovee DT: Wound healing mechanisms. *Am J Nurs* (October) 1982; 82:1544–1550.

Influencing repair and recovery. *Am J Nurs* (October) 1982; 82:1550–1557.

Neuberger GB: A new look at wound care. *Nursing 85* (February) 1985; 15:1 (Canadian ed. pp 34–41).

Nichols RL: Techniques known to prevent postoperative wound infection. *Infect Control* (January/February) 1982; 3:34–37.

Nurse's Reference Library Series: *Procedures.* Intermed Communications, 1983.

Schumann D: Preoperative measures to promote wound healing. *Nurs Clin North Am* (December) 1979; 14(4):683–699.

Simmons BP: CDC guidelines for prevention of surgical wound infections. *Am J Infect Control* (February) 1983; 11(2):133.

Slahetka F: Dakin's solution for deep ulcers. *Geriatr Nurs* (May/June) 1984; 5:168–169.

Taylor DL: Wound healing: Physiology, signs, and symptoms. *Nursing 83* (May) 1983; 13(5):44–45.

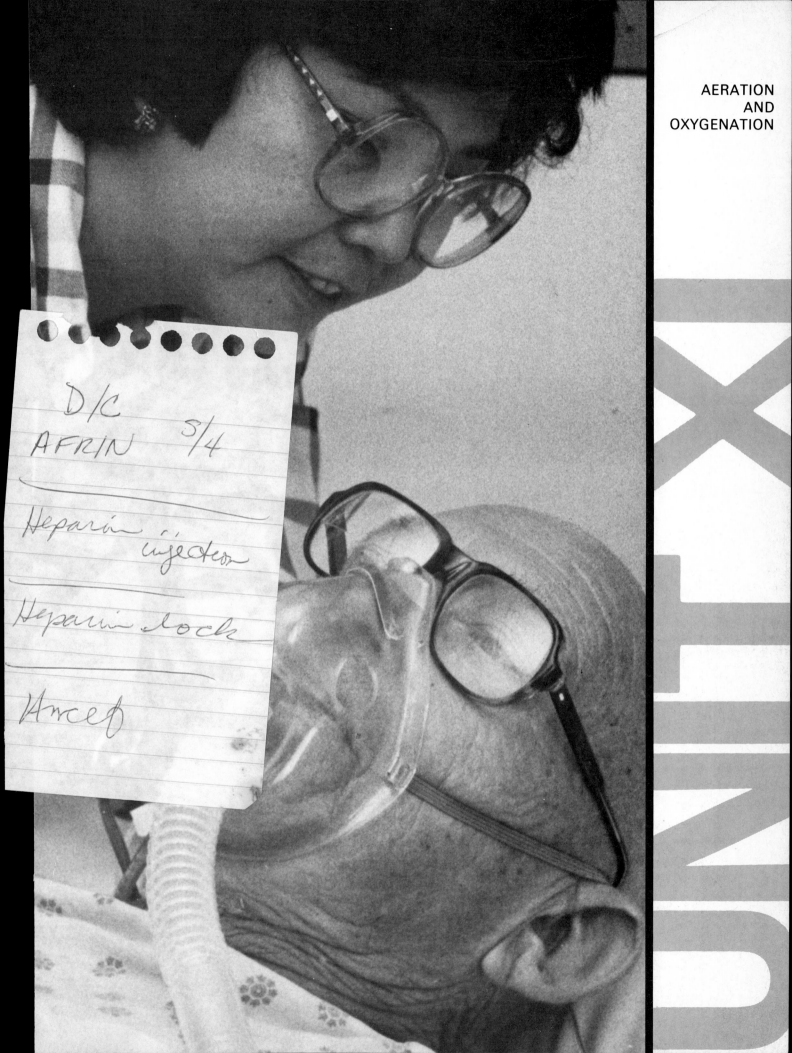

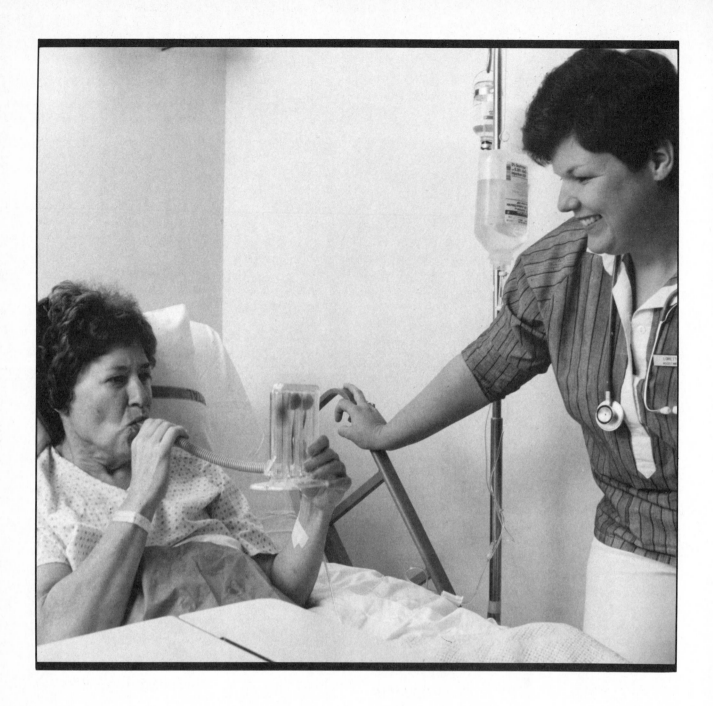

RESPIRATORY ASSISTIVE DEVICES AND POSTURAL DRAINAGE

36

Respiratory assistive devices and postural drainage are used to clear the respiratory tract of secretions and maintain adequate respirations. In a healthy, active person, secretions do not normally accumulate in the lungs. However, when a patient is confined to bed, not all lung tissue may become aerated, and secretions may accumulate. Other conditions that predispose patients to accumulation of lung secretions are chronic lung diseases (eg, emphysema), unconsciousness, and mechanical ventilation of the lungs.

Coughing and deep breathing were described for operative patients in chapter 31. These interventions are also required by other patients who need to clear secretions from the lungs and the respiratory passages. Percussion, vibration, and postural drainage are carried out for nonsurgical and surgical patients; however, the latter often require modified positions, because they have difficulty and discomfort assuming the described positions.

Chapter Outline

Lung Inflation Techniques
- Technique 36–1 Teaching Deep Breathing Exercises
- Technique 36–2 Assisting Patients to Use Blow Bottles or Sustained Maximal Inspiration Devices
- Technique 36–3 Assisting Patients with Intermittent Positive Pressure Breathing (IPPB)

Humidifiers and Nebulizers
- Technique 36–4 Assisting Patients to Use Nebulizers

Chest Physiotherapy
- Technique 36–5 Administering Percussion, Vibration, and Postural Drainage (PVD) to Adults
- Technique 36–6 Administering Percussion, Vibration, and Postural Drainage (PVD) to Infants and Children
- Technique 36–7 Collecting a Sputum Specimen
- Technique 36–8 Obtaining Nose and Throat Specimens

Objectives

Upon completion of this chapter, the student will:

1. Know essential terms and facts about lung inflation techniques, percussion, vibration, and postural drainage
   1.1 Define selected terms
   1.2 Identify essential facts about deep breathing exercises
   1.3 Identify essential facts about respiratory assistive devices
   1.4 Identify essential facts about humidifiers and nebulizers
   1.5 Identify the purposes of percussion, vibration, and postural drainage
   1.6 Identify the positions used for draining all lung segments
   1.7 Describe the procedure for percussion and vibration
   1.8 Identify areas to percuss during postural drainage of various lung segments
2. Understand facts about lung inflation techniques, percussion, vibration, and postural drainage
   2.1 Identify relevant assessment data
   2.2 Identify nursing diagnoses for which the technique may be implemented
   2.3 Identify nursing goals related to the technique
   2.4 Identify expected and unexpected outcomes from assessment data

   2.5 Identify reasons underlying selected steps of the technique
3. Perform lung inflation, percussion, vibration, and postural drainage techniques safely
   3.1 Assess the patient adequately
   3.2 Collect additional data from appropriate sources
   3.3 Select pertinent nursing goals for the patient
   3.4 Establish relevant outcome criteria for the patient following the technique
   3.5 Collect necessary equipment before the technique
   3.6 Implement interventions to enhance the effectiveness of the technique and enhance the patient's comfort and safety
   3.7 Communicate relevant information about the patient to the appropriate persons
   3.8 Determine the evaluative outcomes of the technique
4. Evaluate own performance of specific techniques in a laboratory or clinical setting with the assistance of another
   4.1 Use the performance checklists provided
   4.2 Identify areas of strength and weakness
   4.3 Alter performance in response to own evaluation and that of another

Terms

- adventitious (breath sounds)   abnormal
- alveolus   a saclike dilation or cavity in the body (plural: alveoli)

■ anoxia   systemic absence of oxygen or reduction of oxygen below physiologic levels in body tissues

■ apnea   cessation of breathing

■ atelectasis   collapse of lung tissue

■ bradypnea   abnormally slow breathing

■ bronchus   a large air passage of the lungs (plural: bronchi)

■ bubbling   gurgling sounds as air passes through moist secretions in the respiratory tract

■ Cheyne-Stokes breathing   rhythmic waxing and waning of respirations from very deep breathing to very shallow breathing and temporary apnea; often associated with cardiac failure, increased intracranial pressure, or brain damage

■ cough   a sudden expulsion of air from the lungs

■ creps (crepitation)   a dry, crackling sound like that of crumpled cellophane, produced by air moving through fluid in the alveoli or by air in the subcutaneous tissue

■ cyanosis   a bluish coloring of the mucous membranes, nail beds, or skin due to excessive deoxygenation of hemoglobin

■ deep breathing   inhaling the maximum amount of air possible, then exhaling

■ diaphragm   a dome-shaped muscle between the lungs and the abdomen

■ dullness   a decreased resonance or percussion sound, in contrast to normal resonance, that occurs when large amounts of fluid or pus collect in the alveoli

■ dyspnea   difficult and labored breathing during which the patient has a persistent unsatisfied need for air and feels distressed

■ emphysema   a chronic obstructive lung disorder in which the terminal bronchioles become distended and plugged with mucus

■ exhalation (expiration)   the outflow of air from the lungs to the atmosphere

■ expectorate   to spit out mucus or other materials

■ fissure   a groove or deep fold, such as those that separate the lobes of the lungs

■ flail chest   the ballooning out of the chest wall through injured rib spaces

■ flatness   an absence of resonance

■ friction rub   *see* pleural rub

■ hemoptysis   blood in the sputum

■ hyperventilation   an increase in the amount of air in the lungs, usually brought about by prolonged and deep respirations; an increased ventilation compared to the amount of carbon dioxide produced by metabolism

■ hypoventilation   a reduction in the amount of air in the lungs, usually brought about by shallow respirations; a decreased expulsion of carbon dioxide in relation to the amount produced by metabolism

■ hypoxemia   deficient oxygenation of the blood as measured by laboratory tests

■ hypoxia   diminished availability of oxygen for body tissues, due to internal or external causes

■ inhalation (inspiration)   the intake of air or other substances into the lungs

■ intercostal retractions   indrawing between the ribs

■ lobe   a well-defined portion of an organ, eg, the lung

■ nonproductive cough   a dry, harsh cough without secretions

■ orthopnea   ability to breathe only in upright sitting or standing positions

■ paradoxical breathing   respirations in which the chest wall balloons during expiration and is depressed or sucked inward on inspiration

■ percussion   the act of striking a body area with short, sharp blows

■ pleural rub (friction rub)   a coarse, leathery, or grating sound produced by the rubbing together of the pleura

■ postural drainage   drainage of secretions of various lung segments by the use of specific positions and gravity

■ productive cough   a cough in which secretions are expectorated

■ rales   rattling or bubbling sounds, generally heard on inhalation, as air moves through accumulated moist secretions

■ resonance   a low-pitched, rich-quality sound produced over normal lung tissue when the chest is percussed

■ rhonchi   coarse, dry, wheezy, or whistling sounds, more audible during exhalation, as the air moves through tenacious mucus or a narrowed bronchus

■ stertor   snoring or sonorous respirations, usually due to a partial obstruction of the upper airway

■ stridor   a shrill, harsh sound heard during inhalation with a laryngeal obstruction

■ substernal retractions   indrawing beneath the breast bone

■ supraclavicular retractions   indrawing above the clavicles

■ suprasternal retractions   indrawing above the breast bone

■ tachypnea   rapid, shallow respirations

■ tenacious   sticky, adhesive

■ trachea   a membranous tube, composed of cartilage, descending from the larynx and branching into the right and left bronchi

- tracheal tug   the indrawing and downward pull of the trachea during inspiration
- vibration   a technique of rapid agitation of the hands while pressing on a body area

- wheeze   a whistling respiratory sound on expiration that usually indicates some narrowing of the bronchial tree

LUNG INFLATION TECHNIQUES

Lung inflation techniques include diaphragmatic breathing exercises, apical and basal lung expansion exercises, and use of blow bottles, sustained maximal inspiration (SMI) devices, or intermittent positive pressure breathing (IPPB) apparatuses. While facilitating the patient's lung expansion, these techniques promote the exchange of gases in the lungs and strengthen the muscles used for breathing.

TECHNIQUE 36–1   ■   Teaching Deep Breathing Exercises

Breathing exercises are frequently indicated for patients with restricted chest expansion, ie, people with chronic obstructive pulmonary disease (COPD) or patients recovering from thoracic surgery. Commonly employed breathing exercises are abdominal (diaphragmatic) and pursed-lip breathing, apical expansion, and basal expansion exercises. Deep breathing and coughing exercises for the postoperative patient are discussed in Technique 31–1 on page 755.

■ Assessment

Assess the patient for:

1. Vital signs for baseline data.
2. Breathing patterns, ie, rhythm, ease or effort of breathing, and volume. Note any dyspnea, orthopnea, hyperventilation, hypoventilation, tachypnea, bradypnea, and Cheyne-Stokes breathing.
3. Chest movements such as retractions, flail chest, or paradoxical breathing. Note the specific location of retractions: intercostal, substernal, suprasternal, supraclavicular, or tracheal tug.
4. Secretions and cough. Note whether a cough is productive or nonproductive. If it is productive, determine the amount, kind, color, and odor of sputum (eg, thick, frothy, pink, rusty, or blood-tinged).
5. Normal and abnormal breath sounds that are audible without amplification and those that are best heard with a stethoscope. See Technique 10–10 on page 202 for auscultation of the lungs. Sounds audible without amplification include stridor, stertor wheezing, and bubbling. Sounds audible by stethoscope include rales, rhonchi, creps, and pleural rub.
6. Pallor and cyanosis of the skin and nail beds.
7. Clinical signs of hypoxia or anoxia, such as increased pulse rate, rapid or deep respirations, cyanosis, restlessness, anxiety, dizziness (vertigo), or faintness (syncope).
8. The location of any surgical incision in relation to the muscles needed for breathing. An incision can impede appropriate lung expansion.

Other data include: information from the patient's laboratory records on the presence of hypoxemia or respiratory acidosis or alkalosis.

■ Nursing Diagnosis

Nursing diagnoses that may indicate the need to implement deep breathing exercises include:

1. Ineffective airway clearance related to:
   a. Excessive or thick secretions
   b. Loss of lung elasticity
   c. Edema of upper airway structures
   d. Improper positioning
   e. General anesthesia
2. Ineffective breathing patterns related to:
   a. Loss of lung elasticity
   b. Loss of functioning lung tissue
   c. Anesthesia

d. Incisional pain
3. Impaired gas exchange related to:
   a. Infection
   b. Loss of functioning lung tissue
   c. Decreased oxygen in inspired air

■ Planning

Nursing goals

1. To increase pulmonary ventilation and lung expansion
2. To loosen respiratory secretions
3. To promote breathing deeply with less effort, thereby conserving energy
4. To prevent untoward effects of anesthesia and/or hypoventilation

■ Intervention

Abdominal (diaphragmatic) and pursed-lip breathing

1. Instruct the patient that diaphragmatic breathing can help her or him to breathe more deeply and with less effort.

2. Have the patient assume a comfortable semi-Fowler's position with knees flexed, back supported, and one head pillow, or a supine position with one head pillow and knees flexed. After learning the exercise, the patient can practice first in either supine or semi-Fowler's position and then when sitting upright, standing, and walking.

   Rationale The supine and semi-Fowler's positions with knees flexed help relax the abdominal muscles.

3. Have the patient place one or both hands on the abdomen just below the ribs. See Figure 36–1.

4. Instruct the patient to breathe in deeply through the nose with the mouth closed, to stay relaxed, not to arch the back, and to concentrate on feeling the abdomen rise as far as possible.

   Rationale When the patient breathes in, the diaphragm contracts (drops), the lungs fill with air, and the abdomen rises or protrudes. See Figure 36–2.

5. If the patient has difficulty raising the abdomen, have him or her take a quick, forceful inhalation through the nose.

   Rationale With a quick sniff, the patient will feel the abdomen rise.

6. Instruct the patient to purse the lips as if about to

FIGURE 36–1

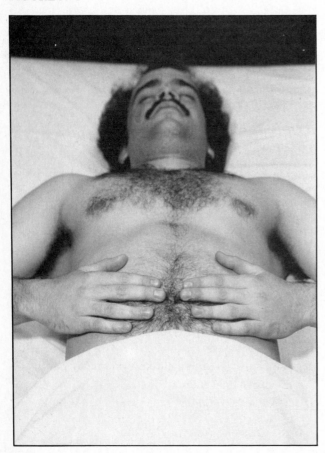

FIGURE 36–2

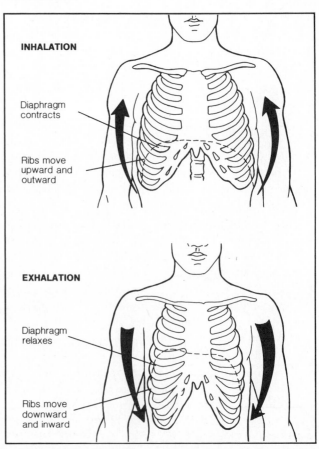

INHALATION

Diaphragm contracts

Ribs move upward and outward

EXHALATION

Diaphragm relaxes

Ribs move downward and inward

whistle, to breathe out slowly and gently, making a slow "whooshing" sound, not to puff out the cheeks, to concentrate on feeling the abdomen fall or sink, and to tighten (contract) the abdominal muscles while breathing out.

Rationale Pursing the lips creates a resistance to air flowing out of the lungs, increases pressure within the bronchi, and minimizes the collapse of smaller bronchioles, a common problem for patients with COPD. While the patient breathes out, the diaphragm relaxes (rises) and the abdomen sinks. See Figure 36–2. Tightening the abdominal muscles helps the patient to exhale more effectively.

7. If the patient has COPD, teach her or him the "double cough" technique. Have the patient:

a. Breathe in through the nose and inflate the lungs to the midinspiration point, rather than to the full deep inspiration point.

b. Simultaneously exhale and cough two or more abrupt, sharp coughs in rapid succession.

Rationale A very forceful cough by a patient with COPD can cause small airway collapse. With two or more abrupt coughs, the first one loosens secretions, while subsequent coughs facilitate movement of secretions toward the upper airways.

8. Instruct the patient to use this exercise whenever feeling short of breath and to increase it gradually to five to ten minutes four times a day.

Rationale Regular practice enables the patient eventually to do this type of breathing without conscious effort.

Apical expansion exercises

Apical expansion exercises are often required for patients who restrict their upper chest movement because of pain from a severe respiratory disease or surgery, eg, lobectomy (removal of a lung lobe) or mastectomy (removal of a breast).

9. Place your fingers below the patient's clavicles and exert moderate pressure, or have the patient place her or his hands over the same area. See Figure 36–3.

Rationale This hand position enables evaluation of the depth of apical inhalation.

10. Instruct the patient to inhale through the nose and to concentrate on pushing the upper chest upward and forward against the fingers.

Rationale This helps to aerate the apical areas of the upper lung lobes.

11. Have the patient hold the inhalation for a few seconds.

Rationale This promotes aeration of the alveoli.

12. Have the patient exhale through the mouth or nose

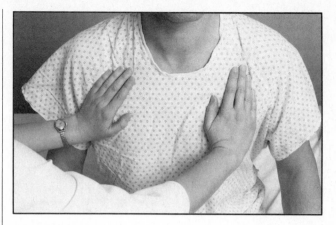

FIGURE 36–3

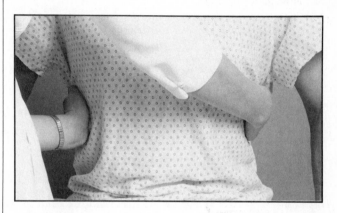

FIGURE 36–4

slowly, quietly, and passively while concentrating on moving the upper chest inward and downward.

13. Instruct the patient to perform the exercise for at least five respirations four times a day.

Rationale Repeating the exercise helps to reexpand lung tissue, eliminate secretions, and minimize flattening of the upper chest wall.

Basal expansion exercises

Basal expansion exercises are often required for patients who have restricted bilateral chest movements because of pain from a respiratory disorder or chest surgery.

14. Place the palms of your hands in the area of the patient's lower ribs along the midaxillary lines, and exert moderate pressure, or have the patient place her or his hands over the same area. See Figure 36–4.

Rationale This hand position enables evaluation and comparison of the depth of bilateral basal inspiration.

15. Instruct the patient to inhale through the nose and to concentrate on moving the lower chest outward against the hands.

16. Have the patient hold the inhalation for a few seconds.

17. Have the patient exhale through the nose or mouth slowly, quietly, and passively. If the patient has COPD, observe the rate and character of the exhalation. Normal exhalation is slow, and the upper chest appears relaxed. If the exhalation appears difficult or there is indrawing of the upper chest, encourage pursed-lip exhalation. See step 6 above.

18. Instruct the patient to perform this exercise for at least five respirations four times a day.

    Rationale Repetition helps to reexpand lung tissue and eliminate secretions.

■ Evaluation

Expected outcomes

1. Stable vital signs
2. Relaxed, quiet, slow breathing pattern
3. Absence of cough, or effective, controlled cough
4. Absence of abnormal breath sounds
5. Pink skin and nail bed color
6. Normal blood gases and pH

Unexpected outcomes

1. Rapid pulse
2. Rapid, shallow breathing
3. Difficult breathing
4. Chest retractions
5. Flail chest or paradoxical breathing
6. Inadequate basal or apical chest expansion
7. Uncontrolled productive or nonproductive cough
8. Audible abnormal breath sounds
9. Cyanosis of lips and/or nail beds
10. Restlessness and apprehension
11. Vertigo or syncope

Upon obtaining an unexpected outcome:

1. Report your findings to the responsible nurse.
2. Adjust the patient's care plan appropriately.

TECHNIQUE 36–2 ■ Assisting Patients to Use Blow Bottles or Sustained Maximal Inspiration Devices

---

Blow bottles are two bottles half filled with water and connected by tubing. They provide feedback about a patient's respiratory *exhalation*. The patient moves the water from one bottle to the other by blowing into a short tube connected to the first bottle. See Figure 36–5. Lung inflation is encouraged by the deep breath the patient needs before blowing into the bottle. After the patient transfers the fluid from the first bottle, the set is reversed, and the procedure is repeated. A single blow bottle may also be used; it is a gallon bottle half filled with water. See Figure 36–6. In this case the patient is asked to "blow bubbles," eg, for five minutes every hour.

Sustained maximal inspiration devices (SMIs) measure the flow of air the patient inhales through the mouthpiece. They therefore offer an incentive to improve *inhalation*. Two general types are the flow-oriented spirometer and the volume-oriented spirometer. The *flow-oriented SMI* consists of one or more clear plastic chambers that contain freely movable, colored balls or discs. The balls or discs are elevated as the patient inhales. The patient is asked to keep them elevated as long as possible with a maximal sustained inhalation. Figure 36–7 shows a Triflo II SMI,

and Figure 36–8 shows a single-chamber spirometer. Flow-oriented SMIs are low-cost devices, are often disposable, and can be used independently by patients. They do not measure the specific volume of air the patient inhales, however.

The more expensive *volume-oriented SMIs* precisely measure the inhalation volume maintained by the patient. These devices contain pistons or bellows that are raised by the patient's inhalation to a predetermined volume. Some volume-oriented devices are designed with an achievement counter or light. The light will not turn on until the patient's inspiration is held at the minimum predetermined volume for a specified time period. See Figure 36–9.

■ Assessment

1. Auscultate the patient's lungs before the technique, for comparative baseline data.
2. See also Technique 36–1 on page 853.

Other data include: the physician's or respiratory thera-

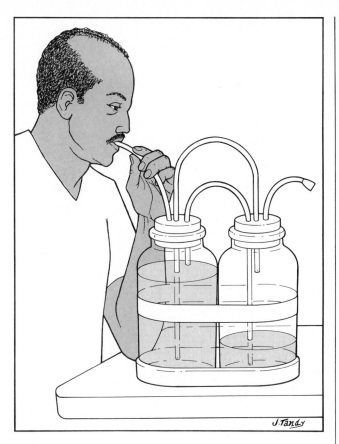

FIGURE 36–5

FIGURE 36–6

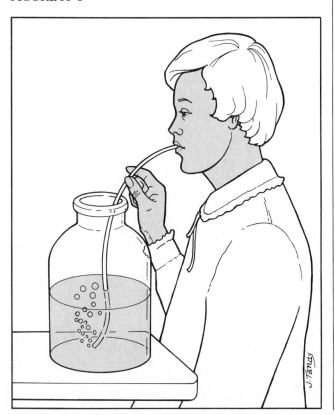

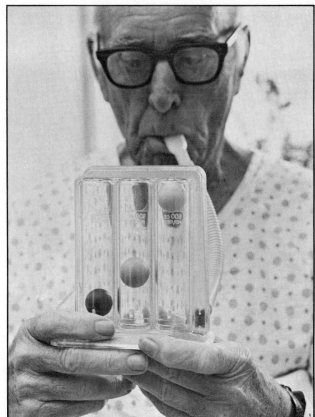

FIGURE 36–7

FIGURE 36–8

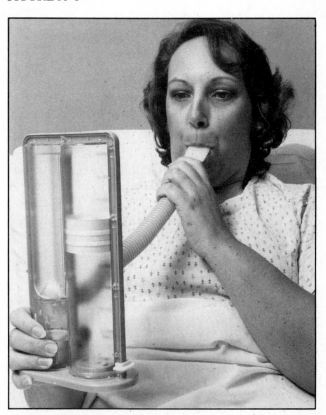

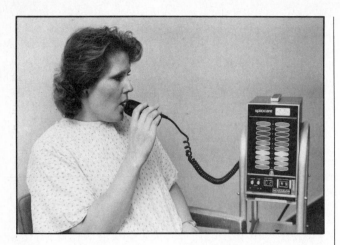

FIGURE 36-9

pist's determination of an inspiratory volume level for the patient.

■ **Nursing Diagnosis**   See Technique 36-1 on page 853.

■ **Planning**

Nursing goals

1.   To improve pulmonary ventilation
2.   To counteract the effects of anesthesia and/or hypoventilation
3.   To loosen respiratory secretions
4.   To facilitate respiratory gaseous exchange
5.   To expand collapsed alveoli

Equipment

1.   Blow bottles
        or
     A flow-oriented SMI
        or
     A volume-oriented SMI
2.   A mouthpiece or breathing tube
3.   A nose clip (optional)

■ **Intervention**

1.   Assist the patient to an upright sitting position in bed or in a chair. If the patient is unable to assume a sitting position for a flow spirometer, have the patient assume any position.
     Rationale   A sitting position facilitates maximum ventilation.

For blow bottles

2.   Instruct the patient to:
     a. Take in a slow, deep breath.

Rationale   A deep breath ensures maximum inflation of the alveoli, which facilitates gaseous exchange.

b. Seal the lips tightly around the mouthpiece, exhale slowly and steadily as long as possible into the bottle, and concentrate on moving the fluid from one bottle to the other.

Rationale   A tight lip seal prevents leakage of exhaled air outside the mouthpiece and ensures adequate movement and measurement of the fluid. As the patient exhales, pressure in the bottle is increased and displaces the water with air. A prolonged exhalation against resistance creates an increase in alveolar pressure, reexpanding collapsed alveoli, preventing atelectasis (collapse of the lung), and strengthening the muscles of expiration.

c. Establish a goal of moving a certain portion of water into the second bottle with each exhalation (eg, ¼, ⅓, ½, ¾). Provide practice periods about five times every hour, and set progressive increases in the volume of fluid to be moved.

Rationale   Initially the patient may be unable to move the entire contents of one bottle to the other with one breath. The nurse and the patient need to establish realistic goals. Practice helps the patient to increase the expiratory volume.

For a flow-oriented SMI

3.   If the spirometer has an inspiratory volume level pointer, set the pointer at the prescribed level. Check the physician's or respiratory therapist's order.

4.   Instruct the patient to:
     a. Hold the spirometer in the upright position.
        Rationale   A tilted spirometer requires less effort to raise the balls or discs.
     b. Exhale normally.
     c. Seal the lips tightly around the mouthpiece, take in a slow, deep breath to elevate the balls, and then hold the breath for 2 seconds initially, increasing to 6 seconds (optimum), to keep the balls elevated if possible. Instruct the patient to avoid brisk, low-volume breaths that snap the balls to the top of the chamber. The patient may use a noseclip if he or she has difficulty breathing only through the mouth.
        Rationale   A slow, deep breath ensures maximal ventilation. Greater lung expansion is achieved with a very slow inspiration than with a brisk, shallow breath, even though it may not elevate the balls or keep them elevated while the patient holds the breath (Luce, Tyler, Pierson, 1984). Sustained elevation of the balls ensures adequate alveolar ventilation.
     d. Remove the mouthpiece, and exhale normally.

e. Cough after the incentive effort.

Rationale   Deep ventilation may loosen secretions, and coughing can facilitate their removal.

f. Relax, and take several normal breaths before using the spirometer again.

g. Repeat the procedure several times and then four or five times hourly.

Rationale   Practice increases inspiratory volume, maintains alveolar ventilation, and prevents atelectasis.

For a volume-oriented SMI

5. Set the spirometer to the predetermined volume. Volume ranges vary from 0 to 5,000 mL depending on the type of spirometer. Check the physician's or respiratory therapist's order.

6. Since some SMIs are battery-operated, ensure that the spirometer is functioning. Place the device on the patient's bedside table.

7. Instruct the patient to:

a. Exhale normally.

b. Seal the lips tightly around the mouthpiece, and take in a slow, deep breath, until the piston is elevated to the preset level. The piston level may be visible to the patient or lights or the word "Hold" may be illuminated to identify the volume obtained.

c. Hold the breath for 6 seconds to ensure maximal alveolar ventilation.

d. Remove the mouthpiece, and exhale normally.

e. Follow steps 4e–g above.

For all devices

8. Clean the mouthpiece with sterile water and shake it dry. Label the mouthpiece and a disposable SMI with the patient's name, and store them in the patient's bedside unit. Only the mouthpiece of a volume SMI is stored with the patient, since volume SMIs are used by many patients. Disposable mouthpieces are changed every 24 hours.

9. Auscultate the patient's lungs to compare with the baseline data.

10. Record the technique, including type of spirometer, number of breaths taken, volume or flow levels achieved, and results of auscultation. For a flow SMI, calculate the volume achieved by multiplying the setting by the length of time the patient kept the balls elevated. For example, if the setting was 500 mL, and the balls were kept suspended for 2 seconds, the volume is $500 \times 2 = 1,000$ mL. For a volume SMI, take the volume directly from the spirometer, eg, 1,500 mL.

Sample Recording

Date	Time	Notes
7/6/86	1100	Instructed in use of Triflo II spirometer. 5 breaths taken at volume of 1,000 mL (500 mL $\times$ 2 sec). Bilateral breath sounds normal on auscultation before and after spirometry.———— Nicholas Coscos, SN

■ Evaluation

Expected outcomes

Blow bottles

1. Moved prescribed amount of fluid from one bottle to the other with one breath

2. Used blow bottles five times hourly

3. Normal breath sounds

Incentive spirometer

4. Moved balls or piston to specified level

5. Used SMI five times hourly

6. Normal breath sounds

Unexpected outcomes

1. Unable to achieve predetermined goal

2. Noncompliant in using device at specified times

3. Abnormal breath sounds before or after technique

Upon obtaining an unexpected outcome:

1. Report your findings to the responsible nurse, physician, and/or respiratory therapist.

2. Adjust the patient's nursing care plan appropriately.

TECHNIQUE 36–3   ■   Assisting Patients with Intermittent Positive Pressure Breathing (IPPB) 🏠

Intermittent positive pressure breathing (IPPB) is the delivery of air or oxygen into the lungs at positive (above

atmospheric) pressure during inspiration and automatic release of the pressure when the predetermined positive pressure level is reached in the air passages, so that expiration occurs passively. Some IPPB machines can exert pressure during expiration, and the abbreviations IPPB/I (inspiratory) and IPPB/E (expiratory) are sometimes used to differentiate the two methods. Generally, however, IPPB refers to positive pressure therapy administered during inspiration, a safer and more common practice.

Use of IPPB therapy has decreased since the advent of incentive spirometers. Advocates of IPPB therapy, however, believe that IPPB devices are more effective in expanding the lungs, moving secretions, promoting coughs, and delivering aerosol medications into the deeper, smaller air passages, while they require less effort by the patient.

Various IPPB machines are marketed. Two commonly used types are the Bird respirator and the Bennett respirator. Assembly and maintenance of respirators is usually done by respiratory therapists. The machine is connected to an oxygen supply and is equipped with an in-line humidifier, which must be filled with distilled water. The patient breathes through a mouthpiece or a mask attached to the end of the respirator tubing. See Figure 36–10.

Usually, IPPB treatments are given by respiratory therapists or by nurses who have had special training. However, the general nurse needs to understand the reason for IPPB therapy and its principles, to assist patients as needed in the absence of special therapists. The nurse must also observe the patient's progress and response to such therapy. This discussion is limited to IPPB therapy that is patient-activated and given on an intermittent basis. Controlled or time-cycled continuous therapy is used for patients unable to initiate inspiration. The breathing of such patients is maintained entirely by machine.

The Bird respirator

There are several types of Bird respirators; however, all are equipped with six basic controls (see Figure 36–11):

1. The *pressure control setting* establishes the pressure that will be received at the height of an inspiration before the patient enters the expiratory phase. It measures the pressure in centimeters of water pressure, from 0 to 60 cm. Usually the pressure is started low, at 15 or 20 cm H_2O, and gradually increased as the patient becomes accustomed to the machine.

2. The *flow rate control* adjusts the inspiratory time and switches the ventilator from *off* to *on*. It is similar to a water tap: The more it is turned on, the faster the flow of gas. Low numbers on this dial indicate slow rates, and higher numbers indicate faster rates. Since the aim of therapy is usually to achieve deep respirations and transfer of gases deep into the alveoli, the flow rate is generally set at 10 or less to coincide with the patient's inspiratory effort. Fast flow rates tend to flood only the upper respiratory tract. Effective flow rates can be assessed by observing the patient's chest expansion during therapy.

3. The *air mix plunger* determines the proportion of oxygen and air delivered to the patient. It has two positions. When the plunger is pushed in, 100% oxygen is delivered. When it is pulled out, a mixture of 40% oxygen and 60% air is delivered. These proportions cannot be varied as they can on more sophisticated respirators. Generally the oxygen/air mixture is used.

4. The *sensitivity control* adjusts the inspiratory effort required by the patient to trigger or trip the machine (start the flow of gas). Once the machine is triggered, the pressure automatically builds to the peak pres-

FIGURE 36–10

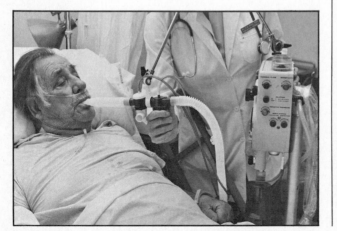

FIGURE 36–11

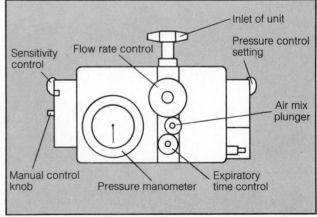

sure that was set by the pressure control knob. The smaller the number set on the sensitivity control, the higher the sensitivity (ie, the less effort required by the patient to start the machine). Patients who are weak often require a high sensitivity control (low number setting) to start the machine, but patients who need to be encouraged to breathe deeply should use a low sensitivity control (high number) that offers more resistance and requires more effort. It is usually set at 15 when starting therapy.

5. The *manual control knob,* a pink knob or pin below the sensitivity control, can be pushed in manually to trigger the ventilator. It is mostly used to check respirator function before applying it to the patient.

6. The *expiratory time control* is turned to *off* for patient-cycled IPPB. It is used only for patients who are apneic or who require continuous assisted ventilation. When the control is turned on, the exhalation times cycle automatically.

The Bennett respirator

This respirator is different in appearance from the Bird respirator (see Figure 36–12), but its operation is similar. The PR-1 model, which is frequently used, has many of the basic controls discussed for the Bird machine:

1. The *pressure control knob,* capable of delivering 0 to 45 cm H_2O pressure, is rotated clockwise and generally set at 15 to 20 cm H_2O for adults or 10 to 12 cm H_2O for children. The initial pressure setting may be lower.

2. The *control pressure gauge* records the pressure that is reached by turning the pressure control knob.

3. The *system pressure gauge* records the pressure that is required by the patient and should equal that measured by the control pressure gauge at the end of inspiration.

4. The *air dilution control* is usually pushed in to allow for an air/oxygen mixture. When it is pulled out, 100% oxygen is delivered.

5. The *sensitivity control* determines the amount of inspiratory effort required to start inspiration and is used only if the patient has difficulty triggering the machine. Indications of difficulty are determined when patients say they are sucking or drawing on the machine to no avail or when the system pressure gauge needle deflects to the negative side. In these instances the sensitivity control should be set higher so that less effort is required by the patient to trigger the machine.

6. The *rate control* regulates the rate of automatic cycling and is turned to the *off* position for patient-cycled IPPB.

7. The *nebulization controls* provide power to the side steam nebulizer to deliver aerosol medications. One

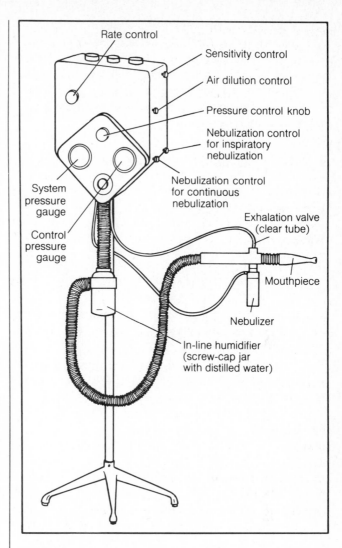

FIGURE 36–12

knob sets the nebulizer for continuous therapy, the other for inspiratory nebulization. If the patient is receiving a medicated treatment, the inspiration knob is generally turned one revolution to ensure adequate nebulization on inspiration. With use of the continuous knob, the medication is delivered immediately upon inspiration.

■ **Assessment**

1. Auscultate the patient's lungs before the therapy for comparative baseline data.

2. Take the patient's vital signs for comparative baseline data.

3. See also Technique 36–1 on page 853.

Other data include:

1. Whether aerosol medications are to be administered during therapy. Check the physician's orders. Bronchodilators, mucolytics, or antibiotics may be ordered.

2. When the IPPB treatments are scheduled. Ensure that they do not conflict with meal hours, if possible. IPPB therapy is generally prescribed for five to six breaths hourly during waking hours. It should not be scheduled right before or after a meal, since it can induce nausea and a full stomach prevents maximum lung expansion.

■ **Nursing Diagnosis** See Technique 36–1 on page 853.

■ **Planning**

Nursing goals

1. To increase the depth of respirations periodically and prevent accumulation of secretions that may result in infections or atelectasis
2. To facilitate the clearing of bronchial secretions in patients who have difficulty coughing or inhaling deeply
3. To provide moisture to the respiratory mucous membranes
4. To administer aerosol medications

Equipment

1. An IPPB machine.
2. A mouthpiece.
3. A noseclip (optional).
4. A mask (to be used only if a mouthpiece and a noseclip are not effective).

5. A source of pressurized air and oxygen if the machine does not have an internal compression unit.
6. Sterile normal saline solution or the prescribed aerosol medication, eg, 1% isoetharine hydrochloride (Bronkosol). Routine measured IPPB medication doses are commercially available in plastic ampules.
7. A 3-mL syringe with a needle to prepare the medication or saline.
8. A Wright respirometer (optional) and an exhaled volume collector.
9. Tissues and a moisture-proof waste bag or other container for expectorated secretions.

■ **Intervention**

1. Explain that the therapy will assist the patient to achieve deep lung expansion and will promote coughing and removal of secretions.
2. Assist the patient to a Fowler's position in bed or to sit upright in a chair.
   Rationale These positions facilitate maximal lung expansion.
3. Teach the patient to breathe normally through the mouth using the mouthpiece and not through the nose. Have the patient practice breathing only through the mouthpiece prior to therapy. Ensure that the patient completely seals the mouthpiece with the lips. Have the patient use a noseclip if she or he has difficulty breathing only through the mouth. See Figure 36–13.
   Rationale Mouth breathing and an airtight seal

FIGURE 36–13

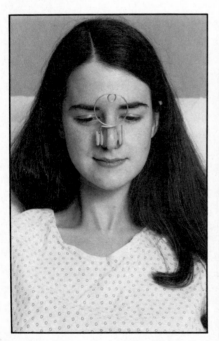

FIGURE 36–14

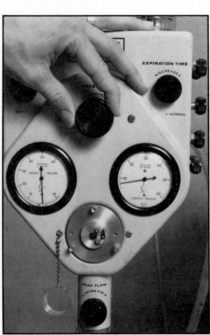

FIGURE 36–15

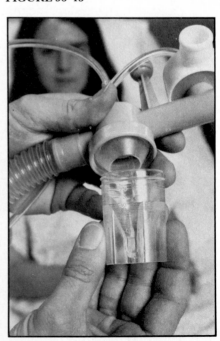

around the mouthpiece are essential for efficient operation of the IPPB system.

4. Adjust the pressure to 10 to 15 cm H₂O. See Figure 36–11 earlier for a Bird respirator, Figure 36–14 for a Bennett respirator (the pressure gauge is the right-hand dial). Permit the patient to cycle, and monitor the volume increase or decrease. Adjust the pressure accordingly.

Rationale   This control sets the pressure that will be received at the height of an inspiration.

5. Fill the nebulizer with sterile saline or prescribed medication, reattach it, and set the nebulization control if necessary. See Figure 36–15. If a medication is used, prepare it before going to the patient.

Rationale   Nebulization delivers prescribed medications and/or moisture to the respiratory mucous membranes. IPPB therapy must be given with medication or sterile saline in the nebulizer unless a mainstream humidifier is used. Air that is not moisturized dries the patient's airways and impedes the mobilization of secretions.

6. Set the oxygen/air mix control as ordered. For a mixture of air and oxygen, pull the knob of a Bird respirator out, push the knob of a Bennett respirator in.

7. Occlude the end of the tubing that will be attached to the mouthpiece, and manually cycle the machine to operate.

Rationale   This ensures that the system is airtight and that it cycles off at the preset pressure. If it does not reach the desired pressure, the nurse needs to check for a leak in the system, eg, a disconnection in the nebulizer.

8. Attach the mouthpiece to the machine's tubing.

9. Have the patient place his or her lips tightly around the mouthpiece, relax, and inhale deeply and slowly through the mouth as the machine cycles on.

Rationale   The machine will not start until the patient breathes in.

10. Encourage the patient not to breathe out until the machine fills the lungs. Explain that the machine will cycle off when the preset pressure is met or when the patient breathes out.

Rationale   By allowing the pressure to reach its peak before exhaling, maximal lung expansion is achieved when the appropriate pressure is set.

11. Optional: After full inspiration, have the patient hold the breath for a few seconds.

Rationale   This provides greater distribution of oxygen, air, and nebulized particles.

12. Instruct the patient to exhale normally in a relaxed and passive manner.

Rationale   Forced exhalation can increase small airway obstructions.

FIGURE 36–16

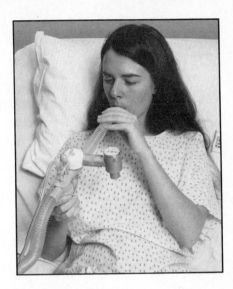

13. Observe the patient for adequate chest expansion with each inhalation and for a relaxed, passive exhalation. Check that the needle gauges reach the preset pressure levels as the patient inhales. See the pressure manometer in Figure 36–11 and the system pressure gauge in Figure 36–12.

Rationale   Although the degree of lung expansion can be observed visually, the gauges on the respirator provide more reliable measures. If the needle gauge on the respirator reaches the preset level as the patient inhales, inhalation is usually satisfactory.

or

It is preferable to attach a Wright respirometer to the expiratory port of the IPPB manifold. See Figure 36–16. The Wright respirometer specifically measures the expired *tidal volume* and/or *inspiratory capacity* and indicates whether the patient is receiving adequate deep lung inflations. *Tidal volume* is the volume of air inspired and expired with a normal breath, about 500 mL. *Inspiratory capacity* is the maximum volume of air inspired after normal exhalation. The Wright respirometer usually has two dials: a large peripheral dial, which measures the volume from 0 to 100 L, and a smaller dial inset at the top, which measures tenths of a liter from 0 to 1 L. See Figure 36–17.

14. If there is inadequate or no deflection of the needle gauges:

a. Check that the system is airtight. The patient may not have sealed the lips around the mouthpiece adequately. If this is the case, decrease the pressure setting until the patient feels comfortable, and then gradually increase the pressure. A noseclip may be necessary.

b. Check that the patient is relaxed. Perhaps the patient is not breathing normally or is blowing back into the mouthpiece before the lungs are filled and needs to be encouraged to breathe

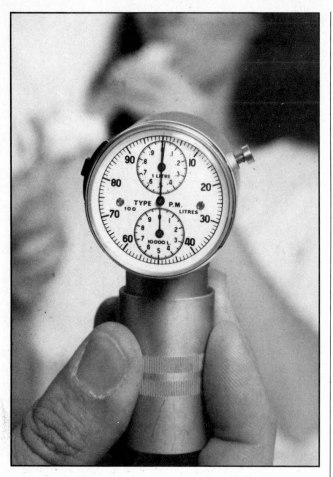

FIGURE 36-17

normally. Some patients have a tendency to force their breathing or to struggle with the apparatus. When advised not to force breaths, to relax, to breathe slowly, and to allow time for expiration (which takes longer than inspiration), patients normally adjust to the therapy readily. Remind the patient that she or he controls the machine: Each time the patient breathes in, he or she starts the machine; each time the patient breathes out, the machine stops at peak inspiration. Extra effort by the patient is not required, because the machine does not dictate breathing.

c. Check that the machine is triggering. Perhaps the patient does not exert sufficient inspiratory effort to start the machine. In that case, adjust the sensitivity gauge to a lower number.

If the needle deflection is negative, the patient may be sucking, or using too much inspiratory effort, or the peak flow could be too low.

15. Take the patient's blood pressure and pulse rate during the therapy, especially at the initial treatment. Stay with the patient throughout the treatment. Stop the treatment and notify the physician if there is a sudden significant increase in pulse rate

(20 or more beats per minute) or a sudden change in blood pressure (10 mm Hg or more). During subsequent IPPB sessions, blood pressure assessment is necessary only if the patient has a history of cardiovascular disease, hypotension, or sensitivity to any medications given during therapy.

Rationale Some bronchodilators, eg, isoproterenol and isoetharine, significantly increase the heart rate. IPPB therapy increases intrathoracic pressure and may cause a temporary decrease in cardiac output and venous return, indicated by hypotension, headache, and tachycardia.

16. If vital signs are stable, continue the IPPB therapy if indicated, until all the medication in the nebulizer is administered, or about 15 to 20 minutes.

17. Following or during the therapy, encourage the patient to expectorate respiratory secretions, as needed. Note the amount of sputum.

18. Auscultate the lung fields, and compare the pretherapy assessment. Note any improvement in aeration and absence of or diminished adventitious breath sounds. See Table 10–15 on page 203.

19. Clean the mouthpiece and nebulizer with sterile water, and dry them thoroughly. Store the mouthpiece in a plastic bag at the patient's bedside or in accordance with agency policy. Generally the mouthpiece is replaced every 24 hours for aseptic reasons.

20. Record the IPPB therapy, its duration, the medication administered, the pressure used, the volume achieved, the breath sounds and vital signs before and after the therapy, the amount of sputum expectorated, and any untoward assessment findings.

Sample Recording

Date	Time	Notes
9/2/86	1500	IPPB administered, 800-mL volume at 15 cm H_2O pressure with sterile normal saline nebulization for 15 min. Adventitious breath sounds absent before and after treatment. BP 120/70, P 78, stable, before and after therapy. No secretions expectorated. ———Constance S. Boyd, RN

■ Evaluation

Expected outcomes

1. Absence of or diminished adventitious breath sounds after therapy

2. Adequate chest expansion during therapy

3. Stable vital signs throughout and after therapy

4. Effective expectoration of secretions, if present
5. Increased inspiratory capacity at least 25%

Unexpected outcomes

1. No change in breath sounds after therapy
2. Inadequate chest expansion during therapy
3. Increase in pulse rate of 20 beats or more during therapy

4. Decrease in blood pressure of 10 mm Hg or more during therapy
5. Ineffective expectoration of secretions
6. Complaints of headache during therapy

Upon obtaining an unexpected outcome:

1. Report your findings to the responsible nurse and/or physician.
2. Adjust the patient's nursing care plan appropriately.

HUMIDIFIERS AND NEBULIZERS

Humidifiers are devices that add water vapor to inspired air. Their purposes are to prevent mucous membranes from drying and becoming irritated and to loosen secretions for easier expectoration. All humidifiers employ the simple method of passing the gas through sterile water so that water vapor is picked up before the gas reaches the patient. The more bubbles are created during this process, the more water vapor is produced. Some humidifiers heat the water vapor, which increases the humidity provided the patient.

There are several kinds of humidifiers; three main types are the room humidifier (for home use most often), the cascade humidifier, and the cold bubble diffuser (humidifier). A *room humidifier* (see Figure 36–18) can provide either cool mist or steam. Some types can be used with gas lines, eg, oxygen, to provide moistened air directly to the patient.

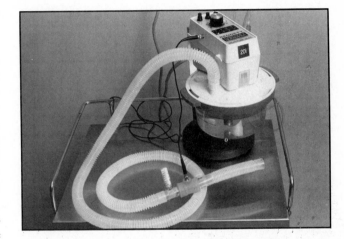

FIGURE 36–19 ■ A cascade humidifier.

A *cascade humidifier* (see Figure 36–19) can deliver 100% humidity at body temperature to a patient. The temperature of the vapor can be controlled, and the machine can be used to provide humidified oxygen to patients on ventilators.

A *cold bubble diffuser* or *humidifier* (see Figure 36–20) is used with all oxygen equipment to moisten the oxygen before it is inhaled by the patient. This device provides 20% to 40% humidity. The oxygen passes through sterile distilled water and then along a line to the device through which the moistened oxygen is inhaled (eg, a cannula, nasal catheter, or oxygen mask). See chapter 38 for additional information.

A *nebulizer* is used to deliver a fine spray of medication or moisture to a patient. *Nebulization* is the production of a fog or mist. There are two kinds: atomization and aerosolization. In *atomization,* a device called an *atomizer* produces rather large droplets for inhalation. When the droplets are suspended in a gas, eg, oxygen, the process is *aerosolization* or *aerosol therapy.* The smaller the droplets, the further they can be inhaled into the respiratory tract. When a medication is intended for the nasal mucosa, it is inhaled through the nose; when it is intended for the trachea, bronchi, and/or lungs, it is inhaled through the mouth.

FIGURE 36–18 ■ A room humidifier.

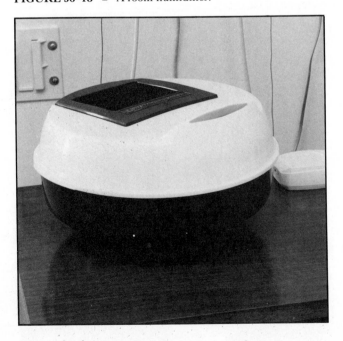

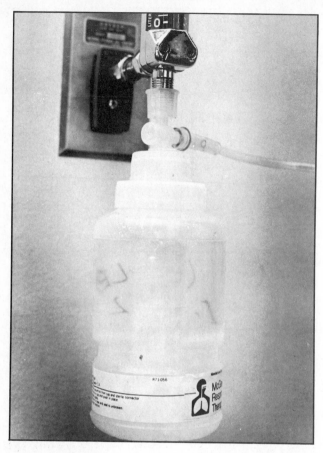

FIGURE 36-20 ■ A cold bubble humidifier.

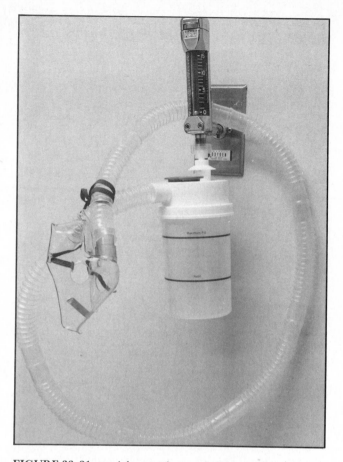

FIGURE 36-21 ■ A large-volume nebulizer.

FIGURE 36-22 ■ An ultrasonic nebulizer.

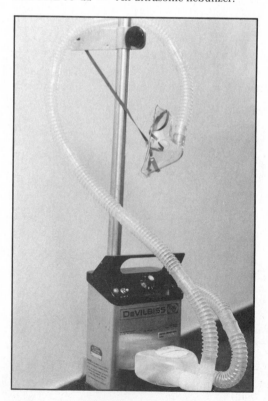

Nebulization can be provided by a large-volume nebulizer, ultrasonic nebulizer, hand nebulizer, mini-nebulizer (Maxi-mist), or side-stream nebulizer. A *large-volume nebulizer* (see Figure 36–21) can provide a heated or cool mist. It is used for long-term therapy, eg, following a tracheostomy. These nebulizers have a 250-mL capacity and deliver oxygen or room air.

The *ultrasonic nebulizer* (see Figure 36–22) provides 100% humidity and can provide particles small enough to be inhaled deeply into the respiratory tract. There are two types: One has a cup that is filled with sterile distilled water; the other requires a continuous supply of sterile distilled water from a bag connected by tubing to the nebulizer bottle.

The *hand nebulizer* (see Figure 36–23) is a container of medication that can be compressed by hand. It then releases the medication through a nosepiece or mouthpiece. The force with which the air moves through the nebulizer causes the large particles of medicated solution to break up into finer particles, forming a mist or fine spray.

The *mini-nebulizer* (see Figure 36–24) is used with oxygen or a pressurized gas source, eg, air. With this device, the patient inhales and exhales independently.

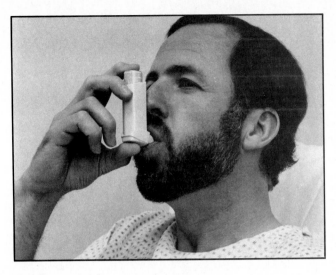

FIGURE 36–23   ■   A hand nebulizer.

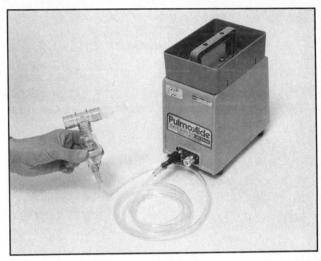

FIGURE 36–24   ■   A mini-nebulizer.

Medication is administered during inhalation. These units are available commercially and are disposable.

A *side-stream nebulizer* provides a medication to a patient who is on a ventilator or receiving IPPB therapy. The gas, eg, oxygen, passes through a device containing the medicated solution and then into the ventilator and to the patient.

TECHNIQUE 36–4   ■   Assisting Patients to Use Nebulizers

■ Assessment

1. Auscultate the patient's lungs to obtain baseline data on lung sounds (eg, rales or rhonchi) and the rate and depth of respirations, to be compared with data after the treatment.
2. Determine whether the patient's cough is productive or nonproductive.
3. Observe the amount, color, and character of expectorated secretions.
4. Observe the patient for dyspnea.
5. Assess the vital signs for baseline data.

Other data include: the type, strength, and amount of medication to be administered, as specified in the order.

■ Planning

Nursing goals

1. To assist the removal of accumulated lung secretions
2. To prevent the accumulation of secretions in patients at risk, eg, patients on mechanical ventilators
3. To relieve dyspnea

Equipment

1. Suction equipment, if necessary

For a large-volume nebulizer

2. The nebulizer
3. A flow meter, an oxygen or air source, oxygen tubing, and a delivery device, eg, a mask
4. An oxygen analyzer
5. Sterile distilled water to fill the water container of the nebulizer to the indicated level
6. A heater if heated water is ordered
7. A thermometer to place in-line between the nebulizer and the patient, to monitor the temperature of the gas if a heater is used

For an ultrasonic nebulizer

8. The nebulizer
9. A flow meter, an oxygen or air source, oxygen tubing, and a delivery device, eg, a mask
10. Sterile distilled water or sterile normal saline to fill the cup of the nebulizer or to connect to the nebulizer unit

For a hand nebulizer

11. The nebulizer, containing the ordered medication

For a mini-nebulizer

12. A mini-nebulizer cup with a lid
13. A flow meter, an oxygen or air source, oxygen tubing, and a mouthpiece, mask, or other delivery device
14. Sterile normal saline or sterile distilled water to dilute the medication
15. The ordered medication
16. A sterile syringe and needle to inject the medication and the saline or water into the cup

For a side-stream nebulizer

17. The nebuilizer with removable cup
18. An oxygen or air source and ventilation machine
19. The ordered medication
20. Sterile normal saline or sterile distilled water to dilute the medication
21. A sterile syringe and needle to add the medication and the saline or water to the medication cup as ordered

FIGURE 36–25

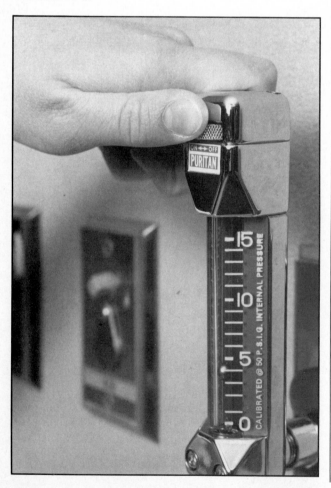

■ Intervention

1. Explain the procedure to the patient and encourage slow, deep breathing to increase lung expansion.
2. Assist the patient to a sitting or high Fowler's position, to encourage lung expansion and facilitate expectoration of secretions
3. Encourage the patient to cough and breathe deeply, or apply suction to remove secretions

For a large-volume nebulizer

4. Attach the flow meter to the oxygen or air source and the nebulizer to the flow meter.
5. Turn on the flow meter to 10 to 14 L/min. See Figure 36–25.

   Rationale A large-volume nebulizer requires at least 10 L/min, and any excess flow will be vented out.
6. Check that mist is emanating from the outflow port.
7. Adjust the setting for the fraction of inspired oxygen (FiO_2) ordered by the physician.
8. Attach the tubing to the outlet port, and attach the delivery device to the tubing.
9. Use an oxygen analyzer to evaluate the percentage of oxygen the patient is receiving.
10. If you are using a heater, install an in-line thermometer near the patient, and monitor it. Warn the patient to report undue warmth, discomfort, or tubing that feels hot.

    Rationale The thermometer will reflect the temperature of the gas going to the patient.
11. Attach the delivery device, eg, a mask, to the patient.
12. Check the water level frequently, and replace the container as needed with another filled with fresh sterile distilled water.

    or

    When reusing the container, empty the old water, and add fresh sterile distilled water.

    Rationale   The remaining water is discarded to reduce the growth of microorganisms.
13. Change the tubing and the nebulizer daily.

    Rationale This reduces the growth of microorganisms and prevents infecting the patient.
14. At the termination of the treatment, auscultate the patient's lungs, and observe the color, amount, and character of the expectorated secretions.
15. Record the duration of the therapy, the type, amount, and strength of any medication, and the FiO_2 if monitored.

For an ultrasonic nebulizer

16. Attach the tubing from the nebulizer to the flow meter on the oxygen or air source.

17. Add sterile normal saline or water, and attach the delivery device to the nebulizer.

18. Turn on the machine, and check for mist from the outflow port.

19. Attach the mask to the patient. Stay with the patient during the treatment, and monitor for dyspnea and bronchospasm.

    Rationale Increased fluid absorption through the respiratory tract can lead to overhydration and subsequent pulmonary edema.

20. Follow steps 14 and 15.

For a hand nebulizer

21. To administer a nasal spray, tilt the patient's head back slightly and close one nostril with the thumb. Insert the nosepiece into the open nostril while holding the nebulizer between the thumb and index finger.

    or

    To administer an oral spray, place the mouthpiece into the mouth.

22. Press the cannister to release the spray.

23. Repeat steps 21–22 two or three times or as ordered by the physician.

24. Follow steps 14 and 15.

For a mini-nebulizer

25. Fill the cup with the appropriate fluid and medication, and attach the oxygen tubing to the oxygen or air source.

26. Turn on the oxygen (or air), and adjust the flow to provide appropriate misting from the port. Usually 5 to 6 L/min of oxygen is satisfactory.

27. Attach the delivery device to the patient. Instruct the patient to hold her or his breath for 2 or 3 seconds on every third inspiration.

    Rationale Holding the breath facilitates inhalation of the medication deeply into the respiratory tract.

28. Remain with the patient during the therapy, and assess for reactions to the medication.

29. Follow steps 14 and 15.

For a side-stream nebulizer

30. Remove the cup, and inject the ordered medication and sterile distilled water as necessary. Replace the cup.

31. Attach the mouthpiece or mask to the ventilator of the IPPB machine.

32. Turn on the machine, and check that an appropriate amount of mist is emanating from the port.

33. Remain with the patient during the therapy (15 to 20 minutes), and assess reactions to the medication.

34. Follow steps 14 and 15.

■ Evaluation

Expected outcomes

1. Decreased rales and/or rhonchi upon auscultation

2. More productive cough

3. Amount, color, and character of expectorated secretions as anticipated from baseline data

4. Dyspnea decreased

5. Vital signs stable or improved

Unexpected outcomes

1. Lung sounds still present and unchanged

2. Coughing nonproductive or less productive

3. Expectorated secretions less in amount and different in color and character than anticipated from baseline data

4. Dyspnea unchanged or increased

Upon obtaining an unexpected outcome:

1. Report your findings to the responsible nurse and/or physician.

2. Adjust the nursing care plan appropriately, eg, assess respirations more frequently.

CHEST PHYSIOTHERAPY

Chest physiotherapy includes chest percussion, vibration, postural drainage, deep breathing, and coughing. Percussion, vibration, and postural drainage are discussed in Technique 36–5.

Deep breathing involves exercises that expand the various segments of the lungs. See Technique 36–1. Coughing here means controlled coughing that removes bronchial secretions. It should be learned by all preoperative patients. See Technique 31–1 on page 755 and Technique 36–1 in this chapter.

TECHNIQUE 36–5 ■ Administering Percussion, Vibration, and Postural Drainage (PVD) to Adults 🏠

Percussing, sometimes called *clapping,* is forcefully striking the skin with cupped hands. To percuss a patient's chest, hold your fingers and thumb together, and flex them slightly to form a cup, as you would to scoop up water. With both hands in this position, alternately flex and extend the wrists rapidly to slap the chest. See Figure 36–26. The hands must remain cupped so that the air cushions the impact, to avoid injuring the patient.

Percussing is usually carried out for only one or two minutes, or up to five minutes over each area, according to the order. It is done over specific congested lung areas, to mechanically dislodge tenacious secretions from the bronchial walls. Percussion is avoided over certain areas, such as the breasts, sternum, spinal column, and kidneys, to prevent injury.

Vibration is a series of vigorous quiverings. It is used after percussion, to increase the turbulence of the exhaled air and thus loosen thick secretions. It is often done alternately with percussion. It can replace percussion if the patient is experiencing chest pain. The orders will specify.

To vibrate, place your hands palms down, one hand over the other, with fingers together and extended, on the chest area to be drained. See Figure 36–27. Alternatively, the hands may be placed side by side. Ask the patient to inhale deeply and exhale slowly. During the exhalation, tense all your hand and arm muscles, and, using mostly the heel of the hand, vibrate (shake) your hands, moving them downward. Stop the vibrating when the patient inhales. Vibration is often done four or five times during postural drainage.

Postural drainage is the drainage of secretions from various lung segments using gravity. Secretions that remain in the lungs or respiratory airways facilitate bacterial growth and subsequent infection. They also can obstruct the smaller airways and can cause atelectasis. Secretions in the major airways, such as the trachea and the right and left main bronchi, are usually coughed into the pharynx, where they can be expectorated, swallowed, or effectively removed by suctioning.

A wide variety of positions is necessary to drain all segments of the lungs, but not all positions are required for every patient. Only those positions that drain specific diseased areas are used. The lower lobes require drainage most frequently, since the upper lobes drain during normal daily activities. The exception occurs in immobilized patients. The sequence for PVD is usually: positioning, percussion, vibration, and removal of secretions by coughing or suction. Each position is usually assumed for

FIGURE 36–26 ■ Percussing the upper posterior chest.

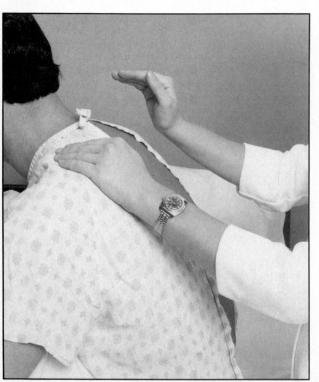

FIGURE 36–27 ■ Vibrating the upper posterior chest.

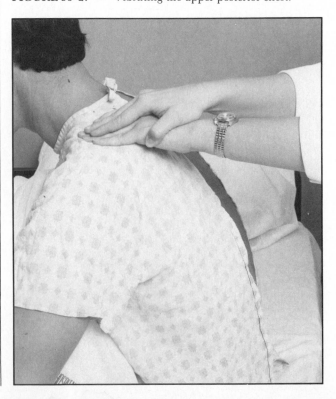

10 to 15 minutes, although beginning treatments may start with shorter times and gradually increase.

■ Assessment

1. Auscultate the patient's lungs to obtain baseline data on lung sounds, eg, rales or wheezes, and the rate and depth of the respirations, to compare with data after the treatment.
2. Determine whether the patient's cough is productive or nonproductive.
3. Observe the amount, color, and character of expectorated secretions.
4. Observe for dyspnea.

Other data include:

1. The lung segments affected.
2. The ordered sequence of percussion, vibration, and postural drainage and the length of time specified.
3. Whether the bronchodilator or moisturizing nebulization therapy is ordered prior to the postural drainage. Secretions are easier to raise after the bronchi are dilated and secretions are thinned.

■ Planning

Nursing goals

1. To assist the removal of accumulated secretions
2. To prevent the accumulation of secretions in patients who are at risk, eg, the unconscious and those receiving mechanical ventilation

Equipment

1. Pillows to support the patient comfortably in the required positions
2. A sputum container for expectorated secretions
3. Tissues for expectorated secretions
4. Mouthwash to clean and freshen the mouth following the treatment
5. A specimen label and requisition, if a specimen is required
6. A hospital bed that can be placed in Trendelenburg's position
7. A hospital gown or pajamas to prevent undue exposure and to protect the skin during percussion and vibration
8. A towel to place over the area to be percussed, if needed, to prevent discomfort

■ Intervention

1. Provide visual and auditory privacy.
   Rationale Coughing and expectorating secretions can embarrass the patient and disturb others.
2. Assist the patient to the appropriate position for postural drainage. See steps 3–11.

Postural drainage

Drainage of the *upper lobes:* The upper lobes consist of three segments—the apical or uppermost segments and the anterior and posterior segments, below them.

3. To drain the *apical segments* of the upper lobes, have the patient lie back at a 30° angle. See Figure 36–28.

FIGURE 36–28

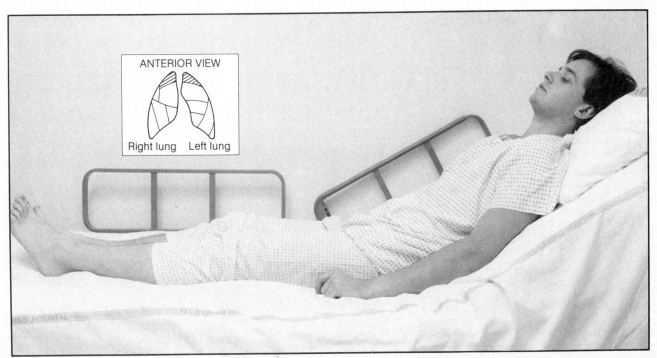

ANTERIOR VIEW

Right lung   Left lung

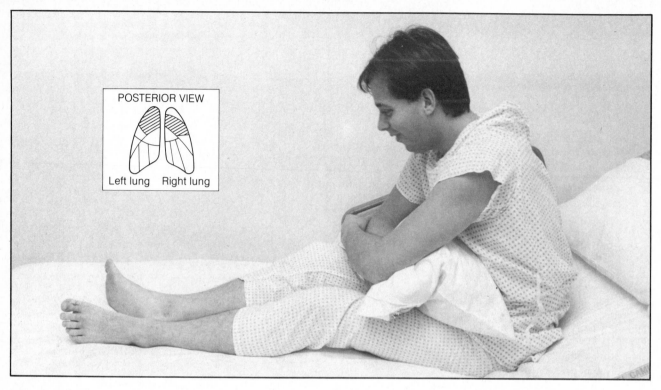

FIGURE 36–29

Percuss and vibrate between the clavicles and above the scapulae.

4. To drain the *posterior segments* of the upper lobes, have the patient sit upright in a chair or in bed with the head bent slightly forward. See Figure 36–29. Percuss and vibrate the area between the clavicles (collarbones) and the scapulae (shoulder blades). For percussion, see steps 12–16; for vibration, see steps 17–20.

5. To drain the *anterior segments* of the upper lobes, have the patient lie on a flat bed with pillows under the knees to flex them. See Figure 36–30. Percuss and vibrate the upper chest below the clavicles down to the nipple line, except for women. The breasts of women are not percussed, because percussion may cause pain.

Drainage of the *right middle lobe and lower division of the left upper lobe:* The right middle lobe has two segments—lateral and medial. The lower division of the left upper lobe, called the *lingula* of that lobe, has two segments—superior and inferior.

FIGURE 36–30

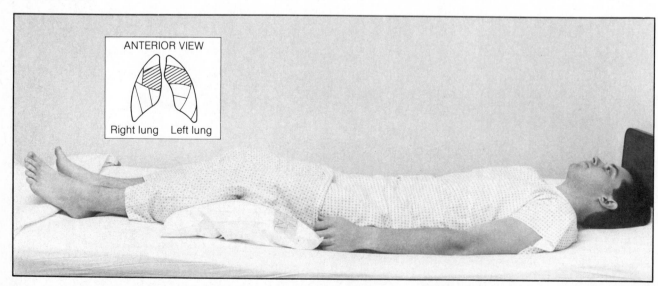

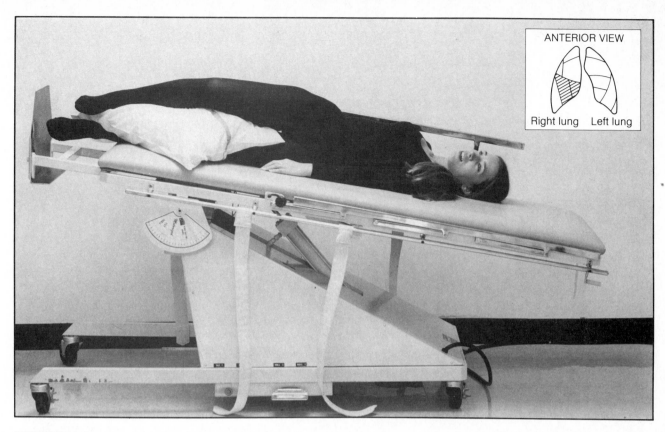

Right lung   Left lung

ANTERIOR VIEW

FIGURE 36–31

6. To drain the *right lateral and medial segments,* elevate the foot of the bed about 15° or 40 cm (15 in), and have the patient lie on the left side. Help the patient to lean back slightly (about a quarter turn) against pillows extending at the back from the shoulder to the hip. See Figure 36–31. If the patient is male, percuss and vibrate over the right side of the chest at the level of the nipple between the fourth and sixth ribs. If the patient is female, position the heel of your hand toward the patient's armpit and your cupped fingers extending forward beneath the patient's breast to percuss and vibrate beneath the breast.

7. To drain the *left lingular segments,* elevate the foot of the bed as in step 6, and have the patient lie as in step 6 except on the right side. See Figure 36–32.

FIGURE 36–32

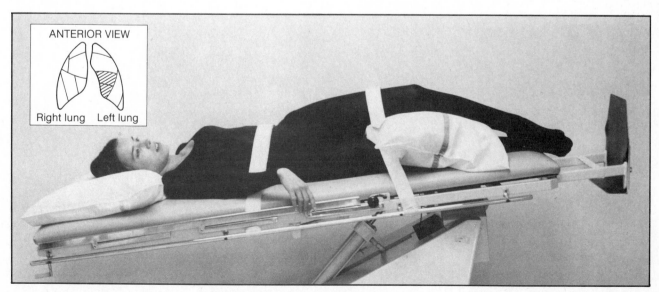

ANTERIOR VIEW

Right lung   Left lung

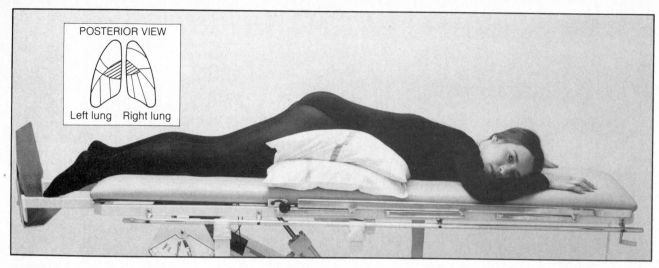

FIGURE 36–33

Percuss and vibrate the right side of the chest as in step 6.

Drainage of the *lower lobes:* The lower lobes have four segments—superior, anterior basal, lateral basal, and posterior basal.

8. To drain the *superior segments,* have the patient lie on the abdomen on a flat bed, and place two pillows under the hips. See Figure 36–33. Percuss and vibrate the middle area of the back (below the scapulae) on both sides of the spine.

9. To drain the *anterior basal segments,* have the patient lie on the unaffected side, with the upper arm over the head. Elevate the foot of the bed about 30° or 45 cm (18 in), or to the height tolerated by the patient. Place one pillow between the patient's knees. Another under the head is optional. See Figure

36–34. Percuss and vibrate the affected side of the chest over the lower ribs, inferior to the axilla.

10. To drain the *lateral basal segments,* have the patient lie partly on the unaffected side and partly on the abdomen. Elevate the foot of the bed about 30° or 45 cm (18 in), or elevate the patient's hips with pillows. See Figure 36–35. Percuss and vibrate the uppermost side of the lower ribs.

11. To drain the *posterior basal segments,* have the patient lie prone. Elevate the foot of the bed about 45 cm (18 in), and elevate the patient's hips on two or three pillows to produce a jackknife position from the knees to the shoulders. See Figure 36–36. Percuss and vibrate over the lower ribs on both sides close to the spine, but not directly over the spine or the kidneys.

FIGURE 36–34

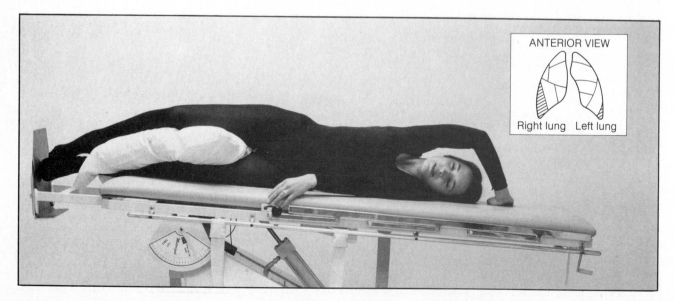

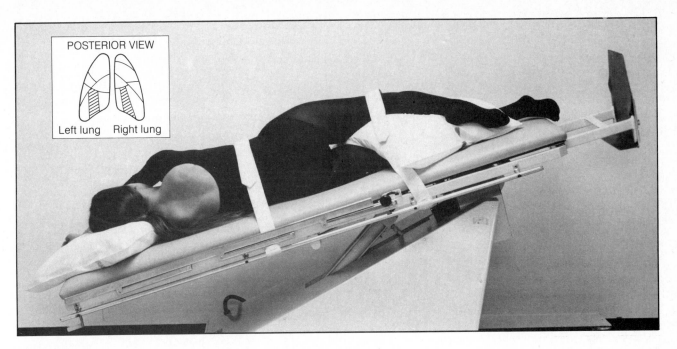

FIGURE 36–35

Percussion

12. Ensure that the area to be percussed is covered, eg, by a gown or towel.

    Rationale   Percussing the skin directly can cause discomfort.

13. Ask the patient to breathe slowly and deeply.

    Rationale   Slow, deep breathing promotes relaxation.

14. Cup your hands so that the fingers are flexed and the thumbs are held against the index fingers.

    Rationale   Cupped hands trap the air against the chest. The trapped air sets up vibrations through the chest wall to the secretions, helping to loosen them.

15. Relax your wrists, and flex your elbows.

    Rationale   Relaxed wrists and flexed elbows help obtain a rapid, hollow, popping action.

16. Alternating hands rapidly, percuss each affected lung segment for one to two minutes. The percussing action should produce a hollow, popping sound when done correctly. See Figure 36–26 earlier.

Vibration

17. Ask the patient to inhale deeply through the mouth and exhale slowly through pursed lips or the nose.

18. During exhalation, press your hands flatly one over

FIGURE 36–36

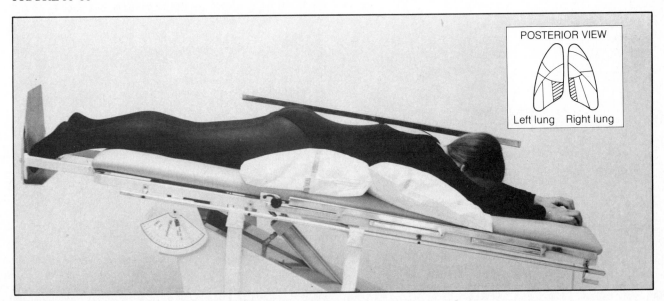

the other (or side by side) against the affected chest area. See Figure 36–27 earlier.

19. Straighten your elbows, and lean slightly against the patient's chest while tensing your arm and shoulder muscles in isometric contractions.

    Rationale Isometric contractions will transmit fine vibrations through the patient's chest wall.

20. Vibrate during five exhalations over one affected lung segment.

21. Encourage the patient to cough and expectorate secretions into the sputum container. Offer the patient mouthwash.

22. Auscultate the patient's lungs, and compare the findings to the baseline data.

23. Note the amount, color, and character of expectorated secretions.

■ Evaluation

Expected outcomes

1. Decreased rales and/or rhonchi upon auscultation

2. Cough more productive

3. Amount, color, and character of expectorated secretions as anticipated from baseline data

4. Dyspnea decreased

Unexpected outcomes

1. Lung sounds still present and unchanged

2. Coughing nonproductive or less productive

3. Expectorated secretions less in amount and different in color and character than anticipated from baseline data

4. Dyspnea unchanged or increased

Upon obtaining an unexpected outcome:

1. Report your findings to the responsible nurse and/or physician.

2. Adjust the nursing care plan appropriately, eg, assess respirations more frequently.

TECHNIQUE 36–6 ■ Administering Percussion, Vibration, and Postural Drainage (PVD) to Infants and Children

---

If a child is too young for hand percussion, a bulb syringe cut in half can be used. Cut the syringe, leaving the nozzle with one half, and tape the cut edge to cushion it. Hold the bulb by the nozzle for percussion. See Figure 36–37.

To make a vibrator for an infant, remove the brush from a portable electric toothbrush and tape padding over the vibrating end.

■ Assessment   See Technique 36–5.

■ Planning   See Technique 36–5.

■ Intervention

Draining the upper lobes

1. *Apical segments.* Assist the child to sit on your lap, with the trunk leaning backward about 30°. A pillow may be used to help support the infant. Percuss and

FIGURE 36–37

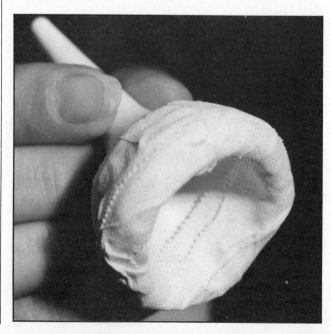

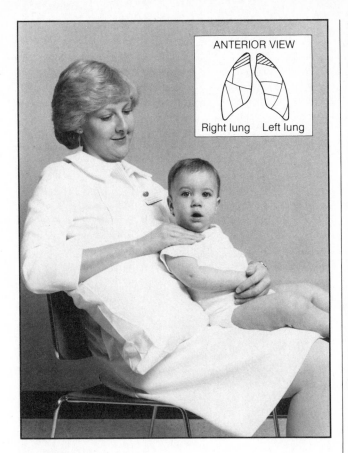

FIGURE 36–38

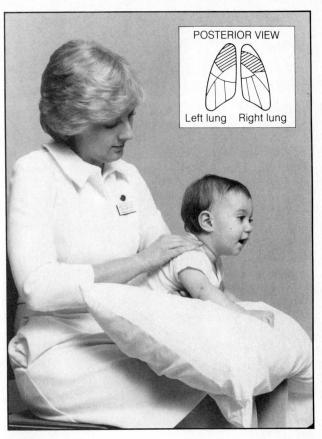

FIGURE 36–39

FIGURE 36–40

vibrate over the area between the clavicles (collarbones) and the scapulae (shoulder blades), using three fingertips flexed and held together. See Figure 36–38.

2. *Posterior segments.* Have the child sit on your lap leaning forward about 20° over a pillow. Percuss and vibrate the upper back on both sides. See Figure 36–39.

3. *Anterior segments.* Have the child lie supine on a flat bed or your lap. Percuss and vibrate the upper chest below the clavicles down to the nipple line. See Figure 36–40.

Draining the middle lobe or lingular segments

4. *Right lateral and medial segments.* Position the child almost supine on your lap, head slanted down about 15°, turned on the left side about a quarter turn, with the right shoulder slightly elevated and the hips higher than the chest. Percuss and vibrate over the right nipple. See Figure 36–41.

5. *Left lingular segments.* Position the child as in step 4 but turned on the right side about a quarter turn. Percuss and vibrate over the left side of the chest at the level of the nipple between the fourth and sixth ribs.

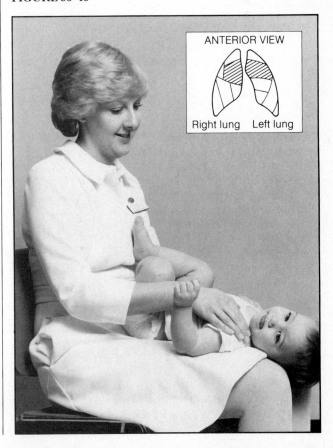

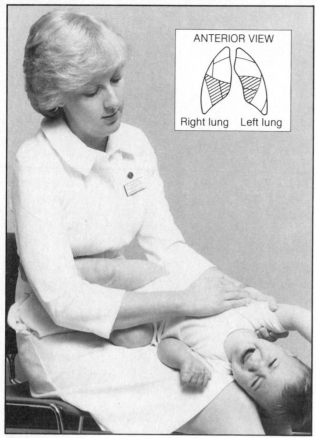

FIGURE 36–41

FIGURE 36–42

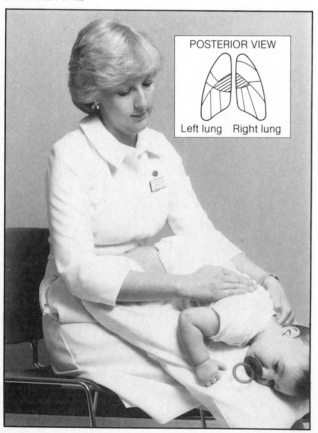

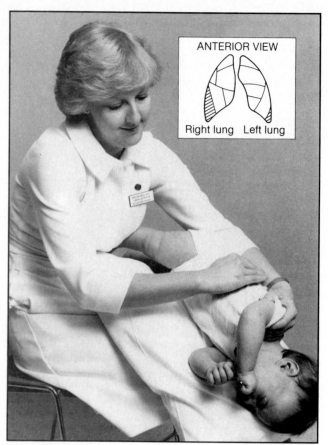

FIGURE 36–43

FIGURE 36–44

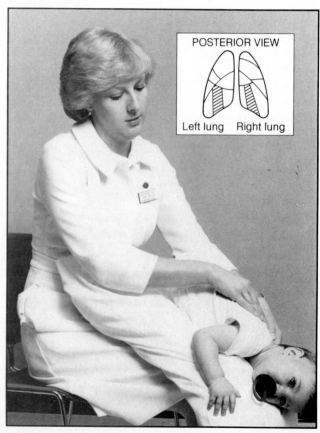

Draining the lower lobes

6. *Superior segments.* Place the infant prone on a pillow over your knees. Elevate the hips slightly. Percuss and vibrate the middle area of the back just below each scapula. See Figure 36–42.

7. *Anterior basal segments.* Position the child on the unaffected side on a pillow over your knees, with the head lowered about 30°. Percuss and vibrate at the side of the chest over the lower ribs beneath the axilla, avoiding the stomach. See Figure 36–43.

8. *Lateral basal segments.* Place the child almost prone on a pillow on your knees, with the head lowered about 30°. Place a pillow under the affected side to elevate it and turn the upper body a quarter turn. Percuss and vibrate the affected side over the lower ribs. See Figure 36–44. Rotate the infant to the opposite side, and repeat the procedure to drain the same segment of the other lung.

9. *Posterior basal segments.* Position the child prone on a pillow over your lap, with the head lowered about 30°. Percuss and vibrate over the lower ribs on both sides close to the spine. See Figure 36–45. Do not percuss directly over the spine or over the kidneys.

■ **Evaluation** See Technique 36–5.

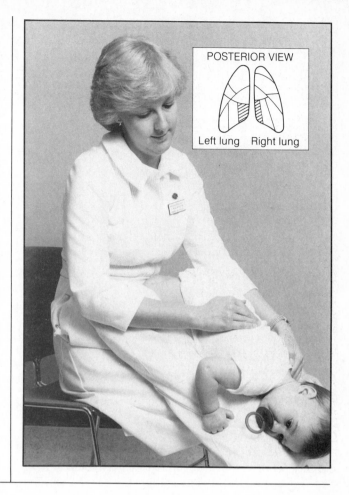

FIGURE 36–45

TECHNIQUE 36–7 ■ Collecting a Sputum Specimen

Sputum is the mucous secretion from the lungs, bronchi, and trachea. It is important to differentiate it from *saliva,* the clear liquid secreted by the salivary glands in the mouth, sometimes referred to as "spit." Healthy individuals do not produce sputum. Patients need to cough to bring sputum up from the lungs, bronchi, and trachea into the mouth, to expectorate it into a collecting container.

■ **Assessment**

Assess the patient's ability to expectorate sputum and the time that sputum is coughed up most readily. Many patients find it easier to expectorate sputum early in the morning after it has collected in the lungs during the night. Other data include:

1. The purpose of the sputum specimen. Check the patient's chart. Sputum specimens ordered for "culture and sensitivity" are obtained to identify a specific microorganism and its drug sensitivities. Specimens for "cytology" often require serial collection of three early morning specimens and are tested to identify cancer in the lung and its specific cell type. Specimens for "acid-fast bacillus (AFB)," which also require serial collection, often for three consecutive days, are obtained to identify the presence of this organism, also known as the tubercle bacillus (TB). Some agencies use a special glass container when the presence of AFB is suspected.

2. Any specific directions on the patient's chart about the specimen, eg, "Collect 30 mL of sputum."

■ **Planning**

Nursing goals

1. To aid in the diagnosis and treatment of a respiratory illness by identifying the microorganisms or cells

present in the sputum and identifying the antibiotic to which the microorganisms are sensitive

2. To confirm the presence or absence of the tubercle bacillus in the sputum

3. To assess the effectiveness of therapeutic measures

Equipment

1. A container with a cover for the sputum. Sputum containers are often made of plastic.

2. Disinfectant and swabs, or liquid soap and water, to clean the outside of the container, and paper towels to dry it.

3. A completed label for the container, with identifying information about the patient.

4. A completed requisition to accompany the specimen to the laboratory.

5. A container, eg, a paper bag, in which to send the specimen to the laboratory. Most agencies have special envelopes or bags for this purpose. This need not be taken to the bedside.

6. Mouthwash.

■ Intervention

1. Inform the patient about the need for the specimen and how to obtain one. If the patient finds it painful to cough, eg, after abdominal surgery, show him or her how to hold a pillow firmly against the affected area while coughing. This provides external support and decreases the discomfort. If the patient needs to assume a postural drainage position to obtain the specimen, explain this, and arrange a time. See Technique 36–5. In some instances pharyngeal suctioning may be required to obtain the specimen. See Technique 37–1 on page 885.

2. Make sure the patient can expectorate the sputum directly into the sputum cup without touching the inside of the container or allowing the sputum to contact the outside of the container. If nursing

FIGURE 36–46

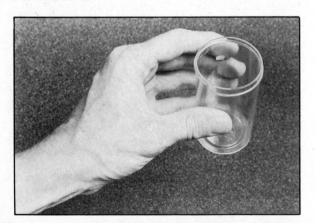

assistance is not required, leave the container with the patient.

3. If nursing assistance is required, ask the patient to hold the sputum cup on the outside, or hold it for a patient who is not able. See Figure 36–46.

4. Ask the patient to breathe deeply and then cough up 1 to 2 tbsp (15 to 30 mL, or 4 to 8 fluid drams). Some agencies may specify another amount.

5. Hold the sputum cup so the patient can expectorate into it, making sure that the sputum does not come in contact with the outside of the container.
Rationale Containing the sputum within the cup restricts the spread of microorganisms to others.

6. Assess the appearance and amount of sputum. Sputum can be described as liquid or thick and white, yellow, blood-tinged, green, or clear in color. The amount can be described as copious, large, small, etc. Cover the container with the lid immediately after the sputum is in the container.
Rationale Covering the container prevents the inadvertent spread of microorganisms to others.

7. Determine the respiration rate, and note any abnormalities or difficulty breathing.

8. Assess the color of the patient's skin and mucous membranes, especially any cyanosis, which can indicate impaired blood oxygenation.

9. Wipe the outside of the container with a disinfectant, if the sputum has contacted the outside surface. Some agencies recommend washing the outside of all containers with liquid soap and water and then drying with a paper towel.

10. Place the completed label on the container.

11. Provide the patient with mouthwash to rinse the mouth.
Rationale This removes any unpleasant taste.

12. Place the labeled container in the envelope or bag to be taken to the laboratory. Attach the completed requisition to the container or to the envelope.

13. Arrange for the specimen to be transported to the laboratory. Specimens that are taken for culture need to be sent directly to the laboratory, where they are placed in a bacteriologic refrigerator. If the specimen is to remain on the nursing unit, it needs to be placed in the refrigerator used for specimens. When 24-hour specimens are collected, they may be sent to the laboratory once the container is about three-fourths full. Containers are only partly filled to ensure that the outside of the container is not in contact with the sputum. In some agencies, the sputum specimens are kept in the specimen refrigerator in separate glass containers, which are numbered in the order in which they were taken. All the specimens collected during the 24-hour period are then sent to the laboratory.

14. Record collection of the sputum specimen on the patient's chart and on the nursing care plan if indicated. Include the color, consistency, and odor of the sputum, any measures needed to obtain the specimen (eg, postural drainage), the general amount of sputum produced, eg, copious (large amount) or scant (small amount), and any discomfort experienced by the patient.

Sample Recording

Date	Time	Notes
6/21/86	0600	Sputum specimen sent to laboratory. Produced large amount of green-yellow thick sputum. States has sharp, knifelike pain in right anterior lower chest when coughing.— Sheila D. Wray, NS

15. On receipt of the report from the laboratory, note which microorganisms were identified and the antibiotic to which they are sensitive. Place the report in the patient's chart, and notify the physician that the report is back. Note if there are changes in the plan of therapy as a result of the report.

■ Evaluation

Expected outcome

Amount, color, and character of expectorated secretions as anticipated from baseline data.

Unexpected outcomes

1. Coughing nonproductive.
2. Expectorated secretions less in amount and different in color and character than anticipated from baseline data.

Upon obtaining an unexpected outcome: Report your findings to the responsible nurse and/or physician.

TECHNIQUE 36–8 ■ Obtaining Nose and Throat Specimens

Nose and throat specimens are collected from the mucosa of the nose and throat and then cultured and examined for the presence of pathogens.

■ Assessment

For assessment of the nose and throat, see Techniques 10–6 and 10–7. Other data include:

1. Whether it is the agency's practice to place specimens on a growing medium at the patient's bedside or whether the swab is inserted into a sterile test tube for transport to the laboratory.
2. Whether the patient is suspected of having a contagious disease, eg, diphtheria. Check the patient's chart. Such a condition requires special precautions.
3. Whether a specimen is required from the nasal cavity, as well as from the pharynx and/or the nostrils. Check the chart.

■ Planning

Nursing goals

1. To identify any pathogenic microorganisms present in the nose and throat and the antibiotics to which they are sensitive

2. To evaluate the effectiveness of antibiotic therapy

Equipment

1. Four sterile swabs or applicators, to obtain the specimens. Swabs are sterilized and then stored in a manner that keeps them from contact with the air and any unsterilized materials.
2. A tongue blade, to depress the patient's tongue and expose the pharynx.
3. Four containers of growing medium or four sterile containers to hold the specimens. Usually glass tubes with securely attachable caps are used. Some agencies use special tubes containing about 2 mL of broth, which keeps the air in the tube moist so that the specimen will not dry out. The swab is suspended without touching the broth.
4. A source of light, to illuminate the inside of the mouth and throat. Some hospital beds have directional lights that can be used. Otherwise a flashlight can be used.
5. An otoscope with a nasal speculum, to light the inside of the nose and provide access to the area to be swabbed.
6. A waste container in which to discard the tongue blade.

7. A container for the nasal speculum, eg, a kidney basin.

8. Completed labels for each specimen container, including identification information about the patient and the exact source of the specimen, eg, right nostril or left tonsil.

9. A completed requisition to accompany the specimens to the laboratory.

10. A container, eg, a bag, in which to send the specimen container to the laboratory. Follow agency practice. This container need not be taken to the bedside.

■ Intervention

1. Assist the patient to a sitting position.

   Rationale This is the most comfortable position for many patients and the one in which the pharynx is most readily visible.

2. Remove the cap from one culture tube and lay the cap on a firm surface, inner side upward.

   Rationale This prevents the inside of the cap from coming into contact with microorganisms on the surface.

3. Remove one sterile applicator from its covering, and hold it carefully by the stick end, keeping the remainder sterile.

   Rationale The swab end is kept from touching any objects that could contaminate it.

Taking a throat specimen

4. Ask the patient to open the mouth, extend the tongue, and say "ah." Assess the pharynx and tonsils for redness, swelling, and discharge.

   Rationale The pharynx is exposed by extending the

FIGURE 36–47

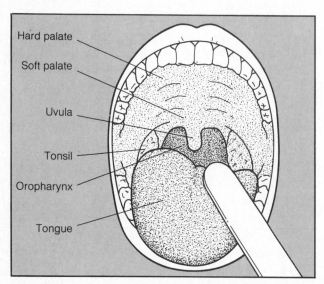

Hard palate
Soft palate
Uvula
Tonsil
Oropharynx
Tongue

tongue. Saying "ah" relaxes the throat muscles and helps minimize contraction of the constriction muscle of the pharynx (the gag reflex).

5. If the posterior pharynx cannot be seen, use a light, and depress the tongue with a tongue blade. Depress the tongue firmly without touching the throat. See Figure 36–47.

   Rationale Touching the throat stimulates the gag reflex.

6. Insert a swab into the mouth, taking care not to touch any part of the mouth or tongue. Quickly run the swab along the tonsils, making sure to contact any areas on the pharynx that are particularly erythematous (reddened) or that contain exudate.

   Rationale The swab should not pick up microorganisms in the mouth. The swab is moved quickly so as not to initiate the gag reflex or cause discomfort. Erythematous areas and areas with exudate will likely have the most microorganisms.

7. Remove the swab without touching the mouth or lips.

   Rationale This prevents the swab from transmitting microorganisms to the mouth.

8. Insert the swab into the sterile tube or container of growing medium without allowing it to touch the outside of the container. Make sure the swab is placed in the correctly labeled tube.

   Rationale Touching the outside of the tube could transmit microorganisms to it and then to others.

9. Place the top securely on the tube, taking care not to touch the inside of the cap.

   Rationale Touching the inside of the cap could transmit additional microorganisms into the tube.

10. Repeat steps 3–9 with the second swab.

11. Discard the tongue blade in the waste container.

Taking a nasal specimen

12. Follow steps 2–3. Gently insert the lighted nasal speculum up one nostril.

13. Observe the inside of the nostril for redness, discharge, and swelling.

14. Insert the sterile swab carefully through the speculum without touching the edges. Wipe along the reddened areas or areas with the most exudate.

15. Remove the swab without touching the speculum, and place it in a sterile tube.

16. Repeat steps 12–15 for the other nostril.

For all specimens

17. Place the specimen tubes in the envelope or bag for transport to the laboratory. Attach the completed requisition to a specimen container or to the bag.

18. Arrange for the specimens to be transported to the laborabory. If they cannot be taken immediately, refrigerate them in the appropriate refrigerator.

19. Record obtaining the nose and throat specimens on the patient's chart and the nursing care plan. Include the appearance of the mucosa of the nares, pharynx, and tonsils; the color, amount, and consistency of any exudate; and any discomfort experienced by the patient.

20. On receipt of the laboratory report, note which microorganisms were identified and the antibiotic to which they are sensitive. Place the report in the patient's chart, and notify the physician that the report is back. Note if there are changes in the plan of therapy as a result of the report.

■ Evaluation

Expected outcome

Redness, swelling, and discharge as anticipated from baseline data.

Unexpected outcome

No discharge present. Upon obtaining an unexpected outcome: Report your findings to the responsible nurse and/or physician.

References

Foss G: Postural drainage. *Am J Nurs* (April) 1973; 73:666–669.

Fuchs PL: Humidifiers. Pages 458–462 in: *The Nurse's Reference Library: Procedures.* Nursing 83 Books, Intermed Communications, 1983.

Fuchs PL: Nebulizers. Pages 462–466 in: *The Nurse's Reference Library: Procedures.* Nursing 83 Books, Intermed Communications, 1983.

Luce JM, Tyler ML, Pierson DJ: *Intensive Respiratory Care.* Saunders, 1984.

Nielsen L: Assessing patients' respiratory problems. *Am J Nurs* (December) 1980; 80:2192–2196.

Nursing 80 Photobook Series: *Providing Respiratory Care.* Intemed Communications, 1979.

Ventilators and how they work. *Am J Nurs* (December) 1980; 80:2202–2205.

Waterson, M (consultant): Teaching your patients postural drainage. *Nursing 78* (March) 1978; 8:51–53.

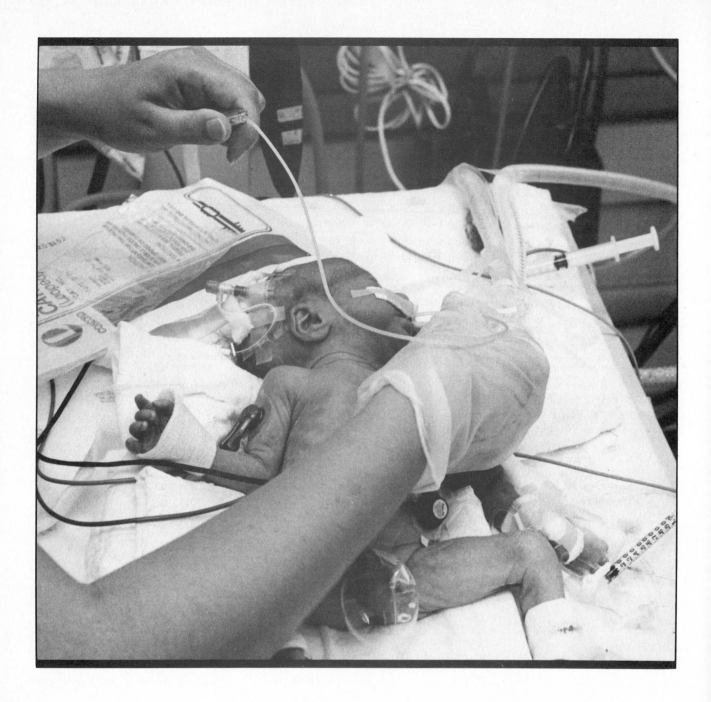

PHARYNGEAL SUCTIONING

37

Nurses must sometimes apply suction to the oropharynx and nasal passages of patients who have difficulty swallowing or expectorating secretions. *Suctioning* is the aspiration of secretions, often through a rubber or polyethylene catheter connected to a suction machine or wall outlet.

Suctioning of the upper respiratory airways is indicated when the patient (a) is unable to expectorate coughed secretions, (b) is unable to swallow, and (c) makes light bubbling or rattling breath sounds that signal the accumulation of secretions. The patient may also be dyspneic or appear cyanotic. Whether and how often to suction a patient are decisions that require judgment on the part of the nurse. Irritation of the mucous mem-

branes by the suction catheter can increase secretions. Suctioning can also cause some hypoxia.

Chapter Outline

■ Technique 37–1 Oropharyngeal and Nasopharyngeal Suctioning

■ Technique 37–2 Bulb Suctioning an Infant

Objectives

Upon completion of this chapter, the student will:

1. Know essential terms and facts about oropharyngeal and nasopharyngeal suctioning
   1.1 Distinguish oropharyngeal and nasopharyngeal suctioning from endotracheal suctioning
   1.2 Identify various types of suction devices
2. Understand facts about techniques used in pharyngeal suctioning
   2.1 Identify relevant assessment data
   2.2 Identify nursing diagnoses for which the technique may be implemented
   2.3 Identify nursing goals related to the technique
   2.4 Identify expected and unexpected outcomes from assessment data
   2.5 Identify reasons underlying selected steps of the technique
3. Perform pharyngeal suctioning techniques safely
   3.1 Assess the patient adequately
   3.2 Collect additional data from appropriate sources

3.3 Select pertinent nursing goals for the patient
3.4 Establish relevant outcome criteria for the patient following the technique
3.5 Collect necessary equipment before the technique
3.6 Implement interventions to enhance the effectiveness of the technique and enhance the patient's comfort and safety
3.7 Communicate relevant information about the patient to the appropriate persons
3.8 Determine the evaluative outcomes of the technique
4. Evaluate own performance of specific techniques in a laboratory or clinical setting with the assistance of another
   4.1 Use the performance checklists provided
   4.2 Identify areas of strength and weakness
   4.3 Alter performance in response to own evaluation and that of another

Terms

■ **bronchus**   a large air passageway of the lungs (plural: bronchi)

■ **cilia**   hairlike projections of the respiratory mucous membrane

■ **cyanosis**   bluish discoloration of the skin and mucous membranes due to a reduced oxygen level in the blood

■ **hypoxemia**   a reduced oxygen supply in the bloodstream

■ **larynx**   a structure composed of nine cartilages guard-

ing the entrance of the trachea and functioning as the voice organ

■ **orthopnea**   the ability to breathe only in the upright sitting or standing position

■ **suctioning**   aspiration of oronasopharyngeal secretions using negative pressure

■ **trachea**   a membranous tube composed of cartilage, connected to the larynx above, and branching into the right and left bronchi below

TECHNIQUE 37–1 ■ Oropharyngeal and Nasopharyngeal Suctioning

Oropharyngeal or nasopharyngeal suctioning removes secretions from the upper respiratory tract. Deeper

suctioning is called *endotracheal suctioning,* and it removes secretions from the trachea and the bronchi. Deep suctioning requires considerably more skill and is usually carried out by a nursing specialist in critical care or an experienced nurse.

It is recommended that sterile technique be used for all suctioning, so that microorganisms are not introduced into the pharynx, where they can multiply and move into the trachea and bronchi. This is particularly important for debilitated patients, who are more susceptible to infection.

■ Assessment

Assess the patient for:

1. Rate, depth, rhythm, and character of respirations. Make special note of noisy, wet respirations, which indicate the presence of secretions in the respiratory tract that are impeding the flow of air. Auscultate the chest with a stethoscope, if necessary, to assess the condition of the airways and the lungs.
2. The color of the skin and mucous membranes. Note cyanosis and pallor.
3. Dyspnea and orthopnea.
4. Ability to cough and produce sputum. Note the color, consistency, amount, and odor of the sputum.
5. Any drainage from the mouth, if the patient is unconscious.

■ Nursing Diagnosis

Nursing diagnoses that may indicate the need to suction a patient's pharyngeal passages include: Ineffective airway clearance related to inability to expectorate or swallow coughed secretions.

■ Planning

Nursing goals

1. To remove secretions that obstruct the airway and to provide a patent airway

FIGURE 37–1 ■ Types of pharyngeal suction catheters: **A,** open-tipped; **B,** whistle-tipped.

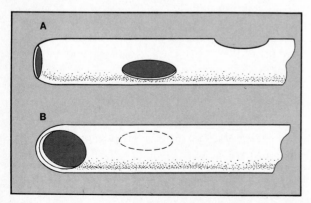

2. To facilitate respiratory ventilation
3. To obtain secretions for diagnostic purposes
4. To prevent infection that may result from accumulated secretions

Equipment

1. A portable suction machine or a gauge to attach to wall suction equipment with tubing and a collection receptacle.
2. A sterile suction package that includes:

   a. A suction catheter. Several types of catheters are available. The open-tipped catheter has an opening at the end and several openings along the sides. See Figure 37–1, *A.* It is effective for thick mucous plugs, but it can irritate tissue. The whistle-tipped catheter has a slanted opening at the tip. See Figure 37–1, *B.* Some catheters have a thumb port on the side, which is used to control the suction. The tip of a suction catheter has several openings along the sides to distribute the negative pressure of the suction over a wide area, thus preventing excesssive irritation of any one area of the respiratory mucous membrane. Catheters used for suctioning vary in size from #12 to #18 Fr. for adults, from #8 to #10 Fr. for children, and from #5 to #8 Fr. for infants. If both the oropharynx and the nasopharynx are to be suctioned, one sterile catheter is required for each.

   b. A glove.

   c. A cup or container for sterile water or sterile normal saline, to lubricate and flush the catheter.
3. Sterile normal saline or water.
4. A Y-connector to regulate the suction system if the catheter does not have a thumb port.
5. Sterile gauzes to wipe the catheter and the patient's mouth or nose (optional).
6. A moisture-resistant bag for disposable catheters and gloves.
7. A towel to protect the patient's gown and pillows.
8. A sputum trap, if a specimen is to be collected during suctioning.

■ Intervention

1. Explain to the patient that suctioning will relieve his or her breathing difficulty and that the procedure is painless but may stimulate the cough, gag, or sneeze reflex.

   Rationale Knowing that the procedure will relieve breathing problems often reassures the patient and enlists cooperation.
2. Position a conscious patient who has a functional gag reflex in the semi-Fowler's position with the

patient's head turned to one side for oral suctioning or with the neck hyperextended for nasal suctioning.

Rationale   These positions facilitate the insertion of the catheter and help prevent aspiration of secretions.

3.   Position an unconscious patient in the lateral position, facing you.

Rationale   This position allows the patient's tongue to fall forward, so that it will not obstruct the catheter on insertion. Lateral position also facilitates drainage of secretions from the pharynx and prevents the possibility of aspiration.

4.   Place the towel over the pillow or under the patient's chin.

5.   Set the pressure on the suction gauge, and turn on the suction. Some suction devices are calibrated to three pressure ranges: high (120 to 150 mm Hg), medium (80 to 120 mm Hg), and low (0 to 80 mm Hg). Generally a pressure of 100 to 120 mm Hg is used for adults and 50 to 75 mm Hg for infants and children.

6.   Open the sterile suction package.

a. Set up the cup or container, touching only its outside.

b. Pour sterile water or saline into the container.

c. Don the sterile glove.

7.   With your sterile gloved hand, pick up the catheter, and attach it to the suction unit. See Figure 37–2.

8.   Make an approximate measure of the depth for the insertion. Mark the position on the tube with the fingers of your gloved hand. An appropriate measure is the distance between the tip of the patient's nose and the earlobe, or about 13 cm (5 in) for an adult.

9.   Moisten the catheter tip by dipping it in the container of sterile water or saline.

Rationale   Moistening reduces friction and eases insertion.

10.   Test the suction and the patency of the catheter by applying your finger to the thumb port or open branch of the Y-connector (the suction control) to create suction.

11.   For a nasopharyngeal suction, insert the catheter gently through one nostril with your thumb away from the suction control (ie, not applying suction). Direct the catheter along the floor of the nasal cavity. If one nostril is not patent, try the other. Never force the catheter against an obstruction.

or

For an oropharyngeal suction, insert the catheter through the mouth along one side into the oropharynx, without applying suction.

Rationale   Gentle insertion and not applying suction during insertion prevent trauma to the mucous membrane. Directing the catheter along the floor of

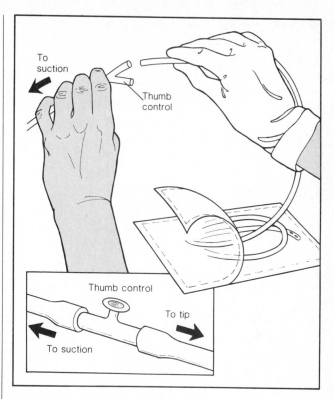

FIGURE 37–2

the nasal cavity avoids the nasal turbinates. Directing the catheter along one side of the mouth prevents gagging.

12.   Apply your finger to the suction control port, and gently rotate the catheter. Apply suction for 5 to 10 seconds, then remove your finger from the control, and remove the catheter. It may be necessary during oropharyngeal suctioning to apply suction to secretions that collect in the vestibule of the mouth and beneath the tongue. A suction attempt should last only 15 seconds. During this time the catheter is inserted, the suction applied and discontinued, and the catheter removed.

Rationale   Placing the finger over the suction control port starts the suction. Gentle rotation of the catheter ensures that all surfaces are reached and prevents trauma to any one area of the respiratory mucosa due to prolonged suction.

13.   Wipe off the catheter with sterile gauze if it is thickly coated with secretions, flush it with sterile water or saline, and repeat steps 9, 11–12, until the air passage is clear, but do not apply suction for more than five minutes in total.

Rationale   Applying suction for too long can decrease the patient's oxygen supply.

14.   Encourage the patient to breathe deeply and cough between suctions.

Rationale   Coughing and deep breathing help carry secretions from the trachea and bronchi into the

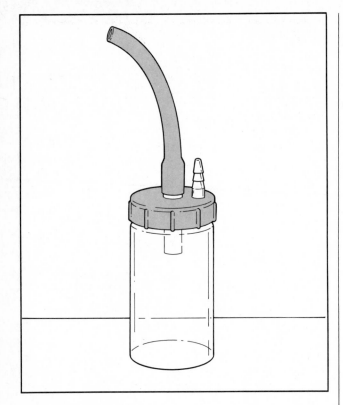

FIGURE 37–3

pharynx, where they can be reached with the suction catheter.

15. If a specimen is required, use a sputum trap (see Figure 37–3):

   a. Attach the suction catheter to the rubber tubing of the sputum trap.

   b. Attach the suction tubing to the sputum trap air vent.

   c. Suction the patient's nasopharynx or oropharynx. The sputum trap will collect the mucus during suctioning.

   d. Remove the catheter from the patient. Disconnect the sputum trap rubber tubing from the suction catheter. Remove the trap air vent from the suction tubing.

   e. Connect the rubber tubing of the sputum trap to its air vent.

   Rationale This prevents the spread of microorganisms from the sputum.

16. When the catheter has been removed, rinse the catheter by flushing it with water.

   Rationale Rinsing the catheter removes secretions from the tubing.

17. Offer, or assist the patient with, oral or nasal hygiene.

18. Dispose of the catheter, glove, water, and waste container.

19. Ensure that equipment is available for the next suctioning. Change suction collection bottles and tubing daily or more frequently as necessary.

20. Record the amount, consistency, color, and odor of sputum, eg, foamy, white mucus; thick, green-tinged mucus; or blood-flecked mucus. Observe the patient's breathing status.

Sample Recording

Date	Time	Notes
5/12/87	0200	Oropharyngeal suctioning for 5 min. 35 mL thick, greenish sputum. Respirations 30/min, wet, difficult. Cyanotic. No response to painful stimuli. Positioned in left Sims's. ——— Rozelle L. Schwartz, RN

If the technique is carried out frequently, eg, q.1h., it may be appropriate to record only once, at the end of the shift.

Sample Recording

Date	Time	Notes
5/12/87	0700	Nasopharyngeal suctioning q.1h. for 3 min. Nares alternated. 175 mL thick, greenish sputum. Respirations remain dyspneic, 30–32/min. No response to verbal stimuli. Position changed q.1h. ——————— Rozelle L. Schwartz, RN

■ Evaluation

Expected outcomes

1. Noiseless respirations
2. Decreased respiratory rate
3. Increased respiratory ventilation
4. Increased ease of respiratory effort
5. Absence of adventitious breath sounds upon auscultation
6. Pink lips and nail beds

Unexpected outcomes

1. Bubbling or rattling breath sounds
2. Respiratory rate unchanged
3. Dyspnea
4. Presence of adventitious breath sounds upon auscultation
5. Pale or cyanotic lips and nail beds

Upon obtaining an unexpected outcome:

1. Report your findings to the responsible nurse and/or physician.
2. Adjust the patient's nursing care plan accordingly.

TECHNIQUE 37–2 ■ Bulb Suctioning an Infant

A bulb syringe is frequently used to suction the oral and nasal cavities of infants and children, particularly when secretions are not severe enough to require deeper suctioning. This technique may be used for a newborn who has amniotic fluid in the air passages or an infant with increased mucus that is causing labored breathing. The technique requires medical aseptic practice rather than surgical asepsis, since only the mouth or nose is entered, not the pharynx.

■ Assessment

Assess the infant for:

1. Rate and depth of respirations, presence or absence of breath sounds, and chest movements
2. Color and pulse rate
3. Color, consistency, and amount of secretions

■ Planning

Nursing goals

1. To establish and maintain a patent airway
2. To prevent or relieve labored respirations

Equipment

1. A bulb syringe. This should be sterile initially, but it can be rinsed and used for subsequent suctions without resterilizing.
2. A kidney basin or other receptacle for removed secretions.
3. A clean towel or bib to place under the infant's chin.

■ Intervention

1. Bundle the infant to restrain the arms, or cradle the child in your arm, tucking the infant's near arm behind your back and holding the other arm securely with your hand. See Figure 37–4. Put the bib or towel under the infant's chin.
2. Compress the bulb of the syringe with your thumb before inserting it. See Figure 37–5.
   Rationale Compressing the bulb while the tip is in the mouth or nose can force secretions deeper into the respiratory tract.
3. Keeping the bulb compressed, insert the tip of the syringe into the infant's nose or mouth.
4. Release the bulb gradually, and slowly move it outward to aspirate the secretions.

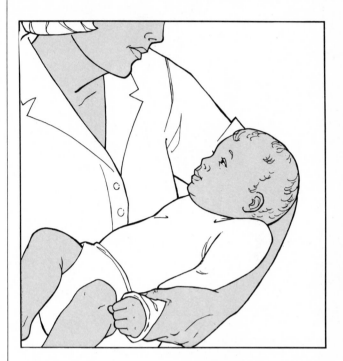

FIGURE 37–4

5. Remove the syringe, hold the tip over the waste receptacle, and compress the bulb again.
   Rationale Compressing the bulb expels the contents into the waste receptacle.
6. Repeat steps 2–5 until the infant's nares and mouth are clear of secretions and the breathing sounds are clear. The same syringe can be used for the nose and the mouth.
7. Cuddle and soothe the infant as necessary, and place the infant in a side-lying position after suctioning.
   Rationale In a back-lying position, the infant is more likely to aspirate secretions.

FIGURE 37–5

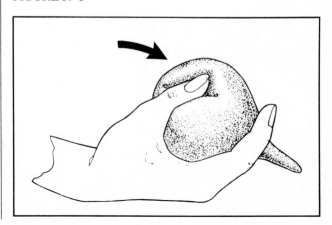

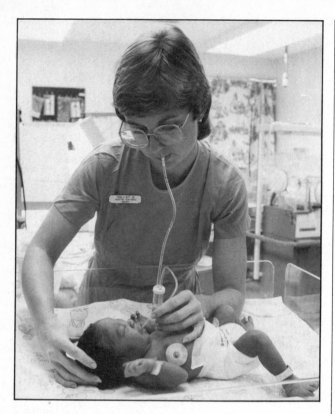

FIGURE 37–6

8. Report to the responsible nurse any problems or untoward response of the infant.

9. Assess the infant's response to the suctioning in terms of breathing pattern, color, and presence of secretions.

10. Rinse the syringe and the waste receptacle. The syringe can be kept in a clean folded towel at the cribside for use as needed.

11. Record the procedure and relevant observations in the appropriate records.

12. Assess the infant's breathing patterns regularly and as frequently as required.

13. Adjust the nursing care plan to include the frequency of suctioning and respiratory assessment.

Variation: The DeLee suction device (mucus trap)

The DeLee mucus trap is a negative-pressure mouth suction device used for infants. See Figure 37–6. To use the device, carefully insert the catheter into the infant's mouth, place the mouthpiece into your mouth, and suck on the mouthpiece.

The DeLee device is commonly used in the delivery room to clear the neonate's nose, mouth, and pharynx of mucus and amniotic fluid and to initiate breathing. Suctioning of the mouth is often needed as soon as the neonate's head presents. The mouth is suctioned before the nose, since nasal stimulation can cause the infant to inhale and aspirate secretions. Suctioning is often repeated after the neonate's first cry.

■ **Evaluation** See Technique 37–1.

References

Fuchs PL: Streamlining your suctioning techniques, part 1: Nasotracheal suctioning. *Nursing 84* (May) 1984; 14:55–61.

Nursing 80 Photobook Series: *Providing Respiratory Care.* Intermed Communications, 1979.

Sandham G, Reid B: Some Q's and A's about suctioning with an illustrated guide to better techniques. *Nursing 77* (October) 1977; 7:60–65.

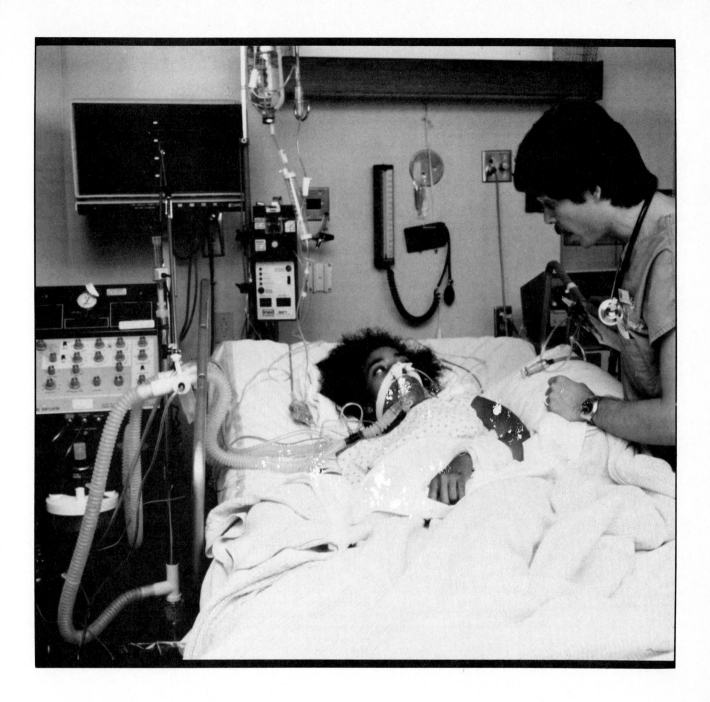

OXYGEN THERAPY

38

Oxygen therapy is administered not only in emergency situations but also when the patient's need is less acute. In emergency situations oxygen is given immediately by whatever method is readily available. In nonemergency situations the route of administration is ordered and takes the patient's special needs into account.

Patients who are dyspneic are frequently anxious. Shortness of breath is frightening, because breathing is necessary for life and because dyspnea may be caused by cardiac disease. A very important aspect of all oxygen therapy is to be supportive of the patient and support persons. The nurse can offer information and reassurance to allay fears about lack of oxygen or about the therapy.

Chapter Outline

Methods of Oxygen Administration

Safety Precautions during Oxygen Administration

Objectives

Upon completion of this chapter, the student will:

1. Know essential terms and facts about oxygen therapy
   1.1 Define selected terms
   1.2 List various methods used to administer oxygen
   1.3 Outline safety precautions necessary during oxygen therapy
2. Understand facts about oxygen therapy techniques
   2.1 Identify relevant assessment data
   2.2 Identify nursing diagnoses for which the technique may be implemented
   2.3 Identify nursing goals related to the technique
   2.4 Identify expected and unexpected outcomes from assessment data
   2.5 Identify reasons underlying selected steps of the technique
3. Perform oxygen therapy techniques safely
   3.1 Assess the patient adequately
   3.2 Collect additional data from appropriate sources
   3.3 Select pertinent nursing goals for the patient
   3.4 Establish relevant outcome criteria for the patient following the technique
   3.5 Collect necessary equipment before the technique
   3.6 Implement interventions to enhance the effectiveness of the technique and enhance the patient's comfort and safety
   3.7 Communicate relevant information about the patient to the appropriate persons
   3.8 Determine the evaluative outcomes of the technique
4. Evaluate own performance of specific oxygen therapy techniques in a laboratory or clinical setting with the assistance of another
   4.1 Use the performance checklists provided
   4.2 Identify areas of strength and weakness
   4.3 Alter performance in response to own evaluation and that of another

Terms

■ bubbling   gurgling sounds as air passes through moist secretions in the respiratory tract

■ Cheyne-Stokes breathing   rhythmic waxing and waning of respirations from very deep breathing to very shallow breathing and temporary apnea, often associated with cardiac failure, increased intracranial pressure, or brain damage

■ cyanosis   a bluish color of the mucous membranes, nail beds, or skin, due to excessive deoxygenation of hemoglobin

■ dyspnea   difficult and labored breathing in which the patient has a persistent unsatisfied need for air and feels distressed

■ flail chest   the ballooning out of the chest wall through injured rib spaces during exhalation and depression or indrawing of the wall during inhalation

■ hypercarbia (hypercapnia)   excess carbon dioxide in the blood

■ hypocarbia (hypocapnia)   reduced carbon dioxide in the blood

■ hypoxemia   deficient oxygenation of the blood measured by laboratory means

■ hypoxia   diminished availability of oxygen for the body tissues, due to internal or external causes

■ nonproductive cough   a dry, harsh cough without secretions

■ orthopnea   ability to breathe only in the upright position, ie, sitting or standing

■ productive cough   a cough in which secretions are expectorated

- **tachycardia**   an excessively rapid heart rate, over 100 beats/min in an adult
- **tachypnea**   rapid respiration marked by quick, shallow breaths
- **tracheal tug**   indrawing and downward pulling of the trachea during inhalation

- **wheeze**   a whistling respiratory sound of exhalation that usually indicates some narrowing of the bronchial tree

METHODS OF OXYGEN ADMINISTRATION

Oxygen is supplied in hospitals in two ways: by liquid portable systems (cylinders) or from wall outlets. Oxygen cylinders are made of steel. Large ones contain 244 cubic feet of oxygen, stored at a pressure of 2,200 pounds per square inch (psi). Smaller cylinders that are readily portable on stretchers are often used. Piped-in oxygen is stored at much lower pressure, usually 50 to 60 psi.

Oxygen that is administered from a cylinder or wall outlet system is dry. When dry gases are given to patients, dehydration of the respiratory mucous membranes occurs. Humidifying devices are thus an essential adjunct of oxygen therapy. See chapter 36.

Using Oxygen Cylinders

Oxygen cylinders are generally encased in metal carriers equipped with wheels for transport and a broad flat base on which the cylinder stands at the bedside to prevent it from falling. A cap on the top protects the valves and outlets. Oxygen cylinders should be placed near the head of the bed and away from traffic areas and heaters. A regulator and a humidifier must be attached before the cylinder is used. The purpose of the regulator is to reduce the pressure in the oxygen cylinder to a safe level. The regulator consists of two parts: a flowmeter and a pressure reducing valve. The flowmeter regulates the gas flow in liters per minute. Two types of regulators are shown in Figure 38–1.

To assemble the oxygen cylinder for use:

1. Remove the protector cap.

2. Remove any dust in the outlets by slightly opening the handwheel at the top of the cylinder. See Figure 38–2. Turn the handwheel clockwise slowly, and then close it quickly. This is called *cracking the cylinder*. People can be frightened if not forewarned of the loud hissing sound that it makes.

FIGURE 38–1 ■ Two types of oxygen regulators: **A,** Thorpe tube; **B,** Bourdon tube.

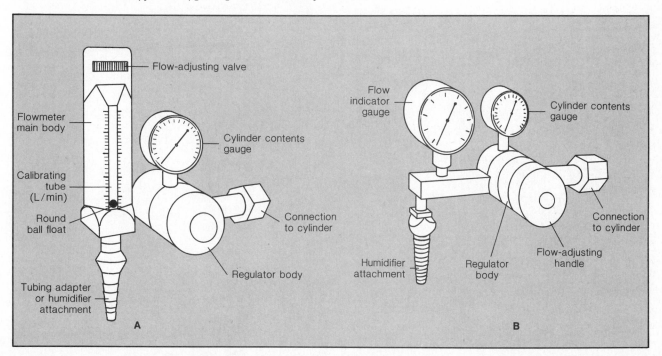

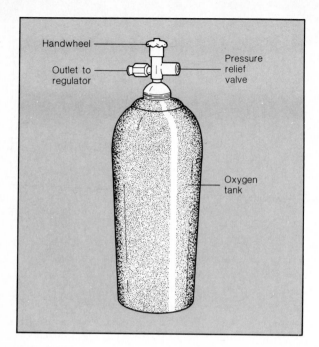

FIGURE 38–2 ■ The basic parts of an oxygen tank.

3. Connect the flow regulator gauge to the cylinder outlet, and tighten the inlet nut with a wrench. This will ensure that the regulator is held firmly.

4. Stand at the side of the cylinder and open the cylinder valve very slowly until it is fully open. Then turn it back one quarter turn.

5. Regulate the flowmeter to the desired rate of flow in

FIGURE 38–3 ■ An oxygen flowmeter attached to a wall outlet.

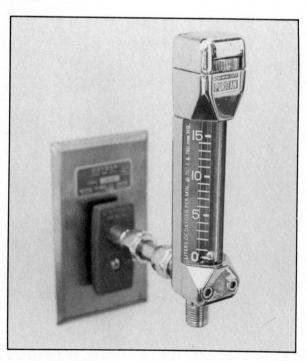

liters per minute. For the Thorpe tube, turn the flow-adjusting valve. For the Bourdon tube, turn the flow-adjusting handle slowly clockwise.

6. Fill the humidifier bottle with distilled water to the mark indicated, and attach it below the flowmeter. On humidifying devices, see chapter 36, page 865.

7. Attach the specific oxygen tubing and equipment prescribed for the patient, eg, nasal catheter, nasal cannula, or face mask.

Using Wall-Outlet Oxygen

For oxygen piped in to a wall outlet, only a flowmeter and a humidifier are required.

1. Attach the flowmeter to the wall outlet, exerting firm pressure. The flowmeter should be in the off position. See Figure 38–3.

2. Fill the humidifier bottle with distilled water. (This can be done before coming to the bedside.)

3. Attach the humidifier bottle to the base of the flowmeter. See Figure 38–4.

4. Attach the prescribed oxygen tubing and delivery device to the humidifier.

5. Regulate the flowmeter to the prescribed level.

FIGURE 38–4 ■ An oxygen humidifier attached to the base of the flowmeter.

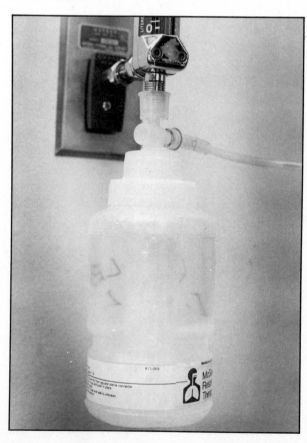

Delivery Devices

Oxygen is administered by either low-flow or high-flow systems. Both systems can deliver oxygen as well as room air. The fraction of inspired oxygen (FiO_2) is variable, depending on the patient's respiratory rate and volume and the oxygen liter flow. A low-flow system is contraindicated where a patient requires a carefully monitored oxygen concentration. Low-flow administration devices include: nasal cannula, simple face mask, nasal catheter, partial rebreathing mask, nonrebreathing mask, Croupette, and oxygen tent.

A high-flow oxygen system delivers all the gas required by the patient. It provides a precise amount of oxygen, regardless of the patient's respirations. The ratio of room air to oxygen is regulated and does not vary with the patient's respirations. High-flow administration devices include the Venturi mask.

Some devices can be used for both low- and high-flow administration, eg, the face tent, oxygen hood, and incubator (Isolette).

Oxygen Analyzers

Oxygen analyzers (see Figure 38–5) measure the concentration of oxygen being received by the patient. The analyzer is first used to measure the concentration of oxygen in the room. It should register 0.21 (21%). If it does not, the nurse adjusts the dial to this calibration. Then the sampling tube is placed next to the patient's nose, and the reading on the analyzer is monitored. The nurse adjusts the oxygen flow rate to obtain the desired fraction of inspired oxygen (FiO_2).

SAFETY PRECAUTIONS DURING OXYGEN THERAPY

Oxygen alone will not burn or explode, but it does facilitate combustion. For example, a bed sheet ordinarily burns slowly when ignited in the atmosphere; however, if saturated with free-flowing oxygen and ignited by a spark, it will burn rapidly and explosively. The greater the concentration of the oxygen, the more rapidly fires start and burn, and such fires are difficult to extinguish. Because oxygen is colorless, odorless, and tasteless, people

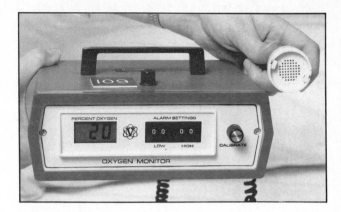

FIGURE 38–5   ■   An oxygen analyzer.

are often unaware of its presence. Safety measures must therefore be taken by the staff, the patient, and visitors. These include:

1. Placing cautionary signs, "No Smoking: Oxygen in Use," on the patient's door, at the foot or head of the bed, and on the oxygen equipment.

2. Removing matches and cigarette lighters from the bedside.

3. Requesting other patients in the room and visitors to smoke in areas provided elsewhere in the hospital.

4. Removing or storing electric equipment, such as razors, hearing aids, radios, televisions, and heating pads, in case short-circuit sparks occur.

5. Avoiding materials that generate static electricity, such as woolen blankets or synthetic fabrics. Cotton blankets are used, and nurses are advised to wear cotton fabrics.

6. Avoiding the use of volatile, flammable materials, such as oils, greases, alcohol, or ether, near patients receiving oxygen. Lip ointments, if required, should have a water-soluble base such as K-Y jelly or glycerin. Alcohol back rubs are avoided, and nail polish removers or the like are taken away from the immediate vicinity.

7. Grounding electric monitoring equipment, suction machines, and portable diagnostic machines. Oxygen therapy should be discontinued temporarily if portable radiographic equipment is required. Monitoring and suction equipment is placed on the bedside opposite the oxygen source.

8. Making known the location of fire extinguishers and making sure personnel are trained in their use.

TECHNIQUE 38–1   ■   Administering Oxygen by Cannula

The nasal cannula (nasal prongs) is the most common device used to administer oxygen. It consists of a rubber or plastic tube that extends around the face, with 0.6- to 1.3-cm (¼- to ½-in) curved prongs that fit into the nostrils. One side of the tube connects to the oxygen tubing and oxygen supply. The cannula is often held in place by an elastic band that fits around the patient's head or under the chin. See Figure 38–6. For patients who are confused or particularly active, it may be helpful to secure the cannula in place with small pieces of tape on each side of the face.

The nasal cannula is easy to apply and does not interfere with the patient's ability to eat or talk. It also is relatively comfortable and permits some freedom of movement. It delivers a relatively low concentration of oxygen (23% to 44%) at flow rates of 2 to 6 L/min. Higher concentrations and flow rates can be administered; however, above 6 L/min there is a tendency for the patient to swallow air and for the nasal and pharyngeal mucosa to become irritated.

■ Assessment

Assess the patient for:

1. Vital signs for baseline data.

FIGURE 38–6 ■ **A,** A nasal cannula; **B,** the cannula in place.

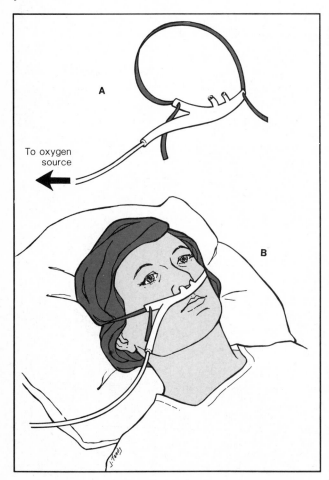

To oxygen source

2. Clinical signs of hypoxia: tachycardia, tachypnea, restlessness, dyspnea, cyanosis, and confusion. Tachycardia and tachypnea are often early signs. Confusion is a later sign of severe oxygen deprivation.

3. Clinical signs of hypercarbia: restlessness, hypertension, headache, lethargy, tremor.

4. Lung sounds audible by auscultating the chest and by ear.

5. Clinical signs of oxygen toxicity: tracheal irritation and cough, dyspnea, and decreased pulmonary ventilation.

Other data include:

1. Levels of oxygen (PaO_2) and carbon dioxide ($PaCO_2$) in the arterial blood. PaO_2 is normally 80 to 100 mm Hg. $PaCO_2$ is normally 34 to 46 mm Hg.

2. The order for the oxygen, including the administering device and the rate (L/min).

3. Whether the patient has chronic obstructive pulmonary disease (COPD). Low-flow oxygen systems are essential for these individuals. A high carbon dioxide level in the blood is the normal stimulus to breathe. However, patients with COPD may have a high carbon dioxide level, and their stimulus to breathe is hypoxemia. Low flows of oxygen (2 L/min) stimulate breathing for such patients by maintaining slight hypoxemia. This is dependent upon the patient's inspiratory flow and normal ventilation. During continuous oxygen administration, PaO_2 and $PaCO_2$ are measured periodically to monitor hypoxemia and adjust the liter flow as needed.

■ Planning

Nursing goal

To deliver a relatively low concentration of oxygen.

Equipment

1. An oxygen supply with a flowmeter
2. A humidifier with sterile distilled water
3. A nasal cannula and tubing
4. Tape, if needed, to secure the cannula in place
5. Gauzes to pad the tubing over the cheekbones

■ Intervention

1. Assist the patient to a semi-Fowler's position if possible.
    Rationale This position permits easier chest expansion and hence easier breathing.

2. Explain that oxygen is not dangerous when safety

precautions are observed and that it will ease the discomfort of dyspnea. Inform the patient and support persons about the safety precautions connected with oxygen use.

3. Set up the oxygen equipment and the humidifier. See page 894.

4. Turn on the oxygen at the flow rate ordered. A relatively low concentration of oxygen (23% to 44%) will be obtained at a flow rate of 2 to 6 L/min for patients who have a regular respiratory pattern, a respiratory rate less than 25 breaths per minute, and a tidal volume of 300 to 700 mL. Higher concentrations and flow rates can be administered, but above 6 L/min there is a tendency for the patient to swallow air and experience irritation of the nasal and pharyngeal mucosa.

5. Check that the oxygen is flowing freely through the tubing. There should be no kinks in the tubing, and the connections should be airtight. There should be bubbles in the humidifier as the oxygen flows through the water. You should feel the oxygen at the outlets of the cannula.

6. Put the cannula over the patient's face, with the outlet prongs fitting into the nares and the elastic band around the head. Some models have a strap to adjust under the chin. Make sure the prongs are turned upward so the oxygen is directed into the nasal passages and not into the tissues at the base of the nares. See Figure 38–7.

7. If the cannula will not stay in place, tape it at the sides of the face. Slip gauze pads under the tubing over the cheekbones to prevent skin irritation.

8. Assess the patient's immediate response to the oxygen, in terms of color, respirations, discomfort, etc, and provide support for adjusting to the cannula.

9. Assess the patient's response to the therapy in 15 to 30 minutes, depending on the patient's condition, and regularly thereafter. Assess vital signs, color, breathing patterns, and chest movements.

10. Make sure that safety precautions are being followed.

11. Check the liter flow and the level of water in the humidifier in 30 minutes and whenever providing care to the patient.

12. Assess the patient regularly for clinical signs of hypoxia: tachycardia, confusion, dyspnea, restlessness, and cyanosis.

13. Assess the patient's nares for encrustations and irritation. Apply a water-soluble lubricant as required to soothe the mucous membranes.

14. Record initiation of the therapy and the patient's response to it.

Sample Recording

Date	Time	Notes
12/5/86	0730	O₂ by cannula at 3 L/min. P 96, R 24. Slightly cyanotic, dyspneic on exertion, and restless. ——— Susan de Camillis, SN
	0800	Cyanosis improved. P 84, R 16. Dyspnea and restlessness reduced.——— ——— Susan de Camillis, SN

■ Evaluation

Expected outcomes

1. Vital signs normal for the patient
2. Absence of clinical signs of hypoxia
3. Absence of clinical signs of hypercarbia
4. Lung sounds improved or normal
5. Blood gas levels normal

FIGURE 38–7

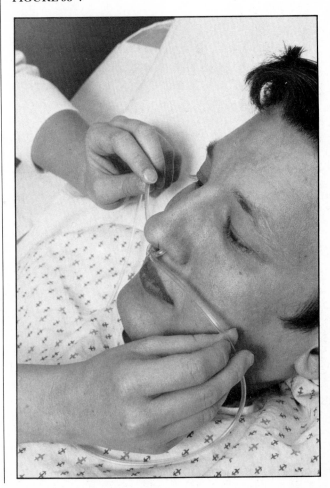

Unexpected outcomes

1. Presence of clinical signs of hypoxia
2. Presence of clinical signs of hypercarbia
3. Decreased blood oxygen level as O$_2$ flow is increased

Upon obtaining an unexpected outcome:

1. Report your findings to the responsible nurse.
2. Adjust the nursing care plan appropriately.

TECHNIQUE 38–2 ■ Administering Oxygen by Mask

Face masks that cover the patient's nose and mouth may be used for oxygen inhalation. Most masks are made of clear, pliable plastic or rubber that can be molded to fit the face. They are held to the patient's head with elastic bands. Some have a metal clip that can be bent over the bridge of the nose for a snug fit. There are several holes in the sides of the mask (exhalation ports) to allow the escape of exhaled carbon dioxide.

Some masks have *reservoir bags,* which provide higher oxygen concentrations to the patient. A portion of the patient's expired air is directed into the bag. Because this air comes from the upper respiratory passages (eg, the trachea and bronchi) where it does not take part in gaseous exchange, its oxygen concentration remains the same as that of inspired air.

A variety of oxygen masks are marketed:

1. The *simple face mask* (low-flow system) delivers oxygen concentrations from 40% to 60% at liter flows of 5 to 8 L/min. See Figure 38–8.
2. The *partial rebreather mask* (low-flow system) delivers oxygen concentrations of 35% to 60% at liter flows of 6 to 15 L/min. See Figure 38–9. The oxygen reservoir bag that is attached allows the patient to rebreathe about the first third of the exhaled air. The partial rebreather bag must not totally deflate during inspiration. If this problem occurs, increase the liter flow of oxygen.
3. The *nonrebreather mask* (low-flow system) delivers the highest oxygen concentration possible by means

FIGURE 38–8 ■ A simple face mask for a low-flow oxygen system.

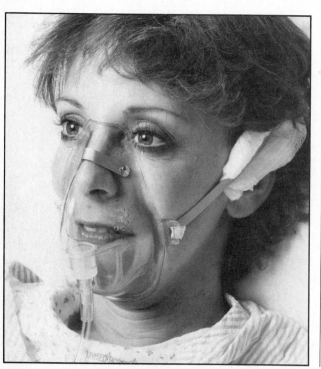

FIGURE 38–9 ■ A partial rebreathing mask for a low-flow oxygen system.

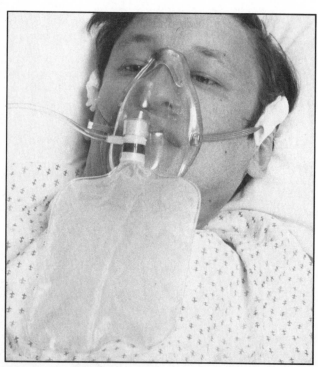

other than intubation or mechanical ventilation, ie, 60% to 90% at liter flows of 6 to 15 L/min. See Figure 38–10. Using a nonrebreather mask, the patient breathes only the source gas from the bag. One-way valves on the mask and between the reservoir bag and the mask prevent the room air and the patient's exhaled air from entering the bag. The nonrebreather bag must not totally deflate during inspiration. If it does, this problem can be corrected by increasing the liter flow of oxygen.

4. The *Venturi mask* (high-flow system) delivers oxygen concentrations precise to within 1% and is often used for patients with COPD. See Figure 38–11. Oxygen concentrations vary from 24% to 40% or 50%, depending on the brand, at liter flows of 4 to 8 L/min. The Venturi mask is designed with wide-bore tubing and various color-coded jet adapters. Each color code corresponds to a precise oxygen concentration and a specific liter flow. For example, a blue adapter delivers a 24% concentration of oxygen at 4 L/min, while a green adapter delivers a 35% concentration of oxygen at 8 L/min. Optional humidification adapters are also available for patients who require them, eg, those receiving oxygen concentrations in excess of 30%.

The Venturi system operates as follows:

1. Oxygen enters the tubing at a prescribed flow rate.
2. When the gas reaches the jet adapter of the Venturi device, which is essentially a restricted orifice, the velocity of the oxygen increases to maintain the same (prescribed) flow rate.
3. As the velocity of the gas increases, less pressure is exerted at the jet outlet.
4. With less pressure, the higher pressure room air is drawn in through the air entrainment ports.
5. This room air dilutes the oxygen to a certain concentration (the percentage specified for the particular jet adapter).

The amount of air drawn in is determined by the size of the orifice (jet adapter). The smaller the orifice, the greater the increase in velocity of oxygen, the greater the decrease in tubing pressure, and the larger the amount of room air drawn in through the entrainment ports. Thus, the narrower the jet adapter, the greater the air dilution, and the lower the concentration of oxygen.

When using a Venturi mask it is important to prevent occlusion of the air entrainment ports by bed linen, clothing, or other objects. Blood gas measurements are taken frequently to monitor the effectiveness of therapy. Changes in the blood gas measurements may necessitate changing the jet adapter and the oxygen concentration.

■ **Assessment**   See Technique 38–1 on page 895.

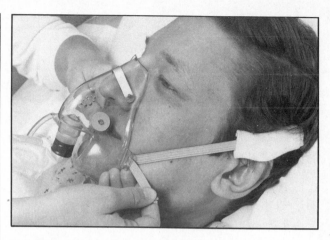

FIGURE 38–10 ■ A nonrebreathing mask for a low-flow or a high-flow oxygen system.

■ **Planning**

Nursing goal

To provide a higher concentration of oxygen and/or humidity to the patient than is provided by cannula or catheter.

Equipment

1. An oxygen supply with a flowmeter
2. A humidifier with sterile distilled water

FIGURE 38–11 ■ A Venturi mask for a high-flow oxygen system.

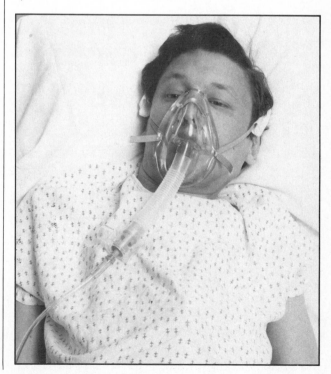

3. A prescribed face mask of the appropriate size for the patient

4. Padding for the elastic band

■ Intervention

1. Follow Technique 38–1, steps 1–3. Encourage the patient to handle the mask.

2. Guide the mask toward the patient's face, and apply it from the nose downward.

3. Turn on the oxygen to the prescribed liter flow.

4. Fit the mask to the contours of the patient's face.
   Rationale The mask should mold to the face, so that very little oxygen escapes into the patient's eyes or around the cheeks and chin.

5. Secure the elastic band around the patient's head so that the mask is comfortable but snug.

6. Pad the band behind the ears and over bony prominences.
   Rationale Padding will prevent irritation from the mask.

7. Assess the patient's immediate response to the oxygen, and provide support for adjusting to the mask.

8. Follow Technique 38–1, steps 9–12 and 14, on page 897.

■ Evaluation   See Technique 38–1 on page 897.

TECHNIQUE 38–3 ■ Administering Oxygen by Face Tent

Face tents can replace oxygen masks when masks are poorly tolerated by patients (eg, children). When a face tent is used alone to supply oxygen, the concentration of oxygen varies; therefore, it is often used in conjunction with a Venturi system.

■ Assessment   See Technique 38–1 on page 896.

■ Planning

Nursing goals

1. To provide high humidity

2. To provide oxygen when a mask is poorly tolerated

FIGURE 38–12 ■ An oxygen face tent.

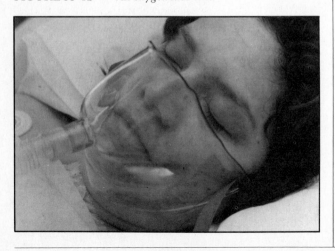

3. To provide a high flow of oxygen when attached to a Venturi system

4. To provide high humidity in conjunction with a nasal cannula

Equipment

1. An oxygen supply with a flowmeter

2. A humidifier with sterile distilled water

3. A face tent of the appropriate size (see Figure 38–12)

■ Intervention

1. Follow Technique 38–1, steps 1–3. Encourage the patient to handle the face tent.

2. Place the tent over the patient's face, and secure the ties around the head.

3. Turn on the oxygen at the prescribed flow rate. Face tents can provide a 30% to 55% concentration of oxygen at 4 to 8 L/min.

4. Assess the patient's immediate response to the oxygen, and provide support for adjusting to the face tent.

5. Follow Technique 38–1, steps 9–12.

6. Inspect the facial skin frequently for dampness or chafing, and dry and treat it as needed.

7. Record initiation of the therapy and the patient's response to it.

■ Evaluation   See Technique 38–1 on page 897.

TECHNIQUE 38–4   ■   Administering Oxygen by Catheter

The nasal catheter (low-flow device) is a rubber or plastic tube about 39 cm (16 in) long, with six or eight holes at the tip to disperse the oxygen. See Figure 38–13. It is used to administer low to moderate concentrations of oxygen, but it can deliver higher concentrations than the nasal cannula. At flows of 1 to 5 L/min, the catheter can deliver concentrations of oxygen of 30% to 35%. It allows the same mobility for the patient as the cannula.

Major problems associated with nasal catheters are laryngeal ulceration, from the constant flow of oxygen into the larynx, and gastric distention, caused by air and oxygen entering the stomach. Gastric distention can be relieved by inserting a nasogastric tube. See Technique 31–3 in chapter 31. Laryngeal ulceration may be prevented by moving the catheter from one nostril to the other every eight hours (Fuchs, 1980, p 39).

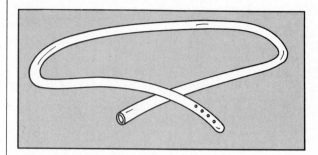

FIGURE 38–13   ■   A nasal catheter.

■ **Assessment**   See Technique 38–1 on page 896.

■ **Planning**

Nursing goals

1. To deliver a low flow of oxygen
2. To prevent irritation of the mucosa of the nares and the larynx

Equipment

1. A nasal catheter of the appropriate size: #8 or #10 Fr. for children; #10 or #12 Fr. for women; #12 or #14 Fr. for men
2. An oxygen supply with a flowmeter
3. A humidifier with sterile distilled water
4. Water-soluble lubricating jelly to facilitate catheter insertion and a gauze square to apply it
5. Adhesive tape (nonallergenic is preferred) to secure catheter to the patient's face
6. A flashlight and a tongue blade for assessing correct placement of the catheter
7. A container of sterile water to test the oxygen flow

■ **Intervention**

1. Follow Technique 38–1, steps 1–3. Test the oxygen flow by turning on the flowmeter to 3 L/min and inserting the tip of the catheter into a container of sterile water. Bubbling indicates that oxygen is flowing.
2. Determine how deeply to insert the catheter by placing the end of the catheter in a straight line

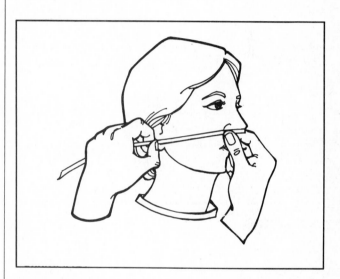

FIGURE 38–14

between the tip of the patient's nose and the earlobe. See Figure 38–14. This distance can be marked with tape.

Rationale   This external distance approximates the distance from the nares to the oropharynx.

3. Lubricate the tip of the catheter with water-soluble jelly. Squeeze the lubricant onto a gauze square, and rotate the catheter tip through it. Do not use mineral oil or petroleum jelly.

Rationale   Lubrication facilitates insertion and prevents injury to the nasal mucosa. If aspirated, mineral oil or petroleum jelly can cause severe lung irritations or lipoid pneumonia.

4. Start the flow of oxygen at about 3 L/min prior to inserting the tube.

Rationale   The flow of oxygen prevents the catheter from becoming plugged by secretions during insertion.

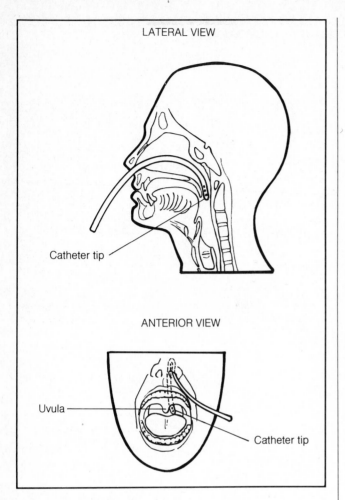

LATERAL VIEW

Catheter tip

ANTERIOR VIEW

Uvula

Catheter tip

FIGURE 38–15

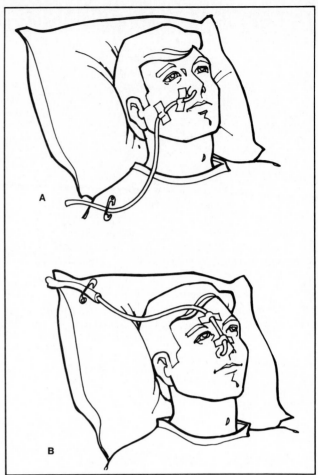

A

B

FIGURE 38–16

5. Introduce the catheter slowly through one nostril until the tip is at the entrance to the oropharynx (the marked distance). See Figure 38–15, *A*. Look into the patient's mouth, using the flashlight and tongue blade, to check placement. The tip of the catheter will be visible through the mouth beside the uvula. See Figure 38–15, *B*.

6. Withdraw the tip slightly so that it can no longer be seen.

    Rationale When the catheter is in this position, the patient is less likely to swallow oxygen.

7. Tape the catheter to the patient's face at the side of the nose and the cheek (see Figure 38–16, *A*) or at the tip of the nose and the forehead (see Figure 38–16, *B*). Pin the tubing to the patient's pillow or gown, leaving slack in the tubing.

    Rationale If taped and pinned, the catheter will not be displaced when the patient moves. Slack allows the patient to move without pulling on the tubing.

8. Adjust the flow to the prescribed rate.

9. Assess the patient's immediate response to the oxygen, and provide support for adjusting to the catheter.

10. Follow Technique 38–1, steps 9–12.

11. Record the initiation of oxygen therapy and the patient's response, including the method and the flow rate.

■ **Evaluation**   See Technique 38–1 on page 897.

TECHNIQUE 38–5   ■   Administering Oxygen by Humidity Tent (Croupette)

A variety of humidity/oxygen tents are available for small children. Each unit generally comes with the manufacturer's instructions for use. However, all have common elements. The tent consists of a rectangular, clear, plastic canopy with outlets that connect to an oxygen or compressed air source and to a humidifier that moisturizes the air or oxygen. The Croupette humidity tent is commonly used. See Figure 38–17. It also has an ice trough that cools the air.

■ Assessment

See Technique 38–1 on page 896. Other data include:

1. Whether the damper valve is to be kept open, kept partially open, or intermittently closed and opened.
2. Whether aerosol medications are to be administered. Check the physician's orders.

■ Planning

Nursing goals

1. To facilitate the patient's breathing by humidifying respiratory membranes and loosening secretions
2. To increase blood oxygenation levels if oxygen is prescribed
3. To cool the body and reduce the fever that accompanies a respiratory infection

Equipment

1. A Croupette tent with frame
2. Ice
3. An oxygen supply and flowmeter
4. Sterile distilled water to moisturize the air or the oxygen
5. A nebulizer, if required, and any aerosol medications
6. Gauze strips
7. Additional gowns and bath blankets

■ Intervention

1. Follow Technique 38–1, steps 1–3. Provide an explanation appropriate to the age of the child, and offer emotional support. Provide the child with a suitable toy, one that will not cause static electricity.
2. Cover the child with a gown or a cotton blanket. Some agencies provide gowns with hoods, or a small towel may be wrapped around the head.

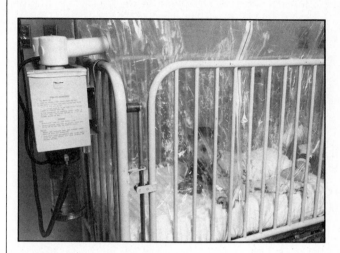

FIGURE 38–17 ■ A Croupette.

Rationale   The child needs protection from chilling and from the dampness and condensation in the tent.

3. Prepare the Croupette before putting the child inside it. Attach the metal frame that supports the canopy to the upper third of the bedsprings, using gauze strips.
4. Close the zippers on each side of the tent.
5. Fanfold the front part of the canopy into the bedclothes or into an overlying drawsheet, and ensure that all sides of the canopy are tucked well under the mattress. See Figure 38–18.
6. Fill the trough with ice to the depth indicated by a line on the trough.
7. Ensure that the drainage tube for the trough is securely in place in the elevated notch or opening provided, until drainage is required.
8. Unscrew the cap on the water jar, and fill the jar with sterile distilled water up to the black line. Reattach the jar.
9. Attach the tube to the oxygen or compressed air source. Attach the other end to the water jar.
10. Flood the tent with oxygen by setting the flowmeter at 15 L/min for about five minutes.
11. Open the damper valve, located on the large tube between the trough and the tent, for about five minutes, to bring the humidity to 100%. This valve controls the mist output. In accordance with the physician's orders, it may be left open for continuous operation, left partially open, or opened periodically and then closed to minimize condensation.
12. Adjust the oxygen flowmeter to deliver the required amount of oxygen.

13. Place the child in the Croupette tent.

14. Make sure that the oxygen safety precautions have been followed.

15. Assess the child's response to the therapy in 15 to 30 minutes, depending on the child's condition, and regularly thereafter. Assess vital signs, color, breathing patterns, and chest movements.

16. Check the liter flow and the level of the water in the humidifier in 30 minutes and whenever providing care to the patient. Monitor the oxygen concentration regularly, ie, at least every four hours, using an analyzer.

17. Assess the child regularly for clinical signs of hypoxia, eg, tachycardia, confusion, dyspnea, restlessness, and cyanosis.

18. Record on the patient's chart initiation of the therapy and the patient's response to it.

Physical care of a child in a Croupette

A child in a Croupette requires protection from chilling, frequent observation, maintenance of the equipment, and safety precautions in using the oxygen (see page 895).

19. Observe the child frequently for signs of hypoxia to assess the child's response to the therapy. See step 17.

20. Change the bed linen and clothing as they become damp.

21. Place a small pillow or rolled towel at the head of the Croupette to prevent bruising or bumping of the child's head. This padding also helps to absorb excess moisture.

22. When administering care, be sure to maintain the humidity of the air and oxygen therapy. The canopy can be moved up around the infant's head and neck and secured under a pillow while providing care.

23. Maintain the equipment regularly. Drain the water from the ice trough. Replenish the ice and the distilled water.

24. Monitor air and oxygen flows frequently to maintain required concentrations, and ensure that all connections are airtight.

25. Maintain the temperature of the Croupette at 20 to 21 °C (68 to 70 °F). Check this by placing a bath thermometer inside the canopy.

FIGURE 38–18

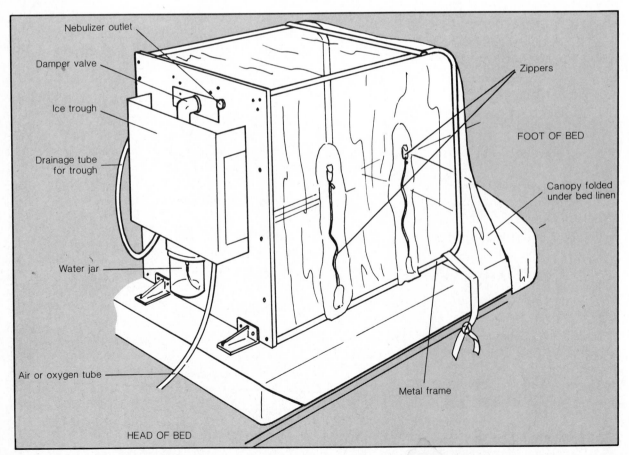

■ Evaluation

Expected outcomes

1. Productive cough
2. Normal temperature

See also Technique 38–1 on page 897.

Unexpected outcomes

1. Dry, nonproductive cough
2. Fever unabated

See also Technique 38–1. Upon obtaining an unexpected outcome:

1. Report your findings to the responsible nurse and/or physician.
2. Adjust the nursing care plan to include regular assessment and appropriate care.

TECHNIQUE 38–6   ■   Administering Oxygen by Incubator (Isolette)

An incubator is a self-contained unit that controls the temperature, humidity, and oxygen concentration for an infant. See Figure 38–19. It is a low-flow or high-flow system, delivering oxygen concentrations of 35% to 40% with the flag up and 80% to 100% with the flag down, depending upon the oxygen liter flow. It can be used with an oxygen hood to provide precise oxygen concentrations. See Technique 38–7.

■ Assessment   See Technique 38–1 on page 896.

■ Planning

Nursing goals

1. To facilitate the patient's breathing by humidifying the inspired air
2. To increase blood oxygenation levels
3. To provide a controlled temperature

Equipment

1. An incubator with a mattress
2. An oxygen supply and flowmeter
3. Ice, if the temperature in the incubator is to be cooled
4. Sterile distilled water to moisturize the air
5. Additional sheets, gowns, and diapers for the infant

■ Intervention

1. Follow Technique 38–1, steps 1–4. Provide an explanation appropriate to the support persons.

Provide the infant with a suitable toy and reassurance.

Rationale   The toy must not produce static electricity, which could cause fire in the presence of oxygen.

FIGURE 38–19   ■   An incubator (Isolette).

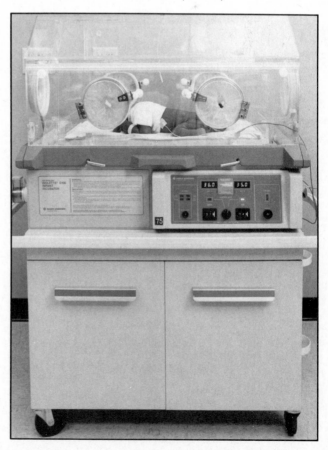

2. Set up the incubator before putting the infant in it. Cover the mattress with a sheet.

3. Plug in the incubator. The light on the front should be on when the incubator is working.

4. Set the temperature control dial to the ordered temperature. Add ice to the ice chamber if the temperature in the incubator is to be below the room temperature.

5. Set the humidity control dial to the ordered setting. Fill the humidity chamber with sterile distilled water. Replenish the water periodically as needed.

6. Connect the oxygen tubing to the outlet, and set the flow rate to the ordered level, usually 6 to 10 L/min. Flood the incubator with oxygen for five minutes to attain the desired concentration. Check the concentration with an oxygen analyzer.

7. If an aerosol mist is ordered, place the medication in the aerosol nebulizer.

8. Place the infant in the incubator.

9. Provide care through the portholes at the sides of the incubator. Open the portholes only when absolutely necessary.

   Rationale Oxygen escapes when the portholes are open, thus lowering the concentration inside the incubator.

10. Change the sheets and clothing as they become damp or soiled.

11. Assess the infant's response in 15 to 30 minutes, depending on the child's condition, and regularly thereafter.

12. Check the oxygen liter flow and monitor the oxygen concentration regularly.

13. Record on the infant's record the initiation of therapy and the patient's response.

■ **Evaluation**   See Technique 38–1 on page 897.

TECHNIQUE 38–7 ■ Administering Oxygen by Hood

An oxygen hood is a rigid plastic dome that encloses an infant's head. See Figure 38–20. It is both a low-flow and a high-flow delivery system and provides precise oxygen levels. It can also provide high humidity.

■ **Assessment**   See Technique 38–1 on page 896.

FIGURE 38–20 ■ An oxygen hood.

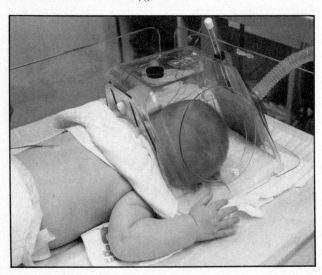

■ **Planning**

Nursing goals

1. To facilitate the patient's breathing by humidifying the inspired air

2. To increase blood oxygenation levels if oxygen is ordered

Equipment

1. An oxygen hood

2. An oxygen source with a flowmeter, tubing, and a nebulizer

3. Sterile distilled water and any medication ordered for the nebulizer

4. A towel or foam rubber to pad the hood

5. Additional diapers, sheets, and towels

■ **Intervention**

1. Follow Technique 38–1, steps 1–4.

2. Fill the nebulizer, and attach it to the oxygen tubing.

3. Turn on the oxygen to the ordered flow rate, and check the mist being produced.

4. Place the hood over the infant's head, and pad the hood with a towel or foam rubber around the neck.
   Rationale The padding prevents oxygen leakage and protects the infant's neck.

5. Assess the infant's response to the therapy in 15 to 30 minutes and regularly as needed thereafter. See Technique 38–1, step 12.

6. Change the bedding around the infant's head whenever it becomes damp.

7. Empty any condensation buildup in the tubing as necessary, eg, every two hours.

8. If a heated nebulizer is used, check the temperature in the hood as necessary, eg, every three hours. The temperature should remain between 34.4 and 35.6 °C (94 and 96 °F).

9. Remove the hood for feeding the infant.

10. Record on the infant's chart initiation of the treatment and the infant's response.

■ **Evaluation**   See Technique 38–1 on page 897.

References

Administering oxygen safely: When, why, how. *Nursing 80* (October) 1980; 10:54–56.

D'Agostino JS: Set your mind at ease on oxygen toxicity. *Nursing 83* (July) 1983; 13:54–56.

Ellmyer P et al: A guide to your patient's safe home use of oxygen. *Nursing 82* (January) 1982; 12:55–57.

Fuchs PL: Getting the best out of oxygen delivery systems. *Nursing 80* (December) 1980; 10:34–43.

Kozier B, Erb G: *Fundamentals of Nursing: Concepts and Procedures,* 2nd ed. Addison-Wesley, 1983.

Swearingen PL: *The Addison-Wesley Photo-Atlas of Nursing Procedures.* Addison-Wesley, 1984.

Worthington L: Hypoxemia. *RN* (May) 1980; 43:48–53.

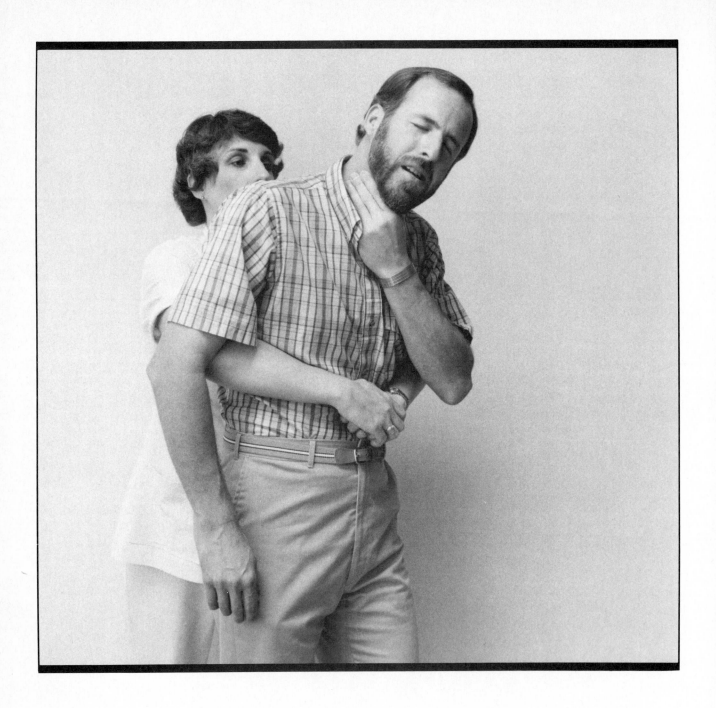

CARDIOPULMONARY RESUSCITATION

39

When a patient's heart and lungs stop functioning, cardiopulmonary resuscitation (CPR) needs to be performed quickly and efficiently. It is a life-saving measure that may be needed in a hospital or anyplace where there are people. A delay of four minutes or more can result in permanent brain damage due to cerebral anoxia. Recognizing the need for CPR and skill in performing it quickly and competently are essential functions of nurses. Increasingly laypersons are also being encouraged to learn CPR. Courses are available at national

Red Cross and Heart Associations throughout the country. Learning to perform these procedures correctly requires instruction from a certified instructor at these associations and supervised practice.

Chapter Outline

Cardiac and Respiratory Arrests

Life Support

CPR in a Hospital

Terminating CPR

■ Technique 39–1 Clearing an Obstructed Airway

■ Technique 39–2 Administering Oral Resuscitation

■ Technique 39–3 Administering External Cardiopulmonary Resuscitation to an Adult in a Health Care Facility

■ Technique 39–4 Administering External Cardiopulmonary Resuscitation to an Infant or Child

Objectives

Upon completion of this chapter, the student will:

1. Know essential terms and facts about cardiopulmonary resuscitation
   1.1 Define selected terms
   1.2 Identify possible causes of airway obstruction
   1.3 Recognize signs indicating an obstructed airway
   1.4 Recognize signs indicating a cardiac arrest
   1.5 Identify various methods of clearing an obstructed airway
   1.6 Identify various methods of providing respiratory resuscitation
   1.7 Identify the location of the carotid pulse
   1.8 Identify the site for cardiac compression in adults, infants, and children
   1.9 Identify the ratio of ventilation to compression for one resuscitator, for two resuscitators, for infants, and for children
2. Understand facts about cardiopulmonary resuscitation techniques
   2.1 Identify relevant assessment data
   2.2 Identify nursing diagnoses for which the technique may be implemented
   2.3 Identify nursing goals related to the technique
   2.4 Identify expected and unexpected outcomes from assessment data

2.5 Identify reasons underlying selected steps of the technique
3. Perform cardiopulmonary resuscitation techniques safely
   3.1 Assess the patient adequately
   3.2 Select pertinent nursing goals for the patient
   3.3 Establish relevant outcome criteria for the patient following the technique
   3.4 Collect necessary equipment before the technique
   3.5 Implement interventions to enhance the effectiveness of the technique and enhance the patient's comfort and safety
   3.6 Communicate relevant information about the patient to the appropriate persons
   3.7 Determine the evaluative outcomes of the technique
4. Evaluate own performance of specific techniques in a laboratory or clinical setting with the assistance of another
   4.1 Use the performance checklists provided
   4.2 Identify areas of strength and weakness
   4.3 Alter performance in response to own evaluation and that of another

Terms

■ airway   a passageway through which air normally circulates; a device that is inserted through the patient's mouth to maintain the patency of an air passage such as the trachea

■ anaphylaxis   an acute allergic reaction

■ anoxia   the absence or a deficiency of oxygen in the tissues

■ cardiac arrest   the cessation of heart function

■ cardiac board   a flat board placed under a patient's

chest when the patient requires cardiac massage while in bed

■ cardiopulmonary resuscitation (CPR)   artificial stimulation of the heart and lungs

■ carotid arteries   major arteries lying on either side of the trachea and larynx

■ pupil   the opening at the center of the iris (colored portion) of the eye

■ respiratory arrest   the sudden cessation of breathing

- **respiratory ventilation** the inhalation of air by artificial means
- **resuscitate** to restore life; to revive
- **sternum** the breastbone, a flat elongated bone lying between the ribs and over the heart
- **xiphoid process** the lower portion of the sternum

CARDIAC AND RESPIRATORY ARRESTS

A *cardiac arrest* is the cessation of cardiac function; the heart stops beating. Often a cardiac arrest is unexpected and sudden. When it occurs, the heart no longer pumps blood to any of the organs of the body. Breathing then stops, and the person becomes unconscious and limp. Within 20 to 40 seconds of a cardiac arrest, the patient is clinically dead. After 4 to 6 minutes, the lack of oxygen supply to the brain causes permanent and extensive damage.

Causes of cardiac arrest are many and include electrocution, myocardial infarction (heart attack), respiratory failure, extensive hemorrhage, and brain injury. The three cardinal signs of a cardiac arrest are apnea, absence of a carotid or femoral pulse, and dilated pupils. The person's skin appears pale or grayish and feels cool. Cyanosis is evident when respiratory function fails prior to heart failure.

A *respiratory* or *pulmonary arrest* is the cessation of breathing. It often occurs as a result of a blocked airway, but it can occur following a cardiac arrest and for other reasons. A respiratory arrest is preceded by short shallow breathing. The breathing becomes increasingly labored. Then the person becomes flushed and disoriented and experiences feelings of suffocation. If the respiratory problem persists, the person becomes cyanotic, becomes comatose, and goes into cardiac arrest. Respiratory arrest leads to cardiac arrest because of the lack of oxygen to vital organs, especially the heart and brain.

LIFE SUPPORT

Resuscitation is restoration to consciousness or life; it includes all measures to revive patients who have stopped breathing due to either respiratory or cardiac failure. *Artificial respiration* (eg, oral resuscitation) is used when the patient's breathing has stopped while the heart continues to beat. *External cardiac compression* or *massage* is used when both the heartbeat and breathing have stopped; then both artificial respiration and external cardiac massage are applied at the same time. These combined measures are often called *cardiopulmonary resuscitation* (CPR) or *basic life support* (BLS). Basic life support must be complemented by a rapid delivery of advanced cardiac life support (ACLS). ACLS includes:

1. Establishing an effective airway: endotracheal intubation is preferable
2. Establishing an IV line
3. Administering epinephrine intravenously
4. Administering sodium bicarbonate
5. Defibrillation
6. Administering other intravenous bolus drug therapy as indicated, eg, atropine, calcium chloride, lidocaine, isoproterenol (Isuprel), norepinephrine (Levophed), or digoxin.

The survival rate from cardiac arrest due to ventricular fibrillation clearly depends upon the promptness of the initiation of CPR and ACLS. Studies show that there is a 43% survival rate if CPR is initiated within four minutes and ACLS within eight minutes. Only 10% survive if ACLS is not initiated until sixteen minutes have elapsed (McIntyre, Lewis, 1983, p 9).

CPR IN A HOSPITAL

Most acute care health agencies have established practices and policies governing cardiopulmonary resuscitation. Nurses need to learn immediately the following information:

1. The agency procedure for external cardiac massage
2. Where the emergency equipment is maintained
3. The agency's method of notification of a cardiac arrest
4. The advised compression rates for adults, children, and infants

Practices commonly include the following:

1. The person who discovers a patient who has had a cardiac arrest is responsible for obtaining assistance. The nurse may simply call out to others or may telephone to the hospital switchboard. The person then starts CPR immediately.
2. Many hospitals have a special team (the crash team) that answers the call. The team usually consists of

physicians and nurses who have had special training in CPR. The team will have a crash cart stocked with the special supplies and equipment required for CPR.

3. Hospitals with a loudspeaker system to summon the special team usually use a code to notify the staff without alarming visitors and patients. Some agencies use a number, such as "99," while others use a color, such as "Blue." The announcement may be "Code Blue West 8" or "Doctor 99 West 8" to tell the members of the team that the cardiac arrest is on the eighth floor of the west wing.

4. When the special team arrives, it takes over the care of the patient. The nursing staff may stay to assist or continue with other nursing responsibilities, depending on the agency's policies.

5. If external cardiac compression does not produce a heartbeat, the physician may decide to defibrillate the patient. There are many types of defibrillators; most function by passing an electric current through the patient's heart to establish normal cardiac rhythm. The two paddles of the defibrillator are lubricated and then placed on the patient's chest: one to the right of the sternum, the other near the apex of the heart along the

left axillary line. The axillary line extends inferiorly from the anterior axillary fold. Before the current is activated, all persons stand away from the patient so as not to receive the electric current from the patient. The effectiveness of the defibrillation can be determined by checking the carotid pulse, the movement of the pupils of the eyes, and the return of respirations.

TERMINATING CPR

A rescuer terminates CPR only when one of the following events occurs:

1. Another person takes over.

2. The patient's heartbeat and breathing are reestablished.

3. Adjunctive life-support measures are initiated.

4. A physician states that the individual is dead and that CPR is to be discontinued.

5. The rescuer becomes exhausted, and there is no one to take over.

TECHNIQUE 39–1   ■   Clearing an Obstructed Airway

There are several possible causes of airway obstruction and, as a result, several different ways of clearing an obstructed airway. Causes include:

1. Aspirated food, mucus plug, or foreign bodies, such as partial dentures or small toys. Food is the most common cause.

2. Unconsciousness or seizures, which cause the tongue to fall back and block the airway.

3. Severe trauma to the nose, mouth, neck, or upper chest.

4. Acute edema of the trachea, from smoke inhalation, facial and neck burns, or anaphylaxis. In these instances, a tracheostomy is often indicated.

■ Assessment

Assess for:

1. Clinical signs that the airway is obstructed: the person clutches at the throat and is unable to speak; wheezes suddenly or has stridor (makes crowing sounds); becomes anxious, restless, and agitated; experiences a feeling of suffocation; has pale or cyanotic skin and/or mucous membranes; has exag-

gerated retractions (indrawing) of the chest wall on inhalation; has tachycardia; is unconscious.

2. Consciousness. Grasp the shoulder of the person who appears unconscious; shake it, and call "Are you all right?" If the patient does not respond, she or he is unconscious. If the person is conscious, determine whether he or she can speak or cough; pinch the earlobe or toes of an infant to determine if he or she can cry.

■ Planning

Nursing goals

1. To permit air to move freely in and out of the lungs

2. To prevent irreversible brain damage from anoxia

■ Intervention

For a conscious person

1. If the conscious person can speak and cough, encourage her or him to keep coughing to expel the object.

Rationale Ability to speak and cough indicates that there is satisfactory air exchange.

2. If the person cannot speak or cough and the airway appears to be obstructed, initiate back blows (see steps 4–7) and abdominal thrusts (see steps 8–11).

    Rationale Inability to speak or cough indicates little or no airway exchange. Back blows loosen the foreign body. Abdominal thrusts increase intrathoracic pressure by exerting pressure against the diaphragm. The increased pressure forces air through the airways, moving the foreign body out with it. Administering both back blows and abdominal thrusts is more effective than either action alone.

3. Call for help.

Removing foreign objects by back blows

4. If the person is sitting or standing:

    a. Position yourself behind the person, slightly to one side, and place one hand on the person's sternum. Have him or her lean forward onto your forearm and hand, until the head is lower than the shoulders. See Figure 39–1.

    b. With the heel of your free hand, deliver four sharp blows to the back over the spine between the scapulae. See Figure 39–2.

       Rationale The blows often dislodge the foreign particle, so that the patient is able to cough it out.

5. If the person is lying down:

    a. Turn the person to a lateral position facing you.

    b. Brace your thighs against the person's chest, and deliver four sharp blows to the back as described in step 4b. See Figure 39–3.

6. If the person is a young child:

    a. Place the child face down over your knees with her or his head lower than the shoulders.

    b. Support the child's head and chest with one hand, if necessary.

    c. Deliver four back blows as in step 4b. See Figure 39–4. Use less severe blows for an infant or child than for an adult, in order not to injure the child.

7. Assess whether the person has effective air exchange. If not, proceed with abdominal thrusts.

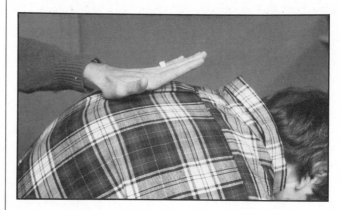

FIGURE 39–2

FIGURE 39–1

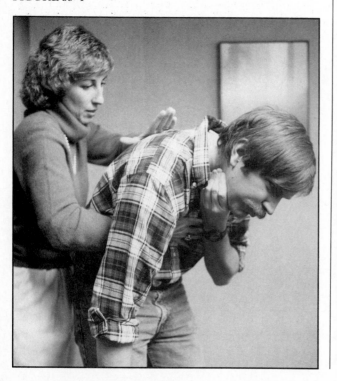

FIGURE 39–3

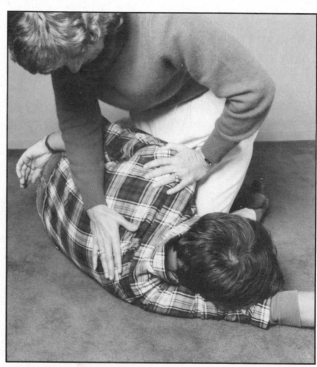

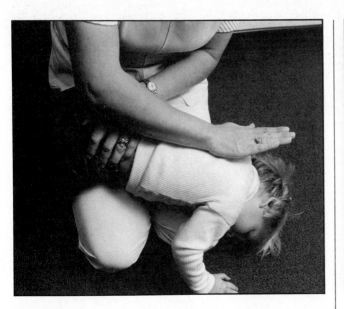

FIGURE 39-4

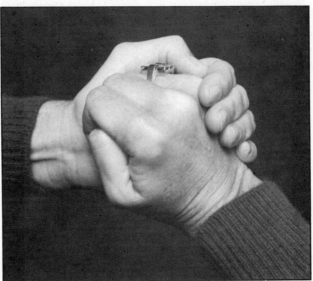

FIGURE 39-5

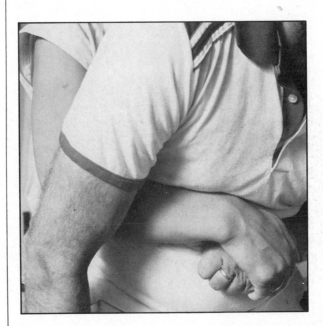

FIGURE 39-6

**Removing foreign objects by abdominal thrusts
(Heimlich maneuver)**

8.   If the person is standing or sitting:

 a. Stand behind the person, and wrap your arms
 around the person's waist.

 b. Make a fist with one hand, tuck the thumb inside the fist, and place the flexed thumb against
 the person's epigastrium, ie, below the xiphoid
 process.

 Rationale   A protruding thumb could injure the
 patient.

 c. With your other hand, grasp the fist (see Figure
 39-5), and press upward with a firm, quick thrust
 (see Figure 39-6). Avoid tightening your arms
 around the rib cage, and thrust in the direction
 of your chin. Deliver four thrusts.

 d. For a very obese or pregnant person, use *chest*
 thrusts: Place your fist on the middle portion of
 the sternum, and thrust backward toward yourself.

 Rationale   The firm thrust against the epigastrium forces exhalation of air through the patient's
 airway. The force of the air may move the
 obstruction.

9.   If the person is lying down:

 a. Kneel beside the person's hips, or straddle the
 person over the hips or one thigh.

 b. Turn the person's head to the side away from you.

 c. Place the heel of one hand over the person's
 epigastric area.

 d. Place your other hand over the first hand. Make
 sure your shoulders are over the person's abdomen

and your elbows are straight. Press the heel of the
first hand firmly toward the patient's head with
a quick thrust. See Figure 39-7.

Rationale   The weight of the nurse's shoulders
and trunk supplies power for the thrust.

 or

Provide chest thrusts:

 e. Kneel beside the person's chest.

 f. Position your hands as for cardiac compression.
 See Technique 39-3.

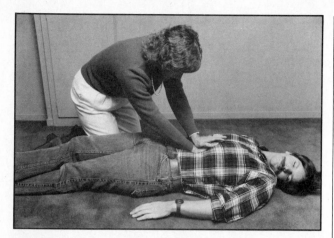

FIGURE 39-7

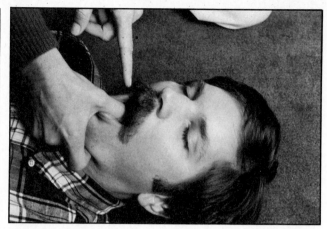

FIGURE 39-10

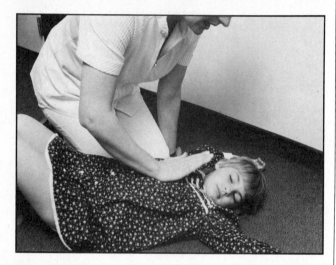

FIGURE 39-8

FIGURE 39-9

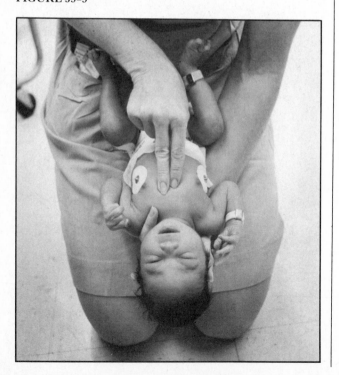

    g. Administer downward thrusts on the lower half of the sternum.

10. If the person is a young child:

    a. Roll the child gently onto his or her back on the floor, positioned horizontally in front of you.

    b. Place the heel of one hand over the middle portion of the child's sternum. See Figure 39-8.

    Rationale Chest thrusts are preferred for children because there is less risk of injuring abdominal organs.

    c. Administer four chest thrusts. The depth of compression should be 2.5 to 3.8 cm (1 to 1½ in).

11. If the person is an infant:

    a. Place the infant on her or his back over your thighs, with the head lower than the trunk.

    b. Place two fingers over the midsternum (ie, between the nipples). See Figure 39-9.

    c. Press downward four times on the sternum. The depth of compression should be 1.2 to 2.5 cm (½ to 1 in).

12. Assess whether the person has effective air exchange. If not, repeat the series of back blows and abdominal or chest thrusts until there is effective air exchange.

13. If there is no effective air exchange and if the person becomes unconscious, do a digital sweep of the mouth (see steps 14–18), and then open the airway using the maneuvers described in Technique 39-2.

    Rationale Unconsciousness relaxes the throat muscles. When the muscles are relaxed, forceful ventilations may bypass the obstruction and provide temporary adequate lung aeration.

Digitally removing foreign material from the mouth

14. Open the person's mouth by grasping the tongue and lower jaw between your thumb and fingers, and lifting the jaw upward. See Figure 39-10.

Rationale   This pulls the tongue away from the back of the throat.

15. Remove loose-fitting dentures.

    Rationale   Dentures can become dislodged and further obstruct the airway.

16. Insert the index finger of your free hand along the inside of the person's cheek and deep into the throat. Using a sweeping motion, attempt to dislodge and lift out the foreign object. If these measures fail, try more back blows and abdominal thrusts.

17. After removing the foreign object, clear out remaining liquid material, such as mucus, blood, or emesis, with a scooping motion, using two fingers or your hand covered with a tissue.

18. After the digital maneuver, assess air exchange. If it is ineffective, proceed with Techniques 39–2 and 39–3.

■ Evaluation

Expected outcomes

1. Pink lips and nail beds
2. Adequate ventilation
3. Patient is conscious

Unexpected outcomes

1. Cyanotic lips and nail beds
2. Absence of breathing
3. Patient remains unconscious
4. Cardiac arrest

Upon obtaining an unexpected outcome: Proceed with artificial respiration and external cardiac compression.

TECHNIQUE 39–2   ■   Administering Oral Resuscitation

Oral resuscitation is achieved in four ways: by mouth-to-mouth, mouth-to-nose, and mouth-to-mouth-and-nose resuscitation, or by the use of a hand-compressible breathing bag. The Ambu resuscitator, frequently supplied in hospitals and ambulances, is the preferred breathing bag. See Figure 39–11.

Mouth-to-mouth resuscitation depends on the large amount of air that a normal person can inhale and therefore breathe into the victim's lungs. Although the oxygen content of expired air is slightly reduced, it is sufficient for revival.

A current problem facing resuscitators relates to the acquired immunodeficiency syndrome (AIDS) epidemic. Some health associations are recommending that health care workers avoid direct contact with the skin, mucous membranes, blood, blood products, excretions, secretions, and tissue of possible AIDS victims. Workers are encouraged to use breathing-bag-and-mask ventilation rather than mouth-to-mouth resuscitation and to wear gloves. Check local policies and recommendations.

■ Assessment

Assess the patient's ability to breathe by:

1. Placing your ear and cheek close to the patient's mouth and nose
2. Looking at the chest and abdomen for rising and falling movement

3. Listening for air escaping during exhalation
4. Feeling for air escaping against your cheek

FIGURE 39–11   ■   An Ambu bag with a face mask.

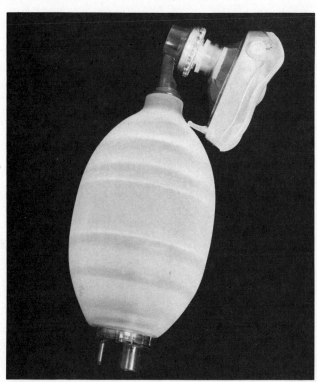

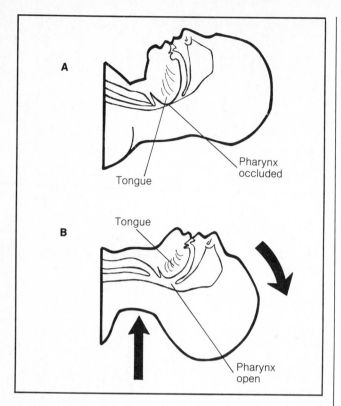

FIGURE 39-12

■ **Planning**

Nursing goals

1. To prevent irreversible brain damage from anoxia
2. To restore a normal breathing pattern

Equipment

A hand-compressible breathing bag and mask, if available or recommended.

FIGURE 39-13

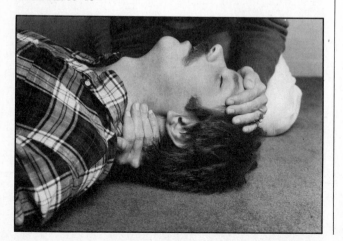

■ **Intervention**

1. Ensure that the patient's mouth and throat are cleared of any obstructive material. See Technique 39-1, steps 14-18.

    Rationale A clear airway prior to resuscitation permits air to move freely in and out of the respiratory passages.

2. If the person is lying on one side or face down, turn her or him onto the back, and kneel beside the head.

3. Tilt the head back (hyperextend the neck) by one of the methods in steps 4-5. These methods are not used for patients with spinal injuries. See step 6 for a method to use with such patients.

    Rationale Tilting the head back ensures an open airway, since the tongue is prevented from falling back. See Figure 39-12. When the patient's neck is *not* hyperextended, the tongue can obstruct the pharynx. When the neck is hyperextended, the tongue does not obstruct the airway. Spontaneous breathing may occur as soon as the airway is opened.

4. *Head-tilt-neck-lift maneuver:*

    a. Place one hand palm downward on the patient's forehead and the other hand palm upward under the patient's neck.

    b. Simultaneously press down on the forehead with one hand, and lift the patient's neck with the other. See Figure 39-13.

    c. For an infant, tilt the head backward only *slightly* while supporting the neck. See Figure 39-14.

    Rationale An infant's breathing passages are more pliable and may be obstructed by forceful extension.

    d. Go to step 7.
       or

5. *Head-tilt, chin-lift maneuver:*

    a. Place one hand palm downward on the forehead.

FIGURE 39-14

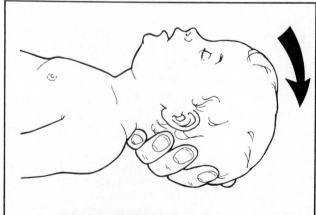

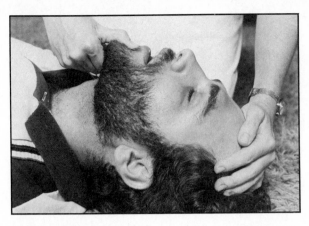

FIGURE 39-15

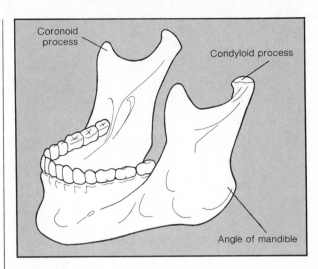

FIGURE 39-16

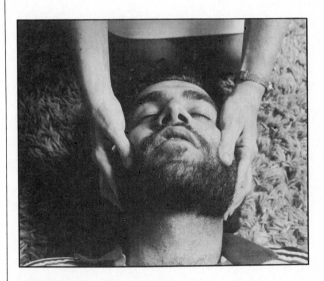

FIGURE 39-17

FIGURE 39-18

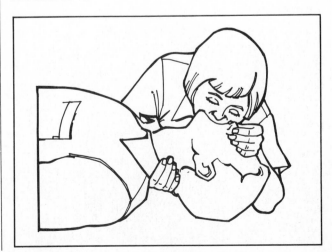

b. Place the fingers of your other hand under the bony part of the chin.

c. Simultaneously press down on the forehead with one hand, and lift the patient's chin upward with the other.

d. Open the patient's mouth by pressing the lower lip downward with your thumb after tilting the head. See Figure 39-15. Go to step 7.

   or

6. If the patient has a spinal injury, do not hyperextend the neck. Instead, use the *modified jaw thrust for a patient with a spinal injury:*

   a. Kneel at the top of the patient's head.

   b. Grasp the angle of the mandible (lower jaw) directly below the earlobe between your thumb and forefinger on each side of the patient's head. See Figure 39-16.

   c. Without hyperextending the neck, lift the lower jaw until it juts forward and is higher than the upper jaw. See Figure 39-17.

   d. Retract the lower lip with your thumbs prior to giving artificial respiration.

7. Check the patient's breathing. See Assessment, steps 1-4.

8. If breathing is not restored, try to blow air into the person's lungs using one of the methods in steps 9-12.

9. *Mouth-to-mouth method:*

   a. Pinch the patient's nostrils with your index finger and thumb of the hand on the patient's forehead.

   Rationale Pinching closes the nostrils and prevents resuscitation air from escaping through them.

   b. Take a deep breath, and place your mouth, opened widely, around the patient's mouth. Ensure an airtight seal. See Figure 39-18.

   c. Blow four quick, full breaths into the patient's

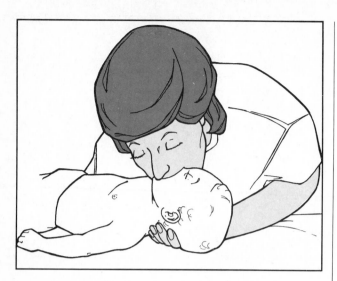

FIGURE 39-19

lungs. At this stage, do not allow the patient's lungs to deflate between breaths. Go to step 13.
or

10. *Mouth-to-nose method:* This method can be used when there is an injury to the mouth or jaw or when the patient is edentulous (toothless), making it difficult to achieve a tight seal over the mouth.

    a. Close the patient's mouth by pressing your thumb over the lips.
    b. Take a deep breath, and place your mouth,

FIGURE 39-20

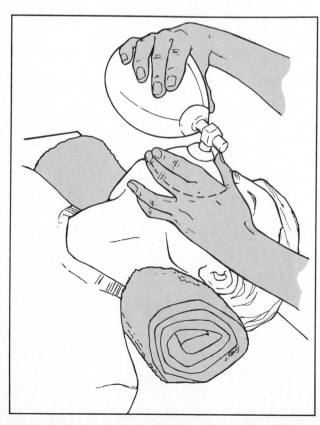

opened widely, over the patient's nose. Ensure a tight seal by making contact with the cheeks around the patient's nose.

    c. Press your cheek against the patient's lips.
    d. Blow four quick breaths into the patient's lungs. Do not allow the patient's lungs to deflate between breaths. Go to step 13.
    or

11. *Mouth-to-mouth-and-nose method:* This method is used for infants and children.

    a. Place your mouth tightly over the infant's nose and mouth. See Figure 39-19.
    b. Puff gently from your cheeks only, once every 3 seconds. Go to step 13.

    Rationale Forceful breathing overinflates the infant's lungs and may also cause gastric distention. To relieve gastric distention, the nurse turns the infant on the side and applies gentle pressure to the epigastrium. The lateral position prevents aspiration of vomitus.
    or

12. *Hand-compressible breathing bag method:* Many agencies use rubberized breathing bags (eg, the Ambu bag) attached to face masks for respiratory resuscitation. The bags are compressed by hand to deliver air into the mask and rapidly self-inflate after compression. Exhaled air is released through an exhaust valve to prevent its entry back into the bag. A significant advantage of the breathing bag is that supplemental oxygen can be attached to it.

    a. Stand at the patient's head and nose.
    b. Use one hand to secure the mask at the top and bottom and to hold the patient's jaw forward. Use the other hand to squeeze and release the bag. See Figure 39-20.
    c. Compress the bag until sufficient elevation of the patient's chest is observed. Then release the bag.

13. Determine whether the patient's breathing is restored. See Assessment, steps 1-4.

14. Determine the patient's carotid pulse by palpating the common carotid artery. See Figure 39-21. (Use the brachial pulse for an infant.) To feel the carotid artery, first locate the larynx, then slide your fingers alongside it into the groove between the larynx and the neck muscles. If you cannot feel a carotid pulse, check for a femoral pulse.

    Rationale Since the carotid arteries carry about one-fourth of the total normal blood flow, bringing it to the brain, a pulse can often be palpated there when more peripheral pulses, such as the radial, are imperceptible.

15. If you feel a carotid pulse, but breathing is not restored, repeat step 8, and inflate the patient's lungs at the rate of 12 breaths per minute (1 breath every 5 seconds). Blow forcibly enough to make the

patient's chest rise. If chest expansion fails to occur, ensure that the head is hyperextended and the jaw lifted upward, or check again for the presence of obstructive material, fluid, or vomitus. For infants and small children provide 1 breath every 3 seconds, using only sufficient force to cause the chest to rise.

16. After each inflation, move your mouth away from the patient's mouth by turning your head toward the patient's chest.

    Rationale This movement allows the air to escape when the patient exhales. It also gives the nurse time to inhale and to watch for chest expansion.

17. Reassess the carotid pulse after every 12 inflations (after one minute). For an infant, reasssess the brachial pulse after every 20 inflations (after one minute). If you cannot locate the pulse, the patient's heart has stopped, and cardiac compression also needs to be provided. See Technique 39–3.

■ **Evaluation** See Technique 39–1 on page 915.

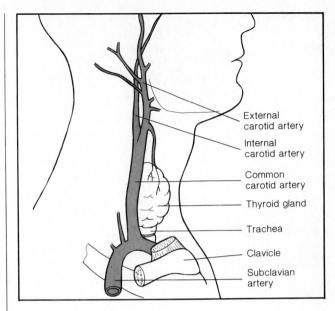

FIGURE 39–21

TECHNIQUE 39–3 ■ Administering External Cardiopulmonary Resuscitation to an Adult in a Health Care Facility

The ABCs of cardiopulmonary resuscitation (CPR) are:

A. Clear the *airways.*
B. Initiate artificial *breathing* (oral resuscitation).
C. Initiate *cardiac* compression or artificial *circulation.*

This sequence is recommended because spontaneous breathing may occur after any one action, such as after the airway is opened or after a few artificial respirations are provided. The purpose of external cardiac compression is to provide artificial circulation. Compression reproduces the normal intermittent heart contractions that pump blood through the body. External cardiac compression is manual, intermittent, rhythmical compression applied to the patient's sternum with the heel of your hand. The heart is squeezed between the sternum and the vertebrae lying posteriorly. Cardiac compression is ineffective unless there is simultaneous artificial respiration to oxygenate the bloodstream.

External cardiac compression should never be practiced on a person with a functioning heart, because it could interfere with the normal cardiac contractions.

■ **Assessment**

Because a cardiac arrest is a sudden occurrence, it is vitally important that an assessment be done quickly and resuscitative measures be implemented immediately.

1. Confirm that the patient has lost consciousness. Grasp the person's shoulder firmly, shake it, and shout, "Are you all right?" If there is no response, the patient is unconscious.

2. Assess the patient's breathing. See Technique 39–2 on page 915.

3. Assess the carotid artery for a pulse. See Technique 39–2, step 14.

4. Assess whether the patient's pupils are dilated.

If the patient does not respond, is apneic, has no palpable pulse, and has dilated pupils, immediately initiate CPR.

■ **Planning**

Nursing goals

1. To maintain blood circulation and prevent irreversible brain damage from anoxia

2. To restore normal cardiac function

Equipment

1. A cardiac board if available. The headboard or footboard of a hospital bed often can be removed and used.

2. An Ambu bag if available.

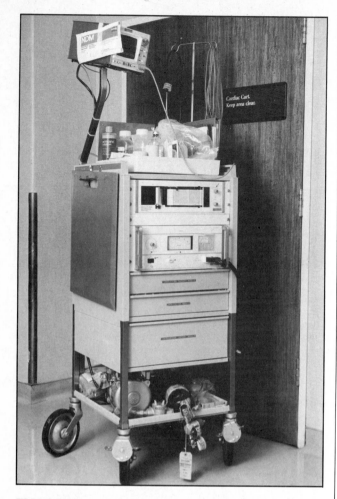

FIGURE 39-22 ■ An emergency (crash) cart.

3. A crash (emergency) cart if available. See Figure 39-22. The cart generally contains a defibrillator, a cardiac monitor, and the following supplies:
   a. Airway equipment.
   b. Prepackaged medications.
   c. Intravenous supplies.
   d. Blood tubes, needles, syringes, and blood gas kits.
   e. Laboratory requisitions.
   f. Suction equipment.

■ Intervention

One rescuer present

1. Call for help.
2. Position the patient on the back on a flat, firm surface. Place a cardiac board, if available, under the back of a bed patient. If necessary, place the person on the floor.
   Rationale A hard surface facilitates compression of the heart between the sternum and the hard surface.
3. Kneel beside the patient's chest. If the patient is in bed, you may have to kneel on the patient's bed.

Airway

4. Clear the airway, if you suspect airway obstruction from food or some other foreign object. See Techniques 39-1 and 39-2 for detailed steps.
   a. Hyperextend the head and lift the chin.
      Rationale This prevents the tongue from occluding the airway.
   b. Ventilate the patient once.
      Rationale If the airway is obstructed, the attempt to ventilate will not be successful.
   c. If ventilation is not successful, deliver four back blows.
   d. Deliver four abdominal thrusts.
   e. Digitally probe for an obstruction and to clear the airway.
   f. Repeat steps a–e until the obstruction is removed.
5. Ensure an open airway. Use the head-tilt and chin- or neck-lift method, if possible. If neck injury is suspected, use the modified jaw thrust.

Breathing

6. Assess breathing: *look* for chest movement; *listen* for exhalation; and *feel* for air flow against your cheek.
7. Ventilate the person, if breathing is not restored. See Technique 39-2 for detailed steps. If dentures were removed, put them in again, to enable you to form a tight mouth-to-mouth seal.
8. Blow four quick full breaths into the person's mouth. Between the breaths, remove your mouth and turn your head to the side, but do not allow the person's lungs to deflate completely.
   Rationale Turning away allows the nurse to take a fresh breath and allows the patient partial exhalation. Not allowing complete lung deflation creates a stair-step air volume effect and increases oxygenation of the lungs.

Circulation

9. Assess the carotid or femoral pulse for 5 seconds.
10. Begin external cardiac compression if the pulse cannot be palpated.
11. Locate the lower end of the sternum (the xiphoid process), by following the lower edge of the near ribs to the notch where the ribs and the sternum join. See Figure 39-23.
12. Measure upward about 4 to 5 cm (1.5 to 2 in) from the lower point of the xiphoid process. You will apply pressure at that location above the xiphoid process.
    Rationale Proper positioning of the hands during cardiac compression prevents injury to underlying organs and the ribs. Compression directly over the xiphoid process can lacerate the patient's liver.

13. Place the heel of one hand on the chest at the point indicated in step 12, and place the heel of the other hand on top of the first hand. The hands should be parallel, with the fingers directed away from you. The fingers should not be pressing against the chest. It may be helpful to interlock the fingers. See Figure 39–24.

    Rationale Compression occurs only on the sternum through the heels of the hands. The muscle force of both arms is needed for adequate cardiac compression of an adult.

14. Lean forward so that your shoulders are directly above the person's chest. Keep your arms extended and your elbows firmly locked.

    Rationale The weight of the nurse's shoulders and trunk supplies power for compression. Extension of the elbows ensures an adequate and even force throughout compression.

15. Using your own weight, press down on the person's chest so that the sternum depresses about 4 to 5 cm (1.5 to 2 in).

    Rationale The pressure compresses the heart between the sternum and the vertebral column and squeezes blood out of the chambers of the heart.

16. Release all pressure, but do not remove your hands. Establish a rhythmic motion, using a rate of 60 to 80 compressions per minute. Maintain the rhythm by counting "one one thousand, two one thousand," etc.

    Rationale Releasing the pressure allows the sternum to return to its normal position and allows the heart chambers to fill with blood. Leaving the hands on the chest prevents taking a malposition between compressions and possibly injuring the patient. The specified compression rate and rhythm simulate normal heart contractions.

17. Give two quick lung inflations after every 15 chest compressions. Continue until the patient revives or until someone relieves you.

18. Check the patient's carotid pulse after one minute of cardiac massage (four sets of 15 compressions, each followed by two lung inflations). If there is no pulse, continue with CPR.

19. Check the person's pulse every four to five minutes thereafter.

Two rescuers present

When help arrives, one rescuer can provide external cardiac compression, and the other can provide pulmonary resuscitation, inflating the lungs once after every five compressions, a 5:1 ratio. The second rescuer follows these initial steps:

20. Tell the first rescuer to "stop compression."
21. Check the carotid or femoral pulse for 5 seconds.

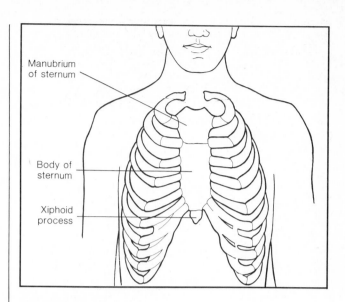

Manubrium of sternum

Body of sternum

Xiphoid process

FIGURE 39–23

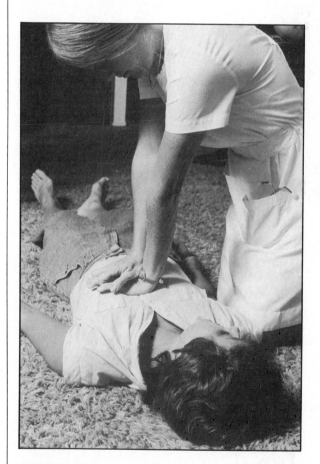

FIGURE 39–24

22. If no pulse is felt, state "No pulse—begin compression."
23. The second rescuer then:

    a. Provides compression.

    b. Sets the pace, counting aloud, "one one thousand, two one thousand, three one thousand, four one thousand, five one thousand, ventilate."

24. The first rescuer:
   a. Provides one ventilation after every five chest compressions.
   b. Observes each breath for effectiveness.
   c. Assesses the carotid pulse frequently between breaths to assess the effectiveness of cardiac compression.
   d. Observes for abdominal (gastric) distention, which can result from overinflation of the lungs. If distention occurs, the rescuer reduces the force of the ventilations, but ensures sufficient ventilation to elevate the ribs.
   e. Assesses the patient's pupils every five minutes (optional). Pupil changes are not the best indicator of restored circulation, however.

25. To initiate a change in positions, the person compressing states, "Change one thousand, two one thousand, three one thousand, four one thousand, five one thousand," moves to the patient's head, and counts the pulse for 5 seconds. CPR should never be interrupted for more than 5 seconds (McIntyre, Lewis, 1983, p 17).

26. The person ventilating gives the breath and moves into position to provide compression.

27. If there is no pulse, the original person compressing states "No pulse—start compression," gives one full breath, and CPR is again initiated.

When relieved from CPR

28. Stand by to assist. Often a person is needed to take notes, document the actions taken, and record the drugs given by the cardiac arrest team.

29. Provide support to the patient's support persons and others who may have witnessed the cardiac arrest. This is often a frightening experience for others, because it is so sudden and so serious.

30. Record on the patient's chart the time CPR was begun, the time a physician arrived, the drugs and techniques employed, the time CPR was terminated, and the response of the patient.

Sample Recording

Date	Time	Notes
12/5/86	0315	CPR initiated by RN and LPN. Patient placed on cardiac board. CPR at 5 compressions to 1 inflation. Code 199 called.——————————— Wayne P. Newman, RN
	0320	No carotid pulse. Pupils dilated. Skin pale, moist.
	0322	Dr. R. Sanduriz and crash team arrived.—
	0340	Femoral pulse 68, regular, good volume.—
	0345	Respirations started 10/min. CPR terminated. Carotid pulse 72. Color good. Reacts to verbal stimuli. BP 100/40. Pupils react and equal.————Wayne P. Newman, RN
	0350	Dr. Sanduriz phoned Dr. Saunders.————
	0355	BP 110/55, P 76. Color good. Condition stable.———— Wayne P. Newman, RN

■ Evaluation

Expected outcomes

1. Restoration of breathing and circulation
2. Absence of permanent neurologic damage

Unexpected outcome

Inability to restore breathing and circulation. Upon obtaining an unexpected outcome:

1. Report your findings to the responsible nurse and/or physician.
2. Follow the practices of the agency regarding death.

TECHNIQUE 39-4 ■ Administering External Cardiopulmonary Resuscitation to an Infant or Child

Resuscitation is most often required for neonates in the first few minutes of life when they are unable to establish adequate ventilation. Conditions that may necessitate CPR include:

1. Airway obstruction due to mucus, blood, meconium, or posterior displacement of the tongue, resulting in asphyxia

2. Respiratory depression resulting from drugs given to the mother, eg, general or local anesthetics, narcotic analgesics, or diazepam

3. Neurologic damage

4. Congenital anomalies of the central nervous system, heart, or respiratory tract

5.   Hypovolemic shock resulting from hemorrhage or cord compression

Primary cardiac arrest in infants and children is rare; it is usually secondary to hypoxia resulting from respiratory arrest. Thus, meticulous attention needs to be paid to appropriate ventilation in infants and children. A prevailing problem during the first year of life, and one of the leading causes of death, is sudden infant death syndrome (SIDS).

Differences in the anatomy and physiology of infants and children compared to adults require different basic life support techniques.

■ Assessment

Assess the infant or child for:

1.   Responsiveness. Shake the child, rub the chest, or slap the bottom of the feet. Try to elicit a cry.
2.   Respiratory function. Look for chest movement, listen for exhalation, and feel for air flow against your cheek.
3.   Circulation. Palpate the *brachial* pulse.

■ Planning   See Technique 39–3 on page 919.

■ Intervention

1.   Call for help.
2.   Place the infant or child on a firm surface.
3.   If you suspect airway obstruction from food or a foreign object, follow Technique 39–1, steps 6, 10, and 11, on pages 912 and 914. Tilt the infant's head only slightly, since hyperextension can cause collapse of the trachea.
4.   Put a rolled towel or your hand under the infant's shoulders.
     Rationale The towel or hand helps to keep the infant or child's chin forward without causing neck hyperextension.
5.   Reassess breathing.
6.   If breathing is not restored, ventilate the infant or child using the mouth-to-mouth-and-nose technique. See Technique 39–2, step 11, on page 918.
     Rationale The infant or child's face is too small to enable a tight mouth-to-mouth seal.
7.   Puff four short breaths into the infant or child's mouth from your cheeks.
     Rationale Short puffs avoid overinflation of the lungs and gastric distention.
8.   Assess the brachial pulse for 5 seconds.
9.   Begin external cardiac compression if the pulse cannot be palpated.

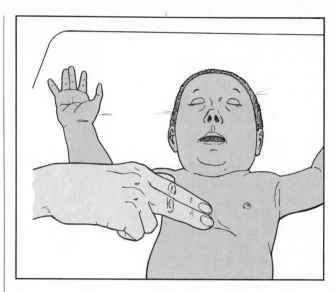

FIGURE 39–25

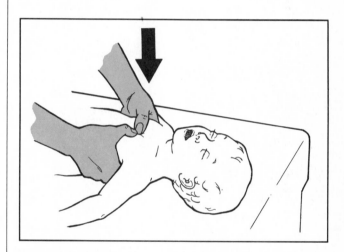

FIGURE 39–26

10.   For an *infant up to 1 year:*
      a. Place two fingers at the middle portion of the sternum. See Figure 39–25.
         or
      b. Encircle the chest, with your fingers over the infant's back and your thumbs over the middle portion of the sternum. See Figure 39–26. This is referred to as the *two-handed chest-encircling method* and is the preferred method for neonates. For very small infants, the thumbs may need to be placed one over the other.

      For a *child 1 to 4 years old,* place the heel of one hand at the junction of the middle and lower thirds of the sternum. For a *child over age 4,* place the heels of both hands over the lower third of the sternum, as for an adult.

11.   For an *infant up to 1 year of age,* compress the sternum

1.5 to 2.5 cm (0.5 to 1 in) 100 times per minute. For a *child from 1 to 8 years of age,* compress the sternum 2.5 to 3.5 cm (1 to 1.5 in) 80 times per minute.

12. Provide cardiac compression and ventilate at the rate of one breath to five compressions (5:1 ratio).

13. Continue CPR as for an adult. See Technique 39–3, steps 17–30.

■ **Evaluation** See Technique 39–3 on page 922.

References

American Heart Association, National Academy of Sciences, National Research Council: Standards and guidelines for cardiopulmonary resuscitation (CPR) and emergency cardiac care (ECC). *JAMA* 1980; 244(5):453–509.

LeFort S: Cardiopulmonary resuscitation (CPR): Step-by-step. *Can Nurse* (February) 1978; 74:38–47.

Manzi CC: Cardiac emergency! How to use drugs and C.P.R. to save lives. *Nursing 78* (March) 1978; 8:30–39.

Mason TN: A hand ventilation technique for neonates. *Am J Maternal Child Nurs* (November/December) 1982; 7(6):366–369.

McIntyre KM, Lewis AJ (editors): *Textbook of Advanced Cardiac Life Support.* American Heart Association, 1983.

Nursing 80 Photobook Series: *Dealing with Emergencies.* Intermed Communications, 1980.

Nussbaum GB, Fisher, JG: A crash cart that works. *Am J Nurs* (January) 1978; 78:45–48.

Ryan MA: Helping the family cope with cardiac arrest. *Nursing 74* (August) 1974; 4:80–81.

Sumner SM, Gran PE: Emergency! First aid for choking. *Nursing 82* (July) 1982; 12:40–49.

Techniques of cardiopulmonary resuscitation in infants. *Am J Nurs* (February) 1978; 78:265.

VanMeter M: Keeping cool in a code. *RN* (March) 1981; 44:29–35.

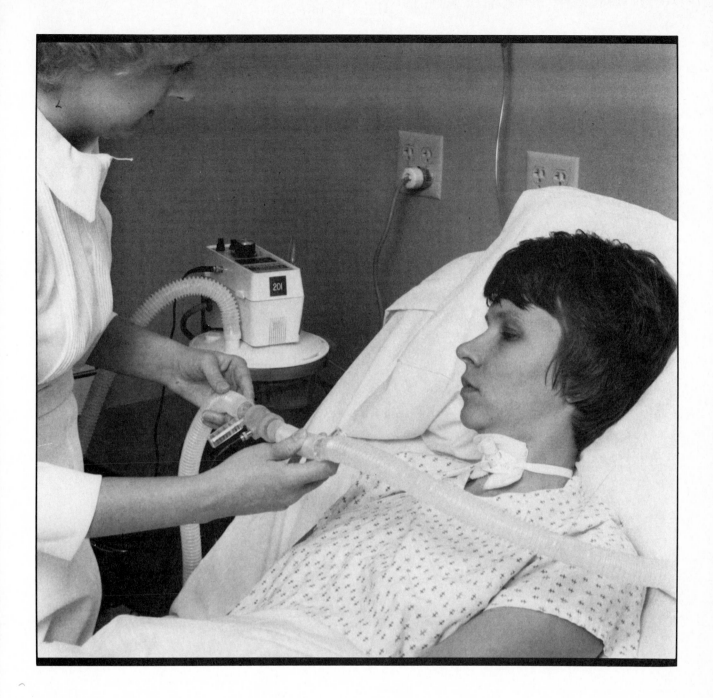

TRACHEOSTOMY CARE

40 Patients sometimes require artificial airways in order to maintain adequate aeration. Care involving artificial airways often provokes considerable anxiety for a patient, since the airway must remain unoccluded for the patient to breathe. Because a tracheostomy is an opening directly into the trachea, the danger of introducing microorganisms must always be considered as well.

A tracheostomy may be a short-term or a long-term therapy. The patient who cares for the tracheostomy independently at home will often have suggestions to make about its care in the hospital. No matter how long a patient has had a tracheostomy, nurses have to remain sensitive to the patient's needs and anxieties about tracheostomy care.

Chapter Outline

Artificial Airways

Objectives

Upon completion of this chapter, the student will:

1. Know essential terms and facts about artificial airways and tracheostomy techniques
    1.1 Define selected terms
    1.2 Identify the different types of artificial airways
    1.3 Identify essential facts about artificial airways
2. Understand facts about techniques for tracheostomy care
    2.1 Identify relevant assessment data
    2.2 Identify nursing diagnoses for which the technique may be implemented
    2.3 Identify nursing goals related to the technique
    2.4 Identify expected and unexpected outcomes from assessment data
    2.5 Identify reasons underlying selected steps of the technique
3. Perform tracheostomy techniques safely
    3.1 Assess the patient adequately
    3.2 Collect additional data from appropriate sources
    3.3 Select pertinent nursing goals for the patient
    3.4 Establish relevant outcome criteria for the patient following the technique
    3.5 Collect necessary equipment before the technique
    3.6 Implement interventions to enhance the effectiveness of the technique and enhance the patient's comfort and safety
    3.7 Communicate relevant information about the patient to the appropriate persons
    3.8 Determine the evaluative outcomes of the technique
4. Evaluate own performance of specific tracheostomy techniques in a laboratory or clinical setting with the assistance of another
    4.1 Use the performance checklists provided
    4.2 Identify areas of strength and weakness
    4.3 Alter performance in response to own evaluation and that of another

Terms

■ airway   a device that is inserted into a patient to maintain the patency of air passages such as the trachea

■ aspirate   to remove gases or liquids from a cavity using suction; to inhale a substance

■ cannula   a tube inserted into the body

■ endotracheal tube   a tube inserted through the mouth and terminating in the trachea

■ intubation   insertion of a tube

■ lavage   irrigation or washing out of a body organ, such as the stomach

■ nasopharyngeal tube   a tube inserted into a nostril and terminating in the pharynx

■ obturator   a disc or instrument that closes an opening; the obturator of a tracheostomy set fits inside and closes off the end of the outer tube

■ oropharyngeal tube   a tube inserted into the mouth and terminating in the pharynx

■ patent   open, unobstructed, not closed

■ tracheostomy   an opening in the anterior neck directly into the trachea

■ tracheostomy button   a very short tube that extends from a tracheostomy stoma to just inside the tracheal wall

■ tracheostomy tube   a tube inserted through a tracheostomy and terminating in the trachea

■ vertigo   dizziness

ARTIFICIAL AIRWAYS

Artificial airways are inserted to maintain a patent air passage for patients who have or may become obstructed. A patent airway is necessary so that air can flow to and from the lungs. Airways are usually inserted by physicians. Four of the more common types of intubation are: oropharyngeal, nasopharyngeal, endotracheal, and tracheostomy.

Oropharyngeal Intubation

Oropharyngeal intubation is done most frequently for patients who have had general anesthesia and for those who are semiconscious and are likely to obstruct their own airways with their tongues. An oropharyngeal tube is inserted in some instances for pharyngeal suctioning. It is not inserted in patients who are conscious, because it stimulates the gag reflex and thus can cause vomiting. This tube may also be inserted in patients who require an orogastric intubation, because the airway facilitates passage of the orogastric tube past the pharynx and into the esophagus.

Oropharyngeal tubes are S-shaped and usually made of plastic. Adult, child, and infant sizes are available. The tube is inserted through the mouth and terminates in the posterior pharynx. See Figure 40–1. For insertion of the tube, the patient should be in a supine position with the neck hyperextended so that the tongue cannot fall back to block the pharynx. This position may be contraindicated for patients with head, neck, and back injuries.

Nursing interventions for intubated patients include:

1. Remove the tube every four hours, or more often if necessary, and provide oral hygiene to maintain the health of oral mucosa.

2. Make sure a bite block is in place if the patient is likely to bite the tube and thus obstruct the airway.

3. Maintain the patient in a lateral or semiprone position, so that blood, vomitus, and mucus will drain out of the mouth and not be aspirated.

4. Remove the airway once the patient has regained consciousness and has the swallow, gag, and cough reflexes.

Nasopharyngeal Intubation

Nasopharyngeal intubation is carried out if the oropharyngeal route is contraindicated, eg, following oral surgery. A nasopharyngeal tube may also be inserted to protect the nasal and pharyngeal mucosa during nasopharyngeal or nasotracheal suctioning. The tube is inserted through a nostril and terminates in the pharynx, below the upper edge of the epiglottis. See Figure 40–2. Tubes vary in size for adults, children, and infants. They are usually made of latex rubber.

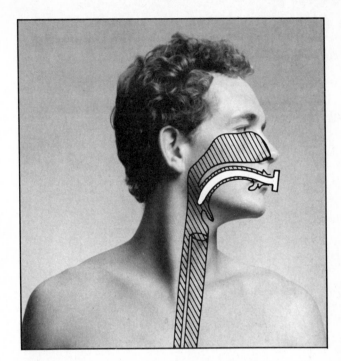

FIGURE 40-1   ■   An oropharyngeal tube in place.

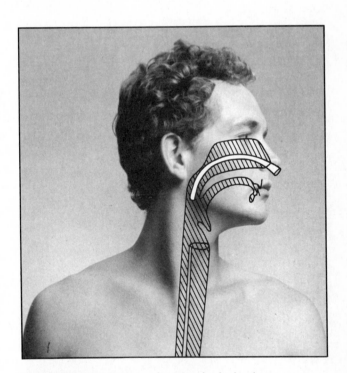

FIGURE 40-2   ■   A nasopharyngeal tube in place.

Nursing interventions include:

1. Lubricate the tube with a water-soluble lubricant and/or a topical anesthetic prior to insertion, to prevent irritation of the nasopharyngeal mucosa and undue discomfort. The local anesthetic will be specified in the order.

2. Remove the tube, and insert it in the other nostril at

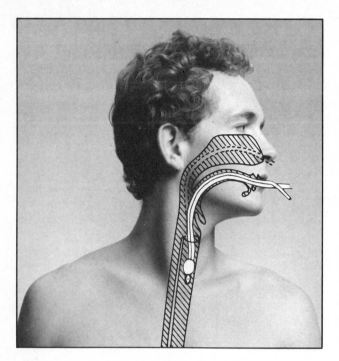

FIGURE 40-3 ▪ An endotracheal tube in place.

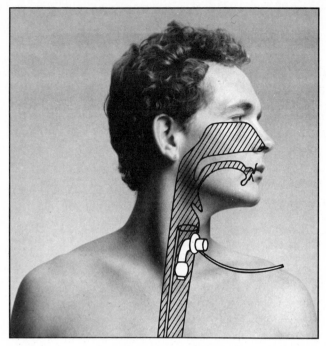

FIGURE 40-5 ▪ A tracheostomy tube in place.

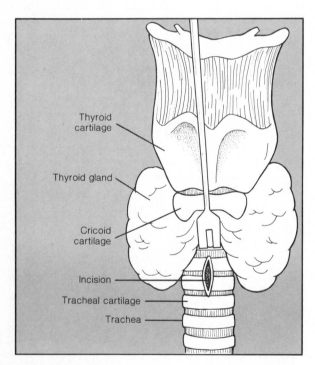

FIGURE 40-4 ▪ The site of a tracheostomy incision.

least every eight hours, or as ordered by the physician, or more often to prevent irritation of the mucosa.

3. Provide nasal hygiene every four hours, or more often if needed.

4. Monitor the patient closely for stimulation of the vagus nerve, if nasotracheal suctioning is carried out. Vagal stimulation can lead to cardiac arrest.

Endotracheal Intubation

Endotracheal tubes are most commonly inserted for patients who have had general anesthetics or in emergency situations where mechanical ventilation is required. An endotracheal tube is a curved polyvinyl chloride tube that is inserted through either the mouth or the nose into the trachea. See Figure 40-3. It terminates just superior to the bifurcation of the trachea into the bronchi. Tubes come in various lengths and diameters. The lengths are measured in centimeters and the inner and outer diameters in millimeters.

Nursing interventions include:

1. Maintain the patient in a lateral or semiprone position so that blood, vomitus, or secretions can drain from the mouth and are not aspirated.

2. Provide oral or nasal hygiene every three hours or as needed.

3. For an oral insertion, provide a bite block so the patient cannot bite the tube and occlude the airway.

4. Change the tube's position to the opposite side of the mouth or to the other nostril every eight hours, or as ordered by the physician, or as needed to prevent irritation of the mucosa.

5. Closely monitor the air pressure in the endotracheal cuff.

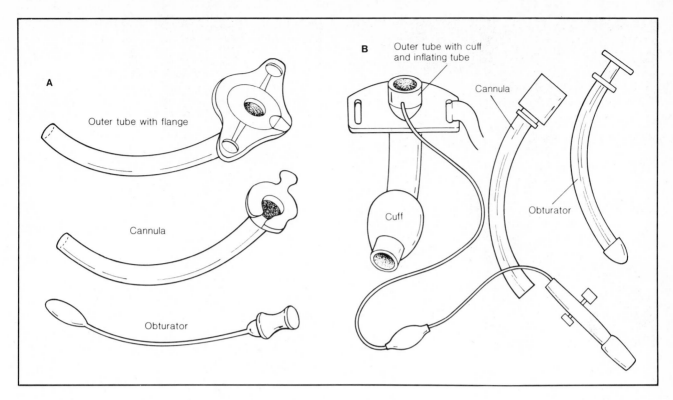

FIGURE 40–6 ■ Two types of tracheostomy sets: **A,** noncuffed; **B,** cuffed.

If it is greater than 20 mm Hg, necrosis of the tracheal tissues can result.

6. Tape the airway in place to prevent accidental slippage or extubation.

7. Provide continuous humidification or aerosol therapy to prevent undue drying and irritation of the mucous membranes, if the tube is left in for more than a short time, eg, for days or weeks.

Tracheostomy Intubation

Tracheostomy tubes are inserted to provide and maintain a patent airway, to remove tracheobronchial secretions from patients unable to cough, to replace endotracheal tubes, to permit the use of positive pressure ventilation, and to prevent unconscious patients from aspirating secretions. A tracheostomy tube is a curved tube that is inserted into a tracheostomy (a surgical incision in the trachea just below the first or second tracheal cartilage). See Figure 40–4. The tube may be metal, plastic, or foam. Plastic tubes are increasingly popular, because they are lightweight, their parts are interchangeable, and crusting from the tissues rarely forms on plastic materials. The tracheostomy tube extends through the tracheostomy stoma into the trachea. See Figure 40–5. Tubes come in different sizes.

The main parts of a tracheostomy set are: the outer tube, the inner tube or inner cannula, and the obturator.

See Figure 40–6. The obturator is used only to insert the outer tube. It is removed once the outer tube is in place. The outer tube usually has ties to secure it around the patient's neck, although many plastic tubes are cuffed with a soft balloon that can be inflated to hold the tube in place. Fitted inside the outer tube is an inner cannula. (Some plastic sets do not have this, because it is unnecessary to change the tube. They are called *single-cannula tubes.*) In double-cannula sets, the inner cannula is inserted and locked in place after the obturator is removed; it acts as a removable liner for the more permanent outer cannula. The inner tube is withdrawn for brief periods to be cleaned. Nursing interventions are described in Techniques 40–1 through 40–5.

An adaptation of the tracheostomy tube is the tracheostomy button. This is a very short tube that extends from the tracheostomy stoma to just inside the tracheal wall. See Figure 40–7. The button enables a patient to breathe and cough more easily than a tracheostomy tube. It has a closure plug, which can be removed for suctioning and/or ventilating. When the plug is inserted, the patient can speak.

Nursing interventions for a tracheostomy button include:

1. Clean the cannula regularly by washing it in hydrogen peroxide solution and rinsing it with sterile water.

2. Clean the stoma regularly to prevent skin irritation and

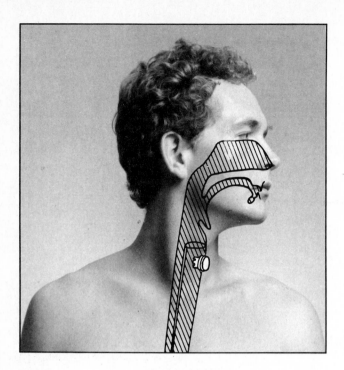

FIGURE 40-7 ■ A tracheostomy button in place.

the formation of crusts. Cleaning is usually done with a solution of hydrogen peroxide. The stoma is then rinsed with sterile water and dried with sterile gauze. It is important that no solution enter the tracheostomy, where it could irritate the mucosal lining and/or be aspirated into the respiratory tract.

TECHNIQUE 40–1 ■ Suctioning a Tracheostomy or Endotracheal Tube

---

Following a tracheostomy, the trachea and surrounding respiratory tissues are irritated and react by producing excessive secretions. Suctioning is necessary to remove these secretions and maintain a patent airway. The frequency of suctioning depends on the patient's condition and how recently the tracheostomy was done.

When suctioning a tracheostomy, use sterile technique to prevent infection of the respiratory tract.

■ Assessment

Assess the patient for:

1. Clinical signs of secretions accumulating in the respiratory tract: restlessness or anxiety, pallor, increased heart rate, increased respiratory rate, bubbling or rattling breath sounds, and/or shallow respirations or dyspnea.

2. The rate, depth, rhythm, and character of respirations. See chapter 8 for further information.

3. Breath sounds that are audible without amplification and those audible by stethoscope. See Technique 10–10 on page 198 for auscultation of the lungs.

4. Clinical signs of hypoxia or anoxia: increased pulse rate, rapid or deep respirations, cyanosis, restlessness, anxiety, vertigo, or syncope (faintness).

5. Pallor and cyanosis of the skin and nail beds.

Other data include:

1. Orders regarding suctioning, eg, to use sterile saline to lavage the trachea

2. Whether the patient's tracheostomy tube has a cuff, and if this needs to be deflated for suctioning

■ Nursing Diagnosis

Nursing diagnoses that may indicate the need to suction a tracheostomy include:

1. Ineffective airway clearance related to:
   a. Ineffective coughing
   b. Fear of pain
   c. Viscous secretions
   d. Fatigue

■ Planning

Nursing goals

1. To maintain a patent airway and prevent airway obstructions

2. To promote respiratory function (optimal exchange

of oxygen and carbon dioxide into and out of the lungs)

3. To prevent pneumonia that may result from accumulated secretions

Equipment

1. Suction equipment, including a collection receptacle. The agency may have wall suction at the bedside, or it may use portable units.

2. A sterile suction catheter. The diameter should be about half the inside diameter of the tracheostomy tube, to prevent hypoxia. Adults often require a #12 or #14 Fr. and children a #8 or #10 Fr. Some catheters have a thumb port on the side to control the suction.

3. A Y-connector to join the catheter to the suction tubing if the cather does not have a thumb port. One arm of the Y is then used to control the suction. A straight connector is used if the catheter has a thumb port.

4. A container with sterile normal saline to lubricate and flush the catheter.

5. A sterile 2- to 10-mL syringe and sterile normal saline without a bacteriostatic preservative for a tracheal lavage, if this is agency practice and/or is ordered. Lavage can liquefy tenacious secretions so that they are more easily suctioned out. The amount used is generally 0.5 to 1 mL for infants, 2 mL for children, and 2 to 5 mL for adults.

6. Sterile gloves.

7. A moisture-resistant bag in which to discard the disposable catheter and gloves.

8. A sterile towel to provide an additional sterile area (optional).

9. An oxygen source and flowmeter with a ventilator, or a manual resuscitator, eg, an Ambu or Laerdal bag.

■ Intervention

1. Inform the patient that suctioning usually causes intermittent coughing and that this assists in removing the secretions.

2. If not contraindicated, place the patient in semi-Fowler's position to promote deep breathing, maximum lung expansion, and productive coughing. Place an unconscious patient in the supine position.
   Rationale Deep breathing oxygenates the lungs, counteracts the hypoxic effects of suctioning, and may induce coughing. Coughing helps to loosen and move secretions.

3. Attach the resuscitation apparatus to the oxygen source. See Figure 40–8.

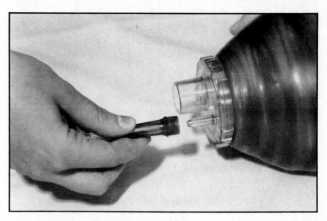

FIGURE 40–8

4. Open the sterile supplies in readiness for use.

5. Place the sterile towel, if used, across the patient's chest below the tracheostomy.

6. Turn on the suction, and set the pressure in accordance with agency policy. Usually 100 to 120 mm Hg pressure is used for adults, and 50 to 75 mm Hg is used for infants and children.

7. Put a sterile glove on your dominant hand. Some agencies recommend putting a sterile glove on the nondominant hand also, to protect you and the patient.

8. Holding the catheter in the dominant hand and the connector in the ungloved hand, attach the catheter to the Y-connector or straight connector. See Figure 40–9.

FIGURE 40–9

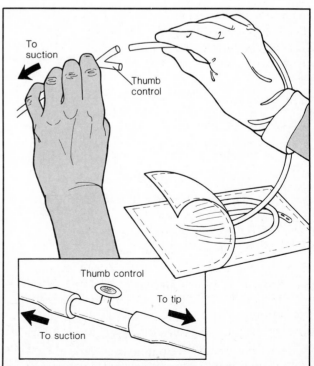

To suction

Thumb control

Thumb control

To tip

To suction

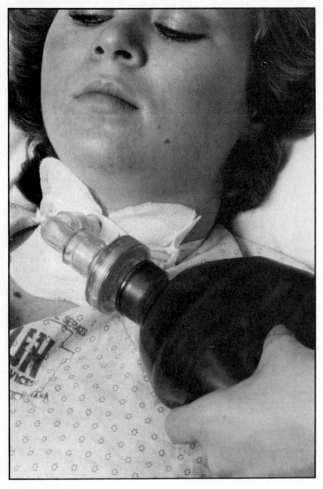

FIGURE 40-10

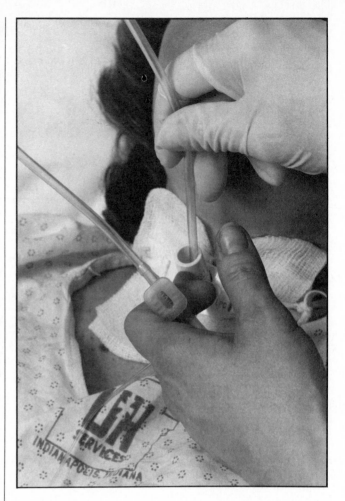

FIGURE 40-11

9. Using the gloved hand, place the catheter tip in the sterile saline solution; using the thumb of the ungloved hand, occlude the thumb control, and suction a small amount of sterile solution through the catheter.

   Rationale This ensures that the suction equipment is working properly and lubricates the outside and the lumen of the catheter. Lubrication eases insertion and reduces tissue trauma during insertion. Lubricating the lumen helps prevent secretions from sticking to the inside of the catheter.

10. If the patient does *not* have copious secretions hyperventilate the lungs with a resuscitation bag before suctioning:

    a. Using your nondominant hand, turn on the oxygen to 12 to 15 L/min.

    b. Attach the tracheostomy adapter of the resuscitator to the tracheostomy or endotracheal tube.

    c. Compress the Ambu or Laerdal bag (see Figure 40–10) as the patient inhales, or every 5 seconds for an adult and every 3 seconds for an infant. This is best done by a second person who can use

both hands to compress the bag, providing a greater inflation volume.

d. Observe the rise and fall of the patient's chest to assess the adequacy of the ventilation.

   or

   If the patient has copious secretions, do not hyperventilate with a resuscitator because the secretions can be forced deeper into the respiratory tract. Instead, keep the patient on the regular wall-outlet oxygen delivery device, and increase the liter flow for a few minutes before suctioning.

11. Remove the oxygen device.

12. With your nondominant thumb off the suction port, quickly but gently insert the catheter into the trachea through the tracheostomy or endotracheal tube. See Figure 40–11. Insert the catheter about 10 to 12.5 cm (4 to 5 in) or until the patient coughs.

    Rationale To prevent tissue trauma and oxygen loss, suction is not applied during insertion of the catheter.

13. Apply suction for 5 to 10 seconds by placing the nondominant thumb over the thumb port. Rotate

the catheter by rolling it between your thumb and forefinger while slowly withdrawing it.

Rationale   Suction time is restricted to 10 seconds or less to minimize oxygen loss. Rotating the catheter as it is withdrawn prevents tissue trauma by minimizing the suction time against any part of the trachea.

14. Withdraw the catheter completely, and release the suction.

15. If secretions are thick, flush the catheter in the sterile solution, and insert 3 to 5 mL of sterile saline solution into the trachea. See Figure 40–12. Then suction.

16. Reapply the patient's source of supplementary oxygen if appropriate. Observe the patient's respirations and skin color, and allow him or her to rest for a few minutes.

17. Encourage the patient to breathe deeply and cough. Repeat steps 10 to 14 until the air passage is clear and the patient's breathing is relatively effortless and quiet. Do not suction for more than three to five minutes in total.

Rationale   Suctioning too long can decrease the patient's oxygen supply.

18. If agency policy indicates, and if the patient's condition warrants it, hyperoxygenate the patient's lungs for a few minutes after each suction attempt and on completion of the suctioning procedure.

Rationale   This relieves hypoxia that may be created by suctioning.

19. Turn off the suction, and disconnect the catheter from the suction tubing.

20. Holding the catheter in your gloved hand, grasp the cuff of the glove with your other hand, and peel the glove off so that it turns inside out over the catheter. See Figure 40–13.

21. Discard the glove and the catheter in the moisture-resistant bag.

22. Provide oral or nasal hygiene for the patient.

23. Observe the amount of secretions obtained by suction, including the color, odor, and thickness.

24. Assist the patient to a comfortable, safe position that aids breathing. If the patient is conscious, a semi-Fowler's position is frequently indicated. If the patient is unconscious, Sims's position can assist the drainage of secretions from the mouth.

25. Replenish the sterile fluid and supplies so that the suction is ready to be used again.

Rationale   Patients who require suctioning often require it quickly, so it is essential to leave the equipment at the bedside ready for use.

26. Record the technique on the patient's chart. Include the suction, the route, the amount and description of suction returns, the amount of sterile saline instilled, and the response of the patient.

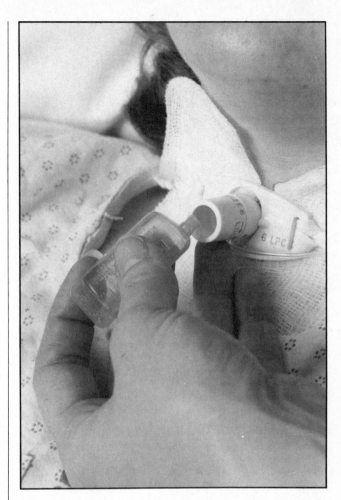

FIGURE 40–12

FIGURE 40–13

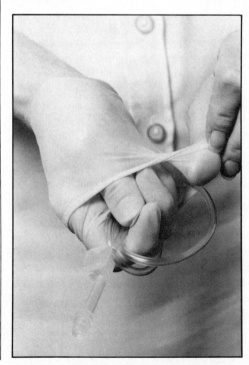

■ Evaluation

Expected outcomes

1. Absence of clinical signs of accumulated secretions, eg, restlessness, bubbling, or rattling breath sounds
2. Respiratory status normal for patient
3. Absence of adventitious breath sounds using stethoscope
4. Normal pulse rate

Unexpected outcomes

1. Clinical signs of accumulated secretions
2. Dyspnea, rales

3. Pulse rate accelerated for patient
4. Pallor, cyanosis

Upon obtaining an unexpected outcome:

1. Report your findings to the responsible nurse and/or physician.
2. Adjust the nursing care plan appropriately, eg, repeat suctioning, and assess the patient every 15 minutes.

TECHNIQUE 40–2 ■ Deflating and Inflating a Cuffed Tracheostomy Tube

Cuffed tracheostomy tubes are tubes surrounded by an inflatable cuff that produces an airtight seal between the tube and the trachea. This seal prevents aspiration of oropharyngeal secretions and air leakage between the tube and the trachea. Cuffed tubes are often used immediately after a tracheostomy in adults and infants and are essential when ventilating a tracheostomy patient with a ventilator. Children do not require cuffed tubes, since their tracheas are resilient enough to seal the air space around the tube.

A variety of tubes are manufactured. Some are disposable plastic, others are metal. Some are high-pressure cuffs, others are low-pressure cuffs, which can be inflated alternately to alter the pressure points on the trachea and prevent tracheal irritation and tissue damage. Alternate inflation also allows uninterrupted respirator function for patients attached to ventilators. Commercially prepared cuffs are available for use on cuffless tracheostomy tubes.

Different tubes have different advantages and disadvantages. Cuffs that are bonded to the tracheostomy tube eliminate the risk of accidental detachment inside the trachea. Low-pressure cuffs, which are more costly than others, distribute a low, even pressure against the trachea, thus decreasing the risk of tracheal tissue necrosis. They do not need to be deflated periodically to reduce pressure on the tracheal wall. Double-cuffed high-pressure tubes may reduce the risk of tissue necrosis with alternate inflation of cuffs but *only* if there is rigid adherence to the alternate inflation schedule. If tracheal damage does occur, a larger area of the trachea is involved with double-cuffed tubes.

A variation of the cuffed tube is the foam cuff. It does not require injected air; instead, when the port is opened, ambient air enters the balloon, which then conforms to the patient's trachea. See Figure 40–14. The physician removes air from the cuff prior to insertion or removal of the tube. See Figure 40–15.

Cuffed tracheostomy tubes are generally inflated in the following situations (check agency practices and policies):

1. During the first 12 hours after a tracheostomy
2. When the patient is being ventilated or receiving IPPB therapy, to prevent air leakage
3. When the patient is eating or receiving oral medications, and for a prescribed period of time following (eg, 30 minutes), to prevent aspiration
4. When the patient is comatose, to prevent aspiration of oropharyngeal secretions

At other times the cuff is deflated. If double-cuffed tubes are used, deflation and inflation must be done at regular intervals according to the manufacturer's directions.

■ Assessment

See Technique 40–1 on page 930. Other data include:

1. The manufacturer's instructions for the particular cuff. Various types are manufactured.
2. The physician's orders and agency policy about the prescribed schedule for deflation and inflation.

■ Planning

Nursing goals

1. To prevent aspiration of oropharyngeal secretions while the patient is comatose or is eating or receiving oral medications
2. To prevent tracheal edema, ulceration, and necrosis

Equipment

1. Equipment needed for suctioning the oropharyngeal cavity (see Technique 40–1 on page 931)
2. A 5- or 10-mL syringe
3. A stethoscope
4. A rubber-tipped hemostat
5. A manual resuscitator (Ambu bag)
6. A manometer specifically designed to measure cuff pressure
7. A sterile three-way stopcock (optional)

■ Intervention

1. Assist the patient to a semi-Fowler's position unless contraindicated. Patients receiving positive pressure ventilation should be placed in a supine position so that secretions above the cuff site are moved up into the mouth.

Deflating a tracheal cuff

2. Suction the oropharyngeal cavity before deflating the cuff. See Technique 37–1 on page 886. Discard the catheter.

   Rationale Suctioning prevents pooled oral secretions from descending into the trachea after the cuff is deflated. The secretions could cause irritation and infection. The first catheter is discarded to avoid introducing microorganisms into the lower airway when it is suctioned in step 6.

3. If a hemostat is clamping the cuff inflation tube, unclamp it. Some tubes have one-way valves that replace the hemostat.

4. Attach the 5- or 10-mL syringe to the distal end of the inflation tube, making sure the seal is tight.

5. Slowly withdraw from the cuff the amount of air indicated by the manufacturer, while the patient inhales and, if agency policy indicates, while providing a positive pressure breath with a manual resuscitator (Ambu bag). Keep the syringe attached to the tubing.

   Rationale Removal of air on inhalation under positive pressure allows secretions to ascend from the bronchi. The syringe is left attached for reinflation of the cuff.

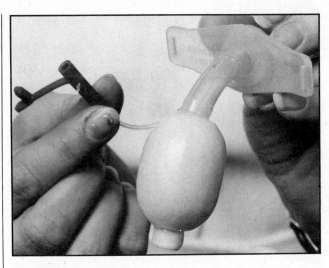

FIGURE 40–14

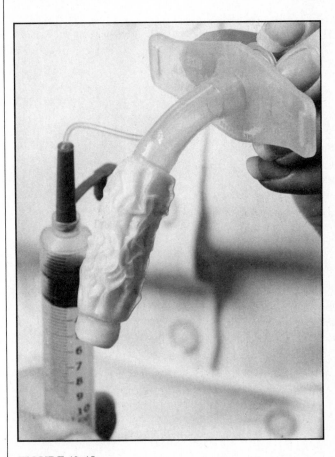

FIGURE 40–15

6. Suction the lower airway with a sterile catheter, if the cough reflex is stimulated during cuff deflation.

   Rationale Cuff deflation can stimulate the cough reflex, which may produce additional secretions.

7. Assess the patient's respirations, and suction the patient as needed. If the patient experiences breathing difficulties, reinflate the cuff immediately.

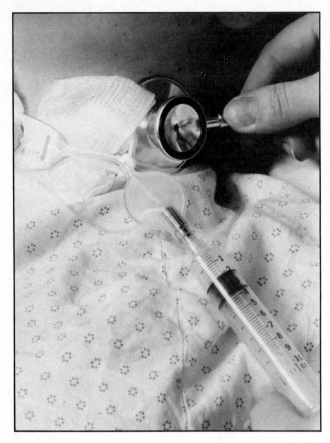

FIGURE 40–16

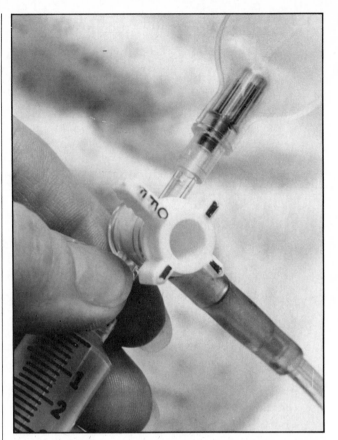

FIGURE 40–17

Inflating a tracheal cuff

8. Add the *least* amount of air following the manufacturer's recommendations, to create a minimal air leak. The minimal leak technique is designed to prevent tracheal damage and is performed as follows:

a. Inflate the cuff on inhalation, and place your stethoscope on the patient's neck adjacent to the trachea. See Figure 40–16.

b. Listen for squeaking or gurgling sounds, which indicate a leak.

c. If no leak is present, slowly remove 0.2 to 0.3 mL more air.

d. Listen again for sounds.

e. The cuff is inflated sufficiently when:

- You cannot hear the patient's voice.
- You cannot feel any air movements from the patient's mouth, nose, or tracheostomy site.
- You hear a slight or no leak from the positive pressure ventilation when auscultating the neck adjacent to the trachea during inspiration.

9. Measure the cuff pressure:

a. Attach the cuff's pillow port to the cuff pressure manometer tubing.

b. Read the dial on the manometer. The pressure should not exceed 15 to 20 mm Hg or 25 cm H_2O. Check agency policy.

Rationale Excessive cuff pressure causes tracheal edema, ulceration, and necrosis. Underinflation may cause inadequate ventilation and may allow aspiration of blood, food, or secretions.

10. Clamp the inflation tube with the hemostat if the tube has no one-way valve.

11. Remove the syringe.

12. Determine the exact amount of air used to inflate the cuff.

Rationale This helps prevent overinflation in subsequent cuff procedures.

13. Record the time of the deflation and/or inflation, the amount of air withdrawn and/or injected, and your assessments.

Variation: Inflating a cuff using a sterile three-way stopcock

14. Attach the ends of the stopcock to the syringe, the manometer tubing, and the inflation balloon. See Figure 40–17.

15. Open all ports of the stopcock.

16. Inject the air into the balloon until the manometer indicates the desired pressure.

17. Clamp the inflation tube if it does not have a one-way valve.

18. Remove the three-way stopcock. Follow step 13.

■ **Evaluation**   See Technique 40–1 on page 934.

TECHNIQUE 40–3   ■   Cleaning a Tracheostomy Tube Using Sterile Technique

Tracheostomy tubes are cleaned whenever necessary but at least once per shift.

■ Assessment

See Technique 40–1 on page 930. Assess the tracheostomy tube and stoma for the presence of secretions.

■ Planning

Nursing goals

1. To prevent infections of the tracheostomy site

2. To prevent airway obstruction by removing encrustations

Equipment

1. Sterile bowls for the cleaning solutions

2. Cleaning solutions: hydrogen peroxide and sterile normal saline

3. A sterile nylon brush or pipe cleaners to clean the lumen of the inner cannula

4. Sterile gauze squares or sterile cotton-tipped applicator sticks to clean the flange of the outer cannula

5. Sterile gloves

6. A clean glove (optional)

■ Intervention

Double-cannula tube

1. Don a sterile glove on your dominant hand.

2. Suction the entire length of the inner cannula prior to its removal. See Technique 40–1 on page 931.
   Rationale   This removes secretions and ensures a patent airway.

3. With your nondominant hand, which is ungloved or wearing a clean glove, remove and discard the patient's tracheostomy dressing.

Rationale   Wearing a clean glove on the nondominant hand is recommended by some agencies, since the dressing may be soiled. The glove maintains the cleanliness of the hand for step 7.

4. With the nondominant hand, unlock the inner cannula by turning the lock about 90° counterclockwise.
   Rationale   The nondominant hand is used to handle the flange of the cannula, which is not sterile.

5. With the nondominant hand, remove the inner cannula by gently pulling it out toward you in line with its curvature.

6. Soak the inner cannula in the hydrogen peroxide solution for several minutes.
   Rationale   This moistens and removes dried secretions.

7. Put a sterile glove on your nondominant hand.
   Rationale   Both hands are needed to clean the tube. To maintain sterile technique, both hands must be gloved.

8. Remove the cannula from the soaking solution. Clean the lumen and entire inner cannula thoroughly, using the pipe cleaners or brush moistened with sterile saline. See Figure 40–18.

9. Agitate the cannula for several seconds in the sterile saline.
   Rationale   This thoroughly rinses the cannula and provides a thin film of moisture to lubricate its insertion.

10. Inspect the cannula for cleanliness by holding it at eye level and looking through it into the light. If encrustations are evident, repeat steps 6, 8, and 9.

11. After rinsing the cannula, gently tap it against the inside edge of the sterile solution bowl.
    Rationale   This removes excess liquid from the cannula and prevents possible aspiration of it by the patient.

12. Dry the inside of the cannula using two or three pipe

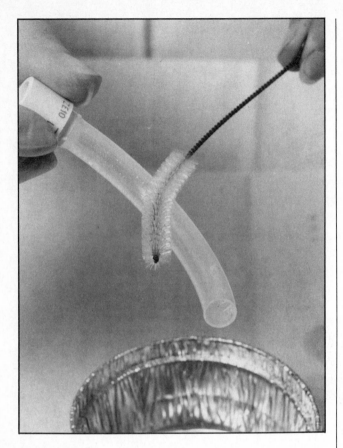

FIGURE 40–18

cleaners twisted together. Do not dry its outer surface.

Rationale A thin film of moisture will lubricate insertion.

13. Suction the outer cannula.

   Rationale Secretions are removed to prevent adherence of the two tubes when the inner cannula is inserted.

14. Clean the flange of the outer cannula if necessary, using cotton-tipped applicators or gauze squares moistened with sterile saline.

15. Grasp the outer flange of the inner cannula, and insert the cannula in the direction of its curvature.

16. Lock the inner cannula in place by turning the lock clockwise about 90° to an upright position.

17. Gently pull on the inner cannula to ensure that it is positioned securely.

18. Clean the tracheostomy site, and apply a new tracheostomy dressing. See Technique 40–4.

19. Record the removal, cleaning, and reinsertion of the cannula and your assessments.

Single-cannula tube

20. Suction the entire length of the cannula. See Technique 40–1.

21. Remove and discard the tracheostomy dressing.

22. Don a sterile glove on your dominant hand.

23. With the gloved hand, saturate a sterile gauze square with sterile normal saline or water, squeeze out excess solution, and clean the patient's neck under the tube flanges.

24. Saturate additional gauze squares as needed, and thoroughly clean the skin surrounding the tracheostomy site and the flanges of the tube. Wipe only once with each gauze square, and then discard it.

   Rationale This avoids contaminating a clean area with a soiled gauze square.

25. For encrustations that are difficult to remove, use sterile cotton-stipped applicators dipped in hydrogen peroxide.

26. Thoroughly rinse the cleaned area, using gauze squares moistened with sterile normal saline.

   Rationale Hydrogen peroxide can be irritating to the skin.

27. Dry the patient's skin and tube flanges with dry gauze squares.

28. Remove and discard the sterile glove.

29. Record the technique. See step 19.

Variation: For the patient on a ventilator

For the patient with a double-cannula tracheostomy tube attached to a ventilator, a spare inner cannula is kept on hand in a sterile container, since ventilation cannot be discontinued long enough to clean the inner cannula. Additional equipment is required: a clean towel, which is placed across the patient's chest (the disconnected ventilator tubing is placed on it); and a hand-held resuscitator.

30. Prepare the tracheostomy suctioning and cleaning equipment.

31. Hyperventilate the patient by using the ventilator's sigh mechanism. If the ventilator does not have a built-in sigh mechanism, use a manual resuscitation bag, such as an Ambu bag, connected to an oxygen source; adjust the oxygen flowmeter to deliver 12 to 15 L/min.

32. Disconnect the ventilator tubing, and place it on the clean towel.

33. Don a sterile glove, and suction the tracheostomy tube.

34. Using the ungloved hand, hyperventilate the patient as required with the hand-held resuscitator.

35. Quickly remove the inner cannula using the ungloved hand, and replace it with the clean cannula:

   a. Use the ungloved hand to remove the lid of the container holding the spare cannula.

Rationale   The lid of the container is exposed to the air and is not sterile.

   b. Use the sterile gloved hand to pick up the cannula and insert it. Lock it in place.

   Rationale   The cannula is sterile and therefore must not be handled by the bare hand.

   c. Use the ungloved hand to reattach the patient to the ventilator.

   d. Clean the soiled cannula. See steps 6–12.

36. Record the technique. See step 19.

■ Evaluation

See Technique 40–1 on page 934.

Expected outcome

Absence of secretions on cannula and tracheostomy tube.

Unexpected outcome

Presence of large amount of foul-smelling, purulent secretions. Upon obtaining an unexpected outcome:

1. Report your findings to the responsible nurse and/or physician.
2. Adjust the nursing care plan appropriately.

TECHNIQUE 40–4 ■ Changing a Tracheostomy Dressing and Tie Tapes

A tracheostomy dressing and the tie tapes need to be changed whenever soiled. Soiled dressings harbor microorganisms and can be a potential source of skin excoriation, breakdown, and infection. Usually the dressing is changed after the cannula is cleaned, but a dressing change may be necessary more frequently.

■ Assessment

Assess the patient for:

1. Secretions from the tracheostomy site
2. Clinical signs of infection at the tracheostomy site, eg, inflammation, purulent discharge, odor
3. Pulse and respiratory rates

Other data include: special orders about the dressing, eg, to apply antibiotic ointment to the stoma after cleaning it.

■ Planning

Nursing goals

1. To prevent infection of the tracheostomy site
2. To provide comfort to the patient

Equipment

1. A moisture-proof bag in which to discard the soiled dressing.
2. Sterile gloves.
3. Cleaning solutions (eg, sterile normal saline and hydrogen peroxide) to clean the wound and surrounding area.
4. Sterile bowls for the cleaning solutions.
5. Sterile non-cotton-filled gauze squares and sterile cotton-tipped applicator sticks to clean the wound. Non-cotton-filled squares are used, since cotton fibers can be pulled off and left in the wound, where they encourage bacterial growth and contamination.
6. Antibiotic ointment for the incision site if ordered or if recommended by agency policy.
7. A commercially prepared dressing or a sterile 4 × 4 gauze square.
8. Cotton twill tape for the ties.
9. A gauze square and tape to pad and cover the knot.

■ Intervention

1. Assist the patient to a semi-Fowler's position to promote lung expansion.
2. If the tracheostomy dressing was not removed previously, remove it and discard it in the moisture-proof bag.
3. Open the sterile equipment, and don the sterile gloves.
4. Clean around the incision site with gauze squares or applicator sticks dampened with sterile normal saline. See Figure 40–19. If encrustations are difficult to remove, use hydrogen peroxide.
5. Rinse the cleaned areas using sterile applicators moistened in normal saline.

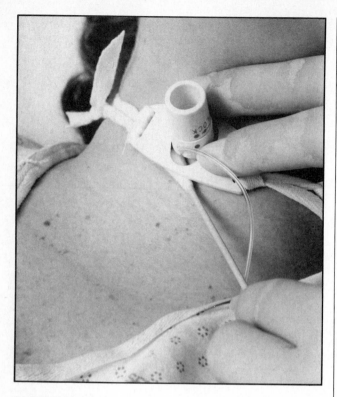

FIGURE 40-19

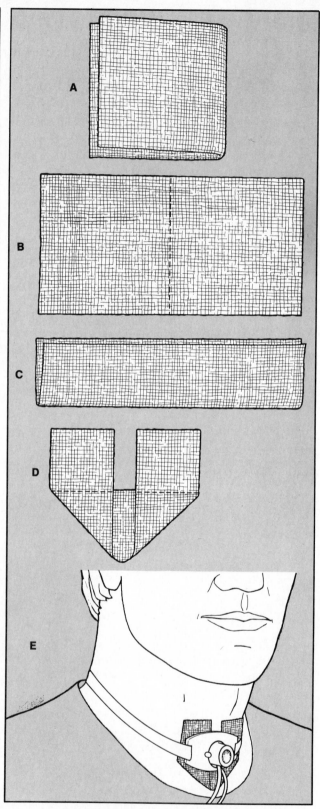

FIGURE 40-20

6. Clean the flange of the tube in the same manner.

7. Thoroughly dry the area with dry gauze squares.

8. Using an applicator stick, apply antibiotic ointment around the incision site if ordered or recommended by agency policy.

9. Apply a dressing around the insertion site. Use a commercially prepared tracheostomy dressing of nonravelling material if available, or open and refold a 4 × 4 gauze as shown in Figure 40-20, *A–D*. Place the gauze as shown in Figure 40-20, *E*, if drainage is heavy; insert the dressing from above if drainage is not heavy. Avoid using cotton-filled gauze squares, and avoid cutting the 4 × 4 gauze.

   Rationale The patient might aspirate cotton lint or frayed fibers, which could subsequently create a tracheal abscess.

10. While applying the dressing, ensure that the tracheostomy tube is securely supported.

    Rationale Excessive movement of the tracheostomy tube irritates the trachea.

11. Change the tie tapes:

    a. Cut two strips of cotton twill tape, one about 25 cm (10 in) long and the other 50 cm (20 in) long.

    Rationale When one tape is longer than the other, they can be fastened at the side of the patient's neck for easy access. A knot at the back of the neck could create pressure and irritate the skin.

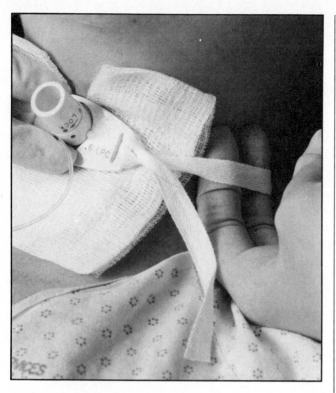

FIGURE 40–21

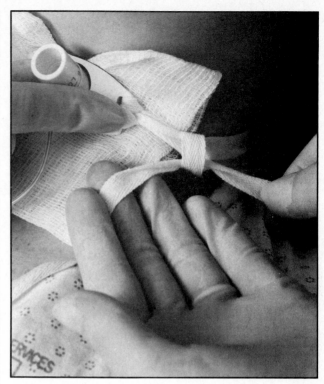

FIGURE 40–22

b. Cut a 1-cm (0.5-in) slit approximately 2.5 cm (1 in) from one end of each strip. This is best achieved by folding the end of the tape back onto itself about 2.5 cm and then cutting a slit in the middle of the tape from its folded edge.

c. Have an assistant don a sterile glove and hold the tracheostomy tube in place while you change the ties. If you do not have an assistant, fasten the clean ties before removing the soiled ties.

Rationale   Holding the tube prevents accidental expulsion of it if the patient coughs or moves.

d. Detach and remove the soiled tapes from the patient. The ties can be cut or untied.

e. Thread the slit end of one clean tape through the eye of the tracheostomy faceplate from the bottom side; then thread the other end of the tie through the slit of the tape, pulling it taut until it is securely fastened to the faceplace.

Rationale   This method avoids the use of knots, which produce pressure, discomfort, and skin irritation.

f. Repeat step e for the second tie.

g. Ask the patient to flex his or her neck, and have your assistant place one or two fingers under the tapes while tying the tapes together at the side of the patient's neck. See Figure 40–21.

Rationale   Flexion of the neck increases neck circumference the way coughing does. The pa-

tient's neck flexion and the assistant's finger placement prevent the nurse from making the ties too tight, which could cause choking or pressure on the jugular veins.

h. Tie the tapes using two square knots. Cut off any long ends. See Figure 40–22.

Rationale   Two square knots will not slip and loosen, allowing the tube to dislodge.

12. Place a folded 4 × 4 gauze square under the tie where it is knotted, and apply tape over the knot.

Rationale   Gauze under the knot prevents skin irritation. Taping over the knot prevents confusing the dressing ties with the patient's gown ties.

13. Frequently check the tautness of the tracheostomy tie, particularly for patients whose neck diameter may increase from swelling (eg, those with radical neck surgery, neck trauma, or cardiac failure) or for patients who are restless and may loosen their ties.

14. Record the dressing change, the application of any ointments, and your assessments.

■ **Evaluation**

Expected outcomes

1. Absence of secretions from the tracheostomy site

2. Absence of clinical signs of infection

3. Pulse and respirations normal for the patient

Unexpected outcomes

1. Tracheostomy site reddened and swollen
2. Large amount of purulent, foul-smelling discharge
3. Site painful

Upon obtaining an unexpected outcome:

1. Report your findings to the responsible nurse and/or physician.
2. Adjust the nursing care plan appropriately.

TECHNIQUE 40–5 ■ Plugging a Tracheostomy Tube 🏠

A tracheostomy plug is usually inserted into a tracheostomy tube for specified lengths of time before the tube is removed. While the tube is plugged, the patient is carefully monitored for signs of respiratory distress. Often the length of time the tube is plugged is increased over a number of days if the patient tolerates the procedure well.

■ Assessment

Assess the patient for:

1. Pulse and respirations before plugging the tube.
2. Excessive secretions in the respiratory tract. Report this finding to the physician. Excessive secretions could indicate the tube should not be plugged.
3. Respiratory status while the tube is plugged. Note breath sounds, respiratory rate, and the use of accessory muscles for breathing.

Additional data include: the order to plug the tube, including the length of time it is to remain plugged.

■ Planning

Nursing goal

To ensure adequate ventilation.

Equipment

1. A sterile tracheostomy plug
2. Suction apparatus
3. Sterile suction catheters
4. Sterile gloves
5. A sterile 10-mL syringe

■ Intervention

1. Assist the patient to a semi-Fowler's position if not contraindicated.

2. Suction the patient's nasopharynx if there are any secretions present. See Technique 37–1 on page 886.
3. Change suction catheters, and suction the tracheostomy. See Technique 40–1 on page 931.
4. Deflate the tracheal cuff if ordered. See Technique 40–2 on page 935.
5. Suction the tracheostomy tube again if secretions are present.
6. Using sterile gloves, fit the tracheostomy plug into either the inner or the outer cannula depending on whether the tracheostomy tube has a double or single cannula.
7. Monitor the patient closely for ten minutes for signs of respiratory distress. At the first signs of distress, remove the tracheostomy plug, and suction the tracheostomy if necessary.
8. Clean the inner cannula, if it was removed, so that it is ready to be reinserted.
9. Observe the patient frequently while the tube is plugged.
10. Remove the plug at the designated time, suction the tracheostomy if indicated, and replace the inner cannula if removed.
11. Reinflate the cuff if ordered.
12. Record the amount, color, and consistency of the secretions, the times the plug was inserted and removed, and your assessments.

■ Evaluation

Expected outcomes

1. Pusle rate unchanged
2. Respirations normal, no signs of dyspnea or cyanosis
3. Absence of secretions in the respiratory tract
4. Breathing effortless while plug in place

Unexpected outcomes

1. Pulse rate increased
2. Dyspneic respirations
3. Large amount of tenacious secretions accumulated in trachea

Upon obtaining an unexpected outcome:

1. Report your findings to the responsible nurse and/or physician.
2. Adjust the nursing care plan appropriately.

References

Albanese AJ et al: A hassle-free guide to suctioning a tracheostomy. *RN* (April) 1982; 45:24–29.

Brown I: Trach care? Take care—infection's on the prowl. *Nursing 82* (May) 1982; 12:44–49.

Fuchs PL: Streamlining your suctioniong techniques, part 3: Tracheostomy suctioning. *Nursing 84* (July) 1984; 14:39–43.

O'Donnell B: How to change tracheostomy ties—easily and safely. *Nursing 78* (March) 1978; 8:66–69.

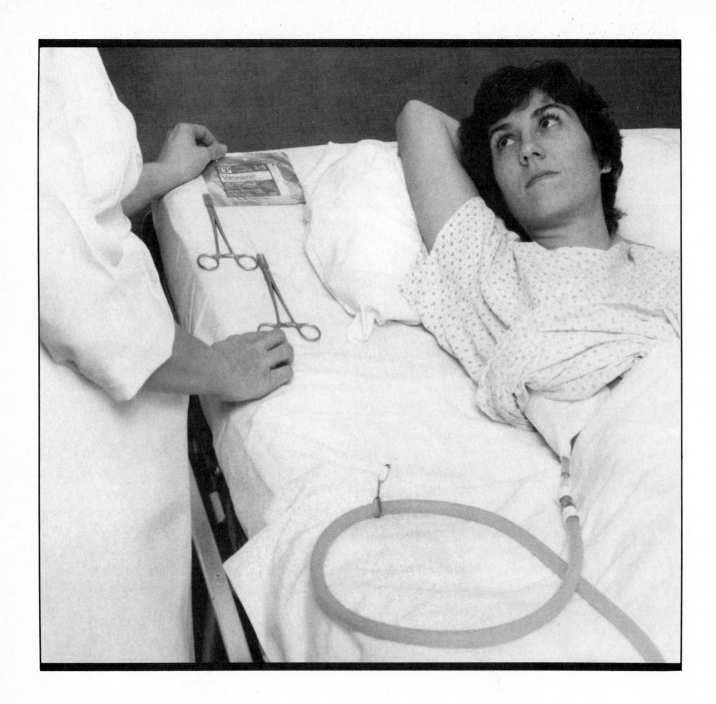

CHEST DRAINAGE

41

Chest drainage is required for patients who have fluid or air in the pleural cavity. Normally the pleural cavity has a negative pressure; this permits the lungs to expand during inhalation. However, because of disease, injury, or surgery, blood or air may accumulate in the pleural cavity. If it is not drained, this liquid or air in the space affects the lungs and their capacity to expand, hence impairing the individual's breathing.

Chest tubes are used to drain blood or air from the pleural cavity. Because of the negative pressure in the cavity, precautions must be taken to prevent air or fluid from being drawn into rather than drawn out of the cavity during drainage. Strict surgical aseptic technique is followed.

Chapter Outline

Chest Tubes

Drainage Systems

■ Technique 41–1 Setting Up a Chest Drainage System

■ Technique 41–2 Assisting with the Insertion and Removal of a Chest Tube

■ Technique 41–3 Monitoring a Patient with Chest Drainage

Objectives

Upon completion of this chapter, the student will:

1. Know essential terms and facts about chest tubes
   1.1 Define selected terms
   1.2 Identify various types of drainage systems
   1.3 Identify clinical signs of pneumothorax
   1.4 Outline safety precautions for patients who have chest tubes
2. Understand facts about techniques associated with chest tubes
   2.1 Identify relevant assessment data
   2.2 Identify nursing diagnoses for which the technique may be implemented
   2.3 Identify nursing goals related to the technique
   2.4 Identify expected and unexpected outcomes from assessment data
   2.5 Identify reasons underlying selected steps of the technique
3. Perform techniques associated with chest tubes safely
   3.1 Assess the patient adequately
   3.2 Collect additional data from appropriate sources
   3.3 Select pertinent nursing goals for the patient
   3.4 Establish relevant outcome criteria for the patient following the technique
   3.5 Collect necessary equipment before the technique
   3.6 Implement interventions to enhance the effectiveness of the technique and enhance the patient's comfort and safety
   3.7 Communicate relevant information about the patient to the appropriate persons
   3.8 Determine the evaluative outcomes of the technique
4. Evaluate own performance of specific techniques associated with chest tubes in a laboratory or clinical setting with the assistance of another
   4.1 Use the performance checklists provided
   4.2 Identify areas of strength and weakness
   4.3 Alter performance in response to own evaluation and that of another

Terms

■ atelectasis   the collapse of lung tissue

■ creps (crepitation)   a dry crackling sound, like that of crumpled cellophane, produced by air in the subcutaneous tissue or by air moving through fluid in the alveoli of the lungs

■ hemopneumothorax   a collection of blood and air or gas in the pleural cavity

■ hemothorax   a collection of blood in the pleural cavity

■ pleural (intrapleural) cavity   the potential space between the visceral and parietal pleurae

■ pneumothorax   an accumulation of air or gas in the pleural cavity

■ stab wound   a small deep wound, made by a sharp instrument such as a scalpel; it is often used for the insertion of drains and tubes

■ subcutaneous emphysema   air or gas in the subcutaneous tissues

■ tube   an elongated cylindrical instrument through which fluid and/or air can flow

CHEST TUBES

Chest tubes are made of pliable plastic or rubber. They are usually inserted through an intercostal space into the pleural cavity. See Figure 41–1. Chest tubes that are used to remove air are usually inserted superiorly, ie, through the second intercostal space, and anteriorly, because air tends to rise in the pleural cavity. Tubes used to drain fluid are inserted more inferiorly, often in the eighth or ninth intercostal space, and more posteriorly. Sometimes a tube used to drain air is inserted inferiorly and threaded superiorly in the pleural space. When a patient requires drainage of both fluid and air, two chest tubes may be inserted. These are sometimes joined externally by a Y-connector.

Chest tubes are inserted during surgery and in nonsurgical situations, eg, in emergency treatment of injuries. When a chest tube is inserted during surgery, it may extrude through the incision or through a stab wound (a small deep wound made with a scalpel for insertion of the tube).

DRAINAGE SYSTEMS

Because the pleural cavity normally has negative pressure, any drainage system connected to it must be sealed,

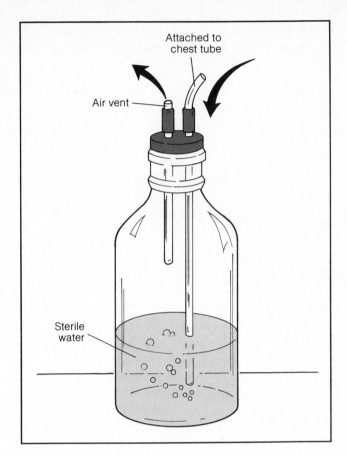

FIGURE 41–2 ■ A one-bottle gravity water-sealed drainage system.

FIGURE 41–1 ■ The pleural cavity is a potential space that lies between the visceral pleura and the parietal pleura. Chest tubes are inserted into this space.

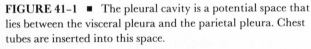
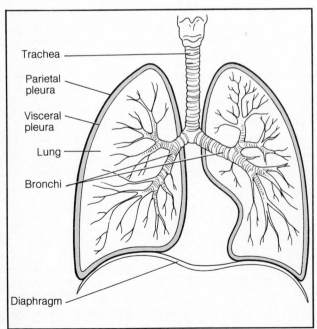

so that air or liquid cannot enter. Such a drainage system is called a *water-sealed (underwater) drainage* or a *disposable pleural drainage system.* In water-sealed drainage, fluid in the bottom of the container prevents air from entering the chest tube and thus entering the pleural cavity. The system must be kept below the level of the patient's chest, so that the fluid in the container is not drawn into the pleural cavity by gravity. It is also very important to maintain the patency of the tubing.

Drainage systems use three mechanisms to drain fluid and air from the pleural cavity: positive expiratory pressure, gravity, and suction. When the pleural cavity contains some air or fluid, a positive pressure develops during expiration. This positive pressure is abnormal, but it does help expel the air and to some extent fluid from the space. Gravity acts as an evacuation force when the tubing is placed so that it descends from the insertion site to the drainage receptacle. Suction is used in conjunction with the other two forces in some drainage systems.

There are several kinds of water-sealed drainage systems: one- and two-bottle gravity systems, two- and three-bottle suction systems, and disposable unit systems.

FIGURE 41–3 ■ A two-bottle gravity water-sealed drainage system.

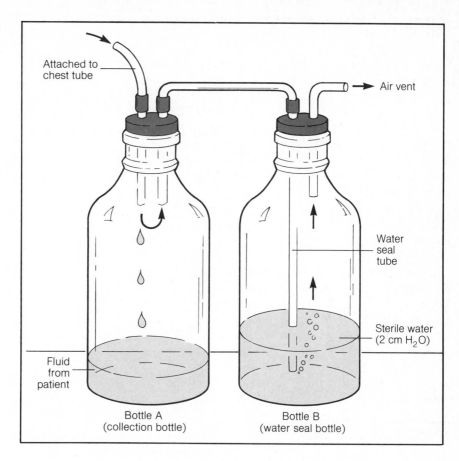

One-Bottle Systems

In a one-bottle system, a single receptacle both receives the fluid and/or air from the patient and seals the system. See Figure 41–2. The patient's air or fluid enters through the collection inlet, which terminates under sterile water, and air exits through the air vent. The fluid in this bottle then is a combination of fluid from the patient and sterile water; it forms the water seal. The one-bottle system depends upon gravity and positive expiratory pressure for drainage.

Two-Bottle Systems

A two-bottle system uses one bottle to receive the fluid or air from the patient and the second bottle to create the water seal. See Figure 41–3. The patient's air or fluid is received into bottle A. The air from bottle A is passed into bottle B. The air then exits from bottle B through the air vent. This system uses gravity and positive expiratory pressure for drainage.

Another type of two-bottle system uses suction as well as positive expiratory pressure and gravity for drainage. See Figure 41–4. In this system, bottle A collects the fluid drainage from the patient and creates the water seal. Bottle B is the suction-control bottle; the depth of the tube below the water level determines the amount of

negative pressure provided (ie, the deeper the tube is submerged in the sterile water, the greater the vacuum).

Three-Bottle Systems

The three-bottle system has a collection bottle (A), a water-seal bottle (B), and a suction-control bottle (C). See Figure 41–5. Fluid from the patient collects in bottle A, which is connected to a tube in bottle B that terminates below the fluid level. Bottle B is then connected to bottle C by a short tube. Bottle C also has a manometer tube submerged in sterile water. The depth to which this tube is submerged determines the amount of suction exerted in the patient's pleural cavity. The suction-control bottle has another inlet, for suction. This system uses positive expiratory pressure, gravity, and suction for drainage.

Disposable Unit Systems

Several types of disposable unit systems are available commercially. Two commonly seen are the Pleur-evac system and the Argyle system. The Pleur-evac system consists of three chambers. See Figure 41–6. Chamber A is the collection chamber. It receives fluid and/or air from the patient and is divided into three subchambers. The patient's fluid remains in this chamber, while air from the patient passes on to chamber B, the water-seal

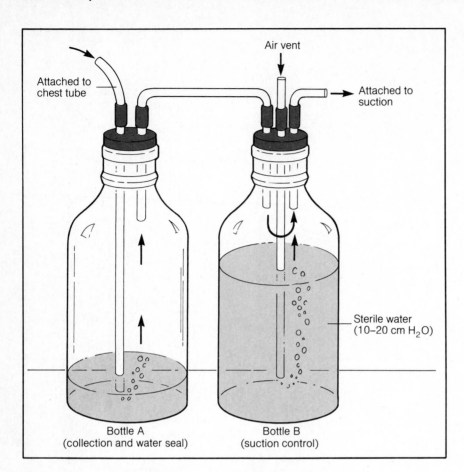

Attached to chest tube

Air vent

Attached to suction

Sterile water (10–20 cm H_2O)

Bottle A
(collection and water seal)

Bottle B
(suction control)

FIGURE 41-4 ■ A two-bottle suction water-sealed drainage system.

FIGURE 41-5 ■ A three-bottle suction water-sealed drainage system.

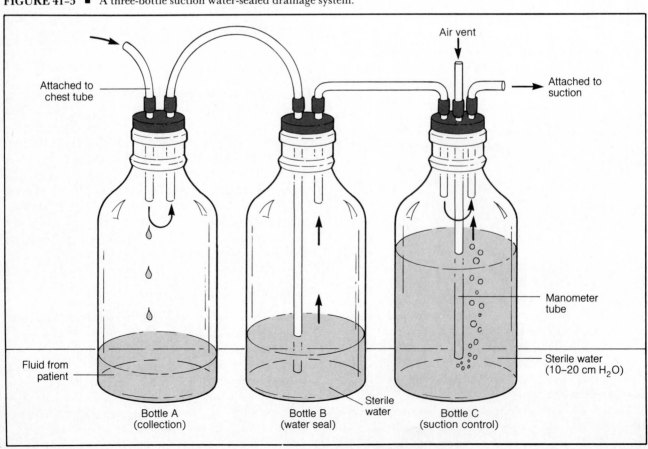

Attached to chest tube

Air vent

Attached to suction

Manometer tube

Sterile water (10–20 cm H_2O)

Fluid from patient

Sterile water

Bottle A
(collection)

Bottle B
(water seal)

Bottle C
(suction control)

chamber. This chamber is U-shaped, and air from the patient passes through the water seal and exits at the suction outlet side of the U. Chamber C, the suction chamber, is also U-shaped. The height of the fluid in chamber C determines the amount of suction pressure exerted upon the patient: Atmospheric air enters on the far left of this chamber, passes through the suction-control water, and joins the air from the patient. These then pass into the suction outlet.

The Argyle double-seal system consists of four chambers. See Figure 41–7. Chamber A is a water-seal chamber with a manometer. Chamber B is the collection chamber. Chamber C is another water seal. Chamber D is for suction control. Normally the patient's air passes from chamber B into chamber C and to the suction source; however, if the suction becomes obstructed, the patient's air can pass to chamber A and to the atmosphere. Chamber A thus serves as a safety vent.

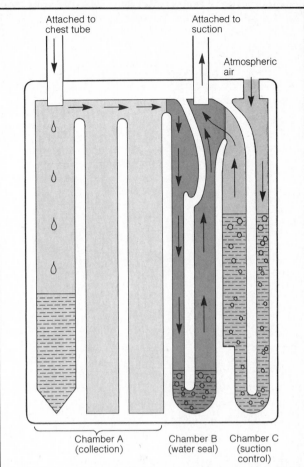

FIGURE 41–6 ■ A Pleur-evac chest drainage system.

FIGURE 41–7 ■ An Argyle chest drainage system.

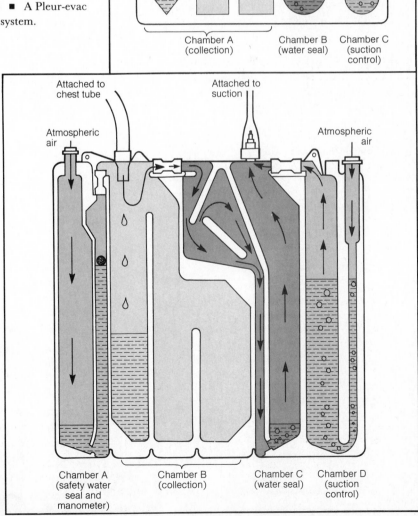

TECHNIQUE 41–1 ■ Setting Up a Chest Drainage System

Before setting up a chest drainage system, check the physician's orders for the type of system to use and whether suction is required. Surgical aseptic technique is followed strictly when setting up chest drainage to prevent microorganisms from entering the system and subsequently entering the patient's pleural cavity.

■ Planning

Nursing goal

To maintain the sterility of the equipment.

Equipment

1. Sterile distilled water.
2. Adhesive tape.
3. Sterile clear plastic tubing.
4. Sterile tubing connectors.
5. A drainage rack. Racks are supplied by the manufacturer for Pleur-evac and Argyle systems.
6. Two rubber-tipped Kelly clamps.
7. Suction apparatus, if ordered.
8. The drainage system. If the agency does not supply partially assembled systems, the following equipment is needed:

For a one-bottle system

a. A sterile 2-L bottle.
b. A sterile short glass tube.
c. A sterile long glass tube.
d. A sterile rubber stopper with two holes.

For a two-bottle gravity system

e. Two sterile 2-L bottles.
f. Sterile clear plastic tubing.
g. Three sterile short glass tubes.
h. One sterile long glass tube.
i. Two sterile rubber stoppers with two holes.

For a two-bottle suction system

j. Two sterile 2-L bottles.
k. Sterile clear plastic tubing.
l. Three sterile short glass tubes.
m. Two sterile long glass tubes.
n. Two sterile rubber stoppers: one with two holes, and one with three holes.

For a three-bottle system

o. Three sterile 2-L bottles.
p. Sterile clear plastic tubing.

q. Five sterile short glass tubes.
r. Two sterile long glass tubes.
s. Three sterile rubber stoppers: two with two holes, and one with three holes.

For a Pleur-evac or Argyle system

t. A sterile 50-mL Asepto (bulb) syringe.

■ Intervention

One-bottle system

See Figure 41–2 on page 946.

1. Fill the bottle with about 300 mL of sterile distilled water.
2. Insert one short glass tube and one long glass tube through the rubber stopper.
3. Attach the rubber stopper with the glass tubes to the bottle. Make sure the long glass tube is submerged in the water about 2 cm (0.75 in).
   Rationale Submersion of the tube creates the water seal.
4. Place the bottle in the drainage rack on the floor beside the patient's bed.
   Rationale A drainage rack prevents accidental breakage or spilling and disruption of the system. Keeping the bottle below the level of the patient's chest prevents the liquid from entering the pleural cavity.
5. Connect the clear plastic tubing to the long glass tube and to the patient's chest tube.
6. Securely tape all tubing connections.
   Rationale Taping prevents tube separation and disruption of the negative pressure system.
7. Place a strip of adhesive tape vertically on the drainage bottle to mark and assess the fluid level at prescribed periods.

Two-bottle gravity system

See Figure 41–3 on page 947.

8. Follow steps 1–3 to set up the water-seal bottle.
9. Insert two short glass tubes through the second rubber stopper, attach the stopper securely to the collection bottle, and place both bottles in the drainage rack on the floor.
10. Connect clear plastic tubing to the long glass tube in the water-seal bottle, and attach it to the nearer short glass tube in the collection bottle.

11. Connect clear plastic tubing to the remaining short glass tube in the collection bottle and to the patient's chest tube.

12. Follow steps 6–7.

Two-bottle suction system

See Figure 41–4 on page 948.

13. Follow steps 1–3 to set up the water-seal (and collection) bottle.

14. Fill the suction-control bottle with sterile distilled water to the level for the required suction.

15. Insert one long glass tube and two short glass tubes through the second stopper, attach the stopper securely to the suction-control bottle, and place both bottles in the drainage rack on the floor.

16. Connect the clear plastic tubing:
    a. Between the short glass tube in the water-seal bottle and one of the short glass tubes in the suction-control bottle.
    b. Between the long glass tube in the water-seal bottle and the patient's chest tube.
    c. Between the remaining short glass tube of the suction-control bottle and the suction source.

17. Follow steps 6–7.

Three-bottle system

See Figure 41–5 on page 948.

18. Follow steps 1–3 to set up the water-seal bottle.

19. Insert two short glass tubes through the remaining two-hole stopper, and attach the stopper securely to the collection bottle.

20. Insert two short glass tubes and one long glass tube through the three-hole rubber stopper.

21. Add sterile distilled water to the suction-control bottle. Make sure the long glass tube will be submerged to the ordered length; then attach the stopper securely to this bottle.

22. Place the bottles on a drainage rack on the floor, with the water-seal bottle in the middle.

23. Connect the clear plastic tubing:
    a. Between the long glass tube of the water-seal bottle and the nearer short glass tube of the collection bottle.
    b. Between the remaining short glass tube of the collection bottle and the patient's chest tube.
    c. Between the short glass tube of the water-seal bottle and the nearer short glass tube of the suction-control bottle.
    d. Between the remaining short glass tube of the suction-control bottle and the suction source.

24. Follow steps 6–7.

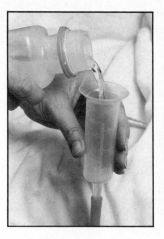 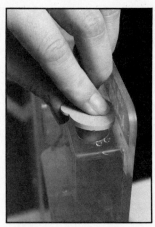

FIGURE 41–8 **FIGURE 41–9**

Pleur-evac or Argyle system

See Figures 41–6 and 41–7 on page 949.

25. Open the packaged unit.

26. Remove the plastic connector from the tube attached to the water-seal chamber. (The Argyle system has two water-seal chambers; do both.)

27. Using a 50-mL Asepto syringe with the bulb removed, fill the water-seal chamber with sterile distilled water up to the 2-cm mark. See Figure 41–8. Then reattach the plastic connector.

28. If the physician has ordered suction, remove the diaphragm (cap) on the suction-control chamber. See Figure 41–9.

29. Using the 50-mL syringe, fill the suction-control chamber with distilled water to the ordered level or 20 to 25 cm, and replace the cap.

30. Place the system in the rack suplied, or attach it to the bedframe (see Figure 41–10).

31. Attach the longer tube from the collection chamber to the patient's chest tube.

FIGURE 41–10

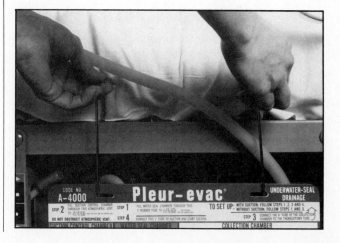

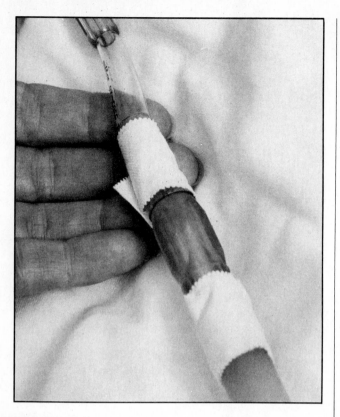

FIGURE 41-11

32. If suction is ordered, attach the remaining shorter tube to the suction source, and turn it on. Inspect the suction chamber for bubbling. Gentle bubbling indicates an appropriate suction level.

33. If suction has not been ordered, keep the shorter rubber tube unclamped.

    Rationale This maintains negative or equal pressure in the system.

34. Tape all tubing connections, but do not completely cover the tubing connectors with tape. See Figure 41-11.

    Rationale Not covering the connectors allows drainage to be seen.

TECHNIQUE 41-2 ■ Assisting with the Insertion and Removal of a Chest Tube

Chest tubes are inserted and removed by the physician with the nurse assisting. Both procedures require sterile technique and must be done without introducing air or pathogens into the pleural cavity. After the insertion, a portable x-ray machine is used to film the chest to confirm the position of the tube. Chest tubes are generally removed within five to seven days. Before removal, the tube is clamped with two large, rubber-tipped clamps for one to two days to assess the patient for signs of respiratory distress and to determine whether air or fluid remains in the pleural space. A chest x-ray film is generally taken two hours after tube clamping to assess full lung expansion. If the patient develops signs of respiratory distress or the film indicates pneumothorax, the tube clamps are removed, and chest drainage is maintained. If neither occurs, the tube is removed. Another chest x-ray film is often taken after removal to confirm full lung expansion.

■ Assessment

Assess the patient for:

1. Vital signs for baseline data.
2. Breath sounds. Auscultate bilaterally for baseline data. Diminished or absent breath sounds indicate inadequate lung expansion.
3. Clinical signs of pneumothorax before and after chest tube insertion. Leakage or blockage of a chest tube can seriously impair ventilation. Signs include: sharp pain on the affected side; weak, rapid pulse; pallor; vertigo; faintness; dyspnea; diaphoresis; excessive coughing; and blood-tinged sputum.

Other data include:

1. The type of chest tube and drainage system ordered
2. Whether suction is required

■ Planning

Nursing goal

To prevent the introduction of air or pathogens into the pleural space.

Equipment

For tube insertion

1. A sterile chest tube tray, which includes:

   a. Drapes

   b. A 10-mL syringe

   c. Sponges to clean the insertion area with antiseptic

   d. A 1-in #22 gauge needle

   e. A ⅝-in #25 gauge needle for the local anesthetic

   f. A scalpel

   g. Forceps

   h. Two rubber-tipped clamps for each tube inserted

   i. Several 4 × 4 gauze squares

   j. Split drain gauzes

   k. A chest tube with a trocar

   l. Suture materials (eg, 2–0 silk with a needle)

2. A pleural drainage system with sterile drainage tubing and connectors

3. A Y-connector, if two tubes will be inserted

4. Sterile gloves for the physician and the nurse

5. A vial of local anesthetic (eg, 1% lidocaine)

6. Alcohol sponges to clean the top of the vial

7. Antiseptic (eg, povidone-iodine)

8. Tape (nonallergenic is preferable)

9. Sterile petrolatum gauze (optional) to place around the chest tube

Set up the drainage system so it is ready for use. See Technique 41–1.

For tube removal

10. Clean gloves to remove the dressing

11. Sterile gloves to remove the tube

12. A sterile suture removal set, with forceps and suture scissors

13. Sterile petrolatum gauze

14. Several 4 × 4 gauze squares

15. Air-occlusive tape, 2 or 3 in wide (nonallergenic is preferred)

16. Scissors to cut the tape

17. An absorbent linen-saver pad

18. A moisture-proof bag

19. Sterile swabs or applicators in sterile containers to obtain a specimen (optional)

■ Intervention

Chest tube insertion

1. Assist the patient to a lateral position with the area to receive the tube facing upward. Determine from the physician whether to have the bed in the supine position or semi-Fowler's position.

   Rationale A supine position is generally preferred for tube insertions into the second or third intercostal space, a semi-Fowler's position for the sixth to eighth intercostal spaces.

2. Open the chest tube tray and the sterile gloves on the overbed table. Pour antiseptic solution onto the sponges. Be sure to maintain sterile technique.

3. While the physician dons the gloves and cleans the insertion area with antiseptic solution, wipe the stopper of the anesthetic vial with an alcohol sponge. Invert the vial and hold it for the physician to withdraw the anesthetic.

4. Attend the patient and assist the physician as necessary, while the physician anesthetizes the area, makes a small incision, inserts the tube, either clamps the tube or immediately connects it to the drainage system, and then sutures the tube to the skin.

5. Optional: Don sterile gloves. Wrap a piece of sterile petrolatum gauze around the chest tube, if the physician prefers this. Place drain gauzes around the insertion site (one from the top and one from the bottom). Place several 4 × 4 gauze squares over these.

   Rationale The gauzes make an airtight seal at the insertion site.

6. Remove your gloves, if donned, and tape the dressings, covering them completely.

7. Tape the chest tube to the patient's skin away from the insertion site.

   Rationale Taping prevents accidental dislocation of the tube.

8. Tape the connections of the chest tube to the drainage tube and to the drainage system.

   Rationale Taping prevents inadvertent separation.

9. Coil the drainage tubing, and secure it to the bed linen ensuring enough slack for the patient to turn and move. See Figure 41–12.

   Rationale This prevents kinking of the tubing and impairment of the drainage system.

10. When all drainage connections are completed, have the patient:

    a. Take a deep breath and hold it for a few seconds.

    b. Slowly exhale.

    Rationale These actions facilitate drainage from the pleural space and lung reexpansion.

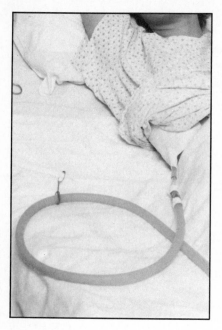

FIGURE 41–12

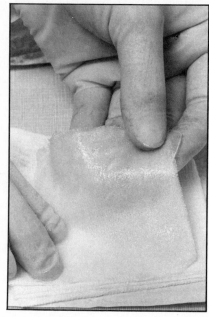

FIGURE 41–13

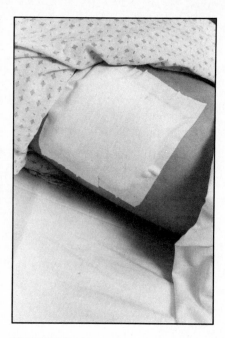

FIGURE 41–14

11. Take the patient's vital signs every 15 minutes for the first hour following tube insertion and then as ordered, eg, every hour for two hours, then every four hours.

12. Auscultate the patient's lungs every four hours to assess breath sounds and the adequacy of ventilation in the affected lung.

13. Place rubber-tipped chest tube clamps at the bedside.

    Rationale These are used to clamp the chest tube and prevent pneumothorax if the tube becomes disconnected from the drainage system or the system breaks or cracks.

14. Observe the patient regularly for signs of pneumothorax and subcutaneous emphysema. Subcutaneous emphysema can result from a poor seal at the insertion site. It is manifested by a "crackling" sound that is heard when the area around the insertion site is palpated. Go to step 29.

Chest tube removal

15. Administer an analgesic, if ordered, 30 minutes before the tube is removed.

16. Ensure that the chest tube is securely clamped.

    Rationale Clamping prevents air from entering the pleural space.

17. Assist the patient to a semi-Fowler's position or to a lateral position on the unaffected side.

18. Put the absorbent pad under the patient beneath the chest tube.

Rationale The pad protects the bed linen from drainage and provides a place for the chest tube after removal.

19. Open the sterile packages, and prepare a sterile field.

20. Wearing sterile gloves, place the sterile petrolatum gauze on a 4 × 4 gauze square. See Figure 41–13.

    Rationale This will quickly provide an airtight dressing over the insertion site after the tube is removed.

21. Remove the soiled dressings, being careful not to dislodge the tube. Don clean gloves to remove the underlying gauzes, which may contain drainage. Discard soiled dressings in the moisture-proof bag.

22. The physician will:

    a. Don sterile gloves.

    b. Hold the chest tube with forceps.

    c. Cut the suture holding the tube in place.

    d. Instruct the patient to either inhale or exhale fully and hold the breath while the physician removes the tube.

    Rationale This prevents air from being sucked into the pleural space during tube removal.

    e. Place the prepared petrolatum gauze dressing over the insertion site immediately after tube removal.

23. While the physician is removing the tube, prepare three 15-cm (6-in) strips of air-occlusive tape.

24. After the gauze dressing is applied, completely cover it with the air-occlusive tape. See Figure 41–14.

    Rationale This makes the dressing as airtight as possible.

25. If a specimen is required for culture and sensitivity, use a swab to obtain drainage from inside the chest tube, while the physician holds the tube.

26. Take the patient's vital signs, and assess the quality of her or his respirations every 15 minutes for the first hour following tube removal and then as ordered.

27. Auscultate the patient's lungs every hour for the first four hours to assess breath sounds and the adequacy of ventilation in the affected lung.

28. Observe the patient regularly for signs of pneumothorax, subcutaneous emphysema, and infection.

29. Record the date and time of chest tube insertion or removal. For insertion, document the insertion site, drainage system used, presence of bubbling, vital signs, breath sounds from auscultation, and any other assessment findings. For removal, document the amount, color, and consistency of drainage, vital signs, and the specimen obtained for culture, if taken.

Sample Recording

Date	Time	Notes
12/6/86	2200	Sudden sharp pain in L chest, diaphoretic, pale, and dyspneic. ———
	2300	BP 100/70, TPR 98.6, 105, 24. Diminished breath sounds in L lung and absence of chest movement. Two chest tubes inserted by Dr. Jung in L 2nd and 8th ICS. Connected by Y-connector and attached to Pleur-evac. Drainage functioning well.——
	2330	BP 110/70, TPR 98.6, 100, 20. Breath sounds present in L lung. ——————————————— Karen P. Smith, RN
12/12/86	1000	Chest tubes removed by Dr. Jung. 100 mL clear pink drainage. BP 120/70, TPR 98.6, 76, 16. Specimen of chest tube drainage taken for culture and sensitivity and sent to lab. ————— Susan March, NS

■ **Evaluation**   See Technique 41–3 on page 959.

TECHNIQUE 41–3   ■   Monitoring a Patient with Chest Drainage

■ **Assessment**

1. Assess the patient's level of comfort, and administer ordered analgesics as needed, especially before the patient moves or does deep breathing and coughing exercises.

2. Assess the patient's vital signs every four hours to check for signs of pneumothorax. For the clinical signs, see Technique 41–2 on page 952.

3. Observe the patient's chest movements. A decrease in chest expansion on the affected side indicates recurrent pneumothorax.

4. Auscultate the patient's lungs for breath sounds. Absent or diminished breath sounds on the affected side indicate recurrent pneumothorax.

5. Inspect the dressing for excessive and abnormal drainage, such as bleeding or foul-smelling discharge.

6. Palpate around the dressing site and listen for a crackling sound indicative of subcutaneous emphysema.

7. Inspect the drainage in the collection container at least every 30 minutes during the first two hours after chest tube insertion and every two hours thereafter.

Every eight hours mark the time, date, and drainage level on a piece of adhesive tape affixed to the container, or directly on a disposable container (see Figure 41–15). Note any sudden change in the amount or color of the drainage. If drainage exceeds 100 mL/hr or if a color change indicates hemorrhage, notify the physician immediately.

8. In gravity drainage systems, check for fluctutation (tidaling) of the fluid level in the water-seal glass tube of a bottle system or the water-seal chamber of a commercial system as the patient breathes. Normally, fluctuations of 5 to 10 cm (2 to 4 in) occur until the lung has reexpanded. In suction drainage systems, the fluid line remains constant.

Rationale   Fluctuations reflect the pressure changes in the pleural space during inhalation and exhalation. The fluid level rises when the patient inhales and falls when the patient exhales. The absence of fluctuations may indicate tubing obstruction from a kink, dependent loop, blood clot, or outside pressure (for example, because the patient is lying on the tubing), or may indicate that full lung reexpansion has occurred.

9. To check for fluctuation in suction systems, tempora-

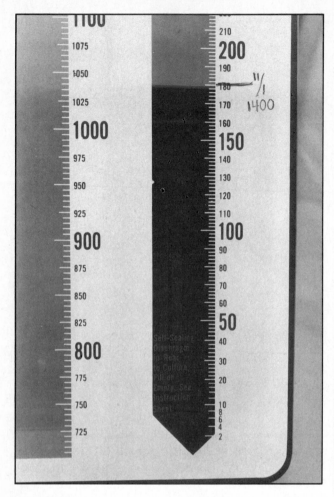

FIGURE 41–15

rily disconnect the system. Then observe for fluctuation.

10. Check for intermittent bubbling in the water of the water-seal bottle or chamber.

    Rationale Intermittent bubbling normally occurs when the system removes air from the pleural space, especially when the patient takes a deep breath or coughs. Absence of bubbling indicates that the pleural space has healed and is sealed. Continuous bubbling or a sudden change from an established pattern can indicate a break in the system and should be reported immediately.

11. Check for gentle bubbling in the suction control bottle or chamber.

    Rationale Gentle bubbling indicates proper suction pressure.

12. Inspect the air vent in the system periodically to make sure it is not occluded. A vent must be present to allow air to escape.

    Rationale Obstruction of the air vent causes an increased pressure in the system that could result in pneumothorax.

13. Inspect the drainage tubing for kinks or loops dangling below the entry level of the drainage system.

■ Planning

Nursing goals

1. To maintain an airtight drainage system and prevent accidental pneumothorax
2. To maintain the patency of the drainage system
3. To facilitate drainage from the pleural space and promote lung reexpansion

Equipment

1. Two rubber-tipped Kelly clamps
2. A sterile petrolatum gauze
3. A sterile drainage system
4. Antiseptic swabs
5. Sterile 4 × 4 gauzes
6. Air-occlusive tape
7. A mechanical chest tubing stripper, if available
8. Specimen supplies, if needed:
    a. A povidone-iodine swab
    b. A sterile #18 or #20 gauge needle
    c. A 3-or 5-mL syringe
    d. A needle protector
    e. A label for the syringe
    f. A laboratory requisition

■ Intervention

Safety precautions

1. Keep two 15- to 18-cm (6- to 7-in) rubber-tipped Kelly clamps within reach at the bedside, to clamp the chest tube in an emergency, eg, if leakage occurs in the tubing.
2. Keep one sterile petrolatum gauze within reach at the bedside to use with an air-occlusive material if the chest tube becomes dislodged.
3. Keep an extra drainage system unit available in the patient's room. In most agencies the physician is responsible for changing the drainage system except in emergency situations, such as malfunction or breakage. In these situations:
    a. Clamp the chest tubes (see step 5).
    b. Reestablish a water-sealed drainage system.
    c. Remove the clamps, and notify the physician.
4. Keep the drainage system below chest level and upright at all times, unless the chest tubes are clamped.

Rationale Keeping the unit below chest level prevents backflow of fluid from the drainage chamber into the pleural space. Keeping the unit upright maintains the glass tube below the water level, forming the water seal.

5. If the chest tube becomes disconnected from the drainage system:

   a. Have the patient exhale fully.

   b. Clamp the chest tube close to the insertion site with two rubber-tipped clamps placed in opposite directions. See Figure 41–16.

   c. Quickly clean the ends of the tubing with an antiseptic, reconnect them, and tape them securely.

   d. Unclamp the tube as soon as possible.

   e. Assess the patient for respiratory distress.

   Rationale Clamping the tube prevents external air from entering the pleural space. Two clamps ensure complete closure of the tube. Having the patient exhale and clamping the tube for no longer than necessary prevent an air or fluid buildup in the pleural space which can cause further lung collapse.

6. If the chest tube becomes dislodged from the insertion site:

   a. Remove the dressing, and immediately apply pressure with the petrolatum gauze, your hand, or a towel.

   b. Cover the site with sterile 4 × 4 gauze squares.

   c. Tape the dressings with air-occlusive tape.

   d. Notify the physician immediately.

   e. Assess the patient for respiratory distress every 15 minutes.

7. Do not empty a drainage bottle unless ordered to do so with specific instructions by the physician. Commercial systems cannot be emptied.

8. If the drainage system is accidentally tipped over:

   a. Immediately return it to the upright position.

   b. Ask the patient to take several deep breaths.

   Rationale Deep breaths help force air out of the pleural cavity that might have entered when the water seal was not intact.

   c. Notify the physician.

   d. Assess the patient for respiratory distress.

Maintaining drainage system patency

9. Check that all connections are secured with tape to ensure that the system is airtight.

10. Milk or strip the chest tubing as prescribed by agency policy. Use a mechanical stripper (see Figure 41–17), or follow these steps:

   a. Lubricate about 30 cm (12 in) of the drainage tubing with lubricating gel, soap, or hand lotion,

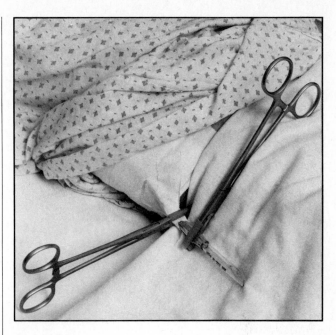

FIGURE 41–16

FIGURE 41–17

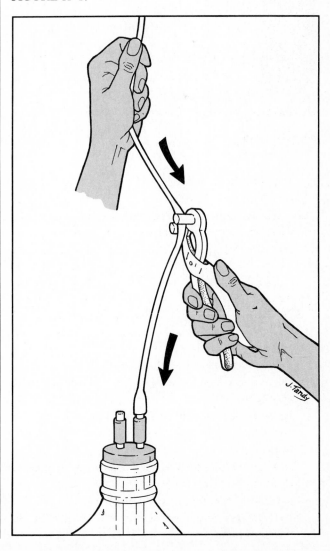

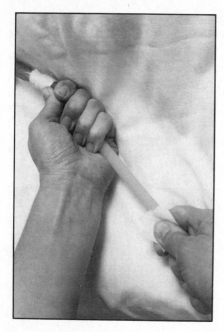

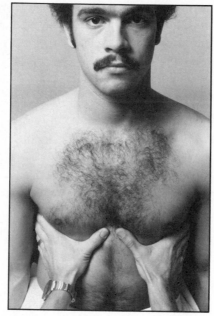

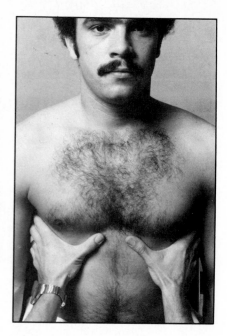

FIGURE 41–18   FIGURE 41–19   FIGURE 41–20

or hold an alcohol sponge between your fingers and the tube (see Figure 41–18).

Rationale Lubrication reduces friction and facilitates the milking process.

b. With one hand, securely stabilize and pinch the tube at the insertion site.

c. Compress the tube with the thumb and forefinger of your other hand and milk it by sliding them down the tube moving away from the insertion site.

Rationale Milking the tubing dislodges obstructions such as blood clots. Milking from the insertion site downward prevents movement of the obstructive material into the pleural space.

d. Reposition your hands farther along the tubing, and repeat steps a–c in progressive overlapping steps, until you reach the end of the tubing.

Patient care

11. Encourage deep breathing and coughing exercises every two hours. Have the patient sit upright to perform the exercises, and splint the tube insertion site with a pillow or with your hand to minimize discomfort.

Rationale Deep breathing and coughing help to remove accumulations from the pleural space, facilitate drainage, and help the lung to reexpand.

12. While the patient takes deep breaths, palpate the chest for thoracic expansion. Place your hands together at the base of the sternum so that your thumbs meet. See Figure 41–19. As the patient inhales, your thumbs should separate at least 2.5 to

5 cm (1 to 2 in). See Figure 41–20. Note whether chest expansion is symmetric.

13. Reposition the patient every two hours. When the patient is lying on the affected side, place rolled towels beside the tubing.

Rationale Frequent position changes promote drainage, prevent complications, and provide comfort. Rolled towels prevent occlusion of the chest tube by the patient's weight.

14. Assist the patient with range-of-motion exercises of the affected shoulder three times per day to maintain joint mobility.

15. When transporting and ambulating the patient:

a. Attach rubber-tipped forceps to the patient's gown for emergency use.

b. Keep the water-seal unit below chest level and upright.

c. If it is necessary to clamp the tube, remove the clamp as soon as possible.

d. Disconnect the drainage system from suction apparatus beforehand, and make sure the air vent is open.

Taking a specimen of chest drainage

16. Specimens of chest drainage may be taken from a disposable chest drainage system, since these systems are equipped with self-sealing ports. If a specimen is required:

a. Use a povidone-iodine swab to wipe the self-sealing diaphragm on the back of the drainage collection chamber. Allow it to dry.

b. Attach a sterile #18 or #20 gauge needle to a 3- or 5-mL syringe, and insert the needle into the diaphragm. See Figure 41–21.

c. Aspirate the specimen, attach the needle protector, label the syringe, and send it to the laboratory with the appropriate requisition form.

■ Evaluation

Expected outcomes

1. Stable vital signs
2. Bilateral equal chest expansion
3. Bilateral breath sounds
4. Dressing dry and intact
5. Clear or slight serosanguineous drainage

Unexpected outcomes

1. Signs of pneumothorax (eleveated pulse, dyspnea, sudden chest pain)
2. Signs of subcutaneous emphysema at insertion site
3. Inadequate chest expansion on affected side
4. Absent or diminished breath sounds on affected side
5. Excessive discharge or bleeding at insertion site
6. Excessive chest drainage (above 100 mL/hr)
7. Bright sanguineous drainage

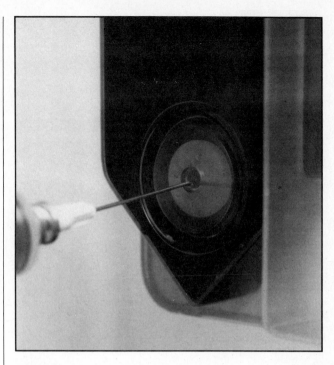

FIGURE 41–21

Upon obtaining an unexpected outcome:

1. Report your findings to the responsible nurse and/or physician.
2. Adjust the patient's nursing care plan appropriately.

References

Bricker PL: Chest tubes: The crucial points you mustn't forget. *RN* (November) 1980; 43:20–26.

Cohen S: How to work with chest tubes . . . programmed instruction. *Am J Nurs* (April) 1980; 80:685–712.

Dalrymple D: Setting up for thoracic drainage. *Nursing 84* (June) 1984; 14:12–14.

Erickson R: Chest tubes: They're really not that complicated. *Nursing 81* (May) 1981; 11:34–43.

Erickson R: Solving chest tube problems. *Nursing 81* (June) 1981; 11:62–67.

Swearingen PL: *The Addison-Wesley Photo-Atlas of Nursing Procedures.* Addison-Wesley, 1984.

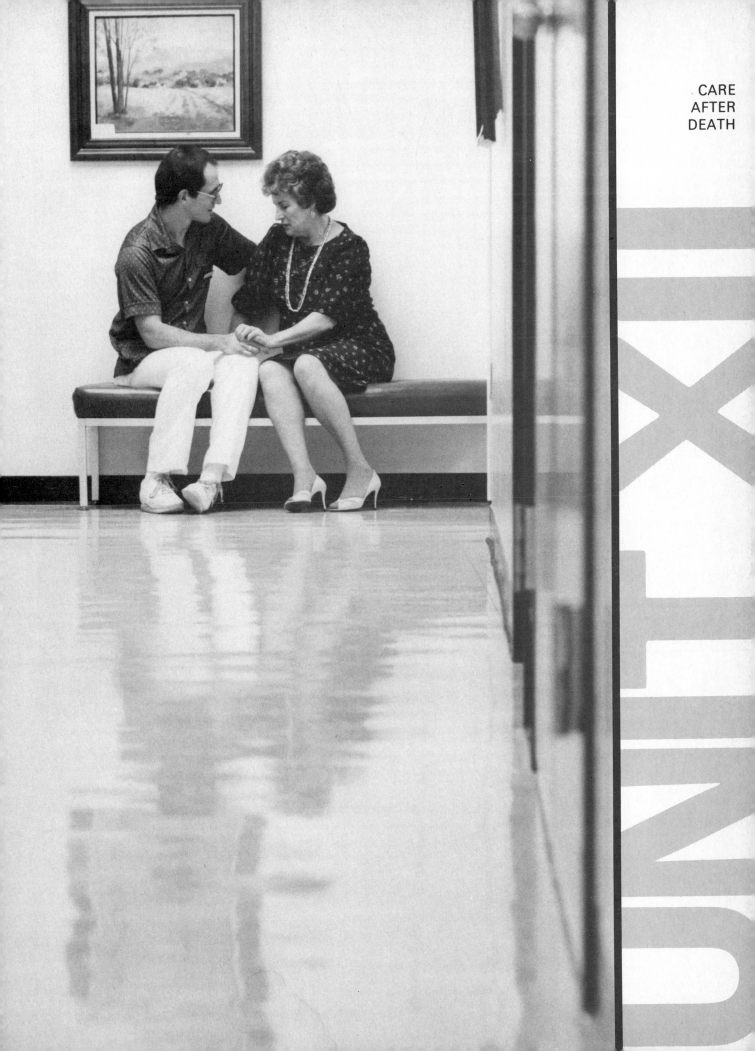

CARE
AFTER
DEATH

UNIT XII

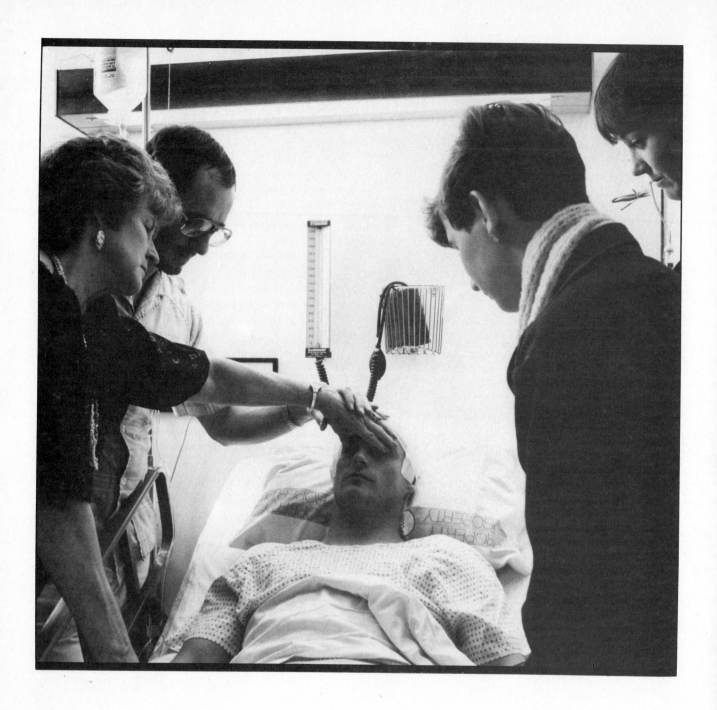

POSTMORTEM CARE

42

Postmortem care is an unpleasant subject for most people and a technique that nurses carry out from necessity, often with considerable feelings. Because so many people in the United States and Canada die in hospitals, nurses encounter death more often than most people. In both countries major causes of death are cardiac disease, cerebrovascular disease, malignancies, and accidents.

Care of the dying and the dead has cultural, social, religious, and legal implications. It is important for nurses to understand how these apply in their own communities. Nurses also need to understand the stages of patients' emotional reactions to

their own death in order to offer emotional support and necessary care.

Chapter Outline

Stages of Dying

Clinical Signs of Impending Death

Nursing Intervention for the Dying Patient

Clinical Signs of Death

■ Technique 42–1 Caring for a Body after Death

Procedures Following Death

Objectives

Upon completion of this chapter, the student will:

1. Know essential terms and facts about death and postmortem care
   1.1 Define selected terms
   1.2 Identify Kübler-Ross's five stages of emotional reactions to death
   1.3 Identify clinical signs of impending death
   1.4 Identify emotional needs of dying patients
   1.5 Identify nursing interventions to meet the physiologic needs of dying patients
   1.6 Identify the clinical signs of death
   1.7 Identify changes that occur in the body after death
2. Understand facts about postmortem care techniques
   2.1 Identify relevant assessment data
   2.2 Identify nursing diagnoses for which the technique may be implemented
   2.3 Identify nursing goals related to the technique
   2.4 Identify expected and unexpected outcomes from assessment data
   2.5 Identify reasons underlying selected steps of the techniques
3. Perform postmortem techniques safely

   3.1 Assess the patient and support persons adequately
   3.2 Collect additional data from appropriate sources
   3.3 Select pertinent nursing goals for the patient and support persons
   3.4 Establish relevant outcome criteria for the patient and support persons following the technique
   3.5 Collect necessary equipment before the technique
   3.6 Implement interventions to enhance the effectiveness of the technique and enhance the support persons' comfort and safety
   3.7 Communicate relevant information about the patient to the appropriate persons
   3.8 Determine the evaluative outcomes of the technique
4. Evaluate own performance of specific postmortem techniques in a laboratory or clinical setting with the assistance of another
   4.1 Use the performance checklists provided
   4.2 Identify areas of strength and weakness
   4.3 Alter performance in response to own evaluation and that of another

Terms

■ algor mortis   postmortem cooling

■ autopsy (postmortem examination)   the examination of a body after death

■ Cheyne-Stokes respirations   rhythmic waxing and waning of respirations, from very deep to very shallow, with periods of apnea

■ coroner   a public official who is responsible for investigating any deaths that appear to be unnatural

■ deceased   dead; a person who is dead

■ embalming   a process of preserving a body chemically

■ expired   dead

■ forensic medicine (legal medicine)   the application of medical knowledge to the law

■ grief   a subjective emotional response of intense sadness; a normal response to loss

■ inquest   a legal enquiry into the cause or manner of a death

■ livor mortis   the discoloration of a body after death

■ medical examiner   a physician who investigates any death that appears to be unnatural

■ morgue   a place where bodies are temporarily detained before release to a mortician; some hospitals have their own morgues

■ mortician   a person who is responsible for the care and disposal of the deceased

■ mourning   a process through which grief is eventually resolved or altered
■ postmortem   after death

■ rigor mortis   a stiffening of the muscles after death
■ shroud   a large rectangle or square of plastic or cotton material used to enclose a body after death

STAGES OF DYING

Elisabeth Kübler-Ross has described five stages of emotional reaction that occur when an individual is told that he or she is dying or will die relatively shortly: denial, anger, bargaining, depression, and acceptance. The five stages do not always occur in an orderly, discrete fashion. An individual often moves back and forth from one stage to another, and stages can overlap. Some individuals never progress through all five stages, and a person may remain, for example, in stage one. A patient who remains in stage one or two while dying often fights death and struggles bitterly.

Denial

Denial is a stage of nonacceptance, when the person thinks, "This is not happening to me. There is a mistake." The individual is not ready to deal with the reality of the illness and often ignores the seriousness of the situation.

Anger

During the anger stage, the person often expresses anger generally. The anger may be directed at nursing personnel, the hospital, or even the patient's support persons. It is not unusual for a patient to blame others or a particular situation. The patient and support persons may be uncharacteristically demanding and find fault with small matters. This is a normal reaction, and it is important that nurses accept it and remain supportive.

Bargaining

The bargaining stage is often learned in childhood. Children bargain to obtain their own way—for example, "I will mow the grass if I can stay overnight at Todd's." The dying patient's bargaining for life is a way of trying to change the inevitable. During this stage, it is important for nurses to listen to the patient and to convey understanding.

Depression

During the depression stage, the individual is sad and dejected. The patient and support persons grieve about what will never be and anticipate the loss. Some patients withdraw and reject people, while others talk freely. Nurses can help by listening when the individual wants to talk and by conveying acceptance and understanding.

Acceptance

The acceptance stage gradually occurs as the individual comes to terms with his or her changed circumstances. At this time the patient often finds it helpful to talk about her or his reactions and make plans. The dying person may be ready to make a will and complete necessary business arrangements. He or she is at peace with the impending death.

CLINICAL SIGNS OF IMPENDING DEATH

The process of dying varies in duration from minutes to hours, days, or weeks. Some people die instantly as a result of injury, but usually the dying process can be assessed, as the cells of the body cease functioning because of anoxia. The clinical signs of impending death are:

1. The reflexes gradually disappear.
2. Respirations become accelerated and dyspneic. Sometimes Cheyne-Stokes respirations occur.
3. The skin feels cold and clammy, but body temperature is elevated.
4. The pupils bcome dilated and fixed.
5. The pulse accelerates and becomes weaker.
6. The blood pressure falls.
7. Mental alertness wanes in some patients.
8. The facial expression becomes pinched, and some cyanosis may appear.

NURSING INTERVENTIONS FOR THE DYING PATIENT

Emotional Interventions

The primary emotional needs of the dying patient involve reassurance. Some of these needs are (Williams, 1976, pp 28–29):

1. Relief from loneliness, fear, and depression. The person requires someone who will spend time with her or him and listen.

2. Maintenance of security, self-confidence, and dignity. The patient should not be neglected or abandoned. Patients fear psychologic abandonment, a situation that occurs, for example, when patients want to talk about dying and their support persons will not permit it, or when support persons gradually lose the physical and emotional energy required to maintain contact with the dying person during a long terminal illness.

3. Maintenance of hope even in the last stages of dying. Hope makes the acceptance of death easier for patients and support persons. Even where death is highly probable, hope is important and not unrealistic. No one really knows what the future holds, and miraculous recoveries have been known to occur.

4. Spiritual needs, which often arise during the night (Gray, 1976, p 18). Frequently, nurses assist patients to meet these needs, particularly when clergy cannot be contacted.

Physiologic Interventions

The physiologic needs of the dying patient are related to the slowing of body processes and physiologic imbalances.

1. The patient may need to have analgesics administered intravenously because of poor blood circulation. The medication may not be effectively absorbed from subcutaneous tissue or muscle.

2. The sphincters that control urination and defecation may relax, and the patient cannot control elimination. Absorbent pads may be used to absorb body excreta, and in some instances a retention catheter is inserted for the urine. See chapter 27.

3. Pharyngeal suctioning (see chapter 37) may be necessary, because, as muscle tone is lost, the patient cannot swallow (dysphagia), and mucus collects in the mouth and pharynx.

4. Sips of water or fruit juices may be needed to lubricate the mucous membranes of the mouth, which become dry due to elevated body temperature. Mouth care is also indicated for this reason. See chapter 13.

5. Physical support becomes increasingly needed for the body to maintain a comfortable position, because there is progressive loss of skeletal muscle tone, starting in the legs and progressing to the arms.

6. Fowler's position is usually indicated for the conscious dying patient, because it eases breathing. If the patient is unconscious, Sims's position will facilitate the drainage of mucus from the mouth.

7. A well-lighted room is usually preferred, because the patient's vision becomes blurred. Hearing is thought to be the last sense to leave the body, so dying patients can often hear what people are saying after they can no longer see or respond. Whispering should be avoided, and care should be taken to speak clearly.

CLINICAL SIGNS OF DEATH

The clinical signs of death have traditionally been the cessation of the apical pulse, respirations, and blood pressure. However, since the advent of artificial means to maintain respirations and blood circulation, identifying death is more difficult. The Harvard decision provides that the absence of electric currents from the brain for at least 24 hours is an indication of death. These electric impulses are measured by an electroencephalogram (EEG). Usually three consecutive flat EEGs (no electric impulses) indicate clinical death. Only a physician can pronounce death, and it is only after this pronouncement that life support systems can be shut off.

Some patients will have expressed a wish that CPR not be initiated once the heart fails. These patients are often designated "no heroics" or "no code" patients, meaning that no resuscitation measures are to be taken. For most patients, however, the nurse is expected to initiate CPR and maintain it until the patient recovers or the physician pronounces that the patient is dead. See chapter 39.

CHANGES IN THE BODY AFTER DEATH

Rigor Mortis

Rigor mortis occurs about two to four hours after death. It results from a lack of adenosine triphosphate (ATP), which is not synthesized because of a lack of glycogen in the body. ATP is necessary for muscle fiber relaxation. Its lack causes the muscles to contract, which in turn immobilizes the joints. Rigor mortis starts in the involuntary muscles (heart, bladder, etc), then progresses to the head, neck, and trunk, and finally reaches the extremities.

Because the deceased's family members often want to view the body, it is important that he or she appear natural and comfortable. Positioning the body, placing the dentures in the mouth, and closing the eyes and mouth must take place before rigor mortis occurs. Rigor mortis usually leaves the body about 96 hours after death.

Algor Mortis

Following termination of the blood circulation and of the function of the hypothalamus, the body temperature falls at a rate of about 1 °C (1.8 °F) per hour, until it reaches room temperature. This cooling is algor mortis. At the same time, the skin loses its elasticity and can easily be broken when removing dressings and adhesive tape.

Postmortem Decomposition

After blood circulation has ceased, the skin becomes discolored, because the red blood cells release hemoglobin when they break down, and the hemoglobin discolors the surrounding tissues. This discoloration, referred to as *livor*

mortis, appears in the lowermost or dependent areas of the body, such as the buttocks in a sitting position.

Tissue softening is another change that takes place after death. Tissues become soft and eventually liquefied by bacterial fermentation. The hotter it is, the more rapidly the change occurs. Therefore bodies are often stored in cool places. Embalming reverses this process by injecting chemicals into the body to destroy the bacteria (Pennington, 1978, p 847).

TECHNIQUE 42-1 ■ Caring for a Body after Death

Generally a nurse is responsible for preparing the body after death and making arrangements for the patient's property. Postmortem care begins after the physician has confirmed death. Although procedures differ among agencies, there are certain common elements.

■ Assessment

1. Assess the body for any bruises, skin discolorations, or injuries.
2. Assess the needs of support persons for support and information.

Other data include:

1. The time of death established by the physician.
2. The local laws and agency policies about:
   a. Identification of the body.
   b. Removal of equipment from the body. In some agencies, the policy is to clamp all tubes and leave them in place if an autopsy is to be performed. In other agencies, tubes are cut 2.5 cm (1 in) from the body and taped to the skin. In still others, tracheostomy or endotracheal tubes are removed, but other tubes, such as IVs and nasogastric tubes, are left in place and clamped. And in some, all tubes are removed and discarded.
   c. Tissue and organ removal and donation.
   d. Autopsy requirements and permission.
   e. The death certificate.
3. The patient's and support persons' cultural beliefs and religious practices regarding death, so that required rituals can be provided.
4. If death occurred following an infectious disease, the precautions to be taken to prevent the spread of the disease to others. Practices depend on the causative organism and its mode of transmission.
5. Whether the deceased's family wishes to view the body.

6. The agency's practices for postioning the patient; handling dentures, hairpieces, etc; and wrapping the body.

■ Nursing Diagnosis

Nursing diagnoses that may indicate the need to assist support persons include:

1. Grieving related to death of a significant other
2. Grieving related to the anticipated loss of a significant other
3. Ineffective individual coping related to death

■ Planning

Nursing goals

1. To maintain the best possible appearance of the body by preventing skin damage and discoloration
2. To maintain the dignity of the deceased by safeguarding belongings and handling the body with respect and care

Equipment

1. A clean gown
2. A valuables list and envelopes for valuables
3. Paper bags or other containers provided by the agency for the patient's clothing
4. A shroud or sheets in which to wrap the body
5. Dressing materials if a wound is present
6. Two identification tags: one to attach to the ankle and one to attach to the shroud or sheet
7. Sheet wadding and gauze (optional) to wrap the ankles and bind them together
8. Absorbent pads or a diaper to place under the buttocks
9. Masking tape to fasten the shroud

■ Intervention

1. Close the room door and/or pull the bed curtains around the bed. If there are other patients in the room, give them an honest explanation.

   Rationale Screening provides privacy for the deceased and the family and is less disturbing to other patients.

2. Identify the body, following agency policy.

3. Position the patient:

   a. Place the body in straight alignment in the supine position, with the arms laid palm down at the patient's sides or according to agency policy. Some agencies prefer the arms to be laid across the abdomen. If this is the case, avoid placing one hand on top of the other, since the underlying hand will become discolored.

   b. Place one pillow under the head and shoulders.

   Rationale This prevents the settling of blood in the face and subsequent discoloration.

   c. Close the eyelids by gently holding your fingertips over each eyelid for a few seconds. Do not use Scotch tape or adhesive tape to close the eyelids, since these are difficult to remove without damaging the tissues. If the eyelids do not remain closed, place a moistened cotton fluff on each eyelid for a few moments.

   Rationale Closed eyelids give the face a natural appearance for viewing.

   d. Put the patient's dentures, if any, in the patient's mouth. If this is not possible, label and store them properly for the mortician to insert.

   e. If the mouth does not remain closed, place a small rolled towel under the chin.

4. Detach bottles, bags, and receptacles from intravenous tubes, nasogastric tubes, urinary catheters, etc, and follow agency policies about whether the tubes are to be removed or clamped and left in place.

5. Using plain water, wash soiled areas of the body. A complete bath is unnecessary, since the body is washed by the mortician. However, excessive soil, such as feces, emesis, or blood, needs to be removed to prevent odor caused by microorganisms.

6. Place absorbent pads under the buttocks if soiling occurs, or apply a diaper according to agency practice.

   Rationale Sphincter muscles relax after death and may release urine or feces.

7. Remove soiled dressings if necessary, and replace them with light gauze dressings.

8. Put a clean gown on the patient if agency policy recommends this.

   Rationale A clean gown is generally put on if the family wishes to view the deceased.

9. Brush and comb the hair. Remove hairpins.

   Rationale The patient should appear nicely groomed for viewing by the family. Hairpins are removed to prevent damage to the scalp or face of the deceased.

10. Remove all jewelry with the possible exception of a wedding band. Family members may request that a wedding band be left on. If a wedding band is not to be removed, check agency policies about whether it is to be taped on or tied with gauze.

11. List all the patient's valuables, label them, and give them to the next of kin or put them in a secure place at the nursing station.

    Rationale The nurse is responsible for preventing the loss of personal items, such as eyeglasses, keys, and religious medals. Generally eyeglasses, dentures, and hair that was shaved for surgery are labeled and sent with the body to the mortician.

12. Assemble the patient's clothing and other personal effects, and place them in a labeled container for the next of kin.

13. Attach identification tags to the body. Leave the wrist identification band in place, and tie another identification tag to the patient's ankle. If the wrist band is restrictive, however, remove it. All identification tags should include the patient's name, hospital number, and physician's name.

    Rationale Appropriate identification cannot be overemphasized. More than one tag is applied in case one becomes detached. Tags tied to the ankles are preferred, since any tissue damage they cause will be concealed by bed linen or clothing.

14. If the support persons are to view the deceased, adjust the top linen as necessary, and cover the patient to the shoulders. Provide soft lighting and chairs for family members.

    Rationale A clean and neat appearance is important to the family, and lowered lighting softens the stark features of the deceased.

15. Stay with the support persons at first, then leave them with the body.

    Rationale Some people may at first want the comfort of the nurse's presence and then privacy with the deceased.

16. After the family leaves, apply a shroud or wrap the body in a sheet. See Figure 42–1. Generally the ankles are first tied together.

    Rationale Wrapping prevents damage to the extremities, avoids unnecessary exposure of the body, and maintains the dignity of the deceased.

17. Securely attach the sheet or shroud in accordance with agency policy. Because safety pins can create pressure and damage the deceased's skin, masking tape is generally preferred to fasten the shroud.

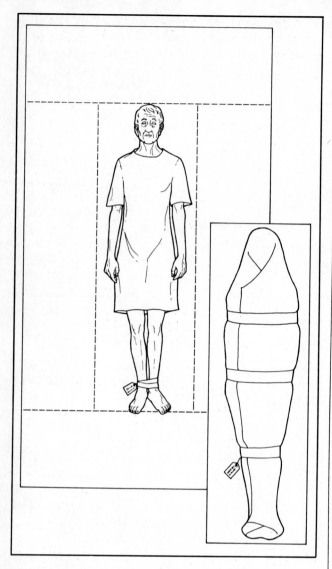

FIGURE 42-1

18. Attach a second identification tag to the outside of the shroud. If the patient had an infectious disease, attach a special tag with that information.

19. Arrange for the body to be transported to the morgue for cooling, if arrangements have not been made for

the mortician to take the body from the patient's room.

20. Move the body gently when transferring it to a stretcher. Ensure that body alignment is maintained.
   Rationale Rough movements could damage the body tissues.

21. Transport the body as inconspicuously as possible. In some agencies other patients' room doors are closed before transporting the deceased through the corridors, and service elevators are used.
   Rationale The sight of a body is often disturbing to patients and visitors.

22. Strip the patient's room.

23. Record the technique, including the date and time of death, the time the physician was notified, who pronounced the death, how valuables and personal belongings were handled, care given the body, any forms signed by the family, visits by any family or clergy, identification attached to the body, disposition of the body, and information given to support persons and their responses.

■ Evaluation

Expected outcomes

1. No injuries, bruises, etc, on the body except those documented on the record previously.
2. Support persons experience grief.
3. Support persons express grief.
4. Support persons share grief with significant others.

Unexpected outcomes

1. Support persons do not express grief.
2. Support persons do not share grief with significant others.

Upon obtaining an unexpected outcome: Report your findings to the responsible nurse and/or physician.

PROCEDURES FOLLOWING DEATH

Autopsy

An *autopsy* or *postmortem examination* is an examination of the body after death. It is performed on only certain bodies. The law describes under what circumstances an autopsy must be performed, eg, when death

is sudden or when it occurs within 48 hours of admission to a hospital. It is the responsibility of the physician or, in some instances, of a designated person in the hospital to discuss an autopsy with the support persons. In some instances the physician may ask the family for permission to perform an autopsy even though one is not required by law, because autopsies contribute a great deal to medical knowledge.

The organs and tissues of the body are examined for several reasons:

1. To establish the exact cause of death
2. To learn more about a disease
3. To assist in the accumulation of statistical data

Inquest

An *inquest* is a legal inquiry into the cause or manner of a death. When a death is the result of an accident, for example, an inquest will be held into the circumstances of the accident to determine any blame. The inquest is conducted under the jurisdiction of a coroner or medical examiner. A coroner is a public official appointed or elected to the position and does not need to be a physician. A medical examiner is a physician who usually has advanced education in pathology or forensic medicine. Agencies have policies about who is responsible for reporting deaths to the coroner or medical examiner.

Death Certificate

By law, a death certificate must be made out when a person dies. It is usually signed by the attending physician and filed with a local health or other government office. The family is usually given a copy to use for legal matters such as insurance claims.

References

Gray VR: Some physiological needs. Pages 15–20 in: *Dealing with Death and Dying.* Nursing 77 Skillbook Series. Intermed Communications, 1976.

Kübler-Ross E: *Death: The Final Stage of Growth.* Prentice-Hall, 1975.

Kübler-Ross E: *On Death and Dying.* Macmillan, 1969.

Pennington EA: Postmortem care: More than ritual. *Am J Nurs* (May) 1978; 78:846–847.

Salter R: The art of dying. *Can Nurse* (March) 1982; 78:20–21.

Williams JC: Allaying common fears. Pages 27–32 in: *Dealing with Death and Dying.* Nursing 77 Skillbook Series. Intermed Communications, 1976.

TECHNIQUE 6–1 ▪ Hand Washing

Equipment

1. Soap (preferably one with bactericidal properties) in a plastic container
2. Five paper towels
3. If running water is unavailable or sanitary conditions are such that medical asepsis would be compromised, use disposable washcloths or alcohol in place of hand washing

▪ Intervention

1. Remove your wristwatch and rings. Open one paper towel and lay it on a flat, dry surface close to the sink, to use as a clean field. Place the soap container and two folded paper towels on the clean field.
2. Wet your hands, apply the soap, and return the container to the clean field.
3. Rub your hand surfaces a minimum of ten times or one minute. If they are grossly contaminated, wash your hands for three minutes.
4. Dry your hands with one paper towel, and turn the faucet off using another paper towel.

   Rationale This prevents contamination of the hands by microorganisms from the faucet knobs.
5. When patient care is completed, return to the sink and repeat steps 1–3.
6. Wash the outside of the soap container.
7. Dry your hands and the clean soap container with one paper towel. Hold the soap container in one hand.
8. Turn the faucet off with the other hand, using the remaining paper towel. Discard all paper towels, including the one used for the clean field.

TECHNIQUE 6–2 ▪ Initiating Protective Aseptic Practices

Medical Asepsis in the Home

Equipment

1. Soap (preferably one with bactericidal properties) in a plastic container
2. Paper towels
3. Newspapers (two thicknesses)
4. A home nursing bag containing nursing supplies; soap and paper towels are kept in an outside pocket

▪ Intervention

1. Before entering the home, obtain newspapers from the family, remove your boots or rubbers, and place them on some of the papers near the doorway.

2. Place other newspapers on a flat, clean, dry surface with adequate working space (preferably close to a faucet), and place your nursing bag on those papers.

   Rationale Newspapers help keep the boots from soiling the patients' home and keep the bag free of microorganisms that could be carried to another home.
3. Remove your coat, folding it so that the lining is protected, and place it on the back of an unupholstered chair away from the wall.

   Rationale An unupholstered chair is less likely to have microorganisms, fleas, ticks, etc.
4. Remove the soap and towels from your nursing bag.
5. Spread one paper towel to establish a clean field for hand washing. See Appendix Technique 6–1.
6. Wash your hands before opening the bag and removing supplies.
7. Proceed with the plan of care, using the patient's equipment whenever possible (eg, the patient's own thermometer). *N.B.:* Patients' families should be encouraged to provide the equipment and supplies regularly used in patient care.
8. If you need to return to your bag once patient contact has been made, repeat a hand wash.

   Rationale This prevents contamination of articles in the bag by microorganisms from the patient.
9. Upon completion of patient care, wash your hands and wash and dry all your articles (soap bottle, instruments, etc.) before returning them to the bag.
10. Teach the patient and family as needed about the nature of the infection and how to prevent it from spreading. Teach them to:

    a. Wash hands thoroughly after contact with any body excreta (urine, feces, sputum, wound drainage, or articles soiled by them) or infective material before handling food or eating.

    b. Use plastic refuse bags for disposable supplies or items contaminated with the patient's body secretions.

    c. Clean soiled articles appropriately.

    ▪ Rinse articles soiled by organic material, such as blood or pus, with cold water.

       Rationale Hot water coagulates the protein of organic material and tends to make it stick to the article.

    ▪ Then wash the article in hot water and soap.

    ▪ Use a stiff-bristled brush to clean articles that have grooves or corners.

    ▪ Rinse and dry the article well.

    d. Thoroughly wash, rinse, and dry dishes that are visibly contaminated with infective material.

    e. Cover the mouth and nose with protective tissue when coughing, sneezing, or blowing the nose.

    f. Avoid talking, coughing, or sneezing over open wounds.

TECHNIQUE 7-3 ■ Establishing a Sterile Field

Teach people who need to carry out sterile techniques (eg, give injections, change dressings) to do the following:

1. Thoroughly wash hands before handling sterile supplies.
2. Place sterile wrapped items on a clean, dry surface.
3. Open sterile packages by handling only the outside of the wrapper or its edges.
4. Use the innermost side of a sterile wrapper as the sterile field.
5. Avoid touching the parts of supplies or equipment that will be inserted into the patient or that will touch an open wound (eg, the shaft of a needle or a cleaning gauze swab).
6. Acquire appropriate supplies. Use of disposable forceps, individually packaged gauzes, etc, is strongly advised to prevent contamination.

TECHNIQUE 8-1 ■ Assessing Body Temperature by Mouth

Teach people who need to monitor an elevated body temperature:

1. How frequently to monitor the temperature. This will depend upon the degree of the fever—eg, for an adult, a fever of 37.7 °C (99.6 °F) might be monitored every four hours; a fever of 39.4 °C (103 °F) might be monitored every hour or more frequently, depending on the patient's condition.
2. Not to measure body temperature by mouth for children under age 6 and for confused or unconscious persons. Explain why.
3. When to notify the home care nurse or physician about changes in the patient's body temperature.
4. About other available temperature measuring devices (eg, chemical disposable thermometers, temperature-sensitive tapes, and automatic digital thermometers), how to use them, and where to obtain them.
5. To allow at least 15 minutes between intake of hot or cold fluids or smoking and the temperature measurement.
6. To shake down a mercury thermometer before using it.
7. Where to place the tip of a thermometer, and how long to keep it in place to ensure an accurate reading.
8. To wash a glass thermometer in tepid, soapy water to remove organic material and then rinse it in cold or tepid (not hot) water to prevent breakage by expansion of the mercury.

TECHNIQUE 8-2 ■ Assessing Body Temperature by Axilla

Teach caregivers the following:

1. That this method of measuring body temperature is the preferred one for children up to age 6 and for persons who

are confused, who have mouth lesions, or who breathe through the mouth.
2. Where to place the thermometer, and how long to keep it in place to ensure an accurate reading.
3. About the availability of automatic digital thermometers.

See also steps 3, 6, and 8 in Appendix Technique 8-1.

TECHNIQUE 8-3 ■ Assessing Body Temperature by Rectum

1. Teach caregivers to use this method of temperature measurement for only those persons who cannot have an oral or axillary measurement.
2. Inform caregivers of the availability of an automatic digital thermometer.
3. Demonstrate a safe method for obtaining the measurement. Include positioning the patient, lubricating the thermometer tip, asking the patient to take a deep breath before you insert the thermometer, *not forcing* insertion of the thermometer, and *holding* the thermometer in place for at least two minutes.
4. See also steps 3, 6, and 8 in Appendix Technique 8-1.

TECHNIQUE 8-4 ■ Assessing a Peripheral Pulse

The pulse may need to be assessed if a patient, for example, is taking certain heart medications or has impaired or potentially impaired circulation to the foot. Teach caregivers:

1. How to locate a radial, pedal, or other peripheral pulse as indicated to assess heart rate and rhythm or arterial circulation to an extremity.
2. To use the index and middle fingers (*not* the thumb) for palpation.
3. How to count the pulse.
4. About the availability of automatic digital pulse rate devices. Some are part of digital blood pressure monitors.

TECHNIQUE 8-8 ■ Assessing Respirations

Home caregivers may need to monitor respirations for patients with an ineffective breathing pattern, alteration in cardiac output, or potential or actual activity intolerance, or patients receiving a medication that influences respirations. Teach the following:

1. The need to assess respirations while appearing to count the pulse.
   Rationale Respirations can be consciously controlled when a patient is aware that they are being assessed.
2. Ways to observe the respirations for rate and depth.

TECHNIQUE 8–9 ■ Assessing Blood Pressure

Teach people who need to monitor their own blood pressure (eg, those who have hypertension) about the following:

1. The availability and cost of various digital blood pressure monitors that do not require alignment of the cuff with the artery or use of a stethoscope. Most monitors show the systolic and diastolic readings in large numerals on the display panel. Some monitors are equipped with the standard bulb for inflation; others have a built-in pump for automatic inflation and a built-in printer that includes the date and time, to keep accurate records at home.

2. The need to avoid eating, smoking, and exertion for 30 minutes before the measurement.

3. The need to assume the same position and use the same arm for each measurement.

TECHNIQUE 14–1 ■ Bathing an Adult

You may need to adjust the bath environment to make a tub bath safer for the patient and to make it easier for caregivers to assist. Teach about:

1. The availability of bath seats that fit in the tub. These are useful for patients whose muscle strength is inadequate for getting into and out of a tub.

2. Installing a hand shower to use with a bath seat. A hand shower is also helpful for shampooing hair.

3. Use of a rubber mat or nonskid surface in the base of the tub to prevent the patient from slipping and falling when going into and out of the tub.

4. Installation and use of hand bars on both sides of the tub to facilitate transfers into and out of the tub.

5. The advisability of measuring the temperature of the water by thermometer before the patient enters the tub, particularly for patients who have sensory impairments and cannot discern temperature variations. Some people find it easier to get into an empty tub. Water temperature is then monitored while the water is running in.

6. The availability of home care nurses to assist patients with baths. Some home care agencies have "bath teams" that visit homes at scheduled times.

TECHNIQUE 15–2 ■ Changing an Occupied Bed

Teach patients who need to remain in bed for long periods about:

1. The availability and sources of equipment that can be rented for use in the home:
    a. Hospital beds
    b. Side rails
    c. Overbed tables

2. The availability and cost of:

    a. A foam "egg crate" mattress to place over the existing mattress, to help prevent pressure areas from developing.
    b. Bed-saver (incontinence) pads to place under the patient's buttocks.

3. Placing a large piece of plastic (eg, a large garbage bag) under the folded sheet or drawsheet to prevent soiling of the bottom sheet.

4. Acquiring a firmer mattress or placing a wooden frame or board under the mattress if more than normal support is required. Good support is essential for the patient in bed for extended periods.

5. Using a firm large box with two ends removed for a leg or foot cradle.

6. Using a rolled blanket at the end of the bed for a foot support. See also the techniques in chapter 17 for position aids and adaptations.

TECHNIQUES 16–2 to 16–9 ■ Moving a Patient in Bed

Teach caregivers:

1. Guidelines for their own body movement such as:
    a. Adjusting the working areas to waist level.
    b. Turning the body as a single unit and pivoting.
    c. Facing the direction of movement of heavy objects or persons.
    d. Pushing or pulling objects, using the body's own weight, rather than lifting them.
    e. Squatting, rather than stooping, when lifting objects.
    f. Using a broad stance to increase balance when moving objects.

2. Safe and effective ways to support the patient in bed while moving him or her.

3. The importance of encouraging the patient to assist in the movement as much as possible.

4. The importance of changing the position of a patient who is unable to move. It should be done at least every three hours and more frequently if warranted. See also Appendix Techniques 17–2 to 17–7.

TECHNIQUES 17–2 to 17–7 ■ Supporting a Patient in Fowler's, Dorsal Recumbent, Prone, Lateral, and Sims's Positions

Teach caregivers about:

1. The essentials and significance of good body alignment in the lying, sitting, and standing positions.

2. The kinds of supportive devices (pillows, towel rolls, foam rubber supports, etc) to place in specified areas according to the patient's position, to maintain body alignment and prevent contractures.

3. A systematic 24-hour schedule of position changes for a bed-confined patient.

4. The skin pressure areas created by the previous position, and the need to massage these areas with lotion whenever the patient is repositioned.

5. The need to keep the bed foundation clean, dry, and free from wrinkles.

6. Measures to keep the bed foundation and pillows dry for incontinent patients, for example, using plastic covers (eg, plastic garbage bags) or incontinence pads.

7. The need to maintain the patient's hydration and nutritional status to preserve skin integrity.

8. The availability of commercial devices to position patients or to protect bony prominences (eg, sheepskins, padded heel protectors, and foot boards).

9. The first stage of cell damage from pressure (redness of intact skin for a prolonged period) and the need to notify the home care nurse so that the positioning schedule can be altered.

10. Use of a wedge or television pillow with arms, for patients with chronic obstructive lung disease, to maintain the patient in an upright sitting position.

TECHNIQUE 18-1 ■ Applying Restraints

Teach caregivers about:

1. The availability of restraints designed especially for people sitting in wheelchairs.

2. Always explaining to the patient the purpose of the restraint, eg, to prevent falling.

3. Applying the restraint so the patient can move as freely as possible without defeating the purpose of the restraint.

4. Padding bony prominences before applying a limb restraint.

5. Monitoring circulation and releasing the restraint at the first sign of impaired circulation, eg, bluish skin color, cool temperature, numbness, tingling, or discomfort.

6. Removing a restraint at least every four hours and exercising the limb before reapplying it. Elderly patients may need limb restraints removed more often because of poorer circulation.

7. Always remaining with a patient when a restraint is removed.

8. Reporting to the home care nurse the first signs of persistent reddened or broken skin areas.

TECHNIQUE 19-3 ■ Assisting a Patient to Walk

Teach caregivers to:

1. Remove scatter rugs on which the patient could slip or trip, and make sure the floor is dry and not slippery.

2. Remove small pieces of furniture from the immediate vicinity, so that the patient will not trip over them.

3. Have the patient wear shoes with nonskid soles for walking.

4. Place a chair for the patient at a point on the walk, eg,

halfway between the bed and the bathroom, if the patient may need to rest on the way.

5. Fold a towel lengthwise and wrap it around the patient's waist as a walking belt to provide stability and support when walking.

6. Choose a time for the walk when the patient is rested.

TECHNIQUE 20-2 ■ Patient Care Immediately after Cast Application

1. Teach patients ways to move effectively with casts, eg, ways to walk with crutches.

2. Give patients and/or caregivers instructions before the patient's discharge (see page 483).

TECHNIQUE 21-1 ■ Applying Nonadhesive Skin Traction

Teach caregivers about:

1. The availability of traction equipment that can be attached to almost any bed (Villalon, Smith, 1982, pp 15-16).

2. Removing and setting up the traction.

3. Assessing circulation to the toes one hour after application of a Buck's boot.

4. Assessing the heels, each time the traction is released, for signs of pressure that could indicate a poorly fitting boot.

5. Using a restraint jacket anchored to the bed for a child who is "pulled" toward the foot of the bed when the ropes are shortened or the foot of the bed is elevated slightly. The restraint is used only then, to prevent the child from slipping (Villalon, Smith, 1982, p 16).

TECHNIQUE 23-1 ■ Monitoring Fluid Intake and Output

Teach the caregivers:

1. The volumes of the glasses, cups, etc, used in the home. You may need to measure these and write a list of their volumes for the caregiver to refer to when recording input.

2. How to measure urine output and record it, if indicated.

3. How to total fluid intake and output at the end of each 24-hour period, if indicated.

4. To report to the home care nurse a discrepancy between fluid intake and fluid output, eg, fluid intake is 1,500 mL more or less than fluid output.

5. To use specially designed drinking cups with nonsplash lids or spouts, if indicated.

TECHNIQUE 24-5 ■ Assisting an Adult to Eat

1. Determine if the patient's diet is appropriate, and, if not, provide recommendations for changes.

2. Determine if the patient has chewing or swallowing difficulties and whether adjustments in food consistency are needed (eg, minced or pureed foods).

3. Determine if special eating aids must be designed or obtained for the patient whose hands are shaky, poorly coordinated, or weak. Examples from Health and Welfare, Canada (1984), include:

   a. Insulated coffee mugs with holders that attach by adhesive to any surface. A straw can be inserted through the steam hole in the lid. These are designed for travelers and intended for use in a car. They can be purchased in places that cater to tourists or truckdrivers.

   b. Two-handled holders for a drinking glass. These are available from medical suppliers.

   c. A pen clip, to attach a straw to a drinking glass.

   d. Special holders for a mug or glass that attach to the arm of a wheelchair.

   e. Adaptations of cutlery to provide a more comfortable grip. Cutlery handles can be wrapped with a thin sponge or a washcloth that is then taped in place. A heavy rubber band or piece of elastic can be looped over each end of the handle and the patient's hand inserted under the loop. Steak knives with wide handles are often easier to grip than ordinary dinner knives. Medical suppliers sell lengths of thick sponge tubing called *rubazote*, which can be cut in lengths and placed over the handles of cutlery, toothbrushes, pencils, etc. The tubing can be taken off before washing the article. A bicycle grip can be used the same way. Specialized cutlery can also be purchased, eg, spoons with swivel handles, angular spoons, and rocking knives.

   f. A dampened washcloth, several folds of dampened paper towel, or a dampened cellulose sponge cloth to place under a dinner plate to keep it from sliding around.

   g. Clip-on rings that fit any size plate, forming an edge that keeps food from being pushed off the plate.

TECHNIQUE 24-6 ■ Administering a Nasogastric Tube Feeding (Gastric Gavage)

1. Ensure that orders by the physician specify the route of administration, type of solution, and amount and rate of infusion.

2. Feedings are generally calculated by a clinical dietitian.

3. Determine whether feeding is to be provided by continuous infusions by a pump, cyclic infusions by a pump, or a bolus method using a syringe.

4. Obtain the mutual consent of the physician, the infusion nurse, and the patient and/or support persons for feedings to be given in the home.

5. Encourage the patient to participate in the planning and implementation of the feedings.

   Rationale Participation enhances confidence and self-esteem.

Teach the caregiver about:

6. The availability of commercial enteral formulas, if appropriate for the patient.

7. The preparation and storage of formulas. A formula can sometimes be thinned with milk, juice, or water if it is viscous (Bayer, Scholl, Ford, 1983, p 1321).

8. Administering the feeding, irrigating the tube, and initiating and disconnecting the pump, if one is used.

9. Giving commercially prepared feedings at room temperature and immediately once the can is opened, because the formula supports the growth of microorganisms. Any formula not used should be stored in the refrigerator in an airtight container. Manufacturers designate how long an opened container can be kept. Usually it must be used within 24 hours.

10. Giving home-prepared formulas within 24 hours after preparation. They should be tightly sealed, dated, and refrigerated (Bayer, Scholl, Ford, 1983, p 1322).

TECHNIQUE 24-7 ■ Administering a Gastrostomy or Jejunostomy Feeding

Teach the caregivers about:

1. Providing peristomal skin care.
2. Available equipment.
3. Administering the feeding.

See also Appendix Technique 24-6.

TECHNIQUE 25-1 ■ Setting Up an Intravenous Infusion

Determine state laws and standards of nursing practice applicable to the delivery of intravenous therapy in the home by nurses. The National Intravenous Therapy Association (NITA) has developed home IV therapy nursing standards of practice (National Intravenous Therapy, 1984, p 93) that include the following:

1. The physician must:

   a. Provide a written, signed, medical order that refers the patient for home IV therapy and initiates and directs home IV therapy.

   b. Routinely review and update the order.

2. The registered nurse must:

   a. Have knowledge and skills to interpret and implement the medical order.

   b. Assess the patient's or caregiver's ability to administer the prescribed home IV therapy safely.

   c. As the primary educator, discuss indications, benefits, methods, and risks of therapy.

   d. Provide specific teaching for the patient and/or caregiver that includes written instructions, verbal explanations, demonstrations, evaluation, and documentation of competence. The teaching should cover proficiency in performing therapy-related procedures, self-monitoring, the scope of physical activities, necessary interventions, safe ways to discard disposable equipment, and specific actions to take in a possible emergency.

e. By the date of the patient's discharge from hospital, perform a home assessment and assist the patient and/or caregiver to determine an appropriate area for clean, safe storage of supplies and equipment, select a suitable area for procedures to be performed, and determine a safe method to discard disposable equipment.

f. Provide ongoing assessment of the patient's and/or caregiver's performance of therapy-related procedures at periodic intervals.

g. Document all communications with and/or site visits to the patient.

h. Communicate to the physician a summary of patient care at regular intervals and report immediately any observation that requires medical intervention.

i. Ensure that all necessary supplies and equipment are available in the home before therapy is initiated and that supply and equipment needs are continuously evaluated and met.

j. Ensure that the patient has 24-hour access to appropriate health care professionals.

3. The patient must:

a. Sign a consent form.

b. Demonstrate a specified level of self-care.

c. Carry and/or wear an identification indicative of therapy.

Determine the policies of the home nursing care agency. For example, many agencies require that:

1. Infusions lasting longer than one hour be given using an infusion pump.

2. The physician's orders include the route of administration (peripheral or central line), type of solution, amount and rate of infusion, additives, and type and frequency of blood tests.

3. IV antibiotics be given using a heparin lock or a central line.

4. Antibiotic medication orders include the dosage, type, and volume of diluent, rate and frequency of administration, and amount of solution and dosage of heparin for the heparin flush.

5. The infusion therapy nurse make no more than three unsuccessful attempts to restart a peripheral IV.

6. Blood tests be ordered weekly to monitor antibiotic effectiveness.

TECHNIQUE 25–2 ■ Monitoring and Maintaining an Intravenous Infusion

Teach patients and/or caregivers:

1. To observe the IV site through the transparent dressing at least four times a day and more often if necessary.

2. To watch for clinical signs of complications and to take the necessary actions listed in Table A-1. Ensure that the patient and/or caregiver understands and can verbalize these signs and demonstrates safe administration of the

TABLE A-1 ■ Signs of IV Complications and Corrective Actions

Complication	Signs	Action
Infiltration	Infusion rate slowed or stopped Swelling, redness, pain, or hardness at needle site Coldness around needle site	1. Stop infusion, remove IV needle, and apply 2 × 2 sterile dressing over site until bleeding stops. 2. Call nurse to restart IV.
IV not running	No evidence of drops	1. Check that roller clamp is open. 2. Check for kinking of tubing.
Phlebitis	Pain and/or tenderness at IV site Red line starting at site and extending up arm	1. Stop infusion, remove IV needle, and apply 2 × 2 sterile dressing over site until bleeding stops. 2. Call nurse to restart IV.
Dislodged catheter	Leaking at site Visibly bent needle	1. Stop infusion, remove IV needle, and apply 2 × 2 sterile dressing over site until bleeding stops. 2. Call nurse to restart IV.
IV plugged	Resistance when injecting saline Infusion rate slowed or stopped Dark blood in adapter or tubing	1. Do not use force to inject saline. 2. Call nurse.

treatment, including initiation and termination of therapy using an infusion pump, before being left unsupervised.

TECHNIQUE 25–5 ■ Starting an Intravenous Infusion Using a Butterfly Needle or Over-the-Needle Angiocatheter

Determine agency policies about:

1. Frequency of rotating the infusion site. The CDC recommends a change every 72 hours. (Centers for Disease Control, 1982, pp 61–72). For patients with poor venous access, some agencies require a less frequent needle change, if the physician approves.

2. Venipuncture sites. Most agencies recommend using the most distal site first, with each subsequent puncture proximal to the previous one. In a prolonged course of treatment, alternating arms is also recommended, to preserve the veins for future use.

TECHNIQUE 25–6 ■ Using an Infusion Pump

1. Determine agency policy regarding the use of pumps. Some agencies use infusion pumps on all home infusions lasting more than one hour.
2. Teach the patient and/or caregiver:
   a. The clinical signs of IV complications. See Table A–1.
   b. The signs of an adverse reaction to the infusion.
   c. How to initiate and terminate an infusion using a pump, when appropriate.

TECHNIQUE 25–9 ■ Establishing and Monitoring TPN (IVH) Therapy

1. Determine that there is a written order from the physician for TPN therapy. The order should include the kind and amount of solution, the rate of infusion, and any medications to be added.
2. Ensure that the patient or a guardian has signed a consent form.
3. Determine that a health care professional is available 24 hours a day (National Intravenous Therapy, 1984, p 93).
4. Explain that a responsible person must be present during TPN therapy.
5. Teach the patient and/or caregiver about:
   a. Keeping the catheter clamped except when flushing or running an infusion.
   b. Changing the injection cap after each infusion. When the cap is off, make sure the patient does not take deep breaths.
      Rationale Deep breaths can draw air into the tubing and subsequently into the bloodstream.
   c. Flushing the catheter using a heparin solution daily and using saline at appropriate times.
   d. Changing the dressing around the catheter every other day. See Appendix Technique 25–11.
   e. Operating an infusion pump. See Appendix Technique 25–6.
   f. Calculating the infusion rate.
   g. Connecting the tubing to the catheter and priming the tubing. See Technique 25–10.
   h. Weighing at the same time each day and recording the weight.
   i. Recording fluid intake and output.
   j. Possible complications and corrective actions to take. See Technique 25–9 in the text.
   k. Monitoring blood values at least every other week.

TECHNIQUE 25–11 ■ Changing a TPN (IVH) Dressing

1. Determine that there is a physician's order for the dressing change, including the type of dressing. Transparent dress-ings are preferred in the home, because they permit periodic assessment by the patient and/or caregiver. Frequently povidone-iodine treatment may be omitted when a transparent dressing is used. Check agency policy.
2. Teach the patient and/or caregiver about:
   a. Inspecting the skin area around the catheter regularly.
   b. Notifying the responsible nurse or physician immediately of the clinical signs of infection, ie, redness, discharge, or swelling.
   c. Changing the dressing using sterile technique. See Technique 25–11 in the text.

TECHNIQUE 25–14 ■ Flushing and Administering a Medication Through a Central Venous Catheter

1. Ensure that there is a responsible caregiver in the home.
2. Determine that the physician's order includes the name of the medication, dosage, type and volume of diluent, rate or frequency of administration, and amount of solution and dosage of heparin for the heparin flush.
3. Ensure that the medication ordered is approved for home care administration by the agency.
4. Arrange for weekly monitoring of therapeutic blood levels of antibiotics.
5. Teach the patient and/or caregiver:
   a. How to administer medications, if appropriate, and how to flush a central line.
   b. Clinical signs of adverse reactions to the medications.
   c. How to store the medications properly.
   d. To contact the nurse if problems arise.

TECHNIQUES 26–1 to 26–2 ■ Giving and Removing a Bedpan or Urinal

Teach caregivers about:

1. Elimination aids that are available from medical suppliers or other agencies, eg, male and female urinals, commodes, and plastic bedpans. Patients confined to bed can easily empty urinals into a pail or commode during the night.
2. Bathroom elimination aids such as removable, elevated toilet seats, toilet arm rests, and grab bars. A physiotherapist can advise caregivers on the best equipment for the patient eg, the kind of grab bars and the level and angle at which they should be installed.

TECHNIQUE 26–3 ■ Administering an Enema

Teach patients and/or caregivers:

1. To administer an enema only when other measures (such as increasing the patient's activity, increasing fiber and

fluid intake) have failed or when the enema is ordered by a physician.

2. To offer prune juice daily and provide a regular time for elimination for the inactive patient.

3. To use laxatives only after consultation with a physician.

4. That disposable enema units are available.

5. How to administer an enema themselves, if indicated:
   a. Assume a back-lying or left lateral position.
   b. Use bed-saver pads beneath the buttocks.
   c. Liberally lubricate the nozzle tip before insertion.
   d. Never force insertion of the nozzle.
   e. Administer the fluid slowly, and retain it for five to ten minutes if possible.

TECHNIQUE 27–1 ■ Female Urinary Catheterization Using a Straight Catheter

Self-Catheterization Using Clean Technique

Sterile technique is necessary for self-catheterization in a hospital because of the danger of nosocomial infection. However, at home, clean technique can be used because of the bladder's natural resistance to the microorganisms normally found at home.

Equipment

1. A supply of rubber catheters
2. A clean washcloth, soap, and water
3. A water-soluble lubricant
4. A drainage container for the urine
5. A plastic bag for the used catheters
6. A good light
7. A hand mirror, if the patient needs one to find the urethral meatus

■ Intervention

Teach the patient the following steps:

1. Try to urinate before starting the catheterization.
2. Wash and dry your hands thoroughly.
3. Separate the vaginal folds (labia majora and labia minora) with one hand.
4. Wash the area thoroughly using downward strokes.
   Rationale This direction washes from the most clean area to the least clean area.
5. Place the hand mirror, if used, to reflect the urinary meatus.
6. Lubricate the first 7.6 cm (3 in) of the catheter. Place the other end of the catheter over the urine drainage receptacle.
7. Hold the catheter as if it were a pencil, about 1 to 2.5 cm (½ to 1 in) from the tip, while holding the vaginal folds apart with the other hand.
8. Slowly insert the catheter into the urethra about 7.6 cm (3 in).
9. Once the urine begins to flow, press down on the abdominal muscles

Rationale The abdominal muscles help to empty the bladder.

10. Withdraw the catheter slowly when the urine stops running.
11. Wash and dry any area where urine spilled.
12. Wash the catheter in warm, soapy water, rinse it, dry it, and place it in the plastic bag.
13. Use each catheter only once. Boil the used catheters for 20 minutes in water, dry them, and store them in a freshly laundered towel (Nursing Photobook Series, 1981a, p 59).
14. Purchase a new supply of catheters each month, or when they become brittle.
    Rationale Repeated use and boiling causes rubber catheters to become brittle and eventually crack.
15. Each day drink the amount of fluid recommended by the physician or home care nurse.
16. Take all medications prescribed by the physician. Medications may be prescribed to prevent bladder infection.
17. Limit the intake of foods rich in phosphorus and calcium, eg, eggs, milk, cheddar cheese, ice cream, organ meats, dark green vegetables.
    Rationale Phosphorus and calcium can form kidney stones.
18. After each catheterization, assess the urine for color, odor, clarity, and the presence of particles or blood.
19. At the first sign of abnormalities in the urine or lower abdominal pain, notify the home care nurse or physician.

TECHNIQUE 27–2 ■ Male Urinary Catheterization Using a Straight Catheter

Self-Catheterization Using Clean Technique

Equipment

1. See Appendix Technique 27–2, items 1–6.
2. A paper towel.

■ Intervention

Teach the patient the following steps:

1. See Appendix Technique 27–1, steps 1–2.
2. Pull back the foreskin if you are not circumcised, and hold it back during the catheterization.
3. Wash the end of the penis with soap and water.
4. Squeeze lubricant onto the paper towel, and lubricate the first 5 to 7 cm (2 to 3 in) of the catheter. Place the other end of the catheter over the drainage receptacle.
5. Hold the penis at a right angle to your body, and hold the catheter as if it were a pencil with the other hand.
6. Insert the catheter into the urethra about 18 to 25 cm (7 to 10 in) until the urine flows, then 2.5 cm (1 in) further.
7. Permit all the urine to drain.
8. When the urine stops, withdraw the catheter, and pull the foreskin forward.
9. See Appendix Technique 27–1, steps 11–19.

TECHNIQUE 27–3 ■ Inserting a Retention Catheter

Teach patients or caregivers:

1. Not to pull on the catheter.
2. To check the tubing for kinks or twists that could impede the flow of urine.
3. To maintain the catheter and tubing intact so that microorganisms cannot enter the system.
4. To keep the drainage bag below the level of the bladder, so that urine will flow out unimpeded.
5. To empty the drainage bag regularly and before it becomes full, eg, q.4h., and to record the amount, appearance, odor, etc, of the urine. Stress the need to maintain the sterility of the drainage tube by not letting it touch the urine receptacle or toilet.
6. After emptying the drainage bag, to swab the end of the drainage tube with povidone-iodine solution before reinserting it into the sleeve of the bag.
7. To use a leg bag that can be attached to the thigh, when up during the day. This bag needs to be emptied more often than the closed-system bag, because it is smaller.
8. To attach a closed-system drainage bag to the catheter at night, as follows:
   a. Empty the leg bag as described in steps 5–6.
   b. Clamp the catheter.
   c. Swab the connection between the catheter and the drainage tubing with povidone-iodine solution.
   d. Disconnect the tubing from the catheter, and attach the tubing from the closed-system drainage bag to the catheter.
   e. Unclamp the catheter.
   f. Tape the drainage tube to the thigh leaving a loop, so the catheter will not pull with movement.
   g. Wash the leg bag with warm, soapy water and rinse it. Then rinse the bag with a solution of 2 quarts water and 1¼ cups white vinegar, to reduce urine odor.
9. To reattach the leg bag, following the procedure in step 8.

TECHNIQUE 27–4 ■ Providing Catheter Care

Teach patients and/or caregivers:

1. To wash the perineum or penis twice a day using soap and water, and to rinse and dry the area well.
2. To wash the rectal area twice a day and after each bowel movement.
3. To notify the home care nurse or physician at the first signs of:
   a. Irritation or infection of the perineum or penis: redness, discomfort, or odor.
   b. Leaking around the catheter.
   c. Discomfort or fullness in the lower abdomen.
   d. Altered urine flow, eg, decreased amount of urine or presence of abnormal constituents in the urine.
4. Not to remove the catheter themselves.

TECHNIQUE 27–7 ■ Applying and Removing a Drainage Condom

Teach the patients and/or caregivers:

1. That commercial drainage condoms are available.
2. That the drainage condom should be changed every day.
3. That they can make a drainage condom that is more economical than the commercial ones:
   a. Obtain from the pharmacy a supply of standard condoms and latex tubing 1 cm (⅜ in) in diameter.
   b. Cut two narrow bands, 0.3 cm (⅛ in) wide, from the tubing (or use two clean elastic bands that fit tightly around the tubing).
   c. Put one band on the tubing about 1.25 cm (½ in) from one end.
   d. Cut off the tip of the condom.
   e. Put the condom on the tubing so that the rolled edge faces inward and the larger open end is beyond the first band on the tubing.
   f. Place a second band over the tubing and the condom between the first band and the end of the tubing.
   g. Invert the condom over the tubing and the second elastic band.
   h. Slide the first elastic band over the second. This will secure the condom firmly to the tubing.
   i. Apply the condom to the penis. Leave a slight gap at the tip of the penis to avoid irritation from the end of the tubing.

TECHNIQUE 27–8 ■ Suprapubic Catheter Care

Teach patients or care givers:

1. To observe the skin around the catheter site for clinical signs of irritation and drainage, and to report these to the home care nurse or physician.
2. To change the dressing around the catheter once a week, or as necessary depending upon drainage. Dry sterile dressings are used unless otherwise ordered by the physician.

TECHNIQUE 27–9 ■ Peritoneal Dialysis

A Silastic catheter, often a Tenchkoff catheter, is surgically implanted in the abdominal cavity. The catheter has two Dacron velour cuffs, one of which rests on the fascia covering the peritoneal membrane; the other is located in the subcutaneous tissue. Tissue growth into these cuffs anchors the catheter and prevents the entrance of microorganisms along the catheter (Binkley, 1984, p 729).

There are three types of peritoneal dialysis for patients at home: intermittent peritoneal dialysis (IPD), continuous ambulatory peritoneal dialysis (CAPD), and continuous cycling peritoneal dialysis (CCPD). With IPD the patient usually requires 40 hours of dialysis per week. This is frequently done at night, eg, four nights for ten hours. The cycle delivers the dialysate and can be regulated to deliver a predetermined number of exchanges, leave the dialysate in for a specified time before it drains by gravity. IPD requires an electric outlet, a floor drain, and ample water. The equipment can be used at night and has an alarm that will ring if there is a problem.

With CAPD, the patient requires only a bag of dialysate and disposable tubing. The patient instills the dialysate, which remains in the abdominal cavity for four to eight hours. The bag is rolled up and carried in the patient's clothing during this time. When it is time for draining, the bag is unrolled, and the used dialysate drains into it by gravity. Another bag of dialysate is then instilled. Often patients require four or five 2-L exchanges each day. The advantages of this system are that no machine, electricity, or water supply is required, and the dialysis is continuous. The main disadvantage is that the system is opened with each exchange, thus increasing the possibility of peritonitis.

CCPD combines IPD and CAPD. Exchanges use a cycling machine. Often three exchanges are done at night and a fourth is instilled and remains in the abdominal cavity during the day. The closed system is opened only twice: once in the morning and once in the evening. This decreases the opportunity for infection.

Teach patients and/or caregivers about:

1. Assessing the skin area around the catheter for clinical signs of infection and assessing for clinical signs of peritonitis, eg, pain, elevated temperature, cloudy drainage fluid.
2. The availability of equipment that includes dialysate, cyclers, and filters.
3. Using sterile technique to carry out peritoneal dialysis.
4. Instilling povidone-iodine solution into the distal end of the catheter after dialysis, to prevent the entrance of microorganisms. The solution is held between the clamp on the catheter and the cap at the end of the filter.
5. Care of the skin around the catheter using sterile supplies.
6. Dietary restrictions, eg, of potassium, sodium, protein, and fluid, if indicated.

Hemodialysis

In hemodialysis, the blood flows through a polyurethane tube to a dialysis machine, or artificial kidney. Through diffusion, filtration, osmosis, and ultrafiltration, the waste products move from the blood through the tubing into the dialysate in the machine. The cleaned blood then returns to the blood circulation. Treatments are frequently required three times a week for four hours or twice a week for five hours (Chambers, 1981, p 750).

To gain access to the patient's circulation, an external shunt or internal fistula is used. With the external arteriovenous shunt, two pieces of Teflon tubing are inserted surgically: one into an artery, eg, the radial artery, and one into a nearby vein, eg, the cephalic vein. The tubes are then attached by a connector. For dialysis, the connector is removed, and each tube is connected to the appropriate tube from the machine. The patient's blood is normally heparinized during hemodialysis.

In an arteriovenous fistula, the vein and artery are connected internally, eg, the radial artery is joined to the cephalic vein under the skin. Two venipunctures are then made for each dialysis session, to carry the blood to and from the hemodialysis machine.

The home care nurse must determine that there is a physician's order for hemodialysis and that 24-hour advice and emergency care is available. Then teach patients and caregivers about:

1. Checking the shunt or fistula for patency. Using a stethoscope, auscultate for a bruit at the venous site or palpate for a thrill. These indicate adequate blood flow in the shunt. If the bruit or thrill is not detected, notify the physician or home care nurse or have the patient go to the dialysis or emergency center. Clotting can occur in the shunt.
2. Assessing the shunt site for infection and injury. Povidone-iodine ointment and sterile dry dressings are applied regularly to external shunt sites.
3. Carrying out the hemodialysis procedure:
   a. Operating the machinery according to the manufacturer's instructions.
   b. Inserting fistula needles.
4. Monitoring temperature, pulse, and blood pressure. The blood pressure should be taken on the arm *not* used for the hemodialysis.
5. Monitoring fluid balance, eg, by assessing daily weight, measuring urine output, and measuring fluid intake.
6. Administering heparin, if indicated.
7. Monitoring electrolyte balance through regular laboratory analysis of the used dialysate, eg, for potassium, sodium, and calcium. Teach the clinical signs of electrolyte imbalance.
8. Monitoring blood cell counts and electrolyte levels as indicated. Teach the clinical signs of defective platelets, eg, bleeding from the mucous membranes.

TECHNIQUE 28-1 ■ Changing a Bowel Diversion Ostomy Appliance

Although the enterostomal nurse-therapist provides instruction for ostomy patients, the home care nurse may teach patients:

1. How to empty the ostomy pouch in the bathroom (Nursing Photobook Series, 1981b, p 107):
   a. Empty the pouch when it is about one-third full.
   b. Place a cup of warm water within reach to rinse the pouch.
   c. Sit either on the toilet with the pouch hanging between your legs or on a chair next to the toilet with the opening of the pouch directed into the toilet.
   d. Turn up the bottom of the pouch and remove the closure clamp.
   e. Place some toilet paper on the surface of the toilet water, or flush the toilet while you direct the pouch contents into the bowl.
      Rationale The toilet paper decreases splashing of the ostomy contents.
   f. Squeeze all the ostomy contents into the toilet by sliding your thumb and fingers down the outside of the pouch.
   g. Using toilet tissue, clean remaining drainage from the outside of the pouch and from the inside of the pouch opening.
   h. Hold the pouch opening upright. Pour the cup of water into the pouch, and swish the water around. Avoid wetting the stoma or the pouch seal, to prevent breaking the seal.
   i. Again, direct the pouch opening into the toilet, and allow it to drain completely.

j. Clean and dry the outside of the pouch, and close it with a clamp or rubber band.

2. How to clean a reusable pouch (ibid, p 108):

a. Remove the double-adhesive disc from the faceplate. It may be necessary to roll some of the adhesive off with your fingertips or to loosen the adhesive with a gauze pad moistened with adhesive solvent. Use solvent sparingly, however.

Rationale Solvent can erode the faceplate.

b. Rinse the pouch under a tap with cool water.

c. Using a long-handled brush, clean the inside of the pouch with water and a mild soap, detergent, or substance recommended by the pouch manufacturer.

d. Rinse the pouch thoroughly with cool water.

e. Either fill the pouch with crumpled paper towels and place it on a flat surface to dry, or use a pouch hook to hang it over the sink. Do not dry the pouch in heat or direct sunlight.

f. When the pouch is dry, remove the paper towels, if used, and store the pouch in a cool, dry place.

TECHNIQUE 29–1 ■ Administering Oral Medications

1. For a blind patient who needs to take a variety of oral medications and who wants to be independent, the following system can be used (Boles, 1984, p 62):

a. Using letters cut from sandpaper, label seven envelopes with the days of the week.

b. Using sandpaper numbers, label small zip-lock plastic bags with the times the pills are to be taken. Label sufficient bags for each day of the week.

c. Place the tablets in the zip-lock bags, and place the zip-lock bags inside the envelopes.

d. File the envelopes in a shoe box, and place it in a convenient place for the patient.

This system can be adapted for patients who have difficulty remembering when to take their medications or whose visual impairments make it difficult for them to read medication labels. Using a black felt pen, label the envelopes and bags with letters and numbers large enough to be easily read by the patient.

2. For patients who need to take antibiotics at prescribed intervals, a medication chart is useful (Yetka, 1984, p 63):

a. Make a cross-off-the-pill chart with a box for each day the antibiotic is to be taken.

b. Inside each box, write the number of pills to be taken each day, eg, "1, 2, 3, 4," and the time for each.

c. Ask the patient to cross off a number after each pill is taken.

TECHNIQUE 30-3 ■ Administering a Subcutaneous Injection

For visually impaired patients who are able to administer injections but who have difficulty loading their syringes with insulin or other medication:

1. Place a piece of tape around the syringe barrel to indicate the unit level to which insulin must be withdrawn.

or

2. Preload two to four insulin syringes, and place them in the refrigerator, maintaining the sterility of the needle. The patient then only needs to take the syringe from the refrigerator and administer the injection.

To help a young diabetic learn proper rotation of insulin injection sites (Emery, 1984, p 63).

1. Trace the child's body outline on brown wrapping paper.

2. After each injection, help the child find and date the site on the paper.

3. Encourage the child to decorate the tracing with yarn and felt pens.

TECHNIQUES 30–6 to 30–9 ■ Adding or Administering an IV Medication

Determine that:

1. The physician's order includes the medication, the dosage, and the method of administration, including the infusion rate if appropriate. Certain medications, eg, vesicants such as Velban, can be given only through a central line, while others can be given through a peripheral intravenous route.

2. If more than one medication is ordered, they are compatible with one another and with the IV solution.

3. Agency policy permits home administration of the medication ordered.

4. Agency policy permits home administration of medications by IV bolus, if ordered.

5. There is a signed consent form.

Teach patients and caregivers about:

1. Inspecting the intravenous site for signs of infection and infiltration.

2. Clinical signs indicating an adverse reaction to the medication.

3. Notifying a health care professional if the signs in step 1 or 2 occur.

4. Administering the medication using sterile technique.

5. Monitoring the IV solution. See Appendix Technique 25–2.

6. Starting and stopping the IV solution. See Techniques 25–3 to 25–5 in the text.

TECHNIQUE 33–2 ■ Basic Bandaging

Applying and Removing an Unna Boot

An unna boot is a paste bandage containing cotton gauze bandage, calamine, zinc oxide, and gelatin.

■ Assessment

Assess the patient for:

1. Edema of the leg. Measure the leg and foot at the calf, ankle, and instep, using a measuring tape. The boot should be applied before the patient is ambulatory or after the legs have been elevated for one to two hours, so that edema is minimal.
2. Appearance of the wound: size, color, depth, and presence of drainage. Assess the drainage for amount, color, viscosity, and odor. Use a measuring tape to assess wound size.
3. Discomfort.
4. Skin color and temperature of the toes of the affected foot.

Other data include:

1. The physician's order for the boot, including the number of layers, and the length of time the boot is to be in place (eg, three to seven days). The time the boot is left in place depends on the adequacy of circulation to the extremity, the amount of edema, and the amount of drainage.
2. Baseline data about edema of the leg and the appearance of the wound.

■ Planning

Nursing goals

1. To facilitate healing of wounds of the lower extremities, eg, varicose ulcers
2. To enhance blood supply to and from the extremity
3. To protect the leg from further injury

Equipment

1. A paste bandage in rolls 7.5 or 10 cm (3 or 4 in) wide.
2. Soap, water, a basin, and a towel to wash and dry the extremity before applying the bandage
3. Bandage scissors
4. A gauze bandage such as Kerlex
5. A measuring tape
6. An elastic bandage
7. Newspapers

■ Intervention

Applying the boot

1. Make sure that the patient's legs have been elevated for at least one to two hours before starting to apply the boot.
2. Place the newspapers on the floor near the patient.
3. Fill the basin with water, and place it on the newspapers.
   Rationale Any water that spills will be absorbed by the newspapers.
4. Wash and dry the leg.
5. Position the leg so that the knee and ankle are flexed.
   Rationale A flexed position minimizes muscle strain.
6. Make a circular turn using the paste bandage at the base of the toes.
   Rationale A circular turn anchors the bandage. Leaving the toes exposed permits assessment of the circulatory status of the foot.
7. Continue bandaging the foot and leg using spiral turns and terminating the bandage just below the knee. Bandage

firmly around the foot, and use less pressure while proceeding up the leg.
   Rationale Spiral turns provide a smooth bandage that is less irritating to the skin than spiral reverse turns. Bandaging from the foot to the knee facilitates venous blood flow.
8. Snip the edges of the bandage or cut the bandage off and start a new turn if the bandage does not fit snugly.
9. With your free hand mold the bandage until it is smooth.
   Rationale Molding should eliminate ridges, which could be irritating to the skin and interfere with blood flow.
10. If necessary make small cuts, 2.5 to 5 cm (1 to 2 in), in the bandage at the knee.
    Rationale The cuts prevent undue pressure on the leg.
11. Apply one to three layers of paste bandage, as required.
12. Cover the bandaged leg with a gauze bandage, eg, Kerlex, applied in the same manner as the paste bandage.
    Rationale The gauze bandage prevents the paste from soiling the patient's clothes.
13. Wrap an elastic bandage over the gauze in the same manner.
14. Leave the boot in place three to seven days depending upon the patient's needs (see Assessment, other data, item 1).
15. Instruct the patient and/or support persons:
    a. To elevate the legs until the bandage dries thoroughly, eg, 30 to 60 minutes.
    b. To check circulation to the leg and foot by assessing the toes for color, temperature, numbness, tingling, discomfort, etc, every hour the first day, and notify the home care nurse immediately if any of these signs occurs.
    c. To elevate the leg and foot regularly during the day, eg, q.2h. for one-half hour, to enhance blood circulation to and from the area.
16. Check the foot yourself for any circulatory impairment later that day.

Removing the boot

17. Soak the bandage in warm water.
    Rationale Water softens the bandage so that it can be removed more readily.
18. Carefully cut the bandage away from the leg while maintaining the intactness of the skin.
19. Assess the appearance of the wound. See Assessment, steps 2–3.
20. Wash and dry the leg.
21. Apply a new bandage if indicated.

■ Evaluation

Expected outcomes

1. Ulcer 5 cm (2 in) in diameter; decreased 1 cm (0.5 in) from previous week
2. Skin around ulcer pink
3. Minimal serous drainage, no odor

Unexpected outcomes

1. Ulcer 5 cm (2 in) in diameter; increased 2 cm (0.7 in) from previous week
2. Skin around ulcer bright red
4. Large amount of thick, white drainage with foul odor

TECHNIQUE 34–1 ▪ Applying a Hot Water Bottle, Electric Heating Pad, or Aquathermia Pad

Teach patients and/or caregivers:

1. The purpose of the heat application. Dry heat is usually applied to improve blood flow to an injured body part, to promote muscle relaxation, and to reduce pain from spasm or stiffness.

2. Guidelines for use of the device.
    a. For a hot water bottle:
    - After filling and capping the bottle, check it for leaks by turning it upside-down.
    - Fill the bottle only two-thirds full, and expel any air at the top, so that the bottle can be more easily molded over the body part.
    - Always cover the bottle with a towel or pillowcase before applying it to the body part.

    b. For an electric heating pad:
    - Check that the pad is functioning and in good repair. The cord should not be cracked, wires should not be frayed, heating components should not be exposed, and temperature distribution over the pad should not be uneven.
    - Do not lie directly on the pad since the surface below the pad does not allow normal heat dissipation. Place the pad over the body part while heat is being applied.
    - Use gauze ties, not safety pins, to hold the pad in place. Safety pins can produce an electric shock.
    - Avoid using the high heat setting, to prevent injury.

    c. For an aquathermia pad:
    - Check for any leak or malfunctions of the pad before use.
    - Cover the pad with a towel or pillowcase.
    - Use tape or gauze ties to hold the pad in place. Never use safety pins, because they can cause leakage.
    - Do not lie directly on the pad (see b, above).

3. To keep the heating appliance in place for 20 to 30 minutes. Prolonged heat, eg, one hour, decreases the blood flow to the area and can damage skin tissue. A timer or clock can help the patient time the application.

4. That tolerance to heat varies with age, physical condition, and duration of the application. The very young and the elderly have the least tolerance to temperature variations. People who have decreased sensation because of a neurologic or vascular impairment may tolerate heat extremely well but are at risk for injury.

5. To avoid adjusting temperature settings during the application. When the heat is first applied, the patient will feel the temperature quite significantly. Soon after, the temperature variation is hardly noticed, since the body's temperature receptors quickly adapt to temperature changes. This adaptive mechanism can lead to tissue injury, especially if the person is insensitive to temperature variations or if the patient adjusts the temperature controls to a higher setting during the application.

6. To avoid applying heat to:
    a. Areas that are bleeding, since heat will increase the bleeding.
    b. Areas that are inflamed, such as a painful appendix, since heat may aggravate the problem.
    c. Large areas of the body, if the patient has a cardiovascular problem, since massive dilation of the blood vessels can divert the blood supply from vital organs and cause fainting.

TECHNIQUE 34–3 ▪ Administering Hot Soaks and Sitz Baths

Teach patients and/or caregivers:

1. The purpose of the heat application. Soaks and baths are usually administered to reduce muscle tension and discomfort, to relieve venous congestion and swelling, to improve blood flow, to clean a wound, and/or to apply a medicated solution to a wound.

2. Guidelines for the procedure.
    a. Hot soak:
    - Administer the soak for 20 minutes.
    - Cover a soak container with a towel to reduce heat loss. The water (or medicated solution) can cool quickly.
    - Add heated solution after 10 minutes. Remove the body part from the solution while the heated solution is being added.
    - Thoroughly dry the body part after the soak, to prevent skin maceration.

    b. Sitz bath:
    - Use disposable sitz baths, available from medical suppliers. Soaking in a tub is not as effective, since it diverts the vasodilation effect to other body parts rather than localizing it in the pelvic area.
    - Wear clothing over the upper body, and drape the legs with a blanket, to prevent chilling.
    - Test the temperature of the water before sitting in the bath. It should feel comfortable to the inner aspect of the wrist.
    - Use the sitz bath for 20 minutes.
    - Add warmer water after 10 minutes. Some disposable units have special attachments that allow the gradual introduction of warmer water.

3. See Appendix Technique 34–1, step 4.

TECHNIQUE 34–4 ▪ Applying an Ice Bag, Ice Collar, Ice Glove, or Disposable Cold Pack

Teach patients and/or caregivers the following:

1. The purpose of the cold application. Dry cold is usually applied to prevent swelling, to control bleeding, and to anesthetize or reduce discomfort.

2. That commercially prepared ice packs are available. The disadvantage of these is that they cannot be frozen for reuse.

3. That a large package of frozen vegetables (peas or corn) can be used instead of an ice pack. It can be frozen for reuse and molds readily to any body part.

4. Guidelines for use of an ice bag or collar:

   a. First fill an ice-bag with water, cap it, invert it, check it for leaks, and then empty it.

   b. Fill the bag only two-thirds full, using crushed ice, and squeeze out excess air, so that the bag can mold more easily over the body part.

   c. Cover the bag with a towel or pillowcase before applying it to the body part.

5. Keep the appliance in place for about 30 minutes and do not reapply it for an hour. Prolonged cold can interfere with circulation, healing, and cell function to a point where severe damage to the tissues results.

6. Avoid applying cold:

   a. To areas that are already swollen, since cold will further impair circulation to the area and prevent absorption of the fluid.

   b. To patients with impaired circulation, eg, with arteriosclerosis.

   c. To people who are shivering, since cold can intensify this problem.

TECHNIQUE 35–1 ■ Changing a Dry Surgical Dressing

Teach patients and/or caregivers:

1. That sterile disposable dressing supplies are available.

2. The type of antiseptic to use to clean the wound.

3. Ways to clean a wound using forceps or disposable gloves and cotton balls. If nondisposable forceps are used to clean a wound, caregivers need to sterilize them by boiling them for 10 minutes before use.

4. To wash hands thoroughly before changing a dressing.

5. Ways to establish a sterile field. See Appendix Technique 7–3.

6. How to make tie tapes from strips of adhesive tape by folding back a portion of the tape onto itself (for the part of the tape that will lie over the dressing), cutting a hole through the tape end and inserting a strip of gauze through the hole to use for tying the tapes together.

7. About expected wound drainage and its appearance.

8. About signs or changes that indicate the need to call the nurse, eg, increased amount of drainage, increased discomfort, bleeding, increased swelling, opening or gaping of wound edges.

TECHNIQUE 36–1 ■ Teaching Deep Breathing Exercises

Teach patients who have chronic obstructive pulmonary disease the following (Weimer, 1983, p 1486):

1. Diaphragmatic breathing. Have the patient expand his or her waist when breathing in, and pull in the waist when breathing out.

2. Pursed-lip breathing and prolonged expiration. To prac-

tice these, have the patient try to bend the flame of a candle placed about 1 foot away.

When patients are proficient in the above breathing patterns, have them incorporate this breathing in the course of daily activities. They should rest while inhaling and perform work when exhaling. For example, when climbing stairs, patients inhale while standing with both feet on a step and then exhale using pursed-lip breathing while ascending two or three steps; when dressing, patients inhale while standing or sitting still and then exhale while putting on a sock, stocking, or shirt; when bathing, patients inhale while sitting in the tub and then exhale while washing or drying an arm, foot, or leg. Control and mastery of this breathing pattern allows patients to perform more activities with less dyspnea.

TECHNIQUE 36–3 ■ Assisting Patients with Intermittent Positive Pressure Breathing (IPPB) or Other Types of Ventilators

For IPPB or aerosol treatments, instruct patients and caregivers about:

1. The equipment to be used. Provide written and oral instructions, present demonstrations, and ensure that patients and/or caregivers understand and can demonstrate how to perform essential procedures.

2. Cleaning procedures for respiratory therapy equipment. Weimer (1983, p 1489) outlines the following steps:

   a. Wipe the surface of the machine with a clean, damp cloth.

   b. Cover the equipment and keep it in a clean area.

   c. After each IPPB or aerosol treatment, rinse the manifold (nebulizer, mouthpiece, exhalation valve) with warm (not hot) running water, and allow it to air dry. Do not wipe it with a towel.

   d. After the last treatment of the day:

   ■ Disassemble the manifold, and remove the large tubing from the IPPB machine.

   ■ Wash all parts in a basin of warm, soapy water, and thoroughly rinse them with warm running water.

   ■ Soak the parts and two smaller tubings in a vinegar-water solution (1 part white distilled vinegar and 4 parts water) for 30 minutes. Use fresh solution each day.

   ■ After soaking them thoroughly, rinse all parts with warm running water.

   ■ Remove water from the tubings by connecting them to the nebulizer outlet on the machine, turning the machine on, and letting air blow the water out.

   ■ Allow all parts to air dry. When they are dry, cover the equipment with a clean towel or store it in plastic bags.

3. Assist the patient to measure all aerosol medications accurately. For those who have poor eyesight, a 3-mL medicine dropper may be easier to use than a syringe. For those who cannot use a dropper, a ½-tsp measure can be substituted.

Home Mechanical Ventilation

Home care of mechanically ventilated patients is a demanding program that requires not only knowledge and skilled abilities of caregivers but also an extraordinary degree of responsibility and commitment. Most patients have permanent tracheostomies, so that caregivers must also learn to do all tracheostomy maintenance procedures (see Appendix Techniques 40–1 to 40–5). Such a home care program often requires the coordinated efforts of the physician, the physical, occupational, and respiratory therapists, a respiratory clinical nurse, registered nurses, a chest physical therapist, a pulmonary laboratory technician, a social worker, a dietitian, and the medical supplier.

Small, lightweight, portable *positive-pressure* ventilators are available for home use. Models vary, but generally they operate on 110-volt alternating current or on a battery for up to 24 hours. The battery provides emergency backup in case of an electric power failure. Built-in alarms sound when the pressure becomes too high or too low, when the voltage is low, and when there is a power failure.

Often *negative-pressure* ventilators are chosen for home use because the patient does not need a tracheostomy and because they are uncomplicated.

Not all ventilator-dependent patients are candidates for independent self-care at home; thus careful selection procedures are needed. Criteria for patient selection include (Sivak, Cordasco, Gipson, 1983, p 43; Gilmartin, Make, 1983, p 1491):

1. The patient could not be weaned from mechanical ventilation after two months, either by intermittent mandatory ventilation or by a graduated T-piece method of nonventilator breathing. In the T-piece method, the patient spends five-minute intervals off mechanical ventilation three times daily. Five minutes are added to each period as long as the respiratory rate remains under 35 breaths per minute. Failure to wean may be determined by the patient's inability to maintain adequate ventilation (eg, a P_{CO_2} less than 50 mm Hg, a P_{O_2} greater than 65 mm Hg for at least ten hours).

2. The patient is medically stable. Other problems, such as pneumonia or urinary tract infections, must be treated and controlled.

3. The patient is motivated and willing to participate in a home care program. Some patients may say they want to go home but do not really mean it.

4. The patient's family members are capable of providing physical and emotional support in the home. Some family members may feel obligated to care for the patient but are not really willing to assume the responsibility demanded.

5. The patient and family are able to initiate and perform independently all required care without staff direction and supervision. Self-care skills include:

   a. Tracheostomy care (suctioning, saline instillation, cuff care, etc.)

   b. Use of a manual resuscitator.

   c. Ventilator care (eg, how to make routine ventilator checks, change and clean the tubing, add water to the humidifier, and deal with problems, such as electric power failure, malfunction of the humidifier or suction machine, holes in the ventilator tubing, or a frozen oxygen gauge).

   d. How to administer aerosol medications.

   e. How to deal rapidly and systematically with shortness of breath.

6. The patient has adequate insurance to cover supplies and equipment. If not, an application for Medicaid or disability should be submitted by the social worker.

Before discharge, plans must be made to increase the patient's mobility, sense of independence, and control over the environment at home, to evaluate the home physical environment, to obtain necessary equipment, and to provide support services.

1. *Increasing the patient's mobility.* Gilmartin and Make (1983, p 1491) outline the following procedure for gradually increasing the patient's time spent off the ventilator, using the T-piece method:

   a. Initially, do not have the patient perform any activities when off the ventilator until he or she is able to remain off for at least one hour.

   b. Next, introduce activities that do not require much energy (eg, eating at the bedside, brushing teeth, performing tracheostomy care, washing at the bedside) while off the ventilator.

   c. When periods off the ventilator lengthen, introduce other ADL, such as walking to the bathroom and using the toilet. Time off the ventilator even if only for an hour gives the patient a sense of independence. Trips out of the patient's room and hospital using a motorized wheelchair with a portable ventilator, if necessary, also help to increase the patient's and family's confidence and independence.

   d. Gradually increase trips in length and distance, from the hospital cafeteria or gift shop to the hospital grounds, to shopping malls or restaurants, and then to day and weekend trips home. Providing the patient and support persons with a list of supplies needed on these trips is helpful.

2. *Home evaluation.* A respiratory therapist, an occupational and/or physical therapist, and a nurse from the home care agency need to visit the patient's home before the discharge date, to assess needed modifications. Home modifications can be expensive and are not covered by medical insurance. Some factors to consider are:

   a. Placement for the respiratory equipment and whether there are enough electric outlets to accommodate the equipment.

   b. Physical access for the patient from outside the house and between rooms. For example, for a wheelchair patient, does a ramp need to be made to the front door, and are doors in the house wide enough to accommodate a wheelchair? For patients who have impaired balance, are there hand rails on the stairs?

   c. Necessary kitchen modifications if the patient plans to prepare meals. For example, is there a kitchen stool for the patient to sit on, to conserve energy while preparing meals? Should a rolling cart be provided to help the patient carry food from the stove to refrigerator, sink, or table?

   d. Necessary bathroom modifications, such as grab bars in the tub and by the toilet, an elevated toilet seat, a shower chair, or a hand-held shower hose.

3. *Equipment.* Equipment and supplies often required for home care of the ventilator-dependent patient include:

   a. A mechanical ventilator and emergency backup ventilator with a humidification device, power source, ventilator alarm, and nondisposable ventilator tubing.

   b. A manual resuscitator.

c. An air compressor.

d. An oxygen supply (eg, tanks, concentrators) and oxygen devices such as tracheostomy masks or T-pieces, connecting tubing, and nasal cannulae.

e. Tracheostomy care supplies, such as tracheostomy tubes, tape, sponges, and brushes; syringes; three-way stopcocks; paper cups; and cotton-tipped applicators.

f. Suctioning supplies, such as suction catheters and connecting tubing; nonsterile gloves; paper cups; and 5-mL vials of normal saline.

g. Miscellaneous supplies, such as disposable hand wipes, tissues, small plastic garbage bags, and white vinegar.

4. *Support services.* Before the patient's discharge, many support services need to be notified. The home care company or the visiting nurse association (VNA) can usually provide home health aides, who can assist the patient and family with personal care, or a homemaker, who can assist with housework, meal preparation, and food shopping. The police and fire departments and the local power company need to be informed that the patient has life-supporting equipment in the home. The patient should place a list of emergency telephone numbers (eg, physician, respiratory company, oxygen company, ambulance, VNA) in a readily accessible spot.

TECHNIQUES 36–5 to 36–6 ■ Administering Percussion, Vibration, and Postural Drainage (PVD) to Adults, Infants, and Children

Instruct patients and/or caregivers in the appropriate technique (Weimer, 1983, p 1487):

1. The technique of postural drainage alone, for patients who live by themselves. This may help the person to clear secretions.

2. The complete technique of PVD for patients and caregivers who can perform the procedures correctly.

3. The correct position(s) to assume. Use pillows to elevate the hips if a slant board or blocks are unavailable to elevate the foot of the bed in the home.

4. The use of mechanical percussors for those who have difficulty providing the necessary force to move secretions or who cannot maintain the proper cupping position of the hands.

5. The use of deep breathing and coughing with the PVD therapy. Have the patient inhale slowly and deeply three times, using diaphragmatic breathing, and then lean forward and cough two or three times using a "huffing" manner. Explain to the patient that deep breathing and coughing help to loosen and move mucus along the respiratory passages.

6. The use of a bean-bag chair to support a child in several comfortable postural drainage positions (Bean, 1984, p 63). This is useful for parents who need to perform daily PVD on a young child with cystic fibrosis.

TECHNIQUE 38–1 ■ Administering Oxygen by Cannula

Check agency policies and procedures about the initiation of home oxygen therapy for the patient:

1. The patient is carefully assessed and selected for this form of therapy, since it is expensive and entails some risk.

2. The physician is responsible for ordering the oxygen therapy and for explaining to the patient the reason for initiating it. The order should specify the flow rate (eg, 2 L/min) and the circumstances under which oxygen is to be used (eg, p.r.n. for shortness of breath and with exercise).

3. Generally the hospital staff provides specific instructions to the patient before discharge, including how to set the correct liter flow, change tanks, fill a portable system, and maintain the equipment.

4. The home oxygen supplier repeats these instructions when the oxygen is delivered to the patient's home.

5. Monthly or more frequent home visits are provided by the oxygen supplier or by home care staff members specially trained in respiratory techniques, to review and reinforce the instructions. Emphasis is placed on return demonstrations from the patient or caregiver to ensure that requisite skills are achieved.

Ensure that the most appropriate type of oxygen delivery system is selected for the patient. Three major oxygen systems are currently available in most communities: cylinders or tanks of compressed gas, liquid (cryogenic) oxygen, and oxygen concentrators.

1. *Cylinders.* These are the system of choice for patients who need oxygen episodically, eg, on a p.r.n. basis. Advantages are that cylinders deliver all liter flows (1 to 15 L/min), and oxygen evaporation does not occur during storage. Two or more cylinders can be manifolded together and stored in the home. Disadvantages are that the 150-pound cylinders are large and awkward to move (smaller portable cylinders are available, however), the supply company must be notified when a refill is needed, and they are costly for the high-use patient. A typical COPD patient consumes 10 to 20 cylinders per month, costing generally $250 to $450 per month for continuous therapy, depending on the locality (Gessner, 1978, p 29).

2. *Liquid oxygen.* Liquid oxygen reservoirs store liquid oxygen at minus 212 °C (minus 350 °F) in a smaller amount of space than compressed gas. The oxygen is vaporized by adding heat from the surroundings. Advantages are that these reservoirs are lighter in weight and cleaner in appearance than cylinders, they are not as difficult to operate, and they are equipped with a walker accessory resembling a Thermos bottle that can be easily filled from the stationary reservoir. The portable unit is beneficial for the patient with COPD who needs continuous oxygen therapy but also needs rehabilitative activities, such as mild exercise, to resume a more normal life-style. Disadvantages of liquid oxygen are that many home care medical supply and service companies are not able to handle it, oxygen evaporation occurs when the unit is not used, only low flows (1 to 4 L/min) can be used or freezing occurs, and the portable unit designed to be carried over the shoulder weighs ten pounds, a burden to the typically weak and emaciated COPD patient. Although wheeled carts are

available from the oxygen manufacturers, the cost factor is significant, since Medicare in the United States does not reimburse the patient for them. A luggage cart or folding grocery cart is a less expensive alternative.

3. *Oxygen concentrators.* Concentrators are electrically powered systems that manufacture oxygen from room air. At 1 L/min, such a system can deliver a concentration of about 95% oxygen, but the concentration drops when the flow rate increases (eg, 75% concentration at 4 L/min). Many models of oxygen concentrators are manufactured. Advantages are that they are more attractive in appearance, resembling furniture rather than medical equipment; they eliminate the need for regular delivery of oxygen or refilling of cylinders; because the supply of oxygen is constant, they alleviate the patient's anxiety about running out of oxygen; they are the most economical system when continuous use is required; and the patient's automobile can be equipped with a special alternator to allow the concentrator to operate from the car battery. The cost of the alternator and its installation is high, however (eg, $900), too expensive for most people. Major disadvantages of a concentrator are that it lacks portability (the smallest unit weighs 45 pounds); it tends to be noisy; it is powered by electricity, and, where the cost of electricity is high, the additional monthly cost can be substantial; an emergency backup unit (eg, an oxygen tank) must be provided for patients for whom a power failure could be life-threatening; and heat produced by the concentrator motor is a problem for those who live in trailers, small houses, or warm climates, where air conditioners are required. The oxygen concentrator must also be checked periodically with an O_2 analyzer to ensure that it is providing an adequate delivery of oxygen. This service is usually provided by the oxygen supplier on a contractual basis.

Another type of oxygen concentrator is the *oxygen enricher.* It uses a plastic membrane that allows water vapor to pass through with the oxygen, thus eliminating the need for a humidifying device. It is also thought to filter out bacteria present in the air. The enricher provides an O_2 concentration of 40% at all flow rates, it tends to be quieter than the concentrator, there is less chance of combustion (since the gas is only 40% oxygen), it has only two moving parts (thus decreasing the risk of something going wrong), and a nebulizer can be operated off the enricher because of the high flow rate.

Ensure that the patient has appropriate help in choosing a reputable home oxygen vendor, since several companies offer home oxygen service. Services furnished should include (McDonald, 1983, p 902):

1. A 24-hour emergency service.
2. Trained personnel to make the initial delivery and instruct the patient in safe, appropriate use of the oxygen and maintenance of the equipment.
3. At least monthly follow-up visits to check the equipment and reinstruct the patient as necessary.
4. A system in which insurance billing is done by the vendor for the patient.
5. A regular cost review to assure that the system is the most cost-effective one for that patient, with routine notification of the physician or home care professional if it seems that another system is more appropriate.

Ensure that the patient knows about the financial reimbursements available from Medicare and Medicaid or other insurance agencies. In the United States, Medicare generally covers 80% of allowable costs, and the patient is expected to pay the remaining 20% of the oxygen costs (McDonald, 1983, p 903). Patients who have supplementary insurance such as Blue Cross may be reimbursed for the additional 20% through this source. Medicaid usually covers 100% of the allowable cost but coverage varies from state to state. Reimbursement from private insurance companies varies, but usually 80% of the cost is covered. Variations exist in reimbursement for home oxygen systems, so specific coverage needs to be checked. For example, Medicare will not reimburse the patient for a wheeled cart for a portable unit with liquid oxygen, a backup device for concentrators/enrichers, the routine servicing of an oxygen concentrator, or the provision of two systems in any one home; Medicaid will pay 100% of the cost of the wheeled cart for portable liquid oxygen; and private insurance companies will pay 80% of the cost. In Canada's system of socialized health care, the cost of home oxygen therapy is fully covered.

TECHNIQUES 40–1 to 40–5 ■ Tracheostomy Care

Teach patients and/or caregivers the following (Jordan, 1979, pp 14–15):

1. The function of each tracheostomy tube part.
2. What supplies and equipment are needed, and the names of drugstores and medical supply houses where they might be obtained. A checklist can be provided to help the patient keep track of supplies that must be replaced.
3. The importance of washing hands especially before handling the tracheostomy. Small alcohol-saturated towels can be used to clean the hands if the patient's physical activity is limited.
4. How to take out the inner cannula, soak it in peroxide, scrub it with a brush, soak it in saline, and insert it into the outer cannula. Cleaning of the inner cannula two or three times a day is recommended.
5. How to clean the tracheostomy site on the neck and apply antiseptic ointment to prevent infection.
6. How to suction their secretions if they experience difficulty coughing secretions up.
7. To observe the secretions for signs of infection, such as a change in color.
8. How to make saline solution by boiling water and adding salt, and how to put saline into the tube to stimulate coughing and to thin the secretions.
9. To use plain paper cups for suctioning rather than a sterile basin. Taking out the bottom cup each time and sealing the box again keeps the cups acceptably clean and dry.
10. To wash suction catheters in soapy water, rinse them, and soak and disinfect them in a vinegar-water solution. It is not necessary to boil and sterilize catheters to eliminate the patient's own bacteria, which are already present on the skin.
11. To avoid contact with people who have colds and to keep the home from becoming too dry or dusty. Patients should use a vaporizer if the air is dry and wear something, eg, a light scarf, over the tube if the air is dusty.
12. Reconditioning exercises to maintain muscle tone of the chest, shoulder, and neck muscles and to prevent tightening or spasm from the increased work of breathing. Examples

include: rotating the head, shrugging the shoulders, swinging the arms, and lifting the arms up when inhaling while pulling them down when exhaling.

References

Aradine CE: Home care for young children with long-term tracheostomies. *Maternal Child Nurs* (March/April) 1980; 5:121–125.

Banaszak EF et al: Home ventilator care. *Respir Care* (December) 1982; 26:1262–1268.

Baptista RJ: Home TPN: Patient identification, formula generation, teaching methods and home vendor selection. *Nutr Support Serv* (February) 1984; 4:71, 74–75.

Bayer LM, Scholl DE, Ford EG: Tube feeding at home. *Am J Nurs* (September) 1983; 83:1321–1325.

Bean S: Home health care tips and timesavers for better patient care: Easier postural drainage. *Nurs Life* (March/April) 1984; 4:63.

Bergers RM, Martin J, Streckfuss BL: A home I.V. antibiotic program. *J Natl IV Ther Assoc* (May/June) 1985; 8:238–239.

Binkley LS: Keeping up with peritoneal dialysis. *Nursing 84* (June) 1984; 14:729–733.

Blagg CR: Problems and solutions for home dialysis in the 1980's. *J Am Assoc Nephrol Nurses Technicians* (February) 1982; 9:9–12.

Boles B: Home health care tips and timesavers for better patient care: Shoebox organizer. *Nurs Life* (March/April) 1984; 4:62.

Boos ML: A program of home traction for congenital dislocation of the hip. *Orthop Nurs* (March/April) 1982; 1:11–16.

Castaldo P: Respiratory home care from the DME point of view . . . durable medical equipment (DME). *Home Health Care Nurse* (March/April) 1985; 3:32–35.

Centers for Disease Control: Guidelines for prevention of intravascular infections. *Infect Control* 1982; 3:61–72.

Chalikian J, Weaver T: Mechanical ventilation: Where it's at. Where it's going. *Am J Nurs* (November) 1984; 84:1373–1379.

Chambers JK: Assessing the dialysis patient at home. *Am J Nurs* (April) 1981:750–754.

Chrystal C: Making the NITA standards work for you . . . home I.V. antibiotic therapy. *J Natl IV Ther Assoc* (September/October) 1985; 8:363–364.

Daeffler RJ, Lewinski J: Home care of the Hickman/Broviac catheter. *Oncol Nurs Forum* (Fall) 1982; 9:59–60.

Daeffler RJ, Lewinski J: Learning to care for your Hickman/Broviac catheter. *Oncol Nurs Forum* (Fall) 1982; 9:61–63.

Decker K: Home parenteral nutrition: Evaluating community services. *Nutr Support Serv* (April) 1984; 4:14–16.

DeMoss CJ: Giving intravenous chemotherapy at home. *Am J Nurs* (December) 1980; 80:2188–2189.

Denniston DJ, Burns KT: Home peritoneal dialysis. *Am J Nurs* (November) 1980; 80:2022–2026.

Dolan MB: If your patient wants to die at home. *Nursing 83* (April) 1983; 13:50–55.

Emery A: Home health care tips and timesavers for better patient care: A trace of fun. *Nurs Life* (March/April) 1984; 4:63.

Feldman J, Tuteur PG: Mechanical ventilation: From hospital intensive care to home. *Heart Lung* (March/April) 1982; 11:162–165.

Fitzgerald BP: TPN: The only road home. *Nursing 82* (September) 1982; 12:44–49.

Frasca C, Weimer M: Establishing a respiratory therapy program in the home: The South Hills program. *Home Health Care Nurse* (March/April) 1985; 3:8–12.

Gaston SF, Jones DR: IV antibiotics at home. *Am J IV Ther Clin Nutr* (February) 1982; 9:21–22.

Gessner DM: New developments in oxygen-therapy equipment for home use. *Respir Ther* (March/April) 1978; 8:29–31.

Gilmartin M, Make BJ: Home care of the ventilator-dependent person. *Respir Care* (November) 1983; 28:1490–1497.

Gilmartin M, Make BJ: Mechanical ventilation in the home. *Curr Rev Respir Ther* 1985; 18(7):139–144.

Glover DW: Going home on an MA-1. *Respir Ther* (January/February) 1978; 8:24–25.

Grant JP et al: A home total parenteral nutrition monitoring system. *Nutr Support Serv* (March) 1985; 5:16–18.

Gross S, Algrim C: Teaching young patients . . . and their families . . . about home peritoneal dialysis. *Nursing 80* (December) 1980; 10:72–73 (Canadian ed. pp 28–29).

Guzman VM, Atcherson E, Roy C: Training for peritoneal self-care options: CAPD, IPD, CCPD. *J Am Assoc Nephrol Nurses Technicians* (August) 1983; 10:33–37.

Hartsell MB et al: Selecting equipment vendors for children on home care. *Maternal Child Nurs* (January/February) 1985; 10:26–28.

Haworth RJ, Nichols PJR: Hoists in the home: Their recommendations and use. *Rheumatol Rehabil* (February) 1980; 19:42–51.

Health and Welfare, Canada: *Help Yourself! Hints from the Handicapped.* Catalog No. H21–95/1984 E., Minister of Supply and Services Canada, 1984.

Holloway VM: Documentation: One of the ultimate challenges in home health care. *Home Health Care Nurse* (January/February) 1984; 2:19, 22.

Home health care: Tips and timesavers for better patient care. *Nurs Life* (March/April) 1984; 4:62–63.

Jenkins EH: Homemakers: The care of home health care. *Geriatr Nurs* (January/February) 1984; 5:28–30.

Jordan DA: Standardizing respiratory care in the home. *Respir Ther* (November/December) 1979; 9:13–16.

Kennedy AH, Johnson WG, Sturdevant EW: An educational program for families of children with tracheostomies. *Maternal Child Nurs* (January/February) 1982; 7:42–49.

Koithan M: Home total parenteral nutrition: Complications. *J Natl IV Ther Assoc* (May/June) 1985; 8:231–237.

Larkin M: Home intravenous care. *J Natl IV Ther Assoc* (January/February) 1984; 7:10–11.

Lemieux GG: Choices: Moral and ethical issues involved with life-support equipment when used in the home . . . personal experience. *Home Health Care Nurse* (January/February) 1984; 2:12–14.

Levine ER: Home therapy and new problems . . . respiratory therapy. *Respir Ther* (May/June) 1985; 15:13.

May C: Antibiotic therapy at home. *Am J Nurs* (March) 1984; 84:348–349.

McDonald GJ: Long-term oxygen therapy delivery systems . . . in the home setting. *Respir Care* (July) 1983; 28:898–905.

The National Intravenous Therapy Association's intravenous nursing standards of practice: Home I.V. therapy. *J Natl IV Ther Assoc* (March/April) 1984; 7:93.

Nursing Photobook Series: *Implementing Urologic Procedures.* Intermed Communications, 1981a.

Nursing Photobook Series: *Performing GI Procedures.* Intermed Communications, 1981b.

Paarlberg J, Balint JP: Gastrostomy tubes: Practical guidelines for home care. *Pediatr Nurs* (March/April) 1985; 11:99–102.

Parfitt DM, Thompson VD: Pediatric home hyperalimentation: Educating the family. *Maternal Child Nurs* (May/June) 1980; 5:196–202.

Pelletier GM: Responding to a need: Home intravenous therapy. *J Natl IV Ther Assoc* (November/December) 1982; 5:383–384.

Pressel P: Total parenteral nutrition: Physician and lifeliner . . . home TPN . . . Lifeline Foundation. *J Enterostomal Ther* (September/October) 1982; 9:27–29.

Quinless F: Teaching tips for T tube care at home. *Nursing 84* (May) 1984; 14:62–64.

Rathlev MC, McNamara MA: Teaching families to give trach care at home . . . a child going home with a tracheostomy. *Nursing 82* (June) 1982; 12:70–71.

Ray R, Samar D: Continuous ambulatory peritoneal dialysis nursing follow-up: How much time does it take? *J Am Assoc Nephrol Nurses Technicians* (June) 1981; 8:26–27.

Roberts C: Renal replacement therapy: Home dialysis, part 2. *Nurs Times* (May 5–11) 1982; 78:752–753.

Rodgers BL: Home parenteral nutrition: Principles and management. *Nurse Practit* (March) 1984; 9:42, 47–48.

Salcedo N: Home peritoneal dialysis: An option for the moribund diabetic patient. *Nephrol Nurse* (May/June) 1983; 5:26–28.

Sivak ED, Cordasco EM, Gipson WT: Pulmonary mechanical ventilation at home: A reasonable less expensive approach. *Respir Care* (January) 1983; 28:42–49.

Smith M: Nursing management of the leg ulcer in the community. *Nurs Times* (July 21–27) 1982; 78:1228–1232.

Stahl SM, Kelly CR, Weill PJ: Effects of home blood pressure measurement on long-term BP control. *Am J Pub Health* (July) 1984; 74:704–709.

Standards for respiratory therapy home care. *AARTimes* (November) 1983; 7:41–42.

Standards for respiratory therapy home care: An official statement by the American Association for Respiratory Therapy. *Respir Care* (November) 1979; 24:1080.

Steiger E: Overview of home parenteral nutrition. *Nutr Support Serv* (January) 1984; 4:8.

Thomson S, Lang K: The I.V. solution: A home care alternative. *J Natl IV Ther Assoc* (September/October) 1984; 7:397–400.

Useful aids for hospital and home nursing. *Nurs Times* (September 27) 1979; 75:1668.

Villalon D, Smith MN: At home with traction . . . Buck's traction at home. *Pediatr Nurs* (January/February) 1982; 8:15–16.

Vogal TC, Meskimming SA: Teaching parents to give indwelling CV catheter care . . . a child going home with an indwelling catheter. *Nursing 83* (January) 1983; 13:54–56.

Weimer MP: Home respiratory therapy for patients with chronic obstructive lung disease. *Respir Care* (November) 1983; 28:1484–1489.

Weinstein SM: The how-to's of home care . . . I.V. therapy. *J Natl IV Ther Assoc* (May/June) 1985; 8:227–230.

Weinstein SM: Intravenous therapy within the scope of home health services. *J Natl IV Ther Assoc* (January/February) 1984; 7:39–41.

Weinstein SM: Specialty teams in home care. *Am J Nurs* (March) 1984; 84:342–345.

Wellerstein J: Home care record systems and the medical record professional. *Med Rec News* (February) 1980; 51:44–46.

Yetka P: Home health care tips and timesavers for better patient care: Medication charts. *Nurs Life* (March/April) 1984; 4:63.

Ziegler JC: Physical conditioning—for the convalescent patient. *Nursing 80* (August) 1980; 10:67–69 (Can ed pp 21–30).

abdominal paracentesis removal of fluids from the peritoneal cavity

ablative surgery surgery to remove a diseased organ or other tissue

abrasion wearing away (erosion) of a structure such as the skin because of friction

accountable answerable

acne an inflammatory disease of the sebaceous glands

acromegaly a disorder caused by excessive growth hormone; characterized by excessive skeletal growth of the hands, feet, nose, jaw, and forehead

adherent sticking together, clinging

adipose fat; of a fatty nature

adventitious sounds sounds not normally heard over the lung fields

aeration the process by which the blood exchanges carbon dioxide for oxygen in the lungs

aerobe an organism that requires oxygen to live

affect the emotional state of a person as it appears to others

airway a passageway through which air normally circulates; a device that is inserted through the patient's mouth to maintain the patency of an air passage such as the trachea

albuminuria the presence of serum in the urine

algor mortis postmortem cooling

alopecia abnormal loss of hair

alveolus a saclike dilation or cavity in the body (plural: alveoli)

ammonia dermatitis diaper rash

ampule a small, sealed, glass flask containing a medication or solution

anaerobe an organism that does not require oxygen to live or requires the absence of oxygen

anal canal the distal portion of the rectum; it joins the rectum proximally and opens to the body surface distally

analgesic a medication used to relieve pain

anaphylaxis an acute allergic reaction

anemia a condition in which the blood is deficient in red blood cells or hemoglobin

anesthesia loss of sensation with or without loss of consciousness

anesthesiologist a physician specializing in the administration of anesthetics

anesthetic a substance that produces anesthesia

anesthetist a person, such as a nurse, who specializes in administering anesthetics

aneurysm localized dilation of the wall of an artery at a weak point in the vessel wall

angiography a diagnostic procedure enabling x-ray visual examination of the vascular system after injection of a radiopaque dye

angle of Louis the angle between the manubrium and the body of the sternum

ankylosis permanent fixation of a joint

annulus a ringlike structure, eg, around the tympanic membrane

anorexia lack of appetite

anoscopy visual examination of the anal canal using an anoscope (a lighted instrument)

anoxia the absence or a deficiency of oxygen in the tissues

antecubital fossa or space the point on the arm located in front of the elbow

anterior of, toward, or at the front

anterior chamber (of the eye) the area immediately behind the cornea and in front of the iris

anthelix the anterior curve on the upper aspect of the auricle of the ear

anthropometry a system of measurement of the size and makeup of the body and specific body parts

antiseptic an agent that inhibits the growth of some microorganisms on skin or tissue

anuria failure of the kidneys to produce urine, resulting in total lack of urination

anus the opening of the anal canal on the body surface

anxiety mental uneasiness

apnea cessation of breathing

appetite a pleasant sensation in which the person desires and anticipates food

appliance a device or bag that is secured to the abdomen to collect either urine or feces through an ostomy

approximate (wound edges) to bring close together

areola the darkened area surrounding the nipple of the breast

arrector pili muscle the erector muscle attached to the hair follicle

arrhythmia a pulse that has an abnormal rhythm

arteriosclerosis a condition in which the walls of the arteries become hardened and thickened

artery forceps *see* hemostat

ascites the accumulation of fluid in the abdominal cavity

asepsis the absence of disease-producing microorganisms

aspirate to remove gases or liquids from a cavity using suction; to inhale a substance

assault an attempt or threat to touch another person unjustifiably

assessment organized collection of data about a patient; the first step of the nursing process

astigmatism a visual refractive error due to differences in curvature of the cornea and the lens

ataxia impairment of position sense; failure of muscular coordination

atelectasis collapse of a lung or portion of it

athlete's foot a fungal infection of the foot

atrioventricular (AV) node the neuromuscular tissue of the heart at the base of the atrial septum that conveys impulses to the ventricles

atrophy a wasting away or decrease in the size of a cell, tissue, body organ, or muscle

auricle (pinna) the visible part of the ear

auscultation the process of listening to sounds produced within the body

autoclave an apparatus that sterilizes, using steam under pressure

autopsy (postmortem examination) the examination of a body after death

axilla the armpit

bactericide an agent capable of destroying some microorganisms

bacteriostatic agent an agent that prevents the growth and reproduction of some microorganisms

bandage a material used to wrap a body part

barium enema x-ray filming of the large intestine using a contrast medium; also called a *lower gastrointestinal series*

barium swallow   x-ray filming of the esophagus, stomach, and duodenum; also referred to as an *upper gastrointestinal series*

barrier (of the skin)   a protective covering for the skin, eg, a liquid, spray, or material such as karaya

barrier technique   *see* reverse protective asepsis

basal metabolic rate   the heat produced through the metabolism (burning) of food

basic human need   something required by human beings in order to maintain physiologic and psychologic homeostasis

Bass method   *see* sulcular technique

battery   the willful or negligent touching of a person (or the person's clothing or even something the person is carrying) without consent, which may or may not cause harm

Beau's line   a transverse white line or groove on the nail associated with an acute and severe illness

bed foundation   the mattress and the frame supporting the mattress

bedpan   a receptacle used to collect urine and feces

Bells palsy   paralysis of the seventh cranial (facial) nerve

bevel   a slanting edge; the slanted part at the tip of a needle

bill of rights   a summary of fundamental rights and privileges guaranteed to people

binder   a type of bandage applied to large body areas, eg, the abdomen or chest

biopsy   the removal and examination of tissue from the living body

biotransformation   the process of deactivating or detoxifying the biologically active chemicals in drugs to more easily excreted forms

bleb   a small, smooth, slightly raised area on the skin, usually filled with fluid; wheal

body mechanics   the efficient and coordinated use of the body during resting activities and movement

borborygmi   gurgling, splashing sounds heard over the large intestine

bradycardia   an abnormally slow heart rate below 60 beats per minute

bradypnea   abnormally slow respirations, usually fewer than 10 respirations per minute

bronchogram   an x-ray film of the bronchial tree taken after injection of

an iodized oil dye, used as a contrast medium

bronchoscopy   visual examination of the bronchi using a bronchoscope

bronchus   a large air passage of the lungs (plural: bronchi)

bruit   a blowing or swishing sound created by turbulent blood flow

bubbling   gurgling sounds as air passes through moist secretions in the respiratory tract

buccal mucosa   the mucous membrane lining the inner surface of the cheeks

bulbar conjunctiva   the mucous membrane over the eyeball

bunion   lateral deviation of the big toe with swelling or callus formation over the metatarsophalangeal joint

cachexia   a state of emaciation, weakness, and malnutrition

calipers   an instrument used to measure the thickness of folds of skin

callus   early bone, formed following fracture of a bone, that is normally ultimately replaced by hard bone; a thickened portion of the skin

cannula   a tube with a lumen (channel) that is inserted into a cavity or duct and is often fitted with a trocar during insertion

canthus   the angular junction of the eyelids at each corner of the eyes

Cantor tube   a single-lumen tube inserted through the mouth into the intestines

cardiac arrest   the cessation of heart function

cardiac board   a flat board placed under a patient's chest when the patient requires cardiac massage while in bed

cardiac output   the amount of blood ejected by the heart with each ventricular contraction

cardiopulmonary resuscitation (CPR)   artificial stimulation of the heart and lungs

carminative   an agent that assists in the passage of flatus from the colon

carotid arteries   major arteries lying on either side of the trachea and larynx

carotid sinus   a dilated portion of the internal carotid artery that contains pressoreceptors that are stimulated by changes in blood pressure

carrier   a mechanism used in traction attached to the rope and upon which weights are placed: a person who carries pathogens but is not ill

caruncle (of the eye)   the red fleshy eminence at the inner canthus of the eye

cast   a stiff cylindrical dressing or casing made of bandages impregnated with hardening material; used to immobilize various parts of the body

caster   a small wheel, often made of rubber or plastic, that permits furniture, such as a bed, to be moved easily

CAT scan   *see* tomography

cataract   an opacity of the lens of the eye

catheter   a tube of plastic, rubber, metal, or other material, used to remove or instill fluids into a cavity such as the bladder

caudal anesthetic   an anesthetic injected into the caudal canal, below the spinal cord

cecum   the dilated pouch that constitutes the first part of the large intestine adjoining the small intestine

cellular fluid   *see* intracellular fluid

Celsius   *see* centigrade

cementum   calcified tissue covering the root of a tooth

center of gravity   the point at which the mass (weight) of the body is centered

centigrade (Celsius)   a thermometer scale used to measure heat; the freezing point of water is 0 °C and the boiling point is 100 °C

central venous line   a catheter inserted into a large vein located centrally in the body, eg, the superior vena cava

central venous pressure (CVP)   a measurement of the pressure of the blood, in centimeters of water, within the vena cava or right atrium of the heart

cerumen   the waxlike substance secreted by glands in the external ear canal

cervix   the lower end of the uterus, which projects into the vagina

Cheyne-Stokes respirations   rhythmic waxing and waning of respirations, from very deep to very shallow, with periods of apnea

cholecystogram (oral cholecystography)   an x-ray film of the gallbladder after the ingestion of a contrast dye

chyme   semifluid material produced by the digestion of food in the stomach; it is found in the small and large intestines

cicatricial tissue   *see* scar tissue

cicatrix   a scar

cilia hairlike projections of the mucous membrane of the respiratory tract

circumference the outer measurement of a rounded body

cisterna a space that is enclosed and serves as a reservoir for body fluid

cisternal puncture insertion of a needle into the subarachnoid space of the cisterna magna

clean free of pathogenic organisms

client a person who seeks help but is neither ill nor injured

closed bed an unoccupied bed with the top covers drawn up to the top of the bed under the pillows

clubbing (of a nail) elevation of the proximal aspect of the nail and softening of the nail bed due to a long-term lack of oxygen

coagulate to clot

cochlea a seashell-shaped structure located in the inner ear; it has numerous apertures for passage of the cochlear division of the auditory nerve

cohesive sticking together

colic paroxysmal cramplike intestinal pain

colitis inflammation of the colon

collagen a gluelike protein found in connective tissue; it is secreted by fibroblasts in granulation tissue, and it forms scar tissue

colon that part of the large intestine that extends from the cecum to the rectum; sometimes used interchangeably with large intestine

colonoscopy visual examination of the interior of the colon with a colonoscope

colostomy a surgically created opening of the colon on the abdomen

colostrum a yellow, milky fluid secreted by the mother's mammary glands a few days before or after childbirth

comedo a blackhead

computerized axial tomography *see* tomography

condom a rubber or plastic sheathlike device applied externally to the penis that can be used to catch urine and direct it to a drainage bag

conduction the transfer of heat from a warm object to a cooler object, or vice versa, by contact

conjunctiva the membrane covering the eyelids and eyeball

conjunctivitis inflammation of the membrane covering the eyelids and eyeball

consent permission given voluntarily by a person in his or her right mind; informed consent implies that the individual is knowledgeable about the consent and understands it

constipation defecation of small, dry, hard stools or passage of no stool for an abnormal period of time

constructive surgery surgery to repair a malformed organ or tissue

contaminated possessing pathogenic organisms

contour position a position with the head and foot sections of the bed elevated, creating a break of about 15°

contract a written or verbal agreement between two or more people to do or not do some lawful act

contraction the normal, active shortening or tensing of a muscle

contracture permanent shortening of a muscle and subsequent shortening of tendons and ligaments

contusion a bruise; an injury to soft tissue produced by a blunt force

convection transfer of heat by movement of a liquid or gas, eg, air currents

convergence a moving together toward a common point

corn a conical, circular, painful, raised area on the toe or foot

cornea a transparent convex avascular structure forming the anterior surface of the eyeball

coroner a public official who is responsible for investigating any deaths that appear to be unnatural

cough a sudden expulsion of air from the lungs

countertraction a force that counteracts the direct pull of traction

cradle cap a yellowish, oily crusting of the scalp of infants

creps (crepitation) a dry, crackling sound like that of crumpled cellophane, produced by air moving through fluid in the alveoli or by air in the subcutaneous tissue

crime an act committed in violation of societal law

crown (of a tooth) the exposed part of a tooth outside the gum

crutch palsy weakness of the hand, wrist, and forearm induced by prolonged pressure of a crutch on the axillary nerves

culture (of cells) the cultivation of microorganisms or cells in a special growth medium

Cushing's syndrome increased production of adrenal hormones

cuticle the flat, thin rim of skin surrounding the nail

cyanosis a bluish coloring of the mucous membranes, nail beds, or skin due to excessive deoxygenation of hemoglobin

cystectomy removal of the bladder

cystocele protrusion of the urinary bladder through the vaginal wall

cystoscopy visual examination of the urinary bladder with a cystoscope

cytology the study of the origin, structure, function, and pathology of cells

dacryocystitis inflammation of the lacrimal sac

Dakin's solution a buffered aqueous solution of sodium hypochlorite used as a bactericide; named after Henry Drysdale Dakin, a New York chemist

dandruff a dry or greasy scaly material shed from the scalp

data base all information known about a patient; it includes the physician's history and physical examination, the nurse's assessment and history, and material contributed by other members of the health team

debridement cleaning of an injured area to remove foreign debris or excessive exudate

deceased dead; a person who is dead

deciduous teeth temporary teeth that are shed

decubitus ulcer a pressure sore or bedsore

deep breathing inhaling the maximum amount of air possible, then exhaling

defamation a communication that is false, or made with careless disregard for the truth, and results in injury to the reputation of a person

defecation the expulsion of feces from the anus

defervescence the stage of abatement of a fever

dehiscence gaping, splitting, or separating of wound edges

dehydration insufficient fluid in the body

delusion a false belief

dental caries tooth decay

dental crown the exposed part of the tooth, covered by enamel

dental plaque deposits on the teeth that serve as a medium for bacterial growth

dental pulp cavity a space in the center of the tooth containing blood vessels and nerves

dental root the part of the tooth that is imbedded in the jaw

dentifrice a paste or powder used to clean or polish the teeth

dentin the chief substance of teeth, forming the body, neck, and roots; it is covered by enamel

dentures a natural or artificial set of teeth; usually the term designates artificial teeth

dependent edema edema of the lowest or most dependent parts of the body

dependent nursing action action carried out by a nurse as a result of a physician's order

depolarize (cardiac muscle) to reduce toward a nonpolarized state; to cause loss of charge

dermatologic relating to the skin

dermis (corium) true skin, containing blood vessels, nerves, hair follicles, and glands

diagnostic surgery surgery performed to confirm a diagnosis

dialysate the water-based solution instilled into the peritoneal cavity during peritoneal dialysis; it contains glucose and normal serum electrolytes

diaphoresis profuse perspiration

diaphragm a dome-shaped muscle between the lungs and the abdomen

diarrhea defecation of liquid feces and increased frequency of defecation

diastasis rectus abdominis separation of the rectus abdominis muscles, often as a result of pregnancy or obesity

diastole the period when the ventricles of the heart are relaxed

diastolic pressure the pressure of the blood against the arterial walls when the ventricles of the heart are at rest

disinfectant an agent that inhibits the growth or reproduction of microorganisms on inanimate environmental surfaces

distal farthest from the point of reference

distention (tympanites) excessive flatus in the intestines or peritoneal cavity

diuresis *see* polyuria

diuretic an agent that increases the production of urine

dorsal of, toward, or at the back

dorsal flexion movement of the ankle so that the toes are pointing up

drain a substance or appliance that assists in the discharge of drainage from a wound

drainage a discharge from a wound or cavity

drawsheet (half sheet) a special sheet, made of cotton, plastic, or rubber, that is placed across the center of the foundation of a bed

dullness a thudlike percussion sound produced from underlying dense tissue

duration (of a sound) the length of a sound heard during auscultation and percussion

dyspnea difficult and labored breathing in which the patient has a persistent unsatisfied need for air and feels distressed

dysuria painful urination

ecchymosis a blotchy area or discoloration of the skin larger than 1 cm in diameter; caused by bleeding into the tissues; a bruise

ectropion eversion; outward turning of the eyelid

edema excess interstitial fluid

effluent urine or feces discharged through a stoma

egocentricity concern about oneself

elective surgery surgery performed for a person's wellbeing but not absolutely necessary for life

electrocardiogram (ECG, EKG) a graph of the electric activity of the heart

electrocardiograph a machine that measures and records the impulses from the heart on an electrocardiogram

electroencephalogram (EEG) a graph of the electric activity of the brain

electroencephalograph a machine that measures and records impulses from the brain on an electroencephalogram

electrolyte (ion) a chemical substance that develops an electric charge and conducts an electric current when placed in water

electromyogram (EMG) a record of the electric potential created by the contraction of a muscle

electromyograph a machine that measures and records impulses from the muscles on an electromyogram

embalming a process of preserving a body chemically

embolus a blood clot (or other substance, such as air) that has moved from its place of origin and is obstructing the circulation in a blood vessel (plural: emboli)

emmetropia normal refraction, in which the eyes focus objects on the retina

emphysema a chronic obstructive lung disorder in which the terminal bronchioles become distended and plugged with mucus

emulsion a liquid that contains another liquid with which it will not mix and in which it will not dissolve

enamel (of a tooth) the covering over the crown of the tooth

endoscope an instrument used for examining the interior of a hollow organ, eg, the bladder, rectum, stomach, or bronchi

endosteum the lining membrane of a hollow bone

endotrachial tube a tube inserted through the mouth and terminating in the trachea

enema a solution that is injected into the rectum and the sigmoid colon

enteric referring to the gastrointestinal system or the organisms that inhabit the system

enterocele any herbia of the intestine through the intact vaginal mucosa

enterostomal therapy (ET) nurse a person who specializes in ostomy care

enterostomy an opening through the abdominal wall into the intestines

entropion inversion; inward turning of the eyelid

enuresis involuntary urination, particularly at night, after the age of 4 years; bedwetting

environmental stimulus anything in the environment that arouses or incites action by a receptor (the terminus of a sensory nerve)

epidermis the outermost, nonvascular layer of skin

epidural block injection of an anesthetic through a lumbar interspace into the spinal canal (external to the dura mater)

epithelial cells cells that cover the surface of the body and line its cavities

epithelialization the formation of skin over a wound

eructation ejection of gas from the stomach through the mouth; (belching)

erythema redness that is associated with a variety of rashes

eschar a slough produced by burning, by a corrosive application, or by death of tissue associated with loss of vascular supply, bacterial invasion, and putrefaction

esophagoscopy visual examination of the interior of the esophagus with a lighted instrument

esophagus the muscular tube that extends from the pharynx to the stomach

ethics the rules or principles that govern right conduct

etiology cause

eupnea normal, quiet breathing

eustachian tube a channel lined with mucous membrane that connects the middle ear and the nasopharynx; it acts as an air pressure stabilizer

evacuator an instrument for removing fluid or small particles from a body cavity

evaporation conversion of a liquid or solid into a vapor

evisceration extrusion of the internal organs

excise to cut off or out

excoriation the loss of the superficial layers of the skin

excretion a waste product produced by the body cells

excursion movement of a part in the performance of a function

exhalation (expiration) the outflow of air from the lungs to the atmosphere

exophthalmus protrusion of the eyeballs with elevation of the upper lids; a staring, startled expression

expectorate to spit out mucus or other materials

expired dead

exploratory surgery surgery performed to confirm the extent of a pathologic process and sometimes to confirm a diagnosis

external auditory meatus the entrance to the ear canal

extinction failure to perceive touch on one side of the body when two symmetric areas are touched simultaneously

extracellular fluid (ECF) fluid found outside the body cells

exudate material, eg, fluid and cells, that has escaped from blood vessels and is deposited in tissues or on tissue surfaces during the inflammatory process

Fahrenheit a thermometer scale used to measure heat; the freezing point of water is 32 °F and the boiling point is 212 °F

fasciculation abnormal contraction of a bundle of muscle fibers

febrile pertaining to a fever; feverish

fecal impaction a mass of hardened feces in the folds of the rectum

fecal incontinence inability to control the passage of feces through the anus

feces the body wastes and undigested food eliminated from the rectum

fenestrated drape a drape with an opening in its center

fibrin an insoluble protein formed from fibrinogen during the clotting of blood; it is produced by fibroblasts during healing

fibrinogen a protein in blood plasma

that by the action of thrombin is converted into fibrin

fibroblast an immature fiber-producing cell

fibrous tissue common connective tissue composed of elastic and collagen fibers

fissure a cleft or groove; cracklike

fistula an abnormal passage between two organs or between an organ and the body surface

flaccid paralysis impaired muscle function with loss of muscle tone

flail chest the ballooning out of the chest wall through injured rib spaces during exhalation and depression or indrawing of the wall during inhalation

flatness (of a sound) an extremely dull sound heard on percussion from very dense tissue

flatulence the presence of excessive amounts of gas in the stomach or intestines

flatus gas or air normally present in the stomach or intestines

flow sheet a record used to record the progress of specific or specialized data such as the vital signs, the fluid balance, or routine medications

fomite an inanimate object that can harbor pathogenic microorganisms

foot drop plantar flexion of the foot with permanent contracture of the gastrocnemius (calf) muscle and tendon

footplate a device that provides both support for a foot and a place to attach the rope of a traction apparatus

forensic medicine (legal medicine) the application of medical knowledge to the law

foreskin a covering fold of skin over the glans of the penis

fovea centralis a tiny pit in the center of the macula of the eye

Fowler's position a bed sitting position with the head of the bed raised to 45°

fracture a break in the continuity of bone

fremitus (tactile, vocal) the vibration felt through the chest wall when a person speaks

frenulum a midline fold connecting the undersurface of the tongue to the floor of the mouth

frequency voiding at frequent intervals

friction rub *see* pleural rub

fundus the larger part, base, or body of a hollow organ

fundus (of the eye) the back portion

of the interior of the eyeball, visible only through an ophthalmoscope

gait the way a person walks

gastric pertaining to the stomach

gastrocolic reflex increased peristalsis of the colon after food has entered the stomach

gastroscopy visual examination of the stomach with a lighted instrument (gastroscope)

Gatch bed a bed fitted with movable joints beneath the hips and knees of the patient

gauge the diameter of the shaft of a needle

gavage administration of nourishment to the stomach through a nasogastric or orogastric tube; tube feeding

gelatinous like jelly

genitals the reproductive organs, usually the external ones

genupectoral (knee–chest) position a position in which the weight is borne by the patient's knees and chest and the body is at a 90° angle to the hips

germicidal possessing the ability to kill microorganisms

germicide an agent that kills some pathogens

gingiva the gum

gingivitis acute or chronic inflammation of the gums

glaucoma an eye disease characterized by increased intraocular pressure, which causes damage to the retina and optic nerve and blindness if left untreated

glossitis inflammation of the tongue

glycosuria abnormally high amounts of glucose in the urine

goal (objective) a hoped-for outcome

goiter an enlargement of the thyroid gland, causing a swelling in the front part of the neck

granulation tissue young connective tissue with new capillaries that is formed extensively in wounds that heal by secondary intention

graphesthesia the act of recognizing a number or letter when it is drawn on the palm of the hand

gravity the force that pulls objects toward the earth

grief a subjective emotional response of intense sadness; a normal response to loss

habitus the body build or body type; it can vary from the slender, wiry body to the heavy, soft body

hair follicle a pouchlike depression in the skin enclosing the root of a hair

hair shaft   the visible part of the hair

halitosis   an unpleasant odor of the breath

hallucination   a distortion of sensory perceptions; hearing voices or seeing things that do not exist

hallux valgus (bunion)   lateral deviation of the big toe with swelling or callus formation over the metatarsophalangeal joint

hammer toe   a flexed proximal toe joint and hyperextended distal toe joint

hangnail   a shred of epidermal tissue at either side of the nail

Harris tube   a single-lumen tube with a metal tip that is inserted through the mouth into the intestines

haustrum   a saclike formation of a part of the colon produced by contraction of the longitudinal and circular muscles (plural: haustra)

height   a vertical measurement extending from the highest point of the head to the surface on which the individual is standing, normally measured in centimeters or inches

helix   the posterior curve on the upper aspect of the auricle of the ear

hemangioma   a large, persistent, bright red or dark purple vascular area of the skin

hematocrit   the percentage of red blood cell mass in proportion to whole blood

hematoma   a collection of blood in a tissue, organ, or body space due to a break in the wall of a blood vessel

hematuria   blood in the urine

hemoglobin   the red pigment in red blood cells, which carries oxygen

hemopneumothorax   a collection of blood and air or gas in the pleural cavity

hemoptysis   the presence of blood in the sputum

hemorrhage   the escape of blood from the blood vessels; bleeding internally or externally

hemorrhoids   distended veins in the rectum

hemostasis   arrest of the escape of blood either by natural (clot formation) or artificial (compression or ligation) means

hemostat (artery forceps)   a small pair of forceps used to constrict blood vessels

hemothorax   a collection of blood in the pleural cavity

heparin   a substance that prevents the coagulation of blood

heparin flush   irrigation of a central venous line using a saline solution containing heparin

heparin lock   the airtight cap covering the end of a patient's intravenous or central venous tubing

hirsutism   abnormal hairiness

histology   the study of the structure and function of tissues

homeostasis   the tendency of the body to maintain a state of balance while continually changing

hordeolum (sty)   an inflammation of one or more sebaceous glands of the eyelid

humidity   the amount of moisture in the air

hydration   the act of combining with water

hydrocephalus   abnormal accumulation of fluid within the ventricular system of the brain; head enlargement

hymen   a thin fold of mucous membrane separating the vagina from the vestibule

hyperalimentation   *see* total parenteral nutrition

hypercarbia (hypercapnia)   excess carbon dioxide in the blood

hyperemia   increased blood flow resulting in redness of the skin

hyperextension position   a position with the head and foot sections of the bed lowered to form a 15° angle in the bed foundation

hyperopia   farsightedness; abnormal refraction in which light rays focus behind the retina

hyperpyrexia   an extremely elevated body temperature

hyperresonance   a booming sound not normally produced by percussion, eg, from emphysematous lung tissue

hypertension   an abnormally high blood pressure

hypertonic   possessing a greater osmotic pressure than another fluid, eg, blood; increased tension, eg, of a muscle

hypertrophy   an increase in the size of a cell, tissue, or body organ such as a muscle

hyperventilation   an increase in the amount of air in the lungs, usually brought about by prolonged and deep breaths; an increased ventilation compared to the amount of carbon dioxide produced by metabolism

hypocarbia (hypocapnia)   reduced carbon dioxide in the blood

hypodermic   *see* subcutaneous

hypodermis   connective tissue beneath the skin; also referred to as *subcutaneous tissue*

hypoesthesia   abnormally decreased sensitivity to stimulation

hypotension   an abnormally low blood pressure

hypothermia   an abnormally low body temperature

hypotonia   diminished tone of skeletal muscles

hypotonic   possessing a lesser osmotic pressure than another fluid, eg, blood; decreased tension, eg, of a muscle

hypoventilation   a reduction in the amount of air in the lungs, usually brought about by shallow respirations; a decreased expulsion of carbon dioxide in relation to the amount produced by metabolism

hypovolemic shock   a state of shock due to a markedly reduced volume of circulating blood and the sudden redirection of the blood flow

hypoxemia   deficient oxygenation of the blood as measured by laboratory tests

hypoxia   diminished availability of oxygen for body tissues, due to internal or external causes

ileocecal valve   membranous folds between the distal ileum and the cecum (entrance to the large intestine)

ileostomy   a surgically created opening of the small intestine on the abdomen

ileum   small intestine

incision   a cut or wound that is intentionally made, eg, during surgery

incompatibility (of medications)   an undesired chemical or physical reaction between a drug and an infusion solution, between two or more drugs, or between a drug and the container or tubing

incontinence   inability to retain urine (urinary incontinence) or feces (anal incontinence)

incus   an anvil-shaped ossicle of the middle ear; it communicates sound waves from the malleus to the stapes

independent nursing action   action carried out by a nurse as a result of the nurse's judgment

infection   the disease process produced by microorganisms or the toxins they produce

inferior   situated below

infiltration   the diffusion or accumulation of substances in tissues or cells

infusion   the introduction of fluid into a vein or other part of the body

infusion controller a device used with intravenous infusions to obtain the desired infusion rate; it regulates gravitational flow by counting drops per minute and compressing the IV tubing

infusion pump a device used with intravenous infusions to obtain the desired infusion rate; it delivers a measured amount of solution at a constant high pressure

ingrown toenail (incurvated nail) penetration of the edges of the nail plate into the surrounding tissues

inhalation (inspiration) the act of breathing in

injection point a site on tubing for the insertion of a needle

inner canthus the corner of the upper and lower eyelids near the nose

inquest a legal enquiry into the cause or manner of a death

inspection (observation) assessment that uses the sense of sight; visual examination

instillation insertion of medication into a body cavity

insufflator an instrument used to blow air into a part of the body, eg, the rectum

insulin a hormone normally formed by the islands of Langerhans in the pancreas; also a preparation for administration

intensity (of a sound) the loudness or softness of a sound as heard during auscultation and percussion

intercostal retractions indrawing between the ribs

interdependent nursing action action carried out by a nurse in association with other health professionals

interstitial fluid fluid found between the body cells

intervertebral between the vertebrae

intracellular fluid (ICF) fluid found within the body cells (cellular fluid)

intradermal within the skin (intracutaneous)

intramuscular within or inside muscle tissue

intrapleural within the pleural cavity

intravascular within a blood vessel

intravenous within a vein

intravenous cholangiogram an x-ray film of the bile ducts after intravenous injection of a contrast dye

intravenous hyperalimentation (IVH) see total parenteral nutrition

intravenous pyelogram an x-ray film of the kidney taken after intravenous injection of a radiopaque dye

intravenous pyelography (IVP) or **intravenous urography (IVU)** x-ray filming of the kidney and ureters after intravenous injection of a radiopaque material

intubation insertion of a tube

iris the colored part of the eye perforated by the pupil

iritis inflammation of the iris

irrigation the washing of a body cavity by a stream of water or other fluid

ischemia deficiency of blood in a part due to constriction or obstruction of a blood vessel

isometric muscle contraction tensing of the muscle against an immovable outer resistance, which does not change muscle length or produce joint motion

isotonic muscle contraction shortening of a muscle in the process of doing work (eg, range-of-motion exercises, weight lifting), which produces joint motion

jaundice a yellowish tinge to the skin and mucous membrane

jejenum the portion of the small intestine that extends from the duodenum to the ileum

Kardex a portable card index file that organizes data about a patient in a concise way and often contains a nursing care plan

keloid a rounded, hard, shiny, white or pink scarlike growth that rises above the skin surface

keratin the type of protein found in epidermis, hair, and nails

keratotic spots horny growths, such as warts or calluses

knotted (referring to veins) knoblike

kyphosis an exaggerated convexity in the thoracic region of the vertebral column

labia the fleshy edges of a structure, usually the female genitals

laceration a tear, rather than a cut, of body tissue

lacrimal canal a passageway from the innermost corner of the eye to the lacrimal sac

lacrimal duct a small passageway from the lacrimal gland draining the tears onto the conjunctiva at the upper outer corner of the eye

lacrimal fluid tears produced by the lacrimal glands that lubricate the eye

lacrimal gland the organ that lies over the upper outer corner of the eye and secretes tears

lacrimal sac a pouchlike structure located in a groove in the lacrimal bone between the inner corner of the eye and the bridge of the nose

lacrimation the secretion and discharge of tears

lanugo fine, woolly hair or down on the shoulders, back, sacrum, and earlobes of the unborn child that may remain for a few weeks after birth

laryngoscopy visual examination of the larynx with a laryngoscope

larynx a structure composed of nine cartilages guarding the entrance of the trachea and functioning as the voice organ

lateral to the side, away from the midline

lavage irrigation or washing out of a body organ, such as the stomach

letdown reflex (milk ejection reflex) a pattern of stimulation, hormone release, and resulting muscle contraction that forces milk into the lactiferous ducts of the breasts, making it available to the infant

leukocytosis an abnormal increase in the number of white blood cells

Levin tube a single-lumen nasogastric tube

libel defamation by means of print, writing, or pictures

lice parasitic insects which infect mammals

license a legal document authorizing an individual to offer knowledge and skills to the public

lithotomy position a back-lying position in which the feet are supported in stirrups

livor mortis the discoloration of a body after death

lobe a well-defined portion of an organ, eg, the lung

lobule small lobe; the earlobe

lordosis an exaggerated concavity in the lumbar region of the vertebral column

lumbar puncture (LP, spinal tap) insertion of a needle into the subarachnoid space at the lumbar region

lymph transparent, slightly yellow fluid found within the lymphatic vessels

macula lutea an irregular, yellowish depression on the retina, lateral to and slightly below the optic disc

malignancy abnormal tissue having a tendency to proliferate and invade other tissues

malleolus a rounded prominence on the distal end of the tibia or fibula

malleus a hammer-shaped ossicle of the middle ear; it is connected to the tympanic membrane and transmits sound waves to the incus

malnutrition any disorder connected with nutrition

malpractice professional misconduct or unreasonable lack of professional skill

manometer an instrument used to measure the pressure of fluids or gases

manubrium a general term for a handlelike structure or part; in relation to the sternum it is the superior portion that joins with the clavicles

mastication the act of chewing

mastitis inflammation of the breast

mastoid breast-shaped; the bony prominence of the temporal bone behind the ear

meatus an opening, such as the opening of the urethra through which urine is excreted

medial toward the middle or midline

mediastinal shift a lateral movement of the organs in the mediastinum, ie, the heart and major blood vessels

medical asepsis practices that limit the transmission of microorganisms; also called *clean technique*

medical examiner a physician who investigates any death that appears to be unnatural

medical record (chart) a written account of a patient's health history, current health status, treatment, and progress

medication (medicine, drug) a chemical or biologic compound administered to humans or animals for disease prevention, cure, or relief, or to affect the structure or function of the body

melanin the dark pigment of the skin

metacarpal referring to the part of the hand between the wrist and the fingers

microcephalus very small head size

microorganism a small (minute) living body visible under a microscope

micturate pass urine from the body (urinate, void)

micturition voluntary discharge of urine; voiding; urination

milia small, white nodules (whiteheads) usually found over the nose and face of newborns

miliaria rubra a prickly heat rash of the face, neck, trunk, or perineal area of infants

Miller-Abbott tube a double-lumen tube inserted through the nose or mouth into the intestine

miosis constriction of the pupil

miter a method of folding the bedclothes at the corners to maintain them securely

mongolian spots blue or black spots of varying size found largely in the sacral area of Oriental or Black infants

mood the emotional state of a person as he or she describes it

morgue a place where bodies are temporarily detained before release to a mortician; some hospitals have their own morgues

mortician a person who is responsible for the care and disposal of the deceased

mourning a process through which grief is eventually resolved or altered

mucin the chief constituent of mucus

multiparous having had two or more pregnancies that resulted in viable fetuses

mydriasis enlargement of the pupil

myelogram an x-ray film of the spinal cord, nerve roots, and vertebrae after injection of a contrast medium into the subarachnoid space

myopia nearsightedness; abnormal refraction in which light rays focus in front of the retina

myxedema hypothyroidism

narcotic a drug that induces insensibility while relieving pain

narrative charting the writing of all information about a patient in descriptive format as it happens

nasogastric tube a plastic or rubber tube inserted through the nose into the stomach

nasolabial folds creases extending from the angle of the nose to the corner of the mouth

nasolacrimal duct the channel between the lacrimal sac and the nose

nasopharyngeal tube a tube inserted into a nostril and terminating in the pharynx

nausea the urge to vomit

negligence the omission of something a reasonable person would do or the doing of something a reasonable person would not do

nerve block chemical interruption of a nerve pathway effected by injecting an anesthetic

nocturia increased urinary frequency at night

nonpathogen a microorganism that does not produce disease under usual conditions

nonproductive cough a dry, harsh cough without secretions

normocephalic normal head circumference

nosocomial associated with or originating in a hospital or similar institution, eg, a nosocomial infection

nulliparous having never given birth to a viable fetus

nursing diagnosis a problem of a patient that the nurse can treat without a physician's order

nursing history a record compiled by nurses by a systematic method, containing data about a patient's past health and current status

nursing process a systematic method used to assess patients' health problems, identify nursing diagnoses, specify plans to solve them, implement the plans or delegate them to others, and evaluate the effectiveness of the interventions

nutrient an organic or inorganic substance in food that is digested and absorbed in the gastrointestinal tract and then used in the body's metabolic processes

nystagmus involuntary rhythmic movements of the eyeball

objective data information about a patient that can be observed or measured by laboratory or other means

obturator a disc or instrument that closes an opening; the obturator of a tracheostomy set fits inside and closes off the end of the outer tube

occult hidden

occupied bed a bed currently being used by a patient

oliguria production of abnormally small amounts of urine by the kidneys

opaque not transparent

open bed a bed not presently being used by its occupant, with the top covers folded back

ophthalmic relating to the eye

ophthalmoscope the instrument used to examine the interior of the eye

optional surgery surgery requested by the patient but not necessary for health

oral referring to the mouth

orifice the external opening of a body cavity, such as the urethra or the anus

oropharyngeal tube a tube inserted into the mouth and terminating in the pharynx

orthopnea the ability to breathe only in the upright position, ie, sitting or standing

osmosis the passage of a solvent (eg, water) through a semipermeable membrane from an area of lesser concentration to an area of greater concentration

ossicles the bones of sound transmission in the middle ear

osteitis deformans (Paget's disease) a disorder in which bony thickness increases

osteoporosis demineralization of the bones

-ostomy a suffix meaning to form an opening or outlet

otic relating to the ear

otitis externa inflammation of the external ear canal

otitis media inflammation of the middle ear

otoscope the instrument used to examine the eardrum and external ear canal

outer canthus the corner of the upper and lower eyelids away from the nose

oval window an opening between the middle and the inner ear

oxytocin a hormone normally produced by the posterior pituitary that is responsible for stimulating uterine contractions and the release of milk into the lactiferous ducts

pace the distance covered in a step when walking or the number of steps taken per minute

Paget's disease *see* osteitis deformans

palate the roof of the mouth

palliative surgery surgery to relieve the symptoms of a disease process

pallor the absence of normal skin color

palpation the act of feeling with the hands, usually the fingers; examination of the body using the sense of touch

palpebral conjunctiva mucous membrane lining the eyelids

palpebral fissure the opening between the eyelids

palpitation a subjective sensation of an irregular or unduly rapid heartbeat

paradoxical breathing respirations in which the chest wall balloons during expiration and is depressed or sucked inward on inspiration

paralytic ileus obstruction of the intestines resulting from inhibition of nerve impulses, which leads to decreased bowel mobility

parasite plant or animal that lives on or within another living organism

paresthesia abnormal sensation such as burning, pricking, or numbness

Parkinson's disease a neurologic disorder characterized by muscle tremor and muscular rigidity

paronychia infection of the tissue surrounding the nail

parotitis inflammation of the parotid salivary gland

parous having borne one or more viable fetuses

passive exercise exercise in which the nurse supplies the energy to move the patient's body part

patent open, unobstructed, not closed

pathogen a microorganism capable of producing disease

patient a person who seeks help because of illness or injury

pediculosis capitis infestation with head lice

penis the male organ of copulation and urinary excretion

Penrose drain a flexible rubber drain

percussion an assessment method in which the body surface is struck to elicit sounds or vibrations

percussion hammer an instrument shaped like a hammer with a head often made of plastic

perfusion the act of pouring over or through; the passage of a fluid through the vessels of a specific organ, eg, passage of blood constituents through blood vessels

pericardium a fibrous sac that surrounds the heart

perineum the area between the vagina and the anus in females and between the scrotum and the anus in males

periodontal disease a general term for a number of inflammatory and degenerative diseases that affect the supporting structures of the mouth

periosteum the connective tissue covering all bones and possessing bone-forming potential

peristalsis wavelike movement produced by circular and longitudinal muscle fibers of the intestines to propel contents onward

peristomal the skin area that surrounds a stoma

peritoneal cavity the area between the layers of the peritoneum in the abdomen; a potential space

peritoneal dialysis instillation and removal of a solution from the peritoneal cavity

peritonitis inflammation of the peritoneum

petechiae pinpoint red areas in the skin

pH a symbol used to express the relative alkalinity or acidity of a solution

phagocyte a cell, eg, a white blood cell, that ingests microorganisms, other cells, and foreign particles

phagocytosis the process by which cells, eg, white blood cells, engulf microorganisms, other cells, or foreign particles

phalanx any bone of the fingers or toes (plural: phalanges)

pharynx the musculomembranous sac behind the nose and mouth that connects with the esophagus and bronchi

phimosis a condition in which the opening of the foreskin of the penis is extremely narrow

phlebitis inflammation of a vein

photophobia abnormal intolerance to light

photosensitive sensitive to light

phrenic referring to the diaphragm

pinna *see* auricle

pitch (of a sound) the frequency of the vibrations; the high or low quality of a sound as heard during auscultation and percussion

pitting edema edema that leaves a small depression or pit after finger pressure is applied to the swollen area

plantar flexion movement of the ankle so that the toes point downward

plantar wart a wart on the sole of the foot

plasma the fluid portion of the blood in which the blood cells are suspended

platelet a disk-shaped blood element with a very fragile membrane; platelets tend to adhere to damaged or uneven surfaces and are involved in blood clotting; they are also called *thrombocytes*

pleura the membrane around the lungs, consisting of an outer layer, the parietal pleura, and an inner layer, the visceral pleura

pleural cavity a potential space between the two layers of the pleura

pleural rub (friction rub) a coarse, leathery, or grating sound produced by the rubbing together of the pleura

pleximeter the finger that is struck during percussion

plexor the finger that strikes during percussion

plexus a network (of nerves, veins, etc)

pneumonia inflammation of the lung tissue

pneumothorax accumulation of air or gas in the pleural cavity

pneumoventriculogram an x-ray film of the ventricles of the brain after the introduction of oxygen

point of maximal impulse (PMI) the point where the apex of the left ventricle touches the anterior chest wall; the point where the apical beat is most clearly palpated or auscultated

polarized (cardiac muscle) electrically charged

polyuria production of abnormally large amounts of urine by the kidneys; diuresis

port an opening or entrance

posterior of, toward, or at the back

postmortem after death

postural drainage drainage of secretions of various lung segments by the use of specific positions and gravity

precordial thump a sharp blow to the sternum by the fist to restore heart function

precordium the area of the chest overlying the heart

preoperative before an operation

presbyopia impaired vision, usually farsightedness, as a result of loss of elasticity of the lens due to aging

primary intention healing healing that occurs in a wound in which the tissue surfaces are or have been approximated and there is minimal or no tissue loss; it is characterized by the formation of minimal granulation tissue and scarring; also called *primary union* or *first intention healing*

privileged communication information given to a professional person such as a physician

problem-oriented medical record (POMR; POR) a patient's record organized according to the patient's problems and recording the reports of several health workers on each problem

proctocele *see* rectocele

proctoscopy visual examination of the interior of the rectum with a proctoscope

proctosigmoidoscopy visual examination of the rectum and sigmoid colon with a proctosigmoidoscope

productive cough a cough in which secretions are expectorated

proprioceptor a sensory nerve terminal in a muscle, a tendon, a joint, or the internal ear that gives information about movements and the position of the body

protective asepsis (isolation) practices setting someone or something apart from others or separating it; practices used to prevent the spread of infections and communicable diseases

protein any of the large, complex compounds of carbon, hydrogen, oxygen, and nitrogen essential to body maintenance

proteinuria protein in the urine

proximal closest to the point of attachment

pruritus itching

ptosis drooping of the eyelid so that one or both lids lie at or below the pupil margin

pulmonary referring to the lungs

pulmonary embolus a blood clot that has moved to the lungs and is obstructing a pulmonary artery

pulp cavity the cavity in the central part of the crown of a tooth that contains pulp

pulse the wave of blood within an artery that is created by contraction of the left ventricle of the heart

pulse deficit the difference between the apical and the radial pulse

pulse pressure the difference between the systolic and the diastolic pressures

pulse rate the number of pulse beats per minute

pulse rhythm the pattern of pulse beats and of the intervals between beats

pulse tension the elasticity of the arteries

pulse volume the force of the blood with each beat produced by contraction of the left ventricle

punctum an extremely small point or spot; the opening into the lacrimal canal

pupil the opening at the center of the iris (colored portion) of the eye

Purkinje's fibers a network of modified cardiac muscle fibers concerned with the conduction of impulses in the heart; dense networks of these fibers form the sinoatrial and atrioventricular nodes

purulent containing pus

pus a thick liquid associated with inflammation and composed of cells, fluid, microorganisms, and tissue debris

pyogenic pus-producing

pyorrhea purulent periodontal disease

pyrexia an elevated body temperature; fever

pyuria pus in the urine

quality (of sound) the subjective description of a sound as heard during percussion and auscultation

radiation the transfer of heat from a warm object to a cooler object by means of electromagnetic waves; electromagnetic waves used in diagnostic tests and some kinds of therapy

rales rattling or bubbling sounds, generally heard on inhalation, as air moves through accumulated moist secretions

range of motion the degree of movement possible for each joint

reconstructive surgery surgery to repair tissues whose function or appearance is damaged

recording (charting) the process of making written entries about a patient on the medical record

rectocele (proctocele) a protrusion of part of the rectum into the vagina

rectum the distal portion of the large intestine

recumbent length the measurement from the soles of the feet to the vertex of the head while the individual is supine; it is often measured in centimeters for accuracy, although inches can also be used

reduction realignment of fractured bone fragments to their normal position

reflex involuntary activity in response to a stimulus

regression reversion to a behavior or state that was acceptable at an earlier age

repolarized (cardiac muscle) reacquiring an electric charge

residual urine the amount of urine remaining in the bladder after voiding

resistive exercise exercise in which the patient contracts a muscle against an opposing force, eg, a weight

resonance a hollow sound produced on percussion from tissue filled with air

respiration the act of breathing

respiratory arrest the sudden cessation of breathing

respiratory ventilation the inhalation of air by artificial means

resuscitate to restore life; to revive

retention accumulation of urine in the bladder

retention (stay) suture a large, plain suture that attaches to underlying tissues of fat and muscle in addition to the skin; retention sutures are used to support incisions

retina the membrane lining the back of the eye that receives the image and is connected to the brain by the optic nerve

retrograde pyelogram an x-ray film taken after a contrast medium is injected through ureteral catheters into the kidneys

retroperitoneal space a space behind the peritoneum

reverse protective asepsis (barrier technique; reverse isolation) practices used to prevent an individual from coming in contact with microorganisms, eg, when a patient has severe burns

reverse Trendelenburg's position a position with the head of the bed raised and the foot lowered, while the bed foundation remains unbroken

rhonchi coarse, dry, wheezy, or whistling sounds, more audible during exhalation, as the air moves through tenacious mucus or a narrowed bronchus

rhythm the pattern of pulse beats and of the intervals between beats

right a matter to which a person has a just claim

rigidity stiffness or inflexibility of a muscle

rigor mortis a stiffening of the muscles after death

rooting reflex an infant's tendency to turn the head and open the lips to suck when one side of the mouth or cheek is touched

rubefacient a substance that reddens the skin

S₁ the first heart sound that occurs, when the atrioventricular valves close; it is a dull, low-pitched sound

S₂ the second heart sound that occurs, when the semilunar (aortic and pulmonary) valves close; it is a high-pitched, snappy sound

sacrum the triangular bone at the base of the spine

Salem sump tube a double-lumen nasogastric tube

sanguineous bloody

satiety a feeling of fullness as a result of satisfying the desire for food

scan a noninvasive type of x-ray procedure capable of distinguishing minor differences in the radiodensity of soft tissues

scar (cicatricial) tissue dense fibrous tissue derived from granulation tissue

sclera a tough white covering over about 75% of the eye; it is continuous with the cornea anteriorly and with the external sheath of the optic nerve posteriorly

scoliosis a lateral curvature of a part of the vertebral column

scored marked with a line or groove

sebaceous gland a gland of the dermis that secretes sebum

seborrheic dermatitis a chronic disease of the skin, characterized by scaling and crusted patches on various body areas, including the scalp

sebum the oily, lubricating secretion of sebaceous glands in the skin

secondary intention healing healing that occurs in a wound in which the tissue surfaces are not approximated and there is extensive tissue loss; it is characterized by the formation of excessive granulation tissue and scarring; also called *secondary union*

secretion the product of a gland, eg, saliva is the secretion of the salivary glands

sedative an agent or drug that tends to calm or tranquilize

semicircular canals passages shaped like half circles in the inner ear that control the sense of balance by the effect of fluid moving against hairlike nerves

sensitivity quick response, often referring to the response of microorganisms to an antibiotic

sensory deprivation lack of sensory stimulation

serous otitis inflammation of the eustachian tube

serum (in blood) the clear liquid portion of the blood that does not contain fibrinogen

shock acute peripheral circulatory failure

shroud a large rectangle or square of plastic or cotton material used to enclose a body after death

sigmoid colon the distal portion, shaped like the letter S, of the colon

sigmoidoscopy visual examination of the interior of the sigmoid colon with a sigmoidoscope

singultus hiccups

sinoatrial (SA) node the pacemaker of the heart; the collection of the Purkinje's fibers in the right atrium of the heart where the rhythm of contraction is initiated

slander unprivileged or false words by which a person's reputation is damaged

smear material spread across a glass slide in preparation for microscopic study

smegma a thick, white, cheeselike secretion that tends to collect between the labia and under the foreskin

SOAP the format used in the POR to record the patient's progress; it has four components: S—subjective data, O—objective data, A—assessment, and P—plan

solute a substance dissolved in a liquid

solvent the liquid in which a solute is dissolved

sordes the accumulation of foul matter (food, microorganisms, and epithelial elements) on the teeth and gums

source-oriented medical record a traditional patient's record, organized according to the source of the entries (that is, the person or department reporting); it includes separate records for the doctor, the nurse, the social worker, etc

spasticity sudden, prolonged involuntary muscle contraction

specific gravity the weight of a substance compared with the weight of an equal amount of another substance used as a standard (eg, water used as a standard has a specific gravity of 1, while urine has a specific gravity of 1.010 to 1.025)

speculum a funnel-shaped instrument used to widen and examine canals of the body, eg, the vagina or nasal canal

sphincter a circular, ringlike muscle that opens and closes an orifice when it relaxes and contracts

sphygmomanometer an instrument used to measure the pressure of the blood within the arteries

spinal anesthesia the introduction of an anesthetic into the subarachnoid space of the spinal canal

splint a rigid bar or appliance used to stabilize a body part

spoon nail a thin nail with a concave profile

spore a round or oval structure resistant to destruction that is formed by some bacterial cells as part of the reproductive process

spreader bar a bar designed to spread traction tape away from the bony prominences of the involved body part, eg, the lateral and medial malleoli of the leg; the bar must be wider than the involved part

stab wound a small deep wound, made by a sharp instrument such as a scalpel; it is often used for the insertion of drains and tubes

stapes a stirrup-shaped ossicle of the middle ear; it transmits sound waves from the incus to the internal ear

stasis stagnation or stoppage of flow of body fluids, such as intestinal fluids, urine, or blood

stature the height or tallness of a person when standing

stenosis constriction or narrowing of a body canal or opening

stereognosis the act of recognizing objects by touching and manipulating them

sterile free from microorganisms and their pathogenic by-products

sterile field a specified area that is considered sterile

sterilization a process that destroys all microorganisms, including spores

sternal angle (suprasternal notch) the point where the clavicles meet

sternum the breastbone

stertor snoring or sonorous respirations, usually due to a partial obstruction of the upper airway

stethoscope an instrument used to listen to various sounds inside the body such as the heartbeats

stoma a surgically created opening in the abdominal wall; it may be permanent or temporary

stomatitis inflammation of the oral mucous membrane

stopcock a valve that controls the flow of fluid or air through a tube

strabismus crossed eyes; squint

stress a physical or psychologic condition or situation that causes tension in the body

striae stretch marks

stridor a harsh, crowing sound made on inhalation due to constriction of the upper airway

stupor a condition of partial or nearly complete unconsciousness characterized by lethargy and reduced response to stimulation

sty *see* hordeolum

stylet a metal or plastic probe inserted into a needle or cannula to render it stiff and to prevent occlusion of the needle by particles of tissue

subarachnoid space the area between the arachnoid membrane and the pia mater

subcostal below the ribs

subcutaneous beneath the layers of the skin (hypodermic)

subcutaneous emphysema air or gas in the subcutaneous tissues

subjective data information about the patient that can be offered only by the patient personally, such as thoughts or feelings

substernal retractions indrawing beneath the breast bone

suctioning aspiration of oronasopharyngeal secretions using negative pressure

sudoriferous gland a gland of the dermis that secretes sweat

sulcular technique (Bass method) a technique of brushing the teeth under the gingival margins

sulcus the groove between the surface of the tooth and the gum

suppository a solid, cone-shaped, medicated substance inserted into the rectum, vagina, or urethra

suppression the sudden stoppage of a secretion or an excretion, such as urine

suppuration the formation of pus

supraclavicular retractions indrawing above the clavicles

suprapubic above the symphysis pubis

suprasternal notch *see* sternal angle

suprasternal retractions indrawing above the breast bone

surgical asepsis measures that render and maintain objects free from microorganisms, ie, that produce sterility

surgical bed (anesthetic, recovery, or postoperative bed) a bed with the top covers fanfolded to one side or to the end of the bed

suspension a preparation of a finely divided, undissolved substance dispersed in a liquid vehicle

suture a surgical stitch used to close accidental or surgical wounds

syncope fainting or temporary loss of consciousness

synthesis the process of putting together; assembling the parts of a whole

syringe an instrument used to inject or withdraw liquids

systole the period when the ventricles of the heart are contracted

systolic pressure the pressure of the blood against the arterial walls when the ventricles of the heart contract

tachycardia an excessively rapid heart rate, over 100 beats/min in an adult

tachypnea abnormally fast respirations, usually more than 24 respirations per minute

tenacious sticky, adhesive

tension the elasticity of the arteries

terminal hair long, coarse, pigmented body hair

thecal whitlow acute inflammation of the tissue surrounding the nail

therapeutic healing; supportive of health

thermometer an instrument used to determine body temperature

thoracentesis (thoracocentesis) insertion of a needle into the pleural cavity for diagnostic or therapeutic purposes

thorax the chest cavity

thought disorganization a condition in which a person has difficulty remembering what he or she is saying, is confused about time (eg, time of day or the day of the week), gives inappropriate verbal responses, and has sensory distortions

thrill a vibrating sensation

thrombophlebitis inflammation of a vein followed by formation of a blood clot

thrombus a solid mass of blood constituents in the circulatory system; a clot (plural: thrombi)

thyroid isthmus the portion connecting the two lobes of the thyroid gland; it lies across the trachea below the cricoid cartilage

ticks parasites that bite into tissue and suck blood

tinea pedis (athlete's foot) a fungal infection of the foot

tissue perfusion passage of fluid, eg, blood, through a specific organ or body part

toe pleat (tuck) a fold made in the top bedclothes to provide additional space for the patient's toes

tomogram an image acquired from a CAT scan

tomography a scanning procedure during which a narrow x-ray beam passes through the body part from different angles; *see also* scan

tonicity the effective osmotic pressure equivalent of a fluid; normal condition of tensity or tone of a muscle

torsion twisting

tort a wrong committed by a person against another person or the other person's property

tortuous twisted

total parenteral nutrition (TPN) (intravenous hyperalimentation) administration of a hypertonic solution of carbohydrates, amino acids, and lipids by an indwelling intravenous catheter placed into the superior vena cava via the jugular or subclavian vein

tourniquet a device, eg, a rugger strip, that is wrapped around a body extremity to compress the blood vessels

trachea a membranous tube, composed of cartilage, descending from the larynx and branching into the right and left bronchi

tracheal tug indrawing and downward pulling of the trachea during inhalation

tracheostomy an opening in the anterior neck directly into the trachea

tracheostomy button a very short tube that extends from a tracheostomy stoma to just inside the tracheal wall

tracheostomy tube a tube inserted through a tracheostomy and terminating in the trachea

traction an apparatus designed to immobilize and to apply a pulling force to an area or areas of the body

traction tape (strap) adhesive or nonadhesive tape, made of various materials (some are elastic and porous), which is applied lengthwise along a limb and attached to a spreader bar

tragus a cartilaginous protrusion at the entrance to the ear canal

transfusion the introduction of whole blood or its components, eg, serum, erythrocytes, or platelets, into the venous circulation

tremor involuntary trembling of a limb or part

Trendelenburg's position a position with the head of the bed lowered and the foot raised, while the bed foundation remains unbroken; in some agencies this position involves elevation of the knees, with the feet lowered and the head lowered

trigone a triangular area at the base of the urinary bladder

trocar a sharp pointed instrument that fits inside a cannula and is used to pierce body tissues

tube an elongated cylindrical instrument through which fluid and/or air can flow

turgor the normal fullness and elasticity of the skin

tympanic membrane the eardrum

tympanites abdominal distention

tympany a musical, drumlike sound produced on percussion from the least dense tissue

ultrasound a noninvasive diagnostic technique that uses sound waves to measure the acoustic density of tissues

umbilicus the navel; the site where the umbilical cord was attached to the fetus

umbo a round projection; eg, the umbo of the tympanic membrane is a slight projection on its external surface

unoccupied bed a bed not currently being used by a patient

unsterile (contaminated) containing microorganisms

ureterostomy a specific type of urostomy in which the ureter opens onto the abdominal wall

urgency a feeling one *must* void immediately

urgent surgery surgery necessary for the patient's health

urinal a receptable used to collect urine

urinalysis laboratory analysis of the urine

urinary retention accumulation of urine in the bladder and inability to void

urine the fluid of water and waste products excreted by the kidney

urostomy (urinary diversion) a surgically created opening into the urinary tract that permits the drainage of urine through the abdomen

uvula a fleshy mass suspended at the midline and back of the palate

vagina the canal of the female reproductive tract

value something of worth; a belief held dearly by a person

vaporization conversion of a solid or liquid into a gas (vapor); evaporation

varicose veins swollen, distended, and knotted veins

vasoconstriction a decrease in the caliber (lumen) of blood vessels

vasodilation an increase in the caliber (lumen) of blood vessels

vasospasm spasm or constriction of the blood vessels

vellus fine, nonpigmented body hair

venipuncture puncture of a vein for collection of a blood specimen or for therapeutic purposes

venous stasis diminished flow of blood in the veins

ventilation the movement of air

ventriculogram an x-ray film of the ventricles of the brain after the introduction of an opaque medium

vernix caseosa the whitish, cheesy, greasy, protective material found on the skin at birth

vertex the top of the head

vertigo dizziness

vesicostomy a surgically created opening of the bladder on the abdomen

vestibule (of the ear) a cavity at the entrance to the ear

vial a small glass bottle with a rubber stopper

vibration a technique of rapid agitation of the hands while pressing on a body area

virulence the degree of pathogenicity of a microorganism as indicated by its ability to invade the tissues of the host and to produce disease

viscosity the quality of being viscous (sticky or gummy)

viscous thick, sticky

visual acuity the degree of detail that the eye can discern in an image

visual field the area an individual can see when looking straight ahead

void urinate; micturate

volatile evaporating readily

volume (of the pulse) the force of the blood with each beat produced by contraction of the left ventricle

weight the heaviness of a body or object, normally measured in kilograms or pounds

wheal *see* bleb

wheeze a whistling respiratory sound of exhalation that usually indicates some narrowing of the bronchial tree

will a person's declaration about how his or her property is to be disposed of after his or her death

xiphoid process the lower portion of the sternum

PHOTOGRAPHIC CREDITS

William Thompson, RN, Limited Horizons

Pages 1, 2, 10, 21, 101, 138, 591, 592, 617, 791, 849, 884

Figures 1–2, 6–2, 6–3, 6–4, 6–6, 7–1, 7–13, 7–14, 7–15, 7–28, 7–29, 7–31, 8–2, 8–12, 8–16, 8–19, 8–27, 9–1, 9–2, 9–3, 9–5, 10–2, 10–3, 10–4, 10–13, 10–14, 10–15, 10–16, 10–18, 10–19, 10–20, 10–21, 10–22, 10–23, 10–27, 10–30, 10–31, 10–32, 10–33, 10–34, 10–35, 10–39, 10–40, 10–44, 10–45, 10–46, 10–54, 10–56, 10–57, 10–73, 10–74, 10–75, 10–76, 10–77, 10–79, 10–80, 10–81, 10–98, 10–99, 10–100A, 10–100B, 10–101, 10–103, 10–106, 10–107, 10–109, 10–110, 10–111, 10–112, 11–3, 11–4, 11–19, 11–20, 13–17, 13–18, 14–9, 14–10, 14–11, 15–18, 15–26, 16–9, 16–18, 16–19, 16–30, 19–66, 19–67, 19–68, 19–69, 19–70, 19–71, 19–72, 19–73, 19–74, 19–75, 19–76, 19–77, 19–78, 19–79, 19–80, 19–81, 19–82, 19–83, 19–84, 19–85, 19–86, 19–87, 19–88, 19–89, 19–90, 19–91, 19–92, 19–93, 19–94, 19–95, 19–96, 19–98, 19–100, 19–102, 19–106, 19–111, 19–112, 20–5, 22–6, 22–8, 22–9, 24–5, 24–9, 24–10, 24–11, 24–12, 24–13, 25–4, 25–5, 25–11, 25–12, 25–16, 25–17, 25–18, 25–26, 25–27, 25–28, 25–36, 25–38, 25–39, 25–40, 27–11, 27–38, 27–43, 28–17, 29–9, 29–13, 29–15, 30–35, 30–39, 30–41, 30–43, 31–5, 31–33, 31–36, 32–3, 34–1, 34–2, 34–3, 34–4, 34–5, 35–1, 35–22, 35–23, 35–24, 35–25, 36–7, 36–10, 36–20, 36–46, 38–3, 38–4, 39–6, 39–15, 39–17, 39–24

Jeffry Collins

Pages 61, 62, 84, 102, 372, 397, 469, 485, 516, 666, 688, 807, 925, 944

Figures 6–15, 7–11, 7–12, 7–26, 7–27, 7–30, 10–63, 10–102, 10–105, 10–113, 19–119, 19–120, 20–2, 20–3, 20–7, 20–8, 20–9, 20–10, 20–11, 20–12, 20–13, 21–2, 21–5, 21–6, 21–7, 21–9, 22–4, 22–11, 24–18, 24–20, 25–3, 25–22, 25–23, 25–24, 25–25, 25–29, 25–30, 25–31, 25–37, 25–42, 25–44, 25–45, 25–46, 25–47, 27–27, 27–28, 27–29, 28–5, 28–6, 28–7, 28–8, 28–9, 28–11, 28–12, 28–13, 28–14, 28–15, 28–19, 28–20, 29–11,

29–12, 29–21, 30–17, 30–30, 30–37, 30–38, 30–44, 30–45, 32–6, 32–7, 32–8, 32–13, 32–14, 33–6, 33–7, 33–8, 33–16, 33–17, 33–21, 33–25, 33–26, 36–1, 36–3, 36–4, 36–8, 36–13, 36–14, 36–15, 36–16, 36–17, 36–19, 36–25, 36–26, 36–27, 36–37, 36–38, 36–39, 36–40, 36–41, 36–42, 36–43, 36–44, 36–45, 38–5, 38–7, 38–8, 38–9, 38–10, 38–11, 38–12, 38–17, 38–19, 40–1, 40–2, 40–3, 40–5, 40–7, 40–8, 40–10, 40–11, 40–12, 40–13, 40–14, 40–15, 40–16, 40–17, 40–18, 40–19, 40–21, 40–22, 41–8, 41–9, 41–10, 41–11, 41–12, 41–13, 41–14, 41–15, 41–16, 41–18, 41–19, 41–20, 41–21

(These photographs originally appeared in PL Swearingen: *The Addison-Wesley Photo-Atlas of Nursing Procedures* [Addison-Wesley, 1984].)

George B. Fry III

Pages 273, 274, 294, 322, 371, 412, 497, 507, 542, 687, 714, 745, 746, 771, 792, 822, 850, 908, 961, 962

Figures 10–108, 12–4, 12–5, 12–6, 12–12, 13–12, 14–12, 14–13, 14–17, 15–25, 15–34, 15–35, 16–27, 16–28, 16–31, 18–2, 18–4, 18–7, 19–3, 19–99, 19–101, 21–10, 22–2, 22–3, 22–5, 22–7, 22–13, 24–7, 24–17, 25–7, 25–13, 25–15, 25–43, 27–30, 27–31, 27–32, 27–33, 27–34, 27–35, 27–36, 28–25, 30–4, 30–9, 30–10, 30–11, 30–12, 31–6, 32–4, 32–9, 32–10, 32–11, 32–12, 33–15, 35–12, 35–13, 35–17, 36–9, 36–18, 36–21, 36–22, 36–23, 36–24, 36–28, 36–29, 36–30, 36–31, 36–32, 36–33, 36–34, 36–35, 36–36, 37–6, 38–20, 39–1, 39–2, 39–3, 39–4, 39–5, 39–7, 39–8, 39–9, 39–10, 39–11, 39–13, 39–22

Stephen McBrady

Pages 29, 153, 246, 351, 508, 891

Paul Fusco

Pages 10, 51, 423

Karen Stafford Rantzman

Figures 7–2, 9–4

INDEX FOR HOME CARE VARIATIONS